handbook of CHRONIC PAIN management

9805
3/10/89

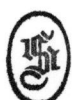 GERALD E. SWANSON M.D.
9601 UPTON ROAD
MINNEAPOLIS, MN 55431
TELE: 881-6869

handbook of CHRONIC PAIN management

EDITED BY
C. DAVID TOLLISON, Ph.D.
President, Pain Therapy Centers
Greenville Hospital System
Greenville, South Carolina

SPECIAL CONSULTANTS

John R. Satterthwaite, M.D.
Anesthesiology, Greenville, South Carolina, Consultant in Anesthesiology,
Pain Therapy Centers, Greenville, South Carolina

Joseph W. Tollison, M.D.
Professor and Chairman, Department of Family Medicine, Medical College of Georgia,
Augusta, Georgia

C. Glenn Trent, M.D.
Orthopedic Surgery, Greenville, South Carolina, Consultant in Orthopedic Surgery,
Pain Therapy Centers, Greenville, South Carolina

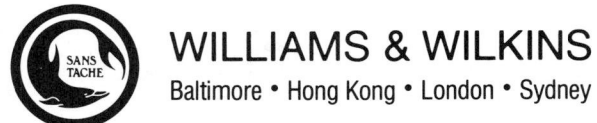

WILLIAMS & WILKINS
Baltimore • Hong Kong • London • Sydney

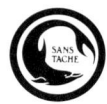

Editor: Nancy Collins
Associate Editor: Carol Eckhart
Copy Editor: Megan Barnard Shelton
Design: Saturn Graphics
Illustration Planning: Joanne Och
Production: Raymond E. Reter

Copyright (c) 1989
Williams & Wilkins
428 East Preston Street
Baltimore, MD 21202, USA

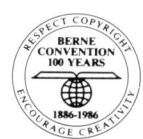

All rights reserved. This book is protected by copyright. No part of this book may be reproduced in any form or by any means, including photocopying, or utilized by any information storage and retrieval system without written permission from the copyright owner.

Accurate indications, adverse reactions, and dosage schedules for drugs are provided in this book, but it is possible that they may change. The reader is urged to review the package information data of the manufacturers of the medications mentioned.

Printed in the United States of America

Library of Congress Cataloging-in-Publication Data

Handbook of chronic pain management / edited by C. David Tollison; special consultants, C. Glenn Trent, John R. Satterthwaite, Joseph W. Tollison.
    p.   cm.
    Includes bibliographies and index.
    ISBN 0-683-08335-X
    1. Intractable pain—Handbooks, manuals, etc.
2. Analgesia—Handbooks, manuals, etc.   I. Tollison, C. David, 1949–   II. Trent, C. Glenn.   III. Satterthwaite, John R.
    IV. Tollison, Joseph W.
    [DNLM: 1. Chronic Disease. 2. Pain—therapy. WL 704 H236]
RB 127.H353 1989
616'.0472—dc19
DNLM/DLC
for Library of Congress   87-31738
                                                                                                                          CIP

88 89 90 91 92
1 2 3 4 5 6 7 8 9 10

To my wife,

Linda Surett Tollison,

and children,

Courtney Louise Tollison

and

Charles David Tollison, Jr.

Foreword

The *Handbook of Chronic Pain Management* is a tribute to progress in medicine. The chapters highlight the tremendous growth of pain research and provide a basis for its clinical application by the many kinds of health professionals who are necessarily involved in treating the chronic pain patient. This text features the complexities of comprehensive multidisciplinary care in such a way that the practitioner can understand and effectively apply this knowledge in the practice of chronic pain management.

Diagnostic and therapeutic difficulties are further complicated by the fact that each patient's problem is unique. This individuality is substantiated by asking, "How many people in the world have the same thumbprint?" The answer, of course, is "None." Not even look-alike twin monkeys have identical thumbprints. This is an anatomic variation. Thus, no two people are alike anatomically, biochemically, or in life-style. Treatment of any diagnosed medical disease or disorder must therefore be tailored to fit each unique individual.

No cookbook recipe for therapy should be employed, nor is the tunnel vision of any single medical specialty adequate, as a rule, for successful chronic pain management. Every practitioner should have the broad background of knowledge that this book supplies.

The superlative chapters of this text review first the classification of pain, its theoretical pathways and mechanisms, and its social, cultural, and psychological aspects. Chapters then focus attention on the diagnosis and management of chronic pain due to many causes, including neurologic lesions of spinal and peripheral nerves, malignancy, visceral and vascular diseases, various forms of joint degeneration and joint locking, and pain as a variant of depression.

One frequent and often overlooked source of chronic pain, the myofascial pain syndrome, receives ample and practical discussion. This condition can be demonstrated objectively by palpation of the muscles for trigger points and by recognition of their related referred pain patterns. The myofascial pain syndrome responds well to specific local therapy if its multiple perpetuating factors are recognized and corrected. Stresses that are both physical and emotional must usually be dealt with if trigger point therapy is to succeed. In addition, systemic perpetuating factors such as chronic infection and parasitic infestation, endocrine disorders (especially marginal (subclinical) hypothyroidism), borderline anemia, vitamin inadequacies, and deficiencies of other nutrients may play a role in maintaining chronicity. Evaluation of these multicausal factors requires unhurried time, detective work, and both skill and humility in communicating with the patient in chronic misery.

The largest organ in the body is the skeletal musculature, comprising nearly half the body weight. The myofascial pain syndrome may be the most common affliction of the human race. Muscles are different from other tissues. When the skin is cut or a bone is broken, it heals. When a muscle is injured or strained, it learns to guard that part. The better the person's athletic ability and coordination, the more likely the muscle is to continue its protective splinting with restricted motion, pain, and weakness for years, until the muscle is taught otherwise. Neuromuscular reeducation may be accomplished by passive stretching to full length during inhibition of reflex contraction, and by other techniques such as the Karel Lewit isometric contraction procedure.

The book's chapters present a large choice of therapeutic modalities, invasive and noninvasive, together with detailed consideration of the pharmacology of anti-inflammatory, analgesic and antidepressant drugs. Prescription of such medications may be necessary, with caution, when other management approaches fail.

The broad range and practical view of the *Handbook for Chronic Pain Management* make it an important working manual for effective clinical care that can improve the quality of life of the suffering patient.

Janet G. Travell, M.D.
Emeritus Clinical Professor of Medicine
The George Washington University
Washington, D.C.

Preface

God whispers to us in our pleasures, speaks in our conscience, but shouts in our pains. . . .

C. S. Lewis
"The Problem of Pain"

Pain is the most basic link between health professional and patient, yet this fascinating phenomenon is generally neglected in medical training, as are some of the most basic elements of the practitioner-patient relationship (i.e., sex and death). Despite recent advances in our understanding of the intricacies of pain, we continue to struggle with basic issues, such as an acceptable definition for the phenomenon of study. Historically, our view of pain has been clouded by the inherent tunnel vision of our educational training. Thus, to the philosopher and theologian pain is perhaps a moralizing force, whereas the sociologist may view pain as an expression of cultural norms. To the physiologist, pain is a perceptual phenomenon based on clinical sensation and to the psychologist it may be learned behavior. To the physician, pain traditionally has been a signal to be decoded for diagnosis and treatment of organic disease, and to the attorney it may be a basis for litigation.

I am reminded of the fable of the three blind men who were asked to describe an elephant. Each man carefully touched and examined a different part of the elephant's anatomy. The conclusion was three totally different descriptions of the same animal! Although each blind man was correct in his partial description, the basic error was essentially a failure of communication—a failure to communicate descriptive knowledge of "parts" into an accurate composite "whole."

Unfortunately, the same holds true for pain. It appears that the ways we have historically perceived, described, and treated human pain have depended, to a great extent, on what part of the phenomenon was emphasized in our educational training and interests. Unfortunately, this approach has retarded our comprehension of pain and, more importantly, our effectiveness in reducing human suffering. Pain is composed of a variety of complex parts, and it is only with acceptance of the total sum of pain that we recognize our personal limitations of competence and collectively strive toward resolving humankind's oldest and most dreaded fear: pain.

Development of a multidisciplinary team approach to the treatment of pain has been a significant, yet incomplete, step in the right direction. The term "multidisciplinary" pain treatment implies only a collection of specialists practicing in a central location. A possible scenario is that each professional independently practices his medical specialty, complete with its limitations inherent in training and human comprehension. Consequently, the factor that then differentiates traditional and multidisciplinary approaches becomes little more than the delivery of clinical services in a central location. Recall, again, the three blind men and the elephant.

Perhaps a preferable approach to pain management may be found in the term "interdisciplinary" and, more importantly, the operational and clinical applications of the term. Interdisciplinary pain management, like the multidisciplinary approach, recognizes pain as a complex omnidimensional phenomenon, and recognizes the valued expertise and knowledge of individual health specialists. However, true interdisciplinary pain management goes on to require implementation of effective and consistent communication between team members with recognition that the synergism of the treatment team is much greater than its discipline membership parts, and with acceptance that the current structure of our health professional training and educational system simply allows no individual or discipline to be all things to all patients in pain. Turk and Stieg (Turk DC, Stieg RL: Chronic pain: the necessity of interdisciplinary communication. *Clin J Pain* 3:163–167, 1987) have summarized the differentiating attributes of an interdisciplinary pain management team as consisting of a core group of individuals who (*a*) share a common conceptualization of patients with chronic pain; (*b*) synthesize the diverse sets of information based on their own evaluations, as well as those of outside consultants, into an intelligent differential diagnosis and treatment plan for each patient; (*c*) work together to formulate and implement a comprehensive rehabilitation plan based on the available data; (*d*) share a common philosophy of disability management; and, perhaps most importantly, (*e*) act as a functional unit whose members are willing to learn from each other and modify, when appropriate, their own opinions based on the combined observations and expertise of the entire group.

This book is an attempt to develop an interdisciplinary text on the management of chronic pain. Drawing on the knowledge and expertise of recognized researchers and clinical leaders, the objective of the text is to respond to the need for an integrated perspective to assist providers in understanding the intricate nature of clinical pain and to guide them in their choices and decisions about its management. As a resource, the text is designed to bridge the present gap between theory and practice by providing a handbook for clinical practice that emphasizes practical information essential for evaluating and treating pain in an interdisciplinary, rather than a partitioned, fashion. As a reference, the text is "user friendly" in that it is organized in a logical manner centering on human anatomy.

Section 1 of the text establishes a required foundation for understanding, diagnosing, and treating pain in an interdisciplinary fashion. Six chapters emphasize the requirement for a universal definition and classification system for pain that accounts for physiologic, sociocultural, and psychological influences and variables. Chronic pain is presented as an omnidimensional phenomenon necessitating attention to both its parts and its sum.

Section 2 is a practical interdisciplinary presentation of an armamentarium of therapeutic modalities utilized in the management of chronic pain. Each chapter presents a major treatment modality, considers the rationale underlying its use, outlines indications and limitations, and emphasizes the value of the technique within an interdisciplinary approach to treatment.

Section 3 comprises the heart of the text by presenting comprehensive interdisciplinary management of painful disorders including headaches, facial pain, back and spinal pain, genitourinary pain, malignant disorders, central-peripheral pain, and musculoskeletal and joint pain. Because the evaluation and treatment of chronic pain consistently cross discipline boundaries, the emphasis throughout these 24 chapters is on comprehensive pain management with attention to the specific contributions of selected disciplines. The unique, yet practical, organization of this section should make this text a convenient resource for the busy clinical practitioner.

The fourth section of the text provides practical information on a collection of ancillary topics carefully chosen based on their impact on comprehensive pain management. Clinicians practicing pain management are acutely aware that such practice involves both clinical and nonclinical issues and may find particularly interesting the chapter on *Legal Aspects of Pain and Social Security Disability* as well as the informative presentation of workers' compensation law.

Section 5 concludes the text with the presentation of the role of pain programs in the evaluation and treatment of chronic pain. During the past 10 years we have witnessed a virtual explosion in the number of pain programs. At first glance these programs appear to vary greatly in their approach to pain management and treatment goals; however, the chapter on *Pain Clinics: A Survey and Analysis of Past, Present, and Future Functioning* may provide some surprises with its presentation of informative and interesting results from a recent survey of leading pain programs.

Patients in pain pose a formidable challenge to all health practitioners, particularly those of us who have elected to target our energies and interests toward delivering effective clinical care to this most deserving population. The increasing number of people living with chronic diseases, disorders, and disabilities suggests that chronic pain and its management will continue to gain importance as we maintain our search for clinical solutions. It is clear that our efforts to assist these individuals in overcoming the multiple ramifications of their pain requires far more than an understanding of pain as a neurophysiologic mechanism.

C. David Tollison, Ph.D.

Acknowledgments

Many individuals have contributed, both directly and indirectly, to the development of this text. First, I would like to express my sincere appreciation to the contributing authors. Seventy-nine authors contributed their time, talents, and considerable expertise to this book.

I would also like to extend my appreciation to Williams & Wilkins. Nancy Collins, Editor, championed this book from the original "idea" stage through completion, and Carol Eckhart, Associate Editor, was of invaluable assistance in coordinating the voluminous details of this project. My thanks are extended to both for their confidence, patience, and support.

I also owe a debt of personal gratitude to many other people, some of whom include: Henry E. Adams, Ph.D., my mentor, who first introduced me to pain management and allowed me to learn from him; Michael L. Kriegel, Ph.D., and his wife, Linda, for their friendship and the important role that he plays in our clinical operations; Frank F. Espey, M.D., for originating the idea of Pain Therapy Centers; Mrs. Melinda Davis, my administrative assistant, for her tireless efforts in the preparation of this book and for her always cheerful efforts in keeping me organized; John R. Satterthwaite, M.D., and C. Glenn Trent, M.D., for serving as consultants for this text; my brother, Joseph W. Tollison, M.D., for serving as a consultant and his family, Betty, Joey, and Julie, who are so important to me; my sister, Ellen T. Hayden, and her husband Walter, for their support and caring; and Dr. Jerry Langley and his family, Sandy, Spencer, and Brittany, for their strong friendship that extends beyond family relations.

I would particularly like to thank my mother, and father, Louise J. and Wade A. Tollison, for deeply instilling in me the values of truth, honesty, concern, caring, and happiness. Without fanfare or great recognition they have devoted much of their lives to the welfare of others and, in doing so, quietly molded similar values in their children. Perhaps there is no greater gift that a parent may offer a child, and certainly there is not a more deeply felt sense of gratitude than that hereby extended to them. Much of my life has been a failed attempt to emulate the human worth of my father—an effort that affords me great personal satisfaction.

Finally, I would be remiss without acknowledging the thousands of patients in pain who have allowed me to learn from them. The contribution of each is sincerely appreciated.

C. David Tollison, Ph.D.

Contributors

Henry E. Adams, Ph.D.
(Chapter 21)
Professor of Psychology
University of Georgia
Athens, Georgia
and
Athens Center for Behavioral Medicine and Pain Management
Athens, Georgia

Eben Alexander, M.D.
(Chapter 11)
Chief Resident
Department of Surgery
Division of Neurosurgery
Duke University Medical Center
Durham, North Carolina

Karen O. Anderson, Ph.D.
(Chapter 45)
Assistant Professor
Section on Medical Psychology
Bowman Gray School of Medicine
Winston-Salem, North Carolina

John Aryunpur, M.D.
(Chapter 26)
Department of Neurosurgery
The Johns Hopkins Hospital
Baltimore, Maryland

J. Hampton Atkinson, Jr., M.D.
(Chapter 8)
Psychiatry Service
San Diego Veterans Administration Medical Center
San Diego, California
and
Department of Psychiatry
University of California at San Diego
School of Medicine
La Jolla, California

Shepard S. Averitt, M.Ed.
(Chapter 21)
Athens Center for Behavioral Medicine and Pain Management
Athens, Georgia

Mahmoud A. Ayoub, Ph.D.
(Chapter 47)
Department of Industrial Engineering
North Carolina State University
Raleigh, North Carolina

Dietrich Blumer, M.D.
(Chapter 16)
Professor of Psychiatry
University of Tennessee
Memphis, Tennessee

David B. Boyd, M.D., F.R.C.P. (C)
(Chapter 2)
Victoria Hospital
London, Ontario, Canada
and
Associate Professor of Internal Medicine and Psychiatry
The University of Western Ontario
London, Ontario, Canada
and
Member of the Taxonomy Subcommittee
The International Association for the Study of Pain

Laurence A. Bradley, Ph.D.
(Chapter 45)
Section of Medical Psychology
Bowman Gray School of Medicine
Wake Forest University
Winston-Salem, North Carolina

Ronald Brisman, M.D.
(Chapter 23)
Department of Neurosurgery
College of Physicians and Surgeons
Columbia University
Columbia Presbyterian Medical Center
New York, New York

Contributors

Kim J. Burchiel, M.D.
(Chapter 22)
Chief, Neurosurgery Service
Veterans Administration Medical Center
University of Washington
Seattle, Washington

Jeffrey A. Burgess, D.D.S., M.S.D.
(Chapter 22)
Senior Resident Fellow
Department of Anesthesiology
Multidisciplinary Pain Center
University Hospital
University of Washington
Seattle, Washington

Jerome D. Buxbaum, D.D.S., F.A.G.D.
(Chapter 24)
Department of Physiology
The University of Maryland
Baltimore College of Dental Surgery
Baltimore, Maryland

Richard L. Byyny, M.D.
(Chapter 43)
Director, Division of General Internal Medicine
Professor of Medicine
University of Colorado School of Medicine
Denver, Colorado

Charles S. Cleeland, Ph.D
(Chapter 33)
Department of Neurology
Clinical Science Center
University of Wisconsin School of Medicine
Madison, Wisconsin

Stephen R. Conway, M.D.
(Chapter 36)
Lahey Clinic Medical Center
Burlington, Massachusetts

David R. Cornblath, M.D.
(Chapter 35)
Associate Professor
Department of Neurology
The Johns Hopkins University School of Medicine
Baltimore, Maryland

Penny Lozon Crook, J.D.
(Chapter 49)
Crook and McDonald
Attorneys at Law
Hudson, Florida

Benjamin L. Crue, Jr., M.D., F.A.C.S.
(Chapter 29)
Medical Director
Durango Pain Rehabilitation Center
Durango, Colorado
and
Emeritus Clinical Professor of Neurological Surgery
University of Southern California School of Medicine
Los Angeles, California

Michael Devlin, M.D., F.R.C.P.C.
(Chapter 13)
Staff Physiatrist
Mount Sinai Hospital
Toronto, Ontario, Canada
and
Assistant Professor
Department of Rehabilitation Medicine
University of Toronto
Toronto, Ontario, Canada

Seymour Diamond, M.D.
(Chapter 19)
Director
Diamond Headache Clinic
Chicago, Illinois
and
Adjunct Professor of Pharmacology
The Chicago Medical School
Chicago, Illinois

Crystal C. Dickerson, M.A.
(Chapter 51)
Assistant Program Director
Pain Therapy Center
Greenville, South Carolina

Thomas B. Ducker, M.D.
(Chapter 26)
Neurological Surgery
Annapolis, Maryland

Theresa Ferrer-Brechner, M.D.
(Chapter 32)
Department of Anesthesiology
Pain Management Center
University of California
Center for Health Sciences
Los Angeles, California

Michael Feuerstein, Ph.D.
(Chapter 1)
Department of Psychiatry
The University of Rochester Medical Center
Rochester, New York
and
Director, Pain Treatment Center
Associate Professor, Department of Psychiatry and Anesthesia
University of Rochester School of Medicine and Dentistry
Rochester, New York

Don E. Flinn, M.D.
(Chapter 15)
Professor and Chairman
Department of Psychiatry
Texas Tech University Health Sciences Center
Lubbock, Texas

Frederick G. Freitag, D.O.
(Chapter 19)
Associate Director
Diamond Headache Clinic
Chicago, Illinois
and
Visiting Lecturer
Department of Family Medicine
Chicago College of Osteopathic Medicine
Chicago, Illinois

Stephen R. Friedberg, M.D.
(Chapter 34)
Chairman, Department of Neurosurgery
Lahey Clinic Medical Center
Burlington, Massachusetts

Larry A. Gaupp, Ph.D.
(Chapter 15)
Chief, Psychology Service
Veterans Administration Medical Center
Newington, Connecticut
and
Assistant Professor
Department of Psychiatry
University of Connecticut School of Medicine
Farmington, Connecticut

J. Leonard Goldner, M.D.
(Chapter 28)
Professor of Orthopaedic Surgery
Division of Orthopaedic Surgery
Duke University Medical Center
Durham, North Carolina

James L. Hall, Ph.D.
(Chapter 3)
Professor of Anatomy
College of Medicine
Department of Anatomy and Cell Biology
University of Cincinnati Medical Center
Cincinnati, Ohio

Lawrence M. Halpern, Ph.D.
(Chapter 7)
Department of Pharmacology
The Pain Center
University Hospital
University of Washington School of Medicine
Seattle, Washington

Mary Heilbronn, Ph.D.
(Chapter 16)
Research Coordinator
Neuropsychiatry
Henry Ford Hospital
Detroit, Michigan

Nelson Hendler, M.D., M.S.
(Chapter 37)
Clinical Director
Mensana Clinic
Stevenson, Maryland

Thomas K. Henthorn, M.D.
(Chapter 44)
Assistant Professor
Department of Anesthesia
Northwestern University Medical School
Chicago, Illinois

Marc Hertzman, M.D.
(Chapter 46)
Department of Psychiatry
George Washington University Hospital
The George Washington University Medical Center
Washington, D.C.

Patricia Howsam, M.D.
(Chapter 28)
Fellow in Hand Surgery
Division of Orthopaedic Surgery
Duke University Medical Center
Durham, North Carolina

Anthony Iezzi, M.S.
(Chapter 21)
Psychology Clinic
University of Georgia
Athens, Georgia
and
Athens Center for Behavioral Medicine and Pain Management
Athens, Georgia

Contributors

J. Greg Johnson, M.D.
(Chapter 30)
Greenville OB/GYN Associates
Greenville, South Carolina

H. Royden Jones, Jr., M.D.
(Chapter 36)
Department of Neurosurgery
Lahey Clinic Medical Center
Burlington, Massachusetts

Tom C. Krejcie, M.D.
(Chapter 44)
Department of Anesthesia
Northwestern University Medical School
Chicago, Illinois

Jerry C. Langley, D.C.
(Chapter 14)
Greenville, South Carolina

Terrence R. Malloy, M.D.
(Chapter 31)
Professor of Urology
Chief, Section of Urology
University of Pennsylvania School of Medicine
Philadelphia, Pennsylvania

G. Wayne McCall, M.Ed., CRC
(Chapter 48)
Vocational Diagnostics Laboratory
Stone Mountain, Georgia

John A. McCulloch, M.D.
(Chapter 27)
Associate Professor of Orthopaedics
Northeastern Ohio University
College of Medicine
Rootstown, Ohio

Barbara Clark Mims, R.N., M.S.N., CCRN
(Chapter 4)
Nurse Internship Coordinator
Department of Nursing Education
Parkland Memorial Hospital
Dallas, Texas

James E. Moore, Ph.D.
(Chapter 6)
Pain Management Program
Section of Physical Medicine and Rehabilitation
Virginia Mason Clinic
Seattle, Washington

Daniel E. Myers, D.D.S., M.S.
Assistant Professor
Orafacial Neuroscience Group
Dept. of Physiology
School of Dentistry, University of Maryland

Norbert R. Myslinski, Ph.D.
Associate Professor
Orafacial Neuroscience Group
Dept. of Physiology
School of Dentistry, University of Maryland

Blaine S. Nashold, Jr., M.D.
(Chapter 11)
Professor, Department of Surgery
Division of Neurosurgery
Duke University Medical Center
Durham, North Carolina

James Nitka, M.D.
(Chapter 28)
Resident, Orthopaedic Surgery
Division of Orthopaedic Surgery
Duke University Medical Center
Durham, North Carolina

Richard B. North, M.D.
(Chapter 12)
Assistant Professor
Department of Neurosurgery
The Johns Hopkins Hospital
Baltimore, Maryland

Robert N. Pilon, M.D.
(Chapter 21)
Athens Center for Behavioral Medicine and Pain Management
Athens, Georgia

Joan M. Romano, Ph.D.
(Chapter 6)
Multidisciplinary Pain Center
Department of Psychiatry and Behavioral Science
University of Washington School of Medicine
Seattle, Washington

Thomas E. Rudy, M.D.
(Chapter 18)
Department of Anesthesiology
Center for Pain Evaluation and Treatment
University of Pittsburgh
School of Medicine
Pittsburgh, Pennsylvania

John D. Rybock, M.D.
(Chapter 10)
Baltimore, Maryland

Steven H. Sanders, Ph.D.
(Chapter 17)
Executive Director
Pain Control and Rehabilitation Institute of Georgia
Decatur, Georgia
and
Clinical Associate Professor of Rehabilitation Medicine
Emory University School of Medicine
Atlanta, Georgia

Joel R. Saper, M.D., F.A.C.P.
(Chapter 20)
Director
Michigan Headache and Neurological Institute
Ann Arbor, Michigan
and
Associate Clinical Professor of Medicine (Neurology)
Michigan State University
Ann Arbor, Michigan

John R. Satterthwaite, M.D.
(Chapter 39)
Medical Director, Pain Therapy Centers
Greenville, South Carolina

David G. Simons, M.D.
(Chapters 41 and 42)
Clinical Professor
Department of Physical Medicine and Rehabilitation
University of California, Irvine
Irvine, California

Lois Statham Simons, M.S., R.P.T.
(Chapter 42)
Physical Therapist
Huntington Beach, California

Bruce M. Smoller, M.D.
(Chapter 46)
Medical Director
Washington Pain Assessment Group
Washington, D.C.

Glen D. Solomon, M.D.
(Chapter 19)
Adjunct Assistant Professor, Pharmacology
The Chicago Medical School
Chicago, Illinois

Rajka J. Soric, M.D., M.Sc., F.R.C.P.C.
(Chapter 13)
Staff Physiatrist
Mount Sinai Hospital
Toronto, Ontario, Canada
and
Assistant Professor
Department of Rehabilitation Medicine
University of Toronto
Toronto, Ontario, Canada

Henry A. Spindler, M.D.
(Chapter 5)
Rehabilitation Medicine
Franklin Square Hospital
Baltimore, Maryland

Blake H. Tearnan, Ph.D.
(Chapter 33)
Sierra Pain Institute
Reno, Nevada
and
University of Nevada School of Medicine
Reno, Nevada

Troy L. Thompson II, M.D.
(Chapter 43)
Director, Division of Consultation-Liaison Psychiatry
Associate Professor of Psychiatry and Medicine
Department of Psychiatry
University of Colorado School of Medicine
Denver, Colorado

Bruce Tobey, M.D.
(Chapter 28)
Fellow in Hand Surgery
Division of Orthopaedic Surgery
Duke University Medical Center
Durham, North Carolina

C. David Tollison, Ph.D.
(Chapter 50)
President, Pain Therapy Centers
The Greenville Hospital System
Greenville, South Carolina
and
Associate Clinical Professor
Medical College of Georgia
Augusta, Georgia

Joseph W. Tollison, M.D.
(Chapter 9)
Professor and Chairman
Department of Family Medicine
Medical College of Georgia
Augusta, Georgia

Roger B. Traycoff, M.D.
(Chapter 40)
Associate Professor of Medicine and Anesthesiology
Division of Rheumatology
Southern Illinois University School of Medicine
Springfield, Illinois

Dennis C. Turk, Ph.D.
(Chapter 18)
Department of Psychiatry
Center for Pain Evaluation and Treatment
University of Pittsburgh School of Medicine
Pittsburgh, Pennsylvania

Judith A. Turner, Ph.D.
(Chapter 6)
Multidisciplinary Pain Center
Departments of Psychiatry and Behavioral Sciences and Rehabilitation Medicine
University of Washington
Seattle, Washington

Clay H. Ward, M.S.
(Chapter 13)
Psychiatry Service
Veterans Administration Medical Center
Reno, Nevada

Clark Watts, M.D.
(Chapter 25)
Professor of Surgery, Neurosurgery
University of Missouri–Columbia
Health Sciences Center
Columbia, Missouri

Richard L. Weddige, M.D.
(Chapter 15)
Associate Chairman and Associate Professor
Department of Psychiatry
Texas Tech University Health Sciences Center
Lubbock, Texas

Tracy Williams, A.B.
(Chapter 45)
Assistant Professor
Section on Medical Psychology
Bowman Gray School of Medicine
Winston-Salem, North Carolina

Peter G. Wilson, M.D.
(Chapter 38)
Department of Psychiatry
Cornell University Medical College
New York, New York

Charles Witten, M.D.
(Chapter 31)
Instructor, Section of Urology
University of Pennsylvania School of Medicine
Philadelphia, Pennsylvania

Larry D. Young, Ph.D.
(Chapter 45)
Assistant Professor
Section on Medical Psychology
Bowman Gray School of Medicine
Winston-Salem, North Carolina

Contents

Foreword by Janet G. Travell, M.D. vii
Preface ix
Acknowledgments xi
Contributors xiii

section 1   foundations

Chapter 1	Definitions of Pain 2
	Michael Feuerstein, Ph.D.
Chapter 2	Taxonomy and Classification of Pain 6
	David B. Boyd, M.D., F.R.C.P.(C.)
Chapter 3	Anatomy of Pain 10
	James L. Hall, Ph.D.
Chapter 4	Sociologic and Cultural Aspects 17
	Barbara Clark Mims, R.N., M.S.N., CCRN
Chapter 5	Medical Electrodiagnostics 26
	Henry A. Spindler, M.D.
Chapter 6	Psychological Evaluation 38
	Joan M. Romano, Ph.D.
	Judith A. Turner, Ph.D.
	James E. Moore, Ph.D.

section 2   therapeutic modalities

Chapter 7	Analgesic and Anti-inflammatory Medications 54
	Lawrence M. Halpern, Ph.D.
Chapter 8	Psychopharmacologic Agents in the Treatment of Pain Syndromes 69
	J. Hampton Atkinson, Jr., M.D.
Chapter 9	Special Considerations in Pharmacologic Pain Management 104
	Joseph W. Tollison, M.D.
Chapter 10	Diagnostic and Therapeutic Nerve Blocks 115
	J. D. Rybock, M.D.
Chapter 11	Neurosurgical Treatment of Deafferentation Pain 125
	Blaine S. Nashold, Jr., M.D.
	Eben Alexander, M.D.

xx Contents

Chapter 12	Neural Stimulation Techniques	136
	Richard B. North, M.D.	
Chapter 13	Role of Physical Medicine	147
	Rajka Soric, M.D., M.Sci., F.R.C.P.C.	
	Michael Devlin, M.D., F.R.C.P.C.	
Chapter 14	Spinal Manipulation and the Reduction of Pain	163
	Jerry C. Langley, D.C.	
Chapter 15	Adjunctive Treatment Techniques	174
	Larry A. Gaupp, Ph.D., ABPP, ABPN, ABCB	
	Don E. Flinn, M.D.	
	Richard L. Weddige, M.D.	
Chapter 16	Dysthymic Pain Disorder: The Treatment of Chronic Pain as a Variant of Depression	197
	Dietrich Blumer, M.D.	
	Mary Heilbronn, Ph.D.	
Chapter 17	Contingency Management in the Reduction of Overt Pain Behavior	210
	Steven H. Sanders, Ph.D.	
Chapter 18	A Cognitive-Behavioral Perspective on Chronic Pain: Beyond the Scapel and Syringe	222
	Dennis C. Turk, Ph.D.	
	Thomas E. Rudy, M.D.	

section 3 pain management in selected disorders

part a headaches

Chapter 19	Differential Diagnosis of Headache Pain	238
	Seymour Diamond, Ph.D.	
	Glen D. Solomon, M.D.	
	Frederick G. Freitag, D.O.	
Chapter 20	Medical Management of Headache Pain	251
	Joel R. Saper, M.D., F.A.C.P.	
Chapter 21	Psychological Management of Headache Pain	264
	Anthony Iezzi, M.S.	
	Henry E. Adams, Ph.D.	
	Robert N. Pilon, M.D.	
	Shepard S. Averitt, M.Ed.	

part b facial pain

Chapter 22	Differential Diagnosis of Orofacial Pain	275
	Kim J. Burchiel, M.D.	
	Jeffrey A. Burgess, D.D.S., M.S.D.	
Chapter 23	Medical/Neurosurgical Management of Orofacial Pain	288
	Ronald Brisman, M.D.	
Chapter 24	Dental Management of Orofacial Pain	297
	Jerome D. Buxbaum, D.D.S., F.A.G.D.	
	Norbert R. Myslinski, Ph.D.	
	Daniel E. Myers, D.D.S., M.S.	

part c back and spinal pain

Chapter 25	Spinal Surgery	317
	Clark Watts, M.D.	

Chapter 26	Differential Diagnosis and Management of Cervical Spine Pain	320
	John Aryanpur, M.D.	
	Thomas B. Ducker, M.D.	
Chapter 27	Differential Diagnosis of Low Back Pain	335
	John A. McCulloch, M.D., F.R.C.S. (C)	
Chapter 28	Painful Arthropathies	357
	J. Leonard Goldner, M.D.	
	James Nitka, M.D.	
	Patricia Howson, M.D.	
	Bruce Tobey, M.D.	
Chapter 29	Painful Neuropathies and Nerve Root Lesions and Syndromes	365
	Benjamin L. Crue, Jr., M.D., F.A.C.S.	

part d genitourinary pain

Chapter 30	Gynecologic Pain	373
	J. Greg Johnson, M.D.	
Chapter 31	Pain in the Male Genitalia	380
	Terrence R. Malloy, M.D.	
	Charles Witten, M.D.	

part e malignant disorders

Chapter 32	Physical Management of Malignant Pain	390
	Theresa Ferrer-Brechner, M.D.	
Chapter 33	Psychological Management of Malignant Pain	402
	Blake H. Tearnan, Ph.D.	
	Clay H. Ward, M.S.	
	Charles S. Cleeland, Ph.D.	
Chapter 34	Neurosurgical Treatment of Pain Related to Cancer	417
	Stephen R. Freidberg, M.D.	

part f central-peripheral pain

Chapter 35	Peripheral Neuropathy	424
	David R. Cornblath, M.D.	
Chapter 36	Entrapment and Compression Neuropathies	430
	Stephen R. Conway, M.D.	
	H. Royden Jones, Jr., M.D.	
Chapter 37	Reflex Sympathetic Dystrophy and Causalgia	444
	Nelson Hendler, M.D., M.S.	
Chapter 38	Phantom Pain	455
	Peter G. Wilson, M.D.	
Chapter 39	Postherpetic Neuralgia	460
	John R. Satterthwaite, M.D.	

part g musculoskeletal and joint pain

Chapter 40	Chronic Joint and Connective Tissue Pain	475
	Roger B. Traycoff, M.D.	
Chapter 41	Single-Muscle Myofascial Pain Syndromes	490
	David G. Simons, M.D.	

Chapter 42	Chronic Myofascial Pain Syndrome *David G. Simons, M.D.* *Lois Statham Simons, M.S., R.P.T.*	509

section 4 selected topics

Chapter 43	Pain Problems in Primary Care Medical Practice *Troy L. Thompson II, M.D.* *Richard L. Byyny, M.D.*	532
Chapter 44	Postoperative Pain Management *Thomas K. Henthorn, M.D.* *Tom C. Krejcie, M.D.*	550
Chapter 45	Psychological Testing *Laurence A. Bradley, Ph.D.* *Karen O. Anderson, Ph.D.* *Larry D. Young, Ph.D.* *Tracy Williams, A.B.*	570
Chapter 46	Early Recognition of the Chronic Pain Patient *Marc Hertzman, M.D.* *Bruce M. Smoller, M.D.*	592
Chapter 47	Ergonomic Considerations in the Workplace *Mahmoud A. Ayoub, Ph.D.*	608
Chapter 48	Legal Aspects of Pain and Social Security Disability *G. Wayne McCall, M.Ed., CRC*	635
Chapter 49	Workers' Compensation *Penny Lozon Crook, J.D.*	644

section 5 pain clinics

Chapter 50	Assessment and Treatment at Pain Therapy Centers Programs *C. David Tollison, Ph.D.*	656
Chapter 51	Pain Centers: A Survey and Analysis of Past, Present, and Future Functioning *Crystal A. Dickerson, M.A.*	664
	Index	685

foundations
section 1

chapter 1
Definitions of Pain

Michael Feuerstein, Ph.D.

Pain, although a common experience to most of us, remains an enigma. Pain is a construct or concept. As a construct, its definition is a function of the theoretical orientation one takes with regard to pain. For example, to some neurosurgeons pain is the description of a sensation by a patient that can best be conceptualized within a strictly neuroanatomic and neurophysiologic framework. Anything that does not fall within this model is not pain but a "psychiatric disorder." Clearly, while secular trends in medicine are moving away from such a position, I am certain many readers have consulted with various surgeons and indeed patients who continue to hold such a "definition" of pain.

In fairness to our neurosurgeon colleagues, there are the proponents of the exclusive psychological definition(s) or conceptualizations of pain who are perhaps equally biased in their viewpoint. These clinicians, frequently psychologists or psychiatrists, often disregard the neurophysiologic, anatomic, or disease process potentially involved in persistent pain because as they conceive it such an approach has not proved useful in the management of many chronic pain disorders. Their definition of pain reflects some integration of psychological and social factors and conceptualizes pain as modulated by a complex set of emotional, environmental, and psychophysiologic variables.

As is the case with most matters, the "truth" probably lies somewhere at the midpoint of this neurophysiologic-behavioral continuum. The purpose of this brief chapter is not to provide a scholarly review of this debate, nor to provide a historic perspective of various views of pain; rather, my intention is to provide the reader with the most recent generally accepted definition of pain proposed by the International Association for the Study of Pain, along with some key definitions related to functional changes associated with pain. Finally, the chapter provides a brief summary of an operational definition of chronic pain that the author has found useful in his practice in providing a framework for conceptualizing the patient with chronic pain.

THE INTERNATIONAL ASSOCIATION FOR THE STUDY OF PAIN DEFINITION

Perhaps the most widely accepted definition of pain by pain specialists is that proposed by the International Association for the Study of Pain (IASP). This definition is as follows:

> **An unpleasant sensory and emotional experience associated with actual or potential tissue damage, or described in terms of such damage.**

Note: Pain is always subjective. Each individual learns the application of the word through experiences related to injury in early life. Biologists recognize that those stimuli which cause pain are liable to damage tissue. Accordingly, pain is that experience which we associate with actual or potential tissue damage. It is unquestionably a sensation in a part or parts of the body, but it is also always unpleasant and therefore also an emotional experience. Experiences which resemble pain, e.g., pricking, but are not unpleasant should not be called pain. Unpleasant abnormal experiences (dysaesthesiae) may also be pain but are not necessarily so because, subjectively, they may not have the usual sensory qualities of pain.

Many people report pain in the absence of tissue

damage or any likely pathophysiological cause; usually this happens for psychological reasons. There is usually no way to distinguish their experience from that due to tissue damage if we take the subjective report. If they regard their experience as pain and if they report it in the same ways as pain caused by tissue damage, it should be accepted as pain. This definition avoids tying pain to the stimulus. Activity induced in the nociceptor and nociceptive pathways by a noxious stimulus is not pain, which is always a psychological state, even though we may well appreciate that pain most often has a proximate physical cause.

Taxonomy Committee of the International Association for the Study of Pain (1)

The emphasis of this definition is on pain as a sensory and emotional experience in which pain is not exclusively defined in terms of nociceptive input but is rather a *psychological state*. This is particularly the case with chronic pain, the focus of this handbook. Indeed, the exclusive emphasis on a nociceptive generator, disease process, and its "associated pain" can impede the pain management process with certain patients. Clearly, the need to assess both nociceptive and psychological processes represents the state of the art approach to pain and its management.

DEFINITIONS OF FUNCTIONAL CAPACITY

Given the recent emphasis in pain management on restoration of functioning with or without reduction of pain itself (2), discussion of definitions of pain should also consider definitions of function. The Committee on Pain, Disability and Chronic Illness Behavior of the Institute of Medicine recently delineated three broad categories that are frequently used to define alterations in functional capacity (3). These terms are *impairment, functional limitation*, and *disability*. Using the World Health Organization's definitions as a framework, the committee defined these terms in the following way:

Impairment: "*Any* loss or abnormality of psychological, physiological or anatomical structure or function" (3). Functions that may be affected by chronic pain include walking, standing, sitting, reaching, lifting, bending, attentional abilities, mood, and social interaction, to name but a few.

Functional Limitation: "*Any* restriction or lack of ability to perform an activity in the manner or within the range considered normal for a human being that results from an impairment (World Health Organization's definition of "disability")" (3). This definition indicates that any loss of capabilities because of an inability to integrate physical and psychosocial functions because of pain, disease, or impairment represents a functional limitation. The limitation can include any combination of physical and psychosocial functions (e.g., housecleaning, operating a drill press, helping one's children get off to school).

Disability: "A disadvantage for a given individual (resulting from an impairment or a functional limitation) that *limits* or *prevents* the fulfillment of a role that is normal (function of age, sex, social and cultural factors) for that individual (World Health Organization's definition of "handicap")" (3). This definition indicates that if pain limits or prevents one from fulfilling an appropriate role in life, the pain is associated with a disability.

The use of such terms as impairment, functional limitation, and disability is found on the numerous forms one is asked to complete daily for patients with chronic pain, yet there remains little consensus as to what these terms mean. Also, each definition includes the term *normal* or *abnormal*, and until there is a sufficient data base to statistically define such terms, the "objective determination" of such states resulting from pain will continue to be influenced by a complex set of social, economic, interpersonal, and medical variables. This current situation places many patients with chronic pain and resultant impairment, functional limitation, or disability in a precarious position. Fortunately, efforts are underway to more carefully define and quantify the functional capabilities necessary to perform various job tasks and activities in daily living that should assist in more definitive determination of these indices of ability.

OPERATIONAL DEFINITION OF PAIN

As will be discussed in Chapter 2 ("Taxonomy and Classification of Pain"), a classification system has been developed by the IASP that defines pain in a given patient along five axes: (*a*) regions, or general anatomic location for pain; (*b*) systems, or the primary organ system in the body associated with the pain (e.g., cardiovascular, nervous); (*c*) temporal characteristics of the pain or its pattern of occurrence (e.g., single episode, recurrent regular, continuous/nonfluctuating); (*d*) time since onset; and (*e*) suspected etiology (e.g., neoplasm, trauma, unknown) (1). Although such a framework should assist with research efforts and provide the clinician with a prognosis and treatment approach, the schema does not consider certain aspects of the presenting complaints.

The components of an operational definition of chronic pain the author uses in practice are presented in Table 1.1. This definition considers pain sensation, pain behavior, functional status at work and home, emotional state, and somatic preoccupation. Various contributors to this handbook will elaborate in detail on certain aspects of these components of chronic pain as they relate to each specific pain problem discussed. However, a brief overview of

Table 1.1
Components of an Operational Definition of Chronic Pain

> Pain sensation
> Pain behavior
> Functional status at work
> Functional status at home
> Emotional state
> Somatic preoccupation

these components should help the clinician place most chronic pain problems within this general framework.

PAIN SENSATION

The pain sensation component of chronic pain is best described as the actual experience of pain as reported by the patient. This category can include actual sensory qualities of the pain as well as its location. A series of measurement devices are available to assist the clinician in evaluating this dimension of pain. However, it is not uncommon to rely on the patient's report of the qualities of pain at certain locations and, when appropriate, to re-create or reproduce the pain sensation during the physical exam. Pain maps are also used for identifying location.

PAIN BEHAVIOR

Pain behavior is a complex set of expressions and overt (observable) behaviors that suggest a patient is experiencing pain. The behaviors can include grimacing, use of supportive devices, vocalizations, continued medication use despite its apparent lack of effectiveness, and avoidance of movement for fear of increased pain, to name but a few. As with pain sensation, there are several direct observation techniques and self-report diaries of pain behavior and activity. Pain behavior represents an important component in defining chronic pain. As one might expect, the variation in such behavior is extensive and its specific manifestations can also vary considerably across patients.

FUNCTIONAL STATUS AT WORK

The area of functional capacity, important to rehabilitation for years, has only recently been a focus of interest in chronic pain. Consideration of this component of chronic pain is essential to its adequate definition. Although in the past much reliance was placed on what the employee and/or supervisor reported, recently direct observation using video techniques at the job site has been used more frequently. In addition, the use of simulated job tasks has represented an area of increased activity, potentially reducing the need for direct observation at the work site. This type of evaluation, coupled with isokinetic strength testing, has been used to provide a more quantitative index of functional abilities related to movements associated with specific job tasks. The influence of pain sensation and emotions in influencing job performance can now be more adequately determined in a given case, and baseline indices of abilities can be used as a point of departure for rehabilitation efforts.

FUNCTIONAL STATUS AT HOME

Consideration of the ability to perform functions related to the home also should be included in a comprehensive definition of chronic pain. Self-report questionnaires, direct observation of home-related functional capabilities, and reports from family members represent sources of data for this component. Although this area is generally limited to physical functioning within the home, such an evaluation should also consider the psychosocial functioning within the family. That is, the different roles that family members play, the communication and problem-solving skills the family possesses, and the role pain and illness plays in the family system should be considered when evaluating functional status at home.

EMOTIONAL STATE

An often-neglected area when considering chronic pain, particularly from the non–pain specialist's perspective, is the emotional component of pain. Many practitioners continue to search for the specific pain generator in patients and if such an "origin" is not found, the patient's pain is considered "not serious" or the patient is said to have psychogenic pain, or some variant of a psychiatric disorder. The all-or-none hypothesis related to chronic pain remains a significant force in health care despite definitions of pain such as that proposed by the IASP.

Emotional factors can play a significant role in the initiation, exacerbation, and maintenance of a variety of chronic pain disorders with or without observable pathophysiologic pain generators. Therefore, it is useful to evaluate the role of emotional factors and include such factors when defining pain.

Anxiety, depression, fatigue, and irritability can all play a complex role in the exacerbation of pain and pain behavior. The clear challenge for the clinician is to differentiate whether the emotional state of the patient is primary or secondary to chronic pain. It is important to obtain as clear a picture as possible as to the long-standing nature of a mood disturbance and/or personality disorder. This information can play an important role in determining various treatment options. As with each of the areas discussed, there are several methods one can use to assess the emotional factors associated with chronic pain.

SOMATIC PREOCCUPATION

Somatic preoccupation represents a cognitive component of chronic pain that can be defined as a heightened sensitivity and/or selective attention to bodily discomfort. This final component of chronic pain is one of the more resistant to modification. Pain reports can be significantly reduced (~ 50% reduction), pain behaviors can be eliminated, and functional status at work and home can be enhanced, while emotional distress can also be significantly reduced. Despite these changes, many patients, particularly those with strong disease convictions, continue to display a persistent sensitivity and selective attention to bodily sensations and discomfort.

Consideration of this component of chronic pain should help the clinician conceptualize the role of different treatment options for the patient. For example, if an overall goal in a treatment program was a reduction in pain, not its elimination, such a goal needs to be made explicitly clear to a patient with a high somatic preoccupation. Otherwise, patient expectations may not be consistent with those of the treating clinician. Another example would be in the area of neural blockade (e.g., epidural steroid injections for back pain with radicular component). A patient with high levels of somatic preoccupation should be clearly informed of what to expect in terms of short-term/long-term pain relief and whether the series of blocks represents a way to help the patient move into a rehabilitation program directed at behavioral pain management or the blocks are in themselves the treatment.

The view the patient has regarding his health and the role this view has taken in influencing his approach to health represents an important area with significant clinical implications. Somatic preoccupation can influence a chronic pain patient's view of the treatment plan, the treatment team, and treatment goals. Assessment of this component of chronic pain, therefore, can be quite important.

SUMMARY

Pain is clearly more than a sensation. Chronic pain should be considered in the context of the patient's abilities and disabilities. An operational definition of chronic pain potentially helpful to the practitioner should include consideration of pain sensation, pain behavior, functional status at work and home, emotional state, and somatic preoccupation. Assessment of these components of chronic pain can provide a working framework for evaluation and management of these complex patients.

References

1. Merskey H: Classification of chronic pain: descriptions of chronic pain syndromes and definitions of pain terms. *Pain* Suppl 3, S217, 1986.
2. Mayer TG, Gatchel RJ, Kishino N, Keeley J, Mayer H, Capra P, Mooney V: A prospective short-term study of chronic low back pain patients utilizing novel objective functional measurement. *Pain* 25:53–68, 1986.
3. Osterweis M, Kleinman A, Mechanic D (Eds): *Pain and Disability: Clinical, Behavioral, and Public Policy Perspectives.* Washington, DC, National Academy Press, 1987.

chapter 2
Taxonomy and Classification of Pain

David B. Boyd, M.D., F.R.C.P.(C)

As interest in chronic pain continues to grow, there is an increasing need to adopt a framework of classification that can be more or less universally accepted. The symptom "pain" is of interest to a wide diversity of students and potential therapists. Each discipline understandably approaches pain problems from its own viewpoint, and with its own body of knowledge, which often leads to several different subspecialized languages being used. At first glance these differing attitudes and jargon seem incompatible, yet everyone involved in the investigation or treatment of patients with chronic pain would agree that a multidisciplinary approach is likely best.

There are many approaches to classifying symptoms, but the author would like to take this opportunity to put forward the "Classification of Chronic Pain" recently published as a supplement of *Pain*, the journal of the International Association for the Study of Pain (IASP) (1). The IASP subcommittee on taxonomy and classification put together this supplement after considerable discussion, taking into consideration a wide range of disciplines and attitudes. The result is not presented with the thought that it is perfect. Any attempt at classification should continue to be remodeled as further information and understanding develop. When discussing classification, it becomes apparent that some people are "lumpers" and others are "splitters." The length and complexity of a classification system have to be reasonably complete but still manageable. The system should have practical applications and, most importantly, it should be adopted and used.

Examine some of the advantages of a unified approach. For research purposes, a homogeneous group of patients lends itself to good study design and more refined results that can reasonably be extrapolated to other patients with the same problem. To say that a patient has "chronic pain" is a start, but it is ludicrous to lump together as if they are the same a patient with metastatic bone pain, a patient with chronic migraine, a patient with postamputation phantom pain, and a patient with psychotic delusional pain. Little wonder that plans to manage pain sometimes, all too frequently, fail. Pain, and especially chronic pain, is a vague and intrinsically difficult subject to measure and categorize. Pain is something everyone knows about regardless of whether we accept the definition of pain as "pain is what hurts" or the more sophisticated definition, by Dr. Harold Merskey, of pain as "an unpleasant sensory and emotional experience associated with actual or potential tissue damage, or described in terms of such damage" (1). Even within disciplines there is much disagreement about any particular pain with respect to etiology, pathophysiology, and treatment. Once different disciplines are trying to compare information, it is even more vital that an accepted pain syndrome is focused upon. For example, "chronic leg pain" might be more clear than simply "chronic pain" but less helpful than "chronic leg pain from diabetic neuropathy." In the ideal situation the presenting pain could be sorted out specifically so that only those therapists who are really likely to be helpful need to become involved. At this point in time the situation is often unclear: Should the patient with low back pain see some or all of the following: physiotherapist, chiropractor, rheumatologist, anesthetist, neurosurgeon, orthopedic surgeon, or psychologist (to name but a few of the potential caregivers)?

If information is collected from all disciplines and put together in a framework that allows accurate comparison then it will be possible to gradually develop a system that expands current knowledge and correlates treatments to

	Biologic	Psychologic	Sociocultural
Predisposing			
Precipitating			
Perpetuating			

Figure 2.1. A sample grid classification often used in psychiatry—an example of a two-dimensional system.

specific situations. Apart from knowledge that is immediately useful clinically, various groups ranging from government statisticians to insurance companies to hospital medical records departments want data about diagnosis, epidemiology, and prognosis. Currently, the position to give much more than speculation about so many aspects of pain is weak. With improving communications systems worldwide and gradual computerization of data, an accepted backbone of structure is needed similar to post office zip codes or telephone books.

Throughout clinical medicine, one is confronted by attempts to classify. There is often a somewhat artificial effort to dichotomize: acute versus chronic, benign versus malignant, mild versus severe, treatable versus intractable. To avoid this oversimplification various one- or two-dimensional systems have been developed as lists or grids, as seen in Figures 2.1 and Table 2.1. Even these approaches leave out a lot, hence the development of systems

Table 2.1
A Sample List Classification Often Used in Internal Medicine—an Example of a One-Dimensional System

Congenital
Acquired
   Infectious (viral, bacterial, fungal, or protozoal)
   Toxic—endocrine-metabolic
   Allergic/autoimmune
   Traumatic
   Collagen vascular
   Vascular
   Neoplastic
   Hematologic
   Neurologic
   Psychiatric
   Degenerative
   Iatrogenic
   Other
      sarcoid
      amyloid

Table 2.2
The IASP Five Axis Pain Taxonomy: Overview

Axis I: Region
Axis II: System
Axis III: Temporal characteristics of pain: pattern of occurrence
Axis IV: Patient's statement of intensity: time since onset of pain
Axis V: Etiology

with axes like that of the IASP Taxonomy, similar to the DSM-III used by the American Psychiatric Association.

The IASP Taxonomy proposes a five-axis system (Table 2.2). Any patient's pain can be described by all five of these axes in sequence, for example, a low back pain (Axis I), of neurologic origin (Axis II), occurring continuously and severely (Axis III) for 6 months (Axis IV) from degenerative disk disease (Axis V). To allow numeric coding, if desired, each axis has been assigned a digit in an order of magnitude (the basic outline is shown in Tables 2.3 through 2.7). For the complete discussions of taxonomy and pain syndromes the reader is referred to *Pain*, Supplement 3, 1986.

The classification takes into account a number of the well-recognized but perhaps poorly standardized approaches to pain: site, system, time course and duration, severity, and etiology. It also allows for further delineation along traditional clinical questioning lines: associated symptoms, aggravating factors, usual course, complications, social and physical disability, pathology, and differential diagnosis.

Table 2.3
Axis I: Regions[a,b]

Head, face, and mouth	000
Cervical region	100
Upper shoulder and upper limbs	200
Thoracic region	300
Abdominal region	400
Lower back, lumbar spine, sacrum, and coccyx	500
Lower limbs	600
Pelvic region	700
Anal, perineal, and genital region	800
More than three major sites	900

[a] From Mersky H: Classification of chronic pain, descriptions of chronic pain syndromes and definitions of pain terms. *Pain* Suppl. 3:S10–S11, 1986.
[b] Record main site first; record two important regions separately. If there is more than one site of pain, separate coding will be necessary.

Table 2.4
Axis II: Systems[a,b]

Nervous system (central, peripheral, and autonomic) and special senses; physical disturbance or dysfunction	00
Nervous system (psychological and social)	10
Respiratory and cardiovascular systems	20
Musculoskeletal system and connective tissue	30
Cutaneous and subcutaneous and associated glands (breast, apocrine, etc.)	40
Gastrointestinal system	50
Genito-urinary system	60
Other organs or viscera (e.g., thyroid, lymphatic, hemopoietic	70
More than one system	80

[a] From Merskey H: Classification of chronic pain, descriptions of chronic pain syndromes and definitions of pain terms. *Pain* Suppl. 3:S10–S11, 1986.

[b] The system whose abnormal functioning produces the pain (e.g., claudication = vascular) is coded. Similarly, the nervous system is to be coded only when a pathologic disturbance in it produces pain. Thus pain from a pancreatic carcinoma = gastrointestinal; pain from a metastatic deposit affecting bones = musculoskeletal.

Table 2.5
Axis III: Temporal Characteristics of Pain: Pattern of Occurrence[a]

Not recorded, not applicable, or not known	0
Single episode, limited duration (e.g., ruptured aneurysm, sprained ankle)	1
Continuous or nearly continuous, nonfluctuating (e.g., low back pain, some cases)	2
Continuous or nearly continuous, fluctuating severity (e.g., ruptured intervertebral disc)	3
Recurring, irregularly (e.g., headache, mixed type)	4
Recurring, regularly (e.g., premenstrual pain)	5
Paroxysmal (e.g., tic douloureux)	6
Sustained with superimposed paroxysms	7
Other combinations	8
None of the above	9

[a] From Merskey H: Classification of chronic pain, descriptions of chronic pain syndromes and definitions of pain terms. *Pain* Suppl. 3:S10–S11, 1986.

Table 2.6
Axis IV: Patient's Statement of Intensity: Time Since Onset of Pain[a]

Not recorded, not applicable, or not known		.0
Mild—	1 month or less	.1
	1 month to 6 months	.2
	more than 6 months	.3
Medium—	1 month or less	.4
	1 month to 6 months	.5
	more than 6 months	.6
Severe—	1 month or less	.7
	1 month to 6 months	.8
	more than 6 months	.9

[a] From Merskey H: Classification of chronic pain, descriptions of chronic pain syndromes and definitions of pain terms. *Pain* Suppl. 3:S10–S11, 1986.

Table 2.8 overviews pain syndromes commonly seen clinically and discussed in greater detail in the IASP Taxonomy and Descriptions of Pain Syndromes.

The ideal classification system would have a specific location for each pain syndrome with no chance of omission or overlap. Clinical medicine rarely lends itself to such precise dissection. Nonetheless, by continual reex-

Table 2.7
Axis V: Etiology[a]

Genetic or congenital disorders (e.g., congenital dislocation)	.00
Trauma, operation, burns	.01
Infective, parasitic	.02
Inflammatory (no known infective agent), immune reactions	.03
Neoplasm	.04
Toxic, metabolic (e.g., alcoholic neuropathy, anoxia, vascular, nutritional, endocrine), radiation	.05
Degenerative, mechanical	.06
Dysfunctional (including psychophysiologic)	.07
Unknown or other	.08
Psychological origin (e.g., conversion hysteria, depressive hallucination). (Note: No physical cause should be held to be present nor any pathophysiological mechanism.)	.09

[a] From Merskey H: Classification of chronic pain, descriptions of chronic pain syndromes and definitions of pain terms. *Pain* Suppl. 3:S10–S11, 1986.

Table 2.8
An Overview of Syndromes as per the IASP Taxonomy[a]

Group	Syndrome
I	Relatively Generalized Syndromes
II	Neuralgias of the Head and Face
III	Craniofacial Pain of Musculoskeletal Origin
IV	Lesions of the Ear, Nose and Oral Cavity
V	Primary Headache Syndromes
VI	Pain of Psychological Origin in the Head and Face
VII	Suboccipital and Cervical Musculoskeletal Disorders
VIII	Visceral Pain in the Neck
IX	Pain of Neurological Origin in Neck, Shoulder and Upper Extremity
X	Lesions of the Brachial Plexus
XI	Pain in the Shoulder, Arm and Hand
XII	Vascular Disease of the Limbs
XIII	Collagen Disease of the Limbs
XIV	Vasodilating Functional Disease of the Limbs
XV	Arterial Insufficiencies in the Limbs
XVI	Pain in the Limbs of Psychological Origin
XVII	Chest Pain
XVIII	Chest Pain of Psychological Origin
XIX	Chest Pain: Referred from Abdomen or Gastrointestinal Tract
XX	Abdominal Pain of Neurological Origin
XXI	Abdominal Pain of Visceral Origin
XXII	Abdominal Pain Syndromes of Generalized Diseases
XXIII	Abdominal Pain of Psychological Origin
XXIV	Disease of Uterus, Ovaries and Adnexa
XXV	Pain in the Rectum, Perineum and External Genitalia
XXIV	Backache and Pain of Neurological Origin in Trunk and Back
XXVII	Back Pain of Musculoskeletal Origin
XXVIII	Back Pain of Visceral Origin
XXIX	Low Back Pain of Psychological Origin
XXX	Local Syndromes in the Leg or Foot—Pain of Neurological Origin
XXXI	Pain Syndromes of Hip and Thigh of Musculoskeletal Origin
XXXII	Musculoskeletal Syndromes of the Leg

[a] From Merskey H: Classification of chronic pain, descriptions of chronic pain syndromes and definitions of pain terms. *Pain* Suppl. 3:S13–S24, 1986.

amination by various groups, even pain gradually becomes more understandable. The IASP pain classification proposed above has several noteworthy advantages. First of all, it was developed by a multidisciplinary association. Second, this association is widely based in terms of both geography and expertise. Third, the association publishes a respected and well-circulated journal and has already published a proposed pain taxonomy. The five axes follow criteria that are currently used in pain problems, and so should be easy to adopt by most clinicians. This classification will be modified as knowledge expands but offers a firm starting point.

Reference

1. Merskey H: Classification of chronic pain, descriptions of chronic pain syndromes and definitions of pain terms. *Pain* Suppl. 3:S217, 1986.

chapter 3
Anatomy of Pain

James L. Hall, Ph.D.

The desired objective of this section is to acquaint the reader with the principal central and peripheral anatomic structures involved in perception of painful stimuli. The mechanisms of pain are perhaps one of the more complex topics in medicine. In many areas complete anatomic and physiologic explanations are not yet known or are inadequate.

This, then, is an attempt by an anatomist to set forth the anatomic substrates that may be more exhaustively dealt with in subsequent sections. It is instructive to note that the word "pain" is derived from a Greek word meaning penalty. We can easily imagine a penalty in the form of pain being visited upon some poor mortal for his affrontries to the Gods of Mt. Olympus.

PERIPHERAL STRUCTURES

RECEPTORS

We are now aware that most receptors on the peripheral endings of afferent nerves respond to a variety of stimuli. However, their shape and location and field of reception indicate that they are able to perceive one type of stimulus more efficiently than many other types. The specific receptor type that is incriminated in the reception of the pain stimulus is said to be an unencapsulated nerve ending. Although this receptor, in many examples, has a thin myelin covering, it is usually referred to as an unmyelinated or naked nerve ending.

The pain receptor is a primitive, unorganized nerve ending and often has a weed-like appearance. It has many branches and often overlaps the territory of other nerve endings from cord segments above and below it. Here, it is important to realize that the strength of the stimulus is a critical factor in the production of pain in this and other types of receptors. When a certain threshold of intensity of the stimulus is surpassed, any stimulus can be interpreted as painful to most receptors. This specific threshold is referred to as a noxious stimulus, one that will elicit tissue damage. At that point the receptor is referred to as nociceptive. Pressure, for example, if increased can become painful, and an encapsulated pacinian corpuscle, which is admirably modified by its onion-like capsule to have a large receptive field for pressure, can at a specific threshold level become a nociceptive receptor and generate an impulse of pain along its afferent nerve.

AFFERENT PAIN FIBERS

All nerve fibers are classified as to their age and conduction rate. They are called A, B, and C fibers, with A fibers being the largest in diameter and most rapid conducting fibers. B fibers are intermediate-sized fibers and have a somewhat slower conducting rate. C fibers are the smallest in caliber and the slowest conducting. There are apparently two types of pain-conducting fibers: an A-delta fiber, which is the most rapid of the pain-conducting fibers but the slowest of the alpha-conducting fibers, and C fibers, which are comparatively the slowest conducting fibers.

The pain conducted by the A-delta fibers is the quick, "bright" pain. It is often described as sharp, shooting, or even intense. C-fiber pain, on the other hand, is described as steady, slow, and constant.

SOMATIC PAIN CLASSIFICATION

Since the days of Henry Head in 1920, two other types of classifications of somatic pain have been used. Head proposed the terms of "epicritic" and "protopathic" to describe somatic pain. Head suggested that epicritic pain supplied with afferent receptors, the pain will be correctly perceived as coming from the appendix.

THE SPINAL CORD

Pain fibers enter the spinal cord in the medial portion of the dorsal roots of spinal nerves. They enter in the dorsolateral funiculus, just dorsal to the dorsal gray horn. Here they usually give off collaterals that descend in the dorsolateral funiculus or the tract of Lissauer for one or two cord segments. The main group of fibers, however, ascend in the tract of Lissauer for about two cord segments before entering the dorsal gray horn to synapse. They do so on cells lying in Rexed's laminae II, III, IV, and V on a group of small neurons called the nucleus proprius. The ascent in the cord prior to synapsing is the anatomic reason given as to why patients perceive somatic pain at a higher level than the origin of the spinal nerve that is involved.

The axons of the cells in the nucleus proprius, following the law of neurobiotaxis, leave diagonally opposite the point of the incoming stimulus and travel across the midline of the cord in the ventral gray and white commissures just below the central canal of the spinal cord.

As these fibers cross just below the central canal they are vulnerable to a condition in which the central canal enlarges or cavitates, known as *syringomyelia*. This would cause a loss of pain and temperature in the patient two cord segments below the cord segment in which the cavitation occurs. Typically this occurs in the cervical cord, and the deficit is a bilateral loss of pain and temperature in the upper extremities; usually other sensory modalities are spared.

The fibers then pass to the ventral lateral portion of the contralateral lateral funiculus, where they form two separate tracks or pathways to the thalamus. These are the classic ventral and lateral spinothalamic pathways. In the current literature these are also referred to as the paleo- and neospinothalamic tracts. The two tracts are joined, and some think that the fibers are mixed in each tract. The neospinothalamic or lateral tract is the more rapidly conducting tract that produces so-called bright, quick pain and the paleospinothalamic or ventral tract elicits dull aching pain. The ventral tract is sometimes thought to be clinically unimportant, but is now receiving more attention.

The spinothalamic tracts are the principal pain-conducting pathways in the cord, but not the only ones. A phylogenetically older tract that conducts visceral pain may be found closely applied to the gray matter of the cord in all funiculi. This is the fasciculus proprius, and its axons travel up or down one cord segment, then synapse in the dorsal gray horn to again travel up one more segment. The reticulospinal tract may also conduct pain impulses, again usually from the viscera, and its axons travel up or down the cord a few segments to eventually reach the thalamus and even the cerebral cortex itself. The fasciculus proprius system ends at the medulla and the impulses conducted by it are conducted rostrally by the reticular formation.

Pain of visceral origin, therefore, can be conducted rostrally in one of three alternative pathways. This is given as the anatomic explanation as to why visceral pain may persist after a surgical procedure to cut the lateral spinothalamic tract, as in a cordotomy.

It should be noted that within the spinal cord the lateral spinothalamic tract is topographically laminated. As the axons from the nucleus proprius in the sacral segments cross the midline and ascend, they take a dorsolateral position in the newly formed tract. Fibers from higher cord segments, as they assume their positions, become more medially placed. The final configuration of the tract would then have sacral segments represented most laterally and cervical segments more ventromedially. A space-occupying extramedullary neoplasm that compresses the ventrolateral spinal cord at any level therefore might compromise the conduction of pain and temperature from the sacral and lumbar regions of the body.

BRAINSTEM PAIN SYSTEMS

An exhaustive treatment of brainstem form systems is not within the intended scope of this chapter. Principal mechanisms and systems are presented with a view to elucidating a very voluminous and complex topic.

SPINOTHALAMIC PATHWAYS IN THE BRAINSTEM

We have seen that there are two spinothalamic tracts, a ventral or paleospinothalamic and a more significant lateral or neospinothalamic tract. Both conduct pain, although of different types, in the spinal cord. These two tracts diverge in the medulla, then come in close proximity in the lateral pons and are eventually associated with the medial lemniscus in either the rostral pons or the caudal mesencephalon. En route to this association both tracts are greatly diminished in size, with the ventral spinothalamic tract probably very modest in the mesencephalon.

The impulse from both tracts ends in the ventrobasal nuclear complex of the thalamus, with most fibers terminating in the ventral posterior lateral nucleus. Many studies have shown that the paleospinothalamic tract is polysynaptic and gives off many collaterals to reticular nuclei in the medulla, chiefly to the nucleus gigantoreticularis and the lateral reticular nucleus. These in turn project to the centromedian nucleus of the thalamus.

There are also many pain-conducting fibers of the reticular formation of both spinal and brainstem origin projecting to the intralaminar nuclei of the thalamus. The reticular formation of the brainstem is a monitoring or modulating mechanism. All modalities pass through its network and are in some way affected by it. It is thought could be discriminated and localized; thus, such pain must usually come from the skin or more superficial areas. Protopathic pain, conversely, can only be discriminated in a generalized way and not definitely localized.

SPINAL OR DORSAL ROOT GANGLIA

Dorsal root ganglia are found on the dorsal or posterior root of all spinal nerves. These are the sensory roots conducting the central process of the spinal ganglion cell into the central nervous system. The spinal or segmental nerve conducts epicritic pain from a specific area of the skin called the *dermatome*.

There may be some individual variation in size and contours of the dermatome, but dermatomic areas are always segmental and have distinct boundaries. A given spinal ganglion supplies a specific dermatome in a one-to-one relationship, but there may be overlap between the sensory roots. A ganglion may carry some information from the dermatome above and below it; this is usually true in the conduction of pain. Thus, when a specific ganglion is destroyed, there may be only a slight loss of pain from the dermatome it supplies.

Protopathic or deep somatic and visceral pain are less rigidly related to the nerve roots. This is at least in part due to the migration of structures during embryonic development (e.g., the diaphragm, supplied by C3–C5 via the phrenic nerve). The segmental division of deep pain is called a *sclerotome*. Because the pain fibers from a sclerotome enter the cord through several posterior roots, a more generalized or nonlocalizing pattern results.

Visceral pain is conducted by the peripheral process of the dorsal root ganglia traveling with the autonomic fibers that supply the target tissue. If they are bound in the same sheath as the sympathetic fibers they may travel some distance from their origin in the spinal ganglia via the white ramus of the sympathetic chain and the very long preganglionic fibers before they reach the specific viscera they supply.

An example of this arrangement is the afferent fibers from spinal ganglia T5–T10 that travel with the greater splanchnic nerve to reach the celiac ganglia in the abdomen. The afferent fibers pass through the celiac ganglia without synapsing and supply the derivatives of embryonic foregut. It is useful to conceptualize the sympathetic innervation of viscera to be somewhat like a cascade or waterfall, with the viscera in the cavities being supplied by sympathetic fibers that originate at higher levels. The afferent fibers to these same viscera accompany the sympathetic fibers. Thoracic fibers cascade down into abdominal viscera, and fibers from lumbar sympathetic ganglia, called lumbar splanchnics, cascade down into pelvic viscera via the hypogastric fibers.

Although this concept also holds for afferents conducted in the parasympathetic vagus nerve, which is also supplying afferent innervation to some structures in the thorax and abdomen from its cranial origin via its two sensory ganglia, it is not entirely true for parasympathetic supply to the embryonic hindgut and pelvic splanchnic nerves. These arise from sacral segments S2–S4 and travel superiorly to supply the embryonic hindgut through the inferior mesenteric plexus. Nevertheless, the axiom that the efferent sympathetic response is regional or widespread and the parasympathetic response is usually local or confined has some validity when applied to afferent impulses as well. Cranial sympathetics, of course, arise at lower levels in the cord and ascend via the anterior and posterior cerebral circulation to higher levels. Thoracic sympathetics, usually above T5 or T6, supply thoracic viscera at those levels even though they may ascend in the chain some distance, as in the case of the cardioaccelerator nerves, to do so.

The relationship between pain-conducting afferent fibers and sympathetic efferent fibers is thought to be involved in the condition known as *causalgia*. The patient complains of a persistent and burning pain usually following the course of the nerve fibers in the region. It is thought that the integrity of the afferent pain fibers has been compromised so that the neurotransmitter of the afferent fibers (in this case, acetylcholine) is noxious to the sympathetic fiber, thus producing the burning sensation. The condition is usually relieved by a sympathectomy.

Receptors of pain are sparse in the viscera, and this generally contributes to a poorly localized sensation from most of the viscera. There are two notable exceptions to this rule. Distention of the gut and pain from the heart can readily be localized by the physician. However, the sensory innervation of the heart is now known to be much more elegant than was previously thought.

REFERRED PAIN

Referred pain is a troublesome topic in the interpretation and diagnosis of pain. In essence, it means that the originating pain from one region of the body is referred to another region of the body that is not receiving the noxious stimulus directly. A classic example is that of pain from the gallbladder being referred to the tip of the right shoulder, because the C3–C5 nerve roots are distributed to both the diaphragm and the shoulder area. Anatomically the usual reason given for referred pain is that the pain-conducting fibers are distributed to different localities by portions of the same spinal nerves. These pain fibers then converge on the same neurons in the dorsal gray horn of the spinal cord. There, based on the patient's past experience and the breakdown of the integrity of the neuronal pool, a message is sent to the cortex that the pain is coming from point "A," which the cortex is preferentially structured to handle with ease, when the pain is really coming from point "B," which it is not so well equipped to handle. The referred pain is finally localized correctly when somatic pain receptors are involved. Pain from the appendix, for example, may initially be perceived as originating from the umbilicus because the T10 nerve supplies both structures. Eventually when the pain involves the peritoneum or the anterior abdominal wall, which are more densely that by its projections to the thalamus and the cortex directly the reticular formation contributes to a better total image of the body and its parts. Certainly, it accentuates or inhibits certain stimuli to produce a focus of attention or awareness of some impulses that are filtered through its all-encompassing network. Some specific reticular mechanisms, such as the nucleus of the median raphe in the pons, play down on other structures, such as the neurons in the IInd, IIIrd, IVth, and Vth lamina of the dorsal gray horn of the cord, to inhibit the transmission of pain. Other reticular nuclei around the periaqueductal gray of the midbrain do the same to the neo- and paleospinothalamic tracts as they pass through the midbrain.

A noteworthy relationship between the spinothalamic tracts and the spinal or descending nucleus of the trigeminal complex is found in the caudal medulla. The spinal nucleus of the trigeminal complex is a pain-conducting nucleus from the ipsilateral face. Its presence usually produces a small, but grossly visible, lateral bulge in the medulla called the tuberculum cinereum. Just ventral to the tuberculum cinereum is another smaller bulge or protuberance, called Monakow's area, that indicates the location of the spinothalamic tracts. At this level, in the medulla the spinothalamic tracts are conducting pain from the contralateral body, because all of the fibers originating from the dorsal gray horn have crossed the midline of the cord and are ascending contralaterally. Both of these areas are supplied by small branches of the posterior inferior cerebellar artery. Both structures are vulnerable to a deficit in the blood supply from the same artery. When this occurs (as the well-known lateral medullary syndrome), the patient complains of a loss of pain and temperature sensation from the ipsilateral face and the contralateral body. Other complaints, such as difficulty in swallowing or loss of taste on the ipsilateral side of the tongue, may also be present if the lesioned area is more extensive and involves the nucleus ambiguous and the nucleus of the solitary tract. This is a classic neuroanatomic deficit and is also known as Weber's syndrome.

THE TRIGEMINAL SYSTEM

Perhaps the most significant neuroanatomic structure involved in pain in the brainstem is the trigeminal system. The trigeminal nuclear complex has components in the midbrain, pons, and medulla, and even extends down into the upper cervical segments of the spinal cord. There are three sensory nuclei and one motor nucleus. The sensory nuclei are a mesencephalic nucleus lying along the cerebral aqueduct that is functionally associated with proprioception; the chief or principal sensory nucleus in the pons, which receives impulses of touch and pressure, but also some impulses of pain; and a long, attenuated spinal or descending nucleus that descends to the upper cervical segments as far as C4 to blend with the substantia gelatinosa of the cervical cord. The spinal nucleus is the nucleus usually associated with pain conduction. The motor nucleus also lies in the pons, and through reflex connections with the spinal nucleus can produce activity of the muscles of mastication (e.g., clenching of the jaw or chattering of the teeth) in response to noxious stimuli to the face.

The sensory nuclei receive their input from the pseudounipolar neurons of the trigeminal gasserian ganglion lying in Meckel's cavity in the middle cranial fossa. The peripheral processes of the ganglion are distributed via the ophthalmic maxillary and mandibular divisions of the trigeminal nerve to those regions of the face anterior to the ears. All three divisions conduct pain from their area of distribution. An irritative lesion of one of these divisions may produce a severe episodic pain in the patient, a condition called *trigeminal neuralgia*. The mandibular division is very commonly affected; the patient would complain of severe pain from the region of the lower lip and jaw. The pain is so severe and debilitating that some patients have contemplated suicide to escape its ravages.

The descending fibers of the pseudounipolar cells in the ganglion descend along the lateral aspect of the spinal nucleus through the pons and the medulla. They enter the spinal nucleus as they descend to synapses on the secondary cells of the nucleus. They, too, descend as far caudally as the C4 segment of the spinal cord.

The spinal nucleus has been described as having a rostral portion called the nucleus oralis, a caudal portion called the caudalis or subcaudalis, and an intermediate portion called the interpolaris. The nucleus appears to be laminated or organized in both a rostral-to-caudal and a dorsal-to-ventral fashion. The nucleus oralis portion would be comprised mainly of secondary neurons receiving pain impulses from the mandibular division of the nerve, whereas the subcaudalis would be receiving much of its input from the ophthalmic division. Hence, the lamination represents an innervated face. Lesions involving the upper cervical cord may sometimes cause production of pain or loss of pain in the ophthalmic region of the face along with other manifestations of spinal cord involvement.

The secondary fibers then sweep caudally from their origin from the neurons in the elongated spinal nucleus and cross the midline. As they cross the midline in the pons and medulla, they are called the ventral central trigeminal tract and are anatomically and physiologically separate from the fibers originating from the principal sensory nucleus conducting primarily impulses of touch and pressure, some of which also cross the midline to ascend to the thalamus as the dorsal central trigeminal tract. The remainder of the fibers originating from the principal sensory nucleus do cross the midline and ascend ipsilaterally. Hence, touch and pressure impulses are found bilaterally represented above the location of the principal sensory nucleus, whereas pain-conducting fibers are found contralaterally only. Touch and pressure perception may often be perceived in a patient with a brainstem lesion because of its bilateral representation, while the pain-conducting pathway may be compromised.

As both pathways ascend to the thalamus they are called the trigeminal thalamic pathways. They will come to be so close to the medial lemniscus in the caudal midbrain that they cannot be anatomically distinguished from it. However, physiologically they maintain their integrity and can be identified. The medial lemniscus is located on the lateral aspect of the midbrain above the level of the inferior colliculus, which is the auditory relay nucleus; above this level the trigeminal thalamic or lemniscal fibers are vulnerable to compromise. They may be severed or compressed by the sharp and firm edge of the dura mater as it forms the incisura to allow the brainstem to pass through. The extensions of the tentorium cerebelli rostrally to the clinoid processes forming the incisura pass alongside the lateral surface of the midbrain to form a formidable presence if there should be any sudden movement of the midbrain such as might occur in some types of trauma. A meningioma at this point could slowly compress the laterally placed medial lemniscus, with the trigeminal fibers at first producing pain through irritation, and eventually causing a contralateral loss of pain in the face as the compression slowly destroyed integrity of the axons to conduct the impulses. The deficit produced by the destruction of the medial lemniscus would be loss of conscious proprioception: position sense, two-point discrimination, and vibratory sense.

The secondary pain and touch axons of the trigeminal thalamic pathway terminate in the posterior ventral medial nucleus of the thalamus. This conforms to a phylogenetic pattern: the older structures in the central nervous system have a more favored position, that is, they are more medially placed. Most neurologic structures concerned with the head and neck are phylogenetically older and more medially placed than others that have to do mainly with body parts.

THE THALAMUS

The two groups of thalamic nuclei that are of interest to us are in the posterior basal complex: the posterior ventral lateral and the posterior ventral medial nuclei. They are mainly concerned with the perception and integration of the pain impulse from the body and from the face, respectively. Other thalamic nuclei may be involved after the impulses reach these primary targets, but which nuclei and to what degree is not clear at the present time. Pain is perceived on a conscious level at the thalamus. However, it is not recognized there as completely as it is in the cortex. Thalamic pain perception is a low-level type of appreciation. The thalamus tends to synchronize all incoming stimuli and place them in some form of order for transmission to the cerebral cortex. Otherwise, much of what we perceive would produce neurologic chaos.

The frailties of the thalamus are known to many. The *thalamic syndrome* can produce amplification of various stimuli so that many innocuous stimuli, such as putting a spoon to the lips, can be interpreted as a very painful experience. Patients may go to great lengths to prevent exposure to these stimuli and protect themselves from the very real pain produced by ordinary events. The thalamic syndrome is thought to be elicited by an altered blood supply to the nuclei involved. The blood supply is in the main from the thalamostriate branch of the posterior cerebral artery. It is presumed to be diminished but not completely absent, thus causing an improper functioning of the nuclei.

Reticular nuclei are found in the external and internal medullary lamina of the thalamus. These nuclei project to the various thalamic nuclei and modulate their activity. The reticular nuclei apparently can excite or inhibit the thalamic nuclei and the various impulses that are received by them. The reticular formation has also been modulating the impulses conducted through it by the specific pain-conducting tracts in the brainstem, that is, the spinothalamic and trigeminothalamic tracts. The attention of the thalamus can thereby be focused in on a specific stimulus or the stimulus could be significantly downgraded both at the brainstem and the thalamic level.

The reticular nuclei also receive input from the corticothalamic fibers arising from the cortex. These fibers are found in the anterior limb of the internal capsule. The thalamic nuclei also receive input from this feedback loop. The cortex then monitors, through this feedback loop, much of the information that comes to it both at the reticular and the thalamic level. The thalamocortical loop could play a major role in the patient's ability to tolerate pain at various thresholds.

INTERNAL CAPSULE

The pain impulse, along with other general sensory impulses, is projected to the cerebral cortex through the posterior limb of the internal capsule. At this point the exquisite orderliness of neurologic organization observed at the brainstem level breaks down. There is little or no organization to the arrangement of the general sensory-conducting fibers in the posterior limb of the internal capsule. The fibers are found alongside the lateral border of the thalamus in the posterior limb. The pain-conducting fibers are spread diffusely in this area. Lesions of the posterior limb of the internal capsule can produce either a diffuse loss of pain or general sensations in the case of irritative lesions such as edema or blood from hemorrhage eliciting the production of pain.

In either instance, the deficit may be puzzling to the diagnostician. The irritated fibers may represent conduction from a knee, a shoulder, a hand, or other widely separated parts of the body. The fact that the patient does have these very unusual deficits may be useful in localizing the lesion to the internal capsule.

It should also be recalled that portions of the optic radiations and the auditory radiations pass through the posterior limb as well as the corticobulbar and cortiocospinal portions of the voluntary motor system. The motor deficits, especially supranuclear facial paralysis, need no elaboration here. However, the possible involvement of the optic radiations, producing visual field deficits, or the auditory radiations, producing hearing deficits or hallucinations, might be useful to keep in mind when presented with patients with seemingly nonlocalizable signs.

THE CEREBRAL CORTEX

The general sensory impulses, including pain, project through the internal capsule and the corona radiata to the postcentral gyrus and posterior paracentral lobule of the cerebral cortex. Other areas of the cerebral cortex have also been incriminated in the pain pathway. The centromedian nucleus is thought to project some pain conducted by the reticular formation to the frontal lobe. Pain is also projected to the parietal operculum just posterior to the postcentral gyrus. It would appear that many cortical areas, not just the primary sensory strip, can be involved in pain. In this respect pain is unique as a general sensory sensation.

Visceral pain is projected to the insular cortex, which is hidden deep to the lateral fissure. The insular cortex, or island of Reil, is known to be associated with the autonomic nervous system and may produce autonomic responses such as nausea and vomiting when stimulated.

The model of the homunculus, or "little man," is laid out on the postcentral gyrus in an inverted fashion. The head, at the base of the gyrus, and the body parts are represented disproportionately as one moves superiorly along the gyrus to the superior longitudinal fissure. For example, the lower extremity below the knee is represented on the medial surface in the posterior part of the paracentral gyrus. The main portion of the lateral convexity of the hemisphere is supplied by the middle cerebral artery and its branches; this would include most of the postcentral gyrus. The superior aspect of the gyrus, however, is supplied by the anterior cerebral artery, as is the postcentral gyrus.

The pariental operculum and the insular cortex as well as the lateral aspect of the frontal lobe are also supplied by branches of the middle cerebral artery. The anterior and middle cerebral arteries are portions of the anterior cerebral circulation and are direct terminal branches of the internal carotid artery. It is worthy of note that cortical areas incriminated in the analytic recognition of pain are supplied by two different branches of the internal carotid, whereas some of the thalamic nuclei involved with relatively crude but conscious recognition of pain are supplied by branches of the posterior cerebral artery.

The thalamic relay nuclei, involved in the projection of pain, project to very specific areas of the cortex on a point-to-point basis. If the nuclei are destroyed there is degeneration of cortical neurons in the specific area to which that nucleus projects its axons.

The pain fibers from the thalamus project to the fourth layer of cortical cells of the postcentral gyrus, the posterior paracentral lobule, and the parietal operculum. Here the impulse is conducted first to the more superficial layers of the cortex for further integration. In a sensory cortex, the layers above the fourth layer or granule layer are perhaps more significant in processing the information that comes to that area of the cortex. Because they are superficial they are more vulnerable to some types of injuries and difficulties within the cranial cavity than the deeper layers (e.g., layers five and six in a mammalian neocortex).

The impulse for pain and other general sensations is then conducted to the superior parietal lobule on the ipsilateral side for integration. This is interpreted to mean the critical recognition of the stimulus, and the specific body part from which that stimulus has been perceived in the other areas of the cortex may be relevant to its significance to a given individual based on his/her past experiences. Interpretation of the stimulus or impulse above and beyond recognition is a function of the parietal lobe. Various forms of aphasia are examples of this type of activity. The primary cortical receptor area is intact, as are the secondary and perhaps tertiary areas. The stimulus is perceived correctly, but when conducted to the parietal lobe, as in the case of pain, its true meaning or significance may not be interpreted correctly.

Impulses are then conducted from the parietal lobe via association bundles in the white matter to other areas of the cortex and specifically to the frontal lobe for further cortical activity and perhaps decision making. The long association bundles of the cerebral hemisphere are very important in the production of a unified activity of the nervous system. The long association bundles involved in transmission, in this case, would be the superior fronto-occipital bundle and the superior longitudinal fasciculus. Lesions of these structures would not alter the perception of the pain or its meaning but would have an effect on the patients' response to it or their attitude toward the pain.

These same association bundles could also send collaterals to the medial portions of the limbic system and evoke an emotional or autonomic response to somatic pain.

DESCENDING PATHWAYS

The periaqueductal gray of the midbrain appears to have an ameliorative effect on pain. When stimulated, these neurons have an analgesic effect on ascending pain pathways.

SUMMARY

The elementary basis of neurologic structures involved in the conduction, recognition, and integration of pain have been identified. A difficulty with understanding the role of each of the anatomic entities involved in the process is that there is a duality or overlap of activities that makes clarification elusive.

There are two pathways for conduction of somatic and visceral pain in the spinal cord, the paleo- and neospinothalamic tracts. A third, the fasciculus proprius, conducts visceral pain. A fourth system, the reticular formation, can conduct either type of pain impulse rostrally or caudally. There are several brainstem structures involved: tracts, both ascending and descending, and cranial nerve nuclei and their secondary nuclear axons. All of these have differing arterial supplies that can, when compromised, involve one structure and spare another, and can cause production of pain or a loss of pain. These entities pass through the reticular formation, which monitors all impulses passing through to all-encompassing networks. This, in turn, can excite or inhibit the production of pain.

Two principal nuclei are involved at the thalamic level, but other nuclei participate. Their role is uncertain; however, they project to areas other than the postcentral gyrus and the paracentral lobule, the classic cortical centers for recognition of pain. In the cortex itself, there are many areas involved in pain perception and their roles differ from recognition to integration to attitudes and response. Even in the white matter two or more association bundles may be involved in even the most straightforward pathway.

An anatomic description of the structures involved in the pain pathway presents a picture that is very different from most other sensory pathways. The structures involved have evolved and been modified and enhanced over a very long period of time and probably are still being modified to deal with a specific type of stimulus that is disturbing to the usual functions of the brain. Yet as we learn more about the structures and their connections their role may become clearer, and more enlightened diagnoses and treatments should be forthcoming.

There cannot be many more causes in medicine more worthy of the attention and efforts of all physicians and scientists than the reflex of pain. The author hopes he has made a contribution to that cause.

Suggested Readings

Adams RD, Victor M: *Principles of Neurology*. New York, McGraw-Hill, 1977, p 1041.

Bond MR: *Pain: Its Nature and Treatment*. New York, Churchill Livingstone, 1979, p 185.

Gilman S, Newman SW: *Manter and Gatz's Essentials of Clinical Neuroanatomy and Neurophysiology*, ed 7. Philadelphia, FA Davis, 1987, p 256.

Hall JL: Peripheral pain pathways. In Lee JF (ed): *Pain Management*. Baltimore, Williams & Wilkins, 1977, pp 1–11.

Holden AV, Winlow N (eds): *The Neurobiology of Pain*. Manchester, England, Manchester University Press, 1983, p 414.

Kandel ER, Schwartz JH: *Principles of Neural Sciences*. New York, Elsevier, 1985, p 979.

Keller JT: The anatomy of central pain pathways. In Lee JF (ed): *Pain Management*. Baltimore, Williams & Wilkins, 1977, pp. 12–24.

Pawl RP: *Chronic Pain Primer*. Chicago, Year Book, 1979, p 106.

chapter 4
Sociologic and Cultural Aspects of Pain

Barbara Clark Mims, R.N., M.S.N., CCRN

Practitioners caring for the patient with chronic pain are faced with a complex, multidimensional problem. Previous research indicates that the etiology of chronic pain involves physiologic, social, psychological, and anthropologic factors (1, 2). There frequently is no discernible organic cause for the pain, and, when there is, the pathology and degree of expressed pain frequently seem incongruent (2, 3). A holistic approach to the patient, in which the practitioner seeks to understand the individual's unique pain experience, is advocated.

Chronic pain is a serious social problem, with substantial consequences for the individual, his family, and the community. Approximately 30–40 million Americans live with chronic pain (4). Low back pain alone affects approximately 8 million Americans annually, and it is the single most common cause of disability in persons less than 45 years of age (5–7). Striking patients during their most productive years, work-related injuries account for approximately 93 million lost work days per year (8). The estimated total cost of chronic pain and its treatment is between $40 and $60 billion per year (9). In light of the recent development of prospective payment systems for health care, the potential economic impact of chronic pain takes on even greater significance.

The social consequences of chronic pain reach far beyond economic concerns. Individuals who live with chronic pain experience tremendous anguish. Roles are altered, income declines, and independence is threatened. Feelings of meaninglessness, helplessness, and hopelessness are common (10). Insomnia occurs, leading to exhaustion and irritability. The patient suffering from chronic pain may focus on his bodily symptoms to the exclusion of work, family, and friends. The boundaries of his world shrink, as he spends hours on end in waiting rooms and pharmacies. Pain is his constant companion, and it takes the place of meaningful social interaction. Depression is inevitable. Interpersonal conflicts develop, and relationships suffer (11). Divorce rates as high as 70% have been reported among couples one member of which suffers from chronic pain (8).

The role of social and cultural factors in both the cause and effect of chronic pain merits consideration by health care practitioners. Since no reliable physiologic measure of pain has been established, the manner in which the practitioner responds to a patient's pain is based largely on his judgment of the patient's description (12). In order to accurately interpret an individual patient's communication, the practitioner needs to have an ethnic and cultural framework from which to draw (13). At the same time, an awareness of intraethnic variability is essential in order to avoid stereotyping. Stereotyping has been defined as "an exaggerated belief associated with a category" (14, p. 1280). By being aware of the range of behaviors to be expected within a group, and the factors that tend to predict variation, the practitioner will be better able to interpret the patient's communication on an individual basis. It will also help the health care practitioner in identifying those members of the ethnic group whose interaction with the health care system is most likely to be affected by cultural beliefs (15).

ETHNIC INFLUENCES: AN OVERVIEW

Ethnicity has been shown to be strongly related to behavior, beliefs, and attitudes associated with pain (16–18). The way in which the individual perceives, responds to, and communicates symptoms is influenced by his ethnic group membership (19, 20). In considering ethnic group influences on pain, two major factors are important. Culture influences the meaning given to symptoms and the treatment individuals seek for health problems. Social factors influence how families and local groups affect people's behavior and relate to illness. Social factors also determine how ethnic expectations affect the relationship between the patient and the health care practitioner (21).

Zborowski was a pioneer in investigating the relationship between ethnicity and the pain experience. In the early 1950s, he interviewed 146 males who were inpatients at a Veterans' Administration Hospital in New York City (17). He was interested in identifying whether or not ethnicity was consistently related to a patient's pain response patterns, attitudes, and beliefs, as well as the meanings attached to the pain symptoms. He hypothesized that responses to pain were learned and patterned as part of the sufferer's heritage. The ethnic groups he studied included Irish, Italian, Jewish, and Old American (white, native born, or Anglo-Saxon origin, usually Protestant, whose grandparents were born in the United States). He found that the Jewish and Italian patients gave a more emotional description of their pain, and tended to "play it up." The Irish and Old American patients were less emotional, and tended to "play it down." The Jewish and Italian patients exhibited pain by crying, complaining, groaning, and being demanding. Irish and Old Americans were more reserved, and tended to withdraw from others when experiencing pain. Zborowski studied interethnic differences, and did not really address intraethnic differences in response to pain. However, he identified type of pathology, generation American, age, and level of education as important factors in the individual's response to pain (17).

Zola performed another well-known study of interethnic differences in the report of responses to and attitudes toward symptoms such as pain (18). He interviewed 196 patients concerning their responses to presenting symptoms. He also asked about their families' response. He found that lower class Irish patients tended to deny pain and emphasize the physical effects of illness. The lower class Italian patients emphasized the importance of their pain. They had diffuse complaints and multiple symptoms, and were vocal and dramatic in describing the effects of pain on their daily lives. The Anglo-Saxon patients fell between the Irish and Italians in their responses, but were more similar to the Irish (18).

Weisenberg studied the relationship between ethnic group and the level of anxiety and attitudes toward pain in the head and oral cavity (16). The ethnic groups included in his study were black, Caucasian, and Puerto Rican. He found that Puerto Rican patients tended to avoid dealing with pain by denying it or getting rid of it quickly. Black and white patients were similar in their attitudes toward pain, but differed from the Puerto Rican patients (16).

Flannery et al. investigated the relationship between pain and ethnic group in 75 women who had recently sustained an episiotomy during childbirth. The ethnic groups included in the study were black, Irish, Jewish, Italian, and Anglo-Saxon. Flannery et al. found no significant differences in pain response between the groups (22).

Lipton and Marbach performed an investigation to determine interethnic differences in the pain experience of black, Irish, Italian, Jewish, and Puerto Rican patients with facial pain (15). After controlling for factors that had been shown by previous studies to influence the pain experience, they found that, although there were some interethnic differences, 66% of reported behavioral and attitudinal responses to pain were similar among the five groups studied. However, significant differences were observed among members of the same ethnic group. In predicting intraethnic variation, the degree of acculturation to American norms for health and illness was one of the most significant factors. Close-knit ethnic groups with strong social relationships within the group were less likely to be acculturated with American norms. Social class, as determined by education, occupation, and income, was a second factor that was found to be important in determining intraethnic differences. The higher socioeconomic classes differed from the lower socioeconomic classes of the same ethnic group. In terms of health behaviors, members of the higher socioeconomic classes tended to be more similar across groups than members of lower socioeconomic classes (15).

An important question concerning the application of the results of the early studies is whether or not the ethnic influences on pain continue to be in effect today, because groups may have become more acculturated since the initial studies were done. To answer this question, Koopman et al., in 1980–1981, replicated the work of Zola (23). They used the same clinic setting and same patient population. Their findings indicate that ethnicity continues to be a very significant factor in the reported pain experience. They also found that, in patients over 60 years of age, Italian-Americans reported pain more frequently than Anglo-Americans. This was not so in younger patients. Age and sex were both found to influence the relationship between ethnicity and the expression of pain. There was no relationship between ethnicity and emotional distress (23).

CULTURAL AND ANTHROPOLOGIC INFLUENCES

Culture consists of customs, traditions, habits, and ethical and moral codes. The ethical and moral codes evolve out of the group's religious system, social organization, and economy (24).

Cultural traditions help the individual know when to anticipate pain. This is beneficial, because the person who is prepared for the sensation of pain is more likely to accept it and will experience less alarm and anxiety. In this country, people are taught to expect pain during childbirth, after surgery, and while participating in some athletic events. People expect to experience minor aches and pains as part of life, and most do not elicit alarm or anxiety. However, when a pain that society associates with serious disease, such as chest pain, occurs, the individual may be very alarmed. In this situation, it is considered acceptable for the individual to display outward behaviors indicative of pain, such as crying and moaning. It is not the intensity of the pain, but rather the potential consequences of it, that determine the patient's behavior (24). Zborowski referred to "pain expectancy" as "the anticipation of pain in association with a specific physical, social, or cultural situation" (24, p. 30). He referred to "pain acceptance" as "the willingness to tolerate this sensation" (24, p. 31). He emphasized that both factors play a part in determining the patient's behavioral and emotional responses to pain.

Society has certain expectations for how people will act during a painful experience. Within a given culture, individual variances in the cultural expectations are granted for such things as age, sex, status, and other social criteria. When the individual does not conform to society's expectations for pain behavior, he may be ridiculed or receive other sanctions. The individual will also punish himself by experiencing feelings of shame, guilt, and decreased self-esteem (24).

Cultural norms and traditions are passed from parent to child by word and by example. These patterns are internalized during childhood, and are reinforced in adult life through interaction with others who have received similar upbringing. Peer pressure and concern over what others might think or say is important in motivating the individual to adhere to cultural norms (24).

The social and cultural meaning applied to pain is an important determinant of how an individual will respond to his pain experience. It is interesting to note that the word pain is a derivative of the Latin word *poena* ("punishment"), which evolves from the Sanscrit root *pu* ("purification") (24). Inflicting pain is a traditional means of administering punishment. It is also viewed as a means toward redemption from sin, or a way the person can pay his debt to God (24). The punitive and purifying significance of pain can be seen in many religious rituals throughout the world.

Pain is also a symbol of grief and mourning. In many societies, mourners mutilate themselves to inflict pain as a demonstration of their grief over loss of a loved one. The way in which the individual responds to pain is an important form of communication (24).

Another cultural variable that may influence the individual's response to pain is the time orientation of the community. In societies that are future oriented, the patient experiencing pain will be most concerned about how the pain will affect his future functioning, such as his ability to make a living. Instead of focusing on the pain sensation itself, he will focus on the effects of the pain. In present-oriented societies, the individual will more likely be concerned with the sensation itself and the relief of the unpleasantness (24).

In the United States today, childbirth is considered to be a very painful experience. A great deal of research has been done in this country to develop methods of alleviating pain during childbirth. This is not the case in many countries. For example, in some South American, African, and Basque cultures, a technique called couvade is practiced. In couvade, the pregnant woman works up until the moment of birth. During delivery, the husband takes to his bed and carries on as if he is experiencing the pain of labor. The wife returns to work in the fields shortly after delivery, and the husband stays home to care for the infant (2).

The Bariba are an ethnic group of 400,000 people inhabiting northern Benin and Nigeria in West Africa. The outstanding characteristic of this ethnic group is the consistent absence of observable behaviors indicative of pain. Stoicism is an integral part of Bariba identify. This culture provides an excellent context for the consideration of the cultural aspects of pain. A Bariba physician responded to questions about postoperative pain by quoting the following Bariba proverb: *sekuru ka go go buram bu* ("between death and shame, death has the greater beauty"). In this culture, any outward manifestation of pain is shameful, because it indicates lack of courage. Members of this culture would rather kill themselves than live in shame. The Bariba display indifference, and they attempt to continue normal activities even in the face of disability and pain. The young Bariba males learn appropriate ways of expressing pain during the ritual of circumcision. The boy sits on a rock with his uncle standing in front of him, staring into his eyes, compelling him not to cry or even to blink. During the actual procedure, the family's praise singer sings praises in tribute to the boy's courage. One Bariba described the ceremony as epitomizing the merging of pain, courage, and honor (25).

In analyzing the cultural aspects of pain, it is useful to consider societies that practice mutilation and deformation as part of rituals and religious rites. In the Aranda tribe, young men must undergo a painful "test" to be admitted to the warrior caste. The scalp is cut with a sharp stick, and one of the elders then lifts it with his teeth. The young man has a chance to demonstrate courage by the absence of complaints or outward signs of suffering. The "hook swinging ceremony" that takes place in India and Latin America is another illustration of the cultural influence on the pain response. In this religious ceremony, an individual is chosen to represent the divine power during the ceremony. Two hooks are inserted in the victim's back, and he is hoisted into the air by a crane connected to the hooks. He is then made to swing in the air so that he appears to fly. He must not display any sign of suffering.

In these cultures, individuals seem to exist in a special state of mind during the rituals. Through the support of the community and a strong desire to be part of a specific culture, the individual is able to raise his pain threshold and create a detached behavior (2).

In addition to rituals and religious ceremonies, numerous other factors contribute to the individual's response to pain. Some of these include parents, school, and work. Others include the level of public health, the type and quality of health service during and after the illness, and the attitude of the community toward the patient (2).

INFLUENCE OF PRACTITIONER'S CULTURE

Just as a patient's cultural background contributes to his response to the pain experience, so the cultural background of the health care practitioner contributes to his beliefs about patient suffering. Davitz et al. reported a situation in which a 45-year-old male was admitted to the emergency room of a large metropolitan hospital (26). Three nurses from different ethnic backgrounds attended to his needs. After the crisis was over, the three nurses were interviewed about their personal reactions to the patient. One nurse was from a Northern European country, and she described the man as very emotional. She thought that he carried on much worse than was appropriate for his condition. She went on to say that in her country, stoicism and self-control were expected when someone was physically hurt or emotionally upset. She recalled that her parents and teachers had taught her emotional restraint from early childhood. She indicated that the degree of injury and the patient's age should partially determine the degree of his reaction to pain.

The second nurse interviewed was Puerto Rican. She indicated that the patient's outbursts were quite understandable, and she wondered if his distress wasn't largely due to concern over his family's welfare.

The third nurse was American. She expressed surprise over the patient's reaction considering his age and background. She expected that an adult male would be stronger and more stoic. She emphasized that her feelings about a patient depend largely on his age and his degree of injury (26).

In this example, three nurses from different cultural backgrounds who cared for the same patient simultaneously had markedly different reactions to the patient's expression of pain. To investigate reasons for such differences, Davitz et al. performed an extensive investigation into the effects of nurses' cultural backgrounds on the judgments they make about patient suffering (27). They found that nurses in different countries differed markedly in the degree of patient suffering inferred. Of six countries studied, nurses in Japan and Korea inferred the greatest degree of patient suffering for both physical pain and psychological distress. This finding was contrary to the popular notion that Orientals are stoic and less sensitive to pain and distress. The following observation reported by Davitz et al. illustrates this stereotype. A Japanese man who was recovering from surgery burst into tears during an interaction with staff. His nurse later commented that the patient's behavior surprised her. She stated, "I thought Japanese could stand pain. They aren't supposed to show emotion" (27).

This stereotype was reflected in a second study by Davitz et al., which showed that, although Americans believe Orientals feel far less pain than do patients from other ethnic backgrounds, Oriental nurses believe that their Oriental patients are especially sensitive to physical pain (28). In fact, they infer more pain in their patients than American nurses do in judging American patients. These findings may be explained by the fact that, in Japan, control of expressive behavior is highly valued. Although Japanese people experience very strong feelings, their feelings are less likely to be expressed in overt behavior (28). It is important for nurses and other health care practitioners to be aware of their cultural stereotypes, because these may interfere with accuracy in assessing the pain their patients are experiencing.

THE SICK ROLE AND CHRONIC PAIN

In the early 1950s, sociologic theorist Talcott Parsons formulated the concept of the sick role. This concept identifies two rights and two responsibilities granted to the sick in our society (29). The first right involves exemption from responsibility for the pathologic condition. Even though the sick person may have brought the condition on himself, he is not held responsible. In fact, the patient is not only absolved from blame, but he is also awarded sympathy and support.

Second, the person in the sick role is relieved from his normal social role responsibilities. These may be related to family, work, or school. The process by which exemption becomes socially recognized has important implications for the patient with chronic pain. The role of the physician in validating the patient's claims is very important. Patients may seek validation for legal reasons, or to convince family members of their need to be exempted from household responsibilities.

Parsons identified two responsibilities of the individual admitted to the sick role. First, the patient must acknowledge the undesirability of the illness, and second, he must make every effort to get well. In so doing, he must seek help from a competent and appropriate practitioner. In modern society, this appropriate source of help is generally considered to be the medical profession. However, some cultures resort to faith healers and other nonconventional disciplines. Once the individual seeks help from the medical profession he becomes a patient, and the expectations for the sick role are extended. In summarizing the rights and responsibilities of the sick role,

Gallagher and Wrobel described it as consisting of a socially legitimized dependency (29).

The sick role as described by Parsons most accurately describes the individual who is suffering an acute illness. The patient with chronic pain presents an interesting deviation from the classic sick role. By definition, chronic illness is ongoing and long term, generally lasting more than 6 months (4). The likelihood of cure is low. The exemptions and social support awarded to the patient with chronic pain are usually long term, but they may fluctuate with the severity of the patient's illness. With chronic illness, adaptation rather than cure is considered to be the goal.

A second feature of the sick role unique to the chronically ill is an increased level of autonomy and responsibility for health maintenance. Although the patient with chronic pain may be suffering and disabled in some areas, he typically has other capacities that are unaffected. Because pain is a subjective experience, the patient may have a difficult time being allowed into the sick role. He may undergo numerous time-consuming and expensive tests in an effort to have his pain diagnosed and legitimized. Frequently, this is important not only for social reasons, but also for litigation following accidents or work-related injuries.

INFLUENCE OF COMPENSATION AND LITIGATION

The individual who experiences chronic pain faces the real or threatened loss of his ability to remain gainfully employed. This creates tremendous anxiety, which can exacerbate the subjective perception of pain. Disability insurance and other forms of remuneration for work-related injuries play a significant role in modifying the patient's pain experience, most notably his decision to return to work.

The first workers' compensation laws were enacted in the United States in 1911. These laws required employers to assume the cost of any disability that was work related, regardless of who was at fault (30). In his address to the Congress on June 8, 1934, President Franklin D. Roosevelt stated: "I am looking for a sound means which I can recommend to provide at once security against several of the great disturbing factors in life—especially those which relate to unemployment and old age" (31, p. 665). Although a pension plan for the elderly came about in the Social Security Act of 1935, it was not until the Eisenhower administration in 1954 that the Social Security Disability Insurance (SSDI) program was established. This legislation has had tremendous economic and social consequences. In 1980, approximately 3 million Americans benefited from the SSDI program, at a cost approaching $13 billion (31).

The literature is replete with allegations that patients who are receiving disability payments, or who have litigation pending from an injury, are less likely to respond positively to medical therapy than patients who do not (30). The term *compensation neurosis* was coined by European physicians in the late 1800s. One of these physicians stated, "many malingerers had been cured by successful suits at law" (30, p. 233). This sentiment is expressed by Kessler, who described workers' compensation as "the etiologic factor responsible for the prolongation of symptoms and the production of the neurotic behavior on which prolonged disability is based" (32).

With less pressure from ethical, religious, and social sources regarding the importance of work, absenteeism and compensation for illness and minor accidents are rapidly on the rise. It is well established that if a self-employed carpenter and a factory worker covered by SSDI sustain the same injury, the carpenter is more likely to keep working and to recover sooner than the factory worker. The worker who pays into the SSDI program is more likely to believe that society should provide for him financially until he feels completely well (2).

In examining the relationship of disability to compensation status in railroad workers, Sander and Meyers found that patients who sustained work-related injuries were disabled for significantly longer than those injured off duty. Patients injured on duty were off work for an average of 14.9 months, compared with 3.6 months for patients sustaining non-work-related injuries (33). These findings are consistent with those reported by the Crozer-Chester Medical Center Low Back Clinic. Six hundred twenty-three patients who were successfully treated for low back pain without surgery were studied. Of the total, 324 patients without secondary gain averaged a total disability of 16 days, whereas the 281 patients with secondary gain averaged 36 days of total disability (34).

A study performed by Guck et al. showed that, among patients who received nonsurgical treatment for chronic pain, one of the factors associated with successful treatment was the absence of financial compensation (9). Trief and Stein obtained similar results among patients with low back pain who were participating in a 6-week behavioral treatment course (1). Scales from the Minnesota Multiphasic Personality Inventory and Sternbach's Health Index were used, along with three behavioral measures of physical mobility. Those patients with current lawsuits for compensation, or unsettled claims for disability benefits, achieved significantly lower results from treatment than those without. Also, patients without pending litigation worried less about their physical problems and had less tendency to use physical symptoms as a means to obtain gratification or to avoid responsibility (1). Recognizing these findings, some chronic pain treatment centers have gone so far as to exclude patients who have litigation pending (35). This is unfortunate, because the data relating compensation or litigation and prognosis are not unequivocal. Dworkin et al. found that employment predicts long-term outcome, whereas compensation and litigation do not (36). They suggested that the poorer outcome among patients receiving compensation or who have litigation pending is due to the fact that the former group is less likely to be employed than the latter group. Instead of focusing on the "compensation neurosis," they recommended focusing on "the role of activity and employment in the treatment and rehabilitation of chronic pain patients" (36, p. 58). Approximately 60% of the patients admitted to the Dallas Spinal Pain Program have pending workers' compensation litigation. This is not considered a contraindication for participation, because the program's experience has shown that the majority of patients will settle their claims once they are convinced that they are not doomed to a lifetime of pain and frustration (8).

In analyzing the role of the current compensation system in relation to continued unemployment, Beals has identified four paradoxes that merit consideration (30). The first is that financial compensation discourages return to work. For example, in 1984, the stipend for temporary total disability in the state of Oregon was two-thirds of gross wages, up to 100% of average wages. For permanent total disability, it was two-thirds of gross wages up to $14,917 per year. This stipend continues until death, not just until age 65. An allowance for dependents is also included. This income is tax free. When the disability payments approach or exceed the income the individual made when employed, in the words of Beals, "any form of treatment is likely doomed to failure" (30, p. 235).

A second paradox is that the appeal process increases disability. In a study performed in Oregon, patients who were dissatisfied with their disability payments and appealed received an average of twice the amount received by patients who did not appeal. There were no organic differences between the two groups.

The third paradox is that an open claim inhibits return to work. Claims remain open as long as the patient is under treatment or is getting better or worse. Patients who are experiencing symptoms hesitate to have their claims closed. They may participate in ineffective treatment programs simply to keep their claims open. A study by Gotten showed that settlement of claims had a positive effect on symptoms (37). It seems logical that patients should be rewarded for return to work, rather than for continued disability.

The fourth paradox is that recovering patients are often unable to return to work. Athletes who are injured fight back to recovery by keeping regular hours, controlling weight, avoiding drugs, and developing strength and motor skills. Although patients who do physical labor for a living should do likewise, the reverse is often true. Workers who are injured become overweight, take drugs, and become undisciplined and unfit. Although gradual return to work would be therapeutic, rules and regulations often prohibit return until the patient is ready to assume his regular workload.

INFLUENCE OF OCCUPATIONAL ROLE

Displacement from the occupational role frequently results in shifting of roles within the family unit (38). This may cause dissonance and dissatisfaction within the family. Members of the family may experience frustration and anger toward the patient, but they displace the anger rather than express it because of the societal mores governing response toward the sick role. Whereas the provider of the family is respected and given status as a result of his ability to provide, perceptions change when the occupational role is dysfunctional. The spouse may now regard the former provider as dependent, similar to the way a child or aged parent is perceived. The disabled family member may be excluded from decision making and family functions, not because he is unable to participate, but because of the way he is perceived by the family members. Redistribution of household responsibilities serves as a further cause of conflict and hostility. These events may lead to mutual role dissatisfaction and potentially to family dissolution.

Displacement from the occupational role also threatens the patient's personal role, which "defines that set of behaviors by which an individual actualizes personal experiences according to sets of personal rules that have been acquired during growth and development" (38, p 54). As the individual lives and works to fulfill his personal expectations, he obtains a sense of mastery or control, leading to personal satisfaction. When the personal role is threatened, the patient may develop regressed behavior. He becomes dependent, clings to family members, complains bitterly of pain, and assumes a defeated and passive position (38).

The goal of rapid return to work in treating patients with chronic pain is consistent with the recommendations of White, made 20 years ago: "Perhaps effective placement of these unfortunate workmen in jobs which are within the limitations imposed by the pain would maintain the morale, avoid concentration of their attention on their complaints, and, while keeping up reasonable body activities, allow passage of sufficient time for the condition to subside" (39, p. 56). In treating patients with the chronic pain syndrome, it has been shown that return to work results in decreased perceived pain level, more manageable pain behavior, and increased self-esteem (40). In treating patients with injuries of the extremities and lower back, Dworkin et al. found that the greater the period of unemployment, the lower the likelihood that the patient will ever return to work (36). In emphasizing the importance of vocational guidance and rapid return to work, David Florence of the Chronic Pain Rehabilitation Unit of the Sister Kenny Institute stated, "Our patients learn that there is no such thing as disability—rather, only varying levels of ability, with a place for each of us in a fast-moving society and a mobile work force" (40, p. 227).

When the woman of the family is the one with chronic pain, a different sort of disequilibrium results (41). Although each family unit delegates household responsibilities in an individual way, the woman typically performs the major portion of nurturing and caretaking. When she is incapacitated, all members of the family experience stress. Being unable to fulfill her role expectations poses a threat to the woman's identity. She feels anxious and guilty.

Society does not readily exempt the woman from her household responsibilities, even in the face of chronic illness. Crook illustrates this point with the example of a woman who offered to help her friend, who was suffering chronic pain. After offering, the friend stated, "I can't afford to get sick; I can't give myself the luxury" (41, p. 71).

PSYCHOLOGICAL CONSIDERATIONS

Although the exact relationship between psychological factors and etiology of pain is still undergoing considerable debate, three mechanisms are recognized as important in the etiology. The first is hallucination, which can occur secondary to schizophrenia or endogenous depression. This is relatively rare. The second mechanism in psychogenic pain involves muscle tension induced by psychological causes. Vascular distention induced by psychological causes, resulting in migraine, is a similar phenomenon. The third psychological mechanism is conversion hysteria. This is a controversial area, because it is difficult to assess and measure. The idea involves pain that arises from psychological events rather than from any physiologic cause (42). The chronic pain syndrome has been defined as a psychological stress state with multiple functional or emotional components, including hysteria, depression, and hypochondriasis (40). The majority of patients with the chronic pain syndrome have few, if any, abnormal physical findings, but they see themselves as severely impaired from a physical standpoint. Patients with this syndrome have unmet psychological, social, economic, and sexual needs, which are thought to contribute to the etiology of the chronic pain syndrome. Florence gives an interesting example of a blue-collar worker with low self-esteem who routinely received little attention from family, friends, and neighbors. After sustaining a back injury, he began to receive more attention. His doctor demonstrated concern by performing numerous tests and treatments. Now when he sees people, they ask, "How is your back?" instead of the perfunctory "How are you?" This is gratifying to the patient, and he perpetuates the chronic pain syndrome (40).

The "inadequacy syndrome" is a type of chronic pain syndrome. The typical patient is male, 25–50 years old, with limited education, who is married to a woman of greater intelligence who works in a more prestigious job. The patient, being a manual laborer, prides himself in his physical ability. When marital problems begin to occur, the patient experiences a minor injury at work. Although the injury is minor, the patient experiences extreme pain, devastation, and disability. He presents a tremendous challenge for the treatment team. This type of patient is typically angry, hostile, and demanding. After careful psychological evaluation, the etiology is usually determined to be psychological, economic, social, and sexual in origin (40). The symptoms are stress related and result from changes mediated by the autonomic nervous system.

Mayer has described a phenomenon called "pain games" that is similar to the chronic pain syndrome (8). This involves an individual with preexisting psychosocial impairments who experiences a stressful period. Perhaps his employer is too demanding, financial problems are occurring, and his friends are unsupportive. He experiences a trivial injury, which results in severe pain and disability. If the patient receives secondary gain in the form of medical attention, family support, relief from social responsibilities, and financial compensation, the pain may become chronic. The patient learns to manipulate the system and maintain the sympathy by playing "pain games." Return to work is critical, because the longer the patient remains off work, the more ingrained the "pain games" become.

Successful management of patients with chronic pain mandates consideration of psychosocial factors that exist before and follow the injury. Although precise psychosocial causes have not been identified, life stresses are known to be important. Meyers found that high scores on the Life Change Unit Value Scale preceded injury in Southern Pacific workers (43). Drug and alcohol abuse preceding the injury is common. In considering psychosocial results of injury, a case for the "accident process" has been made. In this phenomenon, the accident itself and the resulting symptoms serve as a solution to life's problems (43).

A classic example of pain occurring as a result of emotional causes is "effort syndrome" (3). This consists of chest pain, difficulty in breathing, and fatigue. It occurs frequently in soldiers during the stress of war. Chest pain without a physiologic cause is an integral part of this syndrome. A second type of pain that frequently occurs as a result of emotional causes is headache. Studies have shown that patients who experience persistent pain for which there is no organic cause tend to have elevations on the Hypochondriasis, Hysteria, and Depression scales of the Minnesota Multiphasic Personality Inventory (3).

Emotional factors can also have a substantial effect on how acutely the patient feels and responds to pain. A study by Beecher showed that soldiers who were wounded in battle required far less analgesia than civilians with wounds of similar size (44). Although this may be partially due to the mechanism of injury, psychological factors certainly contribute. To the soldier, the wound represents a ticket to safety. To the civilian, it represents an interruption to his normal functioning (11). Pain is sometimes welcomed by the patient, because it may indicate a positive prognosis. For example, pain in a limb whose viability is threatened may be preferable to complete lack of sensation (28).

FAMILY CONSIDERATIONS

The patient who experiences chronic pain spends a great deal of time and money searching for an explanation and cure for his pain. He journeys from practitioner to practitioner, and may see a family physician, orthopedist, neurologist, neurosurgeon, physiotherapist, psychologist, and psychiatrist. The patient frequently feels lost, anxious, and depressed (45). He undergoes numerous tests, which can actually compromise his health and exacerbate his pain. His emotions alternate between hope and despair, resulting in bitterness and anger toward the health care system. The patient with chronic pain frequently fears having a dread disease like cancer, but this fear is rarely openly expressed. He begins to focus more and more on his problem, and he may approach nonconventional practitioners out of desperation. These nonconventional practitioners may include hypnotists and acupuncturists.

The patient with chronic pain frequently becomes depressed as a result of loss of health, loss of enjoyable activities, loss of income, and loss of the ability to fulfill his parental and spousal roles. The patient's family members may also become depressed, and they may respond with pain-reinforcing behavior (46).

Freud was the first to report a relationship between etiology of pain and family problems. It is now believed that the patient's family of origin may influence pain threshold, pain tolerance, pain complaints, and/or the sick role. Patients from large families are more prone to pain, as are firstborn children (46). The results of a study performed in 1978 show that of 63 patients with chronic pain, 40% had not lived their childhood with both parents and 23% had been abandoned. Eighty-two per cent complained of lack of affection during childhood, 63% reported open rejection, and 19% reported lack of physical display of affection from their parents. Thirty-seven per cent of the group had been battered children (45). Most patients with chronic pain have at least one other family member who also suffers from chronic pain. This has been referred to as the "familial pain model." In describing "pain-prone patients," Engel has identified aggression and pain in the family of origin as important contributing factors (47). The patient may have learned that painful attention from his parents was an indication that they cared. As the patient grew up, he developed tremendous guilt feelings, and the experience of pain serves as a punishment that lessens the guilt (47).

SUMMARY

Chronic pain is a complex phenomenon that defies quantitative measurement in scientific terms. The experience of chronic pain is one of extreme importance to health care practitioners because of its financial, social, and personal consequences. In analyzing the impact of chronic pain and in assisting the patient suffering from chronic pain toward adaptation, an interdisciplinary approach, designed uniquely for each individual patient, is essential. Familiarity with the social and cultural aspects of pain, from both a cause and an effect perspective, is a necessary prerequisite for the practitioner facing this complex treatment challenge.

References

1. Trief P, Stein N: Pending litigation and rehabilitation outcome of chronic back pain. *Arch Phys Med Rehabil* 66:95–99, 1985.
2. Beltrutti D: Cultural factors in chronic pain. *Panminerva Med* 26:87–92, 1984.
3. Merskey H: Body-mind dilemma in chronic pain. In Roy R, Tunks E (eds): *Chronic Pain: Psychosocial Factors in Rehabilitation*. Baltimore, Williams & Wilkins, 1982, pp 12, 15.
4. Kotarba J: *Chronic Pain: Its Social Dimensions*. Beverly Hills, CA, Sage, 1983, p 13.
5. Berkson M, Schultz A, Nachemson A, et al: Voluntary strengths of male adults with acute low back syndrome. *Clin Orthop* 129:84–95, 1977.
6. Nordby EJ: Epidemiology and diagnosis in low back injury. *Occup Health Saf* 50:38–42, 1981.
7. White AA, Gordon SL: Synopsis: workshop on idiopathic low back pain. *Spine* 7:141–149, 1982.
8. Mayer T: Rehabilitation of the patient with spinal pain. *Orthop Clin North Am* 14:623–637, 1983.
9. Guck TP, Meilman PW, Skultety FM, et al: Prediction of long-term outcome of multidisciplinary pain treatment. *Arch Phys Med Rehabil* 67:293–296, 1986.
10. LeShan L: The world of the patient in severe pain of long duration. *J Chron Dis* 17:119–126, 1964.
11. Sternbach R: *Pain Patients: Traits and Treatment*. New York, Academic Press, 1974, pp 8, 24.
12. Elton D, Burrows GD, Stanley GV: Clinical measurement of pain. *Med J Aust* 1:109, 1979.
13. Weidman HH: The transcultural view. Prerequisite to interethnic (intercultural) communication in medicine. *Soc Sci Med* 13:85, 1979.
14. Allport G: *The Nature of Prejudice*. New York, Anchor Books, 1958.
15. Lipton JA, Marbach JJ: Ethnicity and the pain experience. *Soc Sci Med* 19:1279–1298, 1984.
16. Weisenberg M, et al: Pain, anxiety, and attitudes in black, white, and Puerto Rican patients. *Psychosom Med* 37:123, 1975.
17. Zborowski M: Cultural components in response to pain. *J Soc Issues* 8:16, 1952.
18. Zola J: Culture and symptoms—an analysis of patients' presenting complaints. *Am Sociol Rev* 31:615, 1966.
19. Kleinman A, Eisenberg L, Good B: Culture, illness, and care. *Ann Intern Med* 88:251, 1978.
20. Mechanic D: *Medical Sociology*. New York, Free Press, 1978.
21. Chrisman N, Kleinman A: Health beliefs and practices. In Thornstrom S (ed): *Harvard Encyclopedia of American Ethnic Groups*. Cambridge, MA, Harvard University Press, 1980.
22. Flannery RB, Sos J, McGovern P: Ethnicity as a factor in the expression of pain. *Psychosomatics* 22:39–51, 1981.
23. Koopman C, Eisenthal S, Stoeckle JD: Ethnicity in the reported pain, emotional distress, and requests of medical outpatients. *Soc Sci Med* 18:487–490, 1984.
24. Zborowski M: *People in Pain*. San Francisco, Jossey-Bass, 1969, pp 30–32, 39, 41, 46.
25. Sargent C: Between death and shame: dimensions of pain in Bariba culture. *Soc Sci Med* 19:1299–1304, 1984.
26. Davitz LL, Davitz JR, Higuchi Y: Cross-cultural inferences of physical pain and psychological distress—1. *Nurs Times* 73:521–523, 1977.
27. Davitz LL, Davitz JR, Higuchi Y: Cross-cultural inferences of physical pain and psychological distress—2. *Nurs Times* 73:556–558, 1977.
28. Davitz LJ, Sameshima Y, Davitz J: Suffering as viewed in six different cultures. *Am J Nurs* 76:1296–1297, 1976.
29. Gallagher EB, Wrobel S: The sick-role and chronic pain. In Roy R, Tunks E (eds): *Chronic Pain: Psychosocial Factors in*

Rehabilitation. Baltimore, Williams & Wilkins, 1982, pp 36–40.
30. Beals RK: Compensation and recovery from injury. *West J Med* 140:233–237, 1984.
31. Hadler NM: Medical ramifications of the federal regulation of the social security disability insurance program. *Ann Intern Med* 96:665–669, 1982.
32. Kessler HH: Low Back Pain in Industry—A Study Prepared for the Special *Committee on Workman's Compensation.* New York, Commerce and Industry Association of New York, 1955.
33. Sander RA, Meyers JE: The relationship of disability to compensation status in railroad workers. *Spine* 11:141–143, 1986.
34. Finneson BE: Psychosocial considerations in low back pain: the cause and cure of industry related low back pain. *Orthop Clin North Am* 8:23–26, 1977.
35. Sternbach RA, Wolf SR, Murphy RW, Akeson WH: Traits of pain patients: low back "loser." *Psychosomatics* 14:226–229, 1973.
36. Dworkin RH, Handlin DS, Richlin DM, et al: Unraveling the effects of compensation, litigation, and employment on treatment response in chronic pain. *Pain* 23:49–59, 1985.
37. Gotten N: Survey of 100 cases of whiplash injury after settlement of litigation. *JAMA* 162:865–867, 1956,
38. Tunks E, Roy R: Chronic pain and the occupational role. In Roy R, Tunks E (ed): *Chronic Pain: Psychosocial Factors in Rehabilitation.* Baltimore, Williams & Wilkins, 1982, pp 54–60.
39. White AWM: Low back pain in men receiving workman's compensation. *Can Med Assoc J* 95:56, 1966.
40. Florence DW: The chronic pain syndrome: physical and psychologic challenge. *Postgrad Med* 70:217–228, 1981.
41. Crook J: Women with chronic pain. In Roy R, Tunks E (ed): *Chronic Pain: Psychosocial Factors in Rehabilitation.* Baltimore, Williams & Wilkins, 1982, p 71.
42. Merskey H: Psychological aspects of pain. In Weisenberg M (ed): *Pain: Clinical and Experimental Perspectives,* St. Louis, CV Mosby, 1975, pp 25–26.
43. Meyers JE: cited by Beals RK: Compensation and recovery from injury. *West J Med* 140:233–237, 1984.
44. Beecher HK: Psychology of the pain experience. In Weisenberg M (ed): *Pain: Clinical and Experimental Perspectives.* St. Louis, CV Mosby Co, 1975.
45. Violin A: The process involved in becoming a chronic pain patient. In Roy R, Tunks E (ed): *Chronic Pain: Psychosocial Factors in Rehabilitation.* Baltimore, Williams & Wilkins, 1982, pp 25, 33.
46. Mohamed S: The patient and his family. In Roy R, Tunks E (ed): *Chronic Pain: Psychosocial Factors in Rehabilitation.* Baltimore, Williams & Wilkins, 1982, pp 145, 146.
47. Engle GL: "Psychogenic" pain and the pain-prone patient. *Am J Med* 26:899–918, 1959.

Suggested Readings

Carron H, DeGood DE, Tait R: A comparison of low back pain patients in the United States and New Zealand: psychosocial and economic factors affecting severity of disability. *Pain* 21:77–89, 1985.
Larkins FR: The influence of one patient's culture on pain response. *Nurs Clin North Am* 12:663–668, 1977.
LeRoy PL: *Current Concepts in the Management of Chronic Pain.* New York, Stratton Intercontinental Medical Book Corp, 1977.
McMahon MA, Miller P: Pain response; the influence of psychosocial-cultural factors. *Nurs Forum* XVII:58–71, 1978.
Spector RE: *Cultural Diversity in Health and Illness.* East Norwalk, CT, Appleton-Century-Crofts, 1979.
Weisenberg M: Pain and pain control. *Psychol Bull* 84:1008–1044, 1977.

chapter 5
Medical Electrodiagnostics

Henry A. Spindler, M.D.

Patients are referred for electrodiagnostic evaluation of a variety of complaints. These include pain, weakness, sensory complaints, gait disturbances, headache, and bowel and bladder dysfunction (1). These electrical studies are frequently of great help in diagnosing acute and chronic pain involving the neck, back, and extremities, whether or not there are positive clinical findings. The most useful tests are electromyography (EMG) and nerve conduction studies (NCS), including H reflex and F wave measurement. Somatosensory-evoked potentials may also sometimes be helpful in evaluating patients with pain syndromes. Older methods of electrodiagnosis (reaction of degeneration, chronaxie, rheobase, galvanic-tetanus ratio, strength-duration curves) are rarely, if ever, used for the evaluation of pain in a modern electrodiagnostic laboratory. However, they are certainly of historic interest, and nerve excitability studies continue to be used for evaluation of Bell's palsy (2, 3).

The primary function of an electrodiagnostic evaluation utilizing EMG and NCS is to evaluate the functional integrity of the motor unit. The term *motor unit* was first used by Liddell and Sherrington in 1925 to describe the functional unit of the peripheral nervous system (4). The motor unit is defined as an anterior horn cell, its axon, and all the muscle fibers innervated by that axon. Electrodiagnostic studies attempt to localize sites of pathology within the motor unit (i.e., root, plexus, peripheral nerve, etc.) to diagnose the presence of a lesion causing the clinical pain syndrome.

ELECTROMYOGRAPHY

Electromyography is the technique of recording voltage changes within a muscle. Resting mammalian muscle fibers have a transmembrane potential of 70–90 mV in the resting state. The inside of the cell is negative with respect to the outside. This resting potential arises since the membrane is impermeable to the large organic anions within the cell and because of the active transport mechanism that maintains the internal Na^+ concentration at a low level. When a nerve impulse reaches the neuromuscular junction, acetylcholine is released across the end plate zone. This initiates an action potential, or reversal of polarity across the muscle membrane, which rapidly spreads over the length of the muscle fiber, initiating contraction. The amplitude of this voltage change may be 100 mV or more when measured with an intracellular electrode.

Intracellular muscle potential recording is technically difficult and unsuited to the clinical situation. Extracellular EMG recordings are performed clinically with a needle electrode. Adrian and Bronk in 1929 introduced the concentric needle electrode (5). This electrode consists of a hypodermic needle serving as the cannula with a wire located centrally in the needle but completely insulated from it. Voltage is recorded as the potential difference between the exposed tip of the central wire and the cannula. Since the recording is made extracellularly at a distance from the muscle fiber, the voltage changes recorded are much smaller, ranging from 500 μV to 5 mV. Also, with standard recording electrodes, the recording surface at the tip is quite large with respect to the muscle fiber, and potentials from several muscle fibers are recorded simultaneously. Specialized electrodes with very small recording areas have been developed for recording single muscle fiber potentials. Single fiber recordings, however, are quite specialized studies, and are not used routinely in the electrodiagnostic examination.

Today, the most commonly used needle electrode is of the monopolar type. This is a small-diameter wire electrode that is coated with insulating Teflon except at the tip, where recording is done. Potential measurements are made between the exposed tip of the needle within the muscle and a surface electrode taped to the skin. This electrode arrangement has largely replaced the concentric electrode in most clinical conditions because of the much greater patient comfort.

Electrical activity measured within the muscle is fed into a suitable amplifier and then displayed on an oscilloscope. The activity is also monitored through a loudspeaker, since the various potential changes encountered have characteristic sound. Electromyographic activity is measured during needle insertion, during complete rest of the muscle without needle movement, and during various grades of active muscle contraction.

INSERTIONAL ACTIVITY

The electrical response seen when a needle electrode is inserted into resting muscle is termed the *insertional activity*. This appears on an oscilloscope as a burst of spike potentials that continues for 100–300 msec after needle motion has ceased. This electrical activity is produced by mechanical damage or deformation of the muscle membrane by the advancing needle. Although the evaluation of insertional activity may appear simple, it is actually a quite difficult procedure. With careful analysis a great deal of information may be gained by an experienced electromyographer.

The duration of insertional activity may be normal, increased, or decreased. The exact duration of normal insertional activity cannot be given since it depends on many factors, including the velocity of needle insertion and the degree of tissue deformation that occurs. Each electromyographer must therefore to some degree determine "normal" insertional activity with his equipment and technique. Increase in the duration of insertional activity may be the first or only sign of neuromuscular disease. Decrease in the duration of insertional activity is also significant. It most commonly indicates a loss of muscle tissue and is usually a late finding in neuromuscular disease.

The character of the electrical discharges seen with needle insertion must also be examined. Occasional positive sharp waves may be seen during insertional activity as the first sign of denervation.

Since abnormal insertional activity may not be uniform throughout the muscle, at least 10–20 needle insertions must be performed at various sites within the muscle. Electromyographers must be aware of the "end plate noise," which is the normal electrical activity seen in the end plate zone of the muscle, and not report this as abnormal insertional activity.

RESTING MUSCLE

With the needle electrode at rest in relaxed muscle, there is normally no electrical activity seen. Resting activity is observed during pauses between needle insertions. During this procedure, the electromyographer is searching for the presence of abnormal spontaneous activity at rest, but he may also encounter normal spontaneous activity, which must be recognized as such.

Normal Spontaneous Activity

Normal spontaneous activity can be recorded if the needle electrode is near the motor end plate region (6). Two types of end plate noise are commonly seen. The first appears as a widening of the baseline, but at closer inspection it is a series of 8–10-μV negative potentials that exhibit a characteristic "seashell" sound over the loudspeaker. This electrical activity corresponds to the miniature end plate potentials caused by acetylcholine release. Occasionally, large spike potentials may be seen superimposed on the end plate noise. These are most likely due to the needle electrode provoking enough acetylcholine release to depolarize the entire muscle membrane, resulting in the recording of a propagated single muscle fiber nerve action potential.

Abnormal Spontaneous Activity

Fibrillation Potentials Fibrillation potentials are the electrical activity recorded from the spontaneous depolarization of single muscle fibers. They are usually bi- or triphasic potentials, 50–500 μV in amplitude, with a duration of less than 1.5 msec. The initial deflection is positive when recording away from the end plate zone. Each muscle fiber depolarizes at a regular rate varying from 1 to 30/sec, but in some cases the firing may be irregular (7). However, since in most cases multiple fibrillations are seen simultaneously, an irregular-appearing pattern appears on the oscilloscope with a characteristic crackling, "rain on a tin roof" sound from the loudspeaker. Fibrillations have been most commonly associated with lower motor neuron disease such as anterior horn cell pathology, radiculopathies, and neuropathies. In these disorders muscle fiber has lost continuity with its motor nerve fiber, allowing spontaneous depolarization. However, it is now known that fibrillations can occur in the presence of myopathies, especially polymyositis, where splitting of the muscle fiber occurs. Fibrillations may also be seen in electrolyte disorders such as hypokalemia or hyperkalemia. Fibrillations have also been reported in spinal cord injury and stroke, but this finding is still controversial (8, 9).

Positive Sharp Waves Positive sharp waves are seen in the same conditions and have the same significance as fibrillation potentials. They are biphasic potentials with an initial sharp positive phase of from 50 μV to 1 mV followed by a low-amplitude, long-duration negative phase commonly exceeding 10 msec before return to baseline. Positive waves fire regularly, commonly at a rate of 2–10/sec. Positive waves are thought to arise from spontaneously depolarizing single muscle fibers that have been damaged by needle insertion.

Fasciculation Potentials Fasciculation potentials are the electrical activity recorded from the spontaneous firing of a motor unit. When these occur near the surface of the muscle, a visible twitch occurs. The neural discharge initiating the fasciculation is most commonly in the anterior horn cell, but it may be anywhere within the motor unit (10). Thus, although they are usually associated with motor neuron disease, fasciculations may be present in radiculopathies or peripheral neuropathies. They may occasionally be seen in otherwise normal muscle, especially with fatigue. Fasciculations are not seen in primary muscle disorders.

Complex Repetitive Discharges Complex repetitive discharges (previously called bizarre high-frequency discharges) can be seen in many forms of lower motor neuron disorders or myopathies. These are trains of potentials that begin and end abruptly. Their amplitude may range from 50 μV to several millivolts. The individual potentials may assume many forms and may be 50–100 msec in duration. They may fire at rates ranging from 5 to 100 cycles/sec. These discharges most likely arise within a group of denervated muscle fibers where one muscle fiber acts as a pacemaker, with spread of depolarization to the neighboring denervated muscle fibers (11). Myotonic discharges are thought to be a distinct repetitive discharge due to muscle membrane instability as seen in disorders such as myotonic dystrophy and myotonia congenita. These discharges wax and wane in frequency and amplitude, whereas complex repetitive discharges display constant rate and amplitude. Myotonic discharges also differ in that the trains of potentials slowly decrease in frequency until they stop, instead of suddenly ceasing.

VOLUNTARY MUSCLE CONTRACTION

After the muscle being examined has been studied at rest, the patient is asked to produce a minimal contraction with the needle electrode in place. The number of motor unit potentials seen is proportional to the strength of contraction; therefore to examine individual motor unit potentials, the contraction must be kept minimal. The normal motor unit potential usually contains up to four phases. A potential with five or more phases is termed polyphasic. A small proportion of normal motor units may be polyphasic (5–15%). An increase in the percentage of polyphasic motor unit potentials is considered abnormal. This may occur either with neuropathic disease or with myopathy. In neuropathy, impaired conduction in the terminal nerve fibers of the motor unit will result in asynchrony of firing and an increase in the number of phases seen on EMG (12). In primary muscle disorders, loss of muscle fibers contributing to the motor unit potential may result in an increased number of phases.

The amplitude of the normal motor unit action potential ranges from 500 μV to 5 mV. This amplitude will vary with the density of the muscle fibers in the region of the tip of the electrode as well as with the synchrony of firing of the individual muscle fibers in the unit. In lower motor neuron disorders, reinnervation frequently leads to increase in fiber density, resulting in increased motor unit potential amplitudes. In myopathy, loss of muscle fibers from the unit will result in decreased amplitude. Normal motor unit potential duration ranges from 5 to 12 msec as defined from the first deviation from the baseline to the final return to baseline. In neuropathy, with slowing in terminal nerve fiber conduction, there will be an increase in the duration of the potential. In myopathy, the common finding is decrease in potential duration.

As the strength of voluntary contraction increases, the number of motor units firing increases proportionally. The first recruited motor unit potentials fire at a rate of approximately 5/sec. As the strength of contraction increases, the initial unit begins firing at a higher rate, and simultaneously other motor units are recruited. In neuropathic disease, when fewer motor units are available for recruitment, the first unit will be seen firing at a higher than normal rate before the second unit appears. In myopathy, where the strength produced by each motor unit is reduced, the second motor unit will be recruited much earlier. With maximal voluntary contraction in normal muscle, the oscilloscope will be obscured by electrical activity, and individual motor units cannot be seen (complete interference pattern). In neuropathic disorders, at maximal contraction there may not be a complete obliteration of the baseline with electrical activity (incomplete interference pattern); or in severe cases, individual motor units may still be discernible (single unit interference pattern). In myopathies, as previously discussed, there is decreased strength produced by contraction by each motor unit. Therefore, for a contraction of fixed strength, more motor units will need to be recruited than in normal muscle. This causes a complete interference pattern with less than maximal effort.

Although evaluation of the interference pattern is important, it must be interpreted with caution since lack of patient cooperation from anxiety or pain may influence the results.

NERVE CONDUCTION STUDIES

Nerve conduction studies are safe, reliable, and reproducible in assessing peripheral nerve function. They are used to determine the presence and type of neuropathy, to localize lesions, and to determine their severity. The nerve is stimulated electrically, and various parameters are measured to determine the nerve's ability to carry the impulse. Stimulation may be done either with needle or surface electrodes. In most laboratories, surface stimulation is the method of choice. However, with deeply placed nerves, such as the sciatic in the gluteal region, near-nerve needle stimulation is easier and more comfortable for the patient. At rest the nerve is charged with a 90 mV transmembrane potential, positive externally. When the negatively applied stimulus exceeds threshold, an action potential is generated. This potential is then self-propagated proximally and distally.

Motor conduction studies are performed by stimulating the nerve and recording the evoked response from a distal muscle. The time from stimulation to the onset of the evoked response is termed the *latency*. Conduction velocity from the distal stimulation site to the muscle cannot be determined because of the presence of the neuromuscular junction. However, if the nerve is stimulated at two points, the velocity between these points is easily determined by subtracting the distal from the proximal latency and dividing this into the distance between the stimulus sites. Conduction velocities can thus be determined over multiple segments of the nerve to localize a lesion.

Sensory conduction studies are performed by placing recording electrodes directly over the sensory nerve being examined. The nerve may be stimulated either proximally (antidromic conduction) or distally (orthodromic conduction) to these electrodes, and the time from the onset of the stimulus to the onset of the action potential that is being recorded is measured. Dividing this time into the distance between the recording and stimulating electrodes yields the sensory conduction velocity. The sensory nerve action potential is usually bi- or triphasic. Latency measurements are frequently made to both the onset and the peak of the first negative phase. As in motor studies, the amplitude of the evoked response is recorded.

Decrease in nerve conduction velocity is most commonly associated with disorders of the myelin. However, this may also occur with diseases affecting the large, rapidly conducting axons. Axonal disorders more commonly cause decrease in the amplitude of the evoked motor and sensory responses since fewer fibers are available to contribute to the response.

Sensory nerves commonly studied include the median, ulnar, radial, medial and lateral antebrachial cutaneous, lateral femoral cutaneous, sural, superficial peroneal, and tibial. Motor studies may be done on the median, ulnar, radial, tibial, peroneal, and sciatic nerves. Motor latency studies may be done on the femoral, axillary, suprascapular, accessory, and facial nerves.

PROXIMAL CONDUCTION STUDIES

The conduction studies discussed thus far allow evaluation of peripheral nerve function in the extremities. Nerve root stimulation, H reflex, and F wave measurements allow examination of proximal segments at the root and plexus level.

Nerve Root Stimulation

Nerve root stimulation may be performed in either the cervical or lumbar region. In the cervical region, the C8 nerve root is the most frequently studied, but C6 and C7 may also be evaluated. In the lumbar region, L4, L5, or S1 may be examined. A stimulating needle cathode is placed into the paraspinal musculature at the proper level. The anode is placed on the skin. Recording to the evoked response from an appropriate muscle in the limb is made in the normal manner. Side-to-side latency comparisons are made to determine abnormality (13).

H Reflex

The H reflex, first discovered by Hoffman in 1918, was later named and further investigated by Magladery and associates in the 1950s (14). Since then hundreds of articles have been published on the further investigation and use of this reflex. Most investigators believe that this is the electrical counterpart of the muscle stretch reflex, but it differs in several ways. In infancy, an H reflex can be obtained from most nerves, but after age 2 it can reliably only be found in the tibial nerve. In spinal shock, when reflexes may be absent, the H reflex may still be present.

The tibial H reflex is normally obtained by stimulating the tibial nerve at the knee with recording from the gastrocnemius or soleus. It is thought that the impulse is carried proximally by the Ia fibers to the spinal cord. There they synapse with the alpha motor neurons and the impulse is conducted back to the muscle, resulting in a muscle twitch. The latency measurement between the stimulus and twitch is therefore a measure of the integrity of both the S1 motor and sensory roots. This study is most commonly used for evaluating S1 radiculopathies, but it is also helpful in evaluating proximal neuropathies such as Guillain-Barré syndrome.

F Wave

The F wave was first described by Magladery and McDougal (14). When any motor nerve is stimulated with recording from a distal muscle, a late response may be seen following the initial muscle response. The amplitude and latency of this late response is quite variable, and it may not be present with each stimulation. In contrast, the H reflex is identical with each stimulus. It is believed that the F wave results from antidromic conduction of the stimulus in the alpha motor neurons to the spinal cord. There they cause firing of the anterior horn cells. These impulses are then carried orthodromically by the alpha motor neurons, causing discharge of the muscle fibers that they innervate. The same alpha motor neurons may not fire with each stimulus, thus resulting in a variable response. Since only alpha motor neurons are involved, the F wave is a measurement of motor function only. F waves are commonly studied in the median, ulnar, peroneal, and tibial nerves. They are most valuable in examining proximal nerve function in neuropathy and thoracic outlet syndrome, but they may also be abnormal in radiculopathy. If distal conduction studies are normal but the F wave latency is prolonged, it may be assumed that a proximal lesion exists.

Somatosensory-Evoked Potentials

Somatosensory potentials may be obtained by stimulating a peripheral nerve, usually the median or ulnar at the wrist or the tibial or peroneal at the ankle, and recording wave forms from the contralateral scalp. It is thought that these potentials are carried by sensory fibers in the peripheral nerves and in the dorsal column–lemniscal system centrally. They can therefore theoretically be used to measure function distally or proximally in the peripheral nervous system or in the spinal cord or brain. They are most commonly used for aid in diagnosing multiple sclerosis (15) along with auditory- and visual-evoked potentials. They have also proven very useful in monitoring spinal cord function during spinal surgery.

Somatosensory-evoked potentials are presently undergoing evaluation as to their clinical usefulness in diagnosing plexus and root lesions, especially when only sensory fibers are involved. Limited success has been achieved thus far, and the clinical usefulness of these studies in radiculopathy is very controversial. Studies in several centers are presently underway to evaluate dermatomal cutaneous stimulation to better localize lesions to a single root, but these studies are still in an experimental stage.

CLINICAL APPLICATIONS

Electrodiagnostic studies were originally developed for evaluation and localization of peripheral nerve injuries. Although this continues to be an important use of these studies, they are more frequently used to diagnose radiculopathies, peripheral neuropathies, entrapment syndromes, and myopathies in patients with acute and chronic pain paresthesias and weakness.

RADICULOPATHIES

Neck and low back pain are the most common forms of musculoskeletal disability. Cervical and lumbar radiculopathies may cause acute and chronic back pain, headaches, extremity pain, numbness, paresthesias, and weakness. Thoracic radiculopathies, although less common, may cause noncardiac chest pain and abdominal pain.

Electrodiagnostic studies have proven very useful in the diagnosis of radiculopathy. Myelography, computed tomography, and magnetic resonance imaging all examine the anatomy of the spine, spinal cord, and roots, but electrical testing is the only widely accepted method of assessing the physiologic function of the nerve roots. Although radiculopathy is usually due to a compressive lesion, such as a herniated disk, it may also be due to a noncompressive lesion, as in diabetic radiculopathy. It has been found that electrodiagnostic studies and myelography are equal in their sensitivity and accuracy in diagnosing compressive root lesions (16). Comparisons with computed tomography have shown electrical studies to be the more accurate in localizing a radiculopathy (17). Most studies have shown that both anatomic and electrical studies have approximately a 75–80% accuracy; however, when a combination of the two types of study is performed, a much higher degree of accuracy will be obtained. Therefore, when evaluating the patient with chronic pain, both imaging and physiologic studies should be employed.

In evaluating for a possible radiculopathy, the examiner performs EMG on multiple muscles innervated by each of the roots supplying the extremity involved. Although this will evaluate function in the anterior primary ramus, the corresponding paraspinal musculature must also be examined to evaluate the posterior primary ramus. If root compression is causing damage to motor fibers within the root, EMG abnormalities will be seen in the muscles supplied by that root, allowing the level of the lesion to be localized. In some cases, EMG abnormalities will be seen only in the paraspinal musculature. This localizes the lesion to the root level, but the exact root involved cannot be determined since there is a large overlap in innervation of the paraspinal musculature. In an acute nerve root lesion, EMG abnormalities in the paraspinal musculature will not occur until approximately 7–10 days after onset. In the extremity musculature, abnormalities such as fibrillations and positive waves may not occur for 3–4 weeks. However, if weakness is present, decrease in motor unit recruitment may be seen in a myotomal pattern during this early phase. Medicolegally, it may be worthwhile performing EMG during the first week after injury to determine if abnormalities are present from a preexisting lesion. This is especially true in the chronic pain patient, who may have had multiple previous injuries or surgery. If no fibrillations are found on this initial examination, but fibrillations are present 3 weeks later, they can be ascribed to the present illness.

Since most peripheral nerves contain fibers from multiple nerve roots, standard peripheral NCS are usually normal. However, they may be abnormal if multiple roots are involved with loss of a large number of nerve fibers. H reflex, F wave, and somatosensory studies in the affected nerve root distribution may be abnormal and aid in the diagnosis.

Cervical Radiculopathy

The C7 nerve root is probably the most commonly involved in cervical radiculopathy, followed by C6, C8, and C5 (18). With *C5 radiculopathies*, pain is usually felt radiating into the shoulder. Weakness may be seen in the deltoid and possibly the biceps. The biceps jerk may be depressed. Sensory complaints are uncommon, but there may be some dysesthesias over the lateral aspect of the forearm. Electromyographic abnormalities may be seen in the rhomboids, supraspinatus, infraspinatus, deltoid, and possibly the biceps. *C6 radiculopathies* give a similar pain pattern, but paresthesias are frequently complained of in the thumb. Electromyographic abnormalities are commonly seen in the biceps, pronator teres, and extensor carpi radialis, but may also be seen in the deltoid and supraspinatus. *C7 radiculopathy* frequently presents with pain radiating into the triceps, forearm, and hand. Paresthesias are commonly present in the index and long fingers. Weakness may be prominent in the triceps with an absent triceps jerk. Electromyographic abnormalities are likely to be found in the triceps, pronator teres, flexor carpi radialis, and extensor digitorum communis. With *C8 radiculopathy*, the patient frequently presents with pain and paresthesias radiating down the ulnar aspect of the arm into the fourth and fifth digits. The triceps tendon jerk may be absent. Electromyographic abnormalities may be seen in the extensor digitorum communis, extensor and flexor carpi ulnaris, and in all the intrinsic hand musculature. Median and ulnar F wave latencies may be prolonged to the thenar and hypothenar musculature, respectively, but these must be interpreted with caution since thoracic outlet syndrome may also cause F wave abnormalities in the C8 distribution.

Although fibrillations and positive waves are the hallmark of an acute radiculopathy, increased insertional activity and an increased number of polyphasic motor unit potentials may be the only abnormalities seen. With chronic radiculopathies, these are commonly the only abnormalities present (19).

Lumbosacral Radiculopathies

Electrodiagnostic studies are of great use in the evaluation of low back and leg pain. They can differentiate radiculopathy from the many other causes of back and leg pain such as vascular lesions, mechanical or muscular low back pain, arthritis of the spine and hip, or disk disease without nerve root compression.

In *L4 radiculopathy*, the patient commonly experiences pain in the hip radiating into the groin, anterior thigh, and knee. Sensory complaints are not common, but paresthesias may be experienced over the medial aspect of the knee. The patient may complain of buckling of the knee on weight bearing. Interestingly, the patient with primary hip pathology will have many of these same complaints. On physical examination, the knee jerk may be decreased and weakness may be appreciated in the quadriceps. Electromyography may show abnormalities in the quadriceps and femoral adductors. Femoral motor conduction should be normal to differentiate this from a femoral neuropathy.

With *L5 radiculopathies*, the patient will commonly complain of pain radiating from the back to the lateral hip and thigh and anterior tibial region. Paresthesias may be felt over the dorsum of the foot, and weakness may be noted in the ankle. On physical examination, weakness in the ankle and toe dorsiflexors may be appreciated. There may also be weakness of hip abduction. The medial hamstring reflex may be reduced. Electrically, EMG abnormalities will be seen in the ankle and toe dorsiflexors, flexor digitorum longus, medial hamstrings, tensor fascia lata, and hip abductors. The peroneal F wave latency recorded from the extensor digitorum brevis may be prolonged on the affected side. Differentiation from peroneal neuropathy is made by normal peroneal conduction and by EMG abnormalities in the proximal L5-innervated musculature at the hip.

In *S1 radiculopathy*, the patient experiences pain radiating to the hip, posterior thigh, and calf. There may be complaints of paresthesias over the lateral aspect of the foot. Weakness is uncommon, but there may be some difficulty with toe standing on the affected side. Electrical abnormalities are most commonly found in the gastrocnemius and soleus. They may also be found in the lateral hamstrings and gluteus maximus as well as the intrinsic foot musculature. However, findings localized to the foot musculature must be interpreted with caution, since the extensor digitorum brevis is subject to much trauma, and tarsal tunnel syndrome may cause abnormality in the tibial innervated foot musculature. The tibial H reflex latency will commonly be prolonged or absent with stimulation of the tibial nerve at the knee and recording from the gastrocnemius or soleus. Normal tibial motor conduction will indicate that this tibial H reflex abnormality is due to a proximal lesion. Normal sural sensory conduction will confirm that the sensory abnormalities on the lateral aspect of the foot are due to a proximal lesion.

In all patients who have undergone spinal surgery, EMG abnormalities found in the paraspinal musculature must be interpreted with caution. Electrical abnormalities may persist in these muscles for years after surgery. Some researchers believe that performing the EMG needle examination at 3 cm from the scar at a 3–5-cm depth will avoid abnormalities due to the trauma of surgery. However, in most circumstances it is safest to avoid examination of these muscles once surgery has been performed. In the distribution of the anterior primary ramus, EMG abnormalities tend to subside faster than clinical abnormalities (20). However, with severe root lesions, EMG abnormalities may persist as long as 3–4 years after surgery. Therefore, in examining a patient with recurrent back or leg pain, it is very helpful to have a preoperative examination for comparison of the distribution of the abnormalities.

Thoracic Radiculopathies

Thoracic radiculopathies are much less common than cervical or lumbosacral radiculopathies. They may be the cause of chest or abdominal pain, which usually begins in the spine and radiates anteriorly, or spinal pain may be the only symptom. Compressive root lesions can occur with a herniated disk or tumor, but the lesion may also be the result of herpes zoster or diabetes. In patients with abdominal pain, but an otherwise normal examination, a radiculopathy must be considered, especially in diabetics. The classic findings in diabetic thoracic radiculopathy include mild peripheral nerve conduction abnormalities with fibrillation in the thoracic paraspinal musculature on the symptomatic side (21).

ENTRAPMENT SYNDROMES

Peripheral nerve entrapment syndromes are a frequent cause of extremity paresthesias, pain, and weakness (22). Median nerve entrapment at the wrist, or carpal tunnel syndrome, is the most commonly encountered nerve entrapment syndrome, but many others have also been described. Both the median and ulnar nerves may be entrapped at the wrist and elbow. The radial nerve may be entrapped at the elbow, and its superficial sensory branch may be entrapped in the forearm. The sensory division of the musculocutaneous nerve may be entrapped at the elbow. The femoral, lateral femoral cutaneous, and tibial nerves may be entrapped in the lower extremities.

The classic electrodiagnostic finding in an entrapment syndrome is segmental slowing of conduction across the area of entrapment. Conduction in segments proximal and distal to the lesion are frequently normal, but with a severe nerve compression, conduction in the distal segment may also be affected. Sensory conduction is commonly affected before motor conduction. Electromyographic abnormalities may be found in the muscle supplied by the entrapped nerve, but this is usually a late finding.

Median Nerve

Median nerve entrapment at the wrist, or *carpal tunnel syndrome*, is by far the most common median nerve entrapment, but it must be differentiated from entrapment at the elbow. Patients with carpal tunnel syndrome usually present with paresthesias in the hand. This should be confined to the thumb, index, long finger, and radial half of the ring finger. However, many patients have difficulty localizing their symptoms and complain of generalized numbness in the entire hand. Although this should alert the examiner to consider other lesions, carpal tunnel syndrome is frequently the only problem found. There may be pain in the hand and wrist with radiation up the arm to the shoulder. Occasionally, shoulder pain may be prominent, and it may be confused with cervical radiculopathy. In a small group of patients, shoulder pain will be the only symptom. There are frequent complaints of weakness in the hand and dropping of small object. Patients commonly complain that their symptoms awaken them at night or are most severe on arising in the morning. The symptoms may be brought on by use of the hand as in knitting, driving, or with any repetitive activity. Complaints are often bilateral, with the dominant hand more involved. Carpal tunnel syndrome may be associated with trauma, arthritis and connective tissue disease, hypothyroidism, and the like. However, it is frequently idiopathic.

Hundreds of articles have been written on the electrodiagnostic evaluation of carpal tunnel syndrome. Many methods exist for evaluating median conduction across the wrist, and each laboratory will have its preferred procedure. Since carpal tunnel syndrome is often bilateral and associated with other entrapment neuropathies, median, ulnar, and radial sensory studies as well as median and ulnar motor conduction studies should be performed in both hands. Slowing of median sensory and motor conduction across the wrist with normal conduction proximal and distal to the transverse carpal ligament is the classic finding in carpal tunnel syndrome. Sensory conduction will be abnormal before motor in the vast majority of patients. Frequently, in early cases, the absolute values of median conduction may be within the normal range, but comparison to the asymptomatic hand or to radial or ulnar conduction in the same hand may yield evidence of relative slowing of median conduction, which may be diagnostic (23). Again, it cannot be emphasized too strongly that when assessing a patient for possible carpal tunnel syndrome, conduction studies should not be limited to the median nerve. In addition to finding other entrapments it is not at all unusual for the electromyographer to discover an unsuspected peripheral polyneuropathy.

Electromyography must always be performed along with NCS for a complete evaluation. Electromyography may sometimes show denervation of the thenar musculature in carpal tunnel syndrome, but usually only in severe cases. In addition to the hand musculature, the entire extremity should be examined to rule out the presence of a radiculopathy simulating carpal tunnel syndrome, or coexisting with it. Persistent symptoms after carpal tunnel release may be due to a root lesion that was not recognized.

In very early or mild carpal tunnel syndrome, all electrical studies may be normal in a small percentage of patients. This occurs since significant demyelinization or axonal damage may not have taken place. Detailed cutaneous sensory testing, when combined with the electrical studies, may improve the diagnostic yield (24), but there still may be the exceptional case with no abnormal findings. In this event, the exam should be repeated at a later date to differentiate psychogenic symptoms from neuropathology.

Median nerve entrapments in the proximal forearm are rare, but they may be confused with carpal tunnel syndrome. At the elbow, the median nerve may be entrapped within the pronator teres (pronator syndrome) or, very rarely, by the ligament of Struthers at the level or the medial epicondyle. Patients with these proximal entrapments may have symptoms very similar to carpal tunnel syndrome, but pain in the forearm is more prominent. These patients frequently perform work that requires repetitive pronation of the forearm, but other cases have been related to fractures, dislocations, and trauma to the elbow. Electrodiagnostically, median conduction slowing may be seen across the elbow or in the forearm. In the pronator syndrome, EMG abnormalities may be seen in the forearm musculature distal to the innervation of the pronator teres. More proximal entrapment at the ligament of Struthers would be necessary for EMG abnormalities to be seen in the pronator teres. In both these elbow entrapments, EMG abnormalities have been reported to be of more diagnostic significance than NCS (25).

The anterior interosseous nerve is a motor branch of the median nerve that arises below the pronator teres. The nerve may be entrapped at this point or, more commonly, may be involved in trauma. Clinically, weakness is found in the pronator quadratus, flexor pollicis longus, and flexor digitorum profundus to digits II and III. Electromyographic abnormalities will be seen in these muscles, while the remainder of the median musculature will be normal. Standard median motor and sensory conduction studies will be normal since they bypass the anterior interosseous nerve. Stimulation of the median nerve at the elbow and recording from the flexor pollicis longus may occasionally reveal a prolonged latency, but this is not frequent (26).

Ulnar Nerve Entrapments

Entrapment of the ulnar nerve at the elbow is the second most common entrapment neuropathy. However, the ulnar nerve may also be entrapped at the wrist and in the palm. Although not truly an entrapment neuropathy, thoracic outlet syndrome commonly causes symptoms primarily in the ulnar distribution.

Ulnar neuropathy at the elbow may be the result of a long-standing deformity of the elbow (*tardy ulnar palsy*) or entrapment of the nerve under the aponeurosis connecting the two heads of the flexor carpi ulnaris (*cubital tunnel syndrome*) (27). Patients commonly complain of pain in the elbow with numbness and paresthesias in the fourth and fifth digits as well as weakness in the hands. These symptoms are often bilateral. Nerve conduction studies will classically show slowing of ulnar motor and/or sensory conduction velocity across the elbow as compared to the proximal and distal segments or as compared to the opposite ulnar nerve. This slowing should be at least 10 m/sec (28). There will usually be decrease in the amplitude of the ulnar sensory nerve action potential recorded from the fifth digit when stimulating at the wrist. In severe ulnar neuropathies, there may be slowing in the distal segments as well as across the elbow as a result of wallerian degeneration. Electromyographic abnormalities in advanced cases will be seen in the ulnar portion of the flexor digitorum profundus and the ulnar innervated intrinsic hand musculature. The flexor carpi ulnaris will be spared since this muscle is innervated by a branch of the ulnar nerve arising above the elbow.

The ulnar nerve may also be compressed at the wrist in Guyon's canal. The sensory complaints and weakness in the hand are similar to lesions at the elbow, but discomfort proximal to the wrist is unusual. Electrical studies will show slowing of ulnar motor and sensory conduction across the wrist, and there may be EMG changes in the ulnar-innervated intrinsic hand musculature. Proximal ulnar conduction studies should be normal.

The deep motor branch of the ulnar nerve may also be traumatized or compressed by a ganglion distal to Guyon's canal. In this case ulnar motor distal latency from the wrist to the abductor digiti quinti may be normal while conduction to the first dorsal interosseous may be prolonged. Sensory conduction to the fifth digit may be normal or abnormal depending on the site of the lesion.

Thoracic outlet syndrome is defined as compression of the neurovascular bundle in the thoracic outlet, which results in pain, dysesthesias, and occasionally weakness in the arm. In most cases this is a vascular syndrome, but in a small percentage neurologic symptoms may be prominent. When this occurs, paresthesias are most prominent in the ulnar distribution and weakness may be seen in the hand. Since this syndrome is most often primarily vascular, electrodiagnostic studies are frequently normal. When there is neurologic involvement, slowing of ulnar conduction through the thoracic outlet may occur. However, the best method to detect this is controversial. It has been proposed that stimulation of the ulnar nerve in the supraclavicular fossa and in the axilla will allow for measurement of ulnar motor conduction velocity through the thoracic outlet (29). However, other authors have found this unreliable since stimulation at the supraclavicular fossa may be distal to the actual area of compression (30). Nerve root stimulation may be a better method of demonstrating slowing of conduction through the thoracic outlet. Well-documented electrical abnormalities found in patients with clear-cut neurogenic thoracic outlet syndrome include reduced ulnar sensory- and motor-evoked amplitudes with denervation of the median- and ulnar-innervated intrinsic hand musculature in the presence of normal distal median and ulnar motor conduction (31). The ulnar F wave latency may also be prolonged on the affected side as compared to the normal side (32).

Thoracic outlet syndrome has classically been considered to be rare, but in recent years this syndrome appears to be being invoked in patients involved in minor trauma, especially when litigation is involved. They usually have vague, poorly documented neck and extremity pain as well as paresthesias. Objective studies are usually normal. Many of these patients are subjected to first rib resection, when conservative treatment until the litigation is resolved would appear to be more appropriate.

Since the ulnar nerve may be injured or entrapped at many points along its course, patients with symptoms in an ulnar distribution should receive segmental conduction studies throughout the course of the nerve to best localize the lesion. Also, studies should be done in both arms since these syndromes are frequently bilateral. Electromyography should also be performed on the extremities and cervical paraspinals to rule out a C8 cervical radiculopathy, which may give a clinical picture identical to an ulnar neuropathy.

Radial Nerve

Although the resulting condition is not a true entrapment neuropathy, the radial nerve is most commonly injured in the spiral groove. Prolonged pressure in this area results in the classic "Saturday night palsy." Triceps strength and the reflex will be normal, while the brachioradialis and all distal radial-innervated muscles will be weak. There may be sensory loss over the radial aspect of the dorsum of the hand. Radial motor conduction studies may show slowing across the spiral groove, and radial sensory conduction may also be abnormal. Electromyographic abnormalities will be found from the brachioradialis distally in the radial distribution.

True entrapments of the radial nerve occur in the region of the elbow. Compression of the recurrent branch of the radial nerve at the elbow gives rise to local pain and is thought to be one of the causes of "tennis elbow." This is a rather small branch, and it cannot be tested electrically.

The *posterior interosseous syndrome* is entrapment of the terminal motor branch of the radial nerve as it passes through the arcade of Froshe between the two heads of the supinator. A lesion at this level will cause weakness of the extensor carpi ulnaris and finger extensors, but the extensor carpi radialis will be spared. Since the superficial radial sensory nerve has already exited the main trunk at this level, there should be no sensory complaints. Motor conduction studies may show slowing in the distal portion with normal proximal conduction. Electromyography will show abnormalities distal to the innervation of the extensor carpi radialis longus and brevis.

Compression of the radial nerve at the wrist (cheiralgia paresthetica) by a wrist band is well documented, and radial sensory conduction studies are useful in demonstrating this lesion (33). Recently, an entrapment of the radial sensory nerve in the forearm has been described (34). These patients usually present with pain or burning over the dorsoradial aspect of the forearm and wrist. The etiology is thought to be local trauma, twisting injuries, or repetitive pronation-supination movements at work. On physical examination, there is usually a positive Tinel's sign over the radial sensory nerve in the distal forearm. There is often a "positive Finklestein's test," which may lead to a misdiagnosis of de Quervain's disease. Sensation may be impaired in the radial distribution of the hand, but strength should be normal. Hyperpronation of the forearm may reproduce the symptoms. It is thought that the superficial radial sensory nerve is compressed between the tendons of the extensor carpi radialis longus and brachioradialis when the wrist is pronated. Radial sensory conduction studies may be abnormal, with slowing of radial sensory conduction in the forearm but with normal conduction from the wrist to the thumb. Comparison to musculocutaneous sensory conduction is often helpful, since they have a similar course. Decrease in the amplitude of the radial sensory nerve action potential may be the only abnormality found. Radial motor conduction studies should be normal, and no EMG abnormalities should be seen.

Suprascapular Nerve

The suprascapular nerve is composed of nerve fibers from the C5 and C6 roots. This nerve leaves the upper trunk of the brachial plexus and passes under the trapezius muscle, eventually passing through the suprascapular foramen to innervate the supra- and infraspinatus muscles. The nerve may be entrapped in this foramen under the transverse scapular ligament, or it may be subjected to a stretch injury at this site. Entrapment of this nerve will result in shoulder pain that may be misdiagnosed as bursitis or cervical radiculopathy. Nerve conduction studies may show prolongation of the suprascapular nerve latency from Erb's point to the supra- or infraspinatus.

Electromyography will show abnormalities confined to the supra- and infraspinatus with no other C5–C6-innervated muscles involved.

Musculocutaneous Nerve

The musculocutaneous nerve is occasionally injured with local trauma, but can also be damaged by heavy exercise. Rarely, the musculocutaneous nerve may be entrapped by the coracobranchialis. Weakness will be seen in the biceps with sensory loss over the lateral aspect of the forearm. The biceps stretch reflex should be absent. This diagnosis may be confirmed by musculocutaneous motor conduction with stimulation in the axilla and at Erb's point. Sensory conduction may also be abnormal. Electromyographic abnormalities will be seen in the biceps, brachialis, and coracobrachialis muscles.

A recently described lesion of the musculocutaneous nerve at the elbow involves only the sensory division, the lateral antebrachial cutaneous nerve. These patients experience pain in the region of the biceps tendon insertion with paresthesias over the radial aspect of the forearm. The biceps tendon jerk and strength will be normal. There is frequently tenderness over the tendon insertion on the biceps, with clinical sensory loss in the distribution of the sensory branch. Musculocutaneous sensory conduction will be abnormal while motor conduction is within normal limits (35, 36). No EMG abnormalities will be present.

Lateral Femoral Cutaneous Nerve

The lateral femoral cutaneous nerve arises from the L2 and L3 nerve roots. It emerges through the inguinal ligament near the anterior superior iliac spine to innervate the skin over the lateral thigh from the hip to the knee. Compression of this nerve in the inguinal ligament results in burning pain and paresthesias over the lateral thigh (meralgia paraesthetica). Objective sensory loss can usually be demonstrated in this area. Since the nerve is purely sensory, there will be no weakness. Nerve conduction studies may show abnormalities in this nerve (37). Comparison should always be made between the symptomatic and asymptomatic legs, since conduction in this nerve is frequently difficult to obtain in obese patients. Electromyography must be performed to rule out a lumbar radiculopathy.

Femoral Nerve

The femoral nerve may be compressed within the pelvis by tumor, psoas abscess, retroperitoneal lymphadenopathy, or hemorrhage into iliopsoas muscle. The nerve may also be entrapped at the level of the inguinal ligament. These patients complain of pain, paresthesias, and weakness in the groin and anterior thigh. Femoral motor conduction studies may show abnormal distal latencies, and slowing may be able to be demonstrated across the inguinal ligament (38). Abnormalities on EMG will be confined to the femoral distribution. Commonly, L3–L4 radiculopathies or plexopathies, especially in diabetics, can mimic femoral neuropathy; EMG of the entire extremity, with emphasis on the quadriceps, femoral adductors, and lumbar paraspinals, should make this differentiation.

Obturator Nerve

The obturator nerve is most commonly injured during labor, but may also be injured with pelvic fractures and pelvic surgery. Obturator hernias may entrap the nerve in the obturator canal. Patients complain of pain in the groin radiating along the medial aspect of the thigh. There may be dysesthesias in the medial aspect of the upper thigh. Reproducible obturator conduction studies have not been reported. However, EMG examination will show abnormalities confined to the femoral adductors.

Peroneal Nerve

The peroneal nerve is commonly injured at the level of the fibular head, where it is very superficial. The nerve may also be compressed at the level of the biceps femoris tendon after prolonged squatting. Pain and numbness may be experienced in the anterior aspect of the leg and foot. Weakness of the ankle and toe dorsiflexors is prominent. Peroneal motor conduction studies may show segmental slowing across the fibular head. With more severe lesions, distal peroneal motor conduction will also be abnormal. Superficial peroneal sensory conduction may also be affected. Electromyographic abnormalities should be confined to the peroneal-innervated musculature. Since this may easily be confused with an L5 radiculopathy, the entire extremity must be examined. Electromyography should always be performed on the short head of the biceps femoris, since this is innervated by a branch from the common peroneal nerve. Involvement of this muscle suggests a lesion proximal to the fibular head.

The deep peroneal nerve is commonly traumatized at the ankle. Many patients may have a prolonged distal peroneal motor latency with no symptoms whatsoever. Fibrillations may be found in the extensor digitorum brevis in approximately 25% of otherwise normal patients, and in older patients the muscle may be completely atrophied. The deep peroneal nerve has been reported to be involved in an entrapment neuropathy at the ankle (39), and this was termed the *anterior tarsal tunnel syndrome*. Patients complain of pain on the dorsum of the foot with numbness between the first and second toes. Since, as previously mentioned, many "normal" individuals have electrical abnormalities in this segment, this diagnosis must only be made when the clinical picture is compatible.

Tibial Nerve

The tibial nerve may be entrapped in the tarsal tunnel, which lies posterior to the medial malleolus and is covered by the lancinate ligament. This entrapment is termed the *tarsal tunnel syndrome* (40). This may be idiopathic or may follow fractures of the ankle. The patient will frequently complain of pain in the ankle, heel, and foot with paresthesias on the sole of the foot and toes. A positive Tinel's sign will be present over the tarsal tunnel. Motor or sensory tibial distal latencies may be abnormal in either the medial or lateral plantar division. However, this is not analogous to carpal tunnel syndrome; very frequently the conduction studies are normal, even when comparing to the asymptomatic side. Electromyography of the abductor hallucis and abductor digiti minimi may help establish this diagnosis (41). Fibrillations confined to these muscles on the involved side with normal extensor digitorum brevis examination (peroneal innervated) and a normal examination of the opposite foot suggest tarsal tunnel syndrome. Positive waves alone are not enough to establish this diagnosis since these are frequently seen in otherwise normal patients. In all patients being evaluated for possible tarsal tunnel syndrome, EMG should be performed on the entire extremity and lumbar paraspinals to rule out a radiculopathy, which may give a similar clinical picture.

PERIPHERAL POLYNEUROPATHY

Peripheral polyneuropathy may be a cause of severe acute or chronic pain, especially in diabetics. However, it may also be a prominent cause of pain with alcoholic neuropathy, vasculitis, or nutritional neuropathies. The clinical and electrical findings may be diffuse and symmetric or more localized. In mononeuritis multiplex, one nerve may be severely abnormal with other nearby nerves relatively spared. If the basic pathology is axonal loss, the EMG will show abnormalities, and NCS will show decreased amplitude of the evoked responses. If the myelin sheath is primarily affected, nerve conduction slowing will be the most prominent finding. Commonly both types of pathology are seen together. Occasionally, small fiber–type neuropathies are seen in which no electrical abnormalities can be demonstrated. This occurs since NCS primarily measure conduction in the large myelinated fibers. In addition to the naturally occurring neuropathies, iatrogenic peripheral neuropathies or plexopathies may be due to chemotherapy or radiation.

MYOPATHIES

Myopathies are generally not considered when evaluating a patient with chronic pain. However, dermatomyositis and polymyositis may result in chronic pain and weakness. Electromyographic examination would demonstrate fibrillations, positive waves, and repetitive discharges at rest. Motor unit action potentials tend to be polyphasic, with decreased amplitude and duration. Proximal muscles are involved more than distal, and the paraspinal musculature is also involved. Myopathy may also be associated with other connective tissue diseases such as scleroderma or rheumatoid arthritis. It may also be secondary to chronic steroid treatment.

THE ELECTRODIAGNOSTIC EXAMINATION

Most patients approach the electrodiagnostic examination with some degree of fear and anxiety, since many have some fear of needle puncture and/or electrical stimuli. Frequently patients have been subjected to "horror stories" involving electrodiagnostic studies by their acquaintances. This may have been either in jest or in an attempt to gain sympathy. Since patient cooperation is important to a successful examination, the electromyographer must be able to allay the patient's fears. Although some complaints of discomfort are to be expected, most patients will agree that their fears were unwarranted and that many other medical diagnostic and therapeutic procedures are much more uncomfortable.

An electrodiagnostic examination, unlike other studies such as electrocardiography or electroencephalography, cannot be performed in a preset, routine manner. Each examination must be individualized according to the clinical picture. In order to properly plan the study, a complete history and physical examination must be done by the physician performing the study. The structure of the examination may be changed several times during the procedure as new information is gained. A patient may initially be thought to have an entrapment neuropathy, but further examination may reveal the presence of a polyneuropathy, radiculopathy, or the like. Screening NCS are performed on the symptomatic extremity as the first step in most examinations. If abnormalities are found, the opposite extremity is also studied. Should abnormal findings again be present, the other limbs may be examined. Electromyography is then conducted on the symptomatic extremity and corresponding paraspinal musculature. Again, other areas will need to be studied if the first limb is abnormal. The results of the examination must then be interpreted in light of the history and clinical findings.

Ideally, the clinical neurophysiologist performing the electrodiagnostic study will have met the minimal training criteria established by the American Association of Electromyography and Electrodiagnosis (42). These criteria recognize that the electrodiagnostic examination is essentially a neuromuscular disease consultation utilizing electrophysiologic methods. The examiner must, therefore, have special expertise in diagnosis of neuromuscular disease. Completion of an approved residency in neurology or physical medicine and rehabilitation is recommended. This training should include adequate instruction in anatomy and physiology of muscle and nerve, electrophysiology, and clinical aspects of neuromuscular disease as they pertain to electrodiagnostic studies. A minimum of 6 months' supervised training with performance of at least 200 examinations is recommended. In spite of these recommendations, one can find electrodiagnostic studies being performed by physicians with little or no formal training. In some states, these studies may legally be performed by technicians. It therefore behooves the physician requesting the electrodiagnostic examination to know the qualifications of the examiner. If an experienced clinical neurophysiologist is to perform the examination, it is best to allow him to plan and carry out the examination as he feels is appropriate to the clinical picture. In this chapter I have specifically not mentioned normal values for most studies since each clinical neurophysiologist will have established these for his own laboratory and will be able to advise the referring physician as to the outcome of his examination. If the electrodiagnostic study is to be performed by a technician, a detailed outline of the examination requested should be given to the technician. All of the diagnostic possibilities should be outlined, and the specific nerves and muscles to be examined must be listed. If a detailed outline is not provided for the technician, an incomplete examination may well be done. This is illustrated by the following case reports.

Case #1 A 54-year-old female received electrodiagnostic studies because of a 1-month history of numbness in the right thumb and index finger. She also complained of pain in the hand and shoulder, but no neck pain. Right median sensory conduction to the index finger could not be obtained, while ulnar sensory conduction and median motor conduction were normal. Electromyography of the thenar musculature was also normal. This was the full extent of the examination, and on the basis of these findings the diagnosis of carpal tunnel syndrome was made.

On admission to the hospital for surgery, a new exam was requested. In addition to the studies outlined above, radial and musculocutaneous conduction were measured, and EMG was performed on the entire extremity and cervical paraspinal musculature. Both median and musculocutaneous sensory conduction were absent while all other conduction studies were normal. Electromyography showed the presence of fibrillations and positive waves in the right biceps, brachialis, and pronator teres with sparing of the paraspinals. These findings indicated that the lesion was in the lateral cord of the brachial plexus, rather than at the wrist. Further workup revealed a metastatic breast carcinoma to the plexus.

This case points out that the study should not be cut short as soon as one abnormality is found, or the clinical impression is "confirmed." Multiple lesions may be missed, or an incorrect diagnosis made.

Case #2 A 62-year-old female patient was referred to a technician for NCS because of weakness. She had fallen on several occasions and had fractured her right hip. Extensive motor and sensory conduction studies were done on the upper and lower extremities with no abnormalities found. This was reported as a "normal study." This patient was later seen in another laboratory where the NCS were confirmed. However, EMG was also done and showed the presence of diffuse fibrillations and fasciculations, which led to the diagnosis of amyotrophic lateral sclerosis.

This case illustrates the need to know your examiner. The initial referring physician assumed his patient would be seen by a physician/clinical neurophysiologist and used the term "nerve conduction study" in a generic sense. Unfortunately the technician took him literally, and hence the inadequate study and delay in diagnosis.

In summary, routine performance of only brief, limited electrical studies is analogous to ordering a limb x-ray and examining only the bones while ignoring the soft tissue structures. Since so much information is to be gained, especially in the evaluation of the patient with chronic pain, the full potential of the electrodiagnostic examination should be utilized.

References

1. Johnson EW: Use of the electrodiagnostic examination in a university hospital. *Arch Phys Med Rehabil* 46:573, 1965.
2. Rogoff J: Traditional electrodiagnosis. In Johnson EW (ed): *Practical Electromyography*. Baltimore, Williams & Wilkins, 1980, p 326.
3. Licht S: History. In Johnson EW (ed): *Practical Electromyography*. Baltimore, Williams & Wilkins, 1980, p 403.
4. Liddell E, Sherrington C: Recruitment and some other features of reflex inhibition. *Proc R Soc Lond (Biol)* 97:488–518, 1925.
5. Adrian E, Bronk D: The discharge of impulses in motor nerve fibers. Part II. The frequency of discharge in reflex and voluntary conduction. *J Physiol (London)* 67:119–151, 1929.
6. Brown W, Varkey G: The origin of spontaneous electrical activity at the endplate zone. *Ann Neurol* 10:557–570, 1981.
7. Buchthal F, Rosenfalk P: Spontaneous electrical activity of human muscle. *Electroenceph Clin Neurophysiol* 20:321–326, 1966.
8. Johnson EW, Denny ST, Kelley JP: Sequence of electromyographic abnormalities in stroke syndrome. *Arch Phys Med Rehabil* 56:468, 1975.
9. Chokroverty S, Medina T: Electrophysiological study of hemiplegia. *Arch Neurol* 35:360, 1978.
10. Wettstein A: The origin of fasciculations in motor neuron disease. *Ann Neurol* 5:295, 1979.
11. Stalberg E, Trontel JV: *Single Fiber Electromyography*. Old Woking, Surrey, U.K., The Mirvalle Press Limited, 1979.
12. Borenstein S, Desmedt J: Range variations in motor unit potentials during reinnervation after traumatic nerve lesions in humans. *Ann Neurol* 8:460, 1980.
13. MacLean I: Nerve root stimulation to evaluate conduction across the brachial and lumbosacral plexuses. *Third Annual Continuing Education Course, American Association of Electromyography and Electrodiagnosis*, Sept. 25, 1980, Philadelphia, Pennsylvania.
14. Magladery JW, McDougal DB: Electrophysiological studies of nerve and reflex activity in normal man: I. Identification of certain reflexes in electromyogram and conduction velocity of peripheral nerve fibers. *Bull Johns Hopkins Hosp* 86:265, 1950.
15. Namerow HS: Somatosensory evoked responses in multiple sclerosis patients with varying sensory loss. *Neurology* 18:1197, 1968.
16. Knutson B: Comparative values of electromyographic, myelographic and clinical-neurological examinations of lumbar root compression syndromes. *Acta Orthop Scand Suppl* 49:1, 1961.
17. Khatri B, Baruah J, McQuillen P: Correlation of electromyography with computed tomography in evaluation of lower back pain. *Arch Neurol* 41:594, 1984.
18. Marinacci A: *Applied Electromyography*. Philadelphia: Lea & Febiger, 1968.
19. Waylonis G: Electromyographic findings in chronic cervical radicular syndrome. *Arch Phys Med Rehabil* 49:407, 1968.
20. Johnson E, Buckhart J, Earl W: Electromyography in postlaminectomy patients. *Arch Phys Med Rehabil* 53:407, 1972.
21. Langstreth G, Newcomer A: Abdominal pain caused by diabetic radiculopathy. *Ann Intern Med* 86:166, 1977.
22. Kopell HP, Thompson WA: *Peripheral Entrapment Neuropathies*. Baltimore, Williams & Wilkins, 1963.
23. Felsenthal G: Median and ulnar distal motor and sensory latencies in the same normal subject. *Arch Phys Med Rehabil* 58:297, 1977.
24. Spindler H, Dellon AL: Nerve conduction studies and sensibility testing in carpal tunnel syndrom. *J Hand Surg* 7:260, 1982.
25. Hartz CR: The pronator teres syndrome: compressive neurology of the median nerve. *J Bone Joint Surg* 63A:885, 1981.
26. Nakano KK: Anterior interosseus nerve syndrome. *Arch Neurol* 34:477, 1977.
27. Feindel W, Stratford J: The role of the cubital tunnel in tardy ulnar palsy. *Can J Surg* 1:287, 1958.
28. Eisen A: Early diagnosis of ulnar nerve palsy. An electrophysiological study. *Neurology* 24:256, 1974.
29. Caldwell JW, Crane CR, Krasen EM: Nerve conduction studies: an aid in the diagnosis of thoracic outlet syndrome. *South Med J* 64:210, 1971.
30. Daube JR: Nerve conduction studies in the thoracic outlet syndrome. *Neurology* 25:347, 1975.
31. Gilliat RW: Peripheral nerve conduction in patients with a cervical rib or band. *J Neurol Neurosurg Psychiatry* 33:615, 1970.
32. Dorfman LJ: F-wave latency in the cervial rib-and-band syndrome. Letter to the Editor. *Muscle Nerve* 2:158, 1979.
33. Dorfman LJ, Jayaram AR: Handcuff neuropathy. *JAMA* 239:957, 1978.
34. Dellon AL, MacKinnon SE: Radial sensory nerve entrapment. *Arch Neurol* 43:833, 1986.
35. Spindler HA, Felsenthal G: Sensory conduction in the musculocutaneous nerve. *Arch Phys Med Rehabil* 59:70, 1978.
36. Felsenthal G, Mondell DL: Forearm pain sensory to compression syndrome of lateral cutaneous nerve of the forearm. *Arch Phys Med Rehabil* 65:139, 1984.
37. Butler ET, Johnson EW, Kaye ZA: Normal conduction velocity in the lateral femoral cutaneous nerve. *Arch Phys Med Rehabil* 55:31, 1974.
38. Johnson EW, Wood P, Pomeus J: Femoral nerve conduction studies. *Arch Phys Med Rehabil* 49:528, 1968.
39. Krause KH, Witt T, Ross A: The anterior tarsal tunnel syndrome. *J Neurol* 217:67, 1977.
40. Delisa JA, Saeed MA: AAEE case report #8: The tarsal tunnel syndrome. *Muscle Nerve* 6:664, 1983.
41. Gatens PF, Saeed MA: Electromyographic findings in the intrinsic muscles of normal feet. *Arch Phys Med Rehabil* 63:317, 1982.
42. *Guidelines in Electrodiagnostic Medicine*. Rochester, MN, American Association of Electromyography and Electrodiagnosis, 1984.

chapter 6
Psychological Evaluation

Joan M. Romano, Ph.D.
Judith A. Turner, Ph.D.
James E. Moore, Ph.D.

Chronic pain of nonmalignant origin remains one of the most prevalent and challenging problems facing the health care system (1). In most cases of chronic pain, evidence of nociceptive input is either absent or insufficient to explain the extent of suffering and disability reported, and one must look to other sources of information to understand why a person's pain has continued beyond normal expected healing time. The psychological evaluation can often provide information critical to such an understanding, as well as to the design and implementation of treatment strategies.

Although psychological evaluation is rarely necessary in cases of acute pain, it is extremely important in the assessment of chronic pain patients. Psychological evaluation has become a standard part of the patient assessment process at the majority of pain clinics in the United States and is now recognized by the Commission on Accreditation of Rehabilitation Facilities as an essential component of pain clinic procedure (2). This evaluation can serve a number of useful functions. First, it can be crucial in identifying psychosocial and behavioral factors that influence the nature, severity, and persistence of chronic pain and disability. Regardless of whether an organic basis for pain can be documented, or whether psychosocial problems preceded or resulted from pain, factors such as depression, anxiety, beliefs about the etiology of pain, and social reinforcement of pain behaviors can contribute to the maintenance of pain and dysfunction. If ignored, these psychological factors can impede the patient's recovery and interfere with his/her response to treatment. Second, psychological evaluation can aid in identifying specific goals for treatment. Often patients, their families, and even health care providers are focused to such an extent on the alleviation of pain that other related problems go unaddressed. Goals for treatment might include increasing activity levels, decreasing depression and family discord, or enhancing stress management and relaxation skills, depending on the needs of the individual patient. The evaluation can also provide information on the extent to which patients may be receptive to different treatment strategies, allowing potential problems in compliance to be identified and perhaps forestalled.

The goal of this chapter is to provide an introduction to the concepts and process of the psychological evaluation of chronic pain patients. This includes a description of the purposes and indications for evaluation and the preparation of patients for the evaluation. Specific components of a psychological evaluation are described in some detail, and relevant applications of the Minnesota Multiphasic Personality Inventory (MMPI) are discussed. Guidelines for the preparation of a report of the psychological evaluation of a chronic pain patient are also presented, along with an example of such a report.

The chapter is written primarily for professionals working in, or referring patients to, multidisciplinary pain clinics. It is assumed that patients have had a complete medical evaluation, that no further medical or surgical treatment is warranted, and that these patients might thus be candidates for a multidisciplinary rehabilitation approach. Despite this primary focus, much of this chapter also applies to other settings, such as hospital consultation services, in which chronic pain patients are seen for psychological evaluation.

CONCEPTS UNDERLYING THE PSYCHOLOGICAL EVALUATION

It has long been recognized clinically that psychological factors play a role in pain perception, but it has only been since Melzack and Wall (3) proposed the *gate control theory* of pain that a scientific model of pain transmission and processing has incorporated cognitive and affective as well as sensory processes in explaining the experience of pain. Briefly, gate control theory posits that complex neurophysiologic mechanisms in both the brain and the spinal cord modulate afferent pain signals (3, 4). Pain is viewed as being a highly complex phenomenon determined by the interaction of sensory-discriminative, motivational-affective, and cognitive-evaluative processes. This multidimensional concept of pain perception has stimulated researchers and clinicians to focus greater attention on psychological factors thought to influence pain. Over the last 20 years, psychological approaches to understanding and treating chronic pain have had an increasing impact on the clinical management of chronic pain problems, especially within the setting of multidisciplinary pain clinics.

Certainly one of the most influential of these approaches has been the operant behavioral model of W. E. Fordyce (5). Fordyce observed that all communication of pain takes place through some form of behavior ("pain behavior," e.g., limping, grimacing, verbal report). Such behaviors are subject to influence by consequences that follow their occurrence. In the language of learning theory, operant conditioning is a form of learning in which a behavior becomes more likely to occur as a result of having been reinforced by positive consequences or the removal of aversive consequences. Thus, pain behaviors may come to be maintained by consequences such as spouse attention and expressions of concern or assumption of aversive tasks. The longer pain persists, the greater are the chances that pain behaviors may come under the control of social/environmental contingencies (5, 6). Fordyce and his colleagues (7) have demonstrated that modification of such contingencies results in a decrease in pain behaviors and dysfunction. It would be predicted from learning theory that pain behaviors will occur most frequently in the presence of discriminative stimuli, such as a solicitous spouse, that signal that pain behaviors are likely to be reinforced if emitted. Subsequent empirical research by Block and his colleagues (8) has supported this hypothesis.

Another trend consistent with concepts of gate control theory is a growing research and clinical emphasis on cognitive factors that influence pain. The specific types of cognitive experiences relevant to pain perception are thought to include focus of attention, beliefs, attributions, expectations, coping self-statements, images, and problem-solving cognitions (9). These can be grouped into thoughts or self-statements when in pain, beliefs about one's medical condition, and appraisals regarding impact of pain on other aspects of life (10). Cognitive theory conceptualizes behavior and emotion as influenced by the interpretation of an event, rather than solely by characteristics of the event itself. Thus, an "event" of pain interpreted as signifying ongoing tissue damage or life-threatening illness is likely to produce considerably more suffering and behavioral dysfunction than is one viewed as being the result of a minor injury, although the amount of nociceptive input in the two cases may be equivalent.

The psychological evaluation of chronic pain patients is predicated on a conceptualization of pain that is multidimensional, and recognizes the interactions among sensory, affective, cognitive, and behavioral processes in producing and maintaining pain and disability. An evaluation of chronic pain problems is incomplete if these complex interactions are ignored and attention is focused solely on identifying or ruling out organic pathology (11). A subsequent section of this chapter describes in detail this assessment of cognitive and behavioral processes.

INDICATIONS FOR PSYCHOLOGICAL EVALUATION

Patients with chronic pain typically are referred for psychological evaluation only in cases where physical findings sufficient to explain the pain are absent. In actuality, however, the psychological evaluation can be useful in all cases in which pain causes significant impairment in normal functioning or has had a negative impact on interpersonal relationships, or in which a patient exhibits signs of significant psychological distress, such as depression or anxiety. A psychological evaluation is also indicated in situations where disability greatly exceeds that expected on the basis of physical findings, when patients excessively use the health care system or persist in seeking diagnostic tests or treatments when not indicated, or when there is excessive or prolonged use of opioid or sedative-hypnotic medications or alcohol for pain control.

PURPOSES OF A PSYCHOLOGICAL EVALUATION

As noted above, the primary purposes of a psychological evaluation are to determine specific psychological and behavioral contributors to patients' pain behaviors, impairment in functioning, and suffering, and to determine appropriate treatment targets and intervention strategies. In addition, psychological assessment can provide pertinent information on aspects of a patient's psychosocial history and current situation that may have a bearing on the pain problem. For example, assessment of factors such as recent life stresses, substance abuse, educational background, vocational history, psychological disorders, and family role models of pain or chronic illness can provide valuable data helpful in interpreting a patient's current complaints and pain behaviors.

It is important to recognize that psychological evaluation cannot provide a definitive etiology for a patient's pain. A common misconception is that pain can be classified as either organic or psychogenic, and that if organic features are not found to explain the pain, a psychogenic etiology is implied. Most chronic pain syndromes represent a combination of contributing components, in which both physical and psychological influences are represented. The fact that significant psychological factors contributing to pain problems can be identified does not preclude the existence of significant physical pathology, nor do positive physical findings necessarily imply the absence of significant psychological or behavioral contributors to pain and disability.

Maintaining a conceptual dichotomy beween organic and psychogenic pain can lead to significant problems in clinical practice. When it is directly stated or implied to patients that pain is psychogenic, they typically interpret this to mean that their pain is not real, or that it is "all in the head." Most patients find this interpretation to be a pejorative one, and react to it with anger and defensiveness. Not only does this have a negative effect on the physician-patient relationship, but may also contribute to a very negative attitude on the part of the patient toward seeing a psychologist.

Another common misconception is that the psychological evaluation can determine if a particular patient is a good or poor candidate for surgery. As is discussed later in the chapter, the precision with which such predictions can be made is not sufficient to warrant reliance on psychological assessment in making surgical decisions in individual cases. These decisions, of course, must be made on the basis of physical findings and indications for such procedures. The psychological evaluation can be quite useful, however, in identifying patients who may be at higher risk for poor surgical outcome because of significant psychological or behavioral factors supporting ongoing pain behaviors and disability. In cases where there are clear physical indications for surgery in addition to strong psychological risk factors, the addition of psychological interventions to medical/surgical management potentially could be of benefit.

PREPARING THE PATIENT FOR A PSYCHOLOGICAL EVALUATION

Most chronic pain patients do not seek out psychological evaluation voluntarily, and many are not receptive to such a referral. Resistance to psychological evaluation may be due to a number of causes. One is that patients may see such a referral as implying that they are "crazy" or that they do not have a legitimate pain problem. Many believe that such an evaluation is not relevant to the assessment of a pain problem, particularly if they have a significant degree of conviction that there is an undiagnosed medical disorder responsible for their pain. Many patients fear that a referral for psychological evaluation implies that they can no longer be helped by the health care system, and are therefore being "dumped" from the care of their physician. When compensation or litigation issues are present, patients may be concerned that they are being viewed as malingerers, and thus see the referral for psychological evaluation as an attempt to "prove" that they do not have a legitimate pain problem.

Given all of the ways in which a referral for psychological evaluation can be misunderstood, it is important that adequate preparation of the patient takes place prior to making such a referral. The provision of accurate preparatory information to patients can serve to minimize the potential for misunderstanding, defensiveness, and non-cooperation on the part of the patient. To facilitate this process, pain programs and psychologists specializing in the evaluation of chronic pain patients can make information available to referral sources outlining the process of evaluation and any testing to be done. Brochures or handouts containing similar information can be sent to patients prior to their appointment for a psychological evaluation. In the brochure and in discussing the referral with the patient, it is often quite helpful to acknowledge directly that such a referral might suggest to the patient that the pain is viewed as "not real" or psychogenic. It can then be emphasized that the validity of the patient's pain complaints is accepted, but that there typically are complex interactions between physical and psychological processes that influence pain, disability, and suffering. It is also important to note that psychological techniques are used with a number of pain syndromes, including those in which there is a well-defined somatic problem such as cancer pain or burn pain. The use of such techniques in no way implies that pain is not "real."

Discussing the devastating effects that chronic pain can have on areas of life other than medical status, such as disruption of vocational, familial, and social functioning, can provide an additional rationale for psychological consultation. Patients are usually willing to acknowledge that chronic pain has indeed caused disruption across a number of areas of functioning. The physician can then suggest that the psychological evaluation may indicate specific treatments to reduce dysfunction and distress.

It is also helpful in preparing patients for the evaluation to describe, in general terms, any psychological testing that might be done and also to discuss the importance of interviewing the family members or significant others as part of the evaluation. Patients generally accept the rationale that information from someone close to them can enhance understanding of their pain problem and of pain-related changes in their functioning over time. In addition, family members often appreciate the opportunity to be included in evaluation and treatment efforts, because they are almost always strongly affected by the patient's pain problem.

OVERVIEW OF THE PSYCHOLOGICAL EVALUATION

The primary components of the initial psychological evaluation are interviews with the patient and spouse (family member or friend if the patient is unmarried) and review of pertinent medical records and activity diaries (cf. ref. 5). In the authors' clinical settings, prior to the initial appointment patients receive a letter describing the process of evaluation in general terms, requesting them to have all pertinent medical records sent to the clinic before the appointment, and asking them to bring their spouse or a "significant other" to participate in the evaluation. (For purposes of simplicity, any "significant other" is referred to as a spouse in the remainder of the chapter.)

A questionnaire and 2 weeks of activity diaries to be completed prior to the appointment can be enclosed with the letter, so that these data are available at the time of evaluation. The activity diaries contain one page for each day of the week, with spaces for recording activities, medication use, and pain intensity each hour of the day. Activities are recorded within categories of walking/standing, sitting, and reclining. There is evidence that such diaries are fairly accurate records of actual behaviors (12), and they can be useful sources of information concerning activity level, medication use, and patterns of pain intensity. Questionnaires are efficient means of obtaining information concerning demographics, history of the pain problem and prior treatments, sources of income, compensation and litigation issues, and medical and psychological treatment history. Perusal of these forms as well as the medical records prior to interviewing the patient and spouse can alert the clinician to areas in need of clarification or elaboration.

At the outset of the interview it is helpful to clarify, as discussed in the previous section, why a psychological evaluation is being conducted, the specific nature of the referral question, how the results will be used, and who will have access to them. Both the patient and spouse are then interviewed, as described in detail later in this chapter. It works well to see the patient and spouse together briefly at first, then to interview them separately. The conjoint interview can be used to clarify what will happen and to discuss the couple's questions and concerns, but behavioral analysis and other components of the evaluation are best performed in separate interviews. It is also recommended that patients complete a Minnesota Multiphasic Personality Inventory (MMPI) at the evaluation appointment.

Following completion of the evaluation, it is important to hold a feedback conference with the patient and spouse to review the findings and discuss recommendations. If a medical evaluation is conducted in parallel with the psychological one (as is often done in multidisciplinary pain clinic), a joint feedback conference, including the patient, spouse, psychologist, and physician, provides a useful opportunity to review results of both evaluations and present an integrated set of recommendations. A well-conducted feedback conference typically can be completed within 15–30 min and can serve evaluative, educational, and even therapeutic functions. It can provide patients with information helpful in understanding the persistence of suffering and disability, and help shape their conceptualization of pain toward a viewpoint that will be compatible with rehabilitation efforts.

A typical feedback conference may begin by again assuring the patient and spouse that the legitimacy of the patient's pain problem is accepted, and that such problems are common and understandable. It is often useful to provide an explanatory model of how chronic pain and excess disability may develop, based on a cognitive-behavioral model. For example, it might be explained that an injury may produce pain and require a period of convalescence to allow healing to occur. Following a period of prolonged inactivity, even mild exercise can be painful since muscles have become tight and deconditioned. Inactivity is frequently extended beyond the normal healing time because of this pain and the patient's concern about reinjury. Continuation of this pattern can result in muscle weakness, avoidance and fear of activity, the development of poor body mechanics, and prolonged pain, as well as psychological distress. By providing patients with such a model, the chronic pain problem is defined as one requiring relearning and rehabilitation, rather than either a purely somatic or purely psychological treatment. This can allow patients to engage in treatment without having to define themselves as either physically or mentally "ill."

The major findings of the evaluation are then described, with a focus on factors seen as contributing to dysfunction and suffering. Potential intervention strategies are outlined, as are realistic expectations for outcome. Typically, it is not the case that patients will be completely pain free following the course of care and remain that way. To help decrease the likelihood of future misunderstanding and disappointment, this should be stated clearly to patients and spouses. It can then be emphasized that the interventions recommended, nonetheless, can be quite helpful in reducing disability and suffering, preventing reinjury, decreasing use of analgesic medications (if this is a problem), and increasing adaptive functioning, despite the fact that some discomfort may persist following treatment. Patients and spouses are encouraged at each step of the conference to raise concerns and questions, which are then discussed. Receptivity of patients and spouses to the feedback from the evaluation and treatment recommendations can be assessed during this discussion.

COMPONENTS OF THE PSYCHOLOGICAL EVALUATION

TAKING A PAIN HISTORY

The sequence in which topics are addressed with patients in the psychological interview can be important. Most patients are primarily concerned with obtaining pain relief and thus are more willing at first to discuss their pain experiences than to focus on more sensitive issues such as family dysfunction and psychological distress. Rapport may be established more easily if the clinician begins the interview by having patients describe when and how their pain began and its course over time in terms of severity, frequency, quality, and location. Such information, of course, must be interpreted in light of physical findings from the medical evaluation and the type of pain problem with which the patient presents, but can be used to identify potential psychological/behavioral contributors to the pain problem. For example, a review of activity diaries and questioning of patients to determine whether any systematic fluctuations in pain level occur in association with certain times of day or situations (such as presence of spouse or family members) may suggest that factors such as environmental reinforcers or stress may be contributing to pain behavior and suffering. This point is covered in more detail in the section on behavioral analysis.

If pain began with a traumatic injury or accident, the interviewer should inquire about the nature of the accident and determine whether the patient experiences anxiety in or avoids situations similar to those in which the trauma occurred (e.g., a patient who was injured in a car accident may avoid driving). It can also be helpful to explore whether environmental stimuli associated with a traumatic injury or accident are linked to changes in pain level.

Another area requiring careful inquiry is response to prior treatments for pain. Patients may report that they have been treated unsuccessfully with a particular modality (e.g., exercise, biofeedback, or antidepressant medication), yet careful questioning concerning the specific type and course of treatment or dosage levels of medications received may suggest that an adequate trial was not conducted. Patients may also reveal that they felt unable to comply with a treatment, such as exercise, due to increased pain. Such "failures" do not necessarily argue against recommending a more adequate trial of an intervention, provided that steps are taken to address patient concerns, provide a strong rational for its use, and structure treatment contingencies to minimize noncompliance.

OBSERVATIONAL ASSESSMENT

Careful observation of patient and spouse interactions and nonverbal behaviors can yield valuable information, supplementing other data obtained during the evaluation. The interviewer should note whether the patient remains seated comfortably throughout the interview, or whether pain behaviors are shown, and if so, what specific behaviors are observed. Do there appear to be antecedent stimuli consistently associated with emission of pain behaviors (e.g., certain topics of discussion)? Are pain behaviors displayed more frequently when the spouse is present? If the spouse is present when pain behaviors occur, how does he/she respond? Are there inconsistencies between patient or spouse report versus interviewer observation of pain behaviors and spouse responses? Although observation of a temporal association between particular situations and increased pain behavior does not establish a definitive relationship between them, it may suggest hypotheses to be explored in more depth. As in any psychological evaluation, behavioral indicators of depression and anxiety should also be noted.

Very frequent and/or very dramatic displays of pain behaviors can suggest the likelihood of social or environmental reinforcers contributing to the maintenance of the pain problem. However, there is evidence (13) that frequency of pain behaviors during physical examination is positively correlated with presence of organic pathology in patients presenting for neurosurgical evaluation, so considerable caution needs to be exercised in interpreting the significance of pain behaviors. Because the meaning of pain behaviors is so complex and because relevant empirical data are lacking, the authors cannot offer hard rules for their interpretation. However, the clinician will usually find it helpful to integrate observational data with other data from the evaluation in forming impressions and treatment recommendations. For example, highly frequent or salient pain behaviors in a chronic pain patient suggest the need for educating the patient about the negative effects of such behaviors and training the patient's family members not to reinforce such behaviors by contingent attention.

EVALUATION OF COGNITIVE ASPECTS OF CHRONIC PAIN

Although the study of cognitive events is not new in psychology, the application of cognitive methods and principles to the assessment and care of medical patients is a relatively recent phenomenon (9). It is increasingly recognized that a patient's interpretation of the meaning of pain and the extent to which pain forms a focus of attention can have profound effects on the patient's responses to pain.

In light of this, it is important to gather information on patients' appraisals of their pain problems, their thoughts and images of what is happening in their bodies when they are experiencing pain, and, similarly, the spouses' explanatory model for the cause and implications of the pain. In many cases, patients have fears based on misinformation or faulty concepts of anatomy and medicine. Information they receive from physicians regarding their medical condition may be easily misinterpreted. For example, some patients believe or have been told that their back pain is the result of degenerative disk disease, and interpret this to mean that their spines are fragile and unstable, and that movement will hasten the process of degeneration and disability. Patients are often convinced that they have a "pinched nerve" or "slipped disk" compressing a nerve and fear that they may damage their spinal cords or even become paralyzed if activity is increased. Given that such patients are interpreting chronic pain as a signal of ongoing tissue damage and physical harm, it is understandable that they avoid activities that increase pain. If spouses have such fears, they are likely to reinforce pain behaviors by overprotecting the patient, and may even sabotage treatment aimed at increasing physical activity.

Although patients may at first state that their only thought during pain is "I hurt," often with some careful questioning they will report that they have "catastrophic" thoughts, such as "I will never get better," "this pain is uncontrollable and unbearable," and "there is nothing I can do but lie still and take medications." This is but a small sample of the types of negative thoughts that can accompany severe pain. A habitual pattern of such maladaptive thoughts may contribute to a sense of hopelessness, dysphoria, and an unwillingness to engage in activity. It has been suggested that such negative thinking patterns may contribute to the maintenance of depression (14), a frequent problem among chronic pain patients (15). For a more complete discussion of this topic and excellent suggestions regarding specific assessment strategies, the reader is referred to Turk, Meichenbaum, and Genest (9).

TREATMENT GOALS AND EXPECTATIONS

Understanding both patient and spouse goals for treatment is also an important part of the evaluation process. It is often the case that the patient or spouse believes that prior diagnostic workups have been incomplete or inadequate, and that further medical testing is necessary, with the likely outcome that surgery will be needed to reduce pain. Such a stance, until addressed in light of the medical evaluation, will make any type of psychological intervention very difficult and probably unproductive. Similarly, if a patient appears to have a firm goal of obtaining or continuing compensation or disability payments, attempts at rehabilitation and return to work are likely to be met with resistance. The evaluation therefore should aim to clarify patient and spouse goals and determine whether some consensus can be reached among patient, spouse, and health care providers as to appropriate treatment goals.

BEHAVIORAL ANALYSIS

An essential part of any psychological evaluation of a chronic pain patient is a behavioral analysis. The objective of this analysis is to specify antecedents and consequences of pain behaviors in order to identify environmental stimuli that either elicit or reinforce pain behaviors. Also in the behavioral analysis, the interviewer aims to determine the potential for modification of environmental reinforcers of pain behaviors, to identify appropriate behavioral goals for treatment, and to assess the likelihood that the patient's social environment will support healthy alternatives to pain behavior and disability. Of course, reinforcement of pain behaviors can be identified in the psychological evaluation only on a presumptive basis. Nonetheless, identification of probable reinforcers through interview of patient and spouse can provide the basis for generating hypotheses to be examined in further interactions with the patient, as well as lay the groundwork for designing treatment strategies. Additional information regarding the operant behavioral approach to chronic pain evaluation can be found in Fordyce (5) and Fordyce and Steger (6).

As noted previously, contingencies maintaining pain behaviors may include the avoidance of aversive situations or activities as well as positive consequences. Contingencies appearing to contribute to the maintenance of pain behaviors and disability may be fairly obvious (e.g., financial rewards, greatly increased attention and affection from family members). In other cases, the interviews may suggest more subtle types of reinforcement. For example, pain may allow the patient "time out" from stressful family situations, provide the patient with increased control over the behavior of family members, or mask sexual or cognitive dysfunction.

Assessment of several major areas forms the basis for determining whether behavioral processes may be contributing to the maintenance of pain behavior and functional impairment. These include changes in patient and spouse activity resulting from the pain problem, patient and spouse learning history, interpersonal relationships and family response to pain behaviors, and work and finance issues. Other topics, of course, may also need to be explored during the behavioral analysis as indicated in individual cases.

Activity Changes

It is usually nonthreatening to start the behavioral analysis by asking the patient to list specific activities he or she is doing less often or no longer doing because of the pain. Often, considerable prompting is needed to obtain a complete list, and the patient may need to be asked specifically about vocational, recreational, home management, and social activities. In order to determine whether these activity changes are positive, negative, or neutral for the patient, questioning should address the frequency of performance of each activity just before pain onset and the extent to which the patient enjoyed the activity. Not infrequently a patient will mention the loss of a certain activity (e.g., hunting or dancing), and then further questioning reveals that the patient had engaged in this activity only occasionally in the years prior to pain onset. The same questions should be asked of the spouse.

When the patient is not currently engaging in activities reported as highly pleasurable and frequently performed prior to pain onset, this information may be quite useful in planning treatment goals. In some cases, however, pleasurable activities may be decreased to a minimal extent or even increased, and/or aversive responsibilities may no longer be required because of the patient's pain. Such situations suggest that operant factors are likely to influence pain behaviors and a behavioral program aimed at contingency modification is indicated. In most cases, the patient's degree of satisfaction with his/her current lifestyle will be consistent with the extent of losses or gains in pleasurable activities. If there is marked incongruence, further questioning of the patient and spouse or (with the patient's permission) of significant others, such as family members, employers, friends, vocational counselors, and attorneys, may reveal additional important information.

It is usually informative to ask the patient and spouse separately what specific activities they would do if the patient had no pain. Fordyce (5) has noted that this information aids in identifying activities that will be reinforcing to the patient and spouse, and thus is useful in selecting treatment goals. Occasionally, both the patient and spouse report, even when prompted to list specific goals, that they would not do anything differently, but that the patient would be "happier." Given the lack of target goals, such patients are usually poor candidates for a behavioral treatment program aimed at improving activity and function. In other cases, a patient would like to be more active but may have difficulty formulating specific behavioral goals because former activities are not available. In these situations, often it is possible to work with the patient over time to develop realistic and desired goals.

Inconsistencies in activities that have been decreased or eliminated because of pain should be noted. For example, when a customary activity is performed but another with similar physical demands is not, it is frequently the case that only the former activity is found pleasurable by the patient. Such a pattern suggests that pain behaviors may be operantly reinforced. This situation should alert the clinician to inquire carefully about characteristics of activities the patient is performing versus avoiding, to help identify potential reinforcers of pain behaviors.

Avoidance Learning

One factor that may contribute to activity changes is avoidance learning. This usually takes the form of persistent avoidance of certain body movements or activities, often for fear of incurring increased pain or tissue damage. This may occur irrespective of other reinforcement processes. As Fordyce, Shelton, and Dundore (7) have described, certain pain behaviors (e.g., limping) may be strongly reinforced by reducing acute pain after an injury. Over time, healing occurs, but these behaviors may continue, with the patient believing that not engaging in them or that using the affected part would result in increased pain and/or body damage. In such cases, a treatment program in which the patient gradually increases performance of correct body movement is needed to overcome the pattern of avoidance learning. When patients have not used a certain part of the body for some time, use of the affected area may cause increased pain initially, but pain is usually reduced over time if activity increases slowly and systematically.

Deactivation

Marked deactivation is commonly seen in pain clinic populations. This may develop because physical activity usually produces increased pain, whereas sitting or lying down reduces discomfort. Because this pain reduction reinforces resting behavior, resting behavior is likely to occur more frequently in the future (6). Excessive resting over time results in decreased physical strength, stamina, and flexibility. Such physical changes are likely to result in increased pain when activities are attempted; this of course punishes activity, reinforces rest, and further convinces the patient that activity is harmful. Inactivity also produces decreased opportunity to engage in pleasurable activities and increased time to focus on pain, which in turn may contribute to depressed mood and withdrawal. Thus a vicious cycle of increasing pain and inactivity may be perpetuated. Activity diaries (5, 12) are helpful in assessing how much time patients spend resting each day. Excessive resting time is a good indicator that a treatment program involving progressive increases in physical activity is needed. A regimen of physical therapy using a baseline and quota system (cf. ref. 5) as well as gradual systematic increases in duration of daily activities are useful methods for reversing deactivation.

Learning History

Questioning concerning whether patients have had significant role models (e.g., parents) for pain and disability and the characteristic responses of the family to health problems may yield important information concerning prior learning experiences related to pain and illness behaviors (16). Similar questioning of the spouse may provide information concerning whether he/she is responding to the patient's pain behaviors in a maladaptive way based on past learning experiences. For example, a spouse may feel guilty about not having been supportive of loved ones with pain in the past and vow to be nurturing "this time." It is also relatively common to find older spouses with a long history of caretaking of ill parents and/or former spouses.

Interpersonal Relationships and Family Response to Pain Behaviors

Several lines of questioning are helpful in assessing the role of social contingencies in reinforcing pain behaviors. The patient and spouse should be asked how others know when the patient has increased pain and exactly how others respond at those times. Detailed questioning of the spouse is often needed to learn how others infer the presence of pain through the patient's verbal and nonverbal behaviors, and what the family then does in response. If family members frequently respond, especially in solicitous ways, to the patient's verbal and nonverbal pain behaviors, it is likely that social reinforcers contribute to maintaining pain behaviors and will need to be addressed in treatment. It is important to note that reinforcement of pain behaviors is defined by the effect that others' responses exert on increasing or decreasing the rate of the patient's pain behaviors. Spouse behaviors that appear "negative" (e.g., expressions of annoyance or withdrawing from the patient) may actually positively reinforce pain behavior. In such cases, a patient's pain behaviors may allow the patient to regulate interpersonal distance from the spouse or other family members.

It is also important to assess the responses of family and friends to "well behaviors," that is, behaviors incompatible with disability. Spouses may discourage patients from engaging in certain physical activities (e.g., certain household chores). Spouses may also withdraw affection or attention, or may increase demands on the patient in response to increased "well behaviors." If this is the case, training spouses to respond more positively to patient well behaviors will be an important component of rehabilitation efforts. Aspects of the patient's pain problem that may be reinforcing to family members (such as changes in roles or responsibilities) also need to be identified. Family members may not be supportive of patients' attempts to resume their former roles and duties if this leads to fewer satisfying activities for them.

In both the patient and spouse interviews, assessment of the quality of the marital relationship is often vital in understanding the pain problem. Because this may be a sensitive area, it can be helpful to start by stating that most people with pain problems find that their marital relationship has been affected by the pain, then asking how the patient and spouse view effects of pain on their marriage. If they indicate the marriage is stressed, it can be informative to inquire about past or discussed separations. It is also useful to ask what they believe would happen to the relationship if the pain were alleviated. In some cases, pain has brought the couple closer together through increased emotional intimacy or increased time together, and successful treatment of the pain and rehabilitation to normal functioning might threaten this satisfactory arrangement. In other cases, a spouse has wanted to terminate the relationship, but does not leave because the patient is "ill" and needs him/her. Thus, alleviation of the pain might bring about an unwanted consequence for the patient. If such issues are present, they will need to be addressed as part of any treatment effort.

Often chronic pain is associated with reductions in the quality and frequency of couples' sexual activity. The interviewer should directly ask about the frequency of sexual activity and the presence of sexual dysfunction currently and prior to the onset of pain. Commonly, sexual activity decreases because pain reduces the patient's level of interest and/or because such activity causes increased pain. However, in some couples, pain complaints are used as an excuse for not engaging in sex, when the real reason is primary sexual dysfunction or marital discord.

Vocational, Financial, and Litigation Issues

In patients who are not retired, thorough assessment of vocational issues is critical in understanding the pain problem and in treatment planning. If the patient is not currently working, additional evaluation and conjoint meetings with vocational counselors, physicians, and physical and occupational therapists are often necessary to determine whether return to work is a desired and realistic goal, and if so, to what type of work, and how this will be accomplished. Nonetheless, it is important during the initial evaluation to inquire about the patient's vocational history and to identify factors that might impede return to work, because often this can shed light on environmental reinforcers of pain and disability. A poor work history with evidence of consistent problems in maintaining employment prior to pain onset may suggest that return to previous work may not be reinforcing and that vocational rehabilitation may be more difficult than in patients with good work histories. Likewise, evidence of few vocational skills or very limited experience may also suggest the need for more vigorous efforts at vocational rehabilitation if working is a desirable goal. It is very useful to assess patient's satisfaction with their jobs, employers, and co-workers prior to pain onset, and to ask patients directly about their specific plans, if any, for return to work, and about potential barriers other than pain to returning to work.

Many patients injured on the job receive workers' compensation or disability payments nearly equivalent to former income. Patients may fear losing this financial support, particularly if the former job is unpleasant or no longer available, if vocational options appear limited, or if the patient fears reinjury or increased pain upon return to work. If decreased disability following treatment implies the loss of compensation income, this issue must be addressed as part of treatment or chances of long-term improvement may be lessened. The interviewer should also inquire about any current or planned applications for disability compensation (e.g., Social Security Disability Insurance), which may likewise form a disincentive to improvement. In cases of patients who receive workers' compensation, elucidation of their understanding of the status of the case with the compensation agency, and of when and how closure of the case will occur, can be highly informative. Often patients have inaccurate or unrealistic perceptions of how long compensation will continue, what constitutes compensable problems, or on what basis cases are settled. When such misperceptions seem likely to interfere with rehabilitation efforts, a conjoint meeting of the patient and spouse, the patient's attorney (if applicable), and the treatment staff can help to clarify these issues and to arrive at mutually agreeable treatment goals.

Similarly, if litigation is pending, the implications of improvement in pain and disability for the suit should be explored prior to making decisions about treatment. The research literature examining whether pending litigation forms a significant barrier to improvement in multidisciplinary pain programs is sparse and has not provided clear guidelines for making such decisions. It has been suggested that pending litigation should constitute grounds for exclusion from a behavioral treatment program if the suit appears to be an important factor in the promotion of continued disability (17). In some studies, however, litigation has not emerged as a significant predictor of outcome

(18, 19) and it has been argued that the effects of litigation per se on treatment outcome have been overemphasized (19).

In individual cases, when litigation is planned or pending, it is very valuable for the clinician to have a frank discussion with the patient's attorney to clarify the nature and status of the litigation and to assess the extent to which the outcome of treatment may affect the lawsuit. If these are judged to be relatively independent, it is usually appropriate to proceed with treatment, assuming other factors support this course of action. If the outcome of a lawsuit is likely to be influenced strongly by treatment outcome, it is frequently recommended that comprehensive pain treatment be delayed until settlement of the suit, unless there are overriding reasons for more immediate intervention. Such interventions may include treatment of depression or drug detoxification, which may be conducted prior to undertaking reactivation and rehabilitation efforts. Considerable care needs to be exercised in making recommendations to pursue or defer treatment when litigation is pending, weighing factors such as patient distress and the potential for increased dysfunction that could occur if treatment is delayed versus the possibility that litigation may form a potent disincentive to improve.

PSYCHOLOGICAL DYSFUNCTION

Psychological disorders are commonly seen in chronic pain populations and should be assessed as part of the psychological evaluation. In some cases, alterations in psychological functioning result from the impact of dealing with chronic pain, disability, and associated life changes; in others, psychological dysfunction can predate pain onset and may be exacerbated by the pain problem or hamper efforts to cope with it. A complete guide to the diagnosis of psychological disorders is, of course, beyond the scope of this chapter. However, disorders most commonly found in chronic pain patients and difficulties related to diagnosis in this population are discussed briefly.

Depression is particularly prevalent in chronic pain patients (15, 20) and should be assessed routinely in the psychological evaluation. The *Diagnostic and Statistical Manual of Mental Disorders, Third Edition* (DSM-III) outlines the criteria specified by the American Psychiatric Association (21) for diagnosis of affective disorders. Assessment of depression should cover the full spectrum of vegetative, affective, and cognitive symptoms, because chronic pain patients often deny or minimize mood disturbance while admitting to other symptoms of depression such as persistent irritability, fatigue, and insomnia. However, these symptoms may be produced by pain, deactivation, and excessive alcohol or opioid or sedative-hypnotic medication use, making diagnosis of depression quite difficult. This may be more of a conceptual than a practical problem because treatments useful for chronic pain also appear to be beneficial for depression. These include medication withdrawal if the patient is taking opioid or sedative-hypnotic medication, cognitive-behavioral therapy, and antidepressant medication.

Anxiety disorders also are seen frequently in chronic pain patients (22). As with depression, many symptoms of anxiety such as muscle tension and sleeplessness also result from chronic pain, making diagnosis difficult. Patients with anxiety disorders occasionally may complain that they cannot work, socialize, or engage in other activities because of their pain, when in actuality anxiety is the primary factor limiting their behavior. Close evaluation of these patients may reveal a generalized anxiety disorder, panic disorder, or specific phobia. Many pain problems begin with traumatic events, such as a motor vehicle accident, a fall, or an industrial accident, and patients sometimes continue to experience intense anxiety when they are in situations similar to that in which the injury occurred. If not treated, these anxiety problems can interfere significantly with rehabilitation.

In older chronic pain patients, previously undiagnosed dementia is not uncommon. Pain may be used as an excuse to avoid certain activities that the patient finds difficult to perform because of intellectual deficits. Although a structured mental status examination such as the Mini-Mental State (23) is a useful screening tool for dementia, subtle impairment may not be detected by the mental status examination, and formal neuropsychological testing (cf. ref. 24) is a more sensitive indicator.

ALCOHOL AND DRUG USE

Many chronic pain patients seen in pain clinic settings have problems with excessive alcohol or opioid or sedative-hypnotic medication use (25). Such use complicates the assessment of the pain problem for a number of reasons. One is that the patient may use his/her pain complaints to legitimize drug and/or alcohol use. Another reason is that patients may mislabel withdrawal symptoms as an increase in "pain" (26). Chronic use of opioid and sedative-hypnotic drugs can produce dysphoria and other symptoms that mimic depression, such as decreased energy, sleep disturbance, and appetite and weight changes.

During the evaluation, the interviewer should routinely ask the patient and spouse independently to specify the patient's current alcohol consumption and pattern of use, as well as whether there is a history of excessive drinking, driving while intoxicated charges, and/or alcohol interference with work, family, or social functioning. A similar inquiry should be conducted as to what medications the patient has been taking recently, the route of administration and dosages used per day, and whether there is a history of street drug abuse or long-term prescription opioid or sedative-hypnotic drug use. Review of activity diaries is helpful in learning types and patterns of medication use, but it should be kept in mind that patients often underreport actual use (25). If patients are hospitalized, the "drug profile" (25), during which patients request medications of the type and amount they were using at home, is a useful method of delineating the nature and amount of current medication use.

Patients evidencing ongoing street drug or alcohol abuse are best referred to a drug or alcohol treatment program before beginning pain treatment. Most pain programs are not equipped to treat such problems, which are very likely to interfere with ability to engage in rehabilitation, as well as with maintenance of gains made in treatment. Prescription opioid and sedative-hypnotic medication dependence, on the other hand, can usually be treated successfully in an inpatient pain treatment program (27, 28).

FAMILY AND SOCIAL HISTORY

No psychological evaluation would be complete without a general inquiry into the patient's family and social background. As mentioned earlier, it is useful to ask about role models for chronic illness behavior and any premorbid learning experiences the patient had with extended illness or disability. A family history of depression, other psychological disorders, or alcohol abuse can alert the clinician to the potential contribution of such factors to the patient's current situation and past development through biologic predisposition and/or learning patterns. Childhood neglect and physical and sexual abuse are frequently reported and may continue to contribute to dysfunction and distress. It is usually necessary to ask direct questions about these experiences. Patients may be reluctant to address them because they do not see them as relevant to their pain problem or because of guilt, embarrassment, or continuing emotional distress. It is also useful to ask about the patient's social and academic adjustment when young, as well as about social and familial adjustment in later years.

STRESS

Researchers have focused considerable attention on the relationship between recent life stress and disease, injury, and illness behavior (cf. ref. 29). Unfortunately, few studies have specifically addressed the relationship between past and ongoing life stress and the onset and persistence of chronic pain problems. In clinical practice, such an association is often seen, although patients may initially deny or minimize the contributions of stress to their pain problems. The spouse can frequently provide additional information about any stressful circumstances surrounding pain onset, and about ongoing stress that may exacerbate pain or be avoided because of pain.

Although in many cases no major stressor can be associated with pain onset, current stressors in the patient's life may contribute to increased levels of muscle tension, illness behavior and disability, and use of medications or alcohol as coping strategies (29). Of course, chronic pain and associated life disruption, as well as worry about the prognosis or cause of the pain, are themselves often sources of severe stress. Identification of major current and past life stressors (e.g., marital or vocational problems, death of a loved one, major financial problems), their effects on pain, and the patient's typical methods of coping with stress frequently indicate directions for treatment. Treatment may aim to modify stress responses by techniques such as relaxation training and/or may aim to alter situations contributing to stress by such methods as marital or family therapy.

MINNESOTA MULTIPHASIC PERSONALITY INVENTORY

The MMPI (30) has been the psychological instrument most widely used in the assessment and study of chronic pain problems. Consisting of 566 true-false items, it yields three validity, 10 clinical, and numerous research scales. Many psychologists use the MMPI routinely in the psychological evaluation of chronic pain patients as a means of assessing psychopathology, mood disturbance, and personality characteristics. Although the MMPI can provide useful information, it can also be used inappropriately.

One misapplication is the use of the MMPI to make a statement about whether a pain problem is "organic" or "functional." Studies that have examined whether patients diagnosed by physicians as having "functional" or "organic" pain differ on MMPI scales have yielded conflicting results (cf. refs. 31–34). Such discrepant findings are not surprising given that, as discussed previously, such a dichotomous conceptualization does not account for the complexity of most chronic pain problems, and that elevations on MMPI scales can occur independent of organic pathology. Although the MMPI can be useful in generating hypotheses and corroborating other evidence concerning possible psychological/behavioral factors maintaining an individual's pain problem, it should never be used to make a statement regarding the extent to which organic features may be involved in the patient's pain.

A second way in which the MMPI can be misused is in predicting patient response to treatment. Various studies have produced no consistent findings with respect to MMPI associations with outcome after nonsurgical treatments for pain (cf. refs. 35–37). Findings have been more consistent with respect to MMPI correlations with outcome after back surgery. Numerous studies have found elevated Hypochondriasis (*Hs*) scores to be associated with poor surgical response (38–42), and other MMPI scales have also been found in some studies to predict outcome (38, 41–44). Several investigators also have found that the Pain Assessment Index (PAI) (45), a measure incorporating several MMPI scales but yielding a single score, can be a moderately good predictor of outcome following surgery (44–46). Although these studies suggest that some relationships exist between MMPI scles (especially *Hs*) and outcome after back surgery, highly accurate predictions regarding a particular patient's response to surgery cannot be made reliably, and considerable caution is needed in clinical decision making in individual cases.

The MMPI, of course, is used primarily to assess psychological disorder in chronic pain patients. One particularly common use of the MMPI has been to assess depression. A study by Turner and Romano (47) suggests that the Depression (D) scale is useful in screening for depression but should not be used to make a clinical diagnosis. Caution should also be exercised in using the Hysteria (Hy) scale to diagnose hysterical personality characteristics in chronic pain patients. Watson (48) found that chronic pain patients, as compared with medical and student groups, acknowledged more physical problems on Hy items but did not differ on denial of psychological problems. Prokop (49) found that low back pain patients were higher than normal subjects on Harris and Lingoes' Lassitude-Malaise and Somatic Complaints subscales but did not differ on Denial of Social Anxiety. Prokop (49) also concluded that the "Conversion V" profile (elevations on Hs and Hy with a relatively unelevated D scale) suggests an unusual focus on physical symptoms, but cautioned against inferring conversion dynamics in the absence of subscale analysis or corroborating evidence from psychological evaluation.

The Schizophrenia (Sc) scale also has potential for misinterpretation. Moore and his colleagues (50) compared Harris and Lingoes' Sc subscales across chronic pain patients, hospitalized psychotics without pain, and nonpsychotic psychiatric outpatients without pain, all of whom had Sc elevations above a T-score of 70. They found pain patients scored significantly lower on Social Alienation, Lack of Ego Mastery–Cognitive, Lack of Ego Mastery–Conative, and Lack of Ego Mastery–Defective Inhibition, but higher on Bizarre Sensory Experiences than did the psychiatric groups. This study suggests that elevations on the Sc scale in chronic pain patient profiles may be misinterpreted as reflecting psychotic symptomatology rather than unusual physical complaints. Inspection of subscale scores may aid in accurate interpretation of the Sc scale with this population.

GUIDELINES FOR REPORT PREPARATION

As is the case for any psychological report, the report of the evaluation of the chronic pain patient needs to be concise and clear, with conclusions anchored to data presented in the report. The audience for such evaluations most frequently will not be psychologists or mental health practitioners, but rather physicians, other health care providers, third-party payers, and attorneys. The use of jargon or psychological terms unlikely to be familiar to those outside the mental health professions should therefore be avoided. The purpose of the report is to summarize psychological and behavioral factors that appear to be involved in the pain problem, and make specific recommendations for treatment.

SAMPLE REPORT OF A PSYCHOLOGICAL EVALUATION OF A CHRONIC PAIN PATIENT

Identification

John Doe is a 45-year-old man with a chief complaint of chronic low back pain, referred by Dr. Jane Smith for psychological evaluation. This evaluation is based on interviews with Mr. Doe and his wife, review of available medical records, a self-report questionnaire, 2 weeks of activity diaries completed by the patient, and the MMPI. Mr. Doe was interviewed and completed the MMPI on January 15, 1987.

Pain History

Mr. Doe states that he was in good health until March 5, 1984, when, while working as a sawmill operator, he experienced the onset of severe lower back and right leg pain when lifting a load of wood. He was taken immediately to the emergency room of a local hospital, where he was diagnosed as having "muscle strain." Conservative treatment, including bed rest and physical therapy modalities of heat, massage, and ultrasound, failed to improve his symptoms. Three months after this injury, Mr. Doe was diagnosed as having a herniated disk at L4–L5, and a laminectomy and diskectomy were performed at that level, followed by considerable improvement in pain. He returned to work in September 1984; however, pain began to increase and he stopped working in December 1984. Mr. Doe reports that he has had constant severe pain in his low back and right leg since that time. A repeat computed tomography scan and myelogram obtained in December 1986 revealed no objective changes that would warrant further surgery.

Mr. Doe describes his pain as dull and aching in quality most of the time, with occasional sharp, shooting pains in his low back and down his right leg. He notes that pain tends to increase over the course of the day. Sitting or standing for more than 15 min at a time causes his pain to worsen, as does any activity involving lifting, bending, or twisting. His pain is decreased by lying down and by medications (currently 6–8 Oxycodone per day).

Functional Limitations

As a result of pain, Mr. Doe is no longer working, hunting, fishing, or engaging in recreational activities (e.g., bowling, taking trips) with his family. He has also decreased performance of household maintenance chores, such as yardwork and cleaning gutters and windows, tasks his three sons now do. He has increased the amount of time spent in sedentary activities such as watching television, with diaries indicating that he spends approximately 20 hr/day lying down or sitting. Mr. Doe states he wants to return to work, although he doubts that he can perform his old job as a sawmill operator, which he describes as very physically demanding. He also wishes to resume hunting and fishing, as well as performing his own yardwork.

Family Relationships

The Does have been married for 20 years and have three sons, ages 17, 14, and 10. Each describes the marriage as basically stable, although both admit that his pain problem has placed a strain on the relationship. Mr. Doe is frequently irritable, often snapping at his spouse or their children. Mrs. Doe became tearful when describing her husband's irritability, stating that she felt discouraged and at a loss as to how to handle his pain problem. When in pain, Mr. Doe will mention that his back hurts and will either sit in his recliner or lie down. His wife responds by sitting with him, and tries to distract him by talking to him, or offers to massage his back. She attempts to keep the children quiet and out of his way when his pain is bad. Both Mr. and Mrs. Doe report that frequency of sexual activity has decreased sharply since his injury. Both state that this is due to increased pain caused by such activity.

Cognitions Related to Pain

Mr. Doe believes that his ongoing pain problem is caused by a recurrence of a herniated disk that is "pinching a nerve" in his spine. He states that he has been told that his pain is likely caused by scar tissue resulting from his operation, but does not understand how this can account for pain in his right leg. He often worries that any increased strain on his back may cause permanent damage to a nerve. He believes that further medical diagnostic evaluation is necessary and that he may need another surgery to completely alleviate his pain. He does not see how it would be possible for him to cope with his pain without opioid medications. He expresses much concern as well about whether he will ever be employable again, and fears not being able to support his family once workers' compensation payments are discontinued.

Vocational History

Mr. Doe worked as a sawmill operator for 22 years prior to his injury. He and his wife report that his job provided him much satisfaction and that he maintained excellent relationships with his coworkers. He has worked for the same company for 22 years and has never missed work for more than a day or two because of illness or injury. Since he stopped work in December 1984, he has received state industrial compensation payments of $1100/month. He does not have an attorney and is not planning litigation related to his injury, but he is considering applying for Social Security Disability Insurance. Prior to his injury, Mr. Doe was making approximately $2200 a month in gross income. His wife has never worked outside the home and they have no other income. Prior to his work in the sawmill, Mr. Doe served in the army for 2 years. He was never in combat and received an honorable discharge.

Alcohol and Drug Use

Mr. Doe reports drinking one to two beers three times a week, and this level of consumption is corroborated by his wife. Both deny that Mr. Doe has abused alcohol or used street drugs. His consumption of Oxycodone has increased in the last few months, and he now uses it on a daily basis.

Psychological Disorders

Mr. Doe denied any history of psychiatric or psychological treatment. He also denies depressed mood, but does admit to frequent irritability and persistent loss of energy, as well as frequent waking during the night and early morning awakening 3–4 days/week. These symptoms have been present to some extent since December 1984, but have increased in the past year. He denies other symptoms of depression, including suicidal ideation. He also denies symptoms consistent with an anxiety disorder or major psychopathology.

Behaviors and Mental Status

Mr. Doe was alert, oriented, and cooperative during the interview and responded appropriately to questions. He was a neatly dressed man, appearing slightly older than his stated age. He walked slowly with a slight limp, favoring his right leg. Despite his report of being unable to sit for more than 15 min at a time, Mr. Doe sat through a 1-hr interview with few pain behaviors noted. He did shift in his chair on several occasions, particularly when discussing the effect of his irritability on the marital relationship. A brief mental status examination revealed no evidence of gross cognitive deficits.

Psychosocial History

Mr. Doe has an 11th-grade education, and received a GED in the army. He grew up in Idaho, and moved to Longview, Washington after leaving the army. His mother is alive and well, but his father died 2 years ago, at the age of 61, of cardiac problems. Mr. Doe's father was described as alcoholic and occasionally abusive toward Mr. Doe's mother when he was a child. His father worked steadily as a millwright until his death, and his mother was a homemaker. His mother continues to live in Idaho. Mr. Doe is the oldest of four children, having two brothers and one sister. He describes himself as not being very close to his family, and sees his mother approximately once a year. He denies any family history of pain problems or psychological disorder other than his father's alcohol abuse.

Stresses

Mr. and Mrs. Doe deny recent significant stresses other than the injury of their oldest son in a car accident 6 months ago. Although this son is now back at school and appears to be doing well, the patient and his wife both state that they were very frightened by this incident. Mr. Doe noted that at times of stress (e.g., during family arguments) his pain appears to be somewhat worse, and that when he can relax or lie down the pain is decreased. He notes that dealing with pain is stressful in itself, and feels that pain causes him to become irritable and snap at his family.

MMPI Welch Code 1″3′207-6895/4 K-L/F

This is a valid MMPI profile, but suggests that in responding to test items, the patient tended to deny problems of a psychological nature. Patients with similar profiles generally are preoccupied with concerns about physical symptoms and health, while tending to minimize emotional distress. Typically, they lack psychological insight. Their focus on health problems and reporting of somatic symptoms, including pain, may escalate at times of increased stress, yet they often fail to perceive this relationship.

It is likely that social and environmental contingencies play an important role in maintaining pain behaviors. For example, pain behaviors may be reinforced by increased attention and care from others and/or by relief from aversive demands. Patients with such profiles often have difficulty directly communicating their needs and wants, and pain behaviors may allow such patients to obtain nurturance and support from others without making direct requests. The profile does not suggest the presence of severe psychopathology. Because such patients may have considerable difficulty acknowledging psychological problems, they typically are not good candidates for traditional insight-oriented psychotherapy.

Summary of Psychological Evaluation

A number of psychological and behavioral factors appear to be contributing to the maintenance of Mr. Doe's suffering and disability. First Mr. Doe appears to have significant concerns about his medical status and fears that activity that produces pain may also cause physical injury. He thus avoids many physical activities for fear of worsening his physical condition. Mr. Doe appears to be significantly deactivated, and disuse and muscle weakness may be contributing to ongoing complaints of pain and fatigue. Second, the evaluation suggests that there may be environmental reinforcement for Mr. Doe's pain behaviors in the form of increased attention and physical contact from his wife at times of pain, as well as a reduction in demands for participation in household chores and responsibilities. Pain behaviors also appear to provide him with some "time out" from dealing with the children when he is stressed and irritable. Third, Mr. Doe appears to be seriously concerned about his ability to function competitively again in the job market. He has few marketable skills other than working as a sawmill operator, and sees himself as having few viable options for returning to work. Fourth, although Mr. Doe does not meet diagnostic criteria for major depression at this time, he does report some symptoms consistent with depression, including irritability, sleep disturbance, and decreased energy. These symptoms may to some extent be due to his medication regimen and pain problem.

Recommendations

Based on the above evaluation, Mr. Doe may likely benefit from a structured pain management program. It is recommended that such a program include: (a) a clear exposition of his medical status, including review of his medical test results, to defuse his illness conviction and fears that increasing activity will damage his back; (b) reactivation through a graded physical reconditioning program, giving Mr. Doe the opportunity to demonstrate to himself in physical and occupational therapy that it is safe for him to be more active; (c) sessions with the family to help them learn to decrease reinforcement of pain behaviors and disability and increase reinforcement of activity; (d) instruction in strategies for relaxation and stress management to help deal with problems of sleep disturbance, managing irritability, and interpersonal stress; and (e) gradual, systematic withdrawal from opioid medication. The program should also include vocational rehabilitation to (a) explore feasible options and goals for return to work; (b) formulate specific vocational rehabilitation plans, including assessment of potential to return to his old employment versus transferring to a new job; and (c) make recommendations concerning whether Mr. Doe would be an appropriate candidate for a work-hardening program.

CONCLUSION

In this chapter, the conceptual basis and procedure for the comprehensive psychological evaluation of the chronic pain patient have been presented. For purposes of exposition and demonstration, each potential area of inquiry in the evaluation has been discussed in detail. In the evaluation of individual patients, each of these areas will not always need to be covered in the same depth. A thorough behavioral analysis and a screening for psychological dysfunction form the core of any chronic pain patient psychological evaluation; however, the clinician will determine which areas require more or less detailed coverage according to the patient's particular situation.

References

1. Bonica JJ: Pain research and therapy. Past and current status and future needs. In Ng L, Bonica JJ (eds): *Pain, Discomfort, and Humanitarian Care*. New York, Elsevier, 1980, pp 1–46.
2. Commission on Accreditation of Rehabilitation Facilities: *Standards Manual for Organizations Serving People with Disabilities*. Tucson, Commission on Accreditation of Rehabilitation Facilities, 1986.
3. Melzack R, Wall PD: Pain mechanisms: a new theory. *Science* 50:971–979, 1965.
4. Melzack R, Wall PD: *The Challenge of Pain*. New York, Basic Books, 1983.
5. Fordyce WE: *Behavioral Methods for Chronic Pain and Illness*. St Louis, CV Mosby, 1976.
6. Fordyce WE, Steger JC: Chronic pain. In Pomerleau OF, Brady JP (eds): *Behavioral Medicine: Theory and Practice*. Baltimore, Williams & Wilkins, 1979.
7. Fordyce WE, Shelton JL, Dundore, DE: The modification of avoidance learning pain behaviors. *J Behav Med* 5:405–414, 1982.
8. Block A, Kremer E, Gaylor M: Behavioral treatment of chronic pain: the spouse as a discriminative cue for pain behavior. *Pain* 9:243–252, 1980.

9. Turk DC, Meichenbaum D, Genest M: *Pain and Behavioral Medicine: A Cognitive-Behavioral Perspective.* New York, Guilford Press, 1983.
10. Turk DC, Rudy TE: Assessment of cognitive factors in chronic pain: a worthwhile enterprise? *J Consult Clin Psychol* 54:760–768, 1986.
11. Keefe FJ, Gil KM: Behavioral concepts in the analysis of chronic pain syndromes. *J Consult Clin Psychol* 54:776–783, 1986.
12. Follick MJ, Ahern DK, Laser-Wolston N: Evaluation of a daily activity diary for chronic pain patients. *Pain* 19:373–382, 1984.
13. Keefe FJ, Wilkins RH, Cook WA: Direct observation of pain behavior in low back pain patients during physical examination. *Pain* 20:59–68, 1984.
14. Beck AT, Rush AJ, Shaw BF, et al: *Cognitive Therapy of Depression.* New York, Guilford, 1979.
15. Ramano JM, Turner JA: Chronic pain and depression: does the evidence support a relationship? *Psychol Bull* 97:18–34, 1985.
16. Violon A, Giurgea D: Familial models for chronic pain. *Pain* 18:199–203, 1984.
17. Follick MJ, Zitter RE, Ahern DK: Failures in the operant treatment of chronic pain. In Foa EB, Emmelkamp PMP (eds): *Failures in Behavior Therapy.* New York, John Wiley & Sons, 1983, pp 312–334.
18. Guck TP, Meilman PW, Skultety FM, et al: Prediction of long-term outcome of multidisciplinary pain treatment. *Arch Phys Med Rehab* 67:293–296, 1986.
19. Dworkin RH, Handlin DS, Richlin DM, et al: Unraveling the effects of compensation, litigation, and employment on treatment response in chronic pain. *Pain* 23:49–59, 1985.
20. Turner JA, Romano JM: Review of prevalence of coexisting chronic pain and depression. In Benedetti C, Moricca G, Chapman CR (eds): *Advances in Pain Research and Therapy.* New York, Raven Press, 1984, vol 7, pp 123–130.
21. American Psychiatric Association: *Diagnostic and Statistical Manual of Mental Disorders*, ed 3. Washington, DC, American Psychiatric Association, 1980.
22. Katon W, Egan K, Miller D: Chronic pain: lifetime psychiatric diagnosis and family history. *Am J Psychiatry* 142:1156–1160, 1985.
23. Folstein MF, Folstein SE, McHugh PR: "Mini-Mental State": a practical method for grading the cognitive state of patients for the clinician. *J. Psychiatr Res* 12:189–198, 1975.
24. Lezak M: *Neuropsychological Assessment*, ed 2. New York, Oxford University Press, 1980.
25. Ready LB, Sarkis E, Turner JA: Self-reported versus actual use of medications in chronic pain patients. *Pain* 12:285–294, 1982.
26. Brodner RA, Taub A: Chronic pain exacerbated by longterm narcotic use in patients with nonmalignant disease: clinical syndrome and treatment. *Mt Sinai J Med* 45:233–237, 1978.
27. Swanson DW, Maruta T, Swenson, WM: Results of behavior modification in the treatment of chronic pain. *Psychosom Med* 41:55–61, 1979.
28. Taylor CB, Zlutnick SI, Corley MJ, et al: The effects of detoxification, relaxation, and brief supportive therapy on chronic pain. *Pain* 8:319–329, 1980.
29. Holroyd KA, Lazarus RS: Stress, coping and somatic adaptation. In Goldberger L, Breznitz S (eds): *Handbook of Stress: Theoretical and Clinical Aspects.* New York, Free Press, 1982, pp 21–31.
30. Hathaway SR, McKinley JC: *The Minnesota Multiphasic Personality Inventory Manual.* New York, Psychological Corporation, 1967.
31. Donham GW, Mikhail SF, Meyers R: Value of consensual ratings in differentiating organic and functional low back pain. *J Clin Psychol* 40:432–439, 1984.
32. Fordyce WE, Brena SF, Holcomb RJ, et al: Relationship of patient semantic pain descriptions to physician diagnostic judgements, activity level measures and MMPI. *Pain* 5:293–303, 1978.
33. Hanvik LJ: MMPI profiles in patients with low back pain. *J Consult Psychol* 15:350–353, 1951.
34. McCreary C, Turner J, Dawson E: Differences between functional versus organic low back pain patients. *Pain* 4:73–78, 1977.
35. McCreary C, Turner J, Dawson E: The MMPI as a predictor of response to conservative treatment for low back pain. *J Clin Psychol* 35:278–284, 1979.
36. Moore JE, Armentrout DP, Parker JC, et al: Empirically derived pain-patient MMPI subgroups: prediction of treatment outcome. *J Behav Med* 9:51–63, 1986.
37. Strassberg DS, Reimherr F, Ward M, et al: The MMPI and chronic pain. *J Consult Clin Psychol* 49:220–226, 1981.
38. Blumetti AE, Modesti LM: Psychological predictors of success or failure of surgical intervention for intractable back pain. In Bonica JJ (ed): *Advances in Pain Research and Therapy.* New York, Raven Press, 1976, vol 1, pp 323–325.
39. Dzioba RB, Doxey NC: A prospective investigation into the orthopaedic and psychologic predictors of outcome of first lumbar surgery following industrial injury. *Spine* 9:614–623, 1984.
40. Long CJ: The relationship between surgical outcome and MMPI profiles in chronic pain patients. *J Clin Psychol* 37:74 4–749, 1981.
41. Pheasant HC, Gilbert D, Goldfarb J, et al: The MMPI as a predictor of outcome in low-back surgery. *Spine* 4:78–84, 1979.
42. Wiltse LL, Rocchio PD: Preoperative psychological tests as predictors of success of chemonucleolysis in the treatment of low-back syndrome. *J Bone Joint Surg* 57:478–483, 1975.
43. Herron LD, Turner J: Patient selection for lumbar laminectomy and discectomy with a revised objective rating system. *Clin Orthop Rel Res* 199:145–152, 1985.
44. Turner JA, Herron L, Weiner P: Utility of the MMPI Pain Assessment Index in predicting outcome after lumbar surgery. *J Clin Psychol* 42:764–769, 1986.
45. Smith WL, Duerksen DL: Personality and the relief of chronic pain: predicting surgical outcome. *Clin Neuropsychol* 1:35–38, 1979.
46. Dhanens TP, Jarret SR: MMPI Pain Assessment Index: concurrent and predictive validity. *Int J Clin Neuropsychol* 6:46–48, 1984.
47. Turner JA, Romano JM: Self-report screening measures for depression in chronic pain patients. *J Clin Psychol* 40:909–913, 1984.
48. Watson D: Neurotic tendencies among chronic pain patients: an MMPI item analysis. *Pain* 14:365–385, 1982.
49. Prokop CK: Hysteria scale elevations in low back pain patients: a risk factor for misdiagnosis? *J Consult Clin Psychol* 54:558–562, 1986.
50. Moore JE, McFall, ME, Kivlahan DR, et al: Risk of misinterpretation of MMPI Schizophrenia scale elevations in chronic pain patients. *Pain* (in press).

therapeutic modalities
section 2

chapter 7
Analgesic and Anti-inflammatory Medications

Lawrence M. Halpern, Ph.D.

This chapter discusses systemic analgesics used to provide pharmacologic solutions to problems of patients who experience pain. The mainstays for drug management in pain control are still the opiates and nonsteroidal anti-inflammatory agents, which comprise the principal groups of systemic analgesics. Administration of these compounds is technically undemanding, relatively inexpensive, uniformly applicable, and widely used in the management of many types of pain. It is precisely these attributes that contribute to uncritical application in day-to-day management of pain of all types, allowing for overmedication (1) with consequent problems, or undermedication with attendant needless suffering (2). This chapter is written with the hope that it will improve the quality of care, especially in relief of suffering, that can be offered to patients in pain.

GUIDELINES FOR USE OF SYSTEMIC ANALGESICS FOR RATIONAL PAIN RELIEF

Specific guidelines that can help provide state-of-the-art pain relief can be outlined succinctly:

1. Choose the drug type to match the pain type: centrally acting drugs for severe pain; peripherally acting drugs for mild to moderate pain; both types if there is an inflammatory component to severe pain.
2. Choose the drug duration to match the pain duration being treated.
3. Choose the route of administration with patient safety and comfort in mind; be sure to provide rapid onset of analgesic activity.
4. Know the detailed pharmacology of the drug to be prescribed; it is generally better to use a drug you know well than to use a newer drug about which little is known.
5. If the drug chosen fails to provide relief do not immediately change drugs. Try increased doses but do not proceed to the point of toxicity.
6. Administer analgesics on a fixed time interval basis to take advantage of pharmacokinetic factors leading to improved analgesia.
7. Administer analgesics on a fixed time interval basis to avoid or minimize the development of chronic phase pain.
8. Treat side effects appropriately or provide a drug that has fewer side effects and is more acceptable to the patient.
9. With long-term pain therapy, if tolerance is observed as a shortening of the duration of analgesia, increase medication to provide adequate analgesia as time progresses.
10. Medication levels must be changed slowly to avoid precipitating uncomfortable withdrawal or increased respiratory depression and other overdose complications. Avoid combining agonists with antagonists.
11. THERE IS NO PLACE FOR PLACEBO MEDICATION IN THE MANAGEMENT OF PAIN.
12. Most physicians undermedicate patients after surgery because of irrational fears of "addiction," and overmedicate their chronic pain patients because they

Chapter 7/Analgesic and Anti-inflammatory Medications 55

do not realize that in chronic pain situations it may be the medicine itself that is responsible for the increased pain. In many cases the development of chronic pain comes from inappropriate and ineffective undertreatment of acute pain.

13. Routine detoxification of chronic pain patients is reasonable for reevaluation of the role of analgesic drugs in the etiology of the patients' chronic pain. There is evidence that patients who fail the detoxification approach can be managed with controlled, nonescalating doses of narcotic analgesics.
14. Patients should never have to beg for relief of pain.

PERIPHERALLY ACTING ANALGESICS

Peripherally acting analgesics are a heterogeneous group of substances that possess the ability to inhibit biosynthetic enzymes in pathways that, when active, result in the formation of prostaglandins and related autocoids (3) (Table 7.1). Prostaglandins are involved in amplification of nociceptive pain, and as messengers in inflammation (4). Inhibitors of synthesizing enzymes reduce pain by direct action, desensitizing nociceptors (5), and indirectly by reducing inflammatory pain. These drugs also possess an antipyretic action also based on their ability to inhibit prostaglandin biosynthesis (6). It has been suggested, for example, that these agents may be useful in management of bone pain due to metastatic carcinoma because they help to reduce osteoclastic and inflammatory prostaglandin-induced responses of bone to the invading tumor.

Aspirin is the prototype agent in this class. It is useful to characterize the potency, spectrum, and frequency of occurrence of side effects and cost of each new nonsteroidal anti-inflammatory drug and compare these to aspirin (7). Because of cost considerations and the observation that there is no convincing evidence that any of these compounds is more effective or less toxic than aspirin, rational use of these agents must include a reasonable assurance that patients can, in fact, no longer tolerate aspirin. Physicians must evaluate the claims made for fledgling drugs as they are marketed and be able to compare these agents pharmacologically and clinically to

Table 7.1
Peripherally Acting Analgesics (Nonsteroidal Anti-inflammatory Agents) Used in the Management of Mild to Moderate Pain

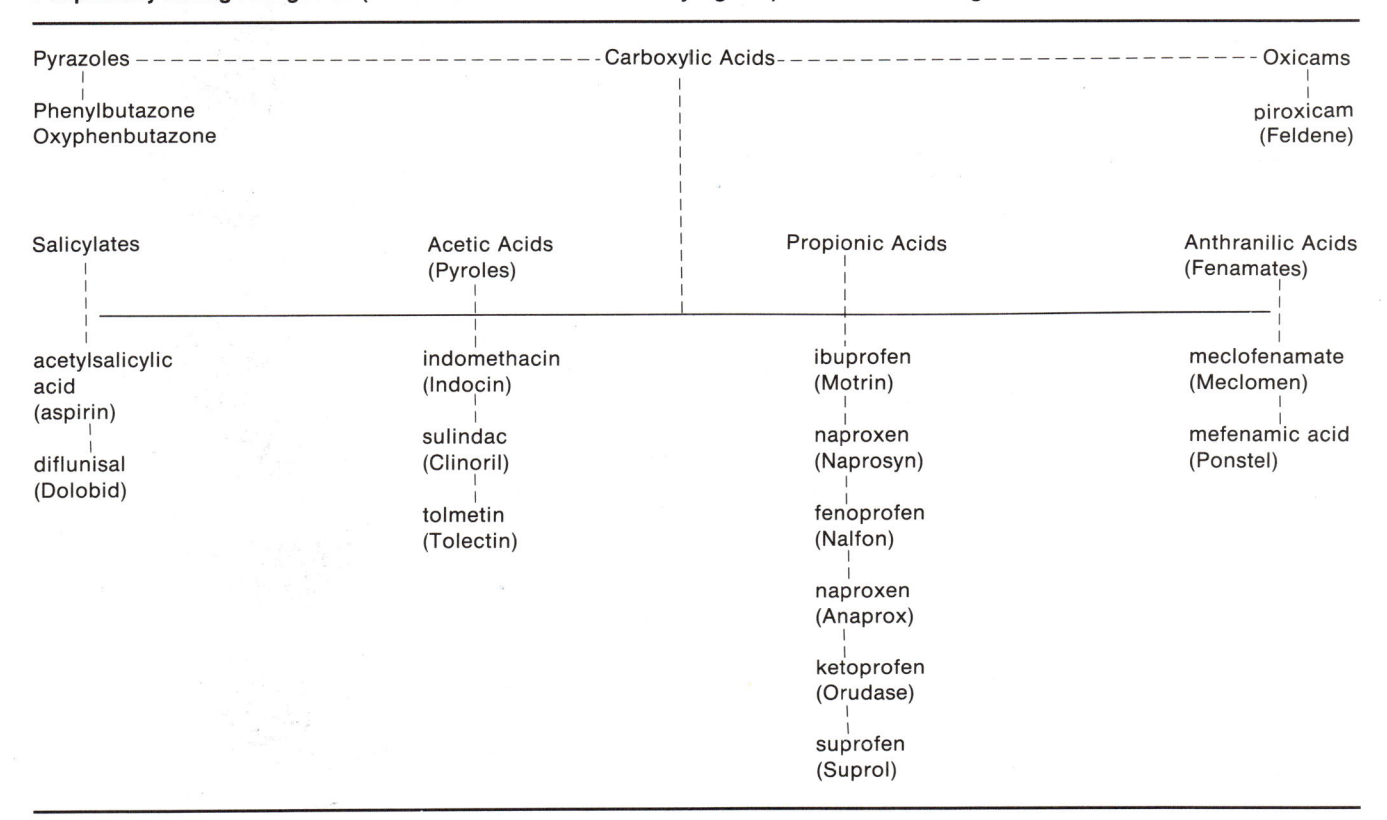

Pyrazoles	Carboxylic Acids			Oxicams
Phenylbutazone Oxyphenbutazone				piroxicam (Feldene)
Salicylates	Acetic Acids (Pyroles)	Propionic Acids		Anthranilic Acids (Fenamates)
acetylsalicylic acid (aspirin)	indomethacin (Indocin)	ibuprofen (Motrin)		meclofenamate (Meclomen)
diflunisal (Dolobid)	sulindac (Clinoril)	naproxen (Naprosyn)		mefenamic acid (Ponstel)
	tolmetin (Tolectin)	fenoprofen (Nalfon)		
		naproxen (Anaprox)		
		ketoprofen (Orudase)		
		suprofen (Suprol)		

aspirin in order to be able to justify their considerable expense. As with aspirin, other nonsteroidal agents are most commonly administered orally for the treatment of mild to moderate pain. In many clinical situations it is important to continue aspirin-like agents as required and as long as possible into the period when narcotics are used. The relief of pain provided by aspirin has been compared to 60 mg of codeine and in some cases, 8 mg of morphine. Thus, by exerting effects via two different mechanisms, peripheral and central, analgesia can be maintained at a lower dose of the opioid and with less exposure to side effects. There is some evidence that antagonism of central prostaglandins increases the analgesic action of the narcotic analgesics.

Tolerance and physical dependence do not develop to nonsteroidal agents, but there is a ceiling past which increasing doses increase side effects and toxicity, which outweighs the benefits of their use. As is well understood in the management of the arthritides, the choice of drug must be individualized for each patient. This may be done on the basis of efficacy, side effects and toxicity, and patient acceptability. Each patient must receive an adequate trial of aspirin before it is abandoned in favor of a newer drug that may not be of any more benefit than the first but may be many times more expensive. An adequate trial consists of administration of aspirin at fixed time intervals, increasing the dosage up to maximum levels tolerated and acceptable to the patient. Should the drug prove to be toxic or not produce adequate analgesia, the patient may be switched to a drug of another chemical class but one that is still an anti-inflammatory agent.

Use of aspirin concomitantly with other nonsteroidals lowers available concentrations of the second drug by displacing it from plasma protein. If pain control after an adequate trial of nonnarcotic analgesics is inadequate or is obtained at a level where toxicity adds to patients' discomfort, these agents can be abandoned and the patient switched to oral, low-ceiling narcotic analgesics. Despite biases to the contrary, narcotic analgesics are sometimes more easily tolerated than nonsteroidal anti-inflammatory agents despite the fact that overall the toxicity of the nonsteroidals is generally lower than that of more potent analgesics.

ACETYLSALICYLIC ACID (ASPIRIN)

Salicylic acid is a simple organic acid with a pK_a of 3. Aspirin (acetylsalicylic acid) has a pK_a of 3.5. It is about 50% more potent than sodium salicylate, although sodium salicylate causes less gastric irritation.

The salicylates are rapidly absorbed from the stomach and upper small intestine, providing a peak plasma level within 1–2 hr of their oral administration. Stomach acid keeps a large fraction of the salicylate in highly absorbable, nonionized form, promoting absorption. When high concentrations of drug get inside the gastric mucosal cell, the drug may damage the mucosal barrier. If gastric pH is raised to 3.5 or higher by means of concomitant administration of a suitable buffer, gastric irritation is minimized.

Aspirin is absorbed and is hydrolyzed to acetic acid and salicylate by esterases in tissue and blood. Salicylate is bound to albumin, but, as serum concentration of salicylate increases, a greater fraction remains unbound and is available to tissues. Ingested salicylate and that generated by hydrolysis of aspirin is converted to water-soluble conjugates that are rapidly excreted by the kidney. Some salicylate may be excreted unchanged, but most is excreted as salicyluric, salicylic phenolic, and acyl glucuronides. When the renal excretion pathway becomes saturated a small increase in aspirin dose results in large plasma levels. Alkalinization of the urine results in a large increase in the rate of excretion of the free salicylate. When aspirin is used in low doses (600 mg) elimination is by first-order kinetics and the serum half-life is 3–5 hr. With higher dosage, zero-order kinetics prevail; at anti-inflammatory doses <4 g/day the half-life increases to 15 hr or more. This effect is related to saturation of hepatic mechanisms that effect the conversion of salicylate to salicylphenyl glucuronide and salicyluric acid.

Major Effects and Uses of Aspirin

Anti-inflammatory Effects The effectiveness of aspirin is primarily due to its ability to inhibit prostaglandin biosynthesis by irreversibly blocking cyclo-oxygenases, which catalyze the formation of endoperoxides from arachidonic acid. In high doses, the drug decreases the formation of prostaglandins and thromboxane A2. Aspirin also interferes with the chemical mediators of the kallicrein system, inhibits granulocyte adherence to damaged vasculature, stabilizes lysosomes, and inhibits the migration of polymorphonuclear leukocytes and macrophages into an inflammation site.

Analgesic Effect Aspirin is most effective in treatment of pain of mild or moderate intensity that arises as a result of prostaglandin mechanisms. It alleviates pain of varying origins (i.e., musculoskeletal, vascular, dental, postpartum, arthritis, and bursitis). In addition to its well-known peripheral actions, aspirin may decrease pain stimuli or pain transmission at a subcortical site in the brain (8). Aspirin is not effective against visceral pain such as myocardial infarction, renal or ureteral colic, pericarditis, or the pain of an acute abdomen.

Antipyretic Effect Aspirin reduces body temperature elevated by pyrogens but has little or no effect on normal body temperature. The fall in body temperature is related to increased heat dissipation through dilated superficial blood vessels, and may be accompanied by profuse sweating.

Fever associated with infection is thought to result from formation of prostaglandins in the central nervous system in response to bacterial pyrogens. Aspirin, by blocking prostaglandin formation, prevents the stimulus to the hypothalamus and causes a facilitation of heat loss back to normal temperature by vasodilation.

Platelet Effects Single doses of aspirin slightly prolong bleeding time. If aspirin is administered for a week, this effect doubles. Aspirin inhibits platelet aggregation secondary to inhibition of thromboxane A2 biosynthesis. Since thromboxane inhibits platelet aggregation, aggregation is inhibited for 8 days or the length of time it takes to manufacture new platelets. This effect of aspirin has a longer duration than other compounds that inhibit platelet aggregation, and there is no relation between platelet effects and gastrointestinal bleeding or real increases in surgical bleeding. There does not seem to be greater surgical risk in patients on aspirin at time of surgery. However, in special circumstances (e.g., plastic surgery or urologic surgery), increased discoloration or discomfort may be observed and attributed to inhibition of thromboxane A2 biosynthesis.

Therapeutic Notes

Analgesia and Anti-inflammatory Actions Aspirin is one of the most frequently used compounds for treating mild to moderate pain of varied origin. There are over 200 over-the-counter products available containing aspirin in combination with other mild analgesics that may be purchased without a prescription. These more expensive combinations have never been shown to be more effective or less effective or toxic than aspirin alone. Poisoning by such combinations is difficult to treat. Phenacetin, for example, which was contained in many of these over-the-counter combinations, has been linked with a toxic interstitial nephritis causing serious renal impairment. The anti-inflammatory properties of aspirin in high doses are well used in the treatment of rheumatoid arthritis, rheumatic fever, and other inflammatory joint conditions. Many patients can be managed with aspirin as their sole medication because it is inexpensive and contributes to patient autonomy and compliance.

Aspirin is the best available drug for the reduction of fever when this is desirable; however, the data on Reye's syndrome, severe hepatic injury and encephalopathy, although not conclusively linking aspirin or other anti-inflammatory agents to the development of this problem (9), give cause to reconsider the use of nonsteroidal antipyretic agents in fever due to virus infections in pediatric patients.

Aspirin reduces the frequency of transient ischemic attacks in men and is used prophylactically for this purpose. It has not proved to be efficacious in preventing myocardial infarction by reducing the incidence of coronary thrombosis but may be helpful in delaying recurrence or severity of thrombosis after the initial attack.

There are preliminary findings indicating that aspirin may prevent cataract formation.

Dosage The optimal dose of aspirin is somewhat less than the 600-mg oral dose commonly used. Larger doses may prolong but not increase aspirin's effects, and after oral doses of 1000 mg toxicity increases dramatically. A dose of 600 mg orally may be repeated every 3 hr; 4000 mg/day can be tolerated by most adults and higher doses can be used if well tolerated by patients.

Blood levels of 15–30 μg/dl are associated with anti-inflammatory effects, and the drug can be titrated to these levels if an anti-inflammatory action is required.

Adverse Effects

Gastrointestinal Side Effects The main adverse effect accompanying the usual dosage of aspirin relates to gastric intolerance. Ingesting aspirin with buffering or with food or water tends to minimize these effects. However, gastroscopy reveals that chronic gastritis is a way of life for arthritics on aspirin or other nonsteroidals. The gastric irritation may be due to direct irritation of the gastric mucosa, to the inhibition of prostaglandins required for healing of gastric mucosa exposed to hydrochloric acid, or to mucosal absorption of un-ionized salicylate. Upper gastrointestinal bleeding is usually the result of erosive gastritis and results in a small increase (1–4 ml) in fecal blood loss as a result of aspirin consumption.

Central Nervous System Salicylism as a result of the central nervous system stimulating effects of aspirin may be manifested after high doses of the compound, and includes vomiting, tinnitus, diminished hearing capacity, and vertigo. However, these symptoms reverse if the dosage is lowered. Salicylates stimulate medullary respiratory rhythm and drive mechanisms, and hyperpnea may result in respiratory alkalosis. Later in salicylate toxicity, acidosis occurs as a result of exhaustion of bicarbonate buffers by renal excretion, accumulation of salicylate derivatives and metabolic end products, and depression of central respiratory drive mechanisms.

Other Effects Low doses of aspirin decrease urate excretion, whereas high doses of aspirin increase uric acid excretion, thereby decreasing serum uric acid levels.

Salicylates may cause reversible decreases in glomerular filtration rates in normal patients or in patients with underlying renal disease. Asymptomatic hepatitis has been reported, and with increasing incidence, in patients with lupus erythematosus and juvenile and adult arthritis. Aspirin in large doses directly affects smooth muscle, and causes peripheral dilation and myocardial depression.

Hypersensitivity to aspirin may occur in patients with nasal polyps or asthma. These leukotriene-mediated reactions have been associated with bronchoconstriction and shock.

Drug interactions include: acetazolamide; ammonium chloride, which enhances toxicity; and alcohol, which increases gastrointestinal bleeding. Tolbutamide, chlorpropamide, nonsteroidal anti-inflammatory agents, methotrexate, phenytoin, and probenecid are all displaced from plasma protein-binding sites by aspirin, and thus have reduced effectiveness. Aspirin antagonizes the effect of heparin, inhibits the uricosuric effects of sulfinpyrazone and probenecid, competes with penicillin for tubular excretion, and reduces the pharmacologic effect of spironolactone.

Diflunisal is a difluorophenyl derivative of aspirin and has a plasma half-life of 8–12 hr. At steady state it has analgesic and anti-inflammatory actions but is not antipyretic. The drug has not been approved for use in rheumatoid arthritis patients.

PYRAZOLES

Phenylbutazone and oxyphenbutazone, derivatives of phenacetin, are potent inhibitors of prostaglandin biosynthesis. For acute musculoskeletal inflammatory conditions (e.g., acute gout, tendonitis, traumatic myopathy), doses to 600 mg/day are tolerated in short courses of up to a week. Two hundred milligrams per day is almost specific for ankylosing spondylitis, juvenile rheumatoid arthritis, and some forms of Reiter's syndrome. Side effects include gastrointestinal and renal toxicity and bone marrow depression, including agranulocytosis. Because of their ability to cause retention of salt and gastrointestinal mucosal irritation, these compounds are contraindicated in peptic ulcer disease, congestive heart failure, and hypertension, as well as in patients with reduction in granulocytes.

PYROLES

Indomethacin (Indocin), tolmetin (Tolectin), and sulindac (Clinoril) comprise this group, and are potent prostaglandin synthetase inhibitors. *Indomethacin* was introduced in 1963 as a potent inhibitor of prostaglandin synthetases. It has a serum half-life of 2 hr. This agent has proven to be highly toxic, but under certain circumstances it is more effective than any of the other nonsteroidal anti-inflammatory agents. *Sulindac* is closely related to indomethacin. Its duration of action is 16 hr, and 400 mg/day is the anti-inflammatory equivalent of 4000 mg/day of aspirin. Stevens-Johnson syndrome, thrombocytopenia, agranulocytosis, and nephrotic syndrome have been reported after use of this agent. *Tolmetin* is similar in effectiveness to aspirin in the arthritides. The drug has a half-life of 60 min, which means that it must be given repeatedly. This is an advantage in some patients in whom toxicity, if observed, can be reversed rapidly by omitting doses or discontinuing the drug altogether.

PROPIONIC ACID DERIVATIVES

Ibuprofen (Motrin), fenoprofen (Nalfon), naproxen (Naprosyn), ketoprofen (Orudase), and suprofen (Suprol) comprise the members of this group, and all are potent prostaglandin synthetase inhibitors. A dose of 2400 mg/day of *ibuprofen* is the equivalent of 4000 mg/day of aspirin as an anti-inflammatory. At lower dosage, the ibuprofen is analgesic but is an inferior anti-inflammatory. Its use results in gastric irritation, but this is reported to be somewhat less than that occurring after aspirin ingestion. Ibuprofen has a half-life of 2 hr. *Naproxen* has a 13-hr half-life and its absorption is impeded by gastric antacids. Naproxen prolongs prothrombin time and competes with aspirin for plasma protein-binding sites. A dose of 750 mg/day is about the equivalent of 4000 mg/day of aspirin. *Fenoprofen* has a 2-hr half-life, and 2400–3200 mg/day compare with 4000 mg/day of aspirin in arthritis. Side effects of fenoprofen and naproxen are similar to those of ibuprofen (e.g., nephrotoxicity, tinnitus, cardiovascular effects, central nervous system effects, peripheral edema, rash and pruritis, and nausea, dyspepsia, and jaundice).

Suprofen is a propionic acid derivative that has structural similarities to the agents discussed above. It is a peripherally acting analgesic with no central opioid-like activity (10). In addition to inhibiting the action of cyclo-oxygenases, suprofen may directly antagonize the actions of prostaglandins on peripheral pain receptors, thus reducing their sensitivity to bradykinin (11). Suprofen has been shown to be effective in dental procedures; general surgical situations and orthopedic surgery; sprains, strains, and fractures; osteoarthritis; dysmenorrhea; and episiotomy pain. The recent finding of unexpected, reversible flank pain, possibly linked to a prominent uricosuric effect, has slowed clinical utilization of this theoretically interesting compound until further information concerning the etiology of this unusual side effect is discovered.

Ketoprofen was recently released for rheumatoid arthritis and osteoarthritis use in the United States, having been used in France and the United Kingdom since 1973. Double-blind trials have established therapeutic equivalence with aspirin, indomethacin, and ibuprofen in rheumatoid arthritis and with aspirin in osteoarthritis. Ketoprofen has a short half-life, a simple metabolism, and a broad therapeutic window and does not accumulate with multiple doses, contributing to a rapid onset of action, flexible dosing, and a reasonable tolerance profile (12).

ANTHRANILIC ACIDS

Mefenamic acid (Ponstel), and meclofenamate (Meclomen) are the only members of this group of prostaglandin synthetase inhibitors currently available. The frequent occurrence of side effects, including diarrhea, rash, elevation of blood urea nitrogen, and bone marrow toxicity, makes these agents somewhat less than ideal for use for long periods. Mefenamic acid is thus heavily promoted for use in dysmenorrhea; however, other peripherally acting analgesics work as well and are less toxic.

OXICAMS

Piroxicam (Feldene) is a new chemical entity unrelated to other chemical families. It is a potent inhibitor of prostaglandin synthetases and has a half-life of 44 hr, permitting once-a-day dosage regimens. At 20 mg/day the incidence of gastrointestinal disturbances is about the same as that following aspirin administration (under 1%). Administration continuously at doses above 20 mg/day leads to a higher incidence of peptic ulcer. For short-term therapy, doses of 60 mg/day for 2 weeks appear to be safe in this regard (13–15). Side effects include gastrointestinal disturbances, dizziness, headache, rash, and tinnitus.

CENTRALLY ACTING ANALGESICS

PRELIMINARY NOTES

The term *opiate* was formerly used to designate agents derived from opium, such as morphine and codeine and the many semisynthetic derivatives of these agents. With the development of synthetic drugs that have morphine-like actions, the term *opioid* was introduced to describe all drugs, natural and synthetic, that share morphine-like effects (Table 7.2).

With discovery of multiple opiate receptors to which agents bind but do not produce morphine-like actions, the term *opioid* has been redefined (16) as a designation for all exogenous substances that bind to opiate receptors and produce agonist actions. Some compounds appear to demonstrate both agonist and antagonist actions. Thus, these compounds are logically divided into three groups: the opioid agonists, opioid antagonists, and opioids with mixed actions, which includes antagonist-agonist and partial-agonist agents.

HISTORY AND USE

The opioids are unsurpassed in relieving pain and have been used as analgesics and for other purposes for hundreds of years. Reference to the use of opiates can be found in the work of Theophrastus, who wrote during the third century B.C. (17). Opium preparations suffered from extreme variability of opium content and variable rates of absorption, with effects varying from inadequate analgesia to overdose and death. When patients became moribund, physicians, lacking potent and effective narcotic antagonists, attempted to revive patients from opium-induced unconsciousness by placing vinegar sponges under their noses or by dripping the juice of an evergreen plant, which produced an acrid, volatile oil, into their ears.

In 1803, the German chemist Surturner isolated the active ingredient in opium, to which he gave the name Morphius after the god of dreams. This compound was significantly more predictable in its absorption and its effects than the parent compound, and was more potent. The problem of accurate administration of morphine was solved in 1853, when Pravaz invented the syringe and Wood developed the hollow needle (18).

Crude opium is prepared by powdering the dried milky substance that exudes from the seed capsules of the opium poppy, *Papaver somniferum*, just before it ripens. The majority of the world's supply of opium comes from Southeast Asia, Southwest Europe, China, India, Iran, Turkey, and the USSR.

Table 7.2
Centrally Acting Analgesics Used in the Management of Moderate to Severe Pain

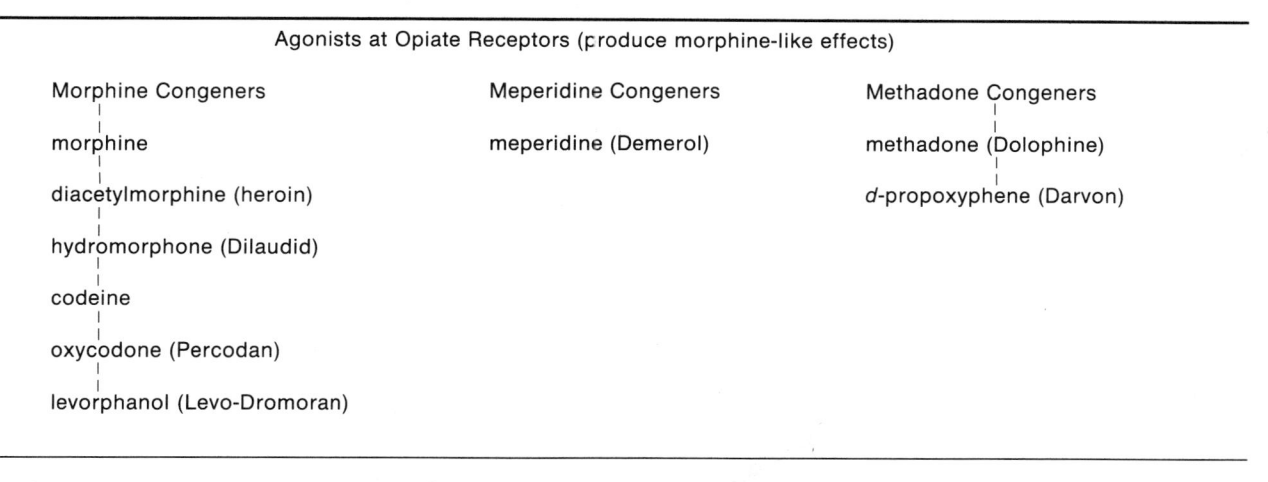

Agonists at Opiate Receptors (produce morphine-like effects)

Morphine Congeners	Meperidine Congeners	Methadone Congeners
morphine	meperidine (Demerol)	methadone (Dolophine)
diacetylmorphine (heroin)		d-propoxyphene (Darvon)
hydromorphone (Dilaudid)		
codeine		
oxycodone (Percodan)		
levorphanol (Levo-Dromoran)		

Antagonists with Agonist Action at the Opiate Receptors (antagonize morphine effects but produce analgesia)

Morphine Type	Nalorphine Type
profadol	pentazocine (Talwin)
propiram	nalbuphine (Nubain)
buprenorphine (Buprenex)	butorphanol (Stadol)

60 Therapeutic Modalities/Section 2

There are over 25 alkaloids in opium, which constitute 25% of the content of opium by weight. Although the total content of alkaloid varies in specimens taken from different regions, the percentage by weight of the most important alkaloids remains relatively constant at approximately 10% morphine, 0.5% codeine, 0.3% thebaine, 1% papaverine, 6% narcotine, and 0.2% narceine (19).

CLINICAL USES OF THE OPIOIDS

The clinical utility of the opioid agents resides in three areas in which one sees biologic activity. Primarily, these agents are analgesic and, as such, are superior to any other class of compound. Second, these agents are potent antitussives and are widely used to suppress cough reflexes. Finally, these compounds cause constipation and are useful for treating diarrhea.

STRUCTURE-ACTIVITY RELATIONSHIPS

Morphine was isolated from opium in 1803, but the structure of morphine was not identified until 1925 by Gulland and Robinson. The relationship between morphine and related compounds is shown in Figure 7.1. It is important to realize that all of these compounds are structurally related. Most therapeutic failures come from imprecise application of these compounds and a desire to find a single "magic" agent. These drugs are available as tools for use in relief of pain and suffering. No one agent is any "better" than any other. Rather, biopharmaceutic

Chemistry:

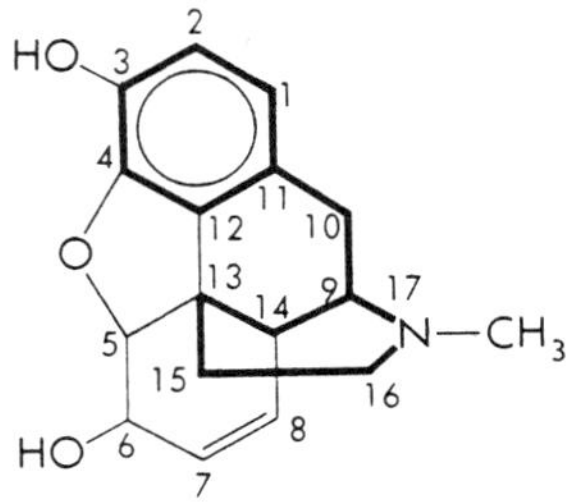

Morphine

Nonproprietary Name	Chemical Radicals at Position #: 3	6	17	Other
Morphine	—OH	—OH	—CH$_3$	—
Heroin	—OCOCH$_3$	—OCOCH$_3$	—CH$_3$	—
Hydromorphone	—OH	=O	—CH$_3$	Single bond C$_7$—C$_8$
Oxymorphone	—OH	=O	—CH$_3$	Single bond C$_7$—C$_8$, OH on C$_{14}$
Levorphanol	—OH	—H	—CH$_3$	Single bond C$_7$—C$_8$, no C$_4$—C$_5$ oxygen
Codeine	—OCH$_3$	—OH	—CH$_3$	—
Hydrocodone	—OCH$_3$	=O	—CH$_3$	Single bond C$_7$—C$_8$
Oxycodone	—OCH$_3$	=O	—CH$_3$	Single bond C$_7$—C$_8$, OH on C$_{14}$
Nalorphine	—OH	—OH	—CH$_2$CH=CH$_2$	—
Naloxone	—OH	=O	—CH$_2$CH=CH$_2$	Single bond C$_7$—C$_8$, OH on C$_{14}$
Naltrexone	—OH	=O	—CH$_2$—◁	Single bond C$_7$—C$_8$, OH on C$_{14}$
Buprenorphine	—OH	—OCH$_3$	—CH$_2$—◁	Single bond C$_7$—C$_8$, C$_6$—C$_{14}$ endetheno C$_7$-hydroxytrimethylpropyl
Butorphanol	—OH	—H	—CH$_2$—◇	OH on C$_{14}$, no C$_4$—C$_5$ oxygen
Nalbuphine	—OH	—OH	—CH$_2$—◇	Single bond C$_7$—C$_8$, OH on C$_{14}$

Figure 7.1. Structures of opioids and opioid antagonists chemically related to morphine.

differences in half-life, duration of action, degree of sedation accompanying analgesia, speed or delay in onset, and relative potency and abuse potential make for rational drug selection and use. No drug will produce satisfactory analgesia unless the appropriate dose is ordered. Failures in analgesic therapy are linked to prescription error and not to the agents used.

Codeine, a naturally occurring opium alkaloid, is methoxy (—OCH$_3$) substituted for a hydroxyl (—OH) group on the morphine ring structure. This compound alleviates moderate pain with fewer side effects than morphine because codeine possesses analgesic effects that are not as great as those of which morphine is capable, and codeine also demonstrates much less in the way of sedative-hypnotic properties. In 1874, the addition of two acetyl (—CH$_3$—COO—) groups produced the compound diacetylmorphine, or heroin. This event was accompanied by great excitement among pharmacologists because it demonstrated that simple modification of the morphine molecule could produce interesting and useful changes in pharmacologic potency.

When heroin was introduced, it was promoted as a more potent and less addicting substitute for morphine sulfate. Today, we know that the sojourn of heroin in the body is only about 20 min (20). The effects of heroin and morphine are identical because heroin is deacetylated to monoacetylmorphine and then to morphine in the brain. Heroin gains access to receptors in the central nervous system more rapidly after administration of the first dose because deacetylation increases lipid solubility, making the drug less polar and, therefore, more readily accessible to the brain. Thus, heroin in not an especially useful agent when compared to morphine or other available opioids.

Synthetic narcotics have been developed almost continuously in attempts to produce more potent analgesic activity and a seemingly futile attempt to decrease liability for physical and psychological dependence.

Four chemical classes of drugs possess pharmacologic activity in humans similar to that of morphine. These are the 4-phenypiperidines such as pethidine; the diphenylpropylamines, such as methadone; the morphinans, such as levorphanol; and the 6,7-benzomorphans, such as pentazocine. These compounds share the ability to produce analgesia, respiratory depression, gastrointestinal spasm, and morphine-like physical dependence. All of these compounds can simulate a piperidine ring structure and possess either nitrogen, methyl groups, or a variety of other bulky groups attached to the ring.

Opiate antagonists are molecules that occupy opiate receptors and have structures similar to other opiates, but do not produce pharmacologic activity of their own. These agents may also prevent or reverse the action of administered opiates because of their ability to occupy opiate receptor sites. Substitution of an allyl group (—CH$_2$—CH=CH) for the methyl group on the nitrogen atom of the morphine molecule produces the narcotic antagonists naloxone and nalorphine. Naloxone has an agonist-antagonist potency ratio so large that it is usually considered to be a pure antagonist. However, most of these agents behave as if they were mixed agonist-antagonist agents.

PHARMACODYNAMICS

Morphine is readily absorbed from most sites of administration. It is most commonly administered subcutaneously or intramuscularly. Oral administration is not uncommon, and the oral/parenteral ratio has been determined to be (60–)30 mg orally/10 mg parenterally. Absorption from the nasal mucosa or lung is known to occur.

Distribution of morphine is fairly uniform in most tissues. Despite the fact that morphine has its greatest effects on the central nervous system, only small quantities pass through the blood-brain barrier and the drug does not concentrate in the brain.

Morphine and most other opiates pass through the placental barrier. Newborn infants may suffer from respiratory depression as a result of an analgesic dose given to the mother or, conversely, may suffer from opioid withdrawal symptoms within several hours of birth if the mother's history included opiate dependence. Opiate withdrawal is not usually considered to be life-threatening in adults. However, the syndrome may have severe consequences for the newborn, especially children born of mothers with inadequate prenatal care and poor nutritional state.

Most administered drug is found in urine within 24 hr of treatment, whereas only 7–10% eventually appears in fecal material. Some morphine is excreted unchanged, but the largest portion is excreted as the glucuronide. This conjugate is filtered more rapidly than unchanged morphine because of the altered ionic state of the molecule.

PHYSIOLOGIC EFFECTS

Central Nervous System Effects

Morphine is usually considered to be the prototype opiate, and the physiologic and pharmacodynamic effects of other drugs are compared to this standard. Related agents have qualitatively similar actions that differ primarily in terms of potency and duration. A real appreciation for the side effects and pharmacokinetics of morphine will make appropriate drug comparison and selection more rational.

Morphine has predominantly central nervous system effects that are dose related. At small doses (5–10 mg) drowsiness is the principal subjective effect, with decreased awareness of external and internal stimuli and loss of anxiety and inhibition. Muscle relaxation follows relief of pain, respiration is depressed in rate, pupils are constricted, and concentration becomes impaired; this is often followed by dreamy sleep.

Street users of opioids frequently refer to the "kick," "bang," or "rush" that occurs immediately after injection of morphine or heroin intravenously. This rush has been likened to an "abdominal orgasm." Patients do not describe a rush. Naive users describe these effects as a sudden flush of warmth, localized in the pit of the stomach. Smoking, nasal inhalation, oral administration, intramuscular administration, or subcutaneous administration are not associated with a rush. The rush does not seem to be the basis for repetition of use because nonintravenous users seem to be just as dependent as intravenous users. It is generally a bad idea to generalize from what we think we know about street users of opiate to the effects of single or repeated doses of opiates to patients in pain (21).

At slightly higher doses, an abnormal state of elation, sometimes called euphoria, may develop. This euphoric effect does not always accompany the administration of morphine or a similar agent. Stable individuals who are free of pain report that the administration of morphine causes restlessness, anxiety, and dysphoria. The elation effect seems to occur in depressed or highly excited patients (22).

Nausea often accompanies the administration of even small therapeutic doses of morphine, increases with higher doses, is more pronounced in patients not in pain than patients in pain, and is in direct response to opiate stimulation of the chemoreceptor trigger zone of the area postrema of the medulla, which contributes vagal input to the gut. Medical students given morphine do not wish to repeat the experience because of the "sick feeling" (23), whereas experienced users report that the nausea and vomiting is thought of as a "good sick" that has secondary reinforcing properties because it signals the onset of euphoria. Vomiting with aspiration may cause patients' deaths at doses lower than those where significant depression of respiratory rate is observed.

At toxic doses morphine depression deepens and unconsciousness ensues. Pupils are further constricted and respiratory rate approaches or becomes zero. At these doses the areas in the medulla that normally are triggered by elevated CO_2 levels to increase the rate and depth of respiration are severely depressed and do not respond to CO_2 stimuli. Respiratory depression may be the ultimate cause of death from narcotics overdosage. In street users an allergic phenomenon has been described in which respiration is depressed by the narcotic and an allergic response of the lungs to one of the agents used to dilute or alter the street narcotic further compromises respiratory function.

Even at the highest doses morphine does not necessarily cause motor uncoordination, slurred speech, nystagmus, or severe mental obtundation, unlike anesthetics and barbiturates, for example, which cause analgesia only when patients are severely confused or unconscious.

Analgesia

Despite a voluminous literature, the mechanism by which opiates produce analgesia is only now beginning to be understood. Of fundamental importance to this problem is the difficulty of quantifying and identifying experimental and pathologic human pain.

Pain is generally considered to be a sensation arising from any tissue-damaging stimulus and is therefore essential to survival. However, a distinction needs to be made between pain as specific sensation and pain as suffering. Polymodal nociceptors can be activated by a variety of stimuli, including radiant heat, cold, electricity, pressure, stretching, tears and cuts, and chemical irritants. Opioids in clinically useful concentrations do not alter receptor or peripheral nerve function (24). The quality of afferent sensory input may vary from slight to intense, but may involve little emotional reaction (25). More severe pain may be accompanied by autonomic responses (e.g., sweating, reduction in blood pressure, nausea, and a strong emotional component). Negative emotional response to somatic afferent pain sensation is not found as definitively in other sensory systems (e.g., auditory or gustatory). The separation of the sensation and emotional components of pain is clearly seen in patients who, after a dose of morphine, maintain that the pain is still present and of the same intensity, yet not aversive. Presumably, the psychophysical response of all patients to the same stimulus is similar, but the emotional reaction process may be widely different in different subjects. Beecher (26) suggested that a patient's reaction process is influenced by the patient's concept of the sensation, by the sensation's significance based on past experience, and by the seriousness of the consequences of that pain for the patient.

The effectiveness of analgesics may be due to (a) reduced sensation, (b) reduced recognition of stimuli, and (c) altered processes of sensory discrimination, memory of past pain events, or judgment that follows recognition (12).

Gastrointestinal Effects

The gastrointestinal effects of morphine are such that opium was used to relieve diarrhea and dysentery even before it was used to produce analgesia. In humans, constipation is a common side effect of opioid use, even in the narcotics-dependent patient. Morphine and other opioids increase tonus and decrease motility of the stomach and intestines, thus slowing the passage of intestinal contents and allowing greater intestinal absorption of water with a corresponding increase in fecal viscosity (constipation). Several opioid agents (e.g., diphenoxylate and loperamide) are used expressly as antidiarrheal compounds because these agents are poorly absorbed, producing few central effects, and yet produce their effects on the intestinal mucosa.

OPIATE RECEPTORS

To explain the variety of actions that distinguish opioid agonist and antagonist agents, it has been hypothesized that at least three subgroups of opiate receptors exist. *Mu receptors* are thought to mediate supraspinal analgesia, respiratory depression, euphoria, and physical dependence; *kappa receptors* mediate spinal analgesia, meiosis, and sedation; and excitation, dysphoria, and hallucinations seem to be mediated by *sigma receptors* (27–29), which also produce respiratory and vasomotor stimulation. Sigma receptors may not be opiate receptors, but rather may be more closely associated with the mechanism of action of phencyclidine and ketamine. These agents produce a peculiar type of dissociative anesthesia with analgesia and seem to work selectively, by some means activating the sigma receptor. Unfortunately pentazocine, butorphanol, and nalbuphine also are capable of activating these receptors, with the resultant production of psychotomimetic effects.

Receptor subgroup information needs to be kept in mind during initial choice of an agent so that undesirable characteristics may be avoided. This information is also useful as an aid in evaluation of risks and benefits of new agents as they appear.

NARCOTIC AGONISTS
Morphine Congeners

Since the isolation of morphine from opium, the analgesic effectiveness of 10 mg of morphine intramuscularly has become the standard against which all other drugs are compared. It is quite useful in pain management to describe the doses of all narcotics in terms of the number of morphine equivalent doses they represent. Table 7.3 is provided to facilitate this comparison.

Morphine is still the drug of choice for moderate to severe pain. Fifty-five to 60 mg of morphine orally is required to produce the same degree of analgesia as a single dose of 10 mg of morphine intramuscularly. Thereafter the oral dose needs to be reduced to 30 mg or the drug will accumulate, leading to sedation, respiratory depression, and even death. For reasons such as rapidity of onset of action, parenteral administration is most commonly used. Despite its reduced oral efficacy, morphine has been used orally (Brompton's cocktail and other oral preparations), and oral morphine produces effective analgesia as long as the concentration in the solution is appropriate.

Heroin is the diacetylated derivative of morphine, and 3–5 mg intramuscularly produces the same analgesia as 10 mg of morphine intramuscularly. The drug is not available in the United States, but was widely used in Great Britain for pain control in terminally ill cancer patients. However, it was found that heroin is similar to morphine in analgesic and mood-altering actions. Cancer patients were unable to discern which drug was being used for pain control. The drug has somewhat better oral efficacy than morphine, its onset of action for the first dose is slightly faster than that of morphine, it is a pro-drug, and its sojourn in the body is approximately 20 min; thereafter, all of its actions are from the morphine to which it is deacetylated, and its duration of action is similar to the morphine it generates. Side effects are similar to those of morphine at equianalgesic doses, and a recent study failed to substantiate the belief that heroin offers any special advantages in the management of cancer pain.

Periodically, there seems to be movement toward legalization of heroin for use in terminally ill patients. Since the

Table 7.3
Morphine Equivalent Doses of Various Narcotics[a]

Drug	Dose (mg) s.c.	Dose (mg) p.o.	Duration (hr)	Withdrawal Symptoms	Comment[b]
Morphine	10	30	4–5		E
Heroin	3	8	3–4	Like morphine	A
Hydromorphone	1.5	7.5	4–5	Like morphine	
Oxymorphone	1.0–1.5	6.0	4–5	Like morphine	
Metopon	3.5		4–5	Like morphine	B
Codeine	120		4–6	See text	
Hydrocodone	—	5–10	4–8	Oral antitussive	C
Dihydrocodeinone	60	—	4–5	between morphine and codeine	
Oxycodone	15	30	4–5	Like morphine	
Levorphanol	2	4	4–5	Like morphine	F
Methadone	101	15–20	4–5	Protracted in dependent patients	E,F,G
Dextromoramide	5–7.5	—	4–5	Like methadone	B,E,G
Meperidine	75–100	300	1–3		D

[a] Data from Beaver and Feise (30), Halpern and Bonica (31), Jaffe and Martin (32), McCaffery (33, 34), Rogers (35, 36), and Twycross (37).
[b] A = illegal in the United States, B = not available in the United States, C = mainly used as antitussive, D = less constipating, E = may accumulate with repeated dosage, F = retains analgesic potency when given orally, and G = irritation at injection sites.

drug offers no special advantages and, indeed, has a shorter duration of action than that of morphine, its use in management of terminal pain is not advocated by this author. Consistency with our current philosophy requires consideration of longer duration of action drugs, not shorter duration ones, as more advantageous for the patient with relentless pain.

Hydromorphone is a potent analgesic congener of morphine. Its onset of action is rapid, similar to that of heroin. Its duration of action is similar to that of morphine. It is somewhat less than ideal for general use, but it does find use in patients with diminished renal or hepatic function for titrating analgesia, and it is useful in elderly patients to avoid the confusion and sedation that may be observed when longer acting drugs are used. Thus, it may be considered as an alternative to morphine that offers advantages only in special situations. It can be used at, and preparations are available for, all portals of entry.

Codeine is a low-ceiling analgesic that is useful as a first approach to patients who cannot tolerate nonnarcotic agents. Side effects of dizziness, nausea and vomiting, and constipation often limit protracted use of the drug at doses high enough to produce analgesia. Thirty milligrams of codeine orally is roughly equivalent to the analgesic effects produced by 600 mg of aspirin orally.

Oxycodone is available in combination with 325 mg of aspirin or 325 mg of acetaminophen, and is now available as a solo agent. It is a short-acting, orally effective agent. Oral administration of 30 mg oxycodone is equivalent to 10 mg or morphine intramuscularly. Because of the combination of ingredients 30 mg of the mixture only contains 5 mg of oxycodone. The full morphine-like narcotic potency of this agent is generally not appreciated, and physical dependence on this drug commonly occurs in chronic nonmalignant pain situations where drug use is not generally desirable. Care must be exercised in elevating the dose of oxycodone lest side effects from nonnarcotic drugs in the mixture lead to undue toxicity. The potency and relatively insidious development of dependence on this agent call for a special caveat that this agent in combination or alone is more like morphine than codeine.

Levorphanol is a narcotic with high potency, good oral efficacy, and a long duration of action. It is useful as an alternative to morphine or methadone because it is active by parenteral and oral routes. Four milligrams orally produces analgesia equal to that of 10 mg of morphine intramuscularly. When used at fixed time intervals the drug tends to be more sedating than morphine; however, after 5 days, the duration of action approaches that of methadone. The half-life of levorphanol is 12–16 hr, and the half-life of methadone is 17–24 hr, whereas that of morphine is only 3–4 hr.

Meperidine Congeners

Meperidine is a short-acting narcotic used for moderate to severe pain. Its poor oral efficacy is not well understood, and it is frequently used, but is usually not very effective when used by, this route of administration. Absorption of small doses via the gastrointestinal route is unpredictable; lower-than-analgesic doses are used, and it is rare that patients are afforded adequate analgesia when the drug is administered by this route. Parenterally, 100 mg intramuscularly, and 200–300 mg orally produce analgesic effects equivalent to 10 mg of morphine intramuscularly. In fact, analgesic threshold does not seem to be reached until at least 70 mg have been administered. Analgesic action of the drug peaks at 90 min and is virtually gone after 2.5–3 hr. This relatively short duration of action is not generally well appreciated, and much needless suffering occurs because this drug is given in homeopathic quantities and at time intervals that are infrequent enough so that patients are without adequate analgesia. Chronic pain states may come about because of undertreatment of acute pain. The major metabolite of meperidine is normeperidine. After accumulation of this metabolite, central nervous system excitation has been a problem, and multifocal myoclonus and major seizures have been observed. When this occurs, it is reasonable to abandon the drug and choose an equianalgesic dose of another narcotic. Treating the seizures with diazepam or clonazepam, then switching to phenobarbital, is usually recommended. Phenytoin given as parenteral loading doses followed by oral phenytoin may be considered because oral phenytoin alone may take up to 4 days for useful antiseizure activity to develop.

Meperidine is contraindicated in patients with compromised renal function.

Methadone Congeners

Propoxyphene Propoxyphene is an optical enantiomorph of methadone that in some studies cannot be distinguished from placebo. It is frequently dispensed in combination with either acetaminophen or aspirin. When combined with aspirin, it has clearly defined analgesic effects that are separate from placebo or aspirin alone, so that it may be useful in certain clinical situations. Respiratory depression, tolerance, and physical dependence develop to propoxyphene, and abstinence syndrome occurs when the drug has been suddenly discontinued. However, dependence on the drug has not been the major problem with its use. Escalated doses of propoxyphene carry escalated doses of either aspirin or acetaminophen that may be in the toxic range. Seizures, tinnitus, and gastrointestinal hemorrhage have been observed in patients taking as high as 40 propoxyphene capsules also containing aspirin each day. Acetaminophen toxicity includes direct hepatotoxicity, and patients have been observed to have elevated transaminase levels after long-term use of high doses of proproxyphene with acetaminophen.

The drug represents a first approach to the management of patients who cannot tolerate nonnarcotics or codeine and should not be escalated past the point where low doses of narcotic would produce analgesia with less risk of disturbing side effects.

Methadone Methadone is a potent, long-acting narcotic analgesic with good oral efficacy. Methadone at 15–20 mg orally is equivalent to 10 mg of morphine intramuscularly or 60 mg of morphine orally. Because of its long half-life (17–24 hr), methadone, after 4 days of regular doses at fixed time intervals, provides long plateau analgesia. Methadone is one of the drugs of choice for acute- and chronic-phase cancer pain.

Methadone is probably not best used for early cancer pain management problems. Experience has shown that when doses of shorter acting, rapid-onset analgesics have approached the point where the patient has been getting the equivalent of 60–100 mg of morphine intramuscularly, then it is appropriate to switch the patient to oral methadone. Care must be taken to switch the patient to the correct equivalent dose so as not to overdose or precipitate abstinence syndrome. Methadone, when used in small doses early in narcotic management, has a duration of action similar to that of morphine. Only when tolerance develops does the half-life of this compound increase.

Caveats to the use of methadone include the warning that because of its long half-life, methadone may tend to accumulate in elderly patients, or in patients with decreased hepatic or renal function. In these cases, excessive sedation or respiratory depression may occur. To prevent excessive sedation or toxicity, the dosage regimen must be decreased appropriately to ensure effective pain relief without excessive side effects. Patients may have doses of methadone reduced as much as 10–20% per day without serious withdrawal symptoms to compensate between excessive sedation and adequacy of pain relief. The appropriateness of the rate of withdrawal can be gauged by observing decreased sedation and increased respiratory rate.

The long half-life of methadone with plateau analgesia makes possible some valuable management strategies for cancer patients with pain. Provision of methadone at fixed time intervals produces sedation and long-duration analgesia. Doses are easily adjusted downward to compensate for the increased sedation.

Patients may be stabilized at much lower doses than were originally anticipated from observation of responses to shorter acting agents previously used. Several reasons have been proposed for this effect. First, patients do not experience periodic episodes of pain or abstinence effects and therefore do not complain as much as the dose is systematically lowered. Second, requests for medication in anticipation of pain are reduced by exposure to protracted analgesia. Patients are less debilitated and feel better as a result of lowering the narcotic dose and pay more attention to their social and physical environment.

Methadone doses may be lowered to the point where some pain may reoccur. If the pain can be localized to peripheral sources, diagnostic regional or local block with local anesthetic may reveal a peripheral nociceptive source that can be eliminated by local anesthetic block or permanent neurolytic procedures. If this is the case, following elimination of peripheral nociceptive sources, dosage of methadone may be further reduced to the end point of the reappearances of pain, then elevated slightly.

Combination of methadone and hydroxyzine provides additional analgesia without increased exposure to narcotic agents. Hydroxyzine 100 mg deep intramuscularly is the equivalent of morphine 10 mg intramuscularly (38). However, analgesia from hydroxyzine is not naloxone reversible, indicating that it produces analgesia by other than opiate receptor mechanisms. When hydroxyzine is added by either oral or parenteral route, sedation increase may again be experienced. Should this happen, further reduction of methadone to the point of reduced sedation with adequate pain control is possible. Further discussion of the antianxiety and sedative components of the action of this useful antihistamine appear below.

Methadone is an ideal agent for substitution-detoxification protocols. It has long been known that withdrawal from methadone produces fewer undesirable effects during abstinence syndrome than those uncomfortable symptoms appearing after withdrawal from morphine or other agonist agents. Thus, use of this agent has provided a stable and reliable method for detoxifying chronic nonmalignant pain patients who have long histories of nonbeneficial use of high-dose opiate agonist agents.

Tricyclic antidepressants may also be combined with methadone for even more improved pain control. Amitriptyline and doxepin (50–150 mg orally before sleep) have provided increased comfort and reduced complaints of pain even where other drugs have failed to do so. This effect occurs within 24–48 hr of onset of use of these agents and is apparently unrelated to the effect of these agents on depression. When sedation occurs following introduction of antidepressant agents in patients receiving methadone and hydroxyzine, even further reduction of the opiate agent may be accomplished.

The use of these techniques, much as the use of small doses of epidural morphine, permits much less restricted patients who may be followed and cared for at home or in less threatening and less expensive environments than the hospital.

Visiting nurse services and hospice nurses have become expert at medication management of the terminally ill patient and provide daily or more frequent feedback about the success or failure of analgesia and treatment of other symptoms.

NARCOTIC ANTAGONISTS AS ANALGESICS

Most of these drugs have only recently become available for clinical use and extensive experience with them is lacking. What information is available suggests that antagonist analgesics of the morphine type possess major advantages over antagonist analgesics of the nalorphine type.

Nalorphine derivatives induce sigma receptor stimulation, producing severe psychotomimetic reactions, and are relatively more deleterious in cardiac patients.

Agonist-Antagonist Analgesics of the Morphine Type

Buprenorphine, the first member of this class of drugs to be released for clinical use, has been used for several years in Great Britain and other countries. Although clinical experience with this agent in the United States is limited, several of its properties are unusual enough to create great excitement about its potential availability here.

Buprenorphine is a semisynthetic derivative of thebaine closely related to etorphine. It is highly lipophilic and binds strongly to mu-class opiate receptors. Theoretically, it is this unusually strong binding to opiate receptors that gives this drug several unique features.

Buprenorphine is 20–30 times as potent as morphine intramuscularly; and 0.3–0.4 mg of Buprenorphine is equivalent to 10 mg of intramuscular morphine. Onset of action, like that of morphine, is from 15 to 60 min, but the duration of action is anywhere from 4 to 14 hr after a single dose. Data indicate that the mean duration of action of this agent is 8.4 hr, and the drug has proven effective in postoperative pain, myocardial infarction pain, pain of neoplastic and orthopedic origin, and labor pain, and as an adjunct to anesthesia. Generally, the drug is as effective as morphine, meperidine, or pentazocine. However, it has side effects much like morphine. Incidence of euphoria has been reported as less than 0.3% and incidence of psychotomimetic reactions at only 0.90%. In only 5 of 9000 patients did systolic blood pressure fall to under 100 mm Hg, and no instances of respiratory depression requiring treatment were reported.

Respiratory depressant activity is slow in onset, but has been reported as being equal to that after equianalgesic doses of morphine. Peak depression of respiration occurs at about 3 hr and lasts for 7 hr after a single dose. There has been some discussion of a plateau or ceiling of respiratory depression occurring at 0.6–1.2 mg buprenorphine, but the degree of respiratory depression does seem to vary directly with the dose.

Buprenorphine has been used as an analgesic after open heart surgery with minimal effects on the cardiovascular system. The small decreases in heart rate and systolic blood pressure noted were of the same magnitude as those seen after morphine.

Unlike other narcotics, the respiratory depressant effect of buprenorphine is only partially reversible even after high doses of naloxone. Paradoxically, buprenorphine has been used as an antagonist of the respiratory depressant effects of other narcotics.

Buprenorphine may induce abstinence syndrome in dependent patients, but may block development of abstinence syndrome. Addicts state that the effects of buprenorphine are like those of morphine; however, it is not particularly reinforcing and is classified as a drug with low abuse potential. Buprenorphine can block the effect of injected morphine for up to 30 hr. Chronic pain patients who received buprenorphine by sublingual administration for weeks or months did not require elevation of the dosage, indicating failure of development of tolerance to the analgesic effects of buprenorphine. Some patients did elect to discontinue the drug because of nausea, but not because of failure of the analgesic effect. Abrupt withdrawal of buprenorphine in dependent patients resulted in a mild-to-moderate abstinence syndrome described as half as severe as after morphine withdrawal. The abstinence syndrome is delayed, peaking at 2 weeks after discontinuance of buprenorphine and lasting for over a week.

Buprenorphine is a useful narcotic with high intrinsic potency, available for parenteral or sublingual routes of administration and possessing an extremely long duration of action. As of this writing the sublingual dosage form has not yet been released for use in the United States. Buprenorphine has a low abuse potential, and tolerance to its analgesia does not seem to develop, but abstinence syndrome is observed after sudden discontinuation of the drug. Side effects are mainly drowsiness, nausea and vomiting, constipation, diaphoresis, respiratory depression, bradycardia, and a lowering of systolic blood pressure. Seventy per cent of an administered dose of buprenorphine is excreted unchanged via the fecal route; thus the drug may be of use in renal failure situations.

Buprenorphine may be given 0.3–0.6 or 0.4–0.8 mg every 6–8 hr parenterally, or by sublingual administration. Major drawbacks, especially in ambulatory patients, are sedation and nausea. It should be used with caution in the presence of other central nervous system depressants, head injury, respiratory problems, and biliary stasis. Cancer patients who are already receiving doses of agonist analgesics may develop precipitated abstinence syndrome when given buprenorphine.

Agonist-Antagonist Analgesics of the Nalorphine Type

Pentazocine, nalbuphine, and butorphanol are the agents of this class that are generally available for clinical use.

Pentazocine Pentazocine has been used for the past 15 years as an analgesic. However, the appearance of psychotomimetic effects with increasing frequency at increasing doses mars the clinical utility of this agent. Pentazocine 50 mg intramuscularly is equivalent to 10 mg morphine intramuscularly. Abstinence syndrome can be precipitated by introduction of pentazocine to a patient dependent on agonist analgesics such as morphine or methadone. The practice of using pentazocine to treat headache in an opiate-dependent patient receiving regular doses of agonist agents such as morphine, methadone, or levorphanol is to be deplored. This agent as well as the other commercially available antagonists agents may well precipitate uncomfortable abstinence syndrome, including nausea and vomiting. In cancer patients this is extremely unfortunate because, in addition to precipitated abstinence syndrome, these patients may reexperience the pain of their primary and/or metastatic lesions, forcing them to lose whatever psychological gains they have made. Tolerance and physical dependence on pentazocine have been observed with some regularity. Although this and the other antagonist agents are generally less of an addiction problem, once again we see that chronic pain patients may well differ from the norm if they become dependent on analgesic, or for that matter, sedative drugs.

Nalbuphine Nalbuphine is an antagonist analgesic with roughly the same potency as morphine, but has a somewhat lesser degree of respiratory depression per dose. Nalbuphine 10 mg intramuscularly induces as much respiratory depression as 10 mg morphine intramuscularly. However, the onset of further increase in respiratory depression is slow to develop.

The drug has been successfully used in the management of pain. Euphoria is observed at 8 mg intramuscularly, and dysphoria and psychotomimetic reactions have generally not been problematic until doses of 70 mg are used.

Nalbuphine is metabolized in the liver and has a plasma half-life of 5 hr. Tolerance and physical dependence have been described, but addicts report that after a week of daily doses of 140 mg/day irritability, inability to concentrate, strange thoughts and dreams, depression, and headaches are experienced.

Nalbuphine may precipitate abstinence syndrome and should be avoided in patients receiving doses of agonist analgesic drugs.

The usual analgesic dose of nalbuphine is 10 mg intramuscularly, intravenously, or subcutaneously every 3–4 hr.

Butorphanol Butorphanol is only available for parenteral administration and is 3–5 times as potent as morphine as an analgesic. It produces satisfactory postoperative analgesia. The utility of this agent for the management of cancer pain is limited since there is a correlation between the frequency of psychotomimetic reactions and the cumulative dose used. Since every attempt should be made to use oral medication in treating cancer, recommendations for use of this agent are reserved to provision of analgesia preoperatively, intraoperatively, and for short times during the postoperative period. For cancer patients who must receive parenteral medication for physical reasons, 2–4 mg every 3–4 hr for up to 8 months provided effective analgesia in 70% of patients with neoplastic disease (39).

References

1. Halpern LM: Psychotropics, ataractics and related drugs. In Bonica JJ, Ventafridda V (eds): *Advances in Pain Research and Therapy*, ed 2. New York, Raven Press, 1979.
2. Marks RM, Sachar EJ: Undertreatment of medical patients with narcotic analgesics. *Ann Intern Med* 78:173–181, 1973.
3. Vane JR: Inhibition of prostaglandin biosynthesis as a mechanism of action for aspirin-like drugs. *Nature [New Biol]* 231:232–235, 1971.
4. Larsen GL, Hensen PM: Mediators of inflammation. *Annu Rev Immunol* 1:335–359, 1983.
5. Perl ER: Sensitization of nociceptors and its relation to sensation. In Bonica JJ, Albe-Fessard D (eds): *Advances in Pain Research and Therapy*, vol 1. New York, Raven Press, 1976, p 17.
6. Ferreria SH, Moncada S, Vane JR: Prostaglandins and the mechanism of analgesia produced by aspirin-like drugs. *Br J Pharmacol* 49:86–97, 1973.
7. [Multiple authors]: Symposium for rational pharmacotherapy: the nonsteroidal anti-inflammatory drugs (NSAID). *Drug Intell Clin Pharm* 18:34–58, 1984.
8. Chen ACN, Chapman CR: Aspirin analgesia evaluated by event-related potentials in man. Possible central action in brain. *Exp Brain Res* 39:359–364, 1980.
9. Committee on Infectious Diseases: Aspirin and Reye's syndrome. *Pediatrics* 69:810–812, 1982.
10. Capetola RJ, Shriver DA, Rosenthale ME: Suprofen, a new peripheral analgesic. *J Pharmacol Exp Ther* 214:16–23, 1980.
11. Dubinsky B, Shupsky JJ: Mechanism of action of suprofen, a new peripheral analgesic, as demonstrated by its effects on several nociceptive mediators. *Prostaglandins* 28:241–252, 1984.
12. Kantor TG: Ketoprofen: a review of its pharmacologic and clinical properties. *Pharmacotherapy* 6(3):93–103, 1986.
13. Simon LS, Mills JA: Drug therapy: nonsteroidal anti-inflammatory agents: Part I. *N Engl J Med* 302:1179–1185, 1980.
14. Simon LS, Mills JA: Drug therapy: nonsteroidal anti-inflammatory agents: Part II. *N Engl J Med* 302:1237–1243, 1980.
15. *AMA Drug Evaluations*, ed 5. Littleton, MA, PSG Publishing Co, 1983.
16. Jaffe JH, Martin WR: Opioid analgesics and antagonists. In Gilman AG, Goodman LS, Rall TW, Murad F (eds): *The Pharmacological Basis of Therapeutics*, ed 7. New York, Macmillan, 1985, p 491.
17. Way EL, Sargent LJ: Morphine and its modifications. In de Stevens G (ed): *Analgetics*. New York, Academic Press, 1965, p 123.
18. Foldes FF, Swerdlow M, Siker CS: *Narcotics and Narcotics Antagonists*. Springfield, IL, Charles C Thomas, 1964.
19. Reynolds AK, Randall LO: *Morphine and Allied Drugs*. Toronto, University of Toronto Press, 1957.
20. Kaiko RF, Wallenstein SL, Rogers A: Analgesic and mood effects of heroin and morphine in cancer patients with postoperative pain. *N Engl J Med* 304:1501–1505, 1981.
21. Halpern LM, Robinson J: Prescribing practices for pain in drug dependence: a lesson in ignorance. In Stimmel B (ed): *Controversies in Alcoholism and Substance Abuse*. New York, The Haworth Press Inc, 1986, p 135.
22. Reynolds AK, Randall LO: *Morphine and Allied Drugs*. Toronto, University of Toronto Press, 1957.
23. Lasagna L: The clinical evaluation of morphine and its substitutes as analgesics. *Pharmacol Rev* 16:47–83, 1964.
24. Senami M, Aoki M, Kitahata L, Collins JG, Kumeta Y, Murata K: Lack of opiate effect on cat polymodal nociceptive fibers. *Pain* 27:81–90, 1986.
25. Winter CA: The physiology and pharmacology of pain relief. In de Stevens G (ed): *Analgetics*. New York, Academic Press, 1965, p 10.
26. Beecher HK: The measurement of pain. *Pharmacol Rev* 9:59–209, 1957.
27. Chang K-J, Quatrecasas P: Heterogeneity and properties of opiate receptors. *Fed Proc* 40:2729–2734, 1981.
28. Martin WR: The pharmacology of opioids. *Pharmacol Rev* 35:283–323, 1983.

29. Snyder SH: Drugs and neurotransmitter receptors in the brain. *Science* 224:22–31, 1984.
30. Beaver WT, Feise GA: Comparison of the analgesic effect of oxymorphone by rectal suppository and intramuscular injection in patients with postoperative pain. *J Clin Pharmacol* 17:276–291, 1977.
31. Halpern LM, Bonica JJ: Analgesics. In Modell W (ed): *Drugs of Choice 1976–1977*. St Louis, CV Mosby, 1976, p 195.
32. Jaffe JH, Martin WR: Opioid analgesics and antagonists. In Gilman AG, Goodman LS (eds): *The Pharmacological Basis of Therapeutics*, ed 6. New York, Macmillan, 1980, pp 491–531.
33. McCaffery M: How to relieve your patients' pain fast and effectively with oral analgesics. *Nursing 1980*, No 10, pp 58–63, 1980.
34. McCaffery M: *Nursing Management of the Patient with Pain*. Philadelphia, JB Lippincott, 1979, p 190.
35. Rogers AG: Pharmacology of analgesics. *J Neurosurg Nurs* 10:180–184, 1978.
36. Rogers AG: Problems in pain control—and ways to solve them. *Your Patient and Cancer* 1:65–75, 1981.
37. Twycross RG: Clinical experience with diamorphine in advanced malignant disease. *Int J Clin Pharmacol* 9:184–189, 1974.
38. Beaver WT, Feise G: Comparison of analgesic effects of morphine sulphate hydroxyzine and their combination in patients with post-operative pain. In Bonica JJ, Ventafridda V (eds): *Advances in Pain Research and Therapy*, vol 1. New York, Raven Press, 1976, pp 553–558.
39. Kouno K, Nakai Y, Ebina A, Sato M, Nagai K, Hayashi I, Ito T: Clinical trial of butorphanol tartrate in cancer patients: evaluation for analgesic effects and safety on the basis of long-term administration. *Gan to Kagaku* 10:1634–1645, 1983.

chapter 8
Psychopharmacologic Agents in the Treatment of Pain Syndromes

J. Hampton Atkinson, Jr., M.D.

This chapter reviews the therapeutic efficacy of psychiatric medications (the antidepressants, neuroleptics, antianxiety drugs, and psychostimulants) in acute and chronic pain syndromes, and provides guidelines for their use. Psychotropic drugs have been used as analgesics, as adjunctive agents to enhance conventional analgesics, and as primary treatment for psychological symptoms or disorders associated with pain. Psychological factors, including anxiety and depression, can profoundly influence pain expression. In addition, the burden of pain itself can produce considerable psychological distress. The use of psychotropics for symptomatic treatment of anxiety, depression, and insomnia is widely practiced.

Despite the importance of the problem of pain, and the abundant literature on psychotropic drugs and pain, few of the available studies can be considered scientifically complete. To rigorously assess the efficacy of an agent in pain management, a clinical trial should include the following criteria: (*a*) a reliable method to measure the intensity of pain and functional impairment; (*b*) an established and appropriate control or reference standard to compare with the experimental drugs; (*c*) differentiation between the analgesic, mood-altering, and sedative components of the drug; (*d*) serum levels of drugs or dose-response curves; and (*e*) double-blind or crossover design trials.

Two additional points must be noted. First, since pain is a multidimensional phenomenon, with emotional and sensory components, an effort should be made to assess which component responds to the drug in question. Second, acute and chronic pain must be considered separately, since their neurophysiologic and psychological aspects may well differ.

This chapter is in two parts. The first critically assesses drug therapy outcomes, mainly from controlled studies. It reviews each major class of psychopharmalogic agent. Following the principle that accurate diagnosis is essential, drug efficacy is discussed in relation to specific pain disorders. Experimentally induced and clinical acute pain are differentiated from their chronic pain counterparts. Where psychiatric disorders complicate the pain syndromes, their response to treatment is also discussed. The second section offers some clinical guidelines for using psychoactive drugs. It describes selecting a drug, preparing and evaluating patients for treatment, and conducting initial and longer term pharmacotherapy. Thus, a clinician considering drug treatment of a particular pain disorder can review selected examples of evidence for efficacy in the text and tables of part one. He can refer to the next section for specifics on treatment.

DRUG THERAPY OUTCOMES OF PSYCHOPHARMACOLOGIC AGENTS

ANTIDEPRESSANTS

Tricyclic antidepressants (TCAs), monoamine oxidase inhibitors (MAOIs), and lithium carbonate have been used as primary or adjunctive agents in pain management. There are four major clinical questions with regard to antidepressants in acute and chronic pain:

1. Are some antidepressants analgesic, and if so, in which pain disorders?
2. Is this analgesia independent of an antidepressant effect?

3. Do antidepressants potentiate narcotic or nonnarcotic analgesics in a clinically relevant manner?
4. Do antidepressants relieve depression associated with chronic pain syndromes?

Crucial to evaluating the role of antidepressant medication is defining what is meant by the term *depression*. It can be used to describe a mood, a symptom, and a syndrome or disorder. Fluctuation in mood or unhappiness as a reaction to life events or physical limitations is not a disorder. Indeed, the symptom of depressed mood or severe sadness may not be present even in patients diagnosed as having a depressive disorder. A diagnosis of a major depressive disorder, as described by the third edition of the *Diagnostic and Statistical Manual of Mental Disorders* (DSM-III) (1), requires an inability to experience pleasure, reduced interest in the environment, and reduced energy. A major depressive episode is thus defined as a period lasting at least 2 weeks that may be marked by a dysphoric mood, and is accompanied by a disorder of sleep and appetite, loss of energy, loss of interest, self-reproach, difficulty concentrating, and thoughts of death or suicide. Major depression differs from depressive symptoms in that the above problems are persistent, interfere with function, and are not explained better by other illness (1). Chronic pain can be associated with intermittent fatigue, withdrawal, insomnia, or other depressive symptoms, and up to 50% of chronic pain patients may suffer a major depressive episode at some point in their pain career.

Tricyclic Antidepressants

Acute Pain

Experimentally Induced and Clinical Pain Treatment outcomes for acute and chronic pain in humans are described in Table 8.1. Studies using animal paradigms demonstrate that TCAs provide species-specific analgesia for acute pain (2). The data with regard to analgesia in humans are contradictory. One careful report noted that single doses of doxepin (Sinequan, Adapin) did not alter laboratory-induced dental pain threshold in 18 normal adult males, who were repeatedly tested in a double-blind, placebo-controlled study over a 4-week period (3). There was no effect on acute anxiety or other mood variables measured by standardized inventories. The authors concluded that doxepin did not have straightforward analgesic properties since it did not alter sensory sensitivity or

Table 8.1
Tricyclic Antidepressants: Populations, Experimental Design, and Treatment Outcome

Authors	Population	N	Interventions	Design	Control	Dependant Measures	Follow-up	Results
	Acute Pain							
Chapman & Butter, 1978 (3)	Experimentally induced dental pain threshold	18	Compared doxepin (150 mg) and placebo	Double-blind, single-dose, crossover	Placebo medication	Sensory sensitivity and detection thresholds	4 wks	Doxepin did not alter sensory sensitivity or detection thresholds or mood variables.
Bromm & coworkers, 1986 (4)	Experimentally induced cutaneous pain	20	Compared imipramine (100 mg), meperidine, and placebo	Randomized, double-blind, crossover	Placebo medication, meperidine	Pain estimates, somatosensory-evoked cerebral potentials, EEG	Hrs	Imipramine reduced pain ratings & somatosensory amplitudes to same extent as meperidine.
Levine & coworkers, 1985	Postoperative dental extraction	30	Compared amitriptyline (25–75 mg), desipramine (25–75 mg), and placebo	Double-blind, group outcome	Placebo medication	Visual analog pain scale	None (single dose)	Desipramine enhanced prolonged morphine analgesia; amitriptyline did not. Neither agent was itself analgesic.
	Chronic Pain							
Kvinesdal & coworkers, 1984 (13)	Diabetic neuropathy	12	Compared imipramine (100 mg) and placebo	Crossover, double-blind	Placebo medication	Clinical assessment of neuropathy & global improvement	5 wks for each arm	Imipramine superior for global improvement.

continued

Table 8.1
Tricyclic Antidepressants: Populations, Experimental Design, and Treatment Outcome (*continued*)

Authors	Population	N	Interventions	Design	Control	Dependant Measures	Follow-up	Results
Turkington, 1980 (14)	Diabetic neuropathy with depression and depressive symptoms	59	Compared amitriptyline (100 mg), imipramine (100 mg), and diazepam (15 mg)	Randomized, double-blind	Diazepam	Kufer-Detre depression inventory; unspecified pain estimates	3 mos	Antidepressants superior to diazepam for relief of pain and mood disorder.
Langohr & coworkers, 1982 (11)	Mixed mono- and poly-neuropathy	48	Compared clomipramine (100 mg) and aspirin	Open label & double-blind, crossover	Aspirin	Rated degree of relief and overall function	5 wks	Clomipramine superior to aspirin. On 14-mo follow-up 41% maintained good relief.
Watson & coworkers, 1982 (12)	Postherpetic neuralgia	24	Compared amitriptyline (75 mg) and placebo	Double-blind crossover	Placebo medication	MMPI, Beck, pain self-report, sleep self-report	Up to 19 mos	Pain reduced in two-thirds of patients, to at least "mild" level; 6/9 with depressive symptoms had mood improvement and pain relief and others had pain relief alone. Fifty per cent had pain return on follow-up.
Couch & Hassanein, 1979 (16)	Migraine headaches	100	Compared amitriptyline (100 mg) with placebo	Randomized, double-blind, group outcome	Placebo medication	Hamilton and Zung depression scales; self-report of headache frequency & duration	Unspecified	Amitriptyline prophylaxis superior to placebo and equivalent to ergotamine.
Lance & Curran, 1964 (21)	Tension headaches	27	Compared amitriptyline (30–75 mg) and placebo	Double-blind, crossover	Placebo medication	Headache severity and frequency	1 mo for each arm, then 12-mo follow-up for amitriptyline	Amitriptyline significantly better than placebo for reducing headache frequency or severity.
Okasha & coworkers, 1978	Tension headaches	80	Compared doxepin (40 mg), amitriptyline (50 mg), and diazepam (10 mg)	Double-blind, group outcome	Diazepam	Hamilton depression and anxiety scores	Unspecified	Doxepin & amitriptyline superior to diazepam. Doxepin reduced headache and mood disturbance; amitriptyline improved mood but not headache.
Mathew, 1981 (17)	Migraine headaches	340	Compared amitriptyline (10–175 mg), propranolol, biofeedback, ergot preparations, and analgesics	Randomized, double-blind, group outcome	Conventional regimen of ergots and analgesics	Zung depression scores, headache severity & frequency	6 mos	Amitriptyline significantly better than conventional therapy, but inferior to propranolol. Combination of amitriptyline with propranolol conferred no added advantage.

continued

Table 8.1
Tricyclic Antidepressants: Populations, Experimental Design, and Treatment Outcome (*continued*)

Authors	Population	N	Interventions	Design	Control	Dependant Measures	Follow-up	Results
Mathew, 1981 (17)	Mixed vascular and muscle contraction headaches	281	Compared amitriptyline (50–75 mg); propranolol; biofeedback; propranolol and biofeedback; amitriptyline and biofeedback; amitriptyline, propranolol, and biofeedback; and ergotamine	Randomized trial	Treatment with ergotamine	Zung depression scores, headache severity & frequency	6 mos	Amitriptyline superior to other agents alone; combination of amitriptyline, propranolol, and biofeedback was most effective therapy.
Feinman & coworkers, 1983	Atypical facial pain	93	Compared dothiepin (150 mg) and placebo	Double-blind, group outcome	Placebo medication	Rigorous psychiatric diagnosis (ICD-9); Montgomery Asberg depression scale	12 mos	Dothiepin superior to placebo. Over 70% had relief of pain at 9 weeks. Pain relief independent of relief of depressive symptoms. Long-term (>1 yr) treatment needed to prevent relapse.
Alcoff & coworkers, 1982 (30)	Chronic low back pain	41	Compared imipramine (150 mg) and placebo	Double-blind, group outcome	Placebo medication	Beck depression scores, activity level, work function, pain severity, analgesic use	8 wks	Imipramine significantly improved activity and work function, but not pain severity, analgesic use, or level of depression.
Jenkins & coworkers, 1976 (34)	Chronic low back pain	44	Compared imipramine and placebo	Double-blind, group outcome	Placebo medication	Standardized personality inventory, Beck depression inventory, self-report of pain and stiffness	4 wks	Imipramine no different from placebo.
Sternbach & coworkers, 1976 (33)	Chronic low back pain	9	Compared chlorimipramine, amitriptyline, and placebo	Double-blind, counterbalanced	Placebo medication	Self-report of pain, pain tolerance on tourniquet test	2 wks	Chlorimipramine reduced pain estimate and increased pain tolerance. Amitriptyline ineffective.
Ward & coworkers, 1979 (25)	Low back pain with major depression	16	Doxepin (150 mg)	Single-blind, group outcome	None	Rigorous (Research Diagnostic Criteria) diagnosis of depression, retrospective self-report of pain before and after treatment, Hamilton depression score	4 wks	Pain "diminished" as depression remitted.

continued

Chapter 8/Psychopharmacologic Agents 73

Table 8.1
Tricyclic Antidepressants: Populations, Experimental Design, and Treatment Outcome (*continued*)

Authors	Population	N	Interventions	Design	Control	Dependant Measures	Follow-up	Results
Ward, 1986 (29)	Low back pain with major depression	35	Compared doxepin (3 mg/kg) and desipramine (3 mg/kg)	Double-blind, group outcome	Placebo responders eliminated from study pool	Hamilton depression, Spielberger anxiety, Profile of Moods, McGill Pain Inventory, Illness Behavior, EMG recording, ice-water pain tolerance	4 wks	Doxepin and desipramine equally reduced pain intensity, frequency, depression, and anxiety. Ice-water pain tolerance unaffected.
Evans & coworkers, 1973	Mixed arthritic disorders	18	Compared doxepin (150 mg) added to analgesic regimen and placebo	Double-blind, group outcome	Placebo medication	Investigator judgment of mood; objective count of analgesic consumption	4 wks	Doxepin improved mood; analgesic use dramatically decreased in both groups.
Gringas, 1976 (37)	Mixed arthritic disorders	55	Compared imipramine (75 mg) and placebo	Double-blind, counterbalanced, crossover	Placebo medication	Self-reported pain and stiffness; objectively assessed grip strength; observer-assessed function and stiffness	4 wks	Treatment group showed significantly less subjective pain and stiffness and improved observer ratings of function and stiffness. Objective grip strength unchanged.
McDonald-Scott, 1969 (38)	Mixed arthritic disorders	22	Compared imipramine (75 mg) added to anti-inflammatory regimen with placebo	Double-blind, crossover	Placebo medication	Patient "preference" of interventions	3 wks	Patient "preferred" imipramine to placebo.
McNeill & Dick, 1976 (36)	Mixed arthritic disorders	29	Compared imipramine with placebo	Double-blind, group outcome	Placebo medication	Pain self-report, objectively determined grip strength, Beck depression inventory	10 wks	No between-group differences in pain report on grip strength; results potentially confounded because imipramine group significantly more depressed at baseline.
Blumer & coworkers 1980 (40)	Mixed chronic pain	129	Compared high-dose (300 mg) and low-dose (unspecified) regimens of amitriptyline, doxepin, imipramine	Open label, group outcome	None	Investigator assessment of mood, pain intensity, activity, sleep	9–16 mos	Investigators rated 55% of high-dose and 32% of low-dose groups as "improved." No statistical comparisons.
Lindsay & Olsen, 1985 (42)	Mixed chronic nonback pain with major depression	25	Maprotiline (75–225 mg)	Open label	None	Self-report of percentage pain reduction	Unspecified	Maprotiline reduced pain by 50% in 72% of sample.

continued

Table 8.1
Tricyclic Antidepressants: Populations, Experimental Design, and Treatment Outcome (*continued*)

Authors	Population	N	Interventions	Design	Control	Dependant Measures	Follow-up	Results
Lindsay & Wycoff, 1981 (26)	Mixed chronic pain with unipolar depression	116	Sequential trials of amitriptyline, imipramine, or doxepin until antidepressant response	Open label, group outcome	None	Rigorous (Feighner) clinical assessment of depression, retrospective self-report of pain decrement	8–12 wks	Significant proportion of those who responded to antidepressant reported pain decrement >50%
Pilowsky & coworkers, 1982 (39)	Mixed chronic pain without organic findings	52	Compared amitriptyline and placebo	Double-blind, crossover	Placebo medication	Illness Behavior Questionnaire, Zung and Levine-Pilowsky depression, Spielberger anxiety, Sickness Impact Profile	6 wks on each arm	Amitriptyline superior to placebo at 2 and 4 weeks. No group differences at 6 weeks. High dropout (40%) and variability of scores may have obscured treatment effect.
Singh & Verma, 1971 (41)	Mixed chronic pain	60	Sequential trials of imipramine, amitriptyline, and chlordiazepoxide	Open label	None	Observer assessment of pain relief and psychiatric symptoms	Unspecified	Imipramine and amitriptyline therapeutically equivalent and superior to chlordiazepoxide for relief of pain and mood disturbance.

detection thresholds, and that it had no detectable effect on pain-induced anxiety at the dosages studied. Another rigorous study reported that single doses of imipramine (Tofranil) reduced pain ratings in response to an intracutaneous electrical stimulus by 40% (4). This reduction was equivalent to oral meperidine (Demerol) and superior to placebo.

With regard to clinical pain, in a double-blind, placebo-controlled study Levine et al. (5) observed that neither amitriptyline (Elavil) nor desipramine (Norpramin, Pertofrane), given for 1 week preoperatively at 25–75 mg daily, provided analgesia after dental extraction.

Chronic Pain Tricyclic antidepressants have been tested in numerous intractable pain syndromes, as summarized in Table 8.1. The data most clearly support their efficacy for neurologic (deafferentation) pain and headache syndromes. Their effectiveness in other chronic pain syndromes, arthritic disorders, and low back pain—which may well represent the diagnosis for which the drugs are most commonly employed—is less certain.

Neurologic Disorders Neuropathic and deafferentation pain etiologically are thought to arise from spontaneous neuronal hyperactivity or disturbed inhibition following central nervous system or peripheral nerve injury. Disorders reported to respond to TCAs include postherpetic neuralgia (6), diabetic peripheral neuropathy (7), persistent postoperative scar pain (8), trigeminal neuralgia (9), thalamic pain (10), and neuralgias from lesions of plexus or peripheral nerves (e.g., postamputation stump pain) (11). Treatment is effective in depressed or nondepressed patients.

For example, in a placebo-controlled study Watson et al. (12) demonstrated a therapeutic effect of amitriptyline (25–150 mg daily) in a sample of elderly patients with persistent postherpetic neuralgia. Minnesota Multiphasic Personality Inventories (MMPIs) and Beck depression scores indicated that the majority of patients had no evidence of depression. In two-thirds of the sample, pain was reduced from "severe" to "mild" within 3 weeks. Nine patients with mild depressive symptoms had good relief of pain, usually along with an antidepressant effect, but some had pain relief without a change in mood. Serum TCA levels were below those associated with antidepressant activity. The authors reported that increases in dosage produced increased pain in some patients, suggesting that there was a "therapeutic window" for dosage. In about half of the subjects who responded initially, there was a later decay of efficacy, casting doubts on the long-term benefits of treatment. Nevertheless several patients were able to discontinue therapy but maintain their improvement beyond 12 months.

Controlled studies indicate that TCAs are effective for the pain of diabetic peripheral neuropathy in patients with and without associated depressive symptoms. Kvinesdal and associates (13) used imipramine (100 mg daily) in insulin-requiring diabetics in good glycemic control with neuropathic symptoms of at least 2 years' duration. None were reported as depressed, although psychometric assessment was not done. Observer ratings of improvement were positively correlated with the plasma concentration of drug. The analgesia did not seem to be mediated by an antidepressant effect since maximum benefit occurred within 2 weeks and was achieved at about one-half the drug concentrations usually required for antidepressant activity. Benefit did not appear to be related to changes in glycemic control.

Turkington (14) studied 59 diabetic patients, all with psychometrically documented depressive symptoms, in a trial comparing amitriptyline (100 mg), imipramine (100 mg), or diazepam (Valium) (15 mg) daily. The antidepressants produced equivalent pain relief (and remission of symptoms of depression) within 8–12 weeks. Diazepam produced no improvement in pain or depression scores. Again, level of control of blood glucose did not appear to mediate the improvement. On 2-year follow-up after discontinuation of therapy, pain recurred in 26% of the patients, and remitted with antidepressants. Taken together these data would indicate that TCAs alleviate diabetic neuropathic pain and depressive symptoms associated with this disorder. Pain relief occurs in 1–2 weeks, whereas an antidepressant effect may take 8–12 weeks.

Bourhis et al. (15) have reported an uncontrolled trial of trimipramine (Surmotil) (50–200 mg) alone and in combination with a phenothiazine, methotrimeprazine (Levoprome), in cancer pain patients. Although pain diagnoses were not stated, patients with head and neck pain syndromes were particularly benefited, and it is likely that postsurgical or postirradiation deafferentation pain states were responsible for the head and neck pain. There was no evidence that psychotropics diminished pain caused by metastasis to bone, or from tumor involvement of viscera, or from other direct effects of neoplasia.

Migraine Headache Syndromes Couch and Hassanein (16) reported that amitriptyline (100 mg daily) was superior to placebo in preventing migraine attacks, and in reducing headache severity in attacks that did occur. The best response occurred in nondepressed patients with severe migraine and in depressed patients with mild headaches; depressed subjects with severe headaches noted little relief. Correlation between improvement in migraine and change in depression was low but significant.

A subsequent study of 340 patients with classic migraine compared amitriptyline, propranolol, and biofeedback in a randomized trial using treatment with ergotamine and conventional analgesics as a comparison control (17). Amitriptyline (50–75 mg) gave significantly better prophylaxis than control therapy but was inferior to propranolol. The combination of amitriptyline and propranolol offered no advantage. The antimigraine action of amitriptyline was relatively independent of its antidepressant effect since even patients with Zung depression scores within the normal range showed significantly more improvement than did control subjects. Uncontrolled studies also report that amitriptyline prevents migraine attacks (18–20).

With regard to mixed migraine-contraction headache prophylaxis, an intriguing study compared ergotamine to: (a) propranolol or amitriptyline (50–75 mg) alone; (b) biofeedback alone; and (c) combinations of drugs and biofeedback (17). Amitriptyline was superior to other single agents and the combination of biofeedback, amitriptyline, and propranolol was overall the most effective regimen. The beneficial effect of amitriptyline alone was significantly correlated with a high initial self-rating depression score, even though the dosage regimen was "subtherapeutic" for depression.

Tension Headaches Several studies suggest that low doses of TCAs may be effective for chronic tension headaches, perhaps more effective than the commonly used antianxiety drugs. In controlled, crossover studies Lance and coworkers demonstrated that amitriptyline was superior to placebo (21) and to imipramine (22) for relief of chronic muscle contraction headache. Amitriptyline was most effective in patients over 60 years old. The majority of patients maintained their improvement for at least 6 months. In an open label study (21) these authors found amitriptyline (30–75 mg daily) and imipramine (30–75 mg daily) superior to barbiturates for overall pain relief. Similarly Okasha et al. (23) reported that amitriptyline (50 mg daily) and doxepin (40 mg daily) were superior to diazepam for tension headache. Interestingly, doxepin relieved headache and diminished anxiety and depression, whereas amitriptyline improved mood without concurrent headache relief.

By comparison, the literature consistently reports that depressed psychiatric clinic patients frequently experience muscle contraction headache (24). Two studies (25, 26) reported that TCAs reduce pain complaints in rigorously diagnosed depressed psychiatric patients whose depression also remitted with treatment. Whether pain remits before mood improves is not documented.

Other Headache There are anecdotal reports of successful use of TCAs for cluster headaches (27). Similar reports suggest that the chronic headache syndrome resulting from closed head injury, which is frequently accompanied by compensation claims, depression, and anxiety, does not respond to TCAs (27).

Atypical Facial Pain This classification contains two conditions. One is the *temporomandibular joint syndrome,* with pain affecting the temporomandibular joint and its musculature. The other, sometimes collectively termed *atypical facial neuralgia*, includes both atypical odontalgia (pain in the teeth) and oral dysesthesia, which features disturbed taste, dry mouth, and a burning tongue, all in the absence of physical disease (28). These conditions are to be distinguished from the typical facial pain due to trigeminal or postherpetic neuralgia, in which pain occurs in superficial tissues, as opposed to the deep vague aches found in atypical facial pain.

Feinmann et al. (28) described a controlled study using dothiepin (150 mg), an analog of doxepin not available in the United States, in patients having temporomandibular joint pain or another atypical facial pain. One-third of the sample met rigorous diagnostic criteria for a depressive disorder. By 9 weeks, drug treatment produced significant reduction in pain (71% pain free) and analgesic use, but not in depression rating scores or overall rating of psychiatric morbidity. Pain diminished equally in depressed and nondepressed patients. Many successfully treated patients who discontinued treatment after 6 months experienced recurrence of pain, which remitted when drug was reinstituted. At 12 months over three-fourths of the sample was pain free on treatment. This study demonstrates that patients with atypical facial pain respond well to antidepressant therapy, but that continuous drug treatment may be required to maintain improvement.

Low Back Pain Two basic groups of chronic low back pain (CLBP) patients have been studied. The first includes those with rigorously diagnosed major affective disorders (unipolar depression or dysthymic disorder) that either precedes or is secondary to pain. The second includes patients with depressive symptoms, but who do not meet criteria for a diagnosable depressive disorder. To a large degree, efficacy of antidepressants depends on the group considered.

Several studies report that CLBP with diagnosable major depression responds well to TCAs. For example, Ward (29) noted that both doxepin and desipramine reduced self-report and objective ratings of depression and anxiety, pain severity, and percentage of day in pain. Clinical pain relief and clinical depression relief were significantly related. The doses achieved were within the usual antidepressant range (3 mg/kg, or at least 150 mg daily for either agent), and the onset of maximum therapeutic response occurred after 3–4 weeks. These factors argued for a primary antidepressant effect. The best clinical predictor of response was a shorter duration of pain complaint; age, number of surgeries, employment status, and orthopedic ratings of the amount of physical impairment were not associated with outcome.

Contradictory effects are reported in CLBP patients having depressive symptoms, but without diagnosed major depression. Alcoff et al. (30) described a group of CLBP patients, 10% of whom had documented depressive symptoms. Those treated with imipramine (150 mg daily) showed significantly higher activity levels and work capacity, but did not differ from those on placebo in pain severity, analgesic use, or degree of change in Beck depression scores after 6 weeks of therapy. This study is particularly informative because the groups were well matched for pain chronicity, prior surgery or injury, and depressive symptoms. Plasma antidepressant concentrations did not correlate with change in depression scores or pain intensity in the subgroup of patients with higher depression scores.

In another controlled study of back pain patients with documented depressive symptoms, Hameroff et al. (31) reported that doxepin (2.5 mg/kg daily) was clearly superior to placebo for improving mood and sleep and reducing muscle tension and the percentage of time patients reported being in pain. Pain intensity, level of activity, and analgesic consumption did not respond to the antidepressant.

Finally, Pheasant et al. (32) reported a controlled, crossover trial of amitriptyline (50–150 mg daily) in CLBP patients with depressive symptoms. Analgesic consumption significantly decreased (by 46%) during treatment with amitriptyline, but mood and activity level were unaltered. A related finding from another controlled trial (33) was that chlorimipramine (Anafranil) (150 mg), an analog of imipramine, significantly decreased verbal pain estimates in low back pain patients and increased tolerance to experimentally induced pain after 2 weeks of therapy. The same study showed, however, that amitriptyline (150 mg) did not differ from placebo. Studies using lower dosages of imipramine (75 mg) reported no significant differences between treatment and control groups in objective or self-reported mood, pain, or stiffness in patients with and without documented depressive symptoms (34).

In summary, it would appear that TCAs are especially effective in CLBP with associated major depression, and that full antidepressant dosages are necessary. In patients not having major depression, such symptoms as insominia or subjective muscle tension may well be improved, but an increase in functional activity and a reduction in analgesic consumption may not occur. Imipramine and desipramine may reduce pain intensity in uncomplicated CLBP, but this is not thoroughly documented.

Arthritic Disorders Intriguing new evidence indicates that TCAs have anti-inflammatory effects in chronic adjuvant-induced arthritis in rats. This effect reduces the physical signs of arthritis itself, increases mobility, and reduces pain-associated behaviors (35).

Three placebo-controlled trials of imipramine have evaluated its use as an adjunct for relief of symptoms of arthritic disorders (rheumatoid arthritis, osteoarthritis, ankylosing spondylitis). In each study imipramine (75 mg) was added to a nonsteroidal anti-inflammatory drug regimen. One study (36) noted no significant drug effect, whereas another (37) showed significant improvement in pain, stiffness, and activity. In the third study (38) patients "preferred" the antidepressant to placebo, but specific dependent variables (mood, pain, grip strength, and physical function) were not assessed. Thus, in humans, imipramine may have therapeutic effects, but more controlled studies are needed to establish its role in arthritic disorders.

Mixed Chronic Pain Syndrome This term describes a heterogeneous group of patients who do not fit into the diagnostic categories discussed previously. The efficacy of TCAs in these patients again appears to depend upon the presence of coexisting major depression.

In a crossover study of amitriptyline, Pilowsky et al. (39) reported the treated group had significantly less pain than the untreated group at weeks 2 and 4, but that pain ratings became equivalent to placebo after 6 weeks of drug treatment. Although amitriptyline generally did not improve daily functioning or symptoms of anxiety and depression, the authors concluded that patients showing clear-cut endogenous depression were the most responsive.

Among the uncontrolled investigations, Blumer et al. (40) addressed the differential effect of high-dose (antidepressant) versus low-dose (analgesic) regimens of amitriptyline, imipramine, or doxepin in a pain clinic population. The high-dose groups had a more favorable outcome (50% versus 30% "improved"), but the clinical and statistical significance of these results is difficult to evaluate.

Singh and Verma (41) reported that imipramine and amitriptyline were superior to chlordiazepoxide for relief of both pain and associated anxiety and depressive symptoms in a sample of patients with pain referred for psychiatric assessment.

In another uncontrolled study Lindsay and Olsen (42) treated 25 non–back pain patients with rigorously diagnosed major depression using maprotiline, a newer TCA structurally similar to imipramine, at doses of 150–300 mg daily. Pain estimates diminished by at least one-half in 72% of patients. Among patients who had received previous unsuccessful antidepressant treatment, 62% had pain reduced by half or more. This finding probably reflects the known antidepressant action of maprotiline.

Tricyclic Antidepressants as Adjuncts to Analgesics Amitriptyline (43), nortriptyline (Aventyl, Pamelor) (43), chlorimipramine (44), desipramine (45), nomifensine (Merital) (46), and doxepin (46) are all reported to potentiate opiate analgesia in animal models, perhaps by increasing opiate receptor sensitivity (43). In human acute clinical pain, chronic administration of desipramine (25–75 mg), but not amitriptyline, potentiates and prolongs morphine analgesia, resulting in 10–20% lower verbal estimates of pain intensity (5).

In chronic pain France et al. (47) and Urban et al. (48) reported that the combination of either doxepin or amitriptyline with a narcotic analgesic reduced pain intensity more than either an antidepressant or a narcotic agent alone in patients with low back (47) and phantom limb (48) pain. Narcotic dose escalation and narcotic abuse did not occur, and no patient required more than the equivalent of 20 mg of methadone (Dolophin) daily. Since these patients also were enrolled in a comprehensive pain management program, the authors speculate that both the program itself and the TCAs may have contributed to the low maintenance dosages of narcotic. Of particular interest is that narcotics generally are ineffective in central pain states such as phantom limb (49), and that TCAs may promote narcotic efficacy in these disorders. Controlled trials assessing combination versus single drug on pain intensity, side effects, functional status (employment, exercise tolerance, etc.), and emotional state are needed.

Mechanisms of Action Tricyclic antidepressants have several actions, including; (a) antidepressant effects; (b) "anticonvulsant" effects; (c) serotonergic or noradrenergic affects with augmentation of endogenous pain-inhibitory mechanisms; (d) anti-inflammatory properties; and (e) central skeletal muscle relaxation. It is possible to speculate that the major therapeutic action depends upon the etiology or etiologies of the pain syndrome. An antidepressant effect would be paramount in pain patients with coexisting major depressive illness. In migraine headache and other neurologic pain from deafferentation disorders, stabilizing aberrantly conducting neurons or inhibiting their afferent transmission at the level of the spinal cord may be crucial. An anticonvulsant mechanism (50, 51) is possible, given the evidence of epileptiform activity in deafferentated neurons, the structural similarity of TCAs to traditional anticonvulsants like carbamazeine, and their ability to suppress firing in polysynaptic neurons (9, 50, 51). Peripheral anti-inflammatory properties may be therapeutic in other pathologic states. Possible sites of action include (a) altering the transport or activity of substances involved in inflammation at the tissue level, such as serotonin; (b) inhibiting prostaglandin synthetase, an enzyme crucial to inflammation; or (c) modifying of blood protein-binding capacity, another property shared with conventional anti-inflammatory drugs (35). Finally, amitriptyline has a chemical structure almost identical to cyclobenzaprine (Flexeril), a centrally acting skeletal muscle relaxant. The centrally acting skeletal muscle relaxants are sedatives and preferentially depress polysynaptic reflexes, without directly relaxing skeletal muscle or depressing neuronal conduction or muscle excitability. Amitriptyline may act by sedative or neuronal mechanisms to reduce muscle tension in selected headache or low back disorders. Of course, an augmentation of serotonergic or other endogenous pain-inhibitory neurotransmitter systems may be fundamental to any therapeutic effect.

Monoamine Oxidase Inhibitors

Acute and Chronic Pain Monoamine oxidase (MAO) is a term for intramitochondrial enzymes widely distributed throughout the body. An intraneuronal MAO deactivates biologically active amines potentially important in pain perception, including norepinephrine, 5-hydroxytryptamine (serotonin), and dopamine. Monoamine oxidase inhibitors (MAOIs) increase intraneuronal pools of these neurotransmitters by inhibiting their degradation. Phenelzine (Nardil) and tranylcypromine (Parnate) are the most commonly prescribed MAOIs.

Monoamine oxidase inhibitors do not appear to have analgesic properties in acute pain. With regard to chronic pain syndromes, the MAOIs show promise for migraine headache, atypical facial pain, and major depression with secondary pain, as noted in Table 8.2. One uncontrolled study using phenelzine for treatment-resistant migraine headache reported that 20 of 25 patients had a reduction in frequency of headache to less than one-half that of the preceding 12-month control period, and 7 of these patients became headache free (52). Although serotonin is thought to be important to the pathogenesis of migraine, no correlation was observed between changes in pain and in platelet serotonin concentrations.

Cyclic migraine, consisting of daily headaches in recurrent episodes lasting 2 weeks or more, also may be a phenelzine-responsive disorder. Uncontrolled studies (53,

Table 8.2
Lithium and Monoaxmine Oxidase Inhibitors: Populations, Experimental Design, and Treatment Outcome

Authors	Population	N	Interventions	Design	Control	Dependant Measures	Follow-up	Results
Anthony & Lance, 1969 (52)	Migraine headache	25	Phenelzine	Case studies, open label	None	Self-report of headache frequency	5–24 mos	Phenelzine reduced headache frequency by 50% in 20/25; 7/25 headache free.
Lascelles, 1966 (55)	Atypical facial pain	20	Compared phenelzine (45 mg) and placebo	Double-blind, group outcome	Placebo medication	Clinical psychiatric diagnosis, Hamilton depression scale, self-report of pain	1 mo	Phenelzine superior to placebo. Pain relief in 15/20. Relief of depression associated with pain relief.
Raft & coworkers, 1981 (56)	Primary unipolar depression, pain secondary to depression	23	Compared phenelzine, amitriptyline, and placebo	Double-blind, group outcome	Placebo medication	Beck depression inventory, Hamilton Rating Scale for Depression	6 wks	Phenelzine (1.5 mg/kg) superior to placebo for relieving depression at 6 wks.
Chazot & coworkers 1979 (59)	Migraine headache	25	Lithium	Case studies, open label	None	Self-report of headache frequency		Lithium decreased number of headache attacks in 50% of patients.
Medina & Diamond, 1981 (54)	Cyclical migraine	22	Lithium	Case studies, open label	None	Self-report of headache frequency & duration	3–4 mos	Nineteen of 22 patients had decreased duration, frequency of attacks.
Peatfield & Rose, 1981 (60)	Migraine headache	5	Lithium	Case studies, open label	None	Self-report of headache frequency & intensity	2 wks	All had more severe, more frequent headache.
Damasio & Lyon, 1980 (61)	Acute cluster headache	8	Lithium	Case studies, open label	None	Self-report of headache frequency & severity	1–5 mos	Headache remitted in 3/8 patients at 2 wks. Lithium prophylactic if initiated during remission.
Ekbom, 1977	Acute cluster headache	7	Lithium	Case studies, open label	None	Self-report of headache frequency & intensity	1–36 mos	No response in 3/7 patients; headache intensity decreased by 20–33% in others. Lithium prophylactic if initiated during remission.

continued

Table 8.2
Lithium and Monoaxmine Oxidase Inhibitors: Populations, Experimental Design, and Treatment Outcome (*continued*)

Authors	Population	N	Interventions	Design	Control	Dependant Measures	Follow-up	Results
Kudrow, 1978	Cluster headache	15	Compared lithium, prednisone and methylsergide	Group outcome, open label	Reference medication	Self-report of headache improvement	1–12 mos	Eighty-seven per cent had 75% improvement with lithium, 50% and 41% improved with prednisone and methylsergide.
Damasio & Lyon, 1980 (61)	Chronic cluster headache	12	Lithium	Case studies, open label	None	Self-report of headache improvement	1–24 mos	Complete remission in 6/12 patients on follow-up.
Ekbom, 1981 (62)	Chronic cluster headache	8	Lithium	Case studies, open label	None	Self-report of headache improvement	1–24 mos	All reported pain decreased 75–100% at 2 wks; 11/12 had return of headache to baseline by 8 mos.
Lieb & Zeff, 1978	Chronic cluster headache	2	Lithium	Case studies, open label	None	Self-report of headache frequency	12–27 mos	Markedly reduced frequency of headache.
Medina & coworkers, 1978 (63)	Chronic cluster headache	12	Lithium	Case studies, open label	None	Self-report of headache improvement	3 mos	Complete remission in all 12 patients.

54) noted complete remission in 20% of patients, and reduced duration of attacks in the remaining patients.

Lascelles (55) described a controlled trial of phenelzine (45 mg) in patients with prolonged atypical facial pain, without detectable organic pathology. This group suffered deep, aching pain in the soft tissues and bone, and diagnostically embraced temporomandibular joint syndrome and atypical facial neuralgias (described earlier). Phenelzine significantly outperformed placebo at 4 weeks in relieving both objectively rated depressive symptoms and facial pain. Three-fourths of the treated patients showed improvement of pain and depression. Pain relief was associated with improvement in depression, and was ascribed to an antidepressant effect.

Raft et al. (56) reported a significant antidepressant effect of phenelzine (1.5 mg/kg) in a controlled study of psychiatric patients with definite primary depression in whom pain was symptomatic of depression and did not precede it. The effect of phenelzine on pain was not reported, but the patients' daily functioning improved. Interestingly, the authors observed that pain clinic populations may contain a high proportion of patients with "atypical" depression. Such patients exhibit reverse vegetative symptoms of depression (e.g., increased sleep, appetite, and libido) and may be specifically responsive to MAOI agents.

Lithium Carbonate

Acute and Chronic Pain Lithium is widely used in psychiatric disorders and has been employed for numerous medical and neurologic conditions (57). The rationale for its use in pain syndromes derives from its postulated effects on central nervous system dopaminergic and serotonergic systems, and its demonstrated efficacy in treating cyclic or recurrent disorders (e.g., bipolar affective disorder). Lithium has been used to treat common migraine, cyclic migraine, and cluster headaches, but its efficacy in these syndromes is not established (see Table 8.2). Uncontrolled reports (54, 58, 59) suggest that lithium diminishes the frequency and severity of common migraine attacks, but there are also indications that the drug precipitates more frequent and severe migraine headaches (60). Lithium has been used to abolish acute attacks of cluster headache but has not been consistently beneficial (61, 62). Several studies (61–66) noted that lithium relieves chronic cluster headache, although in many patients headaches returned to pretreatment levels within 18 months, despite continued lithium therapy (62). Perhaps some subtypes of these headache syndromes, but not others, respond to lithium.

Mechanism of Action of MAOIs and Lithium Carbonate

The therapeutic mechanism of action of MAOI and lithium in headache syndromes is unknown, but probably is not simply a primary antidepressant effect. Their widespread effects on serotonergic and noradrenergic neurotransmission may activate endogenous pain modulating systems.

Summary

In summary, these studies identify promising treatments and also illuminate deficits in our current approach to using antidepressants in treatment of these patients. First, there are no clinical or biologic markers to predict drug responders from nonresponders. Second, the high dropout rate in many studies indicates that antidepressants alone are insufficient to treat these patients and that a more comprehensive approach is required. Finally, improved laboratory methods for detecting major depression may permit the more specific application of these drugs.

NEUROLEPTIC DRUGS

Neuroleptics include the various classes of phenothiazines, butyrophenones, and other compounds used primarily as antipsychotics or "major tranquilizers." Like opiates, they inhibit gross motor activity, and act at higher centers to produce affective indifference and emotional quieting. Neuroleptics are used widely in combination with narcotics to treat postoperative pain and have been employed for chronic pain syndromes. Recently, however, it has been recognized that there is very little evidence that neuroleptics have analgesic effects or that they potentiate opiate analgesia, and a reassessment of their use is in order. Details of these studies are presented in Table 8.3.

Phenothiazines and Related Drugs

Acute Pain

Experimentally Induced Pain The extensive work of Dundee et al. (67–70) assessed the effect of 14 different phenothiazines on pain experimentally induced by pressure on the anterior surface of the tibia, using healthy patients admitted to a gynecologic service for minor surgical procedures. All phenothiazines tested increased sensitivity to pain at 20 min after injection. By 60 min, however, two distinct response patterns emerged. First, some agents showed mild analgesic activity: chlorpromazine (Thorazine), promazine (Sparine), propiomazine (Largon), and methotrimeprazine (Levoprome) (68). Next, some agents moderately amplified pain reports: prochlorperazine (Compazine), perphenazine (Trilafon), and trifluoperazine (Stelazine). Finally, one agent markedly increased pain report over baseline: promethazine (Phenergan) (68). Further observations suggested that the action of certain phenothiazines was biphasic—first antianalgesic and later analgesic. Promethazine, trifluoperazine, and perphenazine, for example, enhanced pain sensitivity at 20 and 60 min after injection but demonstrated some slight analgesic activity by 180 min after administration (67–70).

Table 8.3
Antipsychotic Drugs: Populations, Experimental Design, and Treatment Outcome

Authors	Population	N	Interventions	Design	Control	Dependant Measures	Follow-up	Results
	Acute Pain							
Dundee & coworkers, 1960, 1961, 1963 (68–70)	Patients awaiting minor surgery; experimentally induced pain sensitivity	20–140	Compared effect of 14 different phenothiazines on sensitivity to experimentally induced pain	Group outcome, open label	No treatment	Self-report of sensitivity to experimentally induced pain	3 hrs	All phenothiazines increased sensitivity to pain at 20 min. Methotrimeprazine, chlorpromazine, promazine, and propiomazine slightly analgesic 60 min after injection.
Moore & Dundee, 1961 (67)	Patients awaiting minor surgery; experimentally induced pain sensitivity	42–60	Compared ability of 5 phenothiazines to enhance meperidine	Group outcome, open label	No treatment	Self-report of sensitivity to experimentally induced pain	3 hrs	Promethazine & perphenazine antagonized meperidine analgesia. Promazine slightly enhanced meperidine. Propiomazine and trifluoperazine ineffective.
Siker & coworkers, 1966 (71)	Healthy volunteers; experimentally induced pain threshold	16	Compared promethazine and placebo	Double-blind, group outcome	Placebo medication	Self-report, scale unspecified	Hrs	Promethazine antagonized meperidine analgesia.

continued

Table 8.3
Antipsychotic Drugs: Populations, Experimental Design, and Treatment Outcome (*continued*)

Authors	Population	N	Interventions	Design	Control	Dependant Measures	Follow-up	Results
Keats & coworkers, 1966 (74)	Postoperative patients	13	Compared promethazine and placebo; meperidine with and without promethazine	Double-blind, group outcome	Placebo medication	Self-report of pain improvement	Hrs	Promethazine equivalent to placebo; promethazine did not enhance meperidine.
Lasagna & DeKornfeld, 1961 (72)	Postoperative, postpartum pain.	37–66	Compared methotrimeprazine and morphine; methotrimeprazine and placebo	Double-blind, case control	Placebo, reference analgesic (morphine)	Self-report of pain improvement	Hrs	Methotrimeprazine (15 mg) equivalent to morphine (10 mg).
McZuitty, 1967 (75)	Labor pain	525	Compared promethazine, promazine, or propiomazine with & without meperidine	Double-blind	Placebo medication	Observer rating of pain intensity	Hrs	Promazine, promethazine & propiomazine not analgesic and did not enhance analgesia obtained from meperidine (100 mg).
Minuck, 1972 (73)	Postoperative pain	197	Compared methotrimeprazine, meperidine, & placebo	Double-blind, group outcome	Placebo medication	Observer rating of analgesia as excellent, good, fair, or poor	Hrs	Methotrimeprazine (5–10 mg) equal to meperidine (25–50 mg); both superior to placebo for analgesia.
Powe & coworkers, 1962 (76)	Labor pain	520	Compared (1) meperidine, (2) meperidine with propiomazine, and (3) meperidine with propiomazine	Goup outcome	Reference analgesic (meperidine)	Observer ratings of pain	Hrs	Promethazine and propiomazine combined with meperidine produced "calmer" course of labor. Outcome criteria confounded by sedative effects of phenothiazines.
	Chronic Pain							
Bloomfield & coworkers, 1964	Mixed chronic pain	18	Compared methotrimeprazine with morphine	Group outcome	Placebo medication	Self- and observer ratings	4 hrs	Methotrimeprazine (15 mg) equivalent to morphine for analgesia.
Caviness & O'Brien, 1980 (82)	Cluster headache	13	Chlorpromazine given to patients who had not responded to conventional therapy	Case study, open label	None	Self-report of headache frequency, intensity	Up to 8 mos	Chlorpromazine associated with headache suppression within 2 weeks and 13 patients.
Hakkarainen, 1977 (81)	Tension headache	48	Compared fluphenazine and placebo	Group outcome, double-blind	Placebo medication	Self-report of headache duration, intensity, frequency	2 mos	Fluphenazine (1 mg) produced significant decreases in headache duration, intensity, and frequency.
Montilla & coworkers, 1963 (98)	Mixed chronic pain	105	Compared methotrimeprazine and morphine	Group outcome, double-blind	Reference analgesic (morphine)	Self- and observer pain ratings	4 hrs	Methotrimeprazine (15 mg) equivalent to morphine (10 mg).

continued

Table 8.3
Antipsychotic Drugs: Populations, Experimental Design, and Treatment Outcome

Authors	Population	N	Interventions	Design	Control	Dependant Measures	Follow-up	Results
Beaver & coworkers, 1978	Chronic cancer pain	40	Compared single-dose methotrimeprazine and morphine	Case control, single-blind	Reference analgesic (morphine)	Observer rated pain hourly for 6 hrs	6 hrs	Methotrimeprazine about half as potent as morphine on a milligram basis.
Bourhis & coworkers, 1978 (15)	Chronic cancer pain	100	Methotrimeprazine added to ongoing treatment	Case studies, open label	None	Observer rating of invalidism and of unsolicited pain reports during interview	15 days	Methotrimeprazine contributed to reduced pain disability.
Houde & Wallenstein, 1955 (88)	Severe cancer pain	34	Compared chlorpromazine, morphine, and their combination	Case control, double-blind	Placebo medication, reference analgesic (morphine)	Self-report of pain intensity	Hrs	Chlorpromazine had no analgesic effect and did not potentiate morphine analgesia.
Moertl & coworkers, 1972 (91)	Cancer pain	100	Compared promazine (50 mg), aspirin, and other nonnarcotic oral analgesics	Case control, double-blind	Placebo medication	Self-rated % pain relief for 6 hrs after each drug	6 hrs	Promazine (50 mg) orally had no analgesic activity and did not potentiate aspirin.
Cavenar & Meltabie, 1976 (93)	Cancer pain	2	Haloperidol added to clinical treatment regimen	Open label, case studies	None	Self- and observer report of pain, activity	1 mo	Haloperidol associated with decreased pain report, increased activity.
Daw & Cohen-Cole, 1981 (94)	Cancer pain	1	Haloperidol added to clinical treatment regimen	Open label, case study	None	Self- and observer report of pain, function	6 mos	Haloperidol associated with decreased pain report, improved function.

The Dundee group (68) also explored the ability of phenothiazines to potentiate a narcotic analgesic, meperidine (Demerol). Promazine slightly but significantly increased the analgesic activity of meperidine at 60–90 min after injection. Other phenothiazine derivatives (propiomazine, trifluoperazine) had no effect on meperidine analgesia. An important finding was that perphenazine and promethazine were strongly antianalgesic and diminished the therapeutic effect of meperidine when given in combination with the narcotic.

A later placebo-controlled, crossover trial (71) reported that promethazine, promazine, and propiomazine were not of themselves significantly analgesic and did not enhance meperidine analgesia. This report replicated the finding that promethazine strongly antagonized meperidine analgesia.

Postsurgical Pain Many clinical studies of the analgesic and narcotic-potentiating properties of neuroleptics consist of single-dose trials with limited follow-up. Methotrimeprazine, a congener of chlorpromazine, is the only phenothiazine with replicable analgesic properties in postoperative pain. One double-blind multiple-dose study (72) of 66 postoperative and postpartum patients concluded that 15 mg of methotrimeprazine subcutaneously was equivalent to 10 mg of morphine sulfate. A similar controlled study of 197 postoperative patients (73) yielded equivalent results.

The balance of the controlled investigations on other antipsychotic drugs indicates that promethazine, promazine, and propiomazine have no analgesic activity and do not enhance narcotic analgesia (74, 75) in the clinical setting. The one study reporting a therapeutic effect of these agents confounded analgesia and sedation, making it difficult to assess the results (76). The one placebo-controlled double-blind study of chlorpromazine for postoperative pain (77) is uninterpretable because of the likelihood of a carryover effect from previously administered analgesics and the lack of statistical analysis.

It is important to note that even analgesics of proven efficacy may decrease laboratory-induced pain threshold by no more than 30% over placebo (78, 79). Nevertheless, the data from studies both of experimentally induced and of acute clinical pain demonstrate that most neuroleptic drugs do not provide clinically relevant analgesia. In addition, some of these agents, such as promethazine, which is used commonly in postoperative patients to "potentiate" narcotic analgesia, lack analgesic properties and may antagonize narcotic analgesia. Methotrimeprazine is an exception to this rule. Methotrimeprazine, apaprently alone among the phenothiazines assessed, is analgesic, but it confers no advantage over narcotics in acute pain and has not had widespread clinical acceptance.

Chronic Pain The risk of tardive dyskinesia must be considered before employing antipsychotic agents to treat chronic pain. Although the daily dosages of antipsychotic medications indicated in chronic pain are small, the cumulative amounts pose some risk, and lasting dyskinesias may appear even after brief treatment (80). This problem is discussed in detail later (see "Treatment Approaches"). Investigations of neuroleptic medications for chronic pain syndromes focus on chronic headaches, neuropathic disorders, and cancer-related pain.

Headaches Hakkarainen (81) reported a placebo-controlled trial of fluphenazine (Prolixin) (1 mg daily) for chronic tension headache. Fluphenazine produced significant decreases in self-reports of headache duration, intensity, and frequency.

An open-label study (82) of chlorpromazine in treatment-resistant cluster headache patients reported that oral doses of 75–700 mg daily uniformly induced a remission, and suppression of headache continued for at least 8 months in some patients. Although the lack of placebo control and the possibility of spontaneous remission contaminate these results, the persistent benefit in some patients indicates that more rigorous trials should be considered. Similarly, an uncontrolled trial of intramuscular chlorpromazine (1 mg/kg) for acute migraine attacks demonstrated complete relief of pain, nausea, and emesis within 1 hr in the vast majority of patients (83). A sizable percentage of patients experienced orthostatic hypotension. There is no evidence that chlorpromazine is effective for migraine prophylaxis.

Neurologic Disorders Several anecdotal reports suggest that phenothiazine or butyrophenone antipsychotic agents, when used in combination with TCAs, are effective for deafferentation syndromes (84, 85). In selected cases, diabetic peripheral neuropathy, postherpetic neuralgia, and similar conditions are reported to respond to combination therapy, whereas treatment with a tricyclic agent alone was ineffective (7, 84). Suggested combinations include amitriptyline (25–75 mg) plus fluphenazine (1–3 mg) (7, 8, 84) or imipramine (25–75 mg) with haloperidol (Haldol) (1–3 mg) (10). The use of an antipsychotic agent alone is less likely to be helpful in these conditions.

Cancer Pain Pain in cancer arises from direct effects of tumor (e.g., compression, infiltration) or as a side effect of treatment (e.g., postirradiation neuropathy). Neuroleptics, with the exception of methotrimeprazine (72), lack analgesic properties in pain secondary to direct effects of tumor (15, 88–90). For example, Moertl et al. (86), rigorously compared single doses of promazine, aspirin, acetaminophen, and other nonnarcotic oral analgesics in ambulatory patients suffering mild to moderate cancer-related pain. Promazine was chosen as the reference antipsychotic because it was one of the few phenothiazines to show promise in studies using experimentally induced pain (67). Aspirin was superior to all other tested agents for relief of cancer pain. Oral promazine has no analgesic activity (91), and did not potentiate the effect of aspirin (86).

In addition, the controlled studies by Houde and Wallenstein (88) of hospitalized cancer patients in severe pain demonstrated that chlorpromazine alone had no significant analgesic effect and did not promote the analgesic activity of morphine.

The butyrophenones are neuroleptic drugs structurally related to meperidine. Haloperidol in preliminary animal models augments opiate analgesia (92). Anecdotal reports (93–97) indicate that haloperidol can reduce or eliminate narcotic requirements and reverse clinical depression in cancer pain patients, but controlled trials are not available.

In summary, most neuroleptic drugs have limited efficacy as primary analgesics or as adjuncts to narcotic analgesia. Many studies supporting the use of neuroleptics to potentiate or replace opiate analgesia neither exploit a crossover design (73, 75, 76, 98) nor have a placebo control (71, 75, 76, 90, 98–100), and use low or inadequate doses of a reference analgesic (73, 74, 77) or confound sedation and analgesia (99).

Some of the rationale for using neuroleptics derived from hopes that troublesome aspects of narcotic use (tolerance, addiction, emesis, and respiratory depression) would be avoided. Data suggest, however, that addictive behavior initiated by prescription narcotics is rare (100) and that escalation of narcotic requirements by a cancer patient more often indicates progression of the malignancy rather than drug tolerance. Acute adverse reactions (sedation, restlessness, hypotension) to phenothiazines are more common and severe than those attributed to narcotics (71, 73–75, 90, 92, 98–101) and phenothiazines amplify these side effects of narcotics. Although some chronic headache and deafferentation syndromes may respond to antipsychotics, clinical trials with homogeneous populations would be needed to clarify the efficacy of these drugs, and the risk of tardive dyskinesia argues against their prolonged use.

Mechanism of Action

The therapeutic mechanism of action of neuroleptic medications for pain syndromes is unclear. Antidopaminergic activity may explain the analgesic effects of methotrimeprazine in acute pain, although other neuroleptic agents with similar ability to block dopamine neurotransmission are not analgesics. The membrane-stabilizing properties of antipsychotic drugs may account for their therapeutic effects in some deafferentation syndromes (50,

51). When a TCA is being coadministered, the neuroleptic may simply increase serum concentrations of the TCA, or may provide an independent or synergistic effect. Obviously the ability of neuroleptics to reduce extreme anxiety may be therapeutic when anxiety amplifies their pain complaints.

ANTIANXIETY AND SEDATIVE AGENTS

Three classes of antianxiety drugs are used in pain syndromes. These are the benzodiazepines [chlordiazepoxide (Librium), diazepam (Valium), clonazepam (Clonopin), and others]; the diphenylmethane derivatives [hydroxyzine (Vistaril)], and the barbiturates (phenobarbital, secobarbital, and others). The benzodiazepines have generally replaced the barbiturates in routine clinical care. The rationale for antianxiety agents is to treat anxiety secondary to pain; or to alleviate the painful muscular spasm and muscular contraction in low back pain and tension headache presumed to be a response to anxiety. These medications also show promise in the treatment neuralgias, perhaps by reducing neuron firing rates. An overview of outcome studies is described in Table 8.4.

Benzodiazepines and Hydroxyzine

Acute Pain

Experimentally Induced and Clinical Pain Diazepam has neither primary antinociceptive effects nor ability to potentiate the antinociceptive activity of narcotic analgesics in animal models (102, 103). Nevertheless, diazepam decreases the affective response to pain and potentiates this property of opiates in animal paradigms (104) and in experimentally induced pain in humans (105, 106). Chapman and Feather (105) noted that diazepam (10 mg orally) prolonged tolerance to experimentally induced pain significantly more than did placebo and aspirin, and diminished pain-associated anxiety better than did placebo. Gracely et al. (106) confirmed that diazepam reduced the affective response to experimentally induced pain without altering sensory sensitivity. The use of benzodiazepines as adjuvants for reducing the affective response to acute clinical (e.g., postoperative) pain, however, has not been widely investigated. Clinical experience indicates that benzodiazepines are often useful in anxious postoperative patients, and that reduction of anxiety helps diminish pain complaints.

Hydroxyzine is a diphenylmethane derivative having antihistaminic, antiemetic, spasmolytic, and anxiolytic activity. In animals hydroxyzine, like the benzodiazepines, has minimal analgesic activity and an inconsistent ability to enhance opiate analgesia, but it potentiates opiate reduction of the affective component of pain (104).

Results of studies in clinical pain are equivocal. Hydroxyzine (100 mg orally) is equivalent to placebo in relieving postoperative pain, and does not potentiate oral meperidine (107) or alter meperidine pharmacokinetics or metabolism (108). Hydroxyzine (100 mg parenterally) is reported to be superior to placebo and equivalent to very low dose morphine (8 mg) in patients suffering severe pain (109). Two studies indicate hydroxyzine (100 mg intramuscularly) combined with morphine produced greater pain relief than morphine alone (109, 110). Nevertheless, in these studies the addition of hydroxyzine to morphine did not increase the percentage of patients who reported better than 50% reduction in pain. The combination did, however, produce significantly greater drowsiness, which may have confounded pain reports.

Thus, hydroxyzine (75–100 mg parenterally) may have an analgesic effect equivalent to 8–10 mg of morphine. Hydroxyzine administration causes sedation and marked discomfort at the injection sites, and subcutaneous administration can produce severe tissue damage. Because of these liabilities and the limited data for therapeutic efficacy, the routine use of hydroxyzine to potentiate opiate analgesia in acute pain cannot be recommended.

Chronic Pain In controlled studies Lance and coworkers (21, 22) concluded that both diazepam and chlordiazepoxide were superior to placebo (but inferior to TCAs) for relief of chronic tension headache. A more recent controlled trial (111) also indicated that diazepam (10–15 mg orally) is superior to placebo for relief of chronic tension headache. By comparison, one carefully controlled study of a small, heterogeneous sample of chronic pain patients found neither chlordiazepoxide nor hydroxyzine to be superior to placebo for relieving nonheadache pain or improving mood (112).

Given the extensive use of benzodiazepines it is surprising that there are so few rigorous studies of their efficacy, indications, interactions with other treatments, therapeutic mechanisms, and liabilities. Hollister et al. (113) suggested that diazepam produces extended relief in chronic pain from musculoskeletal disorders and is rarely associated with abuse. Others argue that conventional measures such as heat, rest, and nonnarcotic analgesics are as effective as diazepam, and that even high doses of this drug do not produce clinically detectable skeletal muscle relaxation (114). Furthermore, Hendler et al. (115) reported significantly more evidence of cognitive impairment in chronic pain patients receiving diazepam than in those receiving narcotic analgesics. The clinical impact and reversibility of benzodiazepine-associated deficits in cognitive functioning, memory, and motor-perceptual performance deserves much further investigation. This is especially important since many chronic pain management programs emphasize behavioral approaches that require intact cognitive skills.

A substantial number of uncontrolled trials support the effectiveness of clonazepam for treatment of chronic neuropathic pain, particularly cranial neuralgias (116–118). Responsive syndromes include trigeminal neuralgia, sphenopalatine ganglion neuralgia, and diverse neuropathies (119). These preliminary reports are encouraging, but limitations of the data include their open design, the difficulty in assessing the magnitude of functional improvement, and the limited follow-up (120).

The relative efficacy of benzodiazepines compared to

Table 8.4
Antianxiety Agents: Populations, Experimental Design, and Treatment Outcome

Authors	Population	N	Interventions	Design	Control	Dependant Measures	Follow-up	Results
	Acute Pain							
Chapman & Feather, 1973 (105)	Experimentally induced pain in nonpatients	30	Diazepam compared to aspirin and placebo	Double-blind, group outcome	Placebo and reference analgesic	Self-report of pain (0–4 scale), pain tolerance	Hrs	Diazepam (10 mg p.o.) prolongs tolerance to pain, diminishes pain-associated anxiety; does not alter sensory sensitivity.
Gracely & coworkers, 1978 (106)	Experimentally induced pain in dental patients	16	Compared pain intensity and quality before and after diazepam	Group outcome, within-subject	Within-subject, no treatment	Verbal descriptions of affective & sensory quality of pain; match handgrip force to pain intensity	Hrs	Diazepam reduced affective response to pain without altering sensory perception.
Beaver & coworkers, 1976	Postoperative patients	96	Single dose of hydroxyzine alone and in combination with morphine	Double-blind, group outcome	Placebo medication	Self-report & observer ratings of pain	Hrs	Hydroxyzine (100 mg i.m.) was superior to placebo and equivalent to morphine (8 mg); hydroxyzine analgesia additive to morphine analgesia.
Hupert & coworkers, 1980 (110)	Postoperative patients	82	Compared hydroxyzine (100 mg) in combination with morphine to morphine alone	Double-blind, group outcome	Morphine	Self-report pain intensity (0–3) and pain relief (0–4)	Hrs	Hydroxyzine (100 mg i.m.) with morphine gave significantly greater analgesia than morphine alone; combination did not increase percentage of patients reporting >50% pain reduction; increased drowsiness with hydroxyzine confounded analgesia.
Kantor & Steinberg, 1976 (107)	Postoperative patients	82	Compared oral hydroxyzine (100 mg) with meperidine, and placebo	Double-blind, group outcome	Placebo medication	Self-report pain intensity	Hrs	Hydroxyzine (100 mg p.o.) equivalent to placebo.
	Chronic Pain							
Lance & coworkers, 1964, 1965 (21, 22)	Tension headache	280	Compared chlordiazepoxide, diazepam, amitriptyline, imipramine, placebo	Double-blind, group outcome	Placebo medication	Self-report of improvement	Up to 12 mos	Chlordiazepoxide and diazepam superior to placebo.
Weber, 1983	Tension headache	19	Compared diazepam and placebo	Double-blind, group outcome	Placebo medication	Self-report of improvement	3 wks	Diazepam superior to placebo in producing improvement.
Yosselson-Superstine & coworkers, 1985 (112)	Mixed chronic cancer & noncancer	9	Compared chlordiazepoxide, hydroxyzine, prochlorperazine	Double-blind, group outcome	Placebo	Self-report of pain (0–5), Multiple Adjective Affect Checklist (MAACL)	8 wks	No overall differences between study drugs and placebo on any dependent measure; individual comparisons reveal anxiety and depression lower with chlordiazepoxide vs. placebo.

other drugs for treatment of selected neuropathic pain syndromes is an important therapeutic issue. One controlled report indicated that both imipramine and amitriptyline (100 mg) outperformed diazepam (15 mg) in relieving painful diabetic peripheral neuropathy (13). Additional studies are needed to fully assess the apparently promising role of benzodiazepines in some neuropathic pain states.

Mechanism of Action Benzodiazepines increase the ability of γ-aminobutyric acid (GABA) to inhibit brain and spinal cord neurotransmission; they also inhibit cholinergic and monoaminergic pathways (121). Since GABA is thought to mediate presynpatic and postsynpatic inhibition and facilitate recurrent inhibition (122), benzodiazepines might decrease the central transmission of ascending noxious stimuli, or inhibit firing peripherally in aberrant neurons. The anxiolytic effects are mediated by poorly understood mechanisms, perhaps by inhibitory effects on the limbic system.

CENTRAL NERVOUS SYSTEM

The most common stimulants now in medical use are the amphetamines [d,l-amphetamine (Benzedrine), d-amphetamine (Dexedrine), and methamphetamine (Methedrine)] and the related compound methylphenidate (Ritalin). The amphetamines and methylphenidate are used primarily for attention-deficit disorders and hyperactivity associated with minimal brain dysfunction in children, and in narcolepsy. Cocaine has traditional use as a local anesthetic, and caffeine appears in numerous combinations with analgesics. Evidence with regard to efficacy is described in Table 8.5.

Acute Pain

Psychostimulants lack primary analgesic properties (123). Amphetamines potentiate narcotic and nonnarcotic analgesia in animals (124, 125) and in humans (126–128), presumably by catecholaminergic mechanisms (124). Several laboratories (126, 127) have demonstrated that dextroamphetamine enhances the analgesic effect of morphine in experimentally induced pain in humans. With regard to clinical pain, a single-dose study of postoperative patients concluded that the combination of dextroamphetamine (10 mg parenterally) and morphine (10 mg) was twice as potent as morphine alone, and a combination with 5 mg of dextroamphetamine was one and one-half times as potent as a given dosage of morphine (128). There were minimal effects on blood pressure, pulse, and respiratory rate. Because of the study design, the effects of longer term use of amphetamine on mood, appetite, sensorium, and other aspects of postoperative convalescence could not be addressed.

Cocaine has a long history of use as a primary abortive agent for acute cluster headache, via topical cocainization of the sphenopalatine fossa. Because the therapeutic mechanism depends on local anesthesia, conventional topical anesthetics such as lidoxaine (Xylocaine) are now preferred (129).

Caffeine may be a useful addition to nonsteroidal anti-inflammatory analgesics. A review of the results of single-dose trials in over 10,000 patients suffering from episiotomy pain indicated that caffeine (100–200 mg orally) increased the analgesic potency of aspirin and acetaminophen by 40% (130). Oral dosages up to 600 mg/day of caffeine cause few side effects. Thus caffeine may be a useful adjunct to mild analgesics in acute pain.

Chronic Pain

Brompton's mixture, a variable combination of cocaine with morphine and a phenothiazine, has been advocated for chronic cancer pain (131). There is no systematic evidence that this combination is superior to morphine alone (132). Cocaine retards the gastrointestinal absorption of morphine; since tolerance to the sedating effects of opiates usually develops rapidly, cocaine is not required for its alerting properties.

More recently a placebo-controlled study in cancer patients with persistent pain demonstrated that methylphenidate (15 mg daily) added to a regimen of narcotic analgesia decreased pain intensity by an additional 20% (133). This study evaluated patients only during a 3-day trial. Therefore a recommendation for general longer term use of these adjuvants must await studies assessing effects and benefits.

There is some evidence that psychostimulants are effective antidepressants in depressed psychiatric and medically ill subjects (134). Recent anecdotal reports (135–137) indicate that dextroamphetamine (2–20 mg/day) and methylphenidate (20 mg/day) are effective antidepressants in hospitalized medically ill patients both with depressive symptoms and with major depression related to medical illness. Improved mood, reduced focus on pain, and renewed interest in rehabilitation occurred in about 50% of patients within 2–7 days. The major side effect was confusion, which developed in demented patients. Most patients were treated for about 1 week, although some required longer therapy.

Mechanism of Action

The mechanism of action of stimulants is unclear. The therapeutic effects probably result from activation of monoamine systems important in pain suppression. Amphetamines exert their effects directly by stimulating adrenergic receptors, and indirectly by releasing catecholamines and inhibiting their degradation by the enzyme monoamine oxidase. Cocaine appears to inhibit the neuronal reuptake of norepinephrine, thereby potentiating the activity of this neurotransmitter. Caffeine has direct and indirect effects similar in kind to those of the amphetamines, but obviously less potent.

SUMMARY

In summary, it is important to realize that this review has been conservative. It may well underestimate therapeutic effects of psychotropic agents in many pain syndromes. Several experimental factors may mask actual

Table 8.5
Psychostimulants: Populations, Experimental Design, and Treatment Outcome

Authors	Population	N	Interventions	Design	Control	Dependant Measures	Follow-up	Results
	Acute Pain							
Ivy & coworkers, 1944 (126)	Experimentally induced pain in nonpatients	30	Dextroamphetamine added to morphine	Double-blind, group outcome	Morphine	Self-report of pain intensity	Hrs	Dextroamphetamine improved morphine analgesia.
Evans, 1962 (127)	Experimentally induced pain in nonpatients	24	Dextroamphetamine (10 mg) added to morphine	Double-blind	Morphine	Self-report of pain intensity	Hrs	Dextroamphetamine improved morphine analgesia.
Forest & coworkers, 1977 (128)	Postoperative patients	450	Single dose of dextroamphetamine (5–10 mg) added to morphine	Double-blind, group outcome	Morphine	Observer and self-rated pain intensity	Hrs	Dextroamphetamine (10 mg) doubled analgesic activity of morphine (10 mg).
Johnstone, 1974 (171)	Postoperative patients	60	Single dose of methylphenidate	Open label, anecdotal case studies	None	Self-report of pain intensity	Hrs	Methylphenidate produced analgesia.
Dodson & Fryer, 1980	Postoperative patients	63	Single dose of methylphenidate (0.4 mg/kg parenterally)	Double-blind	Placebo medication	Self-report of pain, observer-rated alertness	Hrs	Methylphenidate did not produce analgesia at 30 or 180 min postoperatively. Alertness improved at 30 min only.
Laska & coworkers, 1984 (103)	Postpartum pain	>10,000	Caffeine added to aspirin, acetaminophen, or salicylamide	Double-blind, group outcome	Aspirin, acetaminophen, salicylamide	Self-rated pain (0–3 scale)	Hrs	Caffeine (100–200 mg p.o.) increased relative potency of analgesic by 40%.
Kaufman & coworkers, 1982 (136)	Hospitalized medically ill patients with major depression secondary to illness, with and without pain	5	Dextroamphetamine or methylphenidate given daily	Open label, case studies	None	Unspecified assessment of mood, activity, pain	4 wks	Dextroamphetamine (2–20 mg/kg daily) and methylphenidate (10–20 mg/kg daily) improved mood, increased activity, and reduced pain report.
Woods & coworkers 1986 (137)	Hospitalized medically ill patients with major depression secondary to illness, with and without pain	66	Dextroamphetamine or methylphenidate given daily	Retrospective chart review	None	Clinical response of depression	1–87 days	Dextroamphetamine (2–20 mg/kg daily) and methylphenidate improved mood, increased activity, and reduced pain report.
	Chronic Pain							
Bruera & coworkers, 1987 (137)	Outpatients and inpatients with advanced cancer and chronic cancer pain	32	Methylphenidate added to narcotic analgesics	Randomized, double-blind, crossover	Placebo medication	Self-rated pain intensity; narcotic intake; self-estimate of anxiety, depression, activity	3 days	Methylphenidate (15 mg daily) significantly improved analgesia and activity, decreased extra doses of narcotic, decreased sedation.

therapeutic effects. First, given the limits of present diagnostic methods, drug-responsive and nonresponsive subtypes of disorders may be lumped under a common name (e.g., low back pain). Benefits for responsive subtypes could be lost when overall group outcome is determined. Second, problems such as extreme variability of outcome scores, small sample size, or pretreatment between-group differences may obscure significant results. In addition, some drugs produce a therapeutic effect only after 6 weeks or more of treatment. Patients not followed longitudinally may appear to be treatment failures. Also, these agents may improve a variable that is not being assessed (e.g., activity level), while not altering a measured variable (e.g., mood or pain report).

In the next section, "Treatment Approaches," I emphasize psychopharmacologic treatments that have solid support in controlled studies, but also indicate less-proven alternatives worth exploring.

TREATMENT APPROACHES

TRICYCLIC ANTIDEPRESSANT AGENTS

The indications for tricyclic antidepressants are described in Table 8.6, and the compounds and dosages in Table 8.7.

Properties and Side Effects

Tricyclic antidepressants (TCAs) were derived from neuroleptics: imipramine, the first TCA, represents a modification of chlorpromazine, and amitriptyline was derived from imipramine. Maprotiline (Ludiomil) and amoxapine

Table 8.6
Diagnostic Indications for Psychotropic Drug Treatment in Acute and Chronic Pain

Treatment	Relatively Well Established Clinical Efficacy[a]	Possible Clinical Efficacy[b]
Tricyclic antidepressants	*Chronic pain* Atypical facial pain Diabetic neuropathy Postherpetic neuralgia Migraine headache Tension headache Mixed migraine-tension Primary major depression with secondary pain Major depression secondary to chronic pain	*Acute pain* Augment narcotics *Chronic pain* Thalamic pain Other neuropathic pain Augment narcotics
MAO inhibitors	*Chronic pain* Atypical facial pain Primary major depression with secondary pain Major depression secondary to chronic pain	*Chronic pain* Migraine headache
Lithium carbonate		*Chronic pain* Chronic cluster headache
Neuroleptics	*Acute pain* Severe anxiety or delirium after surgery *Chronic pain* Psychosis with delusional pain Tension headache[c]	*Acute pain* Acute migraine *Chronic pain* Neuralgia-neuropathy Thalamic pain
Antianxiety agents	*Acute pain* Acute anxiety *Chronic pain* Tension headache	*Acute pain* Muscular-skeletal strain *Chronic pain* Chronic anxiety
Stimulants	*Acute pain* Augment narcotics[c]	*Chronic pain* Depression-pain syndromes

[a] Effectiveness established in controlled trials.
[b] Effectiveness reported in open label studies.
[c] Effective but not recommended for use because of toxicity.

Table 8.7
Commonly Used Antidepressants

Tricyclics	Usual Daily Oral Dose in Pain Treatment (mg)	Usual Daily Antidepressant Dose (mg)
Tertiary amines		
Imipramine (Tofranil)	10–75	150–250
Amitriptyline (Elavil)	10–75	150–250
Doxepin (Sinequan)	10–75	150–250
Secondary Amines		
Desipramine (Norpramin)	10–75	100–250
Nortriptyline (Aventyl)	10–75	100–150
Maprotiline (Ludiomil)	a	150–200
Atypical		
Trazodone (Desyrel)	a	
Monoamine Oxidase Inhibitors		
Tranylcypromine (Parnate)	10–30	10–30
Phenelzine (Nardil)	15–90	45–90
Lithium Carbonate	300–1200	900–2400

[a] Experience insufficient to determine usage. Probably below usual antidepressant dose.

(Asendin) are variations on the basic TCA structure and are clinically and pharmacologically similar to imipramine (138). These agents increase serotonergic and/or noradrenergic tone by blockade of serotonin and norepinephrine reuptake at presynaptic nerve endings, may increase norepinephrine or serotonin receptor density or sensitivity, and may reduce β-adrenergic receptor sensitivity (139). The TCAs also have strong anticholinergic properties, producing autonomic, cardiac, and central nervous system side effects. Autonomic effects include dry mouth, blurred vision, constipation, ileus, and urinary retention. Cardiovascular effects include orthostatic hypotension, increased heart rate, and repolarization abnormalities on the electrocardiogram (Q-T interval prolongation and T wave inversion or flattening). Atrial and ventricular arrhythmias, as well as conduction delay with bundle branch block, may occur. This results from prolongation of the H-V interval, the time from activation of the bundle of His to activation of ventricular myocardium. These effects resemble the properties of Type I cardiac antiarrhythmics, such as quinidine and procainamide (140). The TCAs also can depress myocardial contractility. Central nervous system effects can include agitated states (not uncommon in elderly patients, perhaps because there is less plasma protein binding of the drug in the elderly and higher plasma concentrations) and deliria caused by an anticholinergic brain syndrome. Other common side effects are weight gain, delayed ejaculation, and impotence. Extrapyramidal symptoms are rare.

Selected Drug Interactions

Sympathomimetic Amines Tricyclic antidepressants potentiate the pressor response of direct-acting amines like norepinephrine, epinephrine, and phenylephrine (141), with possible hypertensive crisis characterized by hypothermia, sweating, severe headache, and cerebrovascular accident.

Neuroleptics Since TCAs and neuroleptics compete for the same hepatic metabolic pathways, their anticholinergic and hypotensive properties may be additive or potentiated (142).

Sedative-Hypnotics Tricyclic antidepressants increase the central nervous system and respiratory depressant activity of barbiturates and related sedatives (142, 143) and increase the toxicity and potential lethality of these agents.

Propranolol Tricyclic antidepressants may potentiate propranolol-induced depression of myocardial contractility and hypotension from central vasomotor regulatory centers (145), and patients with migraine headaches treated with these combinations should be monitored closely.

Opiates Tricyclic antidepressants potentiate meperidine-induced respiratory depression in animals (143), and increase anticholinergic activity of opiates.

Pretreatment Evaluation

Patients over the age of 50 or who have a history of cardiovascular disease (stroke, myocardial infarction, angina, congestive heart failure, syncope, or arrhythmias) should have an electrocardiogram (ECG) and standing and supine blood pressures before treatment. Careful assessment of the risk/benefit ratio and cardiology consultation are indicated in the presence of bradyarrhythmias, heart block, or very long Q-T intervals. Orthostatic blood pressure changes of over 10 mm Hg before drug treatment are associated with pronounced postural changes during treatment, and these patients should be carefully observed. A careful drug history should be obtained, not only to assess possible drug interactions, but to determine past response and reactions to TCAs. Additional laboratory investigation should include a complete blood count with differential and liver function tests.

Drug Selection

Amitriptyline, nortriptyline, imipramine, desipramine, and doxepin are probably equally effective in the pain syndromes for which they are indicated. Additionally, these agents all have approximately equivalent antidepressant efficacy. Drug selection therefore depends on side effects. In general, anticholinergic, cardiac, and central nervous system side effects are more common with tertiary amines (amitriptyline, imipramine, and doxepin) than with demethylated secondary amines (nortriptyline, desipramine, and others). Thus desipramine is the least anticholinergic and sedating of the tricyclic drugs. Patients with agitation or insomnia may benefit more from sedating drugs. There is some evidence that nortriptyline is less likely to depress H-V conduction and less likely to produce orthostatic hypotension (at the serum concentrations usually employed to treat depression) than other TCAs (145). Nortriptyline may thus be preferred in patients with bradyarrhythmias, heart block, or prolonged Q-T interval. Doxepin is also thought to be relatively noncardiotoxic, but that is not well documented. All TCAs will increase heart rate secondary to adrenergic and anticholinergic effects. Furthermore, imipramine suppresses ventricular arrhythmias (ectopy), and patients on quinidine may need their dosage of that agent revised.

Some second-generation antidepressants [e.g., trazodone (Desyrel)] are structurally unrelated to and exert their action through mechanisms different from tricyclic drugs. The efficacy of these agents for chronic pain syndromes has not been adequately assessed. Although their antidepressant efficacy approaches that of the first-generation agents (amitriptyline and imipramine), most patients with responsive pain syndromes or depression should be treated initially with a first-line drug. Claims of an improved safety record for second-generation antidepressants await documentation. Indeed, two of these newer drugs, nomifensine (Merital) and buproprion (Wellbutrin), have been withdrawn recently because of serious side effects.

Treatment Technique for Acute Pain

Although desipramine may potentiate opiate analgesia in acute pain, the practical clinical significance of this is undetermined, and there is no present reason to use TCAs in acute pain.

Treatment Technique for Chronic Pain

Initial Treatment of the Nondepressed Pain Patient
Pain patients without evidence of complicating medical or psychiatric disorders are generally started on a dose of amitriptyline or imipramine at 10–25 mg at night, with 10–25-mg increases every 3 days to a maximum of 75 mg daily. The drug is usually given at bedtime to take advantage of any sedating effects, although doses initially may be divided if a single dose produces excessive side effects. Elderly patients or those with cardiovascular disease should receive a 10–25-mg test dose and have orthostatic blood pressure determinations taken 1 hr later.

A therapeutic response usually ensues within 2 weeks, often within 5–7 days. Follow-up appointments are at least every week during the initial month of treatment, with orthostatic blood pressure determinations or ECGs as warranted. Every-other-week appointments are useful in the next month of therapy.

If no benefit appears within 3–4 weeks, or if side effects are unusually severe, a determination of the plasma concentration of the antidepressant is warranted. Plasma concentrations may be used to check compliance, improve efficacy, diminish toxicity, and detect unsuspected drug interactions (146). This allows the clinician to assess if an alternative therapy is indicated, or if an increase or decrease in dose is necessary. The practitioner should use an experienced laboratory and have his own history of interpreting results from this laboratory.

The most effective plasma concentrations of antidepressants for pain syndromes generally are thought to be below those usually therapeutic for depression. Therapeutic levels for treating depression with amitriptyline are 200 ng/ml total TCA (amitriptyline plus nortriptyline); for nortriptyline there may be a therapeutic window of efficacy between 50 and 150 ng/ml. Concentrations below or above this interval may be ineffective for an antidepressant response. With imipramine, concentrations exceeding 225 ng/ml are therapeutic in depression; doxepin therapeutic concentrations are uncertain, but perhaps in the range of 150–250 ng/ml.

Blood samples drawn for plasma concentrations of antidepressants should reflect steady state levels, and a patient's dosage should have been stabilized for at least 1 week. Samples are obtained 10–16 hr after a single dose, or 2–5 hr after the morning dose if a divided dosage regimen is employed.

Other indications for a plasma concentration include patients with cardiovascular disease, who may warrant routine plasma monitoring because of being at increased risk for toxicity.

Maintenance Treatment A positive response warrants treatment for about 5–6 months. The maintenance dose should be the minimum effective level after control is established. Attempts to discontinue the TCA should be made at 6-month intervals thereafter, since some neuropathic syndromes spontaneously remit or no longer require treatment. One important exception appears to be atypical facial pain, which appears to require prolonged treatment (over 1 year) to maintain relief (28). The TCA should be discontinued over a 2–3-week period, to avoid an abstinence syndrome.

Treatment Nonresponse An inadequate response is

defined as less than 50% reduction in pain, providing there is clinical or laboratory evidence of adequate dosage, after a 3–4-week trial. The antidepressant should be changed to a drug of different class (i.e., if a serotonergic agent is used first, then the switch would be a noradrenergic drug) for another 3–4-week trial. Alternatively, an adjunctive neuroleptic drug may be added to the TCA regimen. (This technique is described in the section on "Neuroleptics," below.) The usual neuroleptics used are haloperidol (0.5–3 mg daily) or fluphenazine (0.5–3 mg daily). Results of adjunctive therapy should be evident within 2 weeks. Other combinations reported to be successful are nortriptyline with carbamazepine (Tegretol) or diphenylhydantoin (Dilantin) (126). If this combination therapy is unacceptable because of side effects or concerns about tardive dyskinesia, and if alternative TCAs have not been helpful, a regimen of clonazepam (usually 1–3 mg daily) is indicated. Conventional anticonvulsants (diphenylhydantoin, carbamazepine) are the drugs of third choice for most practitioners because of unfamiliarity with the drug used and need for closer monitoring of plasma drug concentrations.

Initial Treatment of the Depressed Pain Patient All depressed patients should be evaluated for suicidality and the need for hospitalization. Prescriptions for TCAs should be monitored closely according to the concern about suicide, and hospitalization may be indicated. Tricyclic antidepressant overdoses amounting to 1000 mg produce serious side effects and those of 2000 mg of any tricyclic commonly are lethal. If the symptoms do not meet criteria for major depression, the clinician may decide to treat a TCA-responsive pain syndrome at the usual low dosages of TCA recommended for that disorder, with the view that as the patient's pain remits, so might the depressive symptoms. If the patient has a major depression then full antidepressant dosages should be commenced. We usually still begin at a lower initial dosage of, say, 25 mg of imipramine and increase by 25–50 mg every 3 days to a final dose of 150–300 mg daily. Hospitalized patients may receive higher initial dosage with 50-mg increases daily up to the full amount.

An antidepressant effect is evidenced by improved activity, energy, and mood, and should appear within 3–6 weeks. Reduction of pain intensity may lag behind improvement in activity and mood by several weeks, and is not a target symptom in this instance. As above, plasma antidepressant concentrations would be indicated for a poor response after 6 weeks or if severe side effects intervene.

Maintenance Treatment A maintenance dose of a TCA is usually about 25% lower than the acute antidepressant dosage (138). Treatment is maintained for about 5–6 months (the usual length of an affective episode), and the antidepressant is then discontinued (147). Again, tapering off a TCA regimen over several weeks is indicated to avoid an abstinence syndrome.

Treatment Nonresponse Further treatment of the depressed pain patient who does not respond to initial therapy is a complex topic beyond the scope of this handbook. An experienced psychiatric consultation to reevaluate the diagnosis and treatment regimen is indicated. If the treatment of depression is still indicated, the choices include adding liothyronine (Cytomel) (25–50 μg) to the TCA or switching to another antidepressant of a different class, with or without adding liothyronine; considering electroconvulsive therapy; switching to a MAOI; or attempting combination therapy using lithium or a MAOI with a TCA (138).

A Note on the Dexamethasone Suppression Test The dexamethasone suppression test (DST) was developed as a laboratory aid to assist in the diagnosis of depression, based on the finding that approximately 50% of patients with major depression do not suppress plasma cortisol concentrations below 5 μg/dl after receiving dexamethasone (1 mg orally) (148). The procedure involves administering dexamethasone (1 mg) at 11 PM and obtaining blood samples for cortisol concentration at 8 AM, 4 PM, and 11 PM the following day. Any one concentration above 5 μg/dl is regarded as abnormal or positive. The test has a high sensitivity (the percentage of patients with major depression who have a positive test), and a lower specificity (the percentage of patients without major depression who also have a positive test). The proportion of patients with dementia who have an abnormal DST is 40%; agoraphobia, 15–30%; alcohol use and abstinence, 20–30%; and acute psychological stress, up to 30%. Medications and medical illness also confound interpretations of test results. False-positive tests may result from barbiturates, anticonvulsants, fever, other acute medical illness, diabetes mellitus, and discontinuation of TCAs. False-negative tests may occur with indomethacin (Indocin) (149). Chronic pain by itself does not appear to affect the DST (150).

About 40–50% of chronic pain patients with major depression will have a positive DST, if confounding psychiatric and medical illnesses or medications are excluded (151, 152). The clinical utility of the DST is limited because of these confounding factors. Possible uses of the test are to confirm a diagnosis of major depression in pain patients in whom other psychiatric or medical causes have been excluded, or to follow the response of depressed patients being treated with antidepressants. As the patient begins to respond clinically to treatment, the DST should revert to normal. A partial clinical response, but failure of the DST to become normal, may indicate a higher risk of relapse. The DST does not predict which patients are most likely to respond to treatment.

MONOAMINE OXIDASE INHIBITORS

The indications for MAOIs are described in Table 8.6, and the compounds and doses in Table 8.7.

Properties and Side Effects

Monoamine oxidase inhibitors, like the TCAs, enhance the availability of norepinephrine and serotonin in the brain by inhibiting their catabolism. Antidepressant activity may also be related to effects on norepinephrine and serotonin postsynaptic receptor function or sensitivity.

In psychiatric populations the major indications for MAOIs are agoraphobia with or without panic attacks, the so-called atypical depressive disorders with "reversed" vegetative symptoms (increased sleep, weight gain, reactive mood), and depression that has not responded to trials of TCAs. The MAOI side effect profile is similar to that of the TCAs but of a lesser degree, and includes postural hypotension, agitation, confusion, and mild anticholinergic symptoms: blurred vision, dry mouth, constipation, ileus, and urinary retention. The major issue in using these agents is the need to instruct patients to avoid foods or medications containing pressor amines. Because the MAOIs block metabolism of tyramine and other pressor amines, a hypertensive crisis may ensue after their ingestion, manifested by abrupt and severe hypertension and possible subarachnoid hemorrhage. Proscribed foods include cheese (except cottage cheese and cream cheese), pickled foods, beer and red wines, and fava beans (153).

Selected Drug Interactions

Sympathominetic Agents All medication with sympathominetic activity, including phenylephrine and ephedrine (found in cold tablets), can produce a hypertensive crisis.

Narcotic Analgesics The so-called type I interaction is a potentiation of primary narcotic effects (including analgesia, hypotension, respiratory depression, and coma) as a result of MAOI inhibition of hepatic metabolism of narcotics (140, 154). Naloxone (Narcan) reverses this response. Phenelzine may be safer in this regard than other MAOIs.

The type II interaction is similar to that resulting from administration of sympathomimetic amines or tyramine to patients on MAOIs. The concurrent use of MAOIs and meperidine (155, 156) or dextromethorphan (157) produces agitation, excitement, restlessness, hypertension, headache, rigidity, and convulsions. The mechanism of this response is unknown but it may be mediated by increased brain serotonin release (158).

Codeine may be used safely in patients on MAOIs who require moderate analgesia (153). If other narcotics are mandatory only 20–25% of the usual therapeutic narcotic dose should be used and vital signs and level of consciousness should be observed carefully (153). Meperidine should never be used since its interaction with MAOIs is too unpredictable and life-threatening complications can occur rapidly.

Sedative-Hypnotics Monoamine oxidase inhibitor inhibition of microsomal enzymes prolongs the effects of sedative hypnotics, including barbiturates and chloral hydrate (159). Lower doses of sedative hypnotics and close monitoring is advised.

Pretreatment Evaluation

The physical and laboratory evaluation is similar to that used for TCAs, with a special emphasis on drug and dietary history, the patient's ability to comply with the complex dietary restrictions, and cardiovascular status.

Drug Selection

Phenelzine and tranylcypromine are the most commonly prescribed agents. Tranylcypromine is sometimes preferred because it is much shorter acting and will be out of a patient's system within a day. Phenelzine continues to inhibit MAO for over a week after it is discontinued.

Treatment Technique for Chronic Pain

Initial Treatment Monoaxmine oxidase inhibitors are not the drug of first choice for any chronic pain syndrome. They are most often used in complex cases that have failed alternative treatments. It is recommended that appropriate consultations be obtained to reevaluate the patient's diagnosis at the start. Thus, neurologic consultation is indicated to confirm a diagnosis of a facial pain or migraine syndrome and a psychiatric consultation is useful if a depressive or anxiety syndrome complicates the picture. Serious side effects from use of MAOIs are relatively rare, and their danger has probably been overstated.

Most treatment failures are secondary to inadequate dosage. The clinical end point for correct dosage is mild postural hypotension and muscle fasciculations after the second week of treatment. The ususal dosage of phenelzine for initial treatment is up to 90 mg/day. Treatment begins with 15 mg on day 1, 30 mg on day 2, and 15 mg in the morning and 30 mg in the evening on day 3, if the patient is asymptomatic. A dose of 45 mg daily is maintained until day 14 if there are no side effects, and then the dosage is increased to 30 mg each morning and 30 mg in the evening; on day 21 the dosage can be increased to 30 mg in the morning, 15 mg in the afternoon, and 30 mg in the evening; on day 28 the dosage can be increased to 30 mg three times daily if there are no side effects. After adequate or maximum dosage is achieved, the patient should be monitored weekly for another 4–6 weeks (153).

Maintenance Treatment There are few data regarding proper maintenance dosages for pain syndromes. Psychiatric patients with responsive syndromes often experience a relapse of symptoms at dosages below the initial optimal regimen (153). As with other treatments, an attempt should be made every 6 months to discontinue the medication, cutting back by 15 mg every 1–3 weeks until the patient is off the drug.

Treatment Nonresponse Another MAOI may be used. Monoamine oxidase inhibitors have been combined with various medications, including TCAs and L-tryptophan. It is difficult to evaluate the efficacy of these combinations, and both TCAs and tryptophan may provoke a hypertensive crisis. There are no data that such combinations are useful in chronic pain syndromes. The primary indication for combination therapy would be a nonresponsive depressive disorder. A TCA is usually added cautiously to ongoing MAOI therapy.

LITHIUM

The indications for lithium treatment are described in Table 8.6, and the dosages in Table 8.7.

Properties and Side Effects

Lithium is a monovalent cation in the same group in the periodic table of elements as are sodium and potassium. It is excreted by the kidney. The lithium ion has no known physiologic role. It has widespread effects on brain amine metabolism: it inhibits synaptic release of dopamine and norepinephrine, increases the synaptic reuptake and turnover of norepinephrine and serotonin, and inhibits central nervous system adenylate cyclase. It is not known whether any of these actions is associated with its therapeutic effect (138).

The major indication for the use of lithium is in psychiatric patients with bipolar affective disorder, in whom it decreases the severity and frequency of episodes.

Initial treatment is associated with transient and mild gastrointestinal side effects, including diarrhea and nausea, fine motor tremor, and somnolence. Other side effects include polyuria and polydipsia, weight gain, hypothyroidism, edema, and leukocytosis.

Central nervous system effects may include extrapyramidal symptoms, including rigidity and tremor. Cardiovascular effects are repolarization abnormalities (T wave flattening and inversion) and inhibition of conduction at the sinoatrial node. The only cardiac contraindication is the sick sinus syndrome, wherein lithium is associated with severe bradycardia (133). Concern about nephrotoxic effects of lithium (interstitial fibrosis, tubular atrophy, glomerulosclerosis) appears to have been largely unwarranted.

Selected Drug Interactions

Analgesics Phenylbutazone (Butazolidin) and indomethacin increase serum lithium levels and can provoke frank lithium toxicity. Changes in plasma lithium levels with ibuprofen (Motrin) are inconsistent and relatively minor (160). There is no reported lithium interaction with opiates, although both agents can diminish thyroid function and antagonize antidiuretic hormone.

Sedative-Hypnotics Hydroxyzine potentiates lithium's effect on cardiac repolarization and can precipitate cardiovascular toxicity. It is recommended that this combination be avoided (161). At therapeutic lithium levels there are no reported interactions with other sedative-hypnotics.

This describes but a few of the drug interactions pertinent to lithium. More comprehensive sources should be reviewed before prescribing this agent, particularly in the medically ill pain patient (e.g., ref. 138).

Pretreatment Evaluation

The patient's cardiovascular history should be evaluated and an ECG should be obtained. A complete blood count, electrolytes, and creatinine should be obtained since lithium is fully excreted by the kidneys. Lithium toxicity most often is a result of sodium depletion, since lithium and sodium are absorbed at the same site in the proximal renal tubule. Sodium loss secondary to diarrhea, diuretics, excessive perspiration, or dehydration may produce lithium toxicity. Thyroid function tests (triiodothyronine, thyroxine, thyroid-stimulating hormone) should be obtained every 3–6 months. Lithium should not be prescribed to pregnant patients, especially in the first trimester, since it is associated with fetal cardiovascular abnormalities. Lithium is excreted in the breast milk in clinically significant amounts, and is a hazard to nursing infants.

Treatment Technique

Lithium is clearly a second line agent. Recurrent cluster and perhaps migraine headache syndromes constitute the only convincing reports of its effectiveness. The patient should be instructed that close monitoring of blood levels of lithium is necessary and that therapeutic effects may not be apparent for several weeks. For headache syndromes, the dosage indicated is that needed to keep blood levels within a range of 0.4–0.8 mEq/liter. The customary starting dose is 300 mg twice or three times daily. The usual total daily dosage ranges from 600 to 2400 mg/day, usually given in two equal divided doses. Blood samples for lithium concentration should be taken 12 hr after the last dose. At the beginning of treatment, blood levels are monitored twice weekly for several weeks, then once monthly. After the patient has been stable for 6–12 months lithium levels may be obtained as is clinically indicated. Symptoms of lithium toxicity include emesis, diarrhea, tremor, muscle weakness, dysarthria, vertigo, ataxia, and hyperreflexia. The elderly are particularly susceptible to toxicity, and lithium should be kept in the low therapeutic range for older patients. Lithium does not have proven effectiveness in the treatment of unipolar depression and is not indicated as an antidepressant in chronic pain patients with depressive symptoms complicating their illness.

Maintenance Treatment In psychiatric patients treatment with lithium has been maintained for years without loss of efficacy. However, there is evidence that therapeutic efficacy decays after 1–2 years in headache syndromes. The lowest possible dose consistent with a therapeutic effect is indicated. The patient's thyroid and renal status should be monitored every 3–6 months.

Nonresponse to Treatment Carbamazepine has been used in psychiatric patients who have not responded to lithium for bipolar disorder, and in treatment of diverse neuropathic pain disorders (162). It is unknown whether this agent is therapeutic in cyclical headache syndromes nonresponsive to lithium. Some psychiatric patients who do not benefit from lithium alone improve when a TCA, or carbidopa-levodopa (Sinemet), or bromocriptine (Parlodel) is added to lithium to augment the noradrenergic system. L-tryptophan has been added to lithium to augment serotonergic effects (138). The efficacy of these combinations in affective disorders is not well documented, and their value in treating chronic pain syndromes is purely speculative.

NEUROLEPTIC AGENTS

The indications for neuroleptic drugs are described in Table 8.6, and the compounds and dosages in Table 8.8.

Properties and Side Effects

Neuroleptics increase the central arousal threshold by suppressing afferent sensory transmission from the periphery. The most important pharmacologic effect is widespread inhibition of dopaminergic transmission in the central nervous system. Blockade of the nigrostriatal system produces extrapyramidal symptoms (tremor, rigidity, bradykinesia, akathisia, and dystonia). Blockade of the tuberoinfundibular system produces hyperprolactinemia with gynecomastia and lactation, and inhibition of pituitary gonadotropins. Blockade at the chemoreceptor trigger zone of the hypothalamus produces antiemetic properties. Blockade in the limbic system and associated cortex produces antianxiety and antipsychotic effects (163).

Neuroleptics also have anti-α-adrenergic and anticholinergic effects. These properties are most prominent with the aliphatic agents (e.g., chlorpromazine) and less so with piperadine and piperazine agents and the butyrophenones. Cardiovascular effects include increased heart rate and dose-related postural hypotension. Repolarization abnormalities of the electrocardiogram include T wave abnormalities, prolonged PQ-T intervals, and S-T segment depression. Direct myocardial depressant effects result in diminished myocardial contractility in patients with preexisting cardiovascular disease. Neuroleptic agents may alter conduction times and induce potentially fatal ventricular arrhythmias. Cognitive defects on timed tasks include diminished performance on tests of speed, reaction time, and accuracy.

Idiosyncratic allergic responses can occur, with suppression of the hematopoietic system (leukopenia, anemia, or thrombocytopenia). These reactions usually occur within the first 6 weeks of treatment and their clinical hallmark is the sudden onset of painful pharyngitis and fever. Similarly, an allergic hepatotoxicity with mild increases in liver function tests can occur, and cholestatic jaundice is reported.

The most commonly encountered clinical side effects are the extrapyramidal symptoms, the dystonias, and tardive dyskinesia. Extrapyramidal symptoms can be managed with antiparkinsonism agents [benztropine mesylate (Cogentin), trihexphenidyl (Artane)], diphenhydramine (Benadryl), or amantadine (Symmetrel). The antiparkinsonism drug should not be given prophylactically. Extrapyramidal symptoms often do not occur, especially at the low doses of neuroleptics prescribed to pain patients, and the antiparkinsonism agent can produce adverse anticholinergic effects (toxic megacolon, toxic psychosis). If these agents are used, the usual daily dose is 1–6 mg benztropine mesylate daily or 2–10 mg trihexphenidyl daily. Because of anticholinergic toxicity, some clinicians prefer treating extrapyramidal symptoms with diphenhydramine (10–25 mg three times daily) or amantadine (100 mg once to three times daily), reserving the antiparkinsonism drugs for symptoms not responsive to less toxic agents (163). If such symptoms are treated, it is recommended that these drugs be tapered or discontinued after 3 months.

Dystonia (tonic contraction of muscles, especially involving the head and neck with grimaces, posturing, and torticollis) rarely occurs in the low dosages used in pain patients. It can be treated with diphenhydramine (25–50 mg intramuscularly). Akathisia, the sensation of an inability to sit still, responds best to dose reduction of the offending drug (163).

Tardive dyskinesia is a syndrome of involuntary choreiform movements that commence after prolonged treatment with neuroleptics and persist up to years after the neuroleptics are withdrawn. Symptoms can include periodic

Table 8.8
Commonly Used Neuroleptics

Class	Relative Potency	Usual Daily Oral Dose in Pain Treatment (mg)
Phenothiazines		
Chlorpromazine (Thorazine)	Low	10–50
Methotrimeprazine (Levoprome)	Low	10–50
Thioridazine (Mellaril)	Low	10–75
Perphenazine (Trilafon)	High	1–5
Trifluoperazine (Stelazine)	High	1–5
Fluphenazine (Prolixin)	High	1–3
Butyrophenones		
Haloperidol (Haldol)	High	1–3

tongue protrusions, lip smacking, chewing movements of the mouth, athetoid movements of the fingers, and restless shifting from leg to leg. In their severe form such movements can be disabling. The mechanism is unknown but may involve dopaminergic receptor supersensitivity or excessive dopaminergic activity in the basal ganglia. Treatment with various agents has been only sporadically effective. The best approach is prevention (163). Elderly patients appear to be at higher risk for this disorder. Dosages for the neuroleptics should be kept below 5 mg daily of the high-potency agents or the equivalent in the low-potency agents. Treatment should be limited to months and not years.

Selected Drug Interactions

Nonnarcotic Analgesics There are no apparent adverse drug interactions between nonnarcotic analgesics and neuroleptics, although acetaminophen inhibits chlorpromazine metabolism and therefore augments its effects.

Narcotic Analgesics Phenothiazines enhance and prolong the hypotensive and respiratory depressant effect of narcotics. Chlorpromazine also increases serum levels of the neurotoxic and cardiotoxic N-demethylated metabolites of meperidine, which are associated with neuromuscular irritability, seizures, bradycardia, and hypotension.

Pretreatment Evaluation

The medical evaluation is the same as that for candidates for TCAs, including ECG for patients over age 50 or those with preexisting heart disease, and genitourinary assessment for benign prostatic hypertrophy. These drugs are metabolized by the liver, and patients with hepatic disease will need lower dosages. Laboratory assessment should include baseline complete blood count with differential, and liver function tests.

Drug Selection

Drug selection depends upon the side effect profile, since these agents are generally equivalent for major therapeutic effects. The clinician need select only one neuroleptic in each classification and become thoroughly familiar with its properties and usage. There is some concern that thioridazine (Mellaril) is especially cardiotoxic (164).

Treatment Techniques for Acute Pain

Initial Treatment Generally, these agents are used only to manage severe postoperative agitation or anxiety, or disruptive behavior. In a patient with acute pain, the first task should be to assess the analgesic regimen, since agitation may be related to inadequate analgesia. A postoperative delirium must also be considered. Because of their low incidence of autonomic and cardiovascular complications, the high-potency neuroleptics (e.g., haloperidol) are generally preferred. Customary doses are 0.5–2.5 mg haloperidol orally, administered every 30 min to 1 hr until adequate sedation is achieved. As a guide to further dosage, the total dosage needed to sedate the patient is calculated. The next dose should be about one-half this total amount, given 12 hr after sedation is achieved. If severe anxiety or agitation reemerges then this amount is given at that point. After sedation is achieved dosages can be rapidly tapered to 1–3 mg daily (165). Treatment rarely extends beyond 2 or 3 days.

Another acute indication for neuroleptics is the acute management of severe migraine attacks. Because of its sedative effects the usual agent is chlorpromazine (50–100 mg orally or intramuscularly). An acute attack is usually aborted within 1 hr.

Treatment Techniques for Chronic Pain

Initial and Maintenance Treatment There is evidence that neuroleptics are effective for primary treatment of tension headaches, or adjunctive treatment of neuropathic pain (e.g., postherpetic neuralgia, diabetic neuropathy). Because of the risks of tardive dyskinesia, we avoid their use in headache syndromes and use neuroleptics only for treatment-resistant neuropathic pain. We prefer to employ neuroleptics only after a trial of two different classes of TCAs (e.g., desipramine and nortriptyline) has produced unsatisfactory relief. We add a high-potency neuroleptic to the chosen TCA. Generally we use fluphenazine or haloperidol; the starting dose is 0.5–1 mg at night, with an increase to 1 mg twice daily after 3–5 days, or to 1 mg three times daily if there is no improvement after 10 days. Once the maximum dose of 3 mg daily is reached, this is given as a one-time dose at bedtime. There should be a response within 2–3 weeks. If there is no response with a neuroleptic from one drug class (e.g., fluphenazine) the clinician may switch to an agent from a different class (e.g., haloperidol). Some authorities employ low-potency/high-dose aliphatic agents such as methotrimeprazine, a congener of chlorpromazine. The usual dosage is 50 mg or less, given once daily at bedtime (166). At present, assessing neuroleptic plasma drug concentration is not clinically useful.

The patient should be carefully monitored for symptoms of tardive dyskinesia. After 3 months, the dosage should be tapered to the lowest therapeutic amount. At no more than 6 months we taper the patient off the neuroleptic and observe for an increase in pain. If continued treatment is needed the maintenance dosage should be at the lowest possible amounts, with periodic attempts to discontinue the neuroleptic.

Neuroleptics are indicated for psychiatric patients with chronic pain on a delusional basis, such as patients with paranoid schizophrenia, whose pain has been fully evaluated and is thought to represent a hallucinatory experience. The complaint is often phrased in biazarre terms (e.g., originating from electrodes implanted by the FBI, or other similar persecutory ideas). The patient with schizophrenia should be treated with a neuroleptic dosage adequate to control the major features of his psychosis. The delusion of pain may persist, but the patient's emotional distress as evidenced by this discomfort should diminish.

Eradication of the delusion itself should not be the goal of therapy. Additionally, patients with multiple infarct dementia or other dementing illnesses occasionally develop complaints of pain as symptoms of depression, as psychotic delusions, or as fixed ideas upon which they perseverate (167). Neuroleptics may be used in low dosages (e.g., haloperidol, 2–3 mg daily) to reduce the agitation and anxiety associated with pain complaints in demented patients. It goes without saying that physical illness is often silent and undetected in patients with schizophrenia and dementia, and all efforts should be made to determine the etiology of the patient's complaint (167).

Treatment Nonresponse Some clinicians would prefer to use clonazepam if TCAs fail, and to avoid TCA-neuroleptic combinations. The usual dosage range is 1–3 mg daily. A response should occur within 3 weeks. If no response occurs, then a trial of a conventional anticonvulsant (e.g., diphenylhydantoin or carbamazepine) is indicated.

ANTIANXIETY DRUGS

The indications for anxiolytic drugs are described in Table 8.6, and the compounds and dosages in Table 8.9.

Benzodiazepines

Properties and Side Effects The benzodiazepines have a broad spectrum of pharmacologic activity. Their primary effect is to enhance GABA-mediated presynaptic and postsynaptic inhibition. This action occurs in spinal cord, brainstem, cerebellar cortex, cerebral cortex, and other structures. The major properties of these drugs are their antianxiety, anticonvulsant, and sedative effects, along with an ability to produce centrally induced muscle relaxation. Like other sedatives, all benzodiazepines have the potential to produce tolerance, psychological as well as physical dependence, and an abstinence syndrome upon withdrawal. Their effects are additive with those of other central nervous system depressants, and cross-tolerance and cross-dependence develop.

Sudden discontinuation of benzodiazepines after prolonged, uninterrupted use can produce an abstinence syndrome. The syndrome consists of insomnia, nausea, myalgia, muscle twitching, diaphoresis, and potentially major motor seizures. The probability of developing a withdrawal syndrome appears to vary with the length of treatment: patients treated for less than 4 months at the usual therapeutic dosage are unlikely to develop symptoms; about 5% of those treated for up to 1 year may develop symptoms; and those treated for over 1 year run a much higher risk (168).

The most common side effects are sedation, ataxia, and dysarthria. In the elderly these agents may produce confusion and paradoxical excitement. Teratogenic effects (i.e., cleft palate) during pregnancy are postulated but are not thoroughly documented. There are few autonomic side effects, although bradycardia and hypotension can occur. Allergic phenomena are also reported, and include neutropenia and jaundice.

Drug Interactions The most important interactions involve additive effects with other central nervous system depressants. Cimetidine (Tagamet), disulfiram (Antabuse), and oral contraceptives can increase the half-life of benzodiazepines.

Pretreatment Evaluation In patients for whom benzodiazepines are acutely indicated the major concern is for

Table 8.9
Commonly Used Antianxiety Agents

	Usual Daily Oral Antianxiety Dose in Pain Treatment (mg)	Usual Oral Hypnotic Dose (mg)
Benzodiazepines		
Long Half-life		
Clorazepate (Tranxene)	3–15	15–30
Flurazepam (Dalmane)	—	15–30
Intermediate Half-life		
Chlordiazepoxide (Librium)	15–30	50
Diazepam (Valium)	2.5–15	15–30
Short Half-life		
Alprazolam (Xanax)	0.5–3.0	—
Lorazepam (Ativan)[a]	2–5	—
Oxazepam (Serax)[a]	10–50	30–60
Other		
Hydroxyzine	100–400	—

[a] No active metabolites.

the patient's ability to tolerate the central nervous system depressive effects of the drug. The major concern in candidates for prolonged treatment is misuse or abuse. Elderly patients are particularly at risk for falls due to intoxication and ataxia as well as to acute confusional episodes. Such side effects may occur at relatively low dosages because of the elderly patient's reduced rate of drug metabolism and reduced protein binding. A cardiovascular history and ECG should be obtained as indicated: benzodiazepine withdrawal can precipitate angina, elevated blood pressure, or cardiac arrhythmias. Liver function tests should be obtained and patients with liver disease may require a diminished dose.

Drug Selection All benzodiazepines have similar anxiolytic properties, side effect profiles, and potential for dependency and abuse. They differ mainly in their elimination half-life and presence of active metabolites. Those with the longest half-life are clorazepate (Tranxene), prazepam (Centrax), and halazepam (Paxipam). Moderately long-acting agents are diazepam and chlordiazepoxide. The shortest acting are oxazepam (Serax), lorazepam (Ativan), and alprazolam (Xanax). All these drugs have clinically important active metabolites except for oxazepam and lorazepam. The duration of action reflects the presence of active metabolites. Cumulative clinical effects occur with repeated dosage. If drug accumulation or prolonged effects are problems (as in elderly patients or those with hepatic disease), short-acting agents with no active metabolites may be preferred. The problems of drug accumulation also can be met by reducing the dosage of longer acting drugs. Again, the best clinical practice is to choose one or two agents and learn to employ them effectively. Overall the benzodiazepines have a good margin of safety. By themselves they are unlikely to be lethal in overdoses. Nevertheless their depressant effects are dangerous if they are taken with alcohol, barbiturates, or other drugs that depress the central nervous system.

Treatment Technique for Acute Pain In acute pain the indication is for severe postoperative anxiety or acute musculoskeletal strain.

Initial Treatment Acute postoperative anxiety often indicates insufficient analgesia. Assuming analgesia is adequate, situational acute fearfulness usually responds to diazepam (5–20 mg orally). This will usually produce an anxiolytic effect within 1 hr. If repeated dosage is necessary, the physician can follow the regimen described earlier for titration of antipsychotic drugs in the surgical patient. Diazepam is given each hour; the total dosage needed to produce sedation is calculated; then one-half that dosage is given approximately 12 hr later, or at the time anxiety returns. The drug is then tapered rapidly over the next few days. Most patients will do well on diazepam (5 mg two or three times daily). If treatment is needed beyond several days, the dosage required can usually be given once at bedtime: there will be an initial sedative effect, and because of the drug's prolonged half-life, and anxiolytic will persist throughout the following day. For the acute medical setting some authorities prefer a short-acting agent with no active metabolites, such as oxazepam (15 mg four times daily). Diazepam and chlordiazepoxide should be given orally or intravenously since intramuscular absorption is erratic and incomplete.

For the pain associated with muscle spasm, sedation with attendant muscle-relaxing effects can usually be achieved with diazepam (5–10 mg twice to three times daily). Treatment rarely extends beyond 2 weeks.

Treatment Techniques for Chronic Pain

Initial and Maintenance Treatment Trigeminal neuralgia may be responsive to clonazepam. The usual dosage is 1–3 mg daily, and a therapeutic effect is usually evident within 2 weeks. A major problem for many patients, particularly the elderly, has been oversedation on the dosage required for a therapeutic effect (118). Maintenance treatment is not well described, but probably should follow guidelines offered for other therapy of neuropathic pain. The lowest therapeutic dose should be maintained for 3–6 months; then an attempt to slowly discontinue the drug may be entertained.

Anxiety as a Special Problem Many patients with chronic pain appear to be acutely or chronically anxious as well. Chronic tension headaches and chronic back or neck pain, presumably related to painful muscular contraction, are two common clinical examples. We rarely employ antianxiety agents for these patients. Yet if anxiety is believed to be the major etiology of functional disability or of pain, and the clinician decides to institute treatment, then therapy should follow the principles outlined by Hollister (169) and others (170) for the proper use of benzodiazepines. Seven guidelines have been described (169): (a) use benzodiazepines only when indicated; (b) use nondrug methods when possible; (c) drug treatment should be brief and intermittent; (d) doses should be titrated individually; (e) efficacy should be assessed early; (f) avoid benzodiazepines if a history of drug abuse is known; and (g) gradually discontinue the drug after chronic treatment. This approach allows the physician to avoid the pitfalls of overprescribing.

Treatment with benzodiazepines is indicated when anxiety interferes with the patient's performing his usual life activities. Nonpharmacologic measures for managing anxiety include psychotherapy, exercise programs, relaxation training, and biofeedback. These methods are often components of a comprehensive pain management program, and can help reduce reliance on anxiolytics.

Ideal drug treatment is intermittent and brief. Most anxiety related to life stress is resolved within 1 month. Chronic anxiety, like chronic pain, waxes and wanes in intensity. Anxiolytics would be used only during exacerbations of the patient's chronic disorder. In any event, chronically anxious patients should not be treated indefinitely without assessing the need for continuous treatment. If prolonged therapy is needed, the lowest possible dosage consistent with efficacy should be used. In both acutely or chronically anxious individuals, a drug response generally occurs within the first 2–3 weeks of treatment, since state anxiety is usually more responsive than trait anxiety (170). Therefore if there is no improvement after several weeks on a proper regimen, then benefit is unlikely with prolonged therapy and other avenues should be explored. If anxiety is relieved the physician can propose that the drug be discontinued, and reinstituted if symptoms return. Thus tolerance and/or dependence are avoided (169).

Dose titration involves determining the minimum amount of drug necessary to produce mild sedation. Hollister (169) recommended initiating treatment at night, 2–3 hr before normal bedtime. The minimum effective dose is determined as the amount required to produce restful sleep when taken 2–3 hr before bedtime. If the initial dose does not produce effective hypnosis the first night, twice the dose is given the second night, four times the dose is given the third night, and eight times the dose is given the fourth night. The patient can commence with 2.5 mg diazepam and then increase to 5 mg, 10 mg, or 20 mg. The usual minimum effective hypnotic dose is 10 mg or less. As a result, the patient achieves a good night rest, unwanted oversedation is avoided during the daytime, and the anxiolytic effect is retained. If additional amounts are required during the day, usually one-half or one-third of the nighttime dose will suffice. This approach works best for long-acting benzodiazepines and is not suited for short-acting agents.

Treatment efficacy should be assessed within 3 weeks. Failure to respond may indicate an inadequate dosage regimen, or a misdiagnosis. For example, anxiety frequently accompanies depressive syndromes, and an antidepressant would be required to successfully treat this disorder. Alcohol abuse may also be present, and treatment may be undermined by the patient's tolerance to central nervous system depressants (169).

Patients with a past history of abuse of alcohol or other central nervous system depressants generally are not good candidates for benzodiazepines. Some authorities recommend short-term treatment with agents less likely to be abused, such as hydroxyzine.

Maintenance Treatment for Anxiety Some chronically anxious patients may benefit from long-term treatment. Again the minimum effective dose should be used; reevaluation of the regimen should occur at least every 6 months. Tolerance to anxiolytic effects may not occur. The clinician should be alert for requests for escalating the dose.

Patients who have been treated for more than 4 months with diazepam (20–40 mg daily) (or the equivalent) should be withdrawn slowly, usually over 4–6 weeks.

Buspirone (BuSpar) is a new anxiolytic chemically and pharmacologically unrelated to the benzodiazepines. Since maximum benefit emerges only after 3–4 weeks of treatment, it is advocated for chronic anxiety. Preliminary data indicate it has few central nervous system side effects. Its abuse potential is unknown.

CENTRAL NERVOUS SYSTEM STIMULANTS

Indications for psychostimulants are described in Table 8.6, and the compounds and dosages in Table 8.10.

Properties and Side Effects

Central nervous system stimulants include d,l-amphetamine (Dexedrine), methylphenidate (Ritalin), and pemoline (Cylert). They are rapidly absorbed orally. Methylphenidate has a half-life of 2–7 hr and dextroamphetamine 4–21 hr. They are metabolized by hepatic oxidation and conjugating enzyme systems and also are excreted unchanged in the urine. They produce cerebral stimulation and arousal by decreasing neuronal reuptake and deactivation of norepinephrine and dopamine. Physiologic dependence does not seem to occur in the same sense as with central nervous system depressants, although a withdrawal syndrome of inertia and depressed mood appears upon sudden withdrawal after high intake. Tolerance to euphoriant effects occurs rapidly (138). Side effects are those of anorexia, plus sympathomimetic actions. Other untoward effects include catatonia (mute and bizarre behavior), paranoid reactions, and confusion (171). These agents generally are thought to have fewer cardiovascular side effects (e.g., bundle branch block) than TCAs.

Drug Interactions

The ability of psychostimulants to compete for hepatic enzymes reduces the metabolism of TCAs, neuroleptics, antianxiety agents, and many other drugs. There are additive effects with other sympathomimetic drugs.

Pretreatment Evaluation

Patients over age 50 years and those with a history of hypertension or cardiovascular disease are at increased risk for the drug's sympathomimetic effects, and risk/benefit ratios must be carefully appraised. The elderly are particularly vulnerable to acute agitation or confusion. History of substance abuse must be elicited.

Drug Selection

There are few data available to help distinguish among the psychostimulants. Methylphenidate and pemoline may be less subject to abuse than are amphetamines (138). Because of its short half-life methylphenidate may be preferred in the elderly, to reduce duration of any toxic effects.

Table 8.10
Commonly Used Psychostimulants

	Usual Daily Antidepressant and Pain Management Dose (mg)
d-Amphetamine (Dexedrine)	10–20
Methylphenidate (Ritalin)	15–20

Acute and Chronic Pain

Initial and Maintenance Treatment The central nervous system stimulants have limited use in management of acute or chronic pain. Although they augment narcotic analgesia acutely, there really seems to be little advantage to these drugs since simply increasing the dose of analgesic accomplishes the desired goal.

These agents are not recommended for first-line, routine use in depressed pain patients because of their limited efficacy and risk of increasing agitation (138). If a TCA is contraindicated in a pain patient with a major depression, then a central nervous system stimulant may be employed. For pain control or depression the initial dose of dextroamphetamine or methylphenidate is usually 5–10 mg each morning. With its longer half-life dextroamphetamine may be given once daily, whereas methylphenidate is administered in two divided doses at 8 AM and noon. If no response occurs after 2 days, the dose is increased, but more than 20 mg daily is rarely required (137). A response should ensue by 7–10 days.

Maintenance treatment is not well described, and rarely extends beyond several weeks. Reports usually indicate that the agent is discontinued a few days after the patient becomes asymptomatic (137). Given the controversial nature of treatment with central nervous system stimulants the physician should carefully document his reasons for employing these drugs and his explanation to the patient of side effects and risk/benefit ratio. Treatment should be brief, prescription quantities limited in size, and follow-up frequent.

CONCLUSIONS

Pain is a multidimensional phenomenon. We know little about the basic mechanisms that produce or perpetuate the sensory component of pain following tissue damage, or of mechanisms relevant to the affective or behavioral response to the pain experience. A better understanding of these mechanisms is necessary to design specific and more effective psychopharmacologic treatments.

Four issues must be addressed to ensure appropriate use of psychotropic agents. First, as clear an understanding as is possible of the etiology of pain must be established to identify drug-responsive pain syndromes. Psychiatric disorders contributing to pain or disability must also be accurately diagnosed so that appropriate psychiatric target symptoms can be selected for treatment. Second, detoxification from excessive regimens of analgesics or sedative-hypnotic medications is essential for evaluating perceived pain, functional capacity, and treatment outcome. Third, psychopharmacologic medications are adjunctive treatment, and are not a substitute for a comprehensive treatment plan agreed upon with the patient, involving education, physical reconditioning, behavioral assessment, and evaluation of family and occupational roles. Fourth, few studies reporting initial therapeutic gains follow patients beyond the first weeks of treatment. This means that meticulous follow-up is necessary to detect recurrent symptoms or discontinue ineffective treatments. Psychopharmacologic treatment is effective if it leads to observable improvement in daily function, psychological symptoms, or diminished use of analgesics or other medical resources.

Acknowledgment Supported in part by the Veterans Administration and by USPHS Grant MH-30914 from the National Institute of Mental Health.

References

1. American Psychiatric Association: *Diagnostic and Statistical Manual*, ed 3. Washington, DC, American Psychiatric Association Press, 1978.
2. Saarnivaara L, Mattila MJ: Comparison of tricyclic antidepressants in rabbits: antinociception and potentiation of the noradrenaline pressor responses. *Psychopharmacology* 35:221–236, 1974.
3. Chapman CR, Butler SH: Effects of doxepin on perception of laboratory-induced pain in man. *Pain* 5:253–262, 1978.
4. Bromm B, Meier W, Scharein E: Imipramine reduces experimental pain. *Pain* 25:245–257, 1986.
5. Levine JD, Gordon NC, Smith R, McBryde R: Desipramine enhances opiate postoperative analgesia. *Pain* 27:45–49, 1986.
6. Woodforde JM, Dwyer B, McEwen BW, DeWilde FW, Bleasel K, Connelley TJ, Ho CY: Treatment of post-herpetic neuralgia. *Med J Aust* 2:869–872, 1965.
7. Davis JL, Lewis SB, Gerich JE, Kaplan RA, Schultz TA, Wallin JD: Peripheral diabetic neuropathy treated with amitriptyline and fluphenazine. *JAMA* 238:2291–2292, 1977.
8. Clark IMC: Amitriptyline and perphenizine (Triptafen DA) in chronic pain. *Anaesthesia* 36:210–212, 1981.
9. Dalessio DJ: Chronic pain syndromes and disordered cortical inhibition: effects of tricyclic compounds. *Dis Nerv System* 28:325–328, 1967.
10. Kocher R: Use of psychotropic drugs for treatment of chronic severe pain. In Bonica JJ, Albe-Fessard D (eds): *Advances in Pain Research and Therapy*, Vol 1. New York, Raven Press, 1976, pp 579–582.
11. Langohr HD, Stohr M, Petruch F: An open and double-blind cross-over study on the efficacy of clomipramine (Anafranil) in patients with painful mono- and polyneuropathies. *Eur Neurol* 21:309–317, 1982.
12. Watson CP, Evans RJ, Reed K, Merskey H, Goldsmith L, Warsh J: Amitriptyline versus placebo in postherpetic neuralgia. *Neurology* 32:671–673, 1982.
13. Kvinesdal B, Molin J, Froland A, Gram LF: Imipramine treatment of painful diabetic neuropathy. *JAMA* 251:1727–1730, 1984.
14. Turkington RW: Depression masquerading as diabetic neuropathy. *JAMA* 243:1147–1150, 1980.
15. Bourhis A, Boudouresque G, Pellet W: Pain infirmity and psychotropic drugs in oncology. *Pain* 5:263–274, 1978.
16. Couch JR, Hassanein RS: Amitriptyline in migraine prophylaxis. *Arch Neurol* 36:695–699, 1979.
17. Mathew NT: Prophylaxis of migraine and mixed headache. A randomized controlled study. *Headache* 21:105–109, 1981.

18. Friedman AP: The migraine syndrome. *Bull NY Acad Med* 44:45–62, 1968.
19. Mahloudji M: Prevention of migraine. *Br Med J* 1:182–183, 1969.
20. Gomersall JD, Stuard A: Amitriptyline in migraine prophylaxis. *J Neurol Neurosurg Psychiatry* 36:648–690, 1973.
21. Lance JW, Curran DA: Treatment of chronic tension headache. *Lancet* 1:1236–1239, 1964.
22. Lance JW, Curran DA, Anthony M: Investigations into the mechanism and treatment of chronic headache. *Med J Aust* 2:909–914, 1965.
23. Okasha A, Ghaleb HA, Sadek A: A double-blind trial for the clinical management of psychogenic headache. *Br J Psychiatry* 122:181–183, 1973.
24. Sternbach RA: *Pain Patients: Traits and Treatment*. New York, Academic Press, 1974.
25. Ward NG, Bloom VL, Friedel RC: The effectiveness of tricyclic antidepressants in the treatment of coexisting pain and depression. *Pain* 7:331–341, 1979.
26. Lindsay PG, Wyckoff M: The depression-pain syndrome and its response to antidepressants. *Psychosomatics* 22:571–577, 1981.
27. Raskin NH, Appenzeller C (eds): *Headache*. Philadelphia, WB Saunders, 1980.
28. Feinmann C, Harris M, Cawley R: Psychogenic pain: presentation and treatment. *Br Med J* 28:436–438, 1984.
29. Ward NG: Tricyclic antidepressants for chronic low back pain. *Spine* 11:661–665, 1986.
30. Alcoff J, Jones E, Rust P, Newman R: Controlled trial of imipramine for chronic low back pain. *J Fam Pract* 14:841–846, 1982.
31. Hameroff SR, Cork RC, Scherer K, Crago BR, Neuman C, Womble JK, Davis TP: Doxepin effects on chronic pain, depression and plasma opioids. *J Clin Psychiatry* 43:22–27, 1982.
32. Pheasant H, Bursk A, Goldfarb J, Azen SP, Weiss JN, Borelli L: Amitriptyline and chronic low back pain. *Spine* 8:552–557, 1983.
33. Sternbach RA, Janowsky DS, Huey LY, Segal DS: Effects of altering brain serotonin activity on human chronic pain. In Bonica JJ, Albe-Fessard D (eds): *Advances in Pain Research and Therapy*, Vol 1. New York, Raven Press, 1976, pp 601–606.
34. Jenkins DG, Ebbutt AF, Evans CD: Tofranil in the treatment of low back pain. *J Int Med Res* 4(Suppl 2):28–40, 1976.
35. Butler SH, Weil-Fugazza J, Godefoy F, Besson J-M: Reduction of arthritis and pain behavior following chronic administration of amitriptyline or imipramine in rats with adjuvant-induced arthritis. *Pain* 23:159–175, 1985.
36. MacNeill AL, Dick WC: Imipramine and rheumatoid factor. *J Int Med Res* 4(Suppl 2):23–27, 1976.
37. Gringas M: A clinical trial of Tofranil in rheumatic pain in general practice. *J Int Med Res* 4(Suppl 2):41–45, 1976.
38. McDonald Scott WA: The relief of pain with an antidepressant in arthritis. *Practitioner* 202:802–805, 1969.
39. Pilowsky I, Hallett EC, Bassett DL, Thomas PG, Penhall RK: A controlled study of amitriptyline in the treatment of chronic pain. *Pain* 14:169–179, 1982.
40. Blumer D, Heilbronn M, Pedraza E, Pope G: Systematic treatment of chronic pain with antidepressants. *Henry Ford Hosp Med J* 28:15–21, 1980.
41. Singh G, Verma HC: Drug treatment of chronic intractable pain in patients referred to a psychiatry clinic. *J Indian Med Assoc* 56:341–345, 1971.
42. Lindsay PG, Olsen RB: Maprotiline in pain-depression. *J Clin Psychiatry* 46:226–228, 1985.
43. Malseed R, Goldstein FJ: Enhancement of morphine analgesia by tricyclic antidepressants. *Neuropharmacology* 18:827–829, 1979.
44. Lee RL, Spencer PSJ: The effect of clomipramine and other amine-uptake inhibitors on morphine analgesia in laboratory animals. *Postgrad Med J* 53:53–60, 1977.
45. Liu SJ, Wang RIH: Increased analgesia and alterations in distribution and metabolism of methadone by desipramine in rats. *J Pharmacol Exp Ther* 195:94–104, 1975.
46. Gonzalez JP, Sewell RDE, Spencer PSJ: Antinociceptive activity of opiates in the presence of the antidepressant agent nomifensine. *Neuropharmacology* 19:613–618, 1980.
47. France RD, Urban BJ, Keefe FJ: Long-term use of narcotic analgesics in chronic pain. *Soc Sci Med* 19:1379–1382, 1984.
48. Urban BJ, France RD, Steinberger EK, Scott DL, Maltbie AA: Long-term use of narcotic/antidepressant medication in the management of phantom limb pain. *Pain* 24:191–196, 1986.
49. Pagni CA: Central pain due to spinal cord and brain stem damage. In Wall PD, Melzack R (eds): *Textbook of Pain*. London, Churchill Livingstone, 1984, pp 481–495.
50. Anderson LS, Black RG, Abraham J, Ward AA: Neuronal hyperactivity in experimental trigeminal deafferentation. *J Neurosurg* 35:444–452, 1971.
51. Loeser JD, Ward AA, White LE: Chronic deafferentation of human spinal cord neurons. *J Neurosurg* 29:48–50, 1968.
52. Anthony M, Lance JW: Monoamine oxidase inhibitors in the treatment of migraine. *Arch Neurol* 21:263–268, 1969.
53. Medina JL: Cyclic migraine: a disorder responsive to lithium carbonate. *Psychosomatics* 23:625–637, 1982.
54. Medina JL, Diamond S: Cyclical migraine. *Arch Neurol* 38:343–344, 1981.
55. Lascelles RG: Atypical facial pain and depression. *Br J Psychiatry* 112:651–659, 1966.
56. Raft D, Davidson J, Wasik J, Mattox A: Relationship between response to phenelzine and MAO inhibition in a clinical trial of phenelzine, amitriptyline and placebo. *Neuropsychobiology* 7:122–126, 1981.
57. Yung CY: A review of clinical trials of lithium in neurology. *Pharmacol Biochem Behav* 21(Suppl 1):57–64, 1984.
58. Nieper HA: The clinical applications of lithium orotate. A two year study. *Agressologie* 14:407–411, 1973.
59. Chazot G, Chauplannaz G, Biron A, Schott B: Migraines: treatment per lithium. *Nouv Presse Med* 8:2836–2837, 1979.
60. Peatfield RC, Rose FC: Exacerbation of migraine by treatment with lithium. *Headache* 21:140–142, 1981.
61. Damasio H, Lyon L: Lithium carbonate in the treatment of cluster headaches. *J Neurol* 224:1–8, 1980.
62. Ekbom K: Lithium for cluster headache: review of the literature and preliminary results of long-term treatment. *Headache* 21:132–139, 1981.
63. Medina JL, Fareed J, Diamond S: Blood amines and platelet changes during treatment of cluster headache with lithium and other drugs. *Headache* 18:112, 1978.
64. Kudrow L: Lithium prophylaxis for chronic cluster headache. *Headache* 17:15–18, 1977.
65. Mathew NT: Clinical subtypes of cluster headaches and response to lithium therapy. *Headache* 18:26–30, 1978.
66. Peatfield RC: Lithium in migraine and cluster headache: a review. *J R Soc Med* 74:432–436, 1981.
67. Moore J, Dundee JW: Alterations in response to somatic pain

associated with anaesthesia, Part VII: the effects of nine phenothiazine derivatives. *Br J Anaesth* 33:422–431, 1961.
68. Dundee JW, Love WJ, Moore J: Alterations in response to somatic pain associated with anesthesia, Part XV: further studies with phenothiazine derivatives and similar drugs. *Br J Anaesth* 35:597–609, 1963.
69. Moore J, Dundee JW: Alterations in response to somatic pain associated with anaesthesia, V: the effect of promethazine. *Br J Anaesth* 33:3–8, 1961.
70. Dundee JW, Moore J: Alterations in response to somatic pain associated with anaesthesia, I: an evaluation of a method of analgesimetry. *Br J Anaesth* 32:396–406, 1960.
71. Siker ES, Wolfson B, Stewart WD, Schaner PJ: The earlobe algesimeter, Part 2: the effect of pain threshold of certain phenothiazine derivatives alone or combined with meperidine. *Anesthesiology* 2:497–500, 1966.
72. Lasagna L, DeKornfeld TJ: Methotrimeprazine—a new phenothiazine derivative with analgesic properties. *JAMA* 178:887–890, 1961.
73. Minuck R: Postoperative analgesia—comparison of methotrimeprazine and meperidine as postoperative analgesia agents. *Can Anaesth Soc J* 19:87–96, 1972.
74. Keats AS, Telford J, Kurosu Y: "Potentiation" of meperidine by promethazine. *Anesthesiology* 22:34–41, 1966.
75. McZuitty FM: Relief of pain in labour. *J Obstet Gynaecol Br Commonw* 74:925–928, 1967.
76. Powe CE, Kiem IM, Fromhagen C, Cavanagh D: Propiomazine hydrochloride in obstetrical analgesia. *JAMA* 181:290–294, 1962.
77. Jackson GL, Smith DA: Analgesia properties of mixtures of chlorpromazine with morphine and meperidine. *Ann Intern Med* 45:640–652, 1956.
78. Bromm B, Seide K: The influence of tilidine and prazepam on withdrawal reflex, skin resistance reaction and pain rating in man. *Pain* 12:247–258, 1982.
79. Wolff BB, Kantor TG, Jarvik ME, et al: Response of experimental pain to analgesic drugs. I. Morphine, aspirin, and placebo. *Clin Pharmacol Ther* 1:224–238, 1966.
80. Baldessarini RJ: Drugs in the treatment of psychiatric disorders. In Gilman AG, Goodman LS (eds): *The Pharmacological Basis of Therapeutics*, ed 7. New York, Macmillan, 1985, pp 387–445.
81. Hakkarainen H: Fluphenazine for tension headache: a double-blind study. *Headache* 17:216–218, 1977.
82. Caviness VS, O'Brien P: Cluster headache: response to chlorpromazine. *Headache* 22:128–131, 1980.
83. Iserson KV: Parenteral chlorpromazine treatment of migraine. *Ann Emerg Med* 12:756–758, 1983.
84. Taub A: Relief of post-herpetic neuralgia with psychotropic drugs. *J Neurosurg* 39:235–239, 1973.
85. Merskey H, Hester RA: The treatment of chronic pain with psychotropic drugs. *Postgrad Med J* 48:594–598, 1972.
86. Moertel CG, Ahmann DL, Taylor WF, Schwartau N: Relief of pain by oral medications. *JAMA* 229:55–59, 1974.
87. Sigwald J, Bouther D, Solignac P: L'action antalgique des phenothiazines. *Therapie* 14:978–984, 1958.
88. Houde RW, Wallenstein SL: Analgetic power of chlorpromazine alone and in combination with morphine. *Fed Proc* 14:353, 1955.
89. Sadove MS, Levin MJ, Rose RF: Chlorpromazine and narcotics in the management of pain of malignant lesions. *JAMA* 155:626, 1954.
90. Beaver WT, Wallenstein SL, Houde RW, Schwartau N: A comparison of the analgesic effect of methrotimeprazine and morphine in patients with cancer. *Clin Pharmacol Ther* 7:436–446, 1966.
91. Moertel CG, Ahmann DL, Taylor WF: A comparative evaluation of marketed analgesic drugs. *N Engl J Med* 286:813–815, 1972.
92. Head M, Lal H, Puri S: Enhancement of morphine analgesia after acute and chronic haloperidol. *Life Sci* 24:2037–2043, 1979.
93. Cavenar JO Jr, Maltbie AA: Another indication for haloperidol. *Psychosomatics* 17:128, 1976.
94. Daw JL, Cohen-Cole S: Haloperidol analgesia. *South Med J* 74:364–365, 1981.
95. Maltbie AA, Cavenar JO Jr: Haloperidol and analgesia. *Milit Med* 142:946–948, 1977.
96. Maltbie AA, Cavenar JO Jr, Sullivan JL, et al: Analgesia and haloperidol: a hypothesis. *J Clin Psychiatry* 40:323–326, 1979.
97. Maltbie AA, Cavenar JO Jr, Hammett EB: Treatment of pain syndromes with haloperidol. *North Carolina J Ment Health* 8:50, 1977.
98. Montilla E, Frederik WS, Cass IJ: Analgesic effects of methotrimeprazine and morphine. *Arch Intern Med* 111:725–728, 1963.
99. McGee JL, Alexander MR: Phenothiazine analgesia—fact or fantasy? *Am J Hosp Pharm* 36:633–640, 1979.
100. Porter J, Jick H: Addiction rare in patients treated with narcotics. *N Engl J Med* 302:123, 1980.
101. Shader RI, DiMascio A (eds): *Psychotropic Drug Side Effects.* Baltimore, Williams & Wilkins, 1970, p 92.
102. Shannon HE, Holtzman SG, Davis DC: Interaction between narcotic analgesics and benzodiazepine derivatives on behavior in the mouse. *J Pharmacol Exp Ther* 199:387–399, 1976.
103. Weis J: Morphine antagonistic effect of chloridazepoxide (Librium). *Experientia* 25:381, 1969.
104. Morichi R, Pepeu G: A study of the influence of hydroxyzine and diazepam on morphine antinociception in the rat. *Pain* 7:173–180, 1979.
105. Chapman CR, Feather BW: Effects of diazepam on human pain tolerance and pain sensitivity. *Psychosom Med* 35:330–340, 1973.
106. Gracely RH, McGrath P, Dubner R: Validity and sensitivity of sensory and affective verbal pain descriptors: manipulation of affect by diazepam. *Pain* 5:19–29, 1978.
107. Kantor TG, Steinburg FP: Studies of tranquillizing agents (hydroxyzine and meprobamate) and meperidine in clinical pain. In Bonica JJ, Albe-Fessard D (eds): *Advances in Pain Research and Therapy*, Vol 1. New Yrk, Raven Press, 1976, pp 507–572.
108. Stambaugh JE, Wainer IW: Metabolic studies of the interaction of meperidine and hydroxyzine in human subjects. In Bonica JJ, Albe-Fessard D (eds): *Advances in Pain Research Therapy*, Vol 1. New York, Raven Press, 1976, pp 559–565.
109. Beaver WT, Feise G: A comparison of the analgesic effects of morphine, hydroxyzine and their combination in patients with post-operative pain. In Bonica JJ, Albe-Fessard D (eds): *Advances in Pain Research and Therapy*, Vol 1. New York, Raven Press, 1976, pp 553–557.
110. Hupert C, Yacoub M, Turgeon LR: Effect of hydroxyzine on morphine analgesia for the treatment of postoperative pain. *Anesth Analg* 59:690–696, 1980.
111. Weber MB: The treatment of muscle contraction headaches with diazepam. *Curr Ther Res* 15:210–216, 1973.
112. Yosselson-Superstine S, Lipman AG, Sanders SH: Adjunc-

tive anti-anxiety agents in the management of chronic pain. *Israeli J Med Sci* 21:113–117, 1985.
113. Hollister LE, Conley FK, Britt RH, Shuer L: Long-term use of diazepam. *JAMA* 246:1568–1570, 1981.
114. Greenblatt DJ, Shader RI, Abernathy DR: Current status of benzodiazepines. *N Engl J Med* 309:410–416, 1983.
115. Hendler N, Cimi C, Terence MA, Long D: A comparison of cognitive impairment due to benzodiazepines and to narcotics. *Am J Psychiatry* 137:828–830, 1980.
116. Caccia MR: Clonazepam in facial neuralgia and cluster headache. Clinical and electrophysiological study. *Eur Neurol* 13:560–563, 1975.
117. Smirne S, Scarlato G: Clonazepam in cranial neuralgias. *Med J Aust* 1:93–94, 1977.
118. Swerdlow M, Cundill JG: Anticonvulsant drugs used in the treatment of lancinating pain. A comparison. *Anesthesia* 36:1129–1132, 1981.
119. Martin G: Recurrent pain of a pseudotabetic variety after laminectomy for lumbar disc lesion. *J Neurol Neurosurg Psychiatry* 43:283–286, 1980.
120. Maciewicz R, Bouckoms A, Martin JB: Drug therapy of neuropathic pain. *Clin J Pain* 1:39–49, 1985.
121. Haefely WE: Behavioral and neuropharmacological aspects of drugs used in anxiety and related states. In Lipton MA, DiMascio A, Killam KF (eds): *Psychopharmacology: A Generation of Progress*. New York, Raven Press, 1978, pp 1359–1374.
122. Game CJA, Lodge D: The pharmacology of inhibition of dorsal horn neurones by impulses in myelinated cutaneous afferents in the cat. *Exp Brain Res* 23:75–84, 1975.
123. Goetzl FR, Burrill DY, Ivy AC: The analgesic effect of morphine alone and in combination with dextroamphetamines. *Proc Soc Exp Biol Med* 55:248–250, 1944.
124. Notl MW: Potentiation of morphine analgesia by cocaine in mice. *Eur J Pharmacol* 5:93–99, 1968.
125. Sigg EB, Capriob A, Schneider JA: Synergism of amines and anatgonism of reserpine to morphine analgesia. *Proc Soc Exp Biol Med* 97:97–100, 1958.
126. Ivy AC, Goetzl FR, Burril DY: Morphine-dextroamphetamine analgesia. *War Med* 6:67–71, 1944.
127. Evans WO: The synergism of autonomic drugs on opiate or opioid-induced analgesia: a discussion of its potential utility. *Milit Med* 127:1000–1003, 1962.
128. Forest WH, Brown BW, Brown CR, Defalque R, Gold M, Gordon HE, James KE, Katz J, Mahler DL, Schraff P, Teutsch G: Dextroamphetamine with morphine for the treatment of post-operative pain. *N Engl J Med* 296:712–715, 1977.
129. Kittrelle JP, Gouse DS, Seybold ME: Cluster headache. Local abortive agents. *Arch Neurol* 42:496–498, 1985.
130. Laska EM, Sunshine A, Mueller F, Elvers WB, Siegel C, Rubin A: Caffeine as an analgesic adjuvant. *JAMA* 251:1711–1718, 1984.
131. Saunders CM: *The Management of Terminal Disease*. Chicago, Year Book, 1979.
132. Melzack R: The Brompton mixture versus morphine solutions given orally: effect on pain. *Can Med Assoc J* 120:435–438, 1979.
133. Bruera E, Chadwick S, Brenneis C, Hanson J, MacDonald RN: Methylphenidate associated with narcotics for the treatment of cancer pain. *Cancer Treat Rep* 71:67–70, 1987.
134. Silverman EK, Reus VI, Jimerson DC: Heterogeneity of amphetamine response in depressed patients. *Am J Psychiatry* 138:1302–1306, 1981.
135. Katon W, Raskind M: Treatment of depression in the medically ill elderly with methylphenidate. *Am J Psychiatry* 137:963–965, 1980.
136. Kaufman MW, Murray GB, Cassem NH: Use of psychostimulants in medically ill depressed patients. *Psychosomatics* 23:817–819, 1982.
137. Woods SW, Tesar GE, Murray GB, Cassem NH: Psychostimulant treatment of depressive disorders secondary to medical illness. *J Clin Psychiatry* 47:12–15, 1986.
138. Baldessarini RJ: *Chemotherapy in Psychiatry: Principles and Practice*. Cambridge, MA, Harvard University Press, 1985.
139. Charney DS, Menkes DB, Heninger GR: Receptor sensitivity and the mechanism of action of antidepressant treatment: implications for the etiology and therapy of depression. *Arch Gen Psychiatry* 38:1160–1179, 1981.
140. Risch SC, Groom GP, Janowsky DS: Interfaces of psychoparmacology and cardiology, Part I; Part II. *J. Clin Psychiatry* 42:23–34; 47–59, 1981.
141. Boakes AJ, Laurence DR, Teoh PC, Barar FSK, Benedikter LT, Prichard BNC: Interactions between sympathomimetic amines and antidepressant agents in man. *Br Med J* 1:311–315, 1973.
142. Thornton WE, Pray RJ: Combination drug therapy in psychopharmacology. *J Clin Pharmacol* 15:511–517, 1975.
143. Griffin JP, O'Arcy PF (eds): *A Manual of Adverse Drug Interactions*. Bristol, England, John Wright and Sons Ltd, 1975.
144. Bigger JT, Kantor SJ, Glassman AH, Perel JM: Cardiovascular effects of tricyclic antidepressant drugs. In Lipton MA, DeMascio A, Killam KF (eds): *Psychopharmacology: A Generation of Progress*. New York, Raven Press, 1978, pp 1033–1046.
145. Roose SP, Glassman AH, Giardina EG, Walsh TB, Woodring S, Bigger JT: Tricyclic antidepressants in depressed patients with cardiac conduction disease. *Arch Gen Psychiatry* 44:273–275, 1987.
146. Risch SC, Kalin NH, Janowsky DS, Huey LY: Indications and guidelines for plasma tricyclic antidepressant concentration monitoring. *J Clin Psychopharmacol* 1:59–63, 1981.
147. Prien RF, Kupfer DJ: Continuation drug therapy for major depressive episode: how long should it be maintained? *Am J Psychiatry* 143:18–23, 1986.
148. Carroll BJ, Feinberg M, Greden JF, Tarika J, Albala AA, Haskett RF McL, James N, Kronfol Z, Lohr N, Steiner M, deVigne JP, Young E: A specific laboratory test for the diagnosis of melancholia: standardization, validation, and clinical utility. *Arch Gen Psychiatry* 44:273–275, 1987.
149. Arana G, Baldessarini RJ, Ornsteen M: The dexamethasone suppression test for diagnosis and prognosis in psychiatry. *Arch Gen Psychiatry* 42:1193–1204, 1985.
150. Atkinson JH, Kremer EF, Risch SC, Ward HW, Hopper B, Yen SSC: Pre- and post-dexamethasone saliva cortisol determinations in chronic pain patients. *Biol Psychiatry* 19:1155–1159, 1984.
151. France RD, Krishnan KRR: The dexamethasone suppression test as a biologic marker of depression in chronic pain. *Pain* 21:49–55, 1985.
152. Atkinson JH, Kremer EF, Risch SC, Janowsky DS: Pre- and post-dexamethasone cortisol and prolactin concentrations in patients with chronic pain syndromes. *Pain* 25:23–34, 1986.
153. Sheehan DV, Claycomb JB, Kouretas N: Monoamine oxidase

inhibitors: prescription and patient management. *Int J Psychiatr Med* 10:99–121, 1981.
154. Yeh SY, Mitchell CL: Potentiation and reduction of the analgesia of morphine in the rat by pargyline. *J Pharmacol Exp Ther* 179:642–651, 1971.
155. Palmer H: Potentiation of pethidine. *Br Med J* 2:944, 1960.
156. Shee JC: Dangerous potentiation of pethidine by iproniazid and its treatment. *Br Med J* 2:507–509, 1960.
157. Rivers N, Hornes P: Possible lethal reaction between nardil and dextromorphan. *Can Med Assoc J* 103:85, 1970.
158. Roger KJ: Role of brain monoamines in the interaction between pethidine and tranylcypromine. *Eur J Pharmacol* 14:86–88, 1971.
159. Domino E, Sullivan TS, Luby ED: Barbiturate intoxication in a patient treated with a MAO inhibitor. *Am J Psychiatry* 118:941–943, 1962.
160. Frolich JC, Leftwich R, Ragheb M, Oates JA, Reimann I, Buchanan D: Indomethacin increases plasma lithium. *Br Med J* 1:1115–1116, 1979.
161. Hollister LE: Hydroxyzine hydrochloride: possible adverse cardiac interactions. *Psychopharmacol Commun* 1:61–65, 1975.
162. Killian JM, Fromm GH: Carbamazepine in the treatment of neuralgia. Use and side effects. *Arch Neurol* 19:129–136, 1968.
163. Taylor MA, Sierles FS, Abrams R: *General Hospital Psychiatry.* New York, Free Press, 1985.
164. Giles TO, Modlin RK: Death associated with ventricular arrhythmias and thioridazine hydrochloride. *JAMA* 205:108–110, 1968.
165. Cassem NH: The setting of intensive care. In Hackett TP, Cassem NH (eds): *MGH Handbook of General Hospital Psychiatry.* St. Louis, CV Mosby, 1978, pp 319–341.
166. Monks R, Merskey H: Psychotropic drugs. In Wall PD, Melzack RD (eds): *Textbook of Pain.* London, Churchill Livingstone, 1984, pp 526–537.
167. Hackett TP: The pain patient: evaluation and treatment. In Hackett TP, Cassem NH (eds): *MGH Handbook of General Hospital Psychiatry.* St. Louis, CV Mosby, 1978, pp 41–63.
168. Marks J: Benzodiazepines—for good or evil. *Neuropsychobiology* 10:115–126, 1983.
169. Hollister LE: Principles of therapeutic applications of benzodiazepines. In Smith DE, Wesson DR (eds): *The Benzodiazepines. Current Standards for Medical Practice.* Lancaster, England, MTP Press, 1985, pp 87–96.
170. Rickels K, Case WG, Diamond L: Issues in long-term treatment with diazepam therapy. *Psychopharmacol Bull* 18:38–41, 1982.
171. Johnstone M: The effects of methylphenidate on postoperative pain and vasoconstriction. *Br J Anaesth* 46:778–783, 1974.

chapter 9
Special Considerations in Pharmacologic Pain Management

Joseph W. Tollison, M.D.

Nowhere in the broad area of chronic pain management are the proper selection, dosage, and frequency of administration of medication more critical than in those two very special patient populations, children and the elderly. Previous chapters emphasizing the adult from youth to middle age have carefully defined the pharmacologic actions and administration of various medications for control of chronic pain. However, in cases involving elderly patients and children, where the safety margin is often reduced, special pharmacologic, physiologic, and developmental factors must be very carefully considered. For example, among the elderly, who often are on multiple medications, increasingly frequent manifestations of adverse drug reactions and interactions are commonplace. Another area that is particularly troublesome with these two groups is that of compliance (1–3). Although this is somewhat understandable when considering the unique characteristics of these patients, it nonetheless compounds the prescribing difficulties and decisions. Underprescribing by physicians, as well as variable compliance, is especially common among children, although chronic pain as a motivating force may enhance responsiveness to the latter (4). Overprescribing is equally common among the elderly, especially in light of their propensity for drug accumulation at standard younger adult dosages.

As discussed earlier, pain is often the sentinel manifestation of many diseases or disorders and may thus be the triggering motivation for a patient to seek medical assistance. Altered perception of pain, which frequently occurs in elderly patients, may present some difficulty for the patient both in characterizing and describing the location of the pain. It may also be the only presenting complaint a child is able to express or define clearly. With young children, the inability to describe their symptoms is complicated by the fact that chronic pain of the nonneoplastic type is infrequently seen in this patient population and only in recent years has much study been done on its management. Therefore, well-designed therapeutic responses that would aid the physician in managing the patient effectively over time are relatively new or are still being developed.

The remainder of the chapter examines a number of those factors that make these patients unique, and that make their management complex. Factors ranging from the size/body surface area of the younger patient to the absorption, metabolism, and excretion differences of the older patient are addressed. Various pain medications and their applicability to these patients are also discussed.

CHILDREN

Because children are still developing physically and because of the potential deleterious psychological effects that may result, the management of chronic pain in this patient population is a particularly difficult and complex task. The amount of attention health care providers have given to chronic pain in children has been relatively scanty, and much still remains to be learned about appropriate care for these patients. Drug therapy in children has in general been studied infrequently, leading to the use of the term *therapeutic orphan* by Shirkey (5). The key to the approach to the care of the child with chronic pain is individualization of therapy based on an understanding of the expected physiologic and pharmacologic parameters, and a special awareness that these patients are not just smaller adults when it comes to prescribing. The final arbiter remains the individual patient's response to the drug and to his disease (6). An excellent review of chronic pain in children was presented by Lacouture, Gaudreault, and Lovejoy in 1984 in the *Pediatric Clinics of North America* (7).

Nonneoplastic-generated chronic pain in children is uncommon. This adds to the complexity of management for this patient population group, especially when one considers that many of the drugs released on the market have had limited study for use in children, having been primarily investigated for use in the adult population.

DOSE SELECTION

The variables of total body water, as well as percentages of intracellular and extracellular water, are prime determinants of dose selection. In concert with factors of metabolism and excretion, selecting appropriate dosing patterns becomes even more difficult. Figure 9.1 provides an overview of the body water factor (4, 8).

Dosing regimens in children have historically been based on either the patient's age, weight, or body surface area. Although no system of dose selection is fail-safe, the body surface area and body weight approaches have had the most general acceptance. Nomograms have been made available for the health care provider to assist in dosing selections. Table 9.1, a modification of the earlier work of Catzel (9), was developed as a simplified aide by Leach and Wood (6).

Even greater care should be taken with those drugs that

Table 9.1
Dose as Proportion of Adult Dose and in Milligrams per Kilogram for Different Age Groups[a]

Age	Weight lb	Weight kg	Dose as proportion of adult dose	Dose (mg/kg) if adult dose is 1 mg/kg
Adult	145	66	1	1.0
12 years	82	37	¾	1.25
7 years	51	23	½	
3 years	33	15	⅓	1.5
1 year	22	10	¼	
4 months	14	5.5	⅕	2.0
2 weeks	7	3.2	⅛	

[a] After Catzel; modified by Leach and Wood. From Leach RH, Wood BSB: Drug dosage for children. *Lancet* 1 : 1350–1351, 1967.

have a narrow therapeutic/safety index. Precision is difficult at best, and in the final analysis the individual response to the drugs and the disease is a vital factor (6). Therapeutic serum dose level monitoring, as it becomes available, would be of increasing assistance.

DRUGS USED IN PAIN MANAGEMENT IN CHILDREN

Nonsteroidal Anti-inflammatory Agents

Because of their pharmacologic properties, aspirin and nonsteroidal anti-inflammatory agents generally are often selected for adults who are experiencing mild to moderate pain, especially if accompanied by an inflammatory component. However, only a small percentage of physicians continue to use aspirin for chronic disorders in children. Based on the initial findings of Starko in 1979, and subsequent studies, there was an official announcement in 1985 of an association of aspirin with Reye's syndrome (10–13). Because the incidence of viral illness is so common among children, concurrent disease during long-term chronic pain therapy is very likely. In response to this concern the chronic use of aspirin with its proven analgesic, anti-inflammatory, and antipyretic properties is uncommon. Other potential problems with aspirin, even when given at much lower dosages, include adverse effects ranging from gastrointestinal effects to hematologic effects (e.g., delayed clotting time), as well as occasional hypersensitivity. If the decision is made to use aspirin, the dosage is calculated on a base dose of 65 mg/kg/day in 4–6 divided doses, and routine drug level monitoring is strongly recommended to avoid common toxic effects, including salicylism. Dosage forms include tablets, enteric-coated tablets, and suppositories.

The nonsteroidal agents as a group share the analgesic, the anti-inflammatory, and to a degree the antipyretic potential of the aspirin family. However, also like aspirin, nonsteroidal drugs are rarely recommended for use for

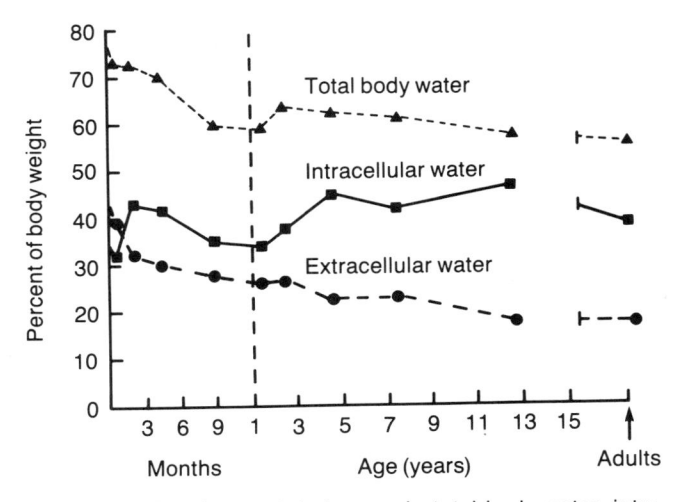

Figure 9.1 Developmental changes in total body water, intracellular water, and extracellular water in infants and children, expressed as percentages of body weight. (From Friis-Hansen B: Body water compartments in children: changes during growth and related changes in body composition. *Pediatrics* 28:169–181, 1961. Reproduced by permission of *Pediatrics*.)

chronic pain in children under age 14. Unlike aspirin, they are expensive. The primary problem is that various metabolic, including renal, concerns have not yet been studied. Therefore, the agents have not been approved for use in children. Currently tolmetin is the only exception to this rule, having been approved primarily for use in juvenile rheumatoid arthritis.

It is important to choose an agent that has proven safe and effective for chronic treatment of mild pain in younger patients while maintaining the essentially similar analgesic effects of aspirin. Acetaminophen meets this criterion and does not appear to have an association with Reye's syndrome. Therefore, there has been a dramatic shift from aspirin by most health care providers in recent years to almost exclusive use of this agent for mild pain (14). Expected side effects and adverse reactions are uncommon with acetaminophen, unless used to excess, at which time this agent becomes very problematic. Any residual of previous or concurrent hepatic disease could reduce the rate of clearance as a result of altered hepatic metabolism, and requires one to choose an increased dosing interval. Overdosage with acetaminophen is potentially life-threatening, and in any case may result in hepatic damage. Acute renal failure also has been reported when acetaminophen has been taken in excessive dosages. The manifestation of renal damage follows that of hepatic by a matter of days, requiring careful follow-up (15). To this point all cases of acute renal failure have been reversible. Acetaminophen comes in various over-the-counter products, including chewable tablets, elixir, drops, and suppositories, with a dosing formula by age as given in Table 9.2 (16, 17).

Opiates and Opioid Compounds

Codeine alone produces excellent analgesia for most patients with moderate pain and is generally the next step in children if acetaminophen therapy alone is insufficient. Dosing levels and frequency for codeine are calculated on a base dose of 3 mg/kg/day administered in 6 divided doses. In combination with acetaminophen, it has an additive and perhaps even a synergistic effect, offering improved analgesia to the younger patient in chronic pain.

Other opiates and associated opioid compounds are all commonly utilized for chronic severe pain, with primary metabolism through the liver. There is a very significant "first pass" effect as the agent passes through the liver, and, therefore, oral doses often range up to 2–6 times that of doses administered parenterally. The oral/parenteral dosage ratios are: methadone, 2:1; meperidine, 4:1; and morphine, 6:1 (18). Meperidine is representative of this class of narcotics, and through its action on the central nervous system creates a level of euphoria and an increase in the pain threshold of as much as 65% (19). Utilized parenterally, meperidine requires an analgesic ratio of 10:1 to morphine (20). It is notably less effective when given orally. Although it has minimal effect on the cardiovascular system, as with morphine, respiratory depression can be a factor (21). Also, because of its propensity for inducing nausea and vomiting, meperidine is often combined with an antihistamine such as promethazine or hydroxyzine, which tends to potentiate the sedative aspects of the drug (20).

A potentially helpful property of these agents is sedation, whereas respiratory depression becomes an increasing concern with the addition of additive or synergistic medications. The increase in the incidence of seizure disorders in patients who have undergone long-term treatment with meperidine is a possible side effect of which health care providers should be cautious (22). However, the overriding disadvantages with these agents are the association of potential tolerance and drug dependence (7). These agents appear to work centrally as contrasted with the agents described earlier, which act largely peripherally. Another possible side effect in children may be the

Table 9.2
Recommended Pediatric Dosing of Acetaminophen by Age and Weight[a]

Age	Weight lb	Weight kg	Single Dose (mg)	Frequency[b]
Under 4 months	6–11	2.5– 5.4	40	every 4 to 6 hr
4 to under 12 months	12–17	5.5– 7.9	80	every 4 to 6 hr
12 months to under 2 years	18–23	8.0–10.9	120	every 4 to 6 hr
2 and 3 years	24–35	11.0–15.9	160	every 4 to 6 hr
4 and 5 years	36–47	16.0–21.9	240	every 4 to 6 hr
6, 7, and 8 years	48–59	22.0–26.9	320	every 4 to 6 hr
9 and 10 years	60–71	27.0–31.9	400	every 4 to 6 hr
11 and 12 years	72–95	32.0–43.9	480	every 4 to 6 hr
	>96	>44	640	every 4 to 6 hr

[a] Data from Korberly (16) and Temple (17).
[b] Not to exceed 5 doses in a 24-hr period.

development of disphoria rather than the euphoria commonly seen in adults (7). This concern alone, aside from the dependence concerns, should lead the health care provider to initially choose nonnarcotic agents when possible. If narcotic agents are required, a longer acting agent such as methadone may be selected. Table 9.3 is a cataloging of narcotic agents and their side effects as developed by Korberly (16). Table 9.4 outlines selected nonnarcotic analgesics as cataloged by Lacouture et al. (7).

Tricyclic Antidepressants

The tricyclic antidepressants, which are frequently utilized in adults as outlined in the previous chapter, may also be chosen for use in children. However, the side effect profile often is great and the therapeutic risk/benefit ratio may therefore be unacceptable. Again, if used, individualization of therapy is in order, as well as adherence to specific indications that tend to be uncommon in childhood chronic pain (7). Potentiation of analgesic is an expected effect. Occasional use of other agents has also been reported with younger patients but these should be very carefully selected and even more carefully monitored. An example is the use of phenytoin in carefully selected patients (lancinating pain) with mild facial pain, and of skeletal muscle relaxants in patients with pain of skeletal muscle origin (7). Significant side effects such as central nervous system (CNS) depression (relaxants) in the short and long term, and CNS depression and hyperplastic changes of the gingiva (phenytoin) over the long term, are possible with these medications.

MANAGEMENT APPROACHES

Of special note is the potential for drug interactions in this age group. Any other medications that are being taken should be carefully considered, and the drug's potential for interaction with the medication chosen for treatment of the chronic pain should be carefully studied.

Table 9.3
The Narcotic Analgesics[a]

Agent	Dosage (oral)	Indication	Side Effects	Comments
Codeine	0.5–60 mg/kg dose q 4 h	Mild to moderate pain	Metabolic; see morphine	Converted to morphine; elevated level of tolerance
Acetaminophen w/codeine elixir (12 mg/5 ml) (Tylenol with Codeine Elixir)	Under 3 yrs: not indicated 3–6 yrs: 5 ml q 3–4 h 7–12 yrs: 10 ml q 3–4 h			
Hydromorphone (Dilaudid)	0.05–5 mg/kg/dose q 6 h	Moderate to severe pain	See morphine	Well absorbed; commonly used in terminal pain
Meperidine (Demerol)	1–100 mg/kg/dose q 4 h	Moderate to severe pain	See morphine	Caution in renal failure; less sedation; may trigger bronchial asthma; may lead to CNS exitation
Methadone (Dolophine)	0.2–10 mg/kg/dose q 6 h	Severe pain	See morphine	Long half-life; minimal euphoria
Morphine	0.5 mg/kg/dose q 6 h	Severe pain	CNS depression; orthostatic hypotension; decreased gastrointestinal motility; mental clouding	Tolerance or dependence may develop
Oxycodone	0.05–10 mg/kg dose q 4–5 h	Moderate pain	See morphine	Short half-life; excellent short-term effects; commonly combined with aspirin (Percodan) or acetaminophen (Percocet)

[a] From Korberly BH: Pharmacologic treatment of children's pain. *Pediatr Nurs* July/August: 292–294, 1985.

Table 9.4
The Nonnarcotic Analgesics[a]

Agent	Dosage (Oral)	Indication	Side Effects	Comments
Salicylates				
Aspirin (multiple)	10–15mg/kg/to 1 g/dose q 4–6 hrs	Mild pain especially with inflammatory processes	Bleeding, hypersensitive, GI distress	Risk of toxicity (metabolism saturation), may enhance effects of oral hypoglycemics; prolonged action. Good therapeutic index
Diflunisal[b]	500 mg q 12 hrs	See Aspirin	Fewer bleeding abnormalities, G. I. upset (low incidence)	
Acetaminophen (multiple)	10–20mg/kg/to 1 g/dose q 4–6 hrs	Mild Pain		
Non-steroidal Anti-inflammatories				
Tolmetin	200–400mg q 6 hrs	Mild Pain, for chronic joint disease	Hypersensitivity; dyspepsia; abdominal discomfort; renal insufficiency; cholestatic hepatitis	Expensive; well absorbed
Motrin[b]	400–800mg q 6 hrs	See Tolmetin	See Tolmetin	
Naprosyn[b]	250–500mg q 8–12 hrs	See Tolmetin	See Tolmetin	
Clinoril[b]	200mg q 12 hrs	See Tolmetin	See Tolmetin	
Indoprofen[b]	50–200mg q 6 hrs	See Tolmetin	See Tolmetin	

[a] From Lacouture PG, Gaudreault P, Lovejoy FH: Chronic pain of childhood: a pharmacologic approach. *Pediatr Clin North Am* 31:1133–1151, 1984.
[b] Use of these drugs in children has not yet been approved.

Another key management approach would be to attempt to maintain these patients on a set, yet reasonable, schedule other than as-needed scheduling, which has been shown to adversely affect pain behavior. Also, the possibility of the child returning to an environment where his learned pain behavior elicits a predictable response may be determined and appropriate adjustments made (7). Another principle is that the pain process should be closely monitored. For example, a child should not be permitted to remain in pain during the latter portion of a "q 4 h" regimen. This requires a careful review of all the variables involved in setting appropriate dosage levels and frequency. A caring response while avoiding the pitfalls of chronic narcotic utilization should be the goal in order to avoid distrust, anger, and other negative emotions. Undertreatment will engender these emotions on the part of the patient, and must be avoided (7).

There are numerous other factor for consideration when selecting an appropriate medication for a child suffering with chronic pain, due in part to the expected differences in psychological impact. For example, in a child who is in the process of developing his self-concept and sense of identity, the health care provider has a challenge of significant magnitude in attempting to select a plan of therapy that will be effective while not having an adverse impact on this critical stage of development. Another challenge is to utilize the selected therapy in the most optimal manner. This makes the diagnostic evaluation of critical importance, since abbreviating the pain process is the ultimate goal, and arriving at a specific diagnosis may predetermine the family of specific agents that can be used. Patterns of chronic pain behavior develop variably. In certain patients relatively healthy coping patterns emerge. However, those patterns of chronic pain behavior expected to develop over time in response to chronic pain have the potential to have an adverse impact on the child's development.

The tragedy of chronic pain in children is no more evident than when attempting to deal constructively with the families of these children. Assessment of the parents' nonverbal as well as verbal communication with the child and with you as the health care provider are critical. The response of the family members to the pain itself is important. Do they attempt to overcompensate? Do they overreact in other ways? What impact does this appear to have upon the child? Does it enhance or promote his response to the pain? The highly complex and yet foundational impact of the interaction with the parents and other family members plays a vital role in the long-term care of these patients. All of this would lead one to study family relationships and interactions and other environmental aspects carefully and to address as many of these as possible prior to selection of medication.

SUMMARY

As stated earlier in this chapter, at this juncture in the history of health care appropriate treatment of children with chronic pain of the nonneoplastic type has drawn precious little attention and emphasis. Most multidisciplinary pain clinics have understandably emphasized care of the adult with chronic pain because of its resultant impact on the work force and economic factors. However, there are unique aspects in the care of children, including the impact of pain on their development and the different physiologic and pharmacologic aspects of selected therapy, that require much more attention than has previously been channeled in that direction. Modification of surrounding factors may alter the pain to some degree, as is also often the case when specific causes of the pain are identified and are addressed rather that treating the resulting pain alone. Again, individualization of care in this age group is paramount. The simplest regimen possible to achieve the desired effect should be undertaken, and, when this involves medication, it should preferably be those drugs with the least dosage, the least frequent dosing interval, and the least toxicity. If possible, the patient should be administered only one medication (7).

Finally, when dealing with children, their trust in the health care provider needs to be honored at all times, and nowhere is this more important than in the relief of pain. A child who presents with chronic pain should be approached with professional concern and constant reassurance. Ambiguity of effort in this regard, albeit unintentional, has deleterious results. Careful and frequent reassessment of children with chronic pain is in order. Under all circumstances, keep in mind that the patient's possible misunderstanding of the health care provider's failure to bring relief may create an environment that makes quality long-term care virtually impossible.

THE ELDERLY

Many perceive pain to be an inevitable by-product of aging (23), occurring with increasing frequency during the aging process. However, with appropriate care, chronic pain in the elderly can be managed effectively over the long term. By almost every diagnostic and therapeutic unit of measurement, including psychosocial, physiologic, and pharmacokinetic, the elderly are the most complex patient group in our society. Those over age 65 are an increasing segment of our population and will comprise well over 20% of the population shortly after the turn of the century, including an expanding percentage of the "older old" (85+ years). The elderly often present with multiple problems, are seen more frequently in the office setting than are younger patients, and generally require longer hospitalizations. Also, the diagnosis and treatment process may be compounded by communication disorders involving reduced vision and/or hearing. With the "older old," increased fragility will also need to be addressed.

The team approach has been helpful in the care of the elderly because it focuses the efforts of all of the health care professionals involved in the patient's total care (whole patient concept) and also is keyed to the various problems of function the patient encounters. Unquestionably, care of the elderly has been greatly improved through the team approach, which is being increasingly utilized in many areas. Enhanced commitment and involvement are the potential benefits to the patient when the various health care professionals sense joint responsibility in the care of the whole patient and not just in their area of expertise. Properly developed, this has a favorable impact on the role of the individual physician, broadening the professional involvement and time commitment to the patient. Improved care will naturally result.

Also, the once infrequently addressed area of preventive health care for the elderly has come into prominence in recent years. The sense of "inevitability" that was once a permanent and commonly encountered attitude among patients as well as among many health care professionals has been modified and has given way to a new emphasis on preventive health care. Proper exercise, nutrition, and activities contributing to emotional health are heavily prescribed, as are routine maintenance and preventive health measures, all of which lead to greater longevity and enhanced health and function during the latter years.

Homeostasis is the goal in caring for the elderly patient with chronic pain. It remains a major goal for the health care provider not to disrupt the delicate physiologic balance in which the patient quite often is maintained. The loss of adaptability becomes the critical factor, followed by a loss of homeostasis with resulting disease in the patient. The body systems become progressively less adaptable over the years and eventually a system failure occurs. Pain syndromes in the elderly frequently present in an atypical manner. A high index of suspicion concerning the presenting problem as well as the pattern of presentation is required. Each of us has encountered in our elderly patient population those with silent or painless myocardial infarctions, afebrile pneumonias, or other processes that do not present in the classic manner more commonly seen in younger adults. One factor at work is thought to be elevation in pain threshold as a result of a degeneration of dorsal column neurons with a resultant reduced sensory awareness (24, 25). Therefore, a preception of pain by the elderly patient may have a heightened significance over that perceived in a younger patient, and indeed may signal a more involved disorder. Proper diagnosis is compounded further by the fact that depression, often resulting in part from the multiple and accelerating emotional losses experienced by the patient, is more common among the elderly, and yet is usually not diagnosed, and therefore not treated, at the suspected rate of prevalence. Depression must be searched for, with a high level of awareness. Is this isolated elderly lady depressed because she is lonely or lonely because she is depressed? Pain, of course, greatly compounds this presentation.

PHARMACOKINETICS OF PAIN MEDICATION IN THE ELDERLY

Pharmacokinetics are of special significance in this age group. There remains much discussion on the effect the aging process has on absorption, with most authorities currently believing that the absorptive process is mildly reduced. Certainly, the rate of absorption is reduced as a patient ages. This is due to various causes ranging from a delayed gastric emptying time to cardiovascular and blood flow determinants, all of which is rather alarming when considering long-term therapy with agents such as aspirin and nonsteroidals, which have the potential of inducing gastric bleeding. The expected reduction in intracellular body water and serum albumin as the patient ages occurs in concert with the previously addressed increase in body fat and reduction of lean muscle mass. This markedly affects drug distribution, and these normal and predictable aspects of biologic aging must be appropriately considered when prescribing medications that have their distribution in various body components.

Table 9.5 defines the normally expected physiologic changes and resulting pharmacokinetic effects of the various aging body systems (26).

Major alterations in percentage of body components occur during aging, and major changes in total body lipid content (appropriate doubling by age 70 from 14% to approximately 30%) take place. Soft tissue and muscle decreases in the range of 25–30%, whereas body water declines approximately 18% (Figure 9.2) (23, 27, 28).

Understanding the expected specific pharmacologic activity of the medication selected is essential. As an example, the medication's lipid solubility is greatly affected. A medication that is highly lipid soluble has increased distribution in body fat, with an expected decrease in the serum level and resultant availability. Correspondingly, those medications that are dependent on protein binding will have an increased concentration of unbound drug in the serum as a result of reduced serum albumin in the elderly patient. Prolongation of activity of the medication and the risk of toxicity or adverse reactions is an increasingly frequent result among elderly patients.

Excretion of various pain medications is another area in which the elderly generally differ from the younger population. The liver is reduced in size and weight, and there is a decrease in activity of the hepatic microsomal enzyme system. There is a tremendous reserve in the human liver, however, and it is debatable whether this in itself will result in clinically apparent biochemical changes (26). However, normal physiologic changes in aging, such as the gradual decrease in cardiac output by approximately 1% per year following age 35–40, and the decrease in the glomerular filtration rate by 40% by age 80, along with many other changes in organ systems, are the norm, and these cellular changes as yet cannot be prevented (29). These expected reductions in the glomerular filtration rate and tubular reabsorption in the aging patient are accompanied by reduced renal blood flow. This reduces the excretion rate and further increases the likelihood of drug toxicity. In general, we should expect accumulation, so prevention of the accompanying toxicity while seeking effective therapy often becomes an elusive goal.

Table 9.5
Physiologic and Pharmacokinetic Changes Associated with Aging[a]

Physiologic Changes	Pharmacokinetic Effects
Cardiovascular	
Decrease in cardiac output	Redistribution of blood flow from liver and kidneys, resulting in prolonged plasma half-life and diminished biotransformation[b]
Decrease in arterial flow	
Alteration of circulation to organ systems	
Gastrointestinal	
Decrease in gastric acidity	Alteration of ionization and solubility
Prolonged gastric emptying	
Decrease in absorptive surface	Decrease in drug absorption
Decrease in liver size and in activity of hepatic microsomal system	Decrease in rate of biotransformation[b] Increase in plasma half-life[b]
Increase in incidence of duodenal diverticula	Increases the potential for malabsorption
Metabolic	
Decrease in intracellular fluid	
Decrease in body weight	Increased effects with standard dosage[b]
Decrease in serum albumin	Increase in free to bound drug ratio[b]
Increase in serum globulin	Increase in storage of lipid soluble drugs[b]
Increase in proportion of: fatty tissue to muscle mass	Increase in plasma half-life[b] Increase in volume of distribution[b]
Neuronal	
Increase in rate of neuron loss	Increased susceptibility to hypoxia[b] Increased sensitivity to central depressants[b] Potential for confusion about drug regimens[b]
Renal	
Decrease in renal clearance	Increase in plasma half-life[b]

[a] From Stimmel B: *Pain, Analgesia, and Addiction: The Pharmacologic Treatment of Pain.* New York, Raven Press, 1983.
[b] Enchances potential for drug toxicity.

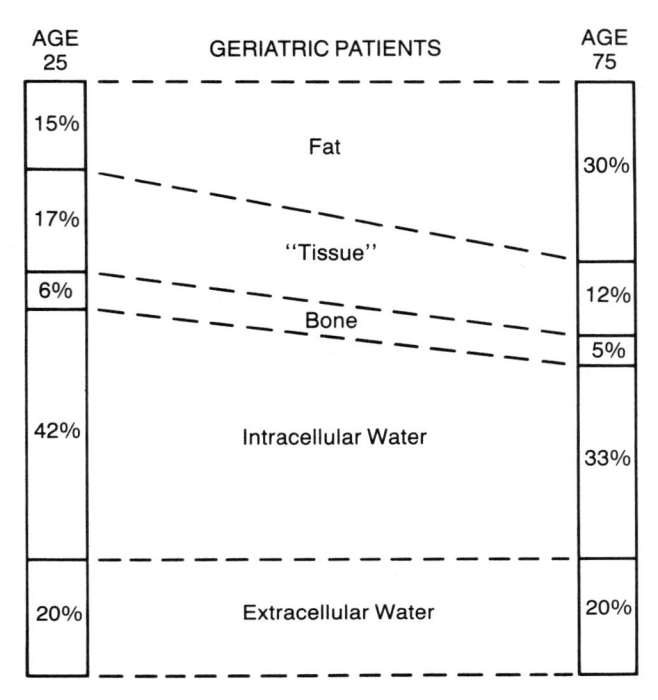

Figure 9.2 Distribution of major body components with age. [Data from Benet et al. (27) and Rossman (28).]

Age 25: Fat 15%, Tissue 17%, Bone 6%, Intracellular Water 42%, Extracellular Water 20%
Age 75: Fat 30%, Tissue 12%, Bone 5%, Intracellular Water 33%, Extracellular Water 20%

DOSAGE AND DRUG INTERACTIONS

Choosing appropriate dosage levels and dosage frequency is extremely important when prescribing medication for elderly patients. As noted above, the elderly are often acutely sensitive both to medication and procedures. This was very clearly illustrated by the study by Reichel on the Stanford Teaching Service of the San Mateo County General Hospital, San Mateo, California (30). The study involved 500 consecutive admissions of elderly patients to the hospital. Of these, 146 patients had 193 reactions, with 54 reactions being to medications, 42 to falls from a bed or chair, and 31 to procedures. Admitting elderly patients to the hospital obviously is frequently necessary, but it should be recognized that it puts them in an unfamiliar environment and subjects them to secondary and perhaps even possibly greater pathology (31). Admission of an elderly patient should be carefully weighed. This is especially true with pain patients, since the occurrence of pain in an unfamiliar environment may increase the patient's inability to function effectively.

In the elderly, who are often on multiple medications and have poorly defined absorptive capability and distribution and excretion differences, drug interactions become an even greater potential hazard. Certain prescribing guidelines for the elderly must be undertaken:

1. Assess very carefully the etiology of the patient's pain and prescribe appropriately.

2. With each visit, reassess the patient's total list of medications (include all over-the-counter medications).
3. Choose the mildest pain medication and simplest regimen possible to achieve the desired effect.
4. Choose the smallest dose possible for initial therapy (a "start low . . . go slow" technique is advised). In general, the elderly often require only one-third to one-half of the initial dose level of younger adults, with a preference for approximately one-third.
5. Because of the above, frequency of dosage should be reduced to avoid the expected accumulation, particularly if the drugs prescribed have extended half-lives of their own, which would compound the patient's excretion difficulties.
6. Be alert to various adverse reactions and drug interactions, which are major deterrents to medication compliance. An example is the constipating effect of codeine. Consider strongly other factors impacting on compliance as well, including the cost of medications.

Well-intentioned physicians may occasionally compound a patient's medical problem by prescribing dosages, frequencies, or specific medications that are inappropriate. A classic example is the elderly patient who suffers increased orthostatic hypotension from a medication, and, on rising, falls and fractures her hip. Culminative anticholinergic effects are of major concern, as may be additive effects of multiple medications or sufficient dosage of a single medication with this propensity (32). Antispasmodics or tricyclic antidepressants, along with other medications including some available over the counter, have this potential. When choosing a tricyclic for an elderly patient one may well consider a medication from the lower end of the anticholinergic scale, such as desipramine (33). Orthostatic hypotension is a leading manifestation of the anticholinergic effect and has the major potential for causing falls that result in fractures or other injuries. Urinary retention is another frequent result of anticholinergic effects from one or a combination of agents. A "start low . . . go slow" approach to dosage selection is almost always indicated in the elderly except in an emergency situation. A broad review of specific medications and factors affecting selection in the elderly was presented by Rhodes et al. in 1985 (34).

Certainly, drug-induced dementia is among the most common of the reversible forms of dementia, and therefore, along with depression, should be high on the list of considered causes. Narcotics, for example, manifest a significantly increased central depressant effect among elderly patients. The decreased respiratory reserve potentially compounds this problem (26). Those experienced in

Figure 9.3 Flow diagram detailing factors leading to unpredictability of drug effects in the elderly. (From Lamy PP: *Prescribing for the Elderly.* Littleton, MA, PSG Publishing, 1980.)

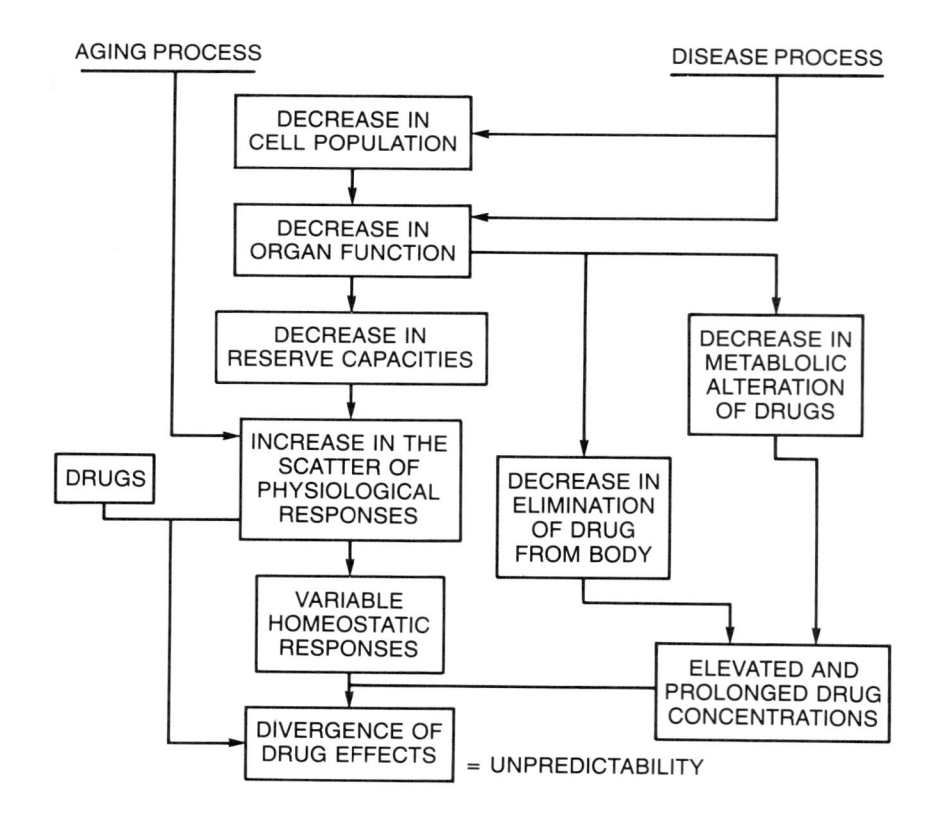

caring for large populations of nursing home patients have long had the impression that physicians have, in general, been more inclined to add medications than to subtract. The less adaptable physiologic systems of the elderly, especially of those most advanced in age, have only compounded the potential of drug-induced dementia. With the increasing attention being given to avoiding adverse reactions and drug interactions, it is hoped that this is becoming a less common occurrence. All of these factors plus others potentially interact to produce unpredictable results (Fig. 9.3).

This unpredictability of drug effects in the aged is heavily compounded not only by wide variation in responsiveness but by the number of medications taken, which tends to average much higher in the elderly. The term *polypharmacy*, used to describe the use of multiple medications in the elderly, refers to both the number of over-the-counter medications the patient is using and those medications prescribed by physicians. The additive and even synergistic effects of many of these medications result in compounding problems, and the potency of medications used for pain adds significantly to the resulting effects. Drug interactions become an increasing problem. Seldom should medications for the elderly be ordered or prescribed in isolation, and the prescribing physician must maintain a constant awareness of the cumulative effect and the potential contained therein.

ADDITIONAL FACTORS IN MANAGEMENT

Decreased mobility is another frequently expected problem, often limiting patient visits. Because of this and other factors associated with aging, the management of medications at home is a critical role. Howard-Ruben discussed this approach well and in breadth in 1985 (35).

CONCLUSIONS

The challenge presented by both the very old and the very young in the area of chronic pain management is truly unique, and requires our most thoughtful and carefully selected approach to achieve an optimal effect with a minimum of problems. Although immensely challenging and difficult to achieve, effective pain management for patients of these two groups remains among our most complex responsibilities and should merit our full professional attention as well as ongoing research.

Acknowledgement Appreciation is extended to A. Thomas Taylor, Pharm. D., for his contribution to the section on pediatric therapeutics.

References

1. Wilson JT: Compliance with instructions in the evaluation of therapeutic efficacy: a common but frequently unrecognized major variable. *Clin Pediatr* 12:333–340, 1973.
2. Becker MH, Drachman RH, Kirscht JP: Predicting mothers' compliance with pediatric medical regimens. *J Pediatr* 81:843–854, 1972.
3. Wilson JT: Drug compliance problems for hospitalized children. In McMahon GF (ed): *Principles and Techniques of Human Research and Therapeutics*. New York, Futura, 1976, vol 10.
4. Rane A, Wilson JT: Clinical pharmacokinetics in infants and children. *Clin Pharmacokinet* 1:2–24, 1976.
5. Shirkey H: Therapeutic orphans. *J Pediatr* 72:119–120, 1968.
6. Leach RH, Wood BSB: Drug dosage for children. *Lancet* 1:1350–1351, 1967.
7. Lacouture PG, Gaudreault P, Lovejoy FH: Chronic pain of childhood: a pharmacologic approach. *Pediatr Clin North Am* 31:1133–1151, 1984.
8. Friis-Hansen B: Body water compartments in children: changes during growth and related changes in body composition. *Pediatrics* 28:169–181, 1961.
9. Catzel P: *Pediatric Prescriber*. Oxford, England, Oxford University Press, 1963 and 1966.
10. Starko KM, et al: Reye's syndrome and salicylate use. *Pediatrics* 66:859–864, 1980.
11. Waldman RJ, et al: Aspirin as a risk factor in Reye's syndrome. *JAMA* 247:3089–3094, 1982.
12. *MMWR* 34:13–16, 1985.
13. United States Food and Drug Administration, Department of Health and Human Services: *Health and Human Services Release*, 10 January 1988.
14. Rahwan GL, Rahwan FG: Aspirin and Reye's syndrome: the change in prescribing habits of health professionals. *Drug Intell Clin Pharm* 20:143–145, 1986.
15. Curry RW, et al: Acute renal failure after acetaminophen ingestion. *JAMA* 247:1012, 1982.
16. Korberly BH: Pharmacologic treatment of children's pain. *Pediatr Nurs* July/August: 292–294, 1985.
17. Temple AR: Pediatric dosing of acetaminophen. *Pediatr Pharmacol* 3:321–327, 1983.
18. Newburger PE, Sallan SE: Chronic pain: principles of management. *J Pediatr* 59:429–432, 1982.
19. Bennett CR: The pharmacology of conscious-sedative agents. In Bennett CR (ed): *Conscious-Sedation in Dental Practice*, ed 2. St. Louis, CV Mosby, 1978.
20. Brandt SK, Bugg JL: Problems of medication with the pediatric patient. *Dent Clin North Am* 28:563–579, 1984.
21. Goodman LS, Gilman A (Eds): *The Pharmacological Basis of Therapeutics*, ed 6. New York, Macmillan, 1980.
22. Barenie JT, et al: *Management of Dental Behavior in Children*. Littleton, MA, PSG Publishing, 1979.
23. Lamy PP: *Prescribing for the Elderly*. Littleton, MA, PSG Publishing, 1980.
24. Procacci P, et al: The cutaneous pain pricking threshold in old age. *Gerontol Clin* 12:213–218, 1970.
25. Andrew W: *The Anatomy of Aging in Man*. New York, Grune & Stratton, 1971.
26. Stimmel B: *Pain, Analgesia, and Addiction: The Pharmacologic Treatment of Pain*. New York, Raven Press, 1983.
27. Benet LZ, et al: Pharmacokinetic considerations in geriatric patients. In *Pharmacokinetic Basis for Drug Treatment*. New York: Raven Press, 1984.
28. Rossman I: *Clinical Geriatrics*, ed 2. Philadelphia, JB Lippincott, 1979.
29. Bender AD: The effect of increasing age on the distribution of peripheral blood flow in man. *J Am Geriatr Soc* 13:192–198, 1965.
30. Reichel W: Complications in the care of 500 elderly hospitalized patients. *J Am Geriatr Soc* 13:973–980, 1965.

31. Vestal RE: Drug use in the elderly: a review of problems and special considerations. *Drugs* 16:358–382, 1978.
32. Muller OF, et al: The hypotensive effect of imipramine hydrochloride in patients with cardiovascular disease. *Clin Pharmacol Ther* 2:300–307, 1961.
33. Thompson TL, et al: Drug therapy: psychotropic drug use in the elderly. *N Engl J Med* 308:134–138, 1983.
34. Rhodes RS, et al: Management of dental pain in the elderly. *Gerodontics* 1:264–273, 1985.
35. Howard-Ruben J: Managing pain medications at home. *Oncol Nurs Forum* 12:78–82, 1985.

chapter 10
Diagnostic and Therapeutic Nerve Blocks

J. D. Rybock, M.D.

Neural blockade, the interruption of a nerve's function by the injection of a local anesthetic agent or other drug, is one of the most powerful tools in the diagnosis of chronic pain problems, and, in many cases, its application can also be a useful form of therapy. Used in a haphazard manner, it can lead to entirely erroneous diagnoses and totally inappropriate treatment.

ROLE OF NERVE BLOCKS IN CHRONIC PAIN MANAGEMENT

Nerve blocks are of no value in many cases of chronic pain. Although virtually any body region can be anesthetized, temporarily abolishing a patient's pain neither adds much insight into the underlying problem nor leads to a long-term solution. Nerve block therapy should be used to answer specific questions resulting from a careful evaluation of the patient's pain problem.

When certain diagnoses seem possible, such as intercostal neuralgia or lumbar facet syndrome, nerve blocks can provide a definitive answer. When there is a discrepancy between the demonstrated pathology and the complaints or findings, such as an L4 disk bulge with an S1 root syndrome, selective blockade will clarify the situation. When multiple sources of pain are present, such as arm pain with both signs of root dysfunction and causalgia-like symptoms, or knee pain with an old knee injury and midlumbar disk disease, selective blocks can help determine the relative contribution of each component. When it is unclear if the pain is central or peripheral, as in leg pain following spinal cord injury, nerve blocks can quickly define the source of the pain.

Careful patient evaluation is necessary not just to pose the questions to be resolved by nerve block, but also to understand the patient's means of describing his pain, as well as how the pain varies over time and with various activities. Such information is necessary to make a meaningful evaluation of the patient's block since it is only through his verbal description that the result can be determined. It must be kept in mind that a patient describing chronic pain is not providing an objective assessment of a noxious sensation but is expressing his suffering in organic terms. The relative contributions of organic dysfunction, psychological abnormalities, and social factors in the patient's complaint of "pain" are only apparent after careful evaluation has been carried out. If the patient's pain complaint is assumed to be a simple description of the nociceptive input, confusion often results from nerve blockade. A successful block, significantly reducing the nociceptive input, may not be reported as giving significant pain relief if significant psychological and social factors are playing a role in the pain. In other cases a block totally ineffective at reducing the pain input may be perceived by a patient as highly effective. To take these results at face value would interfere with future therapy, either causing the true organic lesion to be "ruled out," and therefore ignored once the other factors are dealt with, or leading the patient to further interventional therapy that is inappropriate and ineffective.

Once a patient's complaint of pain is viewed as more than a source of nociceptive input awaiting definition, nerve blockade becomes a much more useful test. It is no longer simply a test to be ordered from an anesthesiologist that returns a yes/no answer; rather, it is a complex interaction between the clinician and the patient that not only explores the specific organic factors but also provides further insight into the patient's sensitivity to pain and means of responding to it. With a fairly brief amount of experience, a clinician can become sensitive to the usual amount of discomfort caused by any particular block and the usual pattern of pain and sensory changes. The response of each subsequent patient can then be measured against this standard, and tendencies toward exaggerated pain behavior, stoicism, or bizarre descriptions of sensations can be recognized. Therefore, rather than a nerve block being a simple test providing a simple answer, it becomes much more a meaningful period of interaction and observation extending from preparation of the patient for the block until the period of complete recovery from its effects.

In addition to careful patient selection, skill in evaluating the results of a block is required. There are two aspects to be evaluated: the adequacy of interruption of nerve function and the effect of that blockade on the patient's pain. The effectiveness of the actual nerve blockade must be evaluated by objective means at the neural level. Even with the best technique, inadequate blockade will occasionally be obtained. With sympathetic nerve blockade, for example, temperature changes in the extremity as well as signs of hyperemia should be documented following the block. With somatic nerve blockade, peripheral motor and sensory loss must be noted and its time course specified.

Once an effective block can be confirmed, then the patient's report of the effect on his pain must be carefully interpreted. If the patient is simply asked to evaluate whether the block helped his pain or not, the result may not be meaningful. For example, even with the best preblock instruction, patients will sometimes report the block to have failed to work if, at the time of questioning, the pain has returned. The best way to carry out evaluation is to either question the patient or have the patient record in writing at 15–30-min intervals following the block the level of his pain, the activities being performed, and any observations concerning weakness, numbness, or other signs of neural blockade. A careful review of these data then allows meaningful interpretation of the result of the block.

It must also be realized that many patients will slant reports of effectiveness in an attempt to please the physician and that the placebo effect does occur with nerve blocks as with other medications. If any doubt exists as to the true effectiveness of the block, the physician should be prepared to repeat the block several times, in some cases using blocking agents of different durations or blocking different nerves on subsequent blocks. In occasional complex cases, it may be helpful to consider the use of placebo injections.

BASIC EQUIPMENT FOR PERFORMING NERVE BLOCKS

ANESTHETIC AGENTS

Although virtually any anesthetic agent can be used for a diagnostic or therapeutic nerve block, a consideration of the goals of the nerve block can lead to the selection of an optimal agent. The large variety of agents and concentrations available are useful in allowing the surgical anesthesiologist to deal with a variety of situations requiring varying durations, varying degrees of muscle paralysis, and differing toxicity risks. The majority of nerve blocks used in chronic pain diagnosis and treatment require only a single injection of a small quantity of medication, and therefore toxicity and absorption rate are minor considerations. Because, in most diagnostic blocks, patient observation and feedback are the means through which the result is assessed, the longer a block is effective the more likely a meaningful evaluation will be made. A short-acting agent may wear off before the patient has adequately recovered from the stress of the injection itself to evaluate the result. In addition, for most blocks, it is desirable to use a concentration that will provide partial to complete motor blockade, since the appearance of a motor deficit is often used to determine the technical adequacy of the block.

Acceptably long durations of action can be obtained by using lidocaine with the addition of epinephrine. The epinephrine, by causing local vasoconstriction, delays the absorption of anesthetic in the area of injection and therefore prolongs the period of time in which nerve fibers are exposed to the active agent. However, some authors believe that such vasoconstriction causes local ischemic necrosis and therefore, at least in injection into muscle, recommend against its use.

Long-acting effects without the use of added epinephrine may be obtained by using bupivacaine (Marcaine, Sensorcaine). This naturally long-acting anesthetic has a rapid onset of action and a duration of action 2–3 times that of lidocaine. Good motor blockade can usually be obtained with a 0.5% concentration, and this is generally the preferred agent for most blocks. For lumbar sympathetic and celiac blocks, requiring large volumes of agent, 0.25% bupivacaine, which will provide good autonomic blockade, is generally used.

In spinal anesthesia, a shorter acting agent may be appropriate since close monitoring is required throughout the entire period of anesthesia. Tetracaine (Pontocaine) is often the preferred agent for spinal anesthesia. It must be kept in mind that, whatever agent is used for spinal (or even epidural) anesthesia, because of the risk of inadvertent intrathecal injection) a single-use vial of drug, with no preservatives, must be used.

NEEDLES

A needle long enough to reach the desired target with length to spare should be selected. For deep blocks, where adjustments in the trajectory have to be made as the needle is advanced, a 21-gauge or larger needle should be used. For more superficial blocks, a 23-gauge needle can be employed. Since many blocks involve advancing the needle to or near a bony prominence, it is best to use a relatively short beveled needle, which is less likely to bend and form a hook that would damage tissue on removal. For the majority of blocks, a disposable 21-gauge 3 ½-inch needle will be quite satisfactory. For lumbar sympathetic and celiac plexus blocks, a 5- or 6-inch needle is required.

NEUROLYTICS

Because of widespread nonspecific and poorly controllable destruction, the caustic lytics used in the past are seldom indicated. Except in very specific circumstances, phenol and absolute alcohol have no role to play in chronic pain therapy.

For reasons not fully understood, depository steroids can be effective in cases in which extremely long-lasting blockade is desired. In some cases, this agent may be effective because of its anti-inflammatory properties, such as in greater occipital nerve entrapment secondary to chronic spasm in the neck muscles. In other situations, where no cause for local inflammation can be easily defined, such as monoradicular pain with negative studies, the observed prolonged effect is more difficult to understand. The possibilities include disruption of a self-perpetuating cycle of inflammation, swelling, and compression or possible minor toxic effects of steroid on small nerve fibers.

In most cases, 40 mg (1 ml) of methylprednisolone acetate (Depo-Medrol, Depo-Predate) suspended in 1 ml of local anesthetic agent is the effective dosage. Although 40 mg is a relatively small dosage and is absorbed over a prolonged period of time, frequent repeated dosage must be avoided to prevent systemic effects. As a basic rule, a dose should not be repeated in less than 30 days.

In cases in which neurolysis is indicated and in which loss of the nerve's function is acceptable, a radiofrequency electrode allows controllable nerve destruction. It is most useful for facet joint denervation but can also be used in difficult cases of greater occipital neuralgia or intercostal neuralgia, and its use has been described in differential denervation of spinal nerve roots.

A radiofrequency electrode is a sharply pointed metal rod approximately the size of an 18-gauge needle. It is insulated except for the very tip, and its hub is connected by cable to a radiofrequency control unit. When a radiofrequency current is passed down the electrode, heating occurs at the interface between the uninsulated tip and the surrounding tissue. The current returns to the machine through a standard patient grounding pad. A thermistor within the tip of the electrode monitors the temperature and provides a continuous readout on the control unit; the operator regulates the tip temperature by adjusting the intensity of current flow. Most control units also allow passage of a stimulating current to provide physiologic confirmation of adequate electrode placement prior to lesion generation.

FLUOROSCOPE

Most nerve blocks can be performed without the use of radiographic control. The early textbooks describe elaborate methods of triangulation based on surface features to allow placement of a needle tip in most locations. However, the use of fluoroscopy, particularly those units with on-line memory storage to provide freeze-frame display, allow for a much more accurate and speedy needle or electrode placement with minimal radiation exposure. Fluoroscopy is now considered essential for properly carrying out nerve root blocks, facet blocks, and lumbar sympathetic and celiac blocks.

SPECIFIC BLOCKS

SPINAL

Subarachnoid

By injecting a substance whose density differs from that of spinal fluid into the subarachnoid space and subsequently positioning the patient appropriately, a region of several contiguous dermatomes can be anesthetized or otherwise affected. Because of the cervical origin of the phrenic nerve, such blockade is generally confined to the midthoracic levels or caudally.

Purpose Diagnostically, this approach may be used to distinguish central from peripheral pain. Such a distinction can usually be made on clinical grounds, but occasionally the clinical signs are too indefinite to yield a firm conclusion. Poorly characterized pain in a leg that is hypesthetic as a result of a stroke might, for example, present such difficulty that a subarachnoid block could be used to clarify the situation.

Therapeutically, subarachnoid injection is generally useful only for malignant pain, because of both its nonspecific destruction of neural tissue and the eventual return of sensation or dysesthesia. The most common use is in pelvic pain due to cancer, especially since midline pain is difficult to control with percutaneous cordotomy.

Anatomy and Technique The injection site and patient position is dependent upon the area to be affected and the agent to be injected. Both tetracaine in distilled water and absolute alcohol are hypobaric to spinal fluid, therefore rising to the top of the subarachnoid space; tetracaine in 5–10% dextrose and phenol and glycerol are hyperbaric, settling to the bottom of the subarachnoid space. The patient must therefore be positioned so that the target area is either uppermost or lowermost, depending upon the agent. Awareness of the slope of the path toward cervical levels is important to prevent dangerous migration of the agent cranialward. Although it seems easier to keep the head and neck higher than the point of injection, making hypobaric agent injection easier, upper lumbar blockade can lead to sympathetic outflow disruption, vasoparalysis in the lower extremities, and a fall in blood pressure. A hypobaric agent, however, prevents treatment by Trendelenburg positioning, so alternatives, including leg elevation without head lowering and fluid infusion, must be available. In fact, it light of the potential widespread effects, desired or otherwise, of subarachnoid agents, such injections are most safely done by or with the assistance of an anesthesiologist, in a fully equipped anesthesia room with the patient screened and prepared as if undergoing general anesthesia. These blocks are not casual undertakings and are inappropriate in the office or clinic block room.

Epidural

Purpose Injection into the epidural space allows blockade of spinal nerve roots over a more limited area than does subarachnoid injection and allows placement of depository agents that can give prolonged effects. Although the risk of penetrating the spinal cord generally limits selection of the site of subarachnoid injection, and hence its area of major effect to the region of L2–L5, epidural drugs can be placed at virtually any point along the spinal axis.

Diagnostically, epidural injection is seldom of use. Although it is easier to confine the medication injected into a limited area, bilateral effects usually occur and controlled manipulation of its area of action is difficult. Unlike subarachnoid drugs, epidural fluids do not flow freely or predictably with changes in the patient position.

Therapeutically, long-lasting relief of nerve root irritation, as occurs in small disk herniations, can be obtained by epidural steroid injection. One theory postulates that the radicular pain of disk herniation is the result of dural irritation due to leakage of the abundant intradiskal degradative enzymes through an anular tear, whereas neurologic deficit results from migration of nuclear fragments through that tear with secondary nerve root compression. Epidural depository steroids, slowly releasing active agent, counter the inflammation, decreasing the pain and increasing mobility.

Although some practitioners recommend epidural steroids as the primary treatment for classic lumbar disk herniation, with definite neurologic deficit and strongly positive nerve root tension signs (straight leg raise test), one must be cautious of increasing the root dysfunction by injecting a volume of nonsoluble material into an already compromised lateral spinal canal. Surgical therapy remains the best solution for clinically classic disk herniation, especially with a stenotic lateral recess or large disk fragment. In less classic cases, where radicular pain is prominent but neurologic findings are minimal, epidural steroids are a reasonable treatment if standard conservative therapy fails. In the latter group of patients, surgical results can be disappointing, and neuroradiologic studies often show only minor structural abnormalities.

Anatomy and Technique A needle can be placed into the epidural space either in the midline or 1 cm lateral to the midline on the side of the affected root. Paramedian insertion is in fact slightly easier as well as more effective at delivering agent to the root desired. The needle is advanced to strike the superior portion of the lamina below the interlaminar space to be injected. It is then advanced cranially to step off the bone. Gentle pressure on a saline-filled syringe will allow detection of the passage of the tip through the dense ligamentum flavum into the nonresistent epidural space. The entrance into the epidural space can also be detected by placing a drop of fluid in the needle hub and observing its disappearance as the negative pressure of the epidural space is encountered. One milliliter of agent is adequate to bathe the target nerve root and the surrounding area.

PERIPHERAL NERVE BLOCK

The need for a well-defined approach and goal is never more apparent than when carrying out blockade of peripheral nerves. Virtually any peripheral nerve or nerve root can be located and blocked, but, in the majority of cases, this serves no useful purpose. Even if blockade of a specific nerve gives temporary pain relief, this seldom leads to any form of useful long-term therapy. If the nerve that is blocked is a major mixed nerve, which is usually the case, the loss of motor function and sensation that would result from permanent interruption is seldom acceptable. Even if sacrifice of the nerve can be justified, surgical section or other maneuvers designed to permanently interrupt its function may fail to provide pain relief and may be followed by the formation of a painful neuroma. If the pain is due to soft tissue or joint injuries in the nerve's peripheral field, dermatomal overlap or subsequent collateral sprouting usually results in return of the painful sensation within 6–12 months. Except in the case of specific syndromes that involve focal nerve root irritation or peripheral nerve entrapment, peripheral nerve blockade has a very minor role in chronic pain therapy.

Selective Root

With the aid of fluoroscopic imaging, it is not difficult to place a needle tip adjacent to the lateral margin of a neuroforamen, allowing selective reproducible blockade of a specific nerve root with a small amount of agent. Any nerve root from C3 through S5 can be selectively blocked utilizing a posterior approach, and the cervical roots can also be blocked by an anterior approach.

Purpose Diagnostically, nerve root blockade is particularly useful in three situations. First, when the patient's pain appears to be due to a classic monoradiculopathy but the neuroradiologic studies fail to provide a structural explanation, selective nerve root blockade will usually clarify the situation. If blocking the suspected nerve root totally abolishes the pain, this provides strong argument that the pain is indeed monoradicular and a closer look at the adjacent disk and neuroforamen would be warranted.

On the other hand, if the patient gets a good pattern of numbness, but some pain persists, this effectively rules out a radicular source of the pain and a search more distally, in both neural and nonneural tissue, needs to be carried out. Second, in some cases of classic monoradicular pain, the radiologic studies may demonstrate an abnormality related to an adjacent nerve root only. Whether this is a false-positive finding or a case of anatomic variation, as occurs in a postfixed plexus, can be determined by selective nerve root blockade. If blockade of the structurally affected nerve root abolishes the pain, this confirms the clinically significant role of the imaged abnormality. If it does not, additional nerve roots should be explored with selective blockade, with the recognition that a neuroradiologic study can be simultaneously falsely positive at one level and falsely negative at another. The third situation in which selective nerve root blockade is useful diagnostically is in those cases in which the clinical picture is suggestive of, but not typical for, both nerve root and distal nerve or joint disease. Blockade of a single root is very unlikely to completely abolish pain with a distal origin because of dermatomal overlap. In this situation, careful questioning of the patient is necessary to make sure that complete pain relief has been obtained before concluding that there is a radicular origin to the pain. A good pattern of sensory and motor loss with some persistence of the pain warrants a further search for a peripheral source.

Therapeutically, selective nerve root blockade is most useful in treating postsurgical radicular pain that is presumed to be due to scarring as well as monoradicular pain, confirmed by diagnostic blockade, in which no surgical lesion can be identified. In both cases, injection of depository steroid will often provide lasting relief. Radiofrequency lesions can be made in the nerve roots, but since the nerve roots commonly affected by surgery or injured by disk herniations contain significant motor components, such destructive lesions are seldom of use.

Anatomy Selective nerve root blockade is carried out by placing a needle tip just lateral to the bony neuroforamen at the desired level. Placement is confirmed fluoroscopically and the patient generally will report paresthesias in the anatomically appropriate region with needle placement or at the beginning of injection.

Technique

Cervical Cervical nerve roots may be blocked by either an anterior or a posterior approach. Although the anterior approach can be performed without x-ray control, using palpation of the transverse processes as landmarks (particularly the bony projection known as Chassaignac's tubercle on the transverse process of C6), the vertebral artery is relatively vulnerable from this approach and we recommend a posterior approach for cervical nerve root blockade. From the back, the vertebral artery is largely protected by the articular masses and, using fluoroscopy control, needle placement lateral to the lateral margin of the neuroforamen can be obtained, so that the needlepoint is in fact well away from the vertebral artery. With the fluoroscope in an anteroposterior direction, local infiltrative anesthesia is obtained directly posterior to the lateral mass on the desired side at approximately the level of the disk space. It should be recalled that in the cervical area, nerve roots exit at approximately the level of the disk above the same numbered vertebral body. Therfore, the C6 nerve root would be exiting at approximately the level of the C5–C6 disk space. The needle is advanced under fluoroscopic control to impinge on the lateral mass at approximately the inferior margin of the appropriate space. The needle is then gradually walked off the lateral edge of the lateral mass. The patient will often report paresthesias in the appropriate area, indicating impingement upon the nerve root, but if he does not, shifting of the fluoroscopic beam toward an oblique position to allow visualization of the neuroforamen will allow precise positioning. Careful aspiration must be carried out, since the subarachnoid space may occasionally continue out the nerve root and be entered by a needle in the described position. Once it is clear that the subarachnoid space has not been entered, 0.5–1 ml of the appropriate agent is injected and the needle removed.

Thoracic In general, selective thoracic nerve root blocks are not carried out, since the problems affecting that region of the body are more commonly distal, in the intercostal nerves, and because intercostal nerve block can be carried out much more easily and safely. If selective thoracic nerve root block is desired, an approach similar to cervical nerve root blockade is performed. In the thoracic area, each numbered root exits through a neuroforamen that is over the superior half of the same numbered body and that also corresponds to the inferior margin of the same numbered rib. Blockade is most easily achieved by inserting the needle toward the junction of the transverse process and lamina at the desired level and then carefully marching the needle caudally and slightly laterally until it drops into the superior portion of the intercostal space. A shift of the fluoroscope to a lateral projection will help control the depth of insertion at this point and minimize the risk of puncturing the pleura with the needle.

Lumbar Selective nerve root block in the lumbar area is simplified by the easy visualization of the pedicle on anteroposterior fluoroscopy. The pedicles appear as oval densities on either side of the upper half of the vertebral body and form the superior margin of the neuroforamen. Each nerve root is closely approximated to the medial surface of the pedicle of the same numbered body and then turns lateralward to enter the neuroforamen. It passes just below the most inferior point on the pedicle and then continues in an approximately 45° angle caudally and laterally to join the lumbar plexus or lumbosacral trunk. Direct insertion of the needle into a position slightly caudal and lateral to the inferior edge of the pedicle will place it in the lateral opening of the neuroforamen. Lateral fluoroscopy should then be used to confirm placement and regulate depth of insertion, since there is a significant amount of variation in the distance from skin to neuroforamen in various patients. One milliliter of agent is adequate for complete root block.

Sacral Selective sacral nerve root blockade is carried out by passing a needle through the appropriate posterior neuroforamen. The foramina can be visualized on fluoroscopy, although at times some repositioning of the patient or reangling of the tube is necessary because of the slope of the sacrum and because of the multiple radiologic lines on the sacrum. The location of the S1 neuroforamen, the one most commonly subjected to selective nerve root block, is approximately the same distance from the inferior margin of the pedicle of L5 as that point is from the inferior margin of the pedicle of L4 and just slightly lateral to a line running through those points. When a needle enters the posterior neuroforamen, a sudden give in resistance can be felt. It should be remembered that this block is in fact carried out in the epidural space and therefore spread of anesthetic to adjacent roots and to contralateral nerve roots may occur. Therefore, injection should be confined to 1 ml of agent.

Greater Occipital Nerve

Occipital neuralgia, resulting from injury to the greater occipital nerve or entrapment of that nerve in its passage to the scalp, is a fairly well-defined cause of headaches. Head pain that radiates from the base of the skull over the posterior two-thirds of the scalp, often with a retro-orbital component, is typical of this condition. The pain may be unilateral or bilateral and may be constant or intermittent. In some cases, occipital neuralgia results from greater occipital nerve injury due to a blow to the back of the head or a direct trauma to the nerve from a scalp laceration. However, in most cases, occipital neuralgia results from entrapment of the greater occipital nerve in its course from this origin from the C2 nerve root to its entrance into the scalp through the midportion of the superior nuchal line. Its course carries it just external to the skull, through the fibrous insertions of the cervical musculature into the pericranium. The passageway through the fibrous tissues forms a tunnel and the nerve is accompanied by the occipital artery.

In some cases, it appears that occipital neuralgia may represent a neurovascular compression syndrome as the result of a continual pulsation of the occipital artery against the nerve. In the majority of cases, however, occipital neuralgia appears to be secondary to chronic spasm of the neck muscles, as a result of either myofascial syndrome or underlying cervical spine disease.

Purpose Diagnostically, blockade of the greater occipital nerve can confirm the clinical impression of occipital neuralgia, particularly if the clinical picture is not entirely typical. Therapeutically, injection of depository steroids along the greater occipital nerve in its course just proximal to its exit from the cervical musculature can give lasting relief, particularly if chronic muscle spasm appears to be present. When pain results from closed or open trauma to the posterior scalp, radiofrequency denervation of the greater occipital nerve can be carried out, although surgical section under direct vision and local anesthesia may be no more difficult and more effective.

Technique In order to carry out injection of the greater occipital nerve, the patient is placed in a seated position with the head flexed forward. The greater occipital nerve exits just below the superior nuchal line, in the interval between the insertion of the trapezius and the sternocleidomastoid muscles. In lean individuals, this location can often be visualized. More commonly, the location can be approximated by selecting the midpoint between the external occipital protuberance in the midline and the mastoid process. Exploration of that region with digital pressure, localizing the area of maximum tenderness, most accurately defines the site for needle placement. For diagnostic block, 2–3 ml of anesthetic agent are injected. If depository steroid is to be injected, 40 mg of methylprednisolone acetate in 1–2 ml of local anesthetic are used. Following injection, the patient should be reassured that a lump palpable in the area for several hours is not unusual. If radiofrequency denervation is to be performed, an anesthetic wheal is raised on the skin overlying the presumed target and the electrode is inserted through the skin. Stimulation is carried out through the electrode while it is moved in a medial and lateral plane until the point of lowest threshold for scalp paresthesias is located. With the electrode held in place, infiltrative anesthesia in the area of its tip is obtained and a radiofrequency lesion at 75°C for 2 min is made.

Suprascapular Nerve

Entrapment of the suprascapular nerve as it passes through the suprascapular notch can produce a syndrome of aching pain within the shoulder in the absence of other evidence of joint dysfunction as well as weakness of the supraspinatus and infraspinatus muscles, characterized by weakness of abduction of the shoulder as well as lateral rotation. The suprascapular nerve, after arising from the superior cord of the brachial plexus, passes posteriorly through the scapular notch, a V-shaped wedge in the superior border of the scapula at the medial border of the coracoid process. An overlying ligament converts the notch into a canal and entrapment can occasionally result. If the diagnosis is suspected, suprascapular nerve block leading to relief of pain can confirm the diagnosis, and injection of depository steroid can sometimes provide lasting relief.

Technique Although there are techniques for injection in the scapular notch based upon trigonometric relationships of the notch to certain palpable landmarks, the block is very easily done under fluoroscopic control. With the patient prone on a fluoroscopy table and a folded sheet placed under the shoulder on the appropriate side, to place the scapula in approximately horizontal position, the scapula can be visualized in an anteroposterior direction. The scapular notch at the base of the coracoid process can then be localized and an anesthetic wheal raised above it. A needle can then be inserted directly into the notch. Since it is difficult to visualize the notch with lateral fluoroscopy, it is preferable to advance the needle to the scapula medial to the notch and then walk the needle into the notch. Once the notch is reached, the needle is advanced to 2–3 mm, aspiration is carried out, and 2 ml of agent are injected.

Intercostal Nerve

Intercostal pain generally results from direct injury to the intercostal nerve, as a result of either a rib fracture or injury from a thoracotomy incision. Although the pain pattern is quite diagnostic, it is sometimes difficult to be certain of which intercostal nerve or nerves are involved, and selective intercostal nerve blockade is useful for completing the definition of the patient's syndrome. Once the specific nerve or nerves has been identified, radiofrequency denervation or surgical section of the nerve can give lasting relief. Intercostal nerve destruction often causes no detectable neurologic deficit, because of the limited motor distribution of the nerve to the intercostal muscles and a small portion of the serratus muscles only, and the marked dermatomal overlap on the thorax.

Anatomy Each intercostal nerve is the main continuation of the ventral primary ramus of the same numbered thoracic nerve root. From its origin at the nerve root to the angle of the rib, the intercostal nerve runs on top of the pleura. At the angle of the rib, the nerve assumes a course between the internal and external intercostal muscles in a groove along the inferior surface of its rib and stays in that position until well past the anterior axilliary line. Therefore, intercostal nerve blockade can usually be carried out anywhere in the interval from the angle of the rib to the anterior axillary line, by placement of the needle into the groove on the inferior surface of the rib.

Technique The appropriate rib is defined by palpation at the point selected for injection. An anesthetic wheal is raised over the lower half of the rib and a needle inserted normal to the skin in order to contact the lower half of the rib. The needle is then walked caudally on the rib until the inferior margin is detected. The needle is then advanced approximately 3 mm under the rib and the injection carried out after a negative aspiration. One to 2 ml of anesthetic agent is satisfactory for blockade. If radiofrequency denervation is to be carried out, the needle is removed and the electrode is inserted in the same manner, first contacting the rib and then being marched caudally until it slips over the inferior edge of the rib and can be advanced several millimeters. A radiofrequency lesion at 75°C for 90 sec is then made. At the time of denervation, a vascular blush may be noted in the field of distribution of the nerve anterior to the electrode. Following completion of the denervation, digital pressure is maintained over the electrode track for 30 sec to allow soft tissue to shift back into place and obliterate the track. This will prevent a pneumothorax in the rare event of a breach in the parietal pleura by the needle or electrode.

Lateral Femoral Cutaneous Nerve

Meralgia paresthetica, a dull aching pain of the anterolateral thigh often associated with dysesthetic cutaneous sensation, results from entrapment of the lateral femoral cutaneous nerve as it traverses a fibrous tunnel in the lateral inguinal region. The diagnosis can usually be easily made on clinical grounds, but blockade of the lateral femoral cutaneous nerve is confirmatory in unclear cases. Lasting relief can often be obtained with injection of depository steroid in the area of entrapment.

Anatomy The lateral femoral cutaneous nerve arises from the ventral primary rami of the second and third lumbar nerve roots and runs internal to the ilium and iliacus muscle until it reaches the anterior superior spine of the iliac crest. The nerve then passes through a fibrous tunnel along the inferior edge of the inguinal ligament just medial to the anterior superior spine, entering the subcutaneum of the thigh in the interval between the inguinal ligament and sartorius muscle insertion. It then distributes to the skin overlying the anterolateral thigh, not quite reaching the knee. Chronic local trauma in the region of the anterior superior spine, as from a corset or belt; chronic traction on the inguinal ligament, as in obesity or pregnancy; or a change in stress on the inguinal ligament, as follows abdominal surgery, can lead to lateral femoral cutaneous nerve entrapment, presumably due to inflammation and edema of the encasing fibrous tissues. Burning or aching pain along with hypesthesia or dysesthesia in the nerve's distribution then results.

When abnormal sensation is present, it is usually very sharply demarcated and can be outlined on the skin. With temporary blockade of the lateral femoral cutaneous nerve, anesthesia is obtained that closely approximates that pattern and relief of the pain occurs. When the symptoms persist despite treatment of the precipitating condition, injection with depository steroids can often give lasting relief.

Technique To carry out blockade of the lateral femoral cutaneous nerve, the anterior superior spine of the iliac crest is palpated. In lean individuals, with the hip extended and slightly rotated internally, the sartorius muscle can often be visualized or palpated, and the triangle formed by the insertion of the inguinal ligament and that muscle can be used as a landmark. Otherwise, a point approximately 2 cm medial and 2 cm inferior to the anterior superior spine is used. A wheal of anesthetic is raised and a needle inserted through the skin. The needle is angled superiorly and laterally, to strike the medial edge of the anterior superior spine of the iliac crest. The needle is then withdrawn a few millimeters and 5 ml of anesthetic, with or without added depository steroid, is injected.

AUTONOMIC NERVOUS SYSTEM
Visceral Efferent (Sympathetic) Blockade

Hyperactivity of sympathetic outflow is demonstrable in a variety of well-defined but poorly understood pain conditions. The most common form is known as causalgia and usually results from a partial penetrating injury of a major mixed nerve. It is thus most commonly a wartime injury. It is characterized by a severe burning pain throughout the affected extremity, usually appearing a short time after the injury. The limb tends to be so hyperpathic that the patient usually cannot bear the contact of clothing on the skin. Even a light breeze blowing across the extremity can elicit severe pain, as does a drop in environmental temperature. The extremity is pale and cool to the touch and the skin quickly loses secondary appendages, becoming shiny and glossy, and occasionally discolored and dusky. The pain relief following sympathetic blockade is usually dramatic, and often a series of three to six sympathetic blocks with local anesthetic alone will give lasting relief. If blocks give only transient relief, sympathectomy is usually curative.

A much more common pain problem is a less dramatic version of causalgia, referred to as causalgia minor or, preferably, post-traumatic sympathetic dystrophy. This condition most commonly comes on after an injury, sometimes trivial, to soft tissues or joints of the extremity. Sympathetic hyperactivity follows, although the findings are generally less dramatic than those in true causalgia. Whereas the diagnosis of true causalgia is easy because of the presence of a functionally useless extremity that the patient is continually protecting, the presence of post-traumatic sympathetic dystrophy may not be recognized until an abnormal thermogram is obtained, documenting the less obvious temperature difference. Although sympathetic blockade can give significant relief, the results are seldom as dramatic as with true causalgia, and much more caution must be taken in proceeding beyond blocks to surgical sympathectomy. In essence, one should make sure that repeated blocks predictably give excellent relief and placebo blocks give no relief before progressing further.

The sympathetic nerve fibers exit the spinal cord along the nerve roots from T1 to L2. After passing laterally a short distance, the fibers leave the nerve roots and enter the paravertebral sympathetic chains, made up of interconnected sympathetic ganglia that traverse the length of the spinal axis, giving up postganglionic fibers to each of the spinal nerves. Therefore, since all sympathetic output to the upper extremity must pass up the sympathetic chain from the thoracic to the cervical region, blockade of the stellate ganglion, a fusion of the inferior cervical ganglion and the first thoracic ganglion, will effectively block all sympathetic output to the limb. Similarly, since all output to the leg arises at L2 and above, blockade of the sympathetic chain at the L3 level will effectively interrupt all sympathetic outflow to the limb.

Anatomy and Technique

Stellate Ganglion Block Although a stellate ganglion block is a technically easy bedside procedure, it has the highest complication rate of any form of nerve block and should therefore be carried out in a facility that is adequately equipped to diagnose and treat the complications.

The complication rate is due to the large number of important structures located in the area of the ganglion. Just lateral to the stellate ganglion are the carotid artery and jugular vein, which must be displaced laterally prior to needle insertion. Deep to the ganglion and sympathetic chain is the vertebral artery. The dome of the pleural cavity often rises close to the stellate ganglion, and the recurrent laryngeal nerve, controlling the vocal cords, and the phrenic nerve, innervating the diaphragm, run nearby.

The block is most easily carried out with the patient supine with a pillow placed under the shoulders so that the head falls back into a gently extended position. The target is approximately two finger-breadths above the sternal notch and two finger-breadths lateral to the midline. The nondominant index and middle finger are applied at that location and the carotid bundle gently displaced laterally. Palpation is used to detect Chassaignac's tubercle, a bony prominence on the transverse process of C6. A wheal is then raised overlying the tubercle and a needle inserted to strike just medial to the tubercle. Bone should be contacted and the needle slightly withdrawn, aspiration carried out, and 3–5 ml of anesthetic agent injected. If there is slight angulation of the needle, the transverse process will be missed and the vertebral artery might be struck. If arterial blood is obtained with aspiration, it is recommended that the procedure be terminated and not reattempted for several hours. If needle placement produces paresthesias down the extremity, this suggests that the needle has passed lateral to the transverse process and is striking the brachial plexus. The needle should then be repositioned before injection.

If sympathetic blockade is obtained, the patient will develop ipsilateral Horner's syndrome, characterized by pupillary miosis and a mild ptosis of the eyelid. If Horner's syndrome is not obtained, it should be concluded that blockade did not occur.

The most common complication is pneumothorax produced by striking the apex of the pleura. In most cases, only a small pneumothorax will occur, producing only mild breathing discomfort and requiring no specific treatment. However, the patient should be alerted to the possibility of an increase in the size of a pneumothorax and should immediately report increasing dyspnea.

Lumbar Sympathetic Block Lumbar sympathetic blockade is obtained by injection of a relatively large quantity of anesthetic agent into the retroperitoneal space anterolateral to the lumbar vertebral column. Since the lowest sympathetic outflow is at the L2 level, injection at the L3 level will effectively block all sympathetic fibers destined for the lower extremity.

With the aid of fluoroscopy, lumbar sympathetic block is easy to perform. The patient is positioned prone on the x-ray table. A wheal of anesthesia is raised over the tip of the L3 transverse process on the side to be blocked. A 6-inch needle is then inserted normal to the skin to contact the transverse process. Depth of insertion is then noted; the final depth achieved will be 3–4 cm deeper. Under fluoroscopic control, the needle is backed out slightly, angled in a slightly caudal direction to pass below the inferior edge of the transverse process, and angled medially 10–15°. There is a tendency to angulate the needle too far medially, causing the tip to strike the posterior half of the vertebral body or enter the neuroforamen. Until one is comfortable with the procedure, it is therefore wise to advance the needle just to the edge of the vertebral body in anteroposterior projection and then to check a lateral view to make sure the tip overlies the anterior half of the vertebral body. The needle is then advanced further until, on lateral view, the tip is even with the anterior surface of the L3 vertebral body.

Careful aspiration needs to be carried out, since the great vessels lie nearby. Ten to 20 ml of anesthetic agent are then injected; there should be minimal resistance to injection. The needle is then removed and the patient placed in a sitting position so that gravitational forces will encourage the anesthetic agent to bathe the lower lumbar sympathetic plexus, maximizing the sympathetic blockade. The extremity is observed for evidence of blockade, in the form of warming to touch and flushing as cutaneous vasodilatation occurs.

In advancing the needle into position, after stepping off the inferior edge of the transverse process, the patient may report paresthesias or pain radiating into the anterolateral thigh, a sign that the needle has impinged upon the L3 nerve root. Slight reangulation in one direction or another should be carried out after the needle is backed out slightly to avoid that sensation. Since the needle does pass close to the L3 nerve root, migration of anesthetic agent along the needle track will occasionally give a partial L3 root block in conjunction with the sympathetic nerve block.

Visceral Afferent Blockade

Visceral pain sensation from the stomach, small intestine, colon, and up to the splenic flexure, liver, gallbladder, pancreas, kidneys, and ureters is conducted through fibers that run along with the sympathetic fibers and traverse the celiac plexus. Temporary relief of abdominal visceral pain can therefore be obtained by blockade of the celiac plexus. This is sometimes most useful diagnostically in sorting out a pain whose characteristics do not allow classification otherwise. A specialized technique, with the injection of a lytic agent into the area of the celiac ganglion, has been used to temporarily treat visceral pain of malignant disease also.

Anatomy and Technique

Celiac Ganglion Block The celiac ganglion is located at the level of the first lumbar vertebra and lies ventral and lateral to the aorta. The technique for celiac plexus block is similar to that of lumbar sympathetic block except that the needle placement is more medial. The skin wheal is therefore raised opposite the body of L1, 10 cm lateral to the midline. The needle is inserted at approximately a 30° angle and advanced under fluoroscopic control to just contact the anterolateral body of L1. The needle is then walked off the body and advanced an additional 2 cm. On anteroposterior filming, the needle point will be just short of the midline. Aortic pulsations may be transmitted through the needle and visible. Very careful aspiration needs to be carried out and a small test injection performed. There should be no resistance to injection; if there is, repositioning of the needle should be carrried out until a resistance-free injection site is identified. Fifteen to 20 ml of anesthetic agent are then injected and the needle withdrawn. Since sympathetic blockade to both lower extremities as well as the abdominal cavity may occur, the patient is only brought gradually to the sitting position because of the possibility of orthostatic hypotension.

Because this technique involves injection of agent into the space surrounding the aorta, it is recommended that the injection of lytic agents such as alcohol be carried out only by those who have been specifically trained in the technique.

FACET JOINT BLOCK AND DENERVATION

Most back and leg pain is not due to disk herniation. Failure to recognize this fact has led to an inordinately high rate of lumbar disk surgery with overall poor results. In the search for other etiologies for back pain, attention became focused upon the facet joints as a possible source. These diarthrodial joints, well supplied with pain fibers, are placed in a state of constant compression with the development of the usual lumbar lordosis early in infancy. Throughout life they are subjected to great forces, and the development of hypertrophic arthropathy of the facet joints is a frequent occurrence in the fifth and sixth decades. It has been postulated that a traumatic arthritis of the facet joints can occur and accounts for some cases of back pain. Furthermore, there appears to be referred pain arising from each of the lower three lumbar facet joints, which explains the occurrence of pain beyond the local area of the facet joint per se. Stimulation of the L3–L4 facet joint often yields sensations rising into the posterior thoracic area; stimulation of the L4–L5 facet produces sensations radiating into the hip and thigh, and L5–S1 facet stimulation produces sensations radiating into the buttock and sacral region.

Facet joint pain is difficult to diagnose, since the joints are not accessible to close examination, and lumbar facet blocks are usually necessary to make the diagnosis. However, the diagnosis can be suspected if the back pain does not have a strong radicular component, does not have associated neurologic deficit, and is aggravated by hyperextension of the spine, which stresses the facet joints. If the diagnosis of facet syndrome is confirmed, long-lasting relief can be obtained by means of lumbar facet denervation using a radiofrequency electrode.

Anatomy and Technique

The technique of lumbar facet denervation has undergone a progressive evolution. The initial procedures used a thin scalpel to make a deep stab incision in the approximate location of the facet joint. The knife was then swept cranially and caudally to interrupt the facet innervation. Finding this excessively traumatic, Shealy developed a technique of insertion of a radiofrequency electrode under fluoroscopic control to the inner transverse ligament, where a heat lesion would be made (1). Anatomic dissections by Bogduk and Long have led to the definition of a more specific target, at the junction of the transverse process and the articular facet (2). Further attempts to refine the target are being made.

Needle placement and electrode placement for facet block and facet denervation, respectively, are identical. The general practice has been to carry out blockade and denervation of the lowest three facet joints bilaterally unless there is specific evidence of injury to a single facet joint. At L4 and L5, the target is the junction of the transverse process with the superior articular process. An anesthetic wheal is raised above the lateral portion of the transverse process and the needle inserted under fluoroscopic control to the above-defined target. A slight medialward angulation of the needle that this approach provides allows the needle to slip under a hypertrophic facet joint and approach the articular branch of the posterior primary ramus directly. At the S1 level, the target is defined by the superior edge of the sacrum at the point where it joins the superior articular process of S1, forming a notch on anteroposterior fluoroscopy. At each location, 1 ml of anesthetic agent is injected. One must avoid injecting large quantities of agent lest blockade of multiple other structures, including the nearby nerve roots, be obtained. If denervation is to be carried out, the needle is removed and replaced by an electrode along the same course. When the tip of the electrode is resting in the proper position, striking the posterior surface of the transverse process, the nerve root itself is shielded from the heat of the electrode. A radiofrequency lesion at 75°C for 90 sec is then made and the electrode removed.

After facet denervation, the patient is advised that he may note some aggravation of his usual pain after the anesthetic wears off. It is normally difficult to draw a definite conclusion as to how helpful a procedure will be until approximately 1 week has elapsed, during which time the associated soft tissue injury will heal and any muscle spasm triggered by needle insertion will have resolved.

References

1. Bogduk N, Long DM: Percutaneous lumbar medial branch neurotomy: a modification of facet denervation. *Spine* 5:193–200, 1980.
2. Shealy CN: Percutaneous radiofrequency denervation of spinal facets. *J. Neurosurg* 43:448–451, 1975.

Suggested Readings

Camins M, O'Leary P: *The Lumbar Spine.* New York, Raven Press, 1987.
Carron H, Korbon GA, Rowlingson JC: *Regional Anesthesia.* Orlando, FL, Grune & Stratton, 1984.
Finneson B: *Low Back Pain,* ed. 2. Philadelphia, JB Lippincott, 1980.
Hendler NH, Long DM, Wise TN: *Diagnosis and Treatment of Chronic Pain.* Littleton, MA John Wright & Sons, 1982.
Rothman R, Simeone F: *The Spine,* ed 2. Philadelphia, WB Saunders, 1982.
Stanton-Hicks M, Boas R: *Chronic Low Back Pain.* New York, Raven Press, 1982.
White JC, Sweet WH: *Pain and the Neurosurgeon.* Springfield, IL, Charles C Thomas, 1969.
Youmans JR: *Neurological Surgery,* ed 2. Philadelphia, WB Saunders, 1982.

chapter 11
Neurosurgical Treatment of Deafferentation Pain

Blaine S. Nashold, Jr., M.D.
Eben Alexander, M.D.

"Doctor, why do I have burning pain in my numb arm?" This question puzzles not only the patient but also the physician. The patient may be describing deafferentation pain if he suffers from brachial plexus avulsion or paraplegia. The diagnosis of deafferentation pain in not difficult, but its cause is unknown and treatment can be difficult. Numerous authors have characterized deafferentation pain as did Tasker et al. (1), whose clinical definition was "a state of dysesthetic pain resulting from neural injury," whereas Wall, a neurophysiologist, defined it as "not only a loss of input but actually degeneration so that the spinal cord cells were free to act in a pathologic way" (2). There remains no adequate pathophysiologic explanation of deafferentation pain. We classify deafferentation pain into three clinical types: (a) a dysesthesia due to lesions that involve the peripheral nerve and/or the dorsal root ganglion, (b) dysesthesia with lesions rostral to dorsal root ganglion but including the spinal cord, and (c) dysesthetic pain with lesions of the spinal axis, brainstem, and/or thalamus. This latter type of pain is often designated as a central pain and was described in the early neurologic literature as associated with the thalamic syndrome. The best clinical examples of the deafferentation pain syndrome include brachial plexus avulsion, avulsion of spinal roots from the conus medullaris, or dysesthesia following spinal cord injury with paraplegia as well as a variety of other pathologic insults of the brainstem and/or thalamus.

The patient with deafferentation syndrome often describes severe pain in a partially or completely anesthetic area of the body. The pains are intractable to treatment. On neurologic examination, there is always alteration of the various sensory modalities, with the pain described as disagreeable and/or burning. The pain may or may not be intensified by cutaneous stimulation of the painful area, but there may exist cutaneous trigger points found in areas of the body at some distance from the original region of dysesthesia. Touching the trigger points will activate the pain. For example, a patient with a brachial plexus avulsion and an associated anesthetic arm may have trigger spots on the skin of the neck or abdomen, usually several dermatomal levels away from the site of the original injury. Touching the trigger spot with excite the pain in the deafferented, anesthetic limb.

Every pathologic lesion involving the central sensory pathways does not necessarily result in a central pain syndrome. In fact, only 10–15% of avulsion injuries to the brachial plexus or spinal cord exhibit this pain syndrome. In the thalamic syndrome, the number of patients who suffer from pain is probably smaller. When the onset of deafferentation pain occurs early in the course of the disease or following trauma, it then becomes intractable, and it is in this group of patients that medical and surgical treatment has been so difficult. In this chapter we confine our discussion to four types of deafferentation pain—the thalamic syndrome and three others due to pathologic changes in the spinal cord: brachial/conus medullaris nerve root avulsions, postherpetic pain involving either the trigeminal or spinal nerve roots, and traumatic paraplegia with pain.

DORSAL ROOT ENTRY ZONE PHYSIOLOGY AND NEUROANATOMY

The successful neurosurgical operation for relief of pain depends on the careful selection of the patient along with the choice of a therapeutic lesion that involves specific neuroanatomic structures, in this case the dorsal entry area. It is well known that a surgical section of the lateral spinothalamic tract will result in the loss of pain and thermal sensation on the contralateral side of the body; therefore, a lateral spinothalamic tractotomy deprives large regions of the body of these two sensory modalities even though the pain may be confined to a smaller region of the body. The ideal pain operation would be made at a specific site in the central nervous system that would result in pain relief only in the area of the body involved with pain. At present no such ideal operation exists; however, lesions of the dorsal root entry zone (DREZ) have certain advantages in that they involve a localized neuroanatomic structure (the DREZ) and can result in pain relief in those restricted regions of the body that are painful (one to several dermatomes). The DREZ operation makes it theoretically possible to confine the pain relief to the painful areas involved. A good clinical example of the DREZ localized effect is in the person with postherpetic pain, which usually involves only one or two dermatomes. If these involved roots are surgically treated, pain relief occurs only in a restricted zone.

The DREZ represents the first spinal cord region where initial integration of sensory information takes place in the central nervous system. We believe that in certain path syndromes (deafferentation) the neural mechanism responsible for the pain originates in the neurons of the damaged dorsal horn. A good example of this are the dorsal root avulsion injuries of paraplegia and postherpetic pain. At present the dorsal horn is under intense study by neurophysiologists. The dorsal horn region was first described by Rolando (3), an Italian anatomist of the 18th century, who identified the region by gross inspection of the spinal cord. Later this dorsal spinal region was named the substantia gelatinosa of Rolando. However, it was Rexed (4) who identified 10 distinctive anatomic layers of the dorsal horn based on its specific cytoarchetectonics (Fig. 11.1). At present neurophysiologists are adding to our knowledge of the neurophysiologic importance of these Rexed zones.

Nonciceptive input from small fiber systems are found in Rexed layer I, sometimes designated as the substantia gelatinosa, and Rexed layer V (Fig. 11.2). The DREZ lesions, using special thermal electrodes, are therefore designed to destroy these five superficial layers of the dorsal horn (Rexed layers I–V). In animal experiments, where deafferentation of the dorsal horn can be experimentally produced, the secondary interneurons in the superficial and deeper Rexed layer (Rexed V) become unstable a few hours after the experimental injury. By monitoring the damaged dorsal horn in these animals with microelectrodes, we have found abnormal electrical activity of the

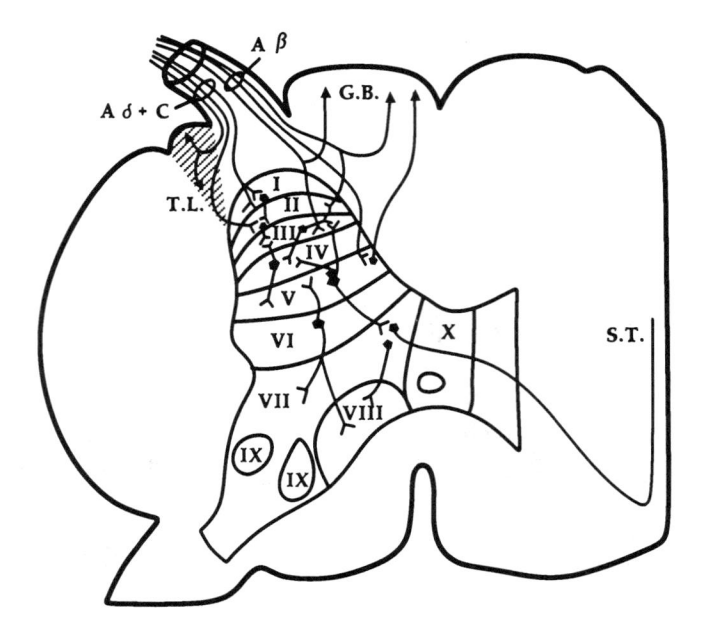

Figure 11.1. Schematic cross-section of spinal cord showing afferent connections and Rexed layers. DREZ lesions destroy layers I–V.

neurons within a few hours of the insult; this electrical abnormality continues for many months. We believe that this abnormal electrical activity (epileptiform) may be the genesis of the pain in both animals and humans. The dorsal horn is rich in a variety of neuropeptides that are altered in the experimental animal model and certainly in humans following injury, but the exact role of these neuropeptides in the pain process is still unknown. We believe that the reduction of pain following lesions of the dorsal horn (DREZ) is the result of destroying the abnormal secondary interneurons and their connections. This was the original theoretical basis for the DREZ operation.

SPINAL ROOT AVULSION

Avulsion of the spinal nerve roots is usually the result of trauma. Years ago it was often due to a fall, with the person striking and depressing the shoulder, causing traction and avulsion of the cervical nerve roots. Today avulsion injuries almost always follow high-speed vehicular accidents with the motorcycle being the main offender, although we have seen it after automobile, snowmobile, and speedboat accidents.

The force of the injury is transmitted to the head and neck along the brachial plexus, avulsing the spinal nerve roots. Both the dorsal and ventral roots can be avulsed with some variation in the number of roots involved, but most of the time in brachial plexus avulsions the dorsal roots from C5 to T1 are involved (Fig. 11.3). Rarely are only one or two roots involved. The person may suffer other serious associated injuries involving the head and neck, so

Chapter 11/Neurosurgical Treatment of Deafferentation Pain   127

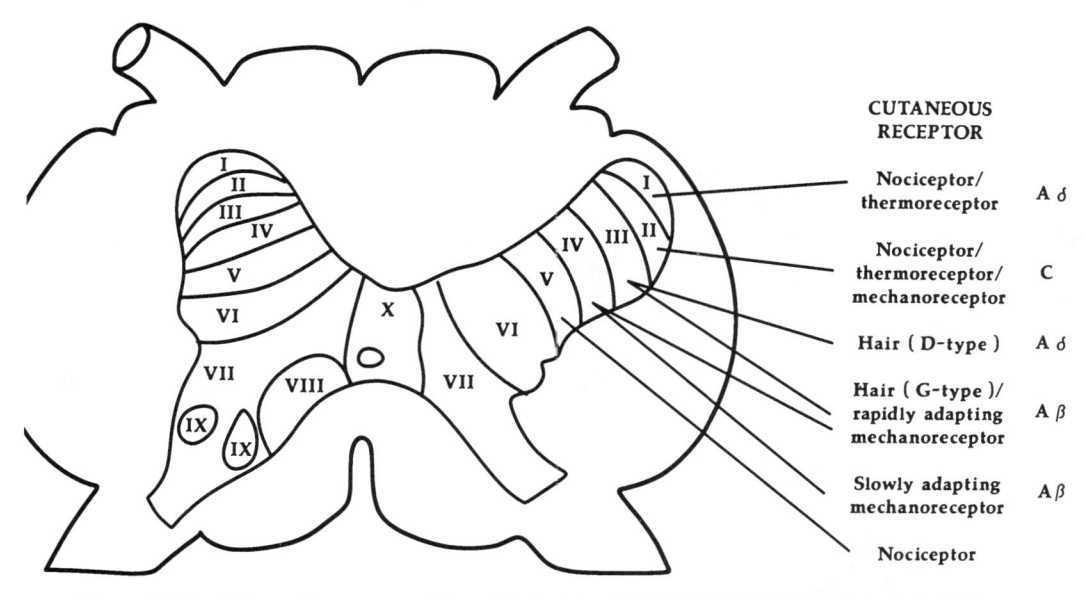

Figure 11.2. Schematic cross-section of spinal cord showing Rexed layers and physiology.

the presence of the avulsion injury may not be evident on the initial examination, particularly if the patient is semiconscious. Intractable pain occurs in about 10% of patients with avulsion, begins very early after the injury, and responds poorly to medical treatment. The DREZ operation has been effective in relief of the pain in about 70% of patients, with the relief lasting over 5 years (5).

The clinical diagnosis of an avulsion injury is not difficult. The patient complains of severe burning and/or electric shock–like pains in the paralyzed analgesic arm or leg. In the arm the pain may be referred along the radial aspect into the thumb or index finger, whereas in the leg it may be confined to a specific dermatomal distribution involving the big toe or the lateral aspect of the foot (L4–S1). It should be recognized that the dorsal spinal roots can also be avulsed from injuries involving the conus medullaris that are the result of severe pelvic trauma (Fig. 11.4). The patients complain of the same types of pain, but the pain is localized to the involved lower extremity. After avulsion the involved arm or leg lies immobile and useless, with atrophic changes of the skin and muscle. Occasionally one finds a patient in whom the paralyzed painful limb has been amputated in order to relieve the pain

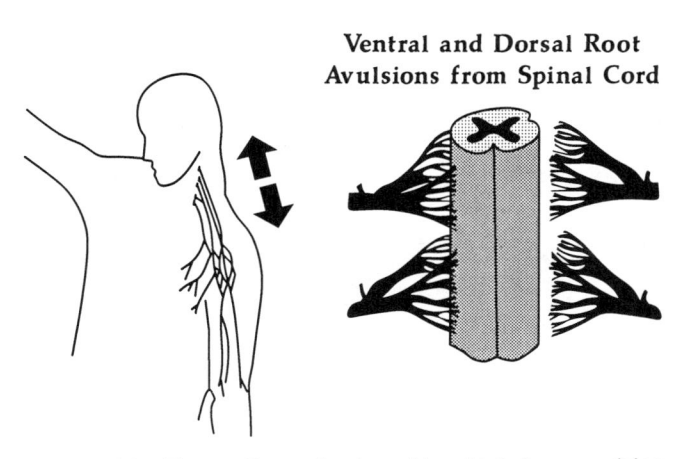

Figure 11.3. Traumatic mechanism of brachial plexus avulsion injury.

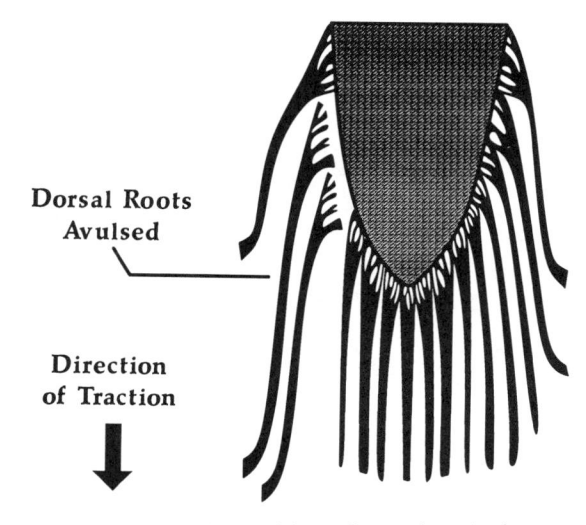

Figure 11.4. Traumatic avulsion of sacral roots from conus medullaris.

128　Therapeutic Modalities/Section 2

and unfortunately the patient now has phantom limb pain. Needless to say, this barbaric treatment is not recommended. Amputation is recommended after relieving the pain, since the lifeless limb is now more of a hindrance than a help to the patient.

Along with the neurologic examination, a myelographic study will help confirm the diagnosis of spinal root avulsion (Fig. 11.5). Traumatic myeloceles of varying size and extent can be seen in the spinal region of the avulsion (cervical/lumbosacral). The number of traumatic myeloceles are not indicative of the extent of the nerve root avulsion, particularly in the cervical region, where it is common for four or five roots to be avulsed with only one or two traumatic myeloceles present (Fig. 11.5). Fewer roots tend to be avulsed in the sacral than in the cervical region, and we have found several paraplegias caused by gunshot wounds with avulsed roots near the site of the spinal cord injury. Additional examination, such as electromyography or the recording of sensory-evoked potentials, is of interest but not diagnostic.

The DREZ operation consists of surgically exposing the region of the spinal cord involved in the avulsion injury and producing small (1–2-mm) thermal lesions in the dorsal horn to destroy the first five Rexed layers of the DREZ (Figs. 11.6 and 11.7). The details of the operation have been reported in the neurospinal literature and are not dealt with here. The complications of the DREZ operation are related to the involvement of neighboring spinal cord structures such as the dorsal columns and/or the descending motor pathways or of the ascending spinocerebellar tract, with lesions in the higher cervical cord. No deaths have occurred in over 400 operations, and the morbidity has been about 5% of the patients who have postoperative ipsilateral arm/leg weakness. Transient bladder and motor disorders have occurred in a few paraplegics.

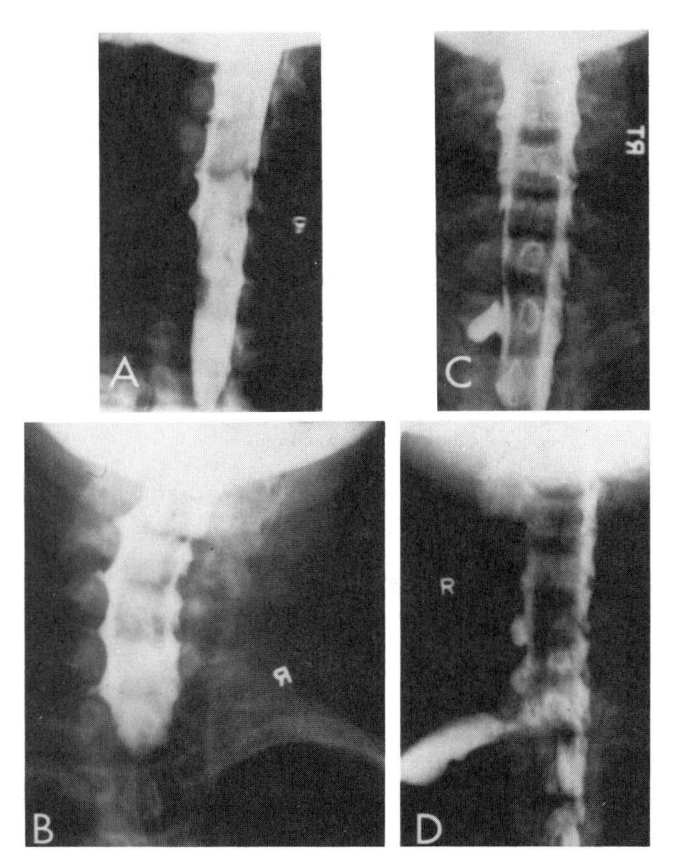

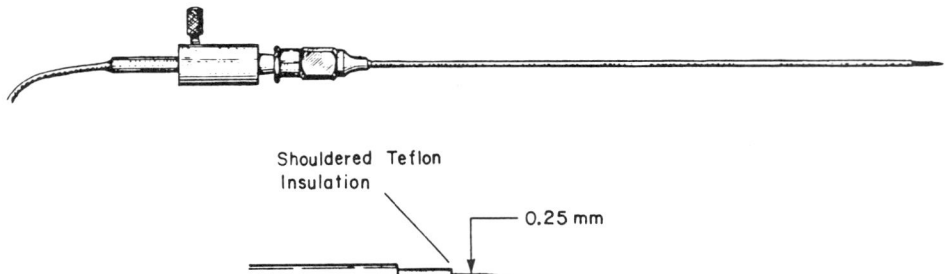

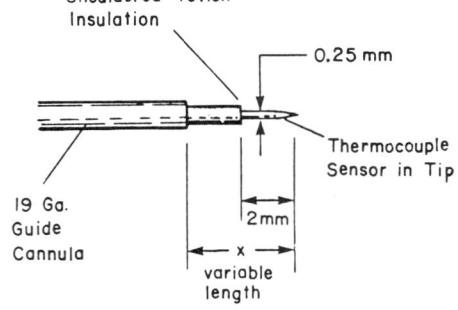

Figure 11.5. Cervical myelograms in patients with brachial plexus avulsion injury.

Figure 11.6. DREZ electrode (Radionics).　　NTCD (0.25) Tip Dimensions

the longer the patient suffers pain the more difficult it is to treat may only be partially true, but early treatment is always preferable.

Two main types of pain are described by the paraplegic patient. One is a diffuse burning pain usually involving widespread areas of the legs and sacrum. The DREZ operation will not relieve this type of pain. Another type of pain is that which occurs in those portions of the body near or just above the cutaneous zone of sensory loss. On sensory examination in these patients one finds a zone of cutaneous sensory change for several dermatomes rostral to the upper anesthetic dermatome. Touching or stroking the skin of this area sets off the patient's pain and is described by him as shooting or electrical discomfort referred into the paralyzed limbs. The pain can also be spontaneously triggered by distention of an abdominal viscera, such as the bladder or the lower bowel. Cutaneous trigger spots in distant dermatomes occur in these paraplegics. Stimulation of the skin will trigger the patient's pain, and it is this pain that responds to the DREZ lesions.

The clinical diagnosis of deafferentation pain in the paraplegic is not difficult. It is helpful to carry out a spinal myelogram to define both the upper and lower limits of the spinal cord pathology as well as to look for the presence of

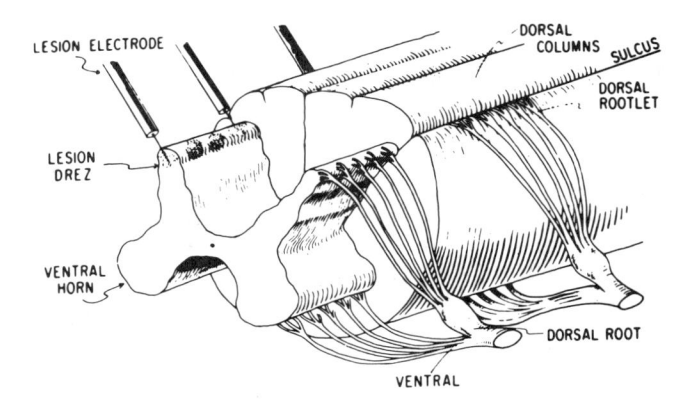

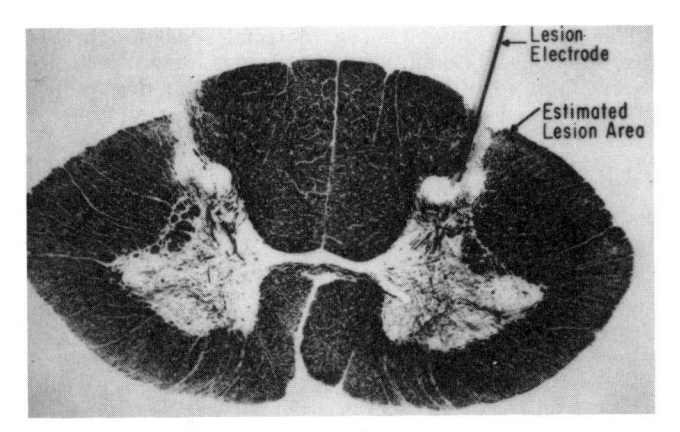

Figure 11.7. Schematic representation of area of dorsal horn involved in DREZ lesion.

PARAPLEGIA

Traumatic paraplegia is associated with chronic deafferentation pain in about 10% of the patients. The onset of pain presents in two ways. In the majority of paraplegics, the pain occurs early after the injury; in another group of paraplegics the pain does not appear for several years after their initial trauma. In these latter paraplegics with a delayed onset of pain, one-third will have an associated spinal cyst at or near the site of spinal cord trauma, visualized either on myelography or at surgery (Fig. 11.8). In our experience, the emptying of the spinal cyst alone may not be sufficient to relieve the patient's pain; in addition, it is necessary to perform the DREZ operation to obtain pain relief. Once the pain syndrome has not responded to medical treatment (6 months), we believe that the DREZ operation should be carried out as early as possible (at 6 months to 1 year). We have had several patients in whom the pain was present for many years; for instance, one man's 30-year pain was finally relieved by the DREZ operation. This suggests that the old idea that

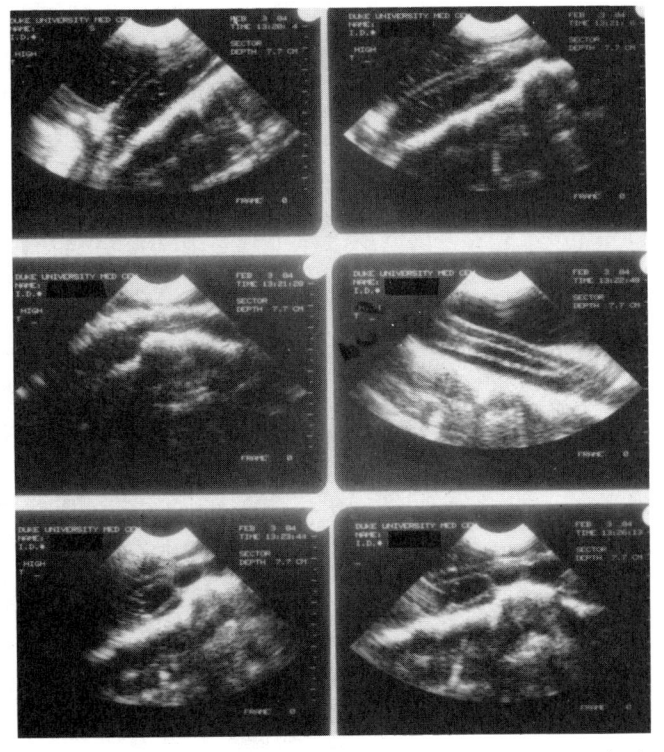

Figure 11.8. Intraoperative ultrasound studies in paraplegic with spinal cord cyst and pain.

one or more spinal cord cysts. The spinal cyst can best be visualized by doing a delayed computed tomography (CT) scan of the spinal cord following the myelogram. After 6 hr, the contrast will have penetrated the cyst cavity sufficiently for good visualization. The use of intraoperative ultrasound studies of the exposed spinal cord at the time of surgery is also very useful in defining the extent of the cyst. At times the spinal myelogram with delayed CT scan does not precisely delineate the cyst, and in several patients, using intraoperative ultrasound, we found two separate spinal cysts that had been missed on the routine myelogram.

The surgical treatment in the paraplegic with deafferentation pain consists of exposing the spinal cord above and below the level of the traumatic lesion (usually two to three vertebral levels). The DREZ lesions are made bilaterally in the DREZ beginning at the level of the trauma and extending rostrally for at least two to three spinal segments. If a cyst is present, it is drained with a permanent catheter into the subarachnoid space. In paraplegics, good relief of pain can be expected in 50% for at least 5 years (6, 7).

POSTHERPETIC PAIN

TRIGEMINAL NUCLEUS CAUDALIS

Chronic facial pain due to postherpetic infection of the gasserian ganglion has been very difficult to treat. The virus initially affects the gasserian ganglion and the skin, with painful cutaneous lesions involving the three divisions of the trigeminal nerve. If there is involvement of the first trigeminal division (V_1) the pain is referred to the eye and forehead and scarring of the involved skin area may be associated with hyperesthesia and/or hyperalgesia (Fig. 11.9). When the cornea is involved, it becomes anesthetic, with the added problem of corneal scarring and the risk of loss of sight. The second and third trigeminal divisions (V_2 and V_3) are similarly involved in some patients (Fig. 11.10).

The anatomic organization of facial sensation in the trigeminal tract (touch and pain) was determined by Soquist and resulted in his sectioning the descending trigeminal tract in the medulla for relief of certain types of facial pain (Fig. 11.11). The facial sensation via the trigeminal system is organized into three separate nuclei located in the medullocervical junction. The pain afferents end in the trigeminal nucleus caudalis, which lies at the medullospinal junction between the lower end of the obex and the second cervical dorsal root. The trigeminal nucleus cau-

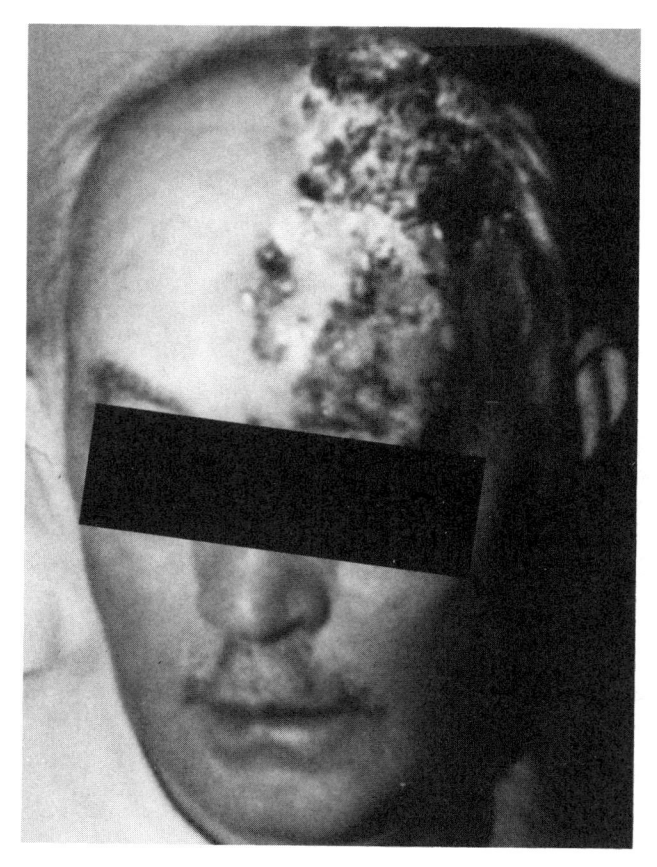

Figure 11.9. Patient with involvement of first division of trigeminal nerve (V_1) during acute phase of herpetic infection.

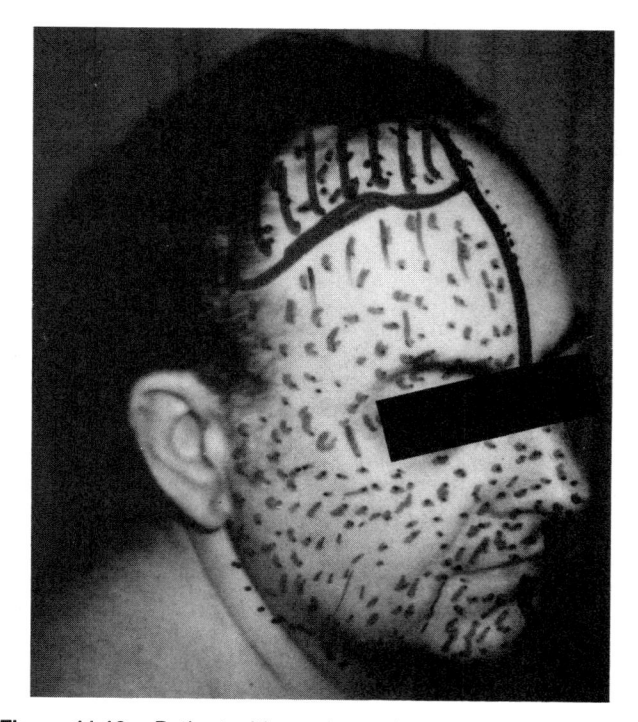

Figure 11.10. Patient with postherpetic pain of the trigeminal nerve, total analgesia over forehead, and remainder of face hyperalgesic to all sensory stimulation. Total relief (3 years pain free) was achieved after caudalis DREZ.

Chapter 11/Neurosurgical Treatment of Deafferentation Pain 131

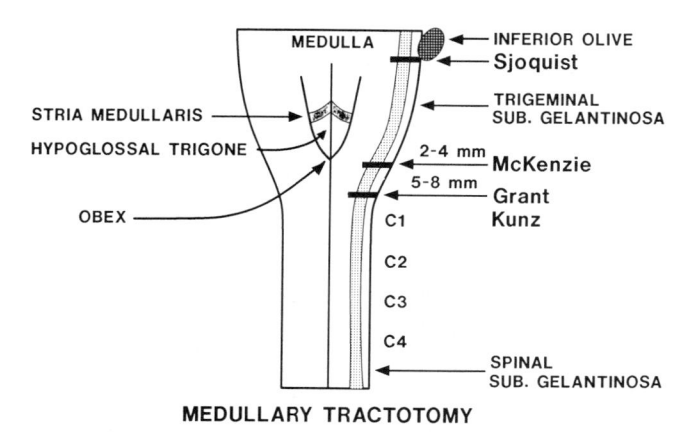

Figure 11.11. Schematic drawing of medullary cervical junction showing extent and merging of substantia gelatinosa from trigeminal system and spinal regions. Levels of section of descending trigeminal tract indicated with names of researchers at suggested DREZ lesion points.

dalis has a neuroanatomic organization similar to that of the spinal dorsal horn (Fig. 11.12). In fact, the dorsal horn merges at the level of the cervical cord with the nucleus caudalis. The nucleus caudalis receives the majority of pain afferents and fibers from the face and oral cavity via the descending trigeminal tract. The nucleus has a unique organization in that the three trigeminal divisions are arranged in a laminar fashion beginning at the level of the medullary obex and extending caudally into the upper cervical cord segments. There is also a dorsoventral lamination of the three divisons, with the eye and forehead division (V_1) situated ventrally near the origin of the roots of the spinal accessory nerve while the jaw and lower cheek division (V_3) is dorsally situated, with the central facial area division (V_2) interposed between the two. Lying along the lateral length of the nucleus caudalis are the ascending fibers of the spinocerebellar tract, which may be involved by the DREZ lesion, causing a transient ipsilateral ataxia of the arm.

Using a special DREZ caudalis electrode, it is possible to destroy the nucleus caudalis at the cervicomedullary junction and, therefore, interrupt not only the descending trigeminal fibers but the secondary trigeminal neurons and their central connections to the midbrain and thalamus. We have successfully reduced the deafferentation pain associated with postherpetic infection of the gasserian ganglion as well as pain of anesthesia dolorosa by destroying the nucleus caudalis. A therapeutic DREZ lesion of this nucleus results in anesthesia over the entire trigeminal distribution of the face and oral cavity. Relief can be expected in half of the patients (8).

The major postoperative complication of a nucleus caudalis lesion is involvement of the adjacent spinocerebellar tract, which may result in ataxia of the ipsilateral arm. This complication has occurred in only a few patients and usually clears in a short time. The caudalis DREZ is a good example of DREZ lesions confined to a specific, well-localized anatomic structure such as the trigeminal system, thus relieving pain in a small, specific area of the face and/or oral cavity.

THORACOABDOMINAL PAIN

Herpetic involvement with pain can also occur in the trunk or abdominal region and is more common than facial involvement. The pain of shingles is one of the most difficult to treat medically or surgically. When the pain becomes chronic (10% of the patients), most therapy has been unsuccessful (9). In those patients with chronic

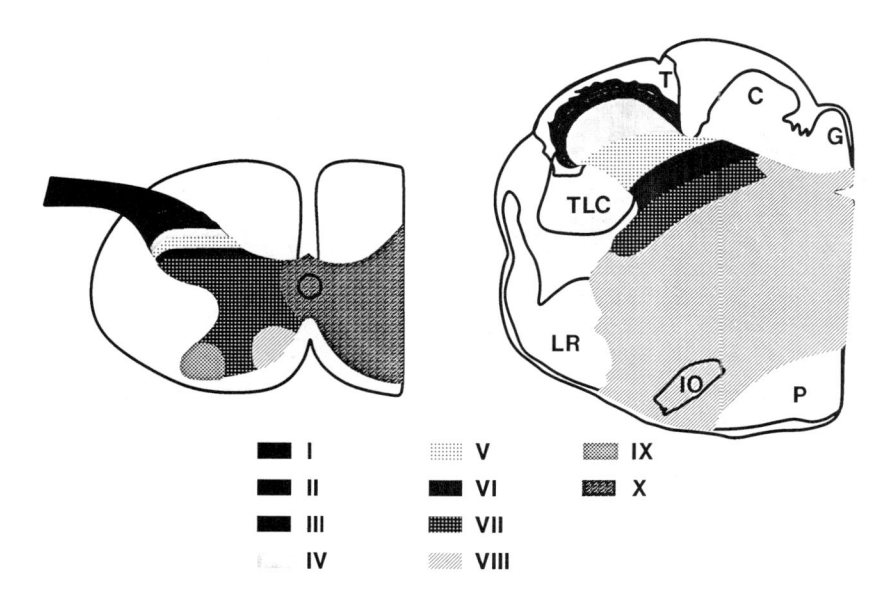

Figure 11.12. Schematic cross-sections of cervical cord and lower medulla. Shows the similarities of the organization of the Rexed layers in spinal cord and medulla. The DREZ lesions in the cord medulla are produced in the Rexed layers I–V.

postherpetic pain, the DREZ operation has been successful in reducing the pain to manageable levels in 60% of patients.

Shingles is the result of a chicken pox infection, which may lie dormant in the dorsal root ganglion of the elderly, who most often suffer from this painful disorder. The viral infection is often triggered by nonspecific stimuli or stress, such as debilitating diseases, surgical operations, and radiation therapy, and by unknown factors. Shingles occurs three times more frequently in the octogenarian. The dermatomal distribution involves most frequently C3, T5, L1, and L2, as well as the ophthalmic division of the trigeminal nerve (V_1). The ophthalmic branch is affected with 20 times the frequency of the other two divisions of the trigeminal nerve.

Originally it was thought that the pathologic process resulting from the viral infection was localized only to the dorsal root ganglion, but it is now apparent that the virus also invades the spinal cord, especially the DREZ region, and at times even the motor neurons in the ventral horn are involved. We believe that the chronic pain syndrome of herpes is due to the dorsal horn involvement, since the DREZ lesion of the involved DREZ area results in good pain relief in a significant number of patients.

The onset of the disease is heralded by a deep, lancinating pain appearing several weeks before the skin rash, which is a vesicular eruption occurring in the involved dermatome (thoracic regions, 65%; facial region, 20%). When healing of the skin occurs, there are large scarred cutaneous regions that are painful. These cutaneously involved dermatomes outlined by the pathologic skin lesions are found to be grossly abnormal on sensory examination. The scarred areas may be hyperalgesic to light touch and pin prick with zones of complete hyperesthesia. Stroking the skin may activate the patient's pain, and patients often protect these skin areas from stimulation. The patient may also complain of another type of pain other than the lancinating pain. This is described as a deep, aching sensation often unaffected by skin stimulation. This deeper pain may not be involved by the DREZ lesion. It is therefore important for the physician to delineate the kinds of pain the patient is suffering before surgery is advised. If at times the patient experiences both the severe lancinating and the deep type of pain, he still may have partial benefit from the DREZ operation.

The DREZ operation for relief of postherpetic pain in the thoracic and/or abdominal region requires careful planning by the neurosurgeon since it is essential that the dorsal roots lesioned are only those involved in the painful syndrome (10). The involvement of the thoracic dermatomes is surgically the most difficult since the anatomic localization of the thoracic dorsal roots is variable (Fig. 11.13). Both intraoperative radiographic and physiologic localization using evoked potentials is important for pre-

Figure 11.13. Postherpetic abdominal involvement with intractable pain. Post-DREZ lesion showing levels of postlesion dermatomes involving dorsal roots T11–L1.

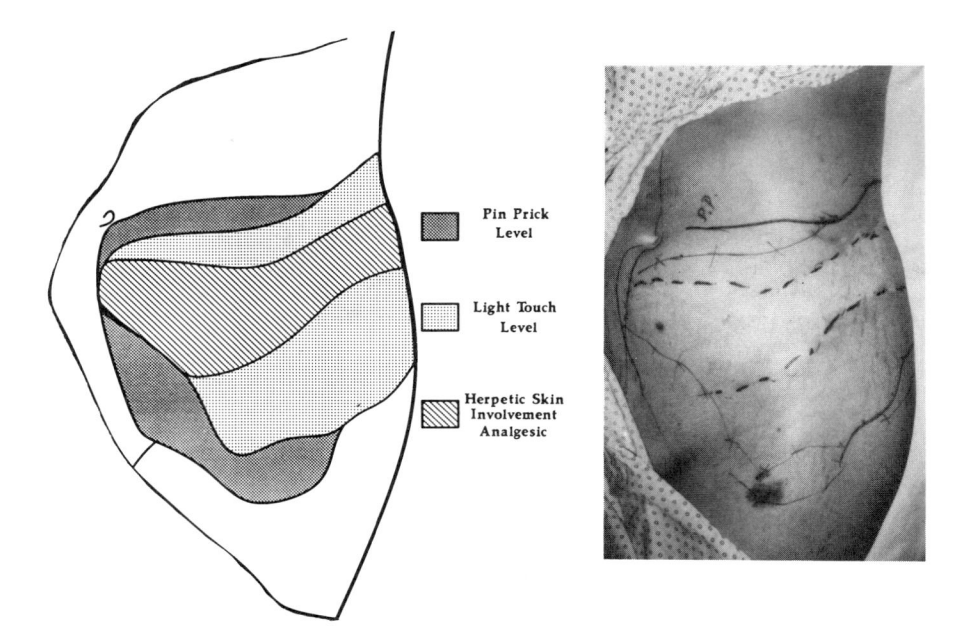

Post Herpetic Pain
DREZ T11 - L1
Post DREZ Sensory Changes

cise placement of the thoracic DREZ lesions. When the appropriate spinal cord segments are surgically exposed, the surgeon inspecting the spinal cord and dorsal roots may find that the involved dorsal roots have an abnormal appearance—atrophied and dullish red in coloration—under the operative microscope. Biopsy of these abnormal dorsal roots reveals specific damage to the larger myelinated sensory fibers with apparent sparing of the smaller (pain) fibers. The entire dorsal root appears to be involved, and we believe this involvement extends into the dorsal horn. For this reason the DREZ lesions are made in the DREZ of the involved painful dermatomes. The thoracic DREZ operation has the greatest potential for postlesion complication since the thoracic cord is sensitive to any type of surgical trauma. The major postoperative risk is weakness in the ipsilateral leg due to encroachment by the DREZ lesions on the pyramidal tract; this occurs in about 5% of patients. The best way to avoid this complication is to carefully control the size of the lesions, which we accomplish by the use of a specially designed thermal DREZ electrode along with the use of steroids in the postoperative period. It is important for the surgeon to warn the patient about this potential complication before the DREZ operation.

THALAMIC SYNDROME

The thalamic syndrome, first described by Dejerine and Roussy in 1906 (11), consists of severe, intractable burning pain with frequent exacerbations, either spontaneous or following mild tactile stimuli, as a sequela of an infarction affecting the thalamus. A similar pain may follow brainstem lesions, including tumors, or ablative neurosurgical procedures (12). The patient initially exhibits a "typical stroke" with a hemiparesis. There may be varying degrees of sensory disturbance on the paretic side of the body. As the hemiparesis clears, the patient begins to experience pain that is most often located in the head and arm on the paretic side. The patient often complains of pain centered deep in the eye. The pain is described as burning in nature and can be aggravated by touching the skin of the involved side. Emotional upsets also can often trigger the pain. Fortunately only 10% of stroke patients develop central pain, but when it is present it is difficult to treat. The pain frequently precedes other facets of the syndrome, and is often ill defined. Pain is constant, although paroxysmal, and frequently described as restricting, burning, or coming in waves. Hyperpathia, with varying degrees of stimulation either locally or at distant points being evocative, commonly occurs, with pain rapidly ascending to a crescendo, followed by a slow diminution. This pain is frequently refractory to medical and behavioral modification therapies.

Of the five principle groups of arteries that supply the thalamus (13), the thalamogeniculate stalk (inferior and posterior group) penetrates between the geniculate bodies to supply the nucleus ventralis posterior, anterior pulvinar, and centrum medianum. Involvement of this group leads to the classic syndrome of Dejerine and Roussy. The hemiparesis is usually transient, leaving hemianesthesia to light touch with profound loss of deep pressure sensation, the severe paroxysms of pain mentioned above, and mild ataxia and astereognosia on the affected side. Choreotaxic movements on the affected side are routinely seen. Vasomotor symptoms, consisting of cyanosis, hyperthermia, pallor, and diaphoresis, are not uncommon (14).

The nucleus ventralis posterior receives the spinothalamic tracts and the medial lemniscus in its pars lateralis, as opposed to the trigeminothalamic tracts, which terminate in the pars medialis. The head is medial with the body lateral in somatotopic organization within the nucleus. Most afferents from this nucleus are directed to the postcentral gyrus.

The pulvinar is mainly an association nucleus with afferents derived from the auditory pathways and nucleus geniculatus lateralis, although this is still under investigation. It has diffuse efferent pathways to the cerebral cortex and probably plays a role in speech formation.

The centrum medianum is divided into a dorsomedial pars magnocellularis, with efferents to the caudate nucleus, and the pars parvocellularis (ventrolateral), which projects to the putamen (14).

The thalamic pain described above has been reported with thalamic lesions in several locations (lateral formation, alone or with the medial nucleus or ventral posterior nucleus, or in the latter alone) (14). Of note, thousands of stereotaxic thalamic lesions have been made with only extremely rare reports of thalamic pain (15). The surgeon defines this by requiring additional lesions in the interal capsule or parietal lobe to explain the "thalamic" pain.

Several forms of surgical therapy for the thalamic pain syndrome have been reported, with varying degrees of success. Extirpation of the postcentral gyrus (16) as well as cervical cordotomy (17) have reportedly been successful. Partial pain relief was noted in one reported case using posteromedial hypothalamotomy (18). The same author has used thermocoagulation of the posterior internal medullary lamina of the thalamus with excellent results (19). Stereotaxic lesions in the pulvinar were completely successful in 3 of 11 cases (20). Pain perception is unaffected by interrupting pathways to the frontal lobes via prefrontal lobotomy (21) or cingulotomy (22), although the "suffering" component may be diminished. Bilateral amygdalectomies have had similar limitations (23). Electrical stimulation of the central gray matter (24), thalamus (25, 26), mesencephalic medial lemniscus (27), and periventricular gray matter have all been reported with varying degrees of success, limited mainly by adaptation, patient compliance, and expense (28, 29). Stereotaxic mesencephalotomy was first reported by Spiegel and Wycis (30), and its success in several series has supported its continued use in certain settings (31–34).

Sixteen of 24 (67%) patients in our series at Duke University Medical Center had long-term relief of their thalamic pain after mesencephalic tractotomy, with two deaths. None of 12 (75%) of those who had lesions made

Figure 11.14. Overall results of DREZ lesions performed at Duke University Medical Center as of 1987.

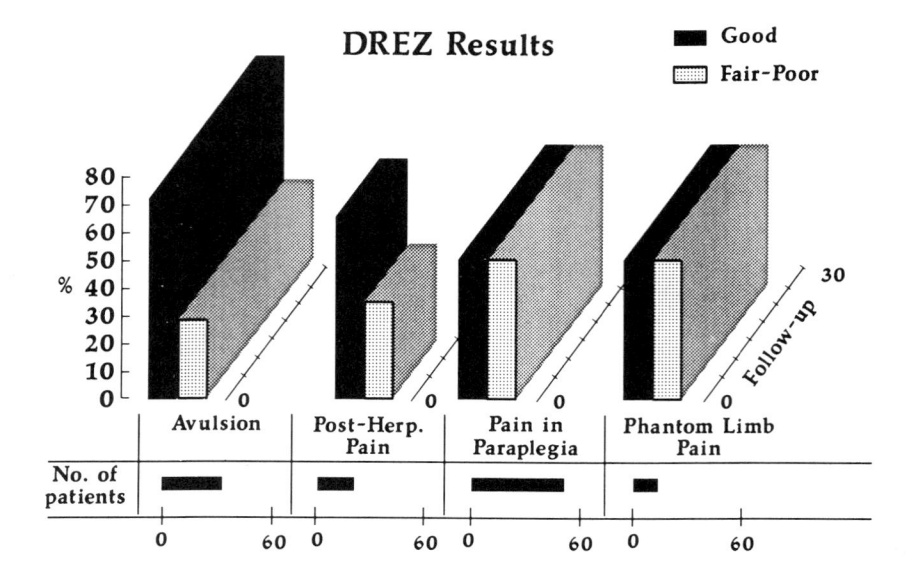

at the "superior colliculus" site reported significant long-term improvement. Seven of 12 (58%) who had surgery at the "inferior colliculus" site reported good pain relief. Postoperative disorders of ocular movement and difficulties with binocular vision have been reduced with recent improvements in technique (Colin Shieff, unpublished information; 35–39).

CHEMICAL HYPOPHYSECTOMY

Chemical hypophysectomy has been used by Levin and colleagues to treat three patients with thalamic syndrome (40). Two patients were significantly relieved of their pain with a follow-up of 19–58 months. The mechanism of pain relief is unknown. The authors suggested several theoretical possibilities. One is that the relief of pain is due to a humoral effect produced by the hypophysectomy on peripheral receptors. Another theory is that the humoral agent acts centrally to relieve pain. The use of pituitary ablation for cancer pain due to prostate and breastbone metastasis is well known, but more clinical studies are needed until hypophysectomy can be applied for the treatment of thalamic pain.

CONCLUSIONS

Our understanding and treatment of deafferentation pain has improved but is far from complete. The goal of the neurosurgeon is to devise surgical treatments that are localized to the site of pathophysiologic changes responsible for the pain, reducing adverse side effects to a minimum. This goal has been in part achieved with the DREZ lesions (Fig. 11.14), but much work is yet to be done in the laboratory and at the bedside.

References

1. Tasker RR, Organ LW, Hawrylyshyn P: Deafferentation and causalgia. In Bonica J (ed): *Pain*. New York, Raven Press, 1980, pp 305–329.
2. Wall P, Devar M: Sensory afferent impulses originate from dorsal root ganglia as well as from the periphery in normal and nerve injured rats. *Pain* 17:321–339, 1983.
3. Rolando L: *Ricerche Anatomiche sulla Struttura del Midollo Spinale*. Torino, Dallas Stamperia Renle, 1824.
4. Rexed B: A cytoarchitectonic atlas of the spinal cord of the cat. *J Comp Neurol* 100:297–380, 1954.
5. Nashold BS, Ostdahl RH: Dorsal root entry zone lesions for pain relief. *J Neurosurg* 51:59–69, 1979.
6. Nashold BS, Bullitt E: Dorsal root entry zone lesions to control pain. *J Neurosurg* 55:414–419, 1981.
7. Friedman AH, Nashold BS: DREZ lesions to relieve pain related to spinal cord injury. *J Neurosurg* 65:465–469, 1986.
8. Bernard EJ, Nashold BS, Caputi F, Moossy J: Nucleus caudalis DREZ lesions for facial pain. *Br J Neurosurg* 1:81–92, 1987.
9. Friedman AH, Nashold BS: Postherpetic neuralgia. In Wilkins RH, Rengachary SS (eds): *Neurosurgery*. New York, McGraw-Hill, 1985 vol 3, pp 2367–2368.
10. Friedman AH, Nashold BS, Ovelmen-Levitt J: Dorsal root entry zone lesions for treatment of post-herpetic neuralgia. *J Neurosurg* 60:1258–1262, 1984.
11. Dejerine J, Roussy G: Le syndrome thalmique. *Rev Neurol (Paris)* 14:521–532, 1906.
12. Currier RD, Giles CL, DeJong RW: Some comments on Wallenberg's lateral medullary syndrome. *Neurology (Minneapolis)* 11:778–791, 1961.
13. Lazorthes G: *Vascularisation et Circulation Cerebrales*. Paris, Masson & Cie, 1961.
14. Martin JJ: Thalamic syndromes. In Vinken PJ, Bruyn GW (eds): *Handbook of Clinical Neurology*, vol 2. Amsterdam, North-Holland, 1969, pp 469–496.
15. Cooper IS: Clinical and physiologic implications of thalamic surgery for disorder of sensory communications, parts I and II. *J Neurol Sci* 2:493–553, 1965.

16. Erickson TC, Bleckwenn WJ, Woolsey CN: Observations on the post-central gyrus in relation to pain. *Trans Am Neurol Assoc* 77:57–58, 1952.
17. Frazier CH, Lewy FH, Rowe SN: The origin and mechanism of paroxysmal neuralgic pain and the surgical treatment of central pain. *Brain* 60:44–51, 1937.
18. Sano K, Sekino H, Hashimoto I, et al: Posteromedial hypothalamotomy in the treatment of intractable pain. *Confin Neurol* 37:285–290, 1975.
19. Sano K, Yoshioka M, Ogashiwa W, et al: Thalamolaminotomy. A new operation for relief of intractable pain. *Confin Neurol* 27:63–66, 1966.
20. Yoshii N, Kudo T, Shimuzu S: Clinical and experimental studies of thalamic pulvinotomy. *Confin Neurol* 37:87–97, 1975.
21. Freeman W, Watts JW: Pain mechanisms and the frontal lobes: a study of prefrontal lobotomy for intractable pain. *Ann Intern Med* 28:747–754, 1948.
22. Foltz EL, White LB: Pain 'relief' by frontal cingulotomy. *J Neurosurg* 19:89–100, 1962.
23. Jelasio P: Relations of the lateral part of the amygdala to pain. *Confin Neurol* 37:53–55, 1966.
24. Gybels JM: Electrical stimulation of the central gray for pain relief in humans: a critical view. In Bonica JJ, Liebeskind JC, Albe-Fessard DG (eds): *Advances in Pain Research and Therapy*, vol 3. New York, Raven Press, 1979, pp 499–508.
25. Hosobuchi Y, Adams JE, Rutkin B: Chronic thalamic stimulation for the control of facial anesthesia dolorosa. *Arch Neurol* 29:158–162, 1973.
26. Richardson DE, Akil H: Pain reduction by electrical brain stimulation in man. *J Neurosurg* 47:176–194, 1977.
27. Mundinger F, Salamao JF: Deep brain stimulation in mesencephalic lamniscus medialis for chronic pain. *Acta Neurochir Suppl* 30:245–258, 1980.
28. Nashold BS, Wilson WP: Central pain. Observations in man with chronic implanted electrodes in the midbrain tegmentum. *Confin Neurol* 27:30–44, 1966.
29. Nashold BS, Wilson WP, Slaughter DG: Sensations evoked by stimulation in the midbrain of man. *J. Neurosurg* 30:14–24, 1969.
30. Spiegel EA, Wycis HT: Mesencephalotomy for relief of pain. In: *Anniversary Volume for O Pitzl*. Vienna, 1948, p 438.
31. Amano K, Iseki H, Notani M, et al: Rostral mesencephalic reticulotomy for pain relief. *Acta Neurochir Suppl* 30:391–393, 1980.
32. Nashold BS, Wilson WP, Slaughter DG: Stereotaxic midbrain lesions for central dysaesthesia and phantom pain. Preliminary report. *J Neurosurg* 30:116–126, 1969.
33. Orthner H, Roeder P: Further clinical and anatomical experiences with stereotactic operations for relief of pain. *Confin Neurol* 27:418–430, 1966.
34. Voris HC, Whisler WW: Results of stereotaxic surgery for intractable pain. *Confin Neurol* 37:86–96, 1975.
35. Nashold BS: Mesencephalotomy. A current appraisal. In Voris HC, Whisler WW (eds): *Treatment of Pain*. Springfield, IL, Charles C Thomas, 1975, pp 121–131.
36. Nashold BS: Brainstem stereotaxic procedure. In Schaltenbrand G, Walker AE (eds): *Stereotaxy of the Human Brain*, ed. 2. Stuttgart, Georg Thieme Verlag, 1982, pp 475–483.
37. Nashold BS, Gills JP: Ocular signs from brain stem lesions. *Arch Ophthalmol* 77:609–618, 1967.
38. Nashold BS, Seaber JH: Defects of ocular motility after stereotactic midbrain lesions in man. *Arch Ophthalmol* 88:245–248, 1972.
39. Nashold BS, Slaughter DG, Wilson WP, et al: Stereotactic mesencephalotomy. In Krayenbuhl H, Sweet WH (eds): *Progress in Neurological Surgery*, vol 8. Basel, Karger, 1977, pp 35–49.
40. Levin AB, Ramirez LF, Katz J: The use of stereotaxic chemical hypophysectomy in the treatment of thalamic path syndrome. *J Neurosurg* 59:1002–1006, 1983.

chapter 12
Neural Stimulation Techniques

Richard B. North, M.D.

Since the late 1960s, electrical stimulation devices have been employed increasingly in the management of pain. Although the underlying mechanisms remain controversial, thousands of spinal, peripheral nerve, and brain implants, and a much larger experience with transcutaneous electrical nerve stimulators, have shown these techniques to be empirically effective in properly selected patients.

The analgesic effects of electrical stimulation have been appreciated since antiquity. In the 1st century BC, Scribonius Largus described the relief of pain by application of a torpedo fish to an injured limb (1). Medical applications were prominent in early investigations of artificially generated electrical current, beginning in the 17th century.

The modern era of pain management with electrical stimulation devices began in the late 1960s. Development of compact, solid-state electronics made portable, and even implantable, devices a practical possibility; techniques for packaging implanted circuitry were already under development for cardiac pacing.

The publication in 1965 of the "gate theory" by Melzack and Wall (2) gave new impetus to this form of treatment. According to this theory, the central transmission of neural activity signaling pain is governed by a spinal "gate" that opens in response to an excess of small fiber activity in the peripheral nervous system. Because the large fibers in a mixed population are more susceptible than small fibers to depolarization by typical rectangular stimulation pulses, they may be recruited selectively, closing the central "gate." Stimulation to achieve this effect might be directed orthodromically, from peripheral nerves, or antidromically, via collateral processes in the dorsal columns of the spinal cord.

The "gate theory" has always been the subject of controversy (3), but the clinical methods it rationalized have succeeded empirically to such a degree that their application continues to grow.

PERIPHERAL NERVE STIMULATION

The first clinical application of the "gate theory," employing stimulation of large-diameter afferents to manage pain, was reported by Wall and Sweet in 1967 (4). Their series of eight patients included those with temporary electrodes implanted directly on peripheral nerve. Sweet and Wepsic (5) later reported on selected patients from a larger series of 18; at extended follow-up in 1976, with chronically implanted devices, sustained benefit was reported in 19 of 31 patients (61%) (6). Comparable results (45–79%) have been reported by other investigators at up to 10-year follow-up (7–12). These series have emphasized the treatment of sequelae of peripheral nerve trauma and entrapment with electrodes implanted proximal to the site of injury as the most consistently successful application of this technique. In general, long-term treatment by peripheral nerve stimulation of pain attributable to a proximal lesion, in particular sciatic nerve stimulation for lumbosacral radiculopathy, has not been successful (7, 13).

In routine clinical practice, candidates for an implanted peripheral nerve stimulator are screened by transcutaneous electrical nerve stimulation (TENS) trial, electrophysiologic testing (12), and diagnostic peripheral nerve blocks (14). Before a permanent device is implanted, peripheral nerve stimulation analgesia is demonstrated in a trial with a temporary percutaneous electrode. For chronic stimulation, electrodes are implanted by open surgical technique, with direct visualization, and under local anesthesia whenever possible, to permit isolation of appropriate sensory fiber populations. Primarily to achieve mechanical stability, electrode arrays backed by cuffs of supporting Silastic and/or Dacron have been used. Although special peripheral nerve electrode and cuff geometries and novel stimulation waveforms have been developed to achieve such effects as unidirectional action potential propagation (15) for functional neural prostheses, these have not been employed to date in clinical pain management. However, multichannel, programmable implants have been employed, yielding the same advantages as in other applications. By noninvasively selecting an appropriate combination of electrodes from a multiple electrode array, stimulation topography may be adjusted after surgery, to isolate and to maintain the desired sensory effect.

TRANSCUTANEOUS ELECTRICAL NERVE STIMULATION

Externally applied electrical stimulation devices have been employed in the management of pain, and available commercially, for over a century (1), but the modern era of their application began two decades ago, when they were investigated as screening devices for candidates for spinal and peripheral nerve implants (16). TENS alone proved to be adequate treatment for a substantial number of patients (17). Controlled trials, using placebo stimulation, have demonstrated a rapid decline in placebo effect shortly after institution of therapy, with profiles and incidence comparable to those seen in pharmacologic studies (18, 19). The art and science of electrode placement, and the necessity for extensive, trial-and-error determination of optimal sites in individual patients, are well documented (20). The applications of TENS have expanded to include postoperative pain (21), and acute as well as chronic pain caused by musculoskeletal, neurologic, and even visceral pathology (20). Although a minority of patients with chronic, intractable pain problems such as "failed back syndrome" will achieve adequate analgesia with TENS alone (22), it deserves a routine trial in a program of conservative management, and in patients who are considered for implanted devices. A failure by such a patient to respond to TENS, although sometimes significant, by no means precludes a favorable response to an implant.

TENS is a benign and reversible form of treatment, with few contraindications or significant adverse effects.

CONTRAINDICATIONS

1. *Implanted cardiac pacemakers.* Demand pacers, depending upon R wave sensing circuitry, may be inhibited by TENS. Any implanted cardiac pacemaker should be considered a contraindication to TENS use.
2. *Pregnancy.* Only limited data (20) are available regarding the safety of TENS in pregnancy, and in labor and delivery; prudence dictates restricting its use in these conditions, pending further investigation.
3. Inability to use the device, because of dementia or psychiatric disease.

PRECAUTIONS

1. Application over the eyes, or in contact with mucous membranes, may be injurious.
2. Application over or near the carotid sinus, particularly in patients with cardiac or cerebrovascular disease, may provoke hypotension and/or bradycardia.
3. Application over the anterior chest of a cardiac arrhythmia patient, although never reported to have caused a complication, should be avoided, as should cephalic application in epilepsy and stroke patients.
4. Skin reactions, due to chemical and mechanical irritation, and sometimes allergy, are common; careful routine hygiene is essential.

MECHANISMS OF STIMULATION ANALGESIA

The analgesic effects of TENS delivered at conventional "low intensity" (12–20 mA) and "high frequency" (50–100 Hz) are not reversible by the narcotic antagonist naloxone in humans (23–25), but analgesia achieved with "acupuncture-like" low-frequency stimulation [2-Hz pulse repetition rate (26) or burst repetition rate (27)] reportedly is reversed. This implies separate mechanisms of action for these stimulation regimens.

The "gate theory" is countered by recent evidence that hyperalgesia is signaled by large fibers (28). The analgesic effects of stimulation, accordingly, might be mediated by an effect such as frequency-related conduction block, acting on this fiber population. Although stimulation parameters employed clinically in peripheral nerves may (29, 30) or may not (31) achieve this effect locally, branch points are particularly vulnerable. The effect of spinal stimulation might involve branch points of primary afferents into dorsal column and dorsal horn fibers. Such a mechanism would not, however, readily explain the prolonged latency and persistence of stimulation analgesia described by many patients with implanted spinal stimulators (32) (Fig. 12.1).

SPINAL CORD STIMULATION

The most common application of implanted neural stimulation devices has been spinal cord stimulation (SCS), typically delivered via longitudinally oriented electrode arrays in the dorsal epidural space, for intractable low back and leg pain. The earliest spinal stimulation electrodes (36) were fixed, flat arrays that required a laminectomy for implantation under direct vision (37, 38). In the typical patient with "failed back syndrome" or "postlaminectomy syndrome," these were implanted at upper thoracic levels, so as to provide stimulation cover-

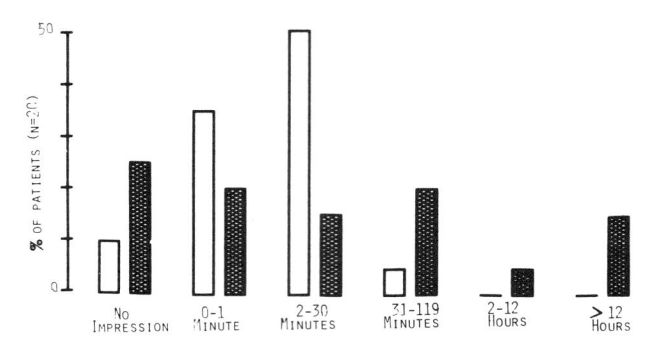

Figure 12.1. Time lags associated with stimulation analgesia (spinal cord stimulation, 8-year follow-up). *Open columns*, latency of analgesia after stimulator is turned off; *shaded columns*, persistence of analgesia after stimulator is turned off. Most patients report that pain relief does not occur instantaneously when stimulation begins, nor does it cease immediately when stimulation ends.

age of all segments below the array (Fig. 12.2). Experience showed, however, that such broad coverage often was accompanied by uncomfortable thoracic radicular stimulation, and that electrode placement more caudally, which afforded more selective stimulation, was more effective. Optimal placement was facilitated with intraoperative stimulation of an awake patient, under local anesthesia, but this was cumbersome when laminectomy was required and when the appropriate level of electrode placement for an individual patient was unknown preoperatively.

In order to determine the proper level of electrode placement in each patient, and to demonstrate analgesic

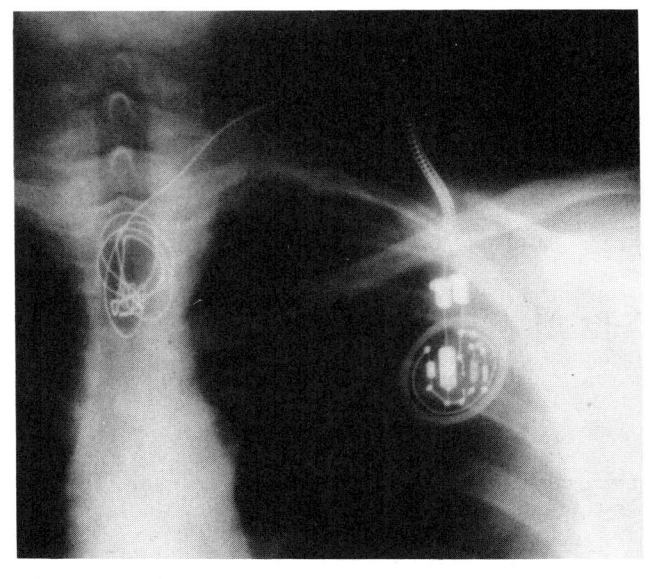

Figure 12.2. Early monopolar spinal stimulation system. High thoracic placement via laminectomy was typical.

effect prior to permanent implantation of a stimulation device, techniques were developed for percutaneous temporary electrode placement (39). These evolved into methods for implantation of permanent electrodes, obviating laminectomy in many patients. Multiple, individually inserted electrodes, however, often migrated spontaneously, requiring surgical intervention in many instances (32). The development of multiple electrode arrays that could be inserted via Tuohy needle ameliorated this problem (40). At the same time, multichannel implanted radiofrequency receivers and pulse generators were developed, to take full advantage of these arrays by noninvasively selecting electrode combinations. The topography of stimulation coverage could then be optimized after surgery. Even hardware failures, such as minor electrode migration, may be amenable to noninvasive correction with these versatile devices.

Under the general criteria described above for implantation of a stimulation device for pain management, the following have emerged as specific indications for SCS; they are listed in decreasing order of application and reported success rates.

1. Lumbar arachnoiditis (lumbosacral spinal fibrosis), a subset of "failed back syndrome" with radiculopathic pain, ideally predominating over axial and mechanical pain
2. Peripheral vascular disease, with ischemic pain (41)
3. Causalgia
4. Phantom limb or stump pain
5. Peripheral neuropathy
6. Spinal cord lesions

Results of SCS for "failed back syndrome," including patients with documented lumbar arachnoiditis, have been reported by a variety of outcome measures, at follow-up periods of up to 8 years: "good" or "excellent" results are obtained in approximately half the patients reported in the literature (42). The long-term results (43) in our earliest series of patients (32) treated with percutaneously inserted electrodes, adapted for chronic implantation, are representative. Figure 12.3 presents the largest subgroup of patients, those with intractable low back and leg pain following multiple lumbar spine surgeries, and myelographically documented arachnoiditis. At 8-year follow-up, 35% maintained excellent (75% or better) pain relief. This decline from our early (6-month mean) follow-up (32) reflects, in large measure, hardware problems: In our first 31 patients, followed over 21 months, we recorded 47 "spontaneous electrode migrations," 9 lead wire fractures, 5 lead insulation failures, and 1 receiver failure (43). Although many electrode migrations were radiographically demonstrable (Fig. 12.4), the total of 47 events includes patients whose topography of stimulation changed following surgery, when they were no longer in the artificial prone position required for implantation. To an extent, this figure reflects the inflexibility of single-channel devices.

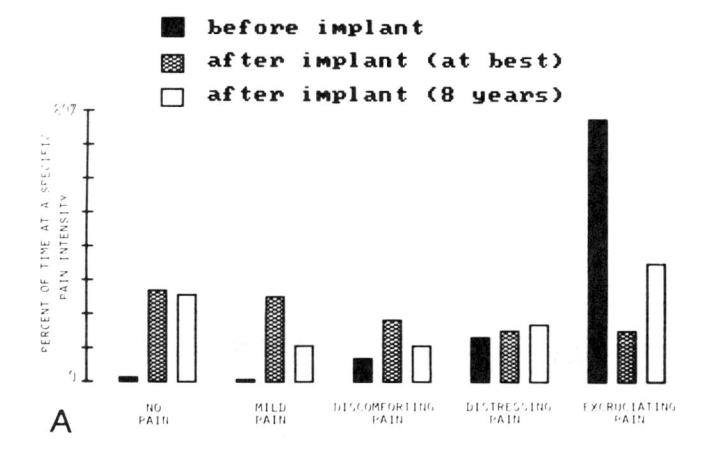

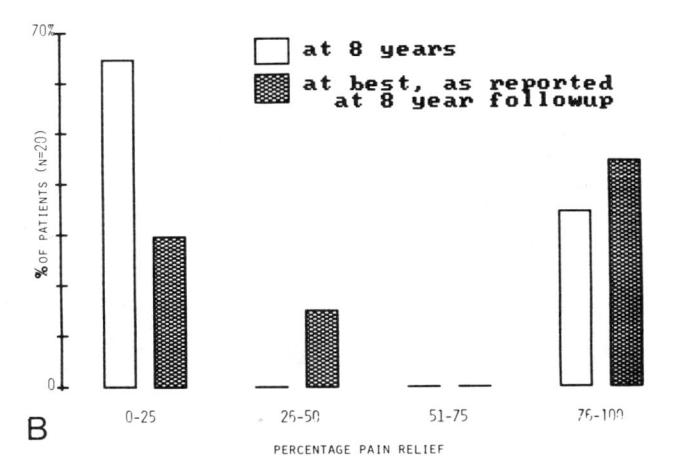

Figure 12.3. Eight-year follow-up on bipolar spinal stimulation systems for pain of lumbar arachnoiditis, expressed as (A) average patient's pain intensity profile, on an analog scale, and (B) direct patient estimates of overall pain relief.

Because of the high incidence, in our experience, of technical difficulties with percutaneously inserted, individual electrodes (typically placed in tandem, for bipolar stimulation), we resumed for some time the implantation of fixed electrode arrays (Fig. 12.5) via laminectomy; the risk of migration of these is inherently minimal. We continue to employ this technique in patients with a prior laminectomy or epidural scarring at the level of proposed electrode placement, in whom the technical difficulty of percutaneous electrode insertion has been confirmed at a trial procedure with a temporary electrode. For the typical "failed back" patient, however, whose postsurgical scarring is caudal to the usual T8–T11 electrode site, percutaneous placement is straightforward. Currently available multiple electrode arrays, designed for insertion via Tuohy needle, are more resistant to migration [and immune, of

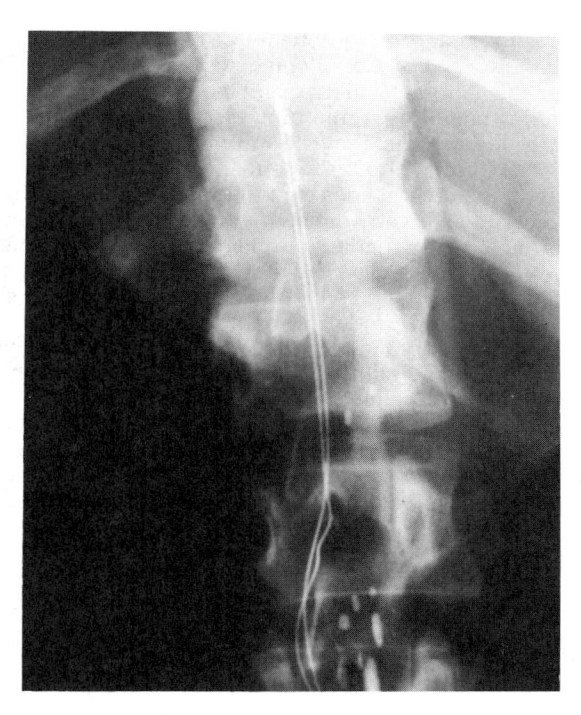

Figure 12.4. Dual, independently inserted spinal electrode systems are vulnerable to migration of either electrode. The result may be a short circuit, as shown.

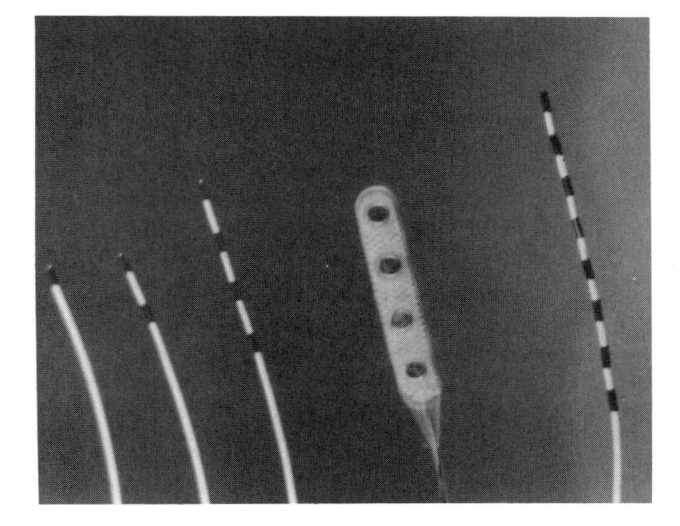

Figure 12.5. Representative spinal stimulation arrays, bearing from one to eight electrodes. Fourth from left is a laminectomy array; the others may be inserted percutaneously, through a Tuohy needle.

course, to migration of one electrode with respect to another (Fig. 12.5)]. Complemented by multichannel, programmable implants that permit noninvasive postoperative adjustments of stimulating electrode location, these rarely require surgical revision in our experience (44).

Prior to implantation of a permanent device, a trial with a temporary percutaneous electrode is undertaken. This is considered technically adequate when stimulation coverage of most of the patient's topography of pain is maintained for at least 3 days, so that its analgesic effects may be assessed fully, and reproducibility established. A simple monopolar electrode suffices for this purpose in most patients; its effects may, however, predict imperfectly the results of bipolar stimulation, which has technical advantages as the routine method of chronic implantation (45).

Electrode placement away from the dorsal midline, and even ventrally, is more difficult technically, and has not been the subject of any recent reports despite encouraging preliminary results (46, 47).

DEEP BRAIN STIMULATION

The analgesic effects of stimulation via stereotaxically implanted brain electrodes (in the human supraoptic nuclei and septal area) were first described 30 years ago by Heath and Mickle (48) and by Pool (49). In 1960, Mazars et al. reported successful treatment of deafferentation pain by stimulation of the spinothalamic fasciculus (50); stimulation of specific sensory nuclei (51, 52) and of internal capsule (52–54) followed.

The antinociceptive effect of periaqueductal gray (PAG) stimulation was reported by Reynolds in 1969 (55), and was given new impetus by the discovery in 1973 of specific opiate receptors in the central nervous system (56), found in high concentration in PAG (57). The phenomenon of "stimulus-produced analgesia" has been found, in animals, to involve a descending inhibitory pathway, extending through the dorsolateral quadrant of the spinal cord; reversal by the narcotic antagonist naloxone, and the development of tolerance, with cross-tolerance to morphine, has been described (58–63). In humans, analgesic effect has been reported to be naloxone reversible (64, 65), and to be associated with elevation of cerebrospinal fluid β-endorphin levels (66, 67), but the latter has been questioned as an artifact produced by contrast ventriculography (68, 69). Mediation of this effect directly by endogenous opiate release, as opposed to other effects of stimulation, remains a matter of controversy, but the method has enjoyed continued clinical success in the management of chronic benign pain as well as cancer pain (35, 70, 71).

Currently recognized indications for the procedure include the following:

1. Deafferentation pain syndromes, treated by thalamic electrode placement:
   a. Thalamic (Déjérine-Roussy) syndrome, if the anatomic substrate remains for stimulation
   b. Anesthesia dolorosa
   c. Postherpetic neuralgia
   d. Phantom limb pain
   e. Postcordotomy dysesthesia
   f. Pain of spinal cord injury
   g. Brachial or lumbosacral plexus lesions
   h. Chronic lumbosacral radiculopathy
2. Pain responsive to narcotics, as determined by a morphine infusion test (35), is considered to be an indication for periaqueductal gray electrode placement:
   a. Chronic low back and leg pain (exclusive of radiculopathic, deafferentation pain)
   b. Cancer pain (exclusive of gross infiltration of the peripheral nervous system, causing deafferentation pain)
   c. Nonmalignant abdominal and perineal pain
   d. Atypical facial pain

Electrode implantation is performed stereotaxically, using standard ventriculographic or computed tomographic techniques, under local anesthesia (Fig. 12.6). Each patient typically receives two electrode arrays. Bilateral PAG/periventricular gray (PVG) electrodes are placed in patients with midline or bilateral pain, particularly when a favorable response to narcotics has occurred; whereas in those with unilateral, deafferentation pain, the

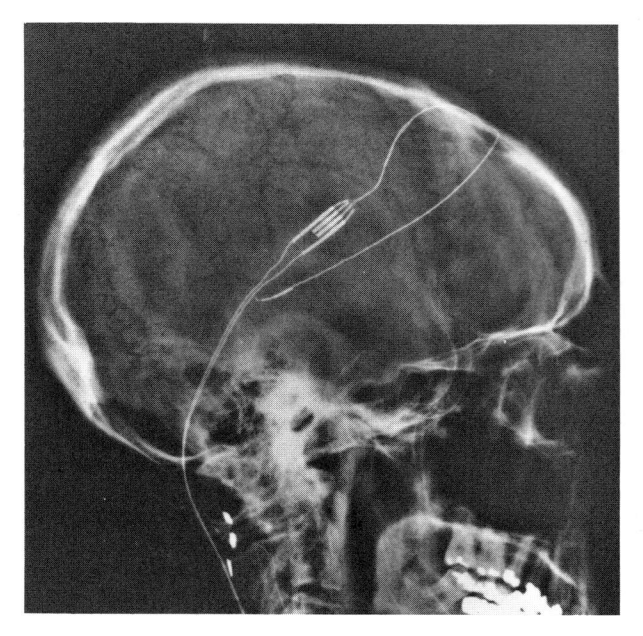

Figure 12.6. A typical deep brain stimulation electrode system, with four available stimulation sites, shown here hardwired in a fixed bipolar configuration.

first electrode is placed in contralateral PAG/PVG, and the second in contralateral sensory thalamus, ventral posterolateral (VPL) nucleus or ventral posteromedial (VPM) nucleus, as appropriate for the topography of a particular patient's pain. Via percutaneous test leads, stimulation is then delivered to representative electrode combinations, in random or pseudorandom order. Because analgesia may persist in some patients for 24 hr or more following stimulation, and a new electrode combination may be assessed only when the patient's pain has returned, the number of combinations that may be tested is limited in this (successful) group. If satisfactory stimulation analgesia is achieved, the system is adapted for chronic use: under general anesthesia, the existing electrodes are connected to subcutaneously implanted electronics. If stimulation is ineffective, the electrode array is easily removed under local anesthesia.

The risks of the procedure, and their frequency of occurrence in the largest published series (35, 71, 72), are as follows:

1. Intracranial hemorrhage (2–4%), which is potentially fatal (0–2%). Accordingly, patients should be screened rigorously for clotting abnormalities, particularly if cancer pain is to be treated in this fashion.
2. Infection (3–6%), which may require removal of implanted hardware. The use of programmable, multichannel implants minimizes the duration of the test phase with percutaneous leads, reducing this risk.
3. Eye movement abnormalities (2–4%) have not occurred when placement of the electrode tip remains rostral to the iter of the aqueduct of Sylvius.
4. Hardware failures (2–12%) range from implanted electrode migration to electromechanical and electronic failures, which may require reoperation. Programmable, multichannel devices permit noninvasive adjustments to correct for certain faults, such as electrode migration or malposition, and to optimize therapeutic effects and minimize the side effects of stimulation.

Histologic analysis of autopsy material has shown no deleterious effect such as gliosis or parenchymal reaction along the trajectories or at the tips of the electrodes (73).

The results of treatment have been reported by a variety of criteria, among them direct estimates of pain relief, and indirect indicators such as analgesic use, patterns of stimulator use, functional capacity, and employment status. As reviewed by Young et al. (71), "success" was reported in the literature from 13 centers in 57% of 698 chronic pain patients treated with electrical stimulation of the brain: from 50 (72) to 80% (74) for thalamic stimulation, and from 0 (75) to 90% (76) for PAG/PVG stimulation. In the most recent literature on the treatment of cancer pain by these techniques, success is reported in 70–76% of patients (35, 77).

Deep brain stimulation is unique as a reversible, nonablative technique for central deafferentation pain states. In patients refractory to peripheral nerve or spinal cord stimulation, although its risks are greater, it represents a worthwhile alternative.

GENERAL CONSIDERATIONS IN PATIENT MANAGEMENT

Concurrently with improvements in hardware and technique, the diagnosis and management of chronic pain syndromes has been refined considerably, and programs specializing in this field have proliferated (33). In particular, the importance of psychological factors in comprehensive management, and in selection for surgical procedures, especially implantation of stimulation devices (34), is widely recognized. Criteria for treatment with an implanted stimulation device have evolved, empirically, as follows.

GENERAL INDICATIONS FOR IMPLANTED STIMULATION DEVICES

1. There is an objective basis for the pain complaint (e.g., myelographically demonstrated arachnoiditis).
2. Alternative therapy has been exhausted or is unacceptable (e.g., decompression, microsurgical lysis of arachnoid adhesions, ablative procedures).
3. Psychiatric clearance has been obtained (demonstrating motivation and long-term commitment, without major issues of secondary gain or a serious drug habituation problem).
4. The topography of pain and its underlying pathophysiology are amenable to stimulation coverage (e.g., by spinal stimulation for radicular thoracic or lumbosacral pain; thalamic nucleus ventralis posteromedialis stimulation for facial anesthesia dolorosa). Periaqueductal gray stimulation will address diffuse, or axial, topographies—particularly, it has been reported, for pain responsive to narcotics (35).

An additional criterion for implantation of a device, required as a condition for reimbursement by some third parties, is that "demonstration of pain relief with a temporarily implanted electrode precedes permanent implantation." This requirement might be met, at least literally, by implantation of a permanent system in a single procedure, if pain relief were reported by the patient intraoperatively; but a higher rate of treatment failures (and explants) would be expected. An extended stimulation trial with a temporary electrode has several advantages beyond simple patient selection (except in deep brain stimulation, where the logistics and the morbidity of insertion of new electrodes must be considered:

1. Its placement affords the physician and patient the opportunity to evaluate a greater number of promising stimulation sites more thoroughly.
2. Assessment of analgesic effect can be made under more

physiologic conditions of activity and body position, away from the time constraints of the operating room.
3. Assuming the temporary electrode is removed (to minimize the risk of infection) rather than internalized for chronic use, this prior experience on the part of physician and patient expedites implantation of the permanent device (again lowering the risk of infection). Multichannel, programmable devices, permitting noninvasive selection of electrodes from an array even after permanent implantation, facilitate this.
4. Observations relevant to hardware choice for a particular patient can be made. For example, if a fully implanted, primary cell device is under consideration, its adequacy may be inferred from measurements of stimulation current requirements and duty cycle.

During percutaneous testing, and at follow-up assessments following implantation of a device, standard outcome measures should be collected, ideally by an evaluator independent of the surgeon, and blinded to parameters of treatment when feasible. Crossover periods without stimulation clarify the cause-effect relationship of treatment and reported relief of pain. Criteria for placement of a permanent implant (and for long-term assessment of the results of treatment) include: direct estimates of analgesic effect, using standard visual analog and similar scales; comparison with effects of prior treatments; and indirect measures such as analgesic use, functional activity levels, and (at long-term follow-up) ongoing health care needs and employment status.

IMPLANTED STIMULATION DEVICES

The typical neural stimulation device (Fig. 12.7), as implanted in a large population of patients over the past two decades, is a passive radiofrequency (RF) receiver. It contains no battery or life-limiting components, and functions only when powered by an external transmitter. The transmitter emits radiofrequency (455-kHz to 2-MHz) bursts, whose amplitude, duration, and frequency (repetition rate) determine the stimulation waveform delivered to the electrodes by the implanted receiver, which functions as a simple AM demodulator. These stimulation parameters are adjusted by physician and patient to optimize analgesic effect.

The latest generation of radiofrequency devices permits selection of stimulating anode(s) and cathode(s) from an array of four electrodes, thereby varying stimulation in the spatial, as well as the temporal, domain. Formerly, with single-channel devices, this could be accomplished only by surgical revision. This feature is invaluable, because electrode position is the major determinant of the topography of stimulation paresthesias, which for peripheral nerve, spinal, and thalamic stimulation should correspond to a patient's painful areas for optimal analgesic effect. In reported clinical applications to date, following manufacturers' recommended strategies, multichannel systems

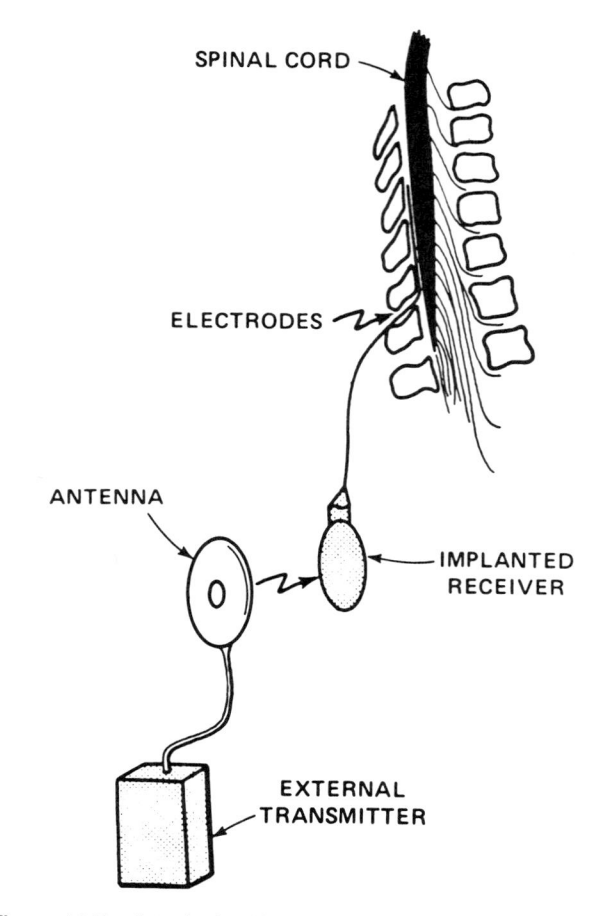

Figure 12.7. A typical radiofrequency-coupled implant, as employed for spinal stimulation.

have been used to vary cathodal position to optimize coverage, but not to achieve specific configurations of anodes and cathodes more complex than dipoles (45), which may yield a specific, favorable current distribution.

Because of the flexibility and redundancy of current multichannel implantable stimulation devices, implantation is expedited, technical success and clinical results are enhanced, and the rate of failures requiring surgical revision has fallen dramatically. As the flexibility and number of stimulation channels of these systems increases, however, the task of adjustment and electrode selection for optimal results grows disproportionately, far in excess of the 50 working combinations of anodes and cathodes possible with four electrodes. A general formula for this relationship may be derived as follows:

> From an array of n electrodes, where $n \geq 2$, the possible combinations of m active and $n - m$ inactive electrodes number $C(n,m) = n! / (n-m)!m!$
>
> For each combination of m active electrodes, there

are 2^m possible selections of anode(s) and cathode(s). This figure includes two open circuit configurations (all anodes, all cathodes); the number of useful configurations, therefore, is $2^m - 2$.

In aggregate, the number of unique electrode combinations is:

$$\sum_{m=2}^{n} n!\,(2^m - 2)/(n - m)!\,m!$$

For example, four electrodes permit:

$$12 + 24 + 14 = 50 \text{ combinations}$$

and eight electrodes permit:

$$56 + 336 + 980 + 1680 + 1736 + 1008 + 254 = 6050 \text{ combinations}$$

If "biphasic" stimulation (alternating complementary electrode combinations) is considered, these figures increase by 50%.

Clearly, as the number of available channels increases, the task of thoroughly evaluating potentially useful electrode combinations to optimize effect may grow tremendously, taxing the capabilities and resources of the physician and his staff. As a practical matter, in determining appropriate commercial transmitter settings for routine clinical practice, exhaustive assessment of all possible combinations is rarely necessary. In theory, and in practice, electrode combinations differing in minor ways (e.g., addition or deletion of one among multiple anodes) are commonly functionally identical, and therefore redundant.

Like the task of postoperative (and even intraoperative) adjustment of stimulation amplitude and pulse repetition rate, electrode selection generally is managed most efficiently by the patient himself, given appropriate means of control, constraints, supervision, and data collection.

For this purpose, we have developed a personal computer interface to standard radiofrequency-coupled implants, with supporting user-friendly, expert system software for direct patient interaction (78). The system incorporates three commercially available radiofrequency transmitters (two four-channel, and one single-channel), in routine clinical use for neurologic stimulation. The range of stimulation pulse parameters nominally available from the system is the same as is available from each commercial transmitter in its usual, freestanding mode of operation. The computer and interface simply allow automatic, rapid switching between standard pulse parameters, to determine the optimal settings for the patient's standard commercial transmitter. The patient controls the system with simple push-button and slide potentiometer controls, designed for greater ease of operation than those of the standard transmitter. Patient responses and impressions are entered through similar controls, and through a simple graphics tablet that conveys topographic data.

Comparisons of the perceived location of stimulation paresthesias with a patient's recorded pain topography may be made rapidly, automatically, and systematically, and psychophysical thresholds may be determined reproducibly. Protocols of varying complexity, which present stimulation parameters in random or pseudorandom order, may be implemented as required for each patient, and for each application.

For research purposes, the system is capable of changing stimulation pulse parameters (electrode combination, amplitude, and duration) in as little as 1 msec. This will permit, for example, interleaving pulses delivered from different electrode combinations whose effects are complementary. The system can continuously vary the interpulse interval as well, in a deterministic, stochastic, or even adaptive fashion. "Modulation" of this parameter in simple, deterministic patterns has been described in the literature on TENS (79).

With advances in lithium battery technology, permitting a life span of a decade for a cardiac pacemaker powered by a primary cell, "totally implanted" neural stimulation devices have been developed. External hardware is still required for control; a permanent magnet commonly is employed for simple adjustments by the patient, and a dedicated programming unit for the full range of adjustment by the physician. Existing devices are limited to fixed menus of stimulation parameters, and lack the flexibility (in accommodating novel stimulation regimes) of passive, radiofrequency-powered implants. For spinal or peripheral nerve applications, whose energy requirements often exceed those of cardiac pacing by two orders of magnitude, currently available primary cell devices may not have acceptable longevity in some patients. Periaqueductal gray stimulation, on the other hand, typically requires a small charge per phase, at a low rate, with a duty cycle of minutes per day, well within the design specifications of these devices for a life span of several years. Automatic cycling on and off, as permitted by the latency of analgesic effect after the stimulator is turned on, and its persistence after the device is turned off, is among the strategies employed to maximize battery life.

STIMULATION WAVEFORMS

In clinical practice with standard peripheral nerve and spinal stimulation hardware, perception by the patient of stimulation paresthesias corresponding to the topography of pain has proven, empirically, to be a necessary condition for analgesic effect. Achieving specific stimulation coverage, without incurring uncomfortable sensory, reflex, or direct motor effects, requires careful attention to the position of surgically implanted electrodes (45). In a given patient, the final choice of stimulation parameters represents a compromise, and stimulation analgesia is often incomplete. At thoracic spinal cord levels, where electrodes are commonly placed to achieve coverage of multiple caudal segments, radicular thoracic effects may predominate. This relates to anatomic factors: (a) the proximity of entering dorsal root fibers to dorsal epidural stimulating electrodes; (b) the relatively superficial location of these fibers in the dorsal columns, within a few segments of their entry (80); and (c) fiber diameter, in that the mean diameter of fibers in fasciculus gracilis decreases at cephalad levels (81).

The effects of "stimulation" are not necessarily excitatory (82); with appropriate electrode geometries and stimulation waveforms, inhibition, blockade, or even unidirectional action potential propagation (15) may be achieved. Likewise, specific subpopulations of different fiber diameters may be selected (83). These effects have been modeled, and observed experimentally, in idealized peripheral nerve preparations, with directly applied and even circumferential electrodes. These are not, however, directly relevant to the most common clinical situation, spinal cord stimulation, which involves an anisotropic medium and electrodes that are neither directly applied nor circumferential.

Finite element modeling of electrical fields applied to the spinal cord and surrounding structures (84) has yielded voltage and current profiles that correspond well to in vitro measurements in primate and cadaver spinal cord (85) for electrode configurations currently in clinical use. This model has addressed only the simple case of cathodal excitatory effects, however; anodal blocking and effects of stimulation waveshape have not been considered.

By superimposing a model of myelinated fiber excitation, the "spatially extended nonlinear nodal" model (86), the effects of waveform permutations might be predicted for representative fiber sizes within the spinal cord tracts of interest. Selective activation of deeper structures while sparing overlying structures, and selective effects on different fiber sizes, are possible. With appropriate modifications to existing radiofrequency transmitters, compensating for the series capacitance in the output of existing receivers, a limited regimen of novel stimulation waveforms might be made available, noninvasively, to patients with existing implants.

CONCLUSIONS

Neural stimulation techniques are employed with increasing success, in properly selected patients, in the management of chronic, intractable pain. The mechanisms by which they act, as presently applied, at different levels of the central and peripheral nervous system, are poorly understood. Simple, monotonic sequences of pulses, of simple rectangular shape, delivered via simple electrode geometries, have been applied to complex neural networks with remarkable empirical success. Further basic and clinical research to optimize this form of treatment may take advantage of (or must contend with) a literally infinite number of possible stimulation regimes. To this end, a computer-based system, permitting direct patient interaction, has been developed for use with existing radiofrequency-coupled implants.

References

1. Stillings D: A survey of the history of electrical stimulation for pain to 1900. *Med Instrum* 9:255–259, 1975.
2. Melzack P, Wall PD: Pain mechanisms: a new theory. *Science* 150:971–978, 1965.
3. Nathan PW: The gate-control theory of pain: a critical review. *Brain* 99:123–158, 1976.
4. Wall PD, Sweet WH: Temporary abolition of pain in man. *Science* 155:108–109, 1967.
5. Sweet WH, Wepsic JG: Treatment of chronic pain by stimulation of fibers of primary afferent neuron. *Trans Am Neurol Assoc* 93:103–107, 1968.
6. Sweet WH: Control of pain by direct electrical stimulation of peripheral nerves. *Clin Neurosurg* 23:103–111, 1976.
7. Campbell JN, Long DM: Peripheral nerve stimulation in the treatment of intractable pain. *J Neurosurg* 45:692–699, 1976.
8. Law JD, Swett J, Kirsch WM: Retrospective analysis of 22 patients with chronic pain treated by peripheral nerve stimulation. *J Neurosurg* 52:482–485, 1980.
9. Long DM, Erickson D, Campbell J, North R: Electrical stimulation of the spinal cord and peripheral nerves for pain control. *Appl Neurophysiol* 44:207–217, 1981.
10. Picaza JA, Cannon BW, Hunter SE, Boyd AS, Guma J, Maurer D: Pain suppress by peripheral nerve stimulation. *Surg Neurol* 4:105–114, 1975.
11. Picaza JA, Hunter SE, Cannon BW: Pain suppression by peripheral nerve stimulation. *Appl Neurophysiol* 40:223–234, 1978.
12. Waisbrod H, Panhans C, Hansen D, Gerbershagen HU: Direct nerve stimulation for painful peripheral neuropathies. *J Bone Joint Surg* 67(B):470–473, 1985.
13. Meyer GA, Fields HL: Causalgia treated by selective large fiber stimulation of peripheral nerve. *Brain* 95:163–168, 1972.
14. Nashold BS, Goldner JL: Electrical stimulation of peripheral nerves for relief of intractable chronic pain. *Med Instrum* 9:224–225, 1975.
15. Van den Honert C, Mortimer J: Generation of unidirectionally propagated action potentials in a peripheral nerve by brief stimuli. *Science* 206:1311–1312, 1979.
16. Long DM: Cutaneous afferent stimulation for relief of chronic pain. *Clin Neurosurg* 21:257–268, 1976.
17. Long D, Hagfors N: Electrical stimulation in the nervous system: the current status of electrical stimulation of the nervous system for relief of pain. *Pain* 1:109–123, 1975.
18. Long D: Electrical stimulation for the control of pain. *Arch Surg* 112:884–888, 1977.
19. Thorsteinsson G, et al: The placebo effect of transcutaneous electrical stimulation. *Pain* 5:31–41, 1978.
20. Mannheimer JS, Lampe GN: *Clinical Transcutaneous Electrical Nerve Stimulation*. Philadelphia, FA Davis, 1984.
21. Vanderark G, McGrath KA: Transcutaneous electrical stimulation in treatment of postoperative pain. *Am J Surg* 130:338–340, 1975.
22. Loeser JD, Black RG, Christman A: Relief of pain by transcutaneous stimulation. *J Neurosurg* 42:308–314, 1975.
23. Abram S, Reynolds A, Cusick J: Failure of naloxone to reverse analgesia from transcutaneous electrical stimulation in patients with chronic pain. *Anesth Analg* 60:81–84, 1981.
24. Woolf CJ, Mitchell D, Myers RA, Barrett GD: Failure of

naloxone to reverse peripheral transcutaneous electroanalgesia in patients suffering from acute trauma. *S Afr Med J* 53:179–180, 1978.
25. Freeman TB, Campbell JN, Long DM: Naloxone does not affect pain relief induced by electrical stimulation in man. *Pain* 17:189–195, 1983.
26. Chapman C, Benedetti C: Analgesia following transcutaneous electrical stimulation and its partial reversal by a narcotic antagonist. *Life Sci* 21:1645–1648, 1977.
27. Sjolund B, Eriksson M: The influence of naloxone on analgesia produced by peripheral condition stimulation. *Brain Res* 173:295–301, 1979.
28. Campbell JN, Meyer RA: Primary afferents and hyperalgesia. In Yaksh TL (ed): *Spinal Afferent Processing*. New York, Plenum, 1986, pp 59–81.
29. Campbell J, Taub A: Local analgesia from percutaneous electrical stimulation. *Arch Neurol* 28:347–350, 1973.
30. Ignelzi RJ, Nyquist JK: Excitability changes in peripheral nerve fibers after repetitive electrical stimulation. *J Neurosurg* 45:159–165, 1976.
31. Swett J, Law J: Analgesia with peripheral nerve stimulation: absence of a peripheral mechanism. *Pain* 15:55–70, 1983.
32. North RB, Fischell TA, Long DM: Chronic stimulation via percutaneously inserted epidural electrodes. *Neurosurgery* 1:215–218, 1977.
33. Bonica JJ: Basic principles in managing chronic pain. *Arch Surg* 112:783–788, 1977.
34. Daniel M, Long C, Hutcherson M, Hunter S: Psychological factors and outcome of electrode implantation for chronic pain. *Neurosurgery* 17:773–777, 1985.
35. Hosobuchi Y: Subcortical electrical stimulation for control of intractable pain in humans. Report of 122 cases (1970–1984). *J Neurosurg* 64:543–553, 1986.
36. Shealy C, Mortimer J, Reswick J: Electrical inhibition of pain by stimulation of the dorsal columns: a preliminary report. *Anesth Analg* 46:489–491, 1967.
37. Nashold BS Jr, Friedman H: Dorsal column stimulation for control of pain: preliminary report on 30 patients. *J Neurosurg* 36:590–597, 1972.
38. Sweet W, Wepsic J: Stimulation of the posterior columns of the spinal cord for pain control. *Clin Neurosurg* 21:278–310, 1974.
39. Erickson DL: Percutaneous trial of stimulation for patient selection for implantable stimulating devices. *J Neurosurg* 43:440–444, 1975.
40. Leclercq TA: Electrode migration in epidural stimulation: comparison between single electrode and four electrode programmable leads. *Pain* 20(Suppl 2):78, 1984.
41. Broseta J, Barbera J, DeVera J, Barcia-Salorio J, March G, Gonzalez-Darder J, Rovaina F, Joanes V: Spinal cord stimulation in peripheral arterial disease. *J Neurosurg* 64:71–80, 1986.
42. De la Porte C, Siegfried J: Lumbosacral spinal fibrosis (spinal arachnoiditis): its diagnosis and treatment by spinal cord stimulation. *Spine* 8:593–603, 1983.
43. North RB, Long DM: Spinal cord stimulation for intractable pain: eight-year followup. *Pain* 20(Suppl 2): 79, 1984.
44. North RB: Spinal cord stimulation for intractable pain: indications and technique. In Long DM (ed): *Current Therapy in Neurological Surgery*. Philadelphia, Brian C. Decker, 1988, vol 2.
45. Law J: Spinal stimulation: statistical superiority of monophasic stimulation of narrowly separated, longitudinal bipoles having rostral cathodes. *Appl Neurophysiol* 46:129–137, 1983.
46. Hoppenstein R: Electrical stimulation of the ventral and dorsal columns of the spinal cord for relief of chronic intractable pain. *Surg Neurol* 4:195–198, 1975.
47. Larson SJ, Sances A, Cusick JF, Meyer GA, Swiontek T: A comparison between anterior and posterior implant systems. *Surg Neurol* 4:180–186, 1975.
48. Heath R, Mickle WA: Evaluation of seven years experience with depth electrode studies in human patients. In Ramey ER (ed): *Electrical Studies on the Unanesthetized Brain*. New York, Hoeber, 1960, pp 214–247.
49. Pool JL: Psychosurgery in elderly people. *J Am Geriatr Soc* 2:456–465, 1956.
50. Mazars G, Roge R, Mazars Y: Results of the stimulation of the spinothalamic fasciculus and their bearing on the physiopathology of pain [in French]. *Rev Neurol* 103:136–138, 1960.
51. Mazars GJ: Intermittent stimulation of nucleus ventralis posterolateralis for intractable pain. *Surg Neurol* 4:93–95, 1975.
52. Hosobuchi Y, Adams JE, Rutkin B: Chronic thalamic and internal capsule stimulation for the control of central pain. *Surg Neurol* 4:91–92, 1975.
53. Adams JE, Hosobuchi Y, Fields HL: Stimulation of the internal capsule for relief of chronic pain. *J Neurosurg* 41:740–744, 1974.
54. Fields HL, Adams JE: Pain after cortical injury relieved by electrical stimulation of the internal capsule. *Brain* 97:169–178, 1974.
55. Reynolds DV: Surgery in the rat during electrical analgesia induced by focal brain stimulation. *Science* 164:444–445, 1969.
56. Pert CB, Snyder SH: Opiate receptor: demonstration in nervous tissue. *Science* 179:405–423, 1973.
57. Kuhar M, Pert C, Snyder S: Regional distribution of opiate receptor binding in monkey and human brain. *Brain* 245:447, 1973.
58. Basbaum AI, Fields HL: Endogenous pain control mechanisms: review and hypothesis. *Ann Neurol* 4:451–462, 1978.
59. Liebeskind JC, Guilbaud G, Besson JM, et al: Analgesia from electrical stimulation of the periaqueductal gray matter in the cat: behavioral observations and inhibitory effects on spinal cord interneurons. *Brain Res* 40:441–446, 1973.
60. Mayer DJ, Wolfe TL, Akil H, et al: Analgesia from electrical stimulation in the brainstem of the rat. *Science* 174:1351–1354, 1971.
61. Mayer DJ, Liebeskind JC: Pain reduction by focal electrical stimulation of the brain: an anatomical and behavioral analysis. *Brain Res* 68:73–93, 1974.
62. Mayer DJ, Hayes RL: Stimulation-produced analgesia: development of tolerance and cross-tolerance to morphine. *Science* 188:941–943, 1975.
63. Mayer DJ, Price DD: Central nervous system mechanisms of analgesia. *Pain* 2:379–404, 1976.
64. Adams JE: Naloxone reversal of analgesia produced by brain stimulation in the human. *Pain* 2:161–166, 1976.
65. Hosobuchi Y, Adams JE, Linchitz R: Pain relief by electrical stimulation of the central gray matter in humans and its reversal by naloxone. *Science* 197:183–186, 1977.
66. Akil H, Richardson DE, Hughes J: Enkephalin-like material elevated in ventricular cerebrospinal fluid of pain patients after analgetic focal stimulation. *Science* 201:463–465, 1978.
67. Hosobuchi Y, Rossier J, Bloom FE, Guilleman R: Stimulation of human periaqueductal gray for pain relief increases immu-

noreactive β-endorphin in ventricular fluid. *Science* 203:279–281, 1979.
68. Dionne RA, Muller GP, Young RF, Greenberg P, Hargreaves KM, Gracely R, Dubner R: Contrast medium causes the apparent increase in β-endorphin levels in human cerebrospinal fluid following brain stimulation. *Pain* 20:313–321, 1980.
69. Fessler RG, Brown FD, Rachlin JR, Mullan S: Elevated β-endorphin in cerebrospinal fluid after electrical brain stimulation: artifact of contrast infusion. *Science* 224:1017–1019, 1984.
70. Richardson DE, Akil H: Pain reduction by electrical stimulation in man (Part I). *J Neurosurg* 47:178–183, 1977.
71. Young RF, Kroening R, Fulton W, Feldman R, Chambi I: Electrical stimulation of the brain in treatment of chronic pain: experience over 5 years. *J Neurosurg* 62:389–396, 1985.
72. Plotkin R: Results in 60 cases of deep brain stimulation for chronic intractable pain. *Appl Neurophysiol* 45:173–178, 1982.
73. Baskin DS, Mehler WR, Hosobuchi Y, Richardson D, Adams J, Flitter M: Autopsy analysis of the safety, efficacy and cartography of electrical stimulation of the central gray in humans. *Brain Res* 371:231–236, 1986.
74. Siegfried J: Monopolar electrical stimulation of nucleus ventroposteromedialis thamami for postherpetic facial pain. *Appl Neurophysiol* 45:179–184, 1982.
75. Amano K, Kitamura K, Kawamura H: Alterations of immunoreactive β-endorphin in the third ventricular fluid in response to electrical stimulation of the human periaqueductal gray matter. *Apply Neurophysiol* 43:150–158, 1980.
76. Boivie J, Meyerson BA: A correlative anatomical and clinical study of pain suppression by deep brain stimulation. *Pain* 13:113–126, 1982.
77. Young RF, Brechner T: Electrical stimulation of the brain for relief of intractable pain due to cancer. *Cancer* 57:1266–1272, 1986.
78. Fowler K, North R: Patient-interactive PC interface to implanted, multichannel stimulators. In *Proceedings of the 39th Annual Conference on Engineering in Medicine and Biology*, Baltimore, 1986, p 380.
79. Mannheimer C, Carlsson CA: The analgesic effect of transcutaneous electrical nerve stimulation (TNS) in patients with rheumatoid arthritis: a comparative study of different pulse patterns. *Pain* 6:329–334, 1979.
80. Dyck PJ, Lais A, Karnes J, Sparks M, Dyck PJB: Peripheral axotomy induces neurofilament decrease, atrophy, demyelination and degeneration of root and fasciculus gracilis fibers. *Brain Res* 340:19–36, 1985.
81. Ohnishi A, O'Brien PC, Okazaki H, Dyck PJ: Morphometry of myelinated fibers of fasciculus gracilis of man. *J Neurol Sci* 27:163–172, 1976.
82. Ranck J: Which elements are excited in electrical stimulation of mammalian central nervous system: a review. *Brain Res* 98:417–440, 1975.
83. Accornero N, Bini G, Lenzi G, Manfredi M: Selective activation of peripheral nerve fibre groups of different diameter by triangular shaped stimulus pulses. *J Physiol* 273:539–560, 1977.
84. Coburn B, Sin W: A theoretical study of epidural electrical stimulation of the spinal cord. Part I: finite element analysis of stimulus fields. *Biomed Eng* 32:971–977, 1985.
85. Sances A, Swiontek TJ, Larson SJ, Cusick JF, Meyer GA, Millar EA, Hemmy DC, Myklebust J: Innovations in neurologic implant systems. *Med Instrum* 9:213–216, 1975.
86. Reilly JP, Freeman VT, Larkin WD: Sensory effects of transient electrical stimulation—Evaluation with a neuroelectric model. *IEEE Trans Biomed Eng* BME-32:1001–1011, 1985.

chapter 13
Role of Physical Medicine

Rajka Soric, M.D., M.Sci., F.R.C.P.C.
Michael Devlin, M.D., F.R.C.P.C.

Physical agents have been used extensively since recorded time in the treatment of painful conditions. The popularity of physical agents has waxed and waned. With increases in medical knowledge about the pathophysiology of pain and the advent of more specific medical treatments, interest in physical modalities declined. With breakthroughs in the technical sciences, on the other hand, newer and more complex modalities have been developed, with an upswing in popularity of physical medicine.

Heat, in a variety of forms, has been employed over the centuries. Hippocrates used warm water in a bag for the treatment of sciatica. Most ancient civilizations used cautery in a variety of guises for treatment of many conditions—a practice that remains today in some cultures (e.g., moxibustion). The Romans promoted the use of baths to treat sciatica as well as paralysis. Spa treatments remain popular today, particularly in Europe. Pliny advocated hot air furnaces to treat arthritis. As technology progressed, particularly after the harnessing of electricity, hot air cabinets became available, and were very popular in the early 1900s.

The invention of the incandescent light bulb led to the use of light cabinets for treatment of many painful conditions. Laser is the more modern counterpart.

The use of cold lagged behind that of heat because of the inability to artificially make ice, which was not overcome until the late 1800s. The use of cold is gaining in popularity, although as early as the mid-1600s the immersion of both legs into cold water was advocated for treating arthritis. In colder countries with plentiful snow, eating snow had been prescribed to treat painful stomach disorders, and it was known in Napoleonic times that snow packed into wounds decreased pain.

Massage is another physical treatment mentioned in Chinese writings from 3000 BC. The Greeks also used it for treatment of pain, and followed it with gymnastics. This has subsequently evolved to the current use of exercise as one approach to pain management.

In times past, physical agents were promoted and used as a treatment in isolation, often with an expectation of a cure. Current practice has altered so that the use of physical modalities is an adjunct to other therapeutic interventions in the management of chronic pain.

The usual goal in treating any condition is to effect a cure. In most patients with chronic pain this is not possible, and so the treatment is directed at controlling the disease process to a degree where there are no symptoms, and no functional limitations. This all too often is not a realistic expectation, and attention must then be directed toward symptomatic pain relief in order to maximize function and to decrease the possibility of developing secondary complications related to deconditioning. In the worst case, even adequate pain control cannot be achieved, but the patient's overall functional level must still be maintained and maximized.

In patients with chronic pain, physical agents should be used with specific goals in mind, which usually can be expressed as:

1. Symptomatic pain relief.
2. Compensation for inadequate or absent structures where such a lack contributes to pain.
3. Allowing a functional activity to be performed in a painless "abnormal" manner, rather than a painful "normal" way.

An example of the first is a hot pack, and of the second the use of a knee orthosis to correct instability due to ligamentous laxity. The use of a wheelchair to travel outdoors in a patient with severe hip arthritis is an illustration of the third.

Countless physical agents and treatments have been developed over the years and marketed for the treatment of a whole host of ailments. Although not explicitly stated, it is often implied that such modalities are disease specific and may effect a long-lasting result. This rarely, if ever, has proven to be the case.

It has become apparent that many different modalities actually have the same physiologic effect, even though this was not initially recognized. Hand in hand with this, an understanding developed that the use of physical modalities in the treatment of the patient with chronic pain must be part of an overall plan of management, and that their use in isolation will not bring about any beneficial result.

Physical agents should be prescribed with the same thought and care as medications or operations. There must be a specific goal, and if that goal is not achieved, and it is obvious that the physical modality is not offering any benefit, its use should be discontinued. Most practitioners would not contemplate performing the same operation on the same patient over and over again, but such common sense is often lacking in the use of physical agents. The initial evaluation and subsequent assessment of the patient's condition is therefore mandatory in determining the efficacy of a used modality.

The following agents are discussed with respect to their utilization in patients with chronic pain, with particular reference to the desired goals, mechanisms of action, and contraindications:

1. Heat
2. Cold
3. Exercise
4. Mobilization
    a. traction
    b. manipulation
    c. massage
5. Electrical stimulation (TENS)
6. Actinotherapy (ultraviolet light, laser)
7. Hydrotherapy
8. Biofeedback
9. Orthotics and assistive devices

THERAPEUTIC HEAT

Over the centuries different methods of heating have been advocated, with claims of superior effect with each new modality that has been developed. Before discussing individual heating devices, the physiologic effects of heat will be outlined. Irrespective of the heating modality used, the effects, in general, of these devices are due to heating itself, and are not a function of the device.

PHYSIOLOGIC EFFECTS OF HEAT

The effects of heat may be divided into those occurring locally and those occurring at a site distant from the area being heated.

Local Effects

At a cellular level, heating increases metabolic activity with increased membrane diffusion, enhanced enzymatic activity, and increased oxygen demand (1–3). As a result, vasodilation occurs to supply more blood to meet the increased energy requirements, and to take away waste products (4). Such an increase in metabolic rate will result in an increase in inflammatory response, nerve conduction velocity, and muscle contractility (5). These responses would be expected to increase pain in situations where the pain is secondary to an inflammatory process. The reason that increased pain is not usually seen with local heating is that the vast majority of heating devices cannot cause an increase in temperature in the structure causing the pain (4). In situations in which the painful area can be heated an increase in pain will result. An example of this is a sunburn, on which a hot shower is painful.

In conditions in which pain is thought to be due to an accumulation of cell metabolites in a relatively ischemic area (e.g., tonically contracted muscle), the vasodilation secondary to heating may allow rapid removal of these substances (4). On the other hand, it can be argued that local acidosis is the most potent vasodilator and heating will not increase blood flow in this situation (6).

Another local effect of heat is a decrease in synovial fluid viscosity (7, 8). This is one explanation for the decrease in joint stiffness in patients with arthritis, because it has been postulated that the stiffness is a result of increased viscosity of synovial fluid. However, most heating agents will not cause an increase in joint temperature, thus making this theory an unlikely explanation for the observed benefit.

Collagen will become more distensible upon being heated, which has led to the use of heating prior to performing stretching exercises in patients with joint contractures (9). The problem of getting heat to the collagenous structure remains largely unsolved, particularly when dealing with large areas, such as the knee capsule.

Another effect that has been claimed is an increase in pain threshold as temperature increases, although the observed change is probably of no clinical significance (10).

In order to achieve a significant change in metabolic rate, collagen distensibility, and blood supply, the temperature in the tissue must rise to between 41°C and 45°C (9). At temperatures greater than this, structural damage may occur, as proteins denature. Most patients will no longer feel a sensation of heat, but rather will feel pain, as tissue temperatures exceed 46°C. Fortunately, pain is usually felt prior to structural damage occurring, thus providing a built-in safety device when using therapeutic heat.

Distant Effects

One of the distant effects of local heating is the consensual vascular response. Heating the skin of the abdomen will reflexly cause vasodilation in the legs, thus causing an increased blood supply. Similarly, heating one leg will cause reflex vasodilation in the opposite leg (11).

Heat is psychologically comfortable, relaxing, and sedating. This aspect of heat is not frequently mentioned in the literature. It is an effect that is so intuitive that it has not warranted much attention.

A third distant effect of heat is that it acts as a sensory stimulus, and thus may function to decrease pain via the gate mechanism (12). This is a nonspecific effect, and does not rely on the heating per se.

Of all the effects of heat that have been discussed, it is likely that the two most important in the treatment of pain are its psychological effects and its counterirritant effects. The other physiologic effects do exist; however, in most clinical situations, the use of heat does not cause a significant rise in temperature in the structure where the pain is originating.

INDICATIONS

The usual indication for the use of heat in patients with chronic pain is for symptomatic pain relief and relaxation. It should not be expected that heat will "cure" the condition, nor that its effects will be long lasting. The pain relief and relaxation may be a goal in its own right, or may be desirable as an adjunct to other physical treatments, such as exercise of manipulation.

CONTRAINDICATIONS

There are a variety of contraindications to the use of heat in general (4). There are some specific, additional contraindications related to specific heating modalities. Any heating device has the ability to burn the patient, and therefore anyone who cannot respond to an impending burn (infants, patients who are mentally confused, those with marked sensory impairment, etc.) should not be exposed to heat as a therapeutic modality. Heat should not be directly applied to ischemic areas, such as in patients with peripheral vascular disease or pressure sores, because the increased metabolic demands may outstrip the blood supply. Reflex vasodilation via the consensual reaction is permissible. Acutely inflamed areas should not be heated, nor should areas with a fresh (less than 24 hr old) hematoma. Heat, as a pain-relieving agent, should not be applied to a tumor, for fear of increasing the tumor's metabolic activity and growth.

COMMON HEATING DEVICES

Heating devices are classified into two major groups, depending upon their depth of penetration. Superficial agents will cause a temperature rise in skin, subcutaneous fat, and occasionally superficial musculature. Deep-heating modalities can cause a temperature increase in joints and deeper muscle layers.

Superficial Heating Devices

Heating Pad The inexpensive, easily available electrically heated pad will heat skin and subcutaneous tissue by conduction. The usual time of application is 20–30 min. These devices should be attached to a timer to prevent longer use, and subsequent burns.

Hot Water Bottle The hot water bottle is the simplest heating device. The major drawbacks with this are scalding caused if the stopper comes out inadvertently, and the rapid heat loss over time. However, this latter drawback also has an advantage in that the duration of heating is self-limited.

Hydrocollator Packs Hydrocollator packs are gel cores surrounded by cotton that conform reasonably well to body contours. The packs are heated to 70–80°C in a water bath and will keep their heat for about 20 min. The heating is via conduction and occurs primarily in the skin. Maximum temperature rise to approximately 42°C occurs after 8 min (13).

Paraffin Wax To achieve heating of very irregular body contours, such as hands and feet, a bath containing paraffin wax and mineral oil at 54°C is used. The hand is dipped into the bath several times until a thick glove is formed, and then wrapped in toweling. This method will cause a temperature rise in the skin to 45°C that can be maintained for 15–20 min (14).

Heating Lamps Heating lamps are usually infrared sources that can be used to heat relatively large areas. The duration of treatment is usually 15–20 min.

Deep-Heating Devices

Because of the limited depth of penetration of the above-mentioned modalities, other devices have been developed in an attempt to achieve deeper heating: shortwave, microwave, and ultrasound. As is discussed below, of these, only ultrasound has proven to be a practical, true deep-heating modality.

Shortwave Diathermy Shortwave diathermy utilizes radiofrequency waves at a frequency of 27.12 MHz that, by conversion, heat tissues. The energy is delivered by plates or coils, with an electric field being set up. The part to be heated is placed into, and becomes part of, the field. Depending on the area to be heated, different coils or plates may be used. The usual treatment time is 20–30 min. There is no method of determining how much energy is being delivered; therefore the current is adjusted until the patient reports a feeling of warmth, but not pain. Even though shortwave diathermy was previously promoted as a deep-heating device, in most applications only skin, subcutaneous fat, and superficial muscles are heated. Small joints, with little soft tissue coverage, may also be heated, but larger, deep-seated joints are not (4).

In most patients with chronic pain, in whom heat is used for symptomatic pain relief and relaxation, there is little advantage to shortwave diathermy over simpler devices, because in both the heating occurs primarily in superficial areas.

There have also been claims for beneficial, nonthermal effects of shortwave diathermy; however, none of these have been adequately documented, particularly with respect to chronic pain (4).

There are specific contraindications to the use of shortwave diathermy. It should not be used in patients with cardiac pacemakers, nor where metallic implants are within the treatment field (15).

Microwave Diathermy Electromagnetic radiation at a frequency of 2456 MHz is beamed at the area to be heated. By conversion, heating will occur. The usual treatment time is 10 min. As with shortwave, dosimetry is not possible, and therefore the power output is determined by the patient's feeling of warmth but not pain. With this frequency, heating of subcutaneous fat and superficial musculature occurs (16).

Generators at 915 MHz are also legally allowed, and will selectively heat muscle if direct contact applicators with skin cooling are used (17). These devices have yet to come into general clinical use.

The usually available microwave diathermy does not offer more therapeutic advantage over simpler conductive heating devices. There are no known nonthermal beneficial effects of microwave.

The same specific contraindications apply to microwave as to shortwave. In addition, microwave should not be used around the eyes or testes (4).

Ultrasound This heating modality uses sonic energy, with a frequency between 0.8 and 1 MHz, which is converted into heat when it interacts with tissues. It is applied to the skin with a small sound head, using an acoustic coupler, usually water or a gel. The head must be continuously moved in a small circular motion, or else standing wave patterns may be created, which will cause cavitation and extreme heating, with subsequent tissue damage. Even though only small volumes may be heated, deep heating will occur, primarily where there are interfaces between tissue types, particularly bone and soft tissue (18). At these interfaces, there is reflection of the sound waves, thus increasing their density and, subsequently, the heating effect. It has been shown that deep structures, such as the hip joint, can be heated with ultrasound (19).

Ultrasound is the one modality where the energy delivered is known, and can be predetermined. It is usually delivered with the initial power level of 0.5 watts/cm^2 for 2–3 min. The maximum safe power output is 4 watts/cm^2, with the level being determined by the patient's feeling of warmth but not pain. The major clinical use of ultrasound is heating smaller, deep-seated structures, such as tendons or joint capsules, prior to stretching exercises. It is also used in chronic tendonitis or bursitis, where some believe the increased temperature will increase circulation and thus help remove toxic metabolites or resorb calcific deposits; others disagree (20).

Pulsed ultrasound, where the energy is constantly interrupted so that a temperature rise is minimized, is also used. It is claimed that when used in this mode, the sound energy will mechanically loosen scar tissue and adhesions, as well as mechanically decrease edema. At a cellular level, it is claimed that ultrasound may increase efficiency of enzyme systems and may alter membrane permeability without a concomitant temperaure rise (1). Most of these claims have not been proven to be exclusively due to mechanical effects (4).

The use of ultrasound is specifically contraindicated over fluid-containing organs, such as eyes or a pregnant uterus. It may be used over metallic implants, because metal and bone are equally dense to ultrasound (21).

SUMMARY

In summary, although there are many different heating devices, with many claims for specific benefit of one device over another, from a practical viewpoint all heating devices, with the exception of ultrasound, heat superficial structures only, and do not heat the tissue where the pain is thought to be originating. The beneficial effects of heating, in most instances, are due to psychological mechanisms, producing relaxation and sedation, and counterirritant phenomena.

THERAPEUTIC COLD

Cryotherapy is becoming increasingly popular in the treatment of pain. Patients and practitioners are becoming more aware of its benefits and more accepting of its use. Although cold may not be particularly comfortable when initially applied, its efficacy as a pain-relieving agent dictates its use in many situations.

PHYSIOLOGIC EFFECTS

The physiologic effects of cold, by and large, are opposite to those of heat (22). Metabolic rate is decreased, thus causing a decrease in inflammatory responses. Blood supply to a cooled area decreases, because of both decreased demand and vasoconstriction (23). Muscle spasm is decreased, since muscle cannot contract effectively as metabolic activity decreases with cooling (24, 25). Nerve conduction velocity and spontaneous discharge also decrease (26).

Because of the induced vasoconstriction, and the insulating properties of fat, muscle will remain cooled for an appreciable length of time, thus explaining why the effects of cold are longer lasting than those of heat, where vasodilation conducts heat away rapidly (27). For these reasons, cryotherapy is an effective pain-relieving agent, when the structure causing pain can be cooled. In addition, there may be benefits via the gate mechanism even when the painful structure is not actually cooled (12).

There are several physiologic effects of cold that may not be beneficial in the treatment of patient with pain. Cooling may increase joint stiffness as the synovial fluid viscosity increases (7). Collagen distensibility is decreased and thus stretching exercises to decrease contractures will not be as effective. However, because such exercises are often painful, the analgesic benefit of cooling may outweigh this disadvantage.

INDICATIONS

Although cryotherapy traditionally has been used in acute painful conditions in which a marked inflammatory response is present, its use in chronic pain should be considered if a pain-producing structure amenable to cooling can be identified.

CONTRAINDICATIONS

There are few contraindications to cryotherapy; presence of Raynaud's phenomenon, cold hypersensitivity, and the presence of cold agglutinins are the major ones, albeit uncommon.

COOLING DEVICES

The usual form of cold application is the use of ice and water in a plastic bag, placed on the skin for 15–20 min. Cooling will occur in skin and fat and up to 2 cm deep in muscle (22).

Other methods of cold application include the use of an ice cube, rubbed over a painful area for 5 min or until the area becomes numb. This can be useful for symptomatic relief of pain where localized muscle spasm or a trigger point is involved.

Vapocoolant sprays are the other major method of applying cold. These are sprayed onto the skin, and by their rapid evaporation cause cooling. This method causes short-lasting, superficial cooling. These are used most frequently in stretch-and-spray techniques in the treatment of myofascial pain syndromes and trigger points.

EXERCISE

Therapeutic exercise is the prescribed movement of body parts or of the body in order to achieve a specific goal. Different exercises are used depending on the patient, his/her problem, and the desired goal. A broad classification distinguishes two major groups: exercises to increase the patient's overall level of activity, and exercises aimed at altering specific aspects of local regions—usually strength, mobility, posture, or endurance.

EXERCISES FOR GENERAL ACTIVITY

Many patients with chronic pain will have a restricted level of overall activity. The reasons for this may be any of the following, alone or in combination:

1. Patient experience shows that activity increases pain.
2. Patients fear that activity will increase pain.
3. Patients are instructed to avoid activity by physicians who fear that activity will increase pain.
4. Patients or physicians fear that pain is a result of injury and that rest must be used until the injury is healed.
5. The underlying condition causing the chronic pain interferes with activity and mobility.

In many situations it is found that many activities that patients with chronic pain have stopped doing are remote from the painful site, do not and could not aggravate the pain, and essentially represent an excessive restriction that is difficult to justify. As a result of decreased activity, patients become deconditioned, become more reliant on others, have decreased social interaction, and tend to have a lessened sense of self-worth and well-being. Generalized activity programs are claimed to counteract these problems.

Patients with chronic pain should be encouraged to participate in general exercise programs, as long as there are no specific contraindications to their participation. The reasons why such a program would be beneficial and why it is thought that no harm will ensue should be carefully explained. The patient should be instructed to start the suggested exercise slowly, increasing first the frequency of participation, and then the duration. Specific goals should be set at the onset and reviewed at regular intervals (28, 29). Depending on the patients, and their requirements, a general exercise program can usually be found. Most programs use low-load, repetitive, and rhythmic activities.

Walking

Walking is easy to prescribe, is easy to perform, and can be done anywhere. Improvement in the patient's condition can be easily monitored by recording the distance walked.

Swimming and Aquatics

Swimming and aquatics exercises are low load with respect to weight-bearing joints, and are particularly appropriate for patients with arthritis. Since they are also soothing and relaxing, swimming and aquatics are also beneficial for patients with any type of chronic pain.

Calisthenics

Although the initial reaction is that these are high-demand exercises, there are many low-level calisthenic exercise routines. These are most commonly found in cardiac or pulmonary rehabilitation books, but can easily be applied to patients with chronic pain (30).

Cycling

Cycling is another rhythmic, repetitive activity that can be done with either a stationary bicycle or a regular one. Although not as universally applicable, particularly in musculoskeletal problems, this can be tolerated by many patients.

GOAL-SPECIFIC EXERCISES

Strengthening Exercises

Specific muscle–strengthening exercises are employed when specific muscle weakness is identified that is believed to be in part, or in whole, responsible for the continuing pain. This is usually found in painful chronic musculoskeletal conditions, where decreased motor control may be contributing to joint instability, thus allowing abnormal stresses to be placed across the joint, resulting in pain. An example of this is the use of quadriceps-strengthening exercises in patients with patellofemoral syndrome, when it is thought that patellar maltracking may be present (31). Another example is the use of abdominal-strengthening exercises in patients with chronic low back pain due to abnormal forces being transmitted through the facet joints. An increase in abdominal strength allows greater weight-bearing loads to be taken through the abdomen. Strengthening exercises can be classified as isometric, isotonic, or isokinetic (32).

Isometric Exercises When performing isometric exercises there is no joint movement, because when the agonist is contracted, movement is prevented either by simultaneous contraction of the agonist or the use of external force. The primary use of isometric exercises is in patients who cannot move their joint (i.e., joint is in a cast, etc.) or where this is undesirable (acute arthritis). Their utility in patients with chronic pain is limited, because often there is no reason why the joint should not move. These exercises are difficult to monitor as far as how much the patient is doing, tend to be boring, and should not be used in patients where there is a concern if their diastolic blood pressure becomes elevated.

Isotonic Exercises Isotonic exercises are the strengthening exercises that most people recognize. The joint is moved through a range, against either no resistance or increasing resistance (against gravity, against weights) (33). Such exercises are easy to do with a minimum of equipment in any location. The patient's progress is easy to monitor with respect to the number of repetitions done each time, and what resistance was used (e.g., the patient did 10 knee extensions from 90° to 0° against a 2-kg weight). These are the most commonly prescribed specific strengthening exercises, and can easily be taught to the patient and performed in a home setting.

Isokinetic Exercises Isokinetic exercises are also done throughout a joint's range, and in addition, at a constant speed and against a constant resistance. The rationale behind such exercises is that strengthening will occur at all lengths of the muscle or throughout the whole joint range, rather than at one length (isometric) or concentrated around one length (isotonic). Such exercises are used primarily for strengthening in subacute or postoperative situations and not in chronic pain. The major disadvantage of this form of exercise is that expensive equipment, such as a Cybex II, must be used in order to perform and monitor the exercise.

Range of Movement Exercises

Range of movement exercises are performed actively by the patient to maintain, or increase, joint mobility. In situations in which it is thought that restricted joint mobility causes abnormal forces across the joint, or in which restricted joint mobility causes abnormal postures elsewhere, it is reasonable to attempt to restore joint mobility to normal. In order to stand upright with hip flexion contractures, the lumbar lordosis must increase, thus increasing weight-bearing forces across the facet joints, creating low back pain. By increasing the range of hip movement in extension, this sequence of events can be reversed.

Another example is the patient with chronic shoulder pain due to recurrent impingement of supraspinatous tendon against the coracoacromial ligament. Often such patients have a decreased range of external rotation, thus preventing the normal clearing of the greater tuberosity behind the acromion while abducting. Having the patient increase his/her movement in external rotation will allow restoration of normal shoulder biomechanics, and relief of the impingement.

Range of movement exercises are usually easy to do and should be utilized where abnormal mobility is thought to contribute to ongoing pain. For specific joints there are specific exercises for specific movements; these details are beyond the scope of this chapter, but are available in standard texts of therapeutic exercises (34).

Stretching Exercises

Stretching exercises are performed to elongate soft tissue structures that have become shortened. Although these exercises may also be considered range of movement exercises and often are indistinguishable from them, stretching exercise usually implies that another person, or a force other than muscles controlling the joint, is used, whereas in range of movement exercise, the patient actively uses the muscle crossing the joint to create the movement. The most common use of stretching exercises is to stretch muscles that have become shortened due to spasm. It is thought that such shortened muscles, when tightened passively by normal movement, respond by contraction, leading to pain and more spasm. A stretching exercise involves a slow, prolonged stretch being placed on the muscle, thus allowing it to relax and elongate, rather than contracting and causing pain.

These exercises are usually preceded by the use of a physical modality such as heat, to allow the patient to relax the muscle in order to perform the stretch more easily. Stretching techniques are primarily used in the treatment of myofascial pain syndromes and chronic back and neck pain, particularly if trigger points are present. With trigger points, stretch-and-spray techniques may be used. Vapocoolant spray is directed onto the skin overlying the muscle to be stretched, starting distal to, and proceeding over, the trigger point in a proximal direction. A slow, passive stretch is then applied to the muscle. The process is repeated several times until full mobility is established.

A rare use of stretching exercises is in the patient with pain due to spasticity—a slow, prolonged stretch will cause the muscle to relax, probably through reflex inactivation from the Golgi tendon organ. Once relaxed, the pain will decrease. Such stretching exercises can often be done by the patient using positioning and gravity as the stretching force. In this situation, stretching will lead to temporary relief of spasticity, but will not have any long-standing effect.

Postural Exercises

Postural exercises are designed to make the patient more aware of his/her posture, and to teach the patient how to correct an abnormal posture. Their major utility is in patients with low back as well as neck and midthoracic pain, in whom it is thought that the abnormal posture is contributing to the pain.

The best known are the pelvic tilt exercises, used when it is believed that an increased lumbar lordosis causes excessive weight-bearing stresses to be placed through the facet joints in the lumbar spine. By instructing the patient to assume a posture in which the pelvis is rotated in a superoposterior/inferoanterior direction greater loads are placed through the vertebral bodies and disk spaces rather than across the facet joints.

Abnormal upper back and neck posture is also frequently seen, in which the shoulders are protracted and the head protruded anteriorly. This posture can cause pain, both by increasing the cervical lordosis and by causing the trapezii to tonically contract in order to support the arms and shoulder girdle. Such patients will commonly have weakness in their shoulder abductors and flexors. These patients can be identified not only by how they look, but also by the fact that reversing their abnormal posture will restore their shoulder strength. Patients may develop this posture as a result of habit, or as a result of a painful neck or shoulder condition. Such a posture appears to be a pain-relieving mechanism in acute conditions, but may lead to chronic pain long after this initial injury has resolved. Patients are instructed about the desired posture, usually in front of mirrors so they can see as well as feel the desired position. This can be reinforced by having them sit with a small sandbag on their head; the bag will stay put with the desired posture, but will fall off with the undesired positioning.

The major problem with such exercises is that they are difficult to monitor and it is difficult to get carryover of the new posture into everyday activities, particularly for people who sit working at a desk. In spite of this, they should be tried, because the patient who finds that the corrected neck posture does decrease pain will continue with it.

Endurance Exercises

Endurance exercises are similar to the general activity programs discussed above as far as what is used, but the goal is different. Whereas general activity programs are designed to gain an overall increase in activity, endurance exercises are designed to increase the patient's ability to perform a given activity over time. The activity must be decided upon prior to starting, according to the patient's needs, because there is less and less crossover benefit as the endurance exercise becomes more dissimilar from the desired activity. For example, a 100% increase in cycling time on a bicycle will not translate into a 100% increase in walking tolerance, even though both involve leg work. Therefore, the best endurance exercise program to increase tolerance for doing a given activity is to perform that activity. An example of such a program would be one in a patient with intermittent claudication due to peripheral vascular disease whose complaint is limited walking distance. By placing the patient on a walking program with instructions to walk until the pain starts, on a repeated basis, an increase in walking endurance will be seen. The mechanism for this is probably a combination of increased muscle oxygen extraction, increased cellular efficiency, and development of collaterals (35).

Such programs usually do not play a large role in the management of patients with chronic pain because the increased ability to perform a stated activity over time is not a common goal.

Relaxation Exercises

When it is thought that chronic muscle contraction is contributing to or causing the patient's pain, exercises designed to teach the patient to relax muscles may be employed. These can be difficult to teach and to learn. The greatest success occurs in patients who will accept that muscle tension is playing a role in their chronic pain.

One method is in a group setting with a live instructor. Another is with a prerecorded cassette tape with an individual patient, in quiet surroundings. The patients are instructed to close their eyes, and to concentrate on their fingers. The instructions continue in a calm, soft manner for the patient to feel his/her fingers relaxing, getting lighter, not resting on the floor as hard, and almost floating. The instructions are then repeated for more and more proximal parts until the patient feels the whole body being loose, relaxed, and almost detached from the mind. When successful, the patient is often asleep by this time. The goal is to teach the patients what it feels like to have their muscles relaxed, and how to achieve relaxation, so that they can now consciously relax tight muscles whenever they want to in order to get pain relief (36). This is essentially a hypnosis-based tool. In situations in which such an approach does not work, other methods of teaching patients how to relax can be used, particularly electromyographic biofeedback.

TRACTION, MASSAGE, AND MANIPULATION

Traction, manipulation, and massage have been used as therapeutic modalities since ancient times in several cultures. In essence, these are all passive exercises directed toward restoration of joint mobility, tissue extensibility, and perfusion.

TRACTION

Traction is a method in which a distracting force is applied in order to stretch soft tissues and separate articulating surfaces in a direction that is not physiologic. Traction is often used as preparation for other mobilization or manipulative procedures, since it is believed that stretching of the muscles will lead to their relaxation, thus improving local circulation and diminishing pain.

As a treatment modality for conditions characterized by chronic pain, traction is most frequently used in the management of neck and low back disorders. Pathogenesis of pain in these disorders is still not well understood. Some believe that in conditions in which a herniated disk or an osteophyte exert pressure on the spinal nerve, pain results from impaired circulation due to stretching of the root and its dural sheath (37). However, this does not explain the pain in patients who do not exhibit any clinical or radiologic evidence of root compression. In these situations, offered explanations for the occurrence of pain include osteoarthritis of the facet joints, capsulitis, and subluxation. Crisp suggested that pain arises as a result of prolapse of the synovial membrane between the two articulating surfaces of the joints (38). Abnormalities of other pain-sensitive structures, such as anterior and posterior longitudinal ligaments, have also been recognized as a cause of chronic back and neck pain (37).

Although the etiology of long-standing pain often cannot be established, traction as a therapeutic modality is frequently used with success. Its main effects on vertebral structures are mechanical, consisting of:

1. Stretching of muscles and ligaments
2. Distraction of vertebral bodies
3. Separation of the facet joints
4. Enlargement of the intervertebral foramina

It is questionable whether distraction of bony elements does actually occur with the traction forces commonly used in clinical practice (39).

An additional explanation for the analgesic effect of traction is the alteration of pain perception and modification of pain response by stimulation of stretch receptors (39).

Before using traction, the patient should be assessed to ensure that there are no contraindications for its use (40). Examples of such contraindications include:

1. Malignancy of the spine
2. Osteomyelitis of the spine
3. Bleeding diathesis
4. Marked osteoporosis
5. Vertebrobasilar insufficiency or severe carotid artery arteriosclerosis
6. Rheumatoid or other inflammatory arthritides

Active peptic ulcer, hiatus hernia, and documented aortic aneurysm are considered relative contraindications for lumbar traction, since it will lead to an increase of the intra-abdominal pressure.

The technique of applying traction is important if one is to achieve the desired therapeutic effect and prevent complications.

Cervical Traction

In treatment of the cervical spine, traction may be applied either manually or by a mechanical apparatus. Although manual traction offers better control of head position, it is more tiresome for the therapist and one cannot precisely control the amount of pulling force applied. With mechanical traction, the head is harnessed in a halter that is attached to a crossbar that is either weighted or connected to a mechanical device. Traction may be applied either in an upright sitting or inclined position using body weight as a counterforce, or with the patient lying supine. In this situation, the necessary counterforce is provided by the friction between the body and the surface on which it lies. The angle of pull is usually maintained at 20–25° of forward flexion, in an attempt to open the intervertebral foramina (41). It is recommended to start the treatment with light weights (2–4 kg), thus allowing the patient to get gradually accustomed to the pulling force (41). This prevents reactive muscle spasm and allows gradual loading of the temporomandibular joints. The weight is then gradually increased, to a maximum of 22 kg.

Traction may be delivered as a constant pulling force for 15–20 min or intermittently, the usual duration of the session being around 30 min (42). Daily treatments for 7–10 days are sufficient in most cases. If the patient's condition does not change during this time, treatments should be considered ineffective and traction should be discontinued. If the patient responds favorably, but returns in the future with a recurrent problem, a home traction apparatus can be suggested (43).

Lumbar Traction

When traction is applied to the lumbar spine, mechanical devices are usually used. The upper half of the body is secured in straps and corsets that anchor the patient, while the traction force is exerted through a pelvic harness. In order to reduce friction between the body of the patient and the surface on which he is lying, elaborate split traction tables may be used. They consist of a fixed (proximal) portion and a mobile (distal) segment on which the lower part of the body lies. The spinal segment to which traction is to be applied rests in between. When the pulling force is applied, the lower part of the body moves together with the mobile part of the table. In order for lumbar traction to be successful, a pulling force of 40 kg or more may have to be used (42, 44).

MASSAGE

Massage is the oldest and probably the most commonly used mobilization technique. Although massage has been known and widely practiced for centuries, it is interesting to note that its therapeutic use has been on a steady decline throughout the North American continent, while in Europe it is still a frequently prescribed modality. The rapid development of pharmaceuticals and inventions of various physical modalities (ultrasound, diathermy, laser therapy, etc.) are greatly responsible for this decline. Nevertheless, massage has an important place among therapeutic modalities for many conditions, including chronic pain.

The physiologic effects of masage are claimed to be:

1. Improved perfusion of soft tissue
2. Rapid elimination of waste products
3. Reduction of soft tissue edema and induration
4. Loosening and stretching of the contracted tissues

Massage also has a soothing effect, producing generalized relaxation and a sense of overall well-being (39, 41). Skin is particularly well adapted for massage. It becomes softer and more supple and its nutrient status improves by virtue of improved circulation. Improved perfusion of the muscles with rapid elimination of waste products and replenishment of nutrients relieves the discomfort of muscle fatigue (37). The effect of massage on the circulatory system largely depends upon the technique used. Deep stroking and kneading leads to increased blood flow through the medium-sized vessels, whereas petrissage causes capillary dilation. When administered in a centripetal direction, massage greatly improves venous return and lymph flow, thus reducing peripheral edema (45).

The "classical massage" includes four different maneuvers (37): petrissage, kneading, effluage, and friction. In *petrissage* one grasps and lifts small areas of skin and subcutaneous tissues, simultaneously applying firm pressure. In *kneading* much larger areas are grasped and lifted (46).

Friction is applied by firm pressure over the tissue in a circular motion (37, 46). Although it may be unpleasant while being done, it will result in a long-term benefit. Its goal is to separate adhesions formed in deep-seated soft tissues that restrict movement and cause pain. It is erroneously assumed that similar effects may be produced by stretching. With the latter maneuver, the fibers parallel to the stretching force are being elongated, while in a transverse plane fibers are approximated (39). In order for friction to be successful the muscle must be relaxed not only during treatment but for a short period afterward so that the broadening effect of deep massage on the tissue fibers can be maintained. Heating the area prior to application of friction will decrease viscosity of the tissue and will further enhance breaking of the adhesions.

Effluage, or stroking, is appropriate for treating larger areas. The therapist uses the palm of the hand, applying firm pressure usually in a centripetal direction. Its major effects are psychological, with no longer lasting benefits (39).

Frequently, various agents (media) are used in conjunction with massage (37). Most commonly used are oil-based substances and powders. In addition to making the skin softer, these agents minimize the friction between the therapist's hand and the patient's skin, which allows the pressure to be transmitted to deeper structures, making massage more effective.

With respect to the clinical application and effectiveness of massage, general opinion among most physicians is that it produces only transient relaxation not worth the therapist's time (39). This may, in fact, be true for superficial stroking of the skin, which results in pleasant sensations but no longer lasting effects.

A major controversy exists amongst the proponents of massage as a therapeutic modality in the treatment of fibrositis (37). James Cyriax considers this condition an absolute contraindication for massage, believing that "trigger points" are simply a manifestation of referred pain from the spine (37, 39). On the other hand, Sjöelund and coworkers believe that deep pressure and massage over the trigger points stimulate proprioceptive endings, facilitating encephalin release that leads to pain modulation (47).

As with any other treatment modality there are contraindications to massage:

1. Infection, for fear of spreading it via enhanced circulation
2. Inflammatory arthritis
3. Nerve entrapment
4. Phlebitis
5. Calcification of the soft tissues

Although massage is by definition a manual treatment, since the earliest days attempts were made to substitute various mechanical devices for the human hand. The most frequently used devices include:

1. Hand-held devices (e.g., vibrator)
2. Stationary devices against which part of the body is moved (e.g., vibrating belt)
3. Alternating pressure mattresses (e.g., air mattress)
4. Hydromassage (e.g., whirlpool)
5. Pneumatic devices (e.g., pneumatic counterpressure pump)

Although vibrating belts and pneumatic counterpressure pumps do have some longer lasting benefits, the rest of these devices produce subjective improvement probably as a result of psychological effect only (45, 48–50).

MANIPULATION

Manipulation consists of a forced passive movement carrying the articular elements beyond their usual physiologic range of movement, often to the limit of their anatomic range. Although it is used primarily for the treatment of spinal disorders, manipulation has its place as a therapeutic modality in the management of peripheral joint disorders as well (39, 51–53). The pathophysiologic basis for manipulation is the presence of a reversible minor intra-articular derangement that may originate from different pathologic conditions (39, 52, 53). Regardless of the cause, in all such derangements there is an element of muscle spasm. It is the relief of this muscle spasm produced by a powerful stretch that is the therapeutic action of manipulation (39). Because manipulation is done to correct mechanical abnormality, it should never be performed unless such an abnormality is present. As with other mobilization techniques, manipulation is absolutely contraindicated in the presence of infection, tumor, fracture, vertebrobasilar insufficiency, and gross articular instability.

Manipulating a patient with a nerve root irritation or a neurologic deficit due to disk herniation remains a controversial issue.

Three steps must be followed during the manipulation:

1. Proper positioning of the patient and therapist
2. Mobilization
3. Manipulative thrust

The need for proper positioning is self-explanatory. The area to be manipulated must be completely relaxed and the therapist must be in a position to take the joint through the anatomic range of movement. Mobilization consists of passive, gentle movement of the joint to the point where the pain is felt, the so-called tension point. From this point, a sudden minimal movement is performed by the therapist—manipulative thrust. When carried out properly, this maneuver is completely painless, although often associated with a cracking sound.

Joints should initially be manipulated in the direction opposite to the one that creates maximal pain (54). For example, in a patient with pain on spinal rotation to the right, manipulation should be carried out first with forced rotation to the left, followed by manipulation to the right at a later stage.

Manipulation can be direct or indirect (37). For indirect manipulation, the patient's body is used as a lever (e.g., forces are applied to the shoulder and pelvic girdles to cause movement in the lumbar spine). In direct manipulation, manipulative thrust is applied directly to the structure involved (e.g., spinous processes of two contiguous vertebrae) (37).

With spinal manipulation, the patient may experience substantial relief even after the first session. More often, however, two or three sessions are required. The interval between manipulations is variable and is determined by the therapist (two manipulations per week or one manipulation every 2 weeks is the most commonly used routine). Patients should be informed about possible reactions to this mode of treatment, particularly after the first session. After the immediate relief that is usually experienced by patients, pain and stiffness may occur, usually lasting up to 24 hr. If the pain lasts longer or if the patient does not experience transient relief immediately after the performed maneuver, it is highly probable that manipulation was done improperly, or the joint that was manipulated was not the source of pain. A number of patients will also experience sympathetic reactions that usually present with increased perspiration. This is most commonly found with cervical spine manipulations (51).

Some physicians advocate the use of adjunctive agents to supplement manipulation. The most frequently used are nonsteroidal anti-inflammatory medications and local steroid injections. These are used prior to manipulation in order to decrease inflammation. Similarly, local heat may enhance relaxation that is required in order to perform successful manipulation. Following manipulation, stretching exercises may be used to further increase the effectiveness of this maneuver.

The following are some of the most frequently encountered chronic painful conditions that may be helped by manipulation:

1. Chronic cervical pain, usually in the presence of degenerative disk disease
2. Chronic headaches for which no other explanation is found
3. Low back pain, particularly with degenerative changes of the facet joints
4. Coccygodynia (55)

When considering manipulation as a treatment modality, the physician should always consider possible adverse effects that may result. Because manipulation is usually done for problems originating in the spine, vascular insults to either the spinal cord or the brain may occur (56–58). Spinal radicular lesions have also been reported to result from manipulation. When done after a thorough patient assessment and by strictly adhering to recommended manipulative techniques such complications are rare.

SUMMARY

As mentioned previously, massage, manipulation, and traction should all be considered types of manipulative techniques. Considering the extent of their use in the treatment of chronic painful conditions it is surprising how little has been done in the way of scientific research to establish the effectiveness of these treatment modalities. Most studies have been poorly designed without adequate control or comparison groups (59). Of the controlled trials that were done over the past 10 years only a few looked at more than one parameter for proving the effectiveness of manipulation (39). A recent trial by Godfrey et al. with more standardized patient selection and well-designed therapeutic protocol did not document any long-term difference in the outcomes of patients treated with different manipulative techniques (60). The question, therefore, remains—are mobilization techniques truly effective or are we dealing with conditions where ultimate recovery represents a natural course of the disease, regardless of the type of therapeutic intervention?

TRANSCUTANEOUS ELECTRICAL NERVE STIMULATION

Since its introduction in 1967, transcutaneous electrical nerve stimulation (TENS) has been extensively used as a pain-relieving modality. The exact mechanism of neuromodulation of pain produced by TENS is still not clear (61). The following hypotheses have been proposed.

1. *Gate Control Theory* The basis for alteration of pain perception is the interaction of large myelinated "A" fibers with small, nonmyelinated "C" fibers that occurs in the substantia gelatinosa in the dorsal horns of the spinal cord. When afferent input via large myelinated fibers is of greater frequency and intensity than afferent input via "C" fibers, the interneurons of the substantia gelatinosa are activated to presynaptically inhibit afferent transmission to suprasegmental levels (i.e., the "gate closes") (12).

2. *Central Biasing Mechanism* The central biasing mechanism theory of pain modulation explains the analgesic effect of TENS in situations in which normal afferent input is diminished or lost (e.g., phantom pain, neuralgias occurring as a result of peripheral nerve damage). By TENS this afferent input is supplemented, providing the central biasing mechanism in the midbrain with adequate stimuli so that pain transmission to higher centers is controlled (62, 63).

3. *Neuropharmacologic Theory* Since the discovery of endorphins and enkephalins in 1975, the effects of electrical stimulation on the formation and release of these substrates has been an area of extensive research. It is believed that TENS increases their concentration, with the end result of elevating the pain threshold (64–67).

4. *Peripheral Blocking Mechanisms* The basis of this theory rests on the ability of TENS to antidromically alter transmission of pain impulses (68).

Various TENS units have been introduced over the last few years. By altering the pulse width, frequency, and current of the electrical stimulus, one can choose the setting that is most efficient for a particular patient (61). The so called HI-TENS units ("conventional TENS"), characterized by pulse widths from 50 to 80 msec and frequencies from 80 to 100 Hz, most likely produce analgesia by raising the cerebrospinal fluid concentrations of enkephalins, as well as operating through the gate mechanism (61). The onset of pain reduction with the use of such units occurs within 10 min and is not blocked by the narcotic antagonist naloxone hydrochloride (61, 69).

The LO-TENS units ("acupuncture TENS"), with larger pulse width (>200 msec) and lower frequencies (0.5–10 Hz), produce analgesia after 15–30 min. Their effect can be reversed by intravenous administration of naloxone, which implies that the analgesic effect of LO-TENS is achieved through the release of β-endorphins (69, 70). This hypothesis has not been unanimously accepted (69, 70).

Sites of electrode placement are most commonly chosen by trial and error, because there is no method to predict the effectiveness of any given placement for any given patient. The most common placements include dermatomes, areas supplied by the peripheral nerve, acupuncture sites, or the painful area itself. Similarly, the stimulus parameters are chosen empirically.

Studies so far have documented that the efficacy of TENS in chronic painful conditions is substantially less than in patients with acute pain (61). Reasons for this observation are still under investigation. One possible explanation is the type of underlying abnormality that is thought to produce pain. Chronic pain is often associated with poorly defined organic pathology. Chronic somatogenic or psychogenic pain is less responsive to TENS treatment than pain of neuropathic origin. Even in situations where TENS is useful in chronic pain, it is often found that over time its efficacy diminishes (61). This may be due to nerve adaptation. Occasionally this problem can be circumvented by changing the stimulation parameters (61).

There are few recognized adverse effects and/or contraindications known for the use of TENS. About 10% of patients will report aggravation of pain as a result of TENS treatments. This problem, thought to result from histamine release, may be controlled by lowering the frequency of stimuli to less than 80 Hz (61). Micropunctate burns and allergic reactions to tape and/or gel are the only other adverse effects recognized. Placement of the electrodes over the carotid sinus and the use of TENS in patients with demand pacemakers have been the only two contraindications recognized (71).

ACTINOTHERAPY

The therapeutic effect of sunlight has been documented as early as 1500 BC in a Sanskrit document worshiping the Indian god of the sun (72). In the late 1800s the first attempts were made to artificially produce ultraviolet rays. In 1903 a Nobel prize was awarded to Niels Finsen for successful treatment of skin tuberculosis with ultraviolet light. Its effectiveness in prevention and treatment of rickets has also been known for years. Claims were made that ultraviolet light could treat an incredible array of conditions, many of which were characterized by pain. It was unclear, however, whether the noted beneficial effects were due to emitted heat or light. The next major breakthrough in the use of therapeutic light occurred in 1916 when Albert Einstein developed the concept of the laser, although it was not until 1960 that the first laser was produced (72).

ULTRAVIOLET LIGHT

The use of ultraviolet light has been declining considerable, so that its application in modern medicine is very limited. Its main current indications rest in the field of dermatology and pediatrics, while its therapeutic use in patients with chronic pain is rare and its efficacy has not been scientifically proven.

LASER

Contrary to ultraviolet light, laser treatment has been gaining in popularity in the treatment of many conditions characterized by acute or chronic pain. Laser is an acronym for *light amplification by stimulated emission of radiation*. It has three unique physical properties (73):

1. Monochromaticity
2. Coherence
3. Lack of divergence

When laser beams come in contact with biologic tissue, reflection, absorption, and dispersion occur. The percentage of radiation that is absorbed, reflected, or dispersed varies according to tissue properties as well as wavelengths, energy, and exposure time to laser beams. Human skin, for example, absorbs 99% of emitted laser radiation.

There are two types of lasers used for therapeutic purposes: high-power ("hot") lasers and low-power ("cold") lasers. The difference between them is based on the optical energy of the device.

High-Power "Hot" Lasers

High-power lasers are the laser systems whose therapeutic effects are not based on the properties of light (72, 73). Once absorbed, light energy is transformed into heat, and, depending upon its energy, reversible or irreversible tissue changes will occur.

The major clinical use of these lasers is in surgery and in the treatment of retinopathy.

Low-Power "Cold" Lasers

Low-power laser systems do not produce any irreversible tissue damage, and the mechanism of their action is not based on conversion of the light energy to heat. Numerous studies have been done in the last 10–15 years using cold lasers for treatment of various conditions. Their use for treatment of pain is rapidly gaining popularity, although the precise mechanism for their action is still unknown (72). Some of the proposed explanations that may have bearing on pain relief include:

1. Relief of arteriolar spasm.
2. Excitation of the mitochondrial membranes.
3. Enhanced activity of superoxide dismutase (SOD), which acts as a scavenger for superoxide radicals that, combined with arachidonic acid, produce prostaglandin E.
4. Enhanced levels of serum serotonin.

The most frequent indications for cold laser therapy include the following:

1. Reduction of pain associated with acute trauma to the tendons and ligaments.
2. Reduction of chronic pain due to various pathologic processes (e.g., osteoarthritis and rheumatoid arthritis).
3. Acceleration of wound healing by stimulating formation of granulation tissue.
4. Reduction of edema.
5. Peripheral nerve regeneration immediately following injury.

Depending upon the surface area that needs to be exposed to laser radiation as well as the nature of the underlying pathologic process, three different techniques of laser applications are available (72).

1. Grid Technique In the grid technique the laser probe is applied perpendicularly onto skin that is previously marked off into small squares, thus ensuring complete coverage of the treatment area. This technique is thought to be useful for local treatment of subcutaneous tissue when the superficial tissue is not involved.

2. Scanning Technique In the scanning technique the laser probe is held 1 cm above the area that is being treated and is moved in a wanding motion. This technique is of benefit when direct contact between the laser probe and the surface of the skin is not desired (e.g., necrotic ulcers, burned tissue).

3. Point Stimulation Technique The point stimulation method of laser application is also known as laser acupuncture. The probe is again in direct contact with the skin, but is angled, so that laser energy may be aimed in various directions. This technique is thought to be of benefit in treating small joints and myofascial pain syndrome (74).

Despite the fact that laser utilization in the management of chronic pain is increasing, convincing scientific evidence for its efficacy in this area is still lacking. So far, no known contraindications or serious side effects are recognized with the use of cold laser therapy. Precautions should be exercised when used in pregnancy and malignancy (72). In addition, care must be taken that patients and therapists do not stare directly into the beam because this may cause permanent retinal changes (72).

HYDROTHERAPY

Hydrotherapy is a treatment modality in which the body, or part of it, is immersed in water. The water is usually heated, and often agitated; the therapeutic effects are the result of a combination of superficial heating, massage-like action, counterirritant phenomena, and buoyancy. Buoyant effects allow weight-bearing loads to be greatly diminished, as well as being comforting and relaxing. For these reasons, hydrotherapy is most commonly used in patients with chronic pain due to arthritis.

The hydrotherapy devices most commonly found in medical settings are therapeutic pools, Hubbard tanks, and whirlpools. The former two are used when the whole body is to be immersed, the latter when only an arm or a leg is to be treated. Hubbard tanks allow the immersion of the whole body when supine, and are used either when a pool is not available, or when hydrotherapy is being used for indications such as cleaning burn wounds, where the risk of crossinfection is significant.

There are few precautions to the use of hydrotherapy. Patients with heart failure may not tolerate being in a heated therapeutic pool because core heating may occur, thus increasing circulatory demand and exacerbating failure.

BIOFEEDBACK

Biofeedback, the use of a device to inform the patient about some unconscious bodily function, has become popular for a variety of conditions, but particularly in chronic pain.

Electromyographic (EMG) biofeedback is used in the treatment of tension headaches, where chronic muscle contracton is thought to be causing pain (75, 76). The device used is a small electromyographic machine, which records EMG signals from surface electrodes taped over the frontalis muscle, and displays these signals as an audio signal, a visual signal on a meter, or both. The threshold for the device to signal can be preset, so that a greater or lesser amount of relaxation is required before the output ceases. This device allows the patient to become aware of the degree of muscle contraction, and the patient can then see, or hear, the results of attempts to achieve muscle relaxation.

The patient is instructed to use a variety of strategies to decrease the machine's output, such as thoughts of pleasant experiences or sensations. When a successful strategy has been found the patient can then be instructed to carry over that same technique even when not hooked up to the biofeedback device, to achieve muscle relaxation and thus pain relief.

Thermal biofeedback is used in the treatment of migraine headache. One factor believed to be playing a role in the etiology of migraine is sympathetic overactivity. In thermal biofeedback hand temperature is monitored and displayed. The patient is instructed, using strategies similar to those in EMG biofeedback, to increase hand temperature. Success is thought to be due to a reduction in sympathetic tone and will result in a decreased frequency of migraine headache (77).

It has been difficult to document the efficacy of biofeedback because of variations in study designs. Nevertheless, it appears that EMG or thermal biofeedback may decrease headache activity by 20% in the majority of patients treated with tension or migraine headaches, respectively (78). These figures are comparable to the results of relaxation exercises.

ORTHOTICS AND ASSISTIVE DEVICES

Orthotics, and related devices, are applied to the body or used in order to:

1. Compensate for inadequate structures
2. Restore normal alignment
3. Provide weight-bearing relief
4. Limit movement

Orthotic devices are used in situations in which any of the above will provide pain relief.

CERVICAL ORTHOSES

Neck collars and braces are frequently used in acutely painful neck conditions, but often their use is continued long past the time when the acute injury has resolved, and the patient has had a painful neck for months or years. There are a whole host of neck braces, ranging from cervical ruffs through soft foam collars to more rigid, plastic devices. The usual rationale behind their use is that they limit neck movement, or relieve weight-bearing stresses through the neck, thus putting neck structures at rest—both of which will relieve pain. These assumptions are, by and large, not true.

The majority of neck orthoses do not significantly restrict neck mobility, and do not afford any degree of stability to the cervical spine. The exception is a halo vest apparatus (79, 80). At best, these devices serve to remind the patient not to move his/her neck to extremes of range (81). Similarly, if no significant restriction of movement can occur, then no significant degree of weight-bearing relief can be provided by these devices.

Although many patients may feel better wearing neck orthoses, the devices are not providing the function that the prescriber and wearer usually think that they do. Other than serving as a reminder and perhaps providing a psychological benefit, there usually is no logical rationale in their use, particularly in patients with chronic pain.

LUMBOSACRAL ORTHOSES

When used in patients with chronic pain, where the goal is pain relief, these devices usually incorporate a corset component as well as some degree of rigidity to prevent movement. None will passively hold the patient in position. The corset component is designed to increase intra-abdominal pressure, thus allowing the abdomen to take more weight-bearing loads, subsequently unloading the lumbar spine (82). The theory is the same as teaching abdominal strengthening exercises—in one situation the muscle does the work and in the other, the corset.

Increasing degrees of rigidity may be built into the orthosis depending on how much "stabilization" is desired (83). It is likely that none of these devices does much more than reminding the patient about his/her position and to avoid extremes of movement (81). If the patient assumes an undesirable posture, or attempts an undesired movement, the orthosis will cause pressure at a contact site, causing pain and leading the patient to resume the desired posture by actively moving away from the painful contact site.

KNEE ORTHOSES

There are a number of orthoses designed to substitute for lax or lacking ligamentous structures around the knee. In situations in which knee instability contributes to pain, such orthoses will increase knee stability, and allow a greater pain-free level of function. The most common examples are braces designed to compensate for anterior cruciate or collateral ligament deficiency.

FOOT ORTHOSES

Foot orthoses are prescribed for a variety of conditions, including painful feet and knee pain. One major group is designed to correct dynamic postural abnormalities in the foot—usually excessive pronation. Such an abnormal alignment may be placing abnormal stresses on the foot, causing metatarsalgia or plantar fasciitis as well as an increased valgus stress about the knee that may aggravate pain due to lateral compartment osteoarthritis or patellofemoral syndrome. A medial longitudinal arch support will passively prevent pronation in a flexible flat foot, and may decrease the pain in these situations.

WRIST ORTHOSES

Patients with chronic painful arthritis of their wrists may benefit from wrist splints, which will help to stabilize their wrist joint while doing activities. If instability is contributing to their pain, most will experience less pain. Similar devices can be fabricated to stabilize the carpometacarpal joint of the thumb, with the same goal (84).

ASSISTIVE DEVICES

In patients with chronic pain, assistive devices may be used. The usual goals are either relief of weight bearing in the lower extremities, where bearing weight contributes to pain, or to allow the patient to perform a functional activity without pain.

Canes or crutches are commonly used in arthritis of knees or hips. The actual type and number of aids is determined by the patient's needs. If only one cane is to be used, it should be used in the hand opposite to the painful joint, because this allows a more normal gait pattern, less energy expenditure, and better weight-bearing relief (85).

The second group of devices are usually used in patients with chronic pain due to arthritis. Two common examples are a long-handled reacher that will allow the patient to pick something up from the floor without bending down to get it and large-handled kitchen utensils, which may be of benefit to patients with arthritic hands. Less grip is required to use these, and therefore less force will cross the joints (86).

SUMMARY

There are many physical modalities available to choose from. Each has its own indications, expected benefit, and contraindications. The choice of the modality is determined by the patient's clinical situation, and by the goals desired. In general, these goals can be divided into symptomatic pain relief, correction of underlying problems that are contributing to pain, and maintenance or restoration of function.

Modalities should be used selectively and intelligently. The same thought and care should be applied to their prescription as is given to medications and operations.

The use of any physical agent in chronic pain should be considered a part of the overall management of the patient, and used in conjunction with other appropriate interventions. Physical modalities are not a panacea, and their indiscriminate use will not be of benefit to the patient with chronic pain.

References

1. Lota MJ, Darling RC: Change in permeability of the red cell membrane in a homogeneous ultrasound field. *Arch Phys Med Rehabil* 36:282–287, 1955.
2. Castor CW, Yaron M: Connective tissue activation: VIII. The effects of temperature studied in vitro. *Arch Phys Med Rehabil* 57:5–9, 1976.
3. Abramson DI, Kahn A, Tuck S Jr, Turman GP, Rejal H, Fleischer CJ, et al: Relationship between a range of tissue temperature and local oxygen uptake in the human forearm. 1. Changes observed under resting conditions. *J Clin Invest* 37:1031–1038, 1958.
4. Lehmann JF, DeLateur BJ: Therapeutic heat. In Lehmann JF (ed): *Therapeutic Heat and Cold*, ed 3. Baltimore, Williams & Wilkins, 1982, pp 404–562.
5. Mense F: Effects of temperature on the discharges of muscle spindles and tendon organs. *Pflugers Arch* 374:159–166, 1978.
6. Ganong WF: *Review of Medical Physiology*, ed 10. Los Altos, CA, Lange Medical Publications, 1981, pp 466–475.
7. Hunter J, Kerr EH, Whillans MG: The relation between joint stiffness upon exposure to cold and the characteristics of synovial fluid. *Can J Med Sci* 30:367–377, 1952.
8. Wright V, Johns RJ: Physical factors concerned with the stiffness of normal and diseased joints. *Bull Johns Hopkins Hosp* 106:215–231, 1960.
9. Lehmann JF, Masock AJ, Warren CG, Koblanski JN, et al: Effect of therapeutic temperatures on tendon extensibility. *Arch Phys Med Rehabil* 51:481–487, 1970.
10. Lehmann JF, Brunner GD, Stow RW: Pain threshold measurements after therapeutic application of ultrasound, microwaves and infrared. *Arch Phys Med Rehabil* 39:560–565, 1958.
11. Fischer E, Solomon S: Physiological responses to heat and cold. In Licht S (ed): *Therapeutic Heat and Cold*, ed 2. Baltimore, Williams & Wilkins, 1965, pp 126–169.

12. Melzack R, Wall PD: Pain mechanisms: a new theory. *Science* 150:971–979, 1965.
13. Lehmann JF, Stonebridge JB, DeLateur BJ, Warren CG, Halar E: Temperature distributions in the human thigh, produced by infrared hot pack and microwave applications. *Arch Phys Med Rehabil* 47:291–299, 1966.
14. Abramson DI, Tuck S Jr, Chu LSW, Agustin C: Effect of paraffin bath and hot fomentations on local tissue temperatures. *Arch Phys Med Rehabil* 45:87–94, 1964.
15. Lehmann JF: Diathermy. In Krusen FH, Kottke FJ, Ellwood AM Jr (eds): *Handbook of Physical Medicine and Rehabilitation*, ed 2. Philadelphia, WB Saunders, 1971, pp 273–345.
16. Lehmann JF, Guy AW, Johnston VC, Brunner GD, Bell JW: Comparison of relative heating patterns produced in tissues by exposure to microwave energy at frequencies of 2450 and 900 megacycles. *Arch Phys Med Rehabil* 43:69–76, 1962.
17. Lehmann JF, Guy AW, Warren CG, DeLateur BJ, Stonebridge JB: Evaluation of microwave contact applicator. *Arch Phys Med Rehabil* 51:143–147, 1970.
18. Horvath SM, Hollander JL: Intraarticular temperature as a measure of joint reaction. *J Clin Invest* 28:469–473, 1949.
19. Lehmann JF, McMillan JA, Brunner GD, Blumberg JB: Comparative study of the efficiency of shortwave, microwave and ultrasonic diathermy in heating the hip joint. *Arch Phys Med Rehabil* 40:510–512, 1959.
20. Flax HJ: Ultrasound treatment of peritendinitis calcarea of the shoulder. *Am J Phys Med* 43:117–124, 1964.
21. Lehman JF, Lane CE, Bell JW, Brunner GD: Influence of surgical metal implants on the distribution of the intensity in the ultrasonic field. *Arch Phys Med Rehabil* 39:756–760, 1958.
22. Lehmann JF, DeLateur BJ: Cryotherapy. In Lehmann JF (ed): *Therapeutic Heat and Cold*, ed 3. Baltimore, Williams & Wilkins, 1982, pp 563–602.
23. Perkins JF, Li M-C, Hoffman F, et al: Sudden vasoconstriction in denervated or sympathectomized paws exposed to cold. *Am J Physiol* 155:165–178, 1948.
24. Lippold OCJ, Nicholls JG, Redfearn JWT: A study of the afferent discharge produced by cooling a mammalian muscle spindle. *J Physiol* 153:218–231, 1960.
25. Coppin EG, Livingstone SA, Kuehn LA: Effects on handgrip strength due to arm immersion in a 10°C water bath. *Aviat Space Environ Med* 49:1322–1326, 1978.
26. Goodgold J, Eberstein A: *Electrodiagnosis of Neuromuscular Diseases*, ed 3. Baltimore, Williams & Wilkins, 1981.
27. Hartvikson K: Ice therapy for spasticity. *Acta Neurol Scand* 38(suppl 3):79–84, 1962.
28. Doleys DM, Crocker M, Patton O: Response of patients with chronic pain to exercise quotas. *Phys Ther* 62:111–114, 1982.
29. Fordyce WE: Behavior concepts in chronic pain and illness. In Davidson PO (ed): *The Behavioral Management of Anxiety, Depression and Pain*. New York, Brunner/Mazel, 1976, pp 147–188.
30. Amundson LR: Rehabilitation exercises for stage II and stage III of the cardiac rehabilitation program. In Amundson LR (ed): *Cardiac Rehabilitation*. New York: Churchill Livingstone, 1981, pp 141–142.
31. Insall J: Current concepts review: patellar pain. *J Bone Joint Surg* 64A:147–152, 1982.
32. DeLateur BJ: Therapeutic exercise to develop strength and endurance. In Kottke FJ, Stillwell GK, Lehmann JF (eds): *Kruson's Handbook of Physical Medicine and Rehabilitation*, ed 3. Philadelphia, WB Saunders, 1982, pp 427–464.
33. Schram DA: Resistance exercise. In Basmajian JV (ed): *Therapeutic Exercise*, ed 4. Baltimore, Williams & Wilkins, 1984, pp 225–235.
34. Basmajian JV (ed): *Therapeutic Exercise*, ed 4. Baltimore, Williams & Wilkins, 1984.
35. Ekroth R, Dahlof AG, Gundevall B, et al: Physical training of patients with intermittent claudication: indications, methods and results. *Surgery* 84:640–643, 1978.
36. *EMG J33 Handbook*. Boston, Cyborg Corporation, 1977.
37. Basmajian JV (ed): *Manipulation, Traction and Massage*, ed 3. Baltimore, Williams & Wilkins, 1985.
38. Crisp EJ: Discussion on the treatment of backache by traction. *Proc R Soc Med (Sec Phys Med)* 48:805, 1955.
39. Swezey RL: The modern thrust of manipulation and traction therapy. *Sem Arthritis Rheum* 12(3):322–333, 1983.
40. Yates DAH: Indications and contraindications for spinal traction. *Physiotherapy* 54:55, 1972.
41. DeLateur BJ: The role of physical medicine in problems of pain. *Adv Neurol* 4:495–497, 1974.
42. Halstead LS, Grabois M: Physical modalities of treatment. In Halstead LS, Grabois M (eds): *Medical Rehabilitation*. New York, Raven Press, 1985.
43. Waylonis GW, Tootle D, Denhart C, Pope Gratton MM, Wapenski JA: Home cervical traction: evaluation of alternate equipment. *Arch Phys Med Rehabil* 63:388–391, 1982.
44. Reilly JP, Gertsten JW, Clinkingbeard JR: Effect of pelvic-femoral position on vertebral separation produced by lumbar traction. *Phys Ther* 59(3):282–286, 1979.
45. Wakim KG: Influence of centripetal rhythmic compression in localized edema of an extremity. *Arch Phys Med Rehabil* 36:98, 1955.
46. Mennell JB: *Physical Treatment by Movement, Massage and Manipulation*, ed 5. Philadelphia, WB Saunders, 1941.
47. Sjöelund B, Terenius L, Eriksson M: Increased cerebrospinal fluid levels of endorphins after electroacupuncture. *Acta Physiol Scand* 100:382–384, 1977.
48. Alexander MA, Wright ES, Wright JB: Lymphedema treatment with a linear pump: pediatric case report. *Arch Phys Med Rehabil* 64:132, 1983.
49. Pflug JJ, Melrose DG: Prevention of thromboembolic disease in surgery. *Vasa* 5:63, 1976.
50. Tracy TM: Hydrotherapy. *J Bone Joint Surg* 52A:180, 1970.
51. Zusman M: Spinal manipulative therapy: review of some proposed mechanisms and a new hypothesis. *Aust J Physiother* 32(2):89–99, 1986.
52. Mennell J: *Back Pain. Diagnosis and Treatment Using Manipulative Technique*. Boston, Little, Brown & Co, 1960.
53. Mennell J: *Joint Pain. Diagnosis and Treatment Using Manipulative Technique*. Boston, Little, Brown & Co, 1964.
54. Maigne R: The concept of painlessness and opposite motion in spinal manipulation. *Am J Phys Med* 44:55, 1965.
55. Greenmann PE: Manipulative therapy in relation to total health care. In Korr J (ed): *The Neurologic Mechanisms in Manipulative Therapy*. London, Plenum Press, 1978.
56. Ford RF, Clark D: Thrombosis of the basilar artery with softenings in the cerebellum and brainstem due to manipulation of the neck. *Bull John Hopkins Hosp* 98:37, 1965.
57. Pratt-Thomas HR, Berger KE: Cerebellar and spinal injuries after chiropractic manipulation. *JAMA* 133:600, 1947.
58. Schwartz GA, Geiger JK, Sapiro AV: Posterior inferior cerebellar artery syndrome of Wallenberg after chiropractic manipulation. *Arch Intern Med* 3:352, 1956.

59. Di Fabio RP: Clinical assessments of manipulation and mobilization of the lumbar spine. *Phys Ther* 66(1):51–54, 1986.
60. Godfrey CM, Morgan PP, Schatzker J: A randomized trial of manipulation for low back pain in a medical setting. *Spine* 9:301–304, 1984.
61. Gersh MR, Wolf SL: Applications of transcutaneous electrical nerve stimulation in the management of patients with pain. *Phys Ther* 65(3):314–322, 1985.
62. Bowsher D: Role of the reticular formation in responses to noxious stimulation. *Pain* 2:361–378, 1976.
63. Mayer DJ, Price DD: Central nervous system mechanisms of analgesia. *Pain* 2:379–404, 1976.
64. Stratton SA: Role of endorphins in pain modulation. *J Orthop Sports Phys Ther* 3:200–205, 1982.
65. Sjöelund BM, Eriksson MB: The influence of naloxone on analgesia produced by peripheral conditioning stimulation. *Brain Res* 173:295–301, 1979.
66. Sjöelund MB, Eriksson MB: Endorphins and analgesia produced by peripheral conditioning stimulation. In *Advances in Pain Research and Therapy*. New York, Raven Press, 1979, vol 3, pp 587–592.
67. Vonkuorring L, Almay BL, Johannson F: Pain perception and endorphin levels in cerebrospinal fluid. *Pain* 5:359–365, 1978.
68. Cambell JN, Taub A: Local analgesia from percutaneous electrical stimulation: a peripheral mechanism. *Arch Neurol* 28:347–350, 1973.
69. Barr JO, Nielsen DN, Soderberg G: Transcutaneous electrical nerve stimulation characteristics for altering pain perception. *Phys Ther* 66(10):1515–1521, 1986.
70. Hughes GS, Lichstein PR, Whitlock D, et al: Response of plasma beta-endorphins to transcutaneous electrical nerve stimulation in healthy subjects. *Phys Ther* 64(7):1062–1066, 1984.
71. Ersek RA: Transcutaneous electrical neurostimulation. *Clin Orthop Rel Res* 128:314–324, 1977.
72. Stillwell GK: *Therapeutic Electricity and Ultraviolet Radiation*, ed 3. Baltimore, Williams & Wilkins, 1983.
73. Kleinhort JA, Foley RA: Laser acupuncture. *Am J Acupunct* 12(1):51–56, 1984.
74. Goldman JA, Chiapella J, Casey H, et al: Laser therapy of rheumatoid arthritis. *Lasers Surg Med* 1:93–101, 1980.
75. Peck CL, Kraft SM: Electromyographic biofeedback for pain related to muscle tension: a study of tension headache, back and jaw pain. *Arch Surg* 112:889–895, 1977.
76. Philips C: The modification of tension headache pain using EMG biofeedback. *Behav Res Ther* 15:119–129, 1977.
77. Sovak M, Kunzel M, Sternbach RA, Dalessio AJ: Mechanism of the biofeedback therapy of migraine: volitional manipulation of the psychophysiological background. *Headache* 29:89–92, 1981.
78. Health and Public Policy Committee, American College of Physicians: Biofeedback for headaches. *Ann Intern Med* 102:128–131, 1985.
79. Colachis SC Jr, Strohm BR, Ganter EL: Cervical spine motion in normal women: radiographic study of effect of cervical collars. *Arch Phys Med Rehabil* 54:161–169, 1973.
80. Johnson RM, Hart DL, Simmons EF, Ramsby GR, Southwick WO: Cervical orthoses: a study comparing their effectiveness in restricting cervical motion in normal subjects. *J Bone Joint Surg* 59A:332–339, 1977.
81. Fisher SV: Spinal orthotics. In Kottke FJ, Stillwell GK, Lehmann JF (eds): *Kruson's Handbook of Physical Medicine and Rehabilitation*, ed 3. Philadelphia, WB Saunders, 1982, pp 530–538.
82. Morris JM, Lucas DB, Bresler B: The role of the trunk in the stability of the spine. *J Bone Joint Surg* 43A:327, 1961.
83. Norton PL, Brown T: The immobilizing efficiency of back braces. *J Bone Joint Surg* 39A:111–138, 1957.
84. Malaick MM: Functional restoration—upper extremity orthotics. In Hopkins HL, Smith HD (eds): *Willard and Spackmans Occupational Therapy*, ed 6. Philadelphia, JB Lippincott, 1983, pp 453–460.
85. Edwards BG: Contralateral and ipsilateral cane usage by patients with total knee or hip replacement. *Arch Phys Med Rehabil* 67:734–740, 1980.
86. May EE, Waggoner NR, Boettke EM: *Homemaking for the Handicapped*. New York, Dodd, Mead and Co, 1966.

chapter 14
Spinal Manipulation and the Reduction of Pain

Jerry C. Langley, D.C.

Throughout history, spinal manipulation has been one of the most maligned and controversial modes of treatment for the reduction of back pain. Much of the controversy revolves around the lack of scientific data to demonstrate the efficacy of manipulative therapy. Ultimately, even the results of clinical trials have been overshadowed by the possibility that results occurred by chance due to spontaneous remission or other phenomena.

Confusion and disagreement surround even the basic definition of manipulation. In recent years, spinal manipulation has been broadly defined. Many times the definition has included all procedures in which the hands are utilized to massage, mobilize, adjust, or manipulate the osseous structures of the body and the surrounding tissue. This broad concept has evolved because most competent manipulators utilize extensive myofascial and soft tissue techniques along with manipulation in the reduction and control of pain syndromes. Further, many authors have construed the terms *manipulation* and *mobilization* to be synonymous, yet there is a distinct difference between the two. Cassidy et al. (1) have provided a very good understanding of this difference. Mobilization involves taking the joint to its limit of passive range of motion, whereas manipulation goes beyond the passive range of motion into the paraphysiologic zone. Of course, extension beyond the paraphysiologic zone induces damage to the articular ligaments.

Further difference of opinion has evolved as a result of the terminology used to describe the primary manipulative lesion. Chiropractic subluxation has been described by Schafer as the alteration of normal dynamic, anatomic, and physiologic relationships of continuous articular structures (2). Schafer indicated that the subluxation is always attended to some degree by articular dysfunction, neurologic insult, and stressed muscles, tendons, and ligaments. Once produced, the lesion becomes a focus of sustained pathologic irritation; a barrage of impulses stream into the spinal cord where internuncial neurons receive and relay the impulses to the motor pathways. The subluxation and joint irritation is thereby reinforced, thus perpetuating both the subluxation and the pathologic process engendered.

Neumann (3) referred to the somatic dysfunction as being a disturbance of any one of the components of an interrelated system, that is, joints, intervertebral disks, muscles, or the nervous system. Johnston (4) cites three cardinal signs of a musculoskeletal dysfunction (which is often referred to as a biomechanical fault). The first sign is palpable muscle tension; second, there is structural or positional irregularity, and finally, there is almost always altered mobility. Other authors use the terms *fixation*, or *blockage*, as well as other broadly described alterations of the spine, to represent a primary manipulatable lesion.

In any of the above-mentioned cases, it is readily accepted that the patient has lost clinical stability of the spine. White and Panjabi (5) have defined clinical stability as the ability of the spine to prevent initial or additional neurologic damage, intractible pain, or gross deformity. With this definition of clinical stability in mind, the primary manipulatable lesion would include not only positional or postural changes but also any aberrant or restricted motion of the spinal segments. The functional characteristics of this lesion would include, of course, the muscle and soft tissue changes. Other factors that have yet to be established by formal research are the neurogenic and nerve compression abnormalities.

PAIN TOLERANCE

Manipulation can be effective in producing relief in low back pain, neck pain, and headaches. Although scientific data have produced evidence of pain relief and manipulators have claimed clinical success, the exact pathway of pain relief is still unknown. Wyke (6) believes that the impact of spinal joint receptor afferentation is a potential component of this pain modulation. Denslow and Hassett (7) and Korr (8) projected the role of muscle spindle afferents in both sustaining and abolishing segmental central fasciculation. These authors believed that spinal manipulation produced short-term bursts of proprioceptive sensory bombardment that could produce secondary effects such as gamma-afferent inhibition and inhibition of the pain pathways. This bombardment would occur as a result of instantaneous stretch of the articular and myofascial receptors as their elastic barriers were exceeded in manipulation. Glover (9) found zones of hyperesthesia lateral to the facet joints at painful segments that he believed were due to fasciculation of cutaneous pain reflexes by nociceptive impulses from the joint receptors. He further found these zones to disappear following rotational manipulation along the involved segment.

Terret and Howard (10) found that a statistically significant elevation of pain tolerance (140%) occurred after manipulation as compared to a control group. These authors concluded that the local paraspinal pain tolerance increased following manipulation. Korr's (8) model of spinal fixation focused on the muscle spindle as the coordinator that may increase or decrease muscle contraction according to the direction of motion of the joint. The reflex muscle contraction can then produce joint motion by this action or prevent joint motion in the area of spinal fixation. Korr proposed two mechanisms whereby manipulation would be successful in reducing pain associated with spinal fixation. First, stretch of the fibers and muscle against its spindle maintained resistance, which would produce a barrage of afferent impulses of sufficient intensity to signal the central nervous system to reduce the gamma motor neuron discharge (muscle contraction). Second, the Golgi tendon organs could be stimulated by manipulation and forced stretch of the skeletal muscles, causing gamma motor neuron inhibition.

GENERAL SPINAL BIOMECHANICS

Even though there is disagreement on the exact mechanism of how spinal manipulative therapy relieves pain, there are specific biomechanical changes along the spine that demonstrate clinical characteristics of a spinal manipulative lesion. Hildebrandt and Howe (11) have listed the following biomechanical changes in accordance with the static and kinetic aspects of the involved vertebral motor units.

Static Vertebral Motor Distortions

1. *Flexion Subluxation* When viewed laterally, the flexion subluxation is characterized by a closing of the vertebral bodies at the anterior and a separation of the vertebral bodies, facets, and spinous process at the posterior. This type of malpositioning may force a posterior bulging of the anular fibers with excursion of the nucleus. There is likely to be stretching of the posterior longitudinal, interspinal, and supraspinal ligaments, along with shearing stress to the synovia of the facets.

2. *Extension Subluxation* When viewed laterally, the extension subluxation is characterized by a separation of the vertebral bodies at the anterior and a closing of the vertebral bodies, facets, and spinous processes at the posterior. This type of distortion may force a bulging of the anulus to the anterior with excursion of the nucleus. There is likely to be stretching of the anterior longitudinal ligament and imbrication or overlapping of the facet articulations with stress to the synovia of the facet articulations.

3. *Lateral Flexion Subluxation* On the anterior to posterior view, the lateral flexion subluxation is characterized by closing of the vertebral bodies and facets on the side of flexion and separation of vertebral bodies and facets on the side of extension. This spinal distortion may indicate imbrication or overlapping of the facets and stress to the synovia of the facets on the side of flexion, with possible bulging of the anulus with excursion of the nucleus toward the side of extension. There may also be stretching of the anterior longitudinal ligament at the lateral aspect on the side of extension.

4. *Rotational Subluxation* On the anterior to posterior view, this subluxation is characterized by rotational displacement of the vertebral bodies laterally and posteriorly on the side of rotation with torsion of the facet articulations in the opposite direction of vertebral body rotation. This distortion is indicative of possible torsion binding of the anulus, decreased resiliency of the intervertebral disk as a result of torsion compression of the anular fibers, and torsion stretching of the anterior and posterior longitudinal ligaments, with rotational overlapping of the facets with reverse shearing stress to the synovia of the facets.

5. *Anterolisthesis Subluxation without Spondylolysis* This spinal distortion is characterized by anteroinferior excursion of the vertebral body at the anterior and by anterosuperior excursion of the vertebral body and facets at the posterior. This distortion may produce forward shearing stress to the anulus and stretching of the anterior and posterior longitudinal ligaments, with overlapping of the facets with forward shearing stress to the synovia of the facets.

6. Anterolisthesis Subluxation with Spondylolysis This spinal distortion is characterized by anterior excursion of the vertebral body, independent of the posterior division of the motor unit, as a result of a separation of the pars. There may be bulging of the anulus with forced excursion of the nucleus pulposus and forward shearing stress to the anular fibers. There may also be stretching of the anterior longitudinal ligaments.

7. Retrolisthesis Subluxation This distortion is characterized by posteroinferior excursion of the vertebral body and facets. With the retrolisthesis, there may be posterior shearing along the anulus with stretching of the anterior and posterior longitudinal ligaments. There may be further overlapping of the facets with posterior stress to the synovia.

8. Laterolisthesis Subluxation This distortion is characterized by lateral, superior, and posterior excursion of the vertebral body on the side of deviation and separation of the facet on the side of deviation with reverse torsion and closing on the side opposite the deviation. Along with this distortion, there may be lateral and posterior shearing stress to the anulus on the side of the deviation and overlapping of the facets with anterior shearing of the synovia of the facets on the side opposite the deviation.

9. Decreased Interosseous Space Subluxation This classification is characterized by narrowing of the intervertebral disk space with narrowing of the vertical intervertebral foramen space and inferior excursion of the facets. There may be traumatic compression of the intervertebral disk with possible herniation of the nucleus through an end plate and an overlapping of the facets with compression shearing to the synovia. There may be further compression of the contents of the intervertebral foramen.

10. Increased Interosseous Space Subluxation This distortion is characterized by superior excursion of the vertebral body and facets. This may be indicative of inflammatory swelling or pathologic enlargement of the intervertebral disk with traction shearing to the anulus and the synovia of the facet articulations. There may also be stretching of the anterior and posterior longitudinal ligaments.

11. Foraminal Encroachment Subluxation This distortion is characterized by findings of possible osteophytic changes along the intervertebral foramen. These changes may produce compression, irritation, and swelling of the foraminal contents with degenerative changes along the vertebral motor unit.

12. Costovertebral-Costotransverse Subluxation In this type of distortion, there is misalignment of the costal processes in relationship to the vertebral bodies and transverse processes independent of vertebral motion; or misalignment of the costal processes in relationship to the vertebral bodies and transverse processes as a result of vertebral subluxation.

13. Sacroiliac Subluxation This distortion is characterized by misalignment of the sacrum in relationship to the ilei. These distortions classically produce biomechanical improprieties of the pelvis.

Kinetic Vertebral Motion Unit Subluxations

1. Hypomobility or Fixation This type of dysfunction is characterized by fixation of vertebral motion in relationship to the supporting structures below. With this classification, there may be stretching along the anterior and posterior longitudinal ligament and spasticity along the muscles of the involved segment, with possible neurologic involvement of both the neural canal and intervertebral foramen.

2. Hypermobility This dysfunction is characterized by an increase in the vertebral motion along the motor unit in relation to the normally functioning unit below. Hypermobility produces increased stress to the anterior and posterior longitudinal ligaments with muscular spasticity and possible neurologic insult to the confines of the neural canal and intervertebral foramen.

3. Aberrant Movement Subluxation This type of distortion is characterized by movement of a vertebra out of the normal phase with the segment above and below the involved unit. This classification may produce occlusion to the intervertebral foramens above and below the aberrant segment and may also produce shearing stress to the intervertebral disk and synovia of the facets along the involved area.

It is important to note that with the above-mentioned classifications there is alteration in the normal vertebral motion. There are at least two reports in which increased vertebral movement following manipulation of the cervical spine has been noted on pre- and postmanipulation x-rays (12, 13).

Commonly, a major criterion for manipulation by many clinicians has become the restriction, fixation, and/or blockage of motion at specific joints of the spine (14). The location and characteristics of the fixation must be determined before manipulation can be given. Motion-palpation of various joints of the spine is an invaluable tool for selecting the site of manipulation as well as the type of procedure to be utilized.

In the hands of a skilled clinician, manipulation is both a safe and an effective alternative for the correction of many musculoskeletal dysfunctions. However, as with any critical procedure (e.g., surgery, medication) manipulation can have harmful effects if it is incorrectly performed or utilized for the wrong reasons. Thorough digital examination of the spinal column is important to the evaluation of the joint dysfunction. Static palpation, however, will determine only the probable locations of the subluxation by the variations in muscular tone, texture, and sensitivity. The clinician must understand that there are several types of joint motion. These motions are described as gliding and angular, flexion, extension, abduction, adduction, rotation, and circumduction. Thorough evaluation of these joint movements by motion palpation will allow the clinician to key in on even minor joint dysfunctions. Since manipulation is employed to attempt to return joints toward a more normal function, it is important for the clinician to fully understand the normal range of motion and the normal limits of the involved joint. Attempts to force a joint beyond its normal limits can be harmful to the integrity of the joint and its surrounding soft tissue structures.

Along with motion palpation, it is important to note the surrounding soft tissue tone. Muscle tissue near a joint dysfunction or subluxation will normally present a spastic condition with localized tenderness. Interestingly, muscle tissue near a subluxation is often active, as shown by electromyelography. Propping the patient in different positions with pillows often increases the electromyelographic activity but does not reduce the palpable firmness of the muscles. This indicates that the decreased tone is not necessarily due to muscle contraction from nociceptive input (15). It has been well established that irritation of the posterior joints and ligaments readily leads to reflex spasms of the erector spinae and other extensors (16). This muscle tone evaluation requires a precise knowledge and extensive practice in palpation. Also, since pain from nerve roots or pathways is referred toward the periphery, the entire nerve leading from the area should be explored. Tenderness, masses, temperature changes, and spasm along the areas of the nerve innervation can also give clues to joint dysfunction if the changes remain dermatomal.

During the examination phase, it is essential for the physician to perform numerous neurologic and orthopedic tests. These tests are significant in forming an opinion as to the type of technique to be employed, as well as detecting contraindications to manipulation. It is important to keep in mind that, along the cervical region, the brachial plexus is comprised of nerve roots from C5 through T1. Involvements along the nerves radiating from the brachial plexus can be examined through reflex changes, muscle weaknesses, and sensation along the areas of distribution of the nerves. Nerve root C5 is responsible for the biceps reflex and innervates the deltoid and biceps muscles. This nerve is responsible for sensations over the lateral arm, primarily along the deltoid area.

Nerve root C6 is primarily responsible for the brachioradialis reflex with contributory factors to the biceps reflex. It innervates the wrist extensors and the biceps muscle. Nerve root C6 is responsible for sensations over the lateral forearm and the thumb side of the hand.

Nerve root C7 is responsible for the triceps reflex. The nerve innervates the wrist flexor muscles, finger extensor muscles, and the triceps. Primary sensory innervation of nerve root C7 is to the middle finger.

Nerve root C8 demonstrates no reflex, but innervates the finger flexor muscles and the hand intrinsics. Sensory innervation is to the medial forearm.

Nerve root T1 has no reflex demonstration. The muscles innervated by T1 include the hand intrinsics, with sensory innervation over the medial arm.

In the lumbar spine, nerve root L4 produces the patellar reflex and innervates the anterior tibialis muscle. It is responsible for sensory innervation to the medial leg and medial foot.

Nerve root L5 has no reflex demonstration. The muscles innervated by L5 include the extensor hallucis longus, with sensory innervation to the lateral leg and dorsum of the foot.

The S1 nerve root is responsible for the Achilles reflex, with innervation to the peroneus longus and brevis muscles. Nerve root S1 gives sensory innervation to the lateral foot. It is important to note that with disk involvement in the lumbar spine, it is typical for the involved nerve to be compressed by the disk one segment below the site of origin.

INDICATIONS FOR MANIPULATION

The determining factor for final selection of the manipulatable patient is based upon the etiology of the primary pathology. Importance lies in determining possible contraindications for manipulation and/or identifying those patients whose conditions preclude manipulation as the primary treatment of choice. A comprehensive examination allows the clinician to clarify not only the nature, but also the extent, of the involved lesion. Differential diagnosis, while excluding some patients from the manipulative mode of treatment, also establishes a basis whereby the clinician is able to assess the progress of the patient and the success or failure of the applied treatment.

Difficulty in selecting the manipulatable patient is further complicated by the poor understanding of the pathogenesis of back pain. Although a breakdown into numerous differential diagnostic categories is possible, many manipulators have found varying results with patients diagnosed as having different symptoms complexes or specifically diagnosed origins of pain (17).

LOW BACK PAIN

A few of the proposed causes of low back pain that respond to spinal manipulative therapy are discussed below. These etiologies have been divided into two categories. Category I findings are definite indication for manipulation. With proper technique and application, excellent results can be expected. Common characteristics found in Category I are (a) absence of radiation of dermatomal pain, (b) little or no alteration in neurologic reflex findings, (c) joint dysfunction, and (d) asymmetric paravertebral muscle spasms. Category II, while responding to the proper application of spinal manipulation, exhibits successful results to a lesser degree.

Category I

1. Uncomplicated Back Pain Uncomplicated back pain is a nonspecific category. The patients in this category present a history of recent onset. There are no sensory changes along the dermatomal tract, with no radiation of pain to the extremities. Potter (16) has noted that patients with uncomplicated acute back pain have a high response rate, with 93% of such patients being fully recovered or much improved following manipulation. Hoehler et al. (18) have indicated that 84% of their manipulated patients experienced a reduction in the amount of pain following the first manipulation. Fisk (19) utilized manipulation to obtain complete recovery in 90% of patients suffering from acute low back pain syndrome. He found patients to have increased spinal mobility and increased straight leg raise ability following treatment.

Glover et al. (20) used rotational manipulation of the trunk to correct a syndrome that was defined as including back pain, skin hyperesthesia, tenderness, and limitation of the trunk in one or more directions of movement. Statistically significant improvement was seen after the first and only manipulation. The patient with uncomplicated back pain is more likely to receive significant relief following the first treatment, and the technique favors that of the long lever rotary manipulation.

2. Uncomplicated Chronic Low Back Pain Statistically, uncomplicated chronic lower back pain responds to a lesser degree than does acute lower back pain. Potter (16) indicated that 71% of patients classified as uncomplicated chronic low back pain sufferers in his study improved following treatment. By the very nature of the pathology, expectations for full recovery of the chronic back pain sufferer are poorer than with uncomplicated acute back pain. Furthermore, spontaneous recovery in this group is rarely seen.

3. Posterior Facet Syndrome The pain of the posterior facet joints begins along the midline of the lower back and may be referred to the buttock, thigh, or leg. The referred pain is nondermatomal. The patient may complain of a generalized achiness over the piriformis muscle. As with other category I–type pain syndromes, there is no major neurologic deficit. In the majority of cases, there are radiographic signs of reduced lumbar mobility or fixation.

Cassidy et al. (1) have divided the posterior facet syndrome into two divisions, the first being the fixed posterior joint syndrome and the second being the unstable posterior joint syndrome. With the fixed posterior joint syndrome, 62% of the patients receiving manipulation had favorable results, whereas only 26% of those patients with unstable posterior joint syndrome showed marked improvement.

4. Fixed Sacroiliac Syndrome The sacroiliac joint, which is an atypical synovial joint with limited range of motion, is susceptible to mechanical derangements. Pain with sacroiliac dysfunction may be local to the lateral aspect of the sacrum or referred to the buttock area. Many times, the patient will complain of symptoms that are relieved by rest and aggravated by activity. As is characteristic of all Category I–type pain syndromes, there is little or no alteration of neurologic reflexes. Jarring at the base of the spine causes sharp localized pain over the affected side. There may be either posterior or anterior torsional displacement.

With the posterior displacement, the patient will have a tendency to stand with the hip, knee, and lower back slightly flexed to the involved side. The posterior superior iliac spine and iliac crest will also be lower on the involved side. The pelvis will be shifted away from the involved side. However, if the patient stands with the leg straight, the posterior superior iliac spine and iliac crest will be lower on the involved side, but the anterior superior iliac spine will be higher. In this case, the pelvis will appear to be rotated forward on the involved side. With anterior torsional displacement of the sacroiliac joint, the patient will have a tendency to stand with the hip and knee in extension on the involved side. The pelvis will likely be shifted toward and inclined away from the involved side. The posterior superior iliac spine and crest of the ileum will be lower on the uninvolved side. If the patient is able to stand erect with anterior torsional displacement, the posterior superior iliac spine and the iliac crest will be higher on the involved side. Cassidy et al. (1) claimed that 71% of patients with fixed sacroiliac syndrome received marked improvement with manipulation of the joint.

5. Muscle Syndrome Manipulators have long recognized the importance of muscle syndrome in the genesis of back pain. Denslow and Hassett (7) studied contracted muscles in individuals shown to have postural abnormalities. Good postural alignment of the body consists of bony structures that are in optimal position for weight bearing to allow the weight of the trunk to be balanced, and further consists of muscles that are adequate in length and balanced in strength. When muscles become shortened, the range of motion in the opposite direction is limited and structural misalignment may be produced. This allows the opposite muscle to stretch and weaken.

Muscle groups of the lower extremities and lower spine are significant because they give foundation for proper postural alignment. Muscles of particular importance include the adductor muscles, which consist of the gracilis, adductor longus, adductor brevis, and adductor magnus muscles. Other muscles to consider are the gluteal, piriformis, psoas, quadriceps, and hamstring muscles. Muscles of importance that act in extension and rotation of the vertebral column include the multifidus and rotatory muscles. Specific manipulative techniques have been developed with the aim of stretching or manually massaging these muscles in an attempt to relax them (14).

Category II

1. Spondylolisthesis Spondylolisthesis should not be considered a contraindication to nontraumatic specific short lever manipulations. Cox (21) found that the presence of such abnormalities did not produce less favorable treatment results. He did, however, note that spondylolisthesis at L4 responded much slower and required more treatments than did L5 spondylolisthesis. Proper manipulative technique will ensure that direct force over the area of slippage is avoided. Manipulation should be directed to the sacroiliac joint or posterior joints above the level of slippage.

   2. **Stenosis** Narrowing of the spinal canal secondary to degenerative changes along the joint and/or disk produce multidermatomal and/or bilateral leg pain. The Achilles reflex may be absent after exercise and present when at rest. Patients may complain of listlessness at night and leg pain that worsens with excessive exercise. A study by Potter (16) found that 70% of patients with stenosis receiving manipulation showed some favorable results. Although very few patients become symptom free, it appears that skilled manipulation may provide at least temporary relief for patients with neurogenic claudication due to spinal stenosis.

   3. **Disk Involvement** Disk involvement many times produces an interesting dilemma for manipulators. The effect of spinal manipulation on degenerative disks is controversial. Some clinicians believe the primary effect of manipulation is the reduction of the nuclear protrusions of the disk (21, 22). Other authors, through clinical trials, have found results of manipulation in patients with disk protrusions on myelography to be much poorer than in patients with normal myelograms (23). These studies were unable to present any evidence of reduction in a positive myelogram finding following manipulation. It should be noted that in the event of frank herniation, competent manipulators exclude the use of rotary movement and use alternative methods such as intermittent distraction and/or reflux-type techniques, which are less traumatic to the disk.

Hirschberg (24) advocates conservative management in the treatment of patients suffering from symptoms of disk herniation. He stated that under favorable circumstances, the protruded portion of the nucleus shrinks by dehydration and the symptoms of the nerve root compression are relieved.

CERVICAL PAIN

Flexion, extension, rotation, lateral flexion, and circumduction are the basic movements of the cervical region (25). Mechanical restrictions may occur as a result of various underlying disorders.

Cervical Strain/Sprain Injuries

Treatment for mild or moderate strain/sprain injuries should include appropriate manipulation to assist in preventing residual joint dysfunction. However, manipulation is not the initial treatment of choice in severe strain/sprain injuries. These severe cases necessitate immobilization, along with physiotherapeutic remedial aid and rest. This regimen of treatment should be followed after several weeks with a series of manipulations to restore the joint function and integrity.

Torticollis

Torticollis can be divided into two types, viral myalgia and acute mechanical. There is little evidence that manipulation can be effective in viral myalgia torticollis; however, proper maneuvers can provide excellent results in acute mechanical torticollis. The manipulative technique used in this instance would be more of a stretching technique in a mild and methodic progressive manner. All maneuvers in this case should be done away from the side of pain.

Acute Cervical Pain

Acute cervical pain may be due to simple mechanical distortions, inflammatory processes, or intervertebral disk lesions. Although simple mechanical distortions respond excellently to manipulation, inflammatory processes and intervertebral disk lesions do not respond as favorably and should not receive harsh manipulation. Many distraction-type techniques with mild stretching and mild mobilization of the area may be effective. Oftentimes, stabilization of the cervical spine with a cervical collar following the treatment is essential.

Headaches of Cervical Origin

Many times headaches will originate in the cervical spine. Normally, these headaches will involve the occipital nerves, which radiate from the posterior branches of C2 and along the anterior branches of C3. Irritation along these nerves can be termed *occipital neuralgia* and may produce headaches along the posterior aspect of the skull, headaches at the base of the skull, and/or radiating pain toward the frontal area. Normally the clinician will find tenderness along the occipital area and at the level of C2 and C3 bilaterally with paravertebral muscle spasms. Many times these headaches will be characteristically associated with increased stress or tension. Quite frequently, proper manipulation will produce favorable results with these headaches in three to five treatments. Vernon (26) found evidence of significant decrease in frequency, duration, and severity of headaches in patients treated by chiropractic manipulation. It should further be noted that additional symptoms of vertigo, nausea, and tinnitus can be effectively treated with manipulation in many cases (27). However, because of the obvious contraindications that are associated with this syndrome, the diagnosis of mechanical malfunction along the cervical spine must be established prior to harsh manipulation.

Radicular Pains of Cervical Origin

Many times mechanical dysfunctions along the cervical spine will produce mild irritation along the brachial plexus that can produce brachial neuralgia. The pain from these dysfunctions can extend across the shoulder and present irritation to the supraspinous, infraspinous, and bicipital areas. These symptoms, which occur in the absence of frank herniation of disks along the cervical region, will readily respond to manipulation and reduce chronic irritation to the corresponding spinal nerves.

THORACIC PAIN
Acute Thoracic Pain

Thoracic pain may be the result of pain originating along the cervical spine and referred to the thoracic region. This occurrence is typical with a patient who has a cervical dysfunction at the level of C5 through C7. Referred pain will typically appear along T5 and T6. Trigger points will occur along the medial border of the scapulae and along the trapezius or the superior margins of the scapulae. These trigger points can be treated with pressure and can effectively be reduced with stretch techniques if there is absence of frank herniation.

Rib Pain

Painful thoracic conditions can be associated with dysfunctions along the costovertebral or costotransverse articulations. Microtraumas or faulty posture can many times initiate this pain. The patient may complain of intense pain along the thoracic region at the costovertebral joints and may further experience radiating pain along the rib cage toward the sternum. This pain is due to an intercostal neuritis and may present symptoms of intense chest pain. Quite frequently, these conditions have a dramatic and instantaneous resolution with proper manipulative care.

TYPES OF MANIPULATION

While researchers are continuing to underscore the positive ramifications of spinal manipulation, clinicians have developed numerous methods and techniques of treatment for musculoskeletal dysfunction. The primary distinguishing factor regarding manipulative methods is the differentiation between general and specific manipulation. General manipulation is a stretch performed to more than one joint and usually more than one spinal segment. Specific manipulation intends to stretch only one segment or one spinal joint (28). Ideally, the use of specific manipulation tends to reduce increased stress to uninvolved segments.

Further distinguishing characteristics of manipulation involve the direction of motion or line of drive. Direct manipulation involves a line of drive into and past the barrier of restricted motion. Indirect manipulation utilizes a line of drive away from the barrier of restricted motion. Generally speaking, indirect manipulation is safer than direct and has less tendency for adverse reaction (14). Usually, manipulators will not attempt direct manipulation until all possibilities of a correction by indirect manipulation have been exhausted. Although direct manipulation may be painful for the patient, there are some specific indications for the utilization of direct manipulation, and in the presence of these indications, the utilization of the technique by the manipulator is both a logical and an effective choice.

The ultimate goal of the manipulator is to correct the musculoskeletal dysfunction and return the patient toward a more normal function. The ideal manipulative procedure should take into account the structural relationship of the vertebral segment being manipulated. This consideration would include any abnormalities or structural asymmetries. With proper manipulative procedures, it is not necessary to regard all bony or structural malformation as contraindications to manipulation. With manipulation, the areas of restricted and fixated joint movements are mobilized, thereby reducing painful and abnormal joint play and eliminating palpable soft tissue fibers with the ultimate correction of muscle spasms along the imbalanced area. The most important goal of the manipulator is to achieve favorable results without inducing trauma to the spine or soft tissues along the spine, so as to allow the patient to receive maximum therapeutic benefit.

A manipulative procedure that is widely used is the short lever, high-velocity thrust, directed specifically at the manipulatable lesion. The proficient clinician must have proper skills to diagnose the clinically significant lesion and develop the ability to direct the manipulative thrust to one vertebra segment in a specific direction.

As opposed to the specific short lever, high-velocity adjustment, the long lever manipulation is an example of a nonspecific manipulation over an entire region of the spine. Without proper care in this type of manipulation, and in the hands of an unskilled manipulator, the segment most often mobilized is the one that is already hypermobile. Nonspecific techniques include what is known as noncontact techniques. These techniques are utilized when greater force is necessary to achieve joint mobility, and the manipulator gains leverage by obtaining contact points away from the manipulative lesion, such as on the chest or the extremity.

Additionally, several authors are proposing the utilization of distraction techniques, specifically for the treatment of intervertebral disk lesions. Cyriax (22) indicated that there are three effects from traction and distraction-type techniques. First, there is an increase in the spacing between vertebral bodies, thus enlarging the space into which the protrusion must recede. Second, there is a tautening of the joint capsule that allows the ligaments joining the vertebral bodies to create a centrifugal force around the joint, which squeezes the disk fibers and the nucleus back into place. Finally, there is suction created within the joint.

Cox utilizes a specific intermittent distraction technique (21) that is designed to provide a push-pull, pumping effect on the intervertebral disk space, creating a milking action of the intervertebral disk and thereby allowing resolution. Proponents of this distraction manipulation are quick to point out the difference between intermittent distraction and static traction. Whereas the distraction technique is designed to pump the intervertebral disk and the nucleus back to a more normal position, static traction actually opens the intervertebral disk space and can allow the nucleus to imbibe fluids, which may increase the intradiskal pressure and cause a worsening of pressure against an already compressed nerve root.

PREPARATION FOR MANIPULATION

In preparation for manipulation, there are a number of general rules one must consider. The patient must be relaxed and comfortable. If there are contracted muscles in the general area where the manipulation is to be applied, a preparatory therapy such as stretching or massage along with a physiotherapeutic modality may be required to assist the patient in obtaining maximum relaxation prior to manipulation.

Additionally, the manipulator must be mentally and physically relaxed. This requires self-assurance and complete confidence in biomechanics, with a mental concept of how the correction is to be made. Furthermore, it is most helpful if the manipulator wears comfortable clothing because manipulation often requires close body contact between the clinician and the patient. It is essential to determine the difference between soft tissue stretch and the pain of muscle guarding. Muscle guarding is a significant sign indicating the clinician is about to move through the point of pain. It is reiterated here that, in general, movement through the point of pain should be avoided. Manipulation through the point of pain requires exact skills and precise techniques that are employed in very selective circumstances.

Consideration must be given to the direction in which the thrust is to be made, which is commonly referred to as the line of drive. The depth and/or velocity of thrust must also be determined. Additionally, skilled manipulators often use torque during the thrust. This torque is a twisting at the wrist of the contact hand to assist in the correction.

VARIATIONS OF MANIPULATIVE TECHNIQUES

Unquestionably, it is impossible to list all of the techniques and variations that have been developed to reduce spinal dysfunction. Some techniques require the patient to be supine; others require the patient to be side-lying or in seated positions. Many techniques require special types of manipulative tables or traction devices. The following examples will illustrate some of the basic principles of spinal manipulation.

The *specific short lever, high-velocity spinal manipulation* would require the patient to be placed in a position that allows movement of the vertebra in the desired position. Normally, contact is made with a small portion of one hand. This could be in the form of a thumb with a pushing action, or it could be the pisiform bone of the contact hand that delivers the thrust. The spinal segment above or below the segment to be manipulated should be stabilized by the clinician's other hand or by moving the

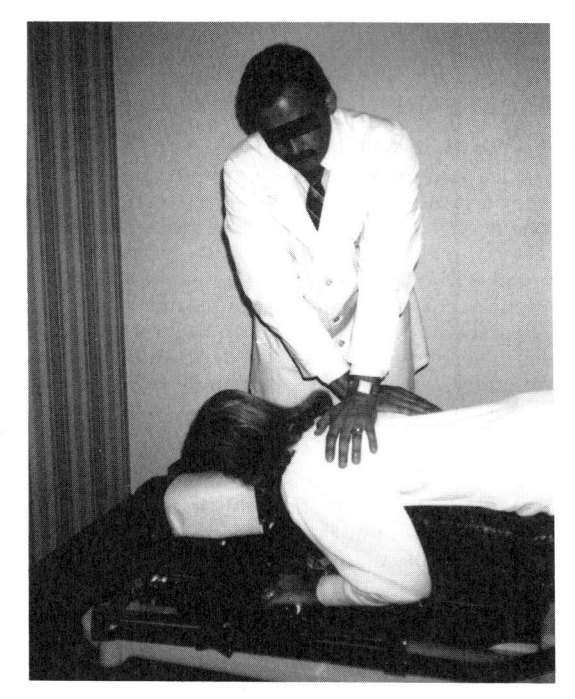

Figure 14.1. Short lever, high-velocity spinal manipulation.

spine to the limit of its passive range of motion. The high-velocity thrust is delivered with the contact hand to the short lever area of the vertebra (i.e., transverse process, spinous process, or mamillary process) in the direction to which the correction should be made (Fig. 14.1).

Lumbar spine manipulation as well as *sacroiliac joint manipulations* are frequently performed with the patient in a side-lying position. The point of contact for the clinician is at the segment to be manipulated in the lumbar spine. The patient's upper body is rotated and laterally flexed downward to the lumbar spine at the point of contact. At this point, the superior knee and hip are flexed, which allows the manipulator to rotate the pelvis and localize the point of counterrotation to the spinal segment to be manipulated. With manipulation of the lumbar spine, the clinician is normally contacting the patient with the pisiform section placed across the mamillary process of the lumbar vertebra or by hooking the spinous process with a cupping action of the fingers. With proper placement of the patient, the force of the manipulation can be localized to higher levels along the lumbar spine, and a skilled manipulator can use this technique to deliver the manipulation to very specific levels of the spine (Fig. 14.2).

A similar technique that allows the patient to receive a different effect is the *side posture manipulation and rotation with extension*. This technique can be effective with patients who have a decrease in the normal lordosis

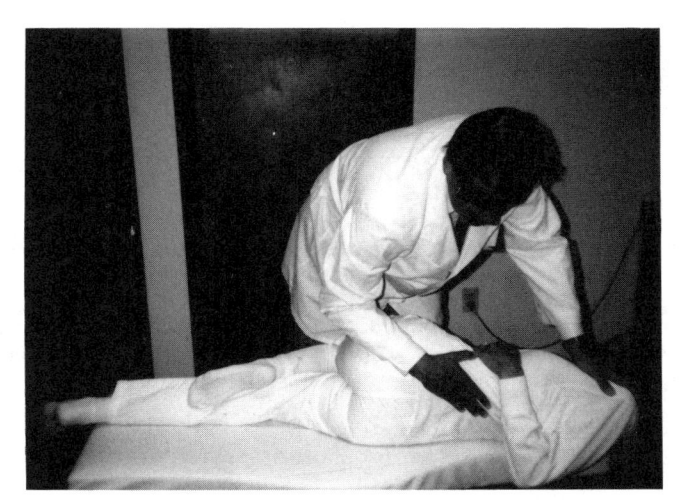

Figure 14.2. Lumbar spine manipulation with patient in side-lying position.

of the lumbar spine. Once again, the patient is on the side with the clinician stabilizing the patient along the shoulder. The patient's inferior leg must be placed posteriorly, bringing the patient's lumbar spine into lordosis. From this position, the contact hand is placed on the anterior superior portion of the ileum. The specific thrust is delivered anteriorly and inferiorly (Fig. 14.3).

Seated positions can be utilized to manipulate even the *lumbar spine*. The patient is seated along the end of the

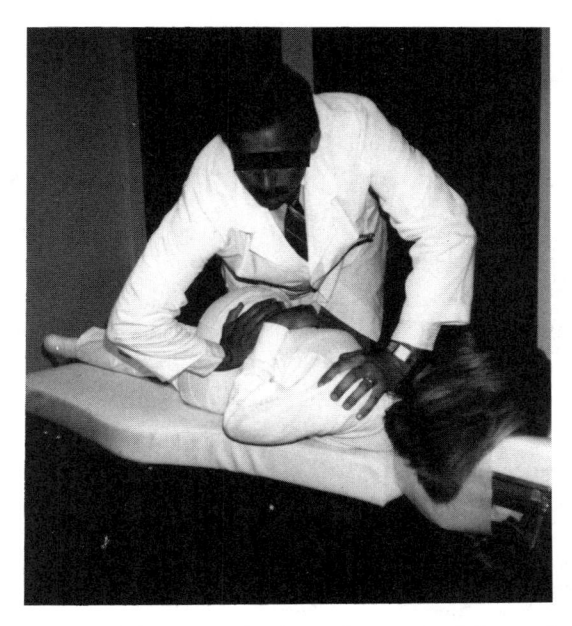

Figure 14.3. Side posture lumbar spine manipulation and rotation with extension.

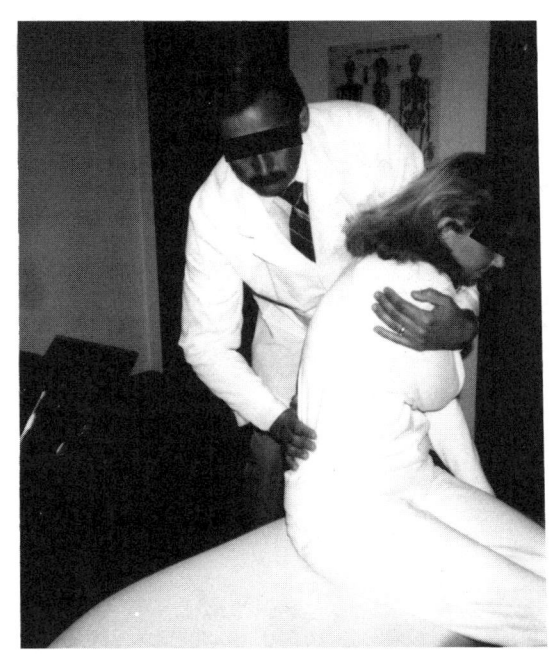

Figure 14.4. Seated position manipulation of lumbar spine.

adjusting table with one arm across the chest and the hand grasping the opposite shoulder. Normally the clinician will contact the spinous process with a thumb. The stabilizing hand is in front of the patient and grasping the patient's shoulder. The manipulator is then able to flex, extend, rotate, or laterally bend the patient. The thrust is delivered with high velocity to the area to be manipulated (Fig. 14.4). This technique is also effective in the thoracolumbar region.

An effective procedure to be performed to the *thoracic spine* is with the patient in a *seated position*. The patient flexes the neck and grasps his hands behind the neck. The manipulator stands behind the patient, placing his forearms under the patient's arms, and grasps the patient's wrists. The contact by the manipulator here is the sternum area against the thoracic spine. The patient's shoulders are brought to tension while the manipulator avoids pressure on the patient's wrists and neck. The thrust is achieved by raising the patient's shoulders while delivering simultaneous thrust with the manipulator's sternum (Fig. 14.5).

An excellent manipulation for *correction of intercostal pain and distortions along the rib cage* is achieved with the patient lying supine. The manipulator stands to the side opposite the pain and extends the hand beneath the patient alongside the spine, contacting the patient's costovertebral articulations. The manipulator stabilizes with the anterior hand against the crest of the opposite ileum. The patient is rotated and the manipulator brings the spine to tension. The thrust is then delivered upward with the

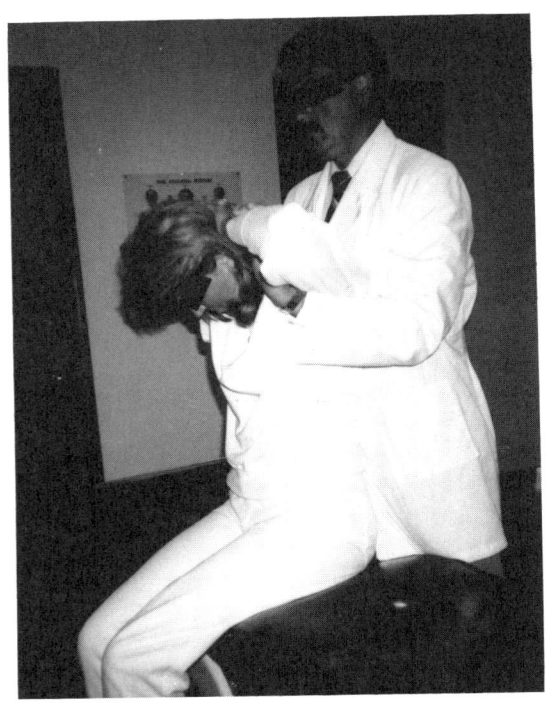

Figure 14.5. Seated position manipulation of thoracic spine.

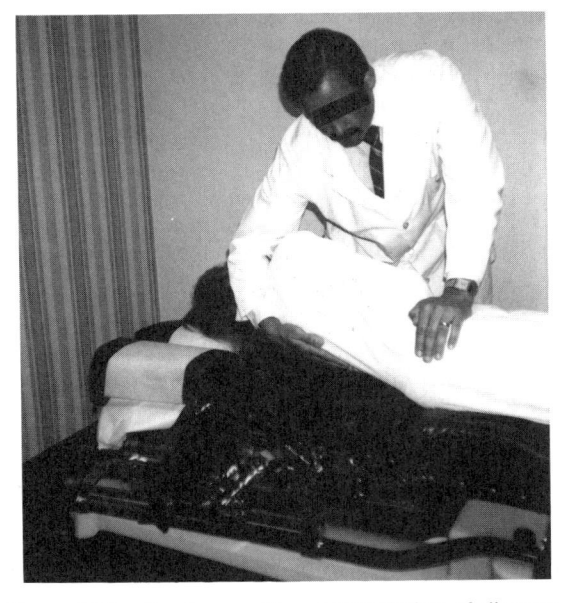

Figure 14.6. Supine position manipulation of rib cage.

contact hand while the stabilizing hand and arm lightly thrust inferiorly (Fig. 14.6).

CONTRAINDICATIONS FOR MANIPULATION

According to rough estimations, based on 50 million manipulations yearly over the past 40 years, the odds of a serious complication occurring as a result of manipulation are 1 in 181 million manipulations. It is safe to say that if proper precautions are taken, and a full understanding of the case at hand is obtained, the frequency of complication is greatly reduced.

The most serious complication to arise is from injury to the cerebral circulation or spinal cord following cervical manipulation. However, there are predisposing factors that greatly increase the risk of cervical manipulation. The most obvious is osteophytic outgrowths, which may obstruct the course of vertebral arteries.

Additionally, degenerative joint disease along the cervical spine may reduce the disk height. This shortens the cervical spine and allows the vertebral arteries to become more tortuous (29).

Yet, the most likely cause of serious injury or complications due to manipulation remains that of an incorrect diagnosis, failure to diagnose, or improper techniques. As with any skilled procedure, the expected results and the resulting complications are dependent upon the skills of the clinician.

References

1. Cassidy JD, Kirkaldy-Willis WH, McGregor M: Spinal manipulation for the treatment of chronic low back and leg pain; an observational study. In Buerger AA, Greenman PE (eds): *Empirical Approaches to the Validation of Spinal Manipulation.* Springfield, IL, Charles C Thomas, 1985, pp 119–148.
2. Schafer RC: *Chiropractic Management of Sports and Recreational Injuries.* Baltimore, Williams & Wilkins, 1982, pp 273–274.
3. Neumann H: A concept of manual medicine. In Buerger AA, Greenman PE (eds): *Empirical Approaches to the Validation of Spinal Manipulation.* Springfield IL, Charles C Thomas, 1985, p 267.
4. Johnston WL: Inter-rater reliability on the selection of manipulable patients. In Buerger AA, Greenman PE (eds): *Empirical Approaches to the Validation of Spinal Manipulation.* Springfield, IL, Charles C Thomas, 1985, p 107.
5. White AA, Panjabi M: The role of stabilization in the treatment of cervical spine injuries. *Spine* 9:229–238, 1984.
6. Wyke BD: Articular neurology. A review. *Physiologist* 58:94–100, 1973.
7. Denslow JS, Hassett CC: The central excitatory state associated with postural abnormalities. *J Neurophysiol* 5:393–402, 1942.
8. Korr IM: Proprioceptors and the discussion of mechanisms of manipulative therapy. In Korr IM (ed): *Neurolobiologic Mechanisms in Manipulative Therapy.* New York, Plenum, 1978.
9. Glover JR: Back pain and hyperasthesia. *Lancet* 1:1165–1169, 1980.

10. Terrett AC, Howard V: Manipulation and pain tolerance. *Am J Phy Med* 63:217–223, 1984.
11. Hildebrant RW, Howe JW: *Spinal Biomechanics and Subluxation Classification*. Lombard, IL, National College of Chiropractic, 1974.
12. Hviid H: The influence of chiropractic treatment on the rotary mobility of the cervical spine. *Ann Swiss Chirop Assoc* V:31–44, 1971.
13. Jirout J: The effect of mobilization of the segmental blockage on the sagittal component of the cervical spine. *Neuroradiology* 3:210–215, 1972.
14. Halderman S: Spinal manipulative therapy in the management of low back pain. In Finnesan BE (ed): *Low Back Pain*. Philadelphia, JB Lippincott, 1980, pp 245–273.
15. Schafter RC: *Clinical Biomechanics: Musculoskeletal Actions and Reactions*. Baltimore, Williams & Wilkins, 1983.
16. Potter GE: A study of 744 cases of neck and back pain treated with spinal manipulation. *J Can Chirop Assoc* 21(4):154–156, 1977.
17. Dyck P, Pheasant HC, Doyle JB, Rieder JJ: Intermittent cauda equina compression syndrome. *Spine* 261:75, 1977.
18. Hoehler F, Tobis JS, Burger AA: Spinal manipulation for back pain. *JAMA* 245:1835–1838, 1981.
19. Fisk JW: An evaluation of manipulation in the treatment of the acute low back pain syndrome in general practice. In Buerger AA, Greenman PE (eds): *Empirical Approaches to the Validation of Spinal Manipulation*. Springfield, IL, Charles C Thomas, 1985, pp 228–273.
20. Glover JR, Morris JG, Khosla T: Back pain; a randomized clinical trial of rotational manipulation of the trunk. *Br J Ind Med* 31:59–64, 1974.
21. Cox J: *Low Back Pain: Mechanism, Diagnosis and Treatment*, ed 4. Baltimore, Williams & Wilkins, 1985.
22. Cyriax J: *Textbook of Orthopedic Medicine*, ed 3. Baltimore, Williams & Wilkins, 1969.
23. Chrisman OD, Mittnacht A, Snook GA: A study of the results following rotatory manipulation in the lumbar intervertebral disc syndrome. *J Bone Joint Surg* 46(A):517–524, 1964.
24. Hirschberg GG: Treating lumbar disc lesions by prolonged continuous reduction of intradiscal pressure. *Tex Med* 70:58–68, 1974.
25. Schafer RC: *Clinical Biomechanics: Musculoskeletal Actions and Reactions*. Baltimore, Williams & Wilkins, 1983.
26. Vernon H: Chiropractic manipulative therapy in the treatment of headaches: a retrospective and prospective study. *J Manipulative Physiol Ther* 5:109–112, 1982.
27. Strange VV: *Essential Principles of Chiropractic*. Davenport, IA, Palmer College of Chiropractic, 1984.
28. Maigne R: Manipulations of the spine. In Basmajian UV (ed): *Mobilization, Traction and Massage*, ed 3. Baltimore, Williams & Wilkins, 1985, pp 71–134.
29. Loach AA: *The Chiropractic Theories*, ed 2. Baltimore, Williams & Wilkins, 1986.

chapter 15
Adjunctive Treatment Techniques

Larry A. Gaupp, Ph. D., ABPP, ABPN, ABCB
Don E. Flinn, M.D.
Richard L. Weddige, M.D.

HYPNOSIS

Hypnoanalgesia and hypnoanesthesia are among the earliest applications of hypnosis, and among the most enduring methods of pain reduction in the clinical setting. The impressive clinical reports of Rejamier (1821), Clouqet (1829), Elliotson (1834), Ward (1842), and Esdaile (1865) of painless surgery under mesmeric sleep fostered a belief in the efficacy of hypnosis in the relief of pain that has prevailed despite an often hostile scientific climate and the discovery of chemical anesthetics (for a review of current applications of hypnosis in surgery and anesthesia, see refs. 1, 2).

Fortunately, the efficacy of hypnosis in the relief of the acute pain of surgery garnered support from the laboratory, where reasonably good laboratory analogues (e.g., cold pressor pain, ischemic pain) permitted the investigation of hypnosis in the reduction of acute pain under controlled conditions. This body of research has repeatedly demonstrated the reality of pain reduction through hypnosis and that the ability to reduce acute pain in the laboratory through hypnosis is related to the level of hypnotic susceptibility as measured by standardized tests of hypnotic susceptibility (e.g., Stanford Hypnotic Susceptibility Scales). The greater the level of hypnotic susceptibility the greater the likelihood of pain reduction (1, 3–6). It has been demonstrated that hypnoanalgesia reduces both the sensory pain and suffering components of acute pain (7). Further, the reduction of acute pain in the laboratory is not attributable to anxiety reduction (1, 3, 8, 9), or to hypnotic induction procedures or suggestion alone (1, 5, 9, 10, 11), or to demand characteristics or expectancy (3, 8). Finally, it has been carefully demonstrated that the reduction of acute pain in the laboratory through hypnosis is not attributable to a placebo effect (12). Hypnoanalgesia acts like a placebo for low hypnotic susceptibles only; for high hypnotic susceptibles, the reduction of pain through hypnosis greatly exceeds the reduction via placebo.

The support that these laboratory findings have given to the clinical reports of the successful reduction of acute pain through hypnosis has been bolstered by experimental studies conducted within the clinical setting. These findings have historically mirrored those of laboratory testing. Gottfredson (13), in a well-designed investigation of hypnoanesthesia as the sole anesthetic in the clinical dental context as it relates to hypnotic susceptibility, found that the more hypnotizable the patient, the less pain the patient experienced. Additionally, the effectiveness of hypnoanesthesia in reducing acute dental pain was comparable to that of chemoanesthesia for the high hypnotic susceptibles. The award-winning research of Wakeman and Kaplan (14) demonstrated the efficacy of hypnoanalgesia and hypnoanesthesia in the treatment of painful burns (i.e., daily tanking, debridement, and dressing changes) in children, adolescents, and adults.

Although laboratory-induced pain has provided a satisfactory experimental framework for the investigation of hypnosis in the reduction of acute pain, does this body of work apply equally well to chronic clinical pain? Does chronic clinical pain with its attendant biopsychosocial contaminants respond like acute pain insofar as hypnosis is concerned? Extant evidence suggests that its does; the only difference between the reduction of acute pain and chronic pain through hypnosis is that the latter, because of its ongoing and/or recurrent nature, requires that the patient learn self-hypnosis so that self-reliance can be achieved.

As is the case with acute pain, there are abundant clinical reports and methodologically compromised studies attesting to the efficacy of hypnosis in the reduction of chronic clinical pain. Examples of these reports include the successful application of hypnoanalgesia to various types of headache (15–40), back pain (28, 32, 37, 41–47), cancer pain (1, 43, 48–69), phantom pain (43, 70–76), facial pain (37, 77, 78), neck and shoulder pain (79, 80), myofibrositis (81), herpes (82), lupus (83), gastrointestinal pain (29, 84), bruxism (85), tic douloureux (86), vaginismus (87), arthritis (43, 88–90), and peripheral nerve pain (43).

In addition to these reports of the use of hypnosis in the reduction of chronic pain, there are several methodologically satisfactory studies that support the assertion that the findings reported for acute pain in the laboratory are pertinent to chronic pain. For example, in a well-controlled outcome study with 1-year follow-up, Friedman and Taub (91) concluded that hypnosis was a cost-effective treatment for migraine headache, especially for patients exhibiting a high level of hypnotic susceptibility. Similarly, L.A. Gaupp and F.J. Magnavito (unpublished information), using hypnotic dissociation to promote hypnoanalgesia, found that hypnoanalgesia was effective in reducing both the sensory pain and suffering components of chronic pain for patients exhibiting medium and high levels of hypnotic susceptibility. This study was conducted with a group of unselected patients with chronic pain of mixed etiology (i.e., low back pain, headache, shoulder pain, neck pain, and chest pain). A significant correlation between standardized measures of hypnotic susceptibility (e.g., Stanford Hypnotic Clinical Scale) and the reduction of chronic pain through hypnosis has been found for headache (91), facial pain (78), and chronic pain of mixed etiology (L.A. Gaupp and F.J. Magnavito, unpublished information). Thus, although further research is desirable, these systematic investigations of hypnosis in the relief of chronic pain, like those for acute pain in the clinical setting, have mirrored the findings for the relief of laboratory-induced pain through hypnosis.

The well-documented relationship between hypnotic susceptibility and the reduction of pain through hypnosis led Gaupp and Magnavito to suggest that a medium level of hypnotic susceptibility should serve as the minimum criterion for attempting hypnoanalgesia in the clinical setting. The formal assessment of hypnotic susceptibility in the clinical setting has become time efficient since the development of brief clinically relevant scales such as the Stanford Hypnotic Clinical Scale (1). This allows for an exploration of the kinds of hypnotic experiences the patient may have (versus simply the absolute level of hypnotic susceptibility), and brings scientifically validated procedure into the clinical setting. This is not to state that the practitioner, workload permitting, should not attempt hypnoanalgesia with low hypnotic susceptibles, because some are able to reduce pain. However, given that the single most important determinant of the patient's ability to reduce pain through hypnosis is level of hypnotic susceptibility (1, 92), it would seem prudent to limit such attempts to two to three sessions unless success is clearly evident.

The practitioner's approach to hypnoanalgesia does not differ substantially from hypnotherapy generally. Care must be given to prepare the patient, especially those naive to the experience of hypnosis, by establishing rapport, gaining the patient's trust and cooperation, enhancing and binding the patient's motivation, exploring the patient's expectations and attitudes, and exploring the patient's knowledge of hypnosis so that any misconceptions can be corrected and attendant apprehension alleviated. Specific to the preparation of the chronic pain patient is the correction of the belief that the successful use of hypnosis to alleviate pain means that the pain is psychological or emotional or imaginary, thereby challenging the veracity of the pain complaint and the integrity of the patient. A brief history of hypnoanalgesia coupled with a graphic description of the use of hypnosis to control painful burns can readily correct this misconception. Finally, it is important that the patient conceptualize hypnosis as a long-term chronic pain management strategy versus a brief intervention that will completely and forever abolish the pain. The ultimate goal of the hypnotic intervention is to teach the patient self-hypnosis so that the patient may become self-reliant in managing the pain and thereby minimize the pain's adverse impact on daily functioning.

HYPNOANALGESIA STRATEGIES

Numerous strategies and variations thereof have been used to promote hypnoanalgesia, reflecting the ingenuity and resourcefulness of the practitioner and the patient as they work collaboratively to reduce the pain. The approaches described below are neither inclusive nor mutually exclusive, and do not include the almost unlimited variations and combinations the practitioner may realize in adapting to what the patient can do and finds congenial. The practitioner should discuss openly with the patient the rationale for the strategy(ies) being used because they may appear unscientific and bizarre to the patient. An explanation that metaphoric and imaginal suggestions mediate neurophysiologic and/or neurochemical processes that alleviate pain will generally be acceptable.

Direct Hypnotic Suggestion

Direct hypnotic suggestion involves giving the patient the direct suggestion that the pain will no longer be experienced. This is not considered to be a very useful strategy in that it may be perceived by the patient as authoritarian and thus create resistance, may limit the effectiveness of other strategies, and is likely to be successful only for high hypnotic susceptibiles with extant cognitive coping strategies that can be creatively utilized to mediate the direct suggestion.

Indirect Hypnotic Suggestion

Indirect hypnotic suggestion is similar to direct suggestion but is worded and offered in a manner conducive to receptiveness and responsiveness, for example, ". . . as you enjoy . . . the comfort of this deeply relaxed state . . . you notice that you gradually lose awareness of your body and how it feels . . . like the many moments throughout each day when you become so involved in things outside yourself . . . you have little or no awareness of your body . . . or that it even exists . . ." This approach is generally considered more effective than direct suggestion, and is applicable to a broader range of hypnotic susceptibility.

Hypnotic Dissociation

Hypnotic dissociation involves transporting the patient away from the present to an imagined pleasing, relaxing, and absorbing place or activity (e.g., walking through a meadow, engaging in some adventure real or imagined), or to an earlier and happier time via age regression. Another approach to this strategy is to suggest a partial or complete out-of-body experience. For example, a patient with a painful foot may be able to imagine disconnecting the painful foot. Or, the patient might be asked to float out of the body and leave the person experiencing the pain behind.

Hypnotic Time Disorientation

Hypnotic time disorientation involves reorientation in time to an earlier stage of the illness or to an earlier time when the pain was of minor consideration. For example, reorientation to a time predating the illness or pain problem can be suggested, along with restoration of normal sensations or of pleasant feelings/sensations and the projection of these into the present to nullify the pain and/or some subjective quality(ies) of the pain experience. Another approach is to suggest reorientation to a time during the course of the illness or pain problem when a medical/surgical intervention successfully relieved the pain (e.g., nerve block), with restoration of attendant sensations or normal sensations and the projection of these into the present.

Hypnotic Replacement or Substitution of Sensations

Hypnotic replacement or substitution of sensations involves the selective, partial, or complete modification of the pain experience through the substitution of or conversion to some other sensation or symptom. Perhaps the most common approach to this strategy is to suggest glove anesthesia, beginning with suggested feelings of coolness or warmth in a hand that gradually develops into a pleasant numbness. The glove anesthesia can then be demonstrated by pinching or pricking the hand, enhancing the patient's sense of efficacy regarding the control over bodily sensations. Then, it is suggested that the numbness be "transferred" from the anesthetic hand to the site of pain by having the patient gently rub or massage the painful part of the body with the hand, as a symbol of the transfer. Another approach to this strategy is to suggest that the patient experience a pleasant sensation (e.g., tingling) at or near the site of the pain to absorb attention along with suggested feelings of warmth, heaviness, or coolness where the pain is experienced. In contrast, an unpleasant and annoying yet bearable sensation (e.g., itching, burning, pain of minor cut) may be suggested to absorb attention along with hypnotic suggestions of warmth and so forth. Or, it may be suggested that the pain be converted to some other annoying yet tolerable symptom (e.g., twitching, cough). One additional approach is to hypnotically promote synesthesia, or the utilization of sensory images such that pleasure from one sensory modality (e.g., visual, auditory) is shifted to another (e.g., nocioceptive perceptions), for example, ". . . the pleasant rhythmic sound of the waves rolling gently onto the shore becomes one with the throbbing in your head."

Hypnotic Displacement

Hypnotic displacement involves displacing the pain or selected qualities thereof from one area of the body to another where it does not carry the same threatening significance or does not as readily interfere with daily functioning (e.g., disabling back pain may be displaced to the little finger of the nonpreferred hand), or where it is simply more tolerable, giving the usually painful area a rest. This strategy is also useful for pain that is not well localized and thus seemingly more difficult to manage. It is suggested that the patient consolidate the pain into a smaller area before moving it.

Hypnotic Reinterpretation

Hypnotic reinterpretation and/or dissociation of the meaning attributed to the pain can alleviate pain. This approach requires full awareness of the meaning attributed by the patient to the pain experience, and is especially useful when the pain experience harbors affectual or metaphoric significance. For example, the pain of an old war injury might come to represent the courage and pride of defending Freedom's Frontier. Or, the pain of child abuse fused with traumatic back pain acquired in adulthood can be differentiated and dealt with as separate experiences.

Hypnoplasty

Hypnoplasty involves hypnotically altering the anatomic site of the pain in a manner that counters the pain experience. A patient might imagine installing circuit breakers, switches, or a rheostat that can be readily manipulated to turn off or lower the level of pain. Or, the patient might shore up a structurally compromised vertebral body so as to relieve compression effects.

Hypnotic Amnesia

Hypnotically suggested amnesia is a useful strategy for pain that is episodic or constant with intermittent exacerbations. Suggestions can be given for partial or complete amnesia of the pain that has been experienced, or for selective subjective qualities and attributes of the pain experience as described by the patient. Forgetting the pain experience can ameliorate the anticipation and dread of future episodes or exacerbations that may increase interepisode discomfort and exacerbate the episode when and if it occurs. Suggestions that any episodes of pain will seem completely transient usually accompany the suggestions for amnesia. Therefore, neither remembered nor anticipated, the experience will seem to have no appreciable duration and thus be more easily tolerated. *Hypnotic time distortion* can be a useful adjunct to this strategy. Once amnesia is developed for all past episodes of pain, hypnotically developed time distortion can be suggested so that the duration of an episode may be experienced as markedly shortened. For example, it may be suggested that each episode of pain will come as a complete surprise; that when an episode occurs it will cue a hypnotic state during which the patient will experience the enjoyment of a surprise party; that because time is relative, the time will seem to fly by because of the fun; that the party, during which the entire episode of pain will be experienced, will seem to last only a matter of seconds or minutes; and that on arousal from this hypnotic surprise, amnesia for the entire experience will occur.

Additional Considerations

Regardless of the strategy or strategies the practitioner employs, it is necessary to be sensitive to the patient's experience so that adjustments can be made. For example, for the patient who believes the chronic pain reflects and serves as a marker of occult disease it can be suggested that the pain be only partially relieved, leaving the patient with a way to monitor health status. Other patients may need to be reassured that the relief of pain through hypnosis will not abolish the ability to experience acute pain indicative of the need for medical attention.

SELF-HYPNOSIS TECHNIQUES

As previously noted, self-hypnosis is generally essential to the long-term management of chronic pain via hypnoanalgesia. Rarely is chronic pain completely abolished through hypnosis; more commonly, partial or complete relief is attained for varying amounts of time. Once a patient has allowed a practitioner to guide him/her into hypnosis, the patient can readily follow the same induction, deepening, hypnoanalgesic strategies, and termination procedures. For the high hypnotic susceptibles, a self-induced cue can be used to enter hypnosis. Fortunately, many patients can readily learn to utilize self-hypnosis with little difficulty following this procedure and with essentially the same results (1). For those who have difficulty, a personalized tape recording of a heterohypnotic session can be made and used by the patient. Many patients can realize effective pain relief within 10 min through self-hypnosis, and should utilize self-hypnosis at least once daily if not as often as is necessary.

Some patients will report that at times the pain is too severe to concentrate sufficiently to induce self-hypnosis. Two induction techniques that have been useful in effectively dealing with this eventuality are fractionation (29) and pain induction. With the *modified fractionation technique* the patient is asked to follow the same induction procedure previously learned, but without any concern as to the depth of hypnosis achieved. Rather, after eye closure, the patient is to simply notice whatever is experienced at the moment of maximal relaxation, no matter how minimal or slight that may be. Next, the patient should rouse up from the hypnosis with a readiness to reexperience hypnosis, knowing that with each rehypnotization a deeper state of relaxed hypnosis will be attained. The patient then induces hypnosis again, paying close attention to those relaxing sensations noted during the previous induction. This procedure is repeated again and again, until a level of hypnosis is achieved that allows the patient to proceed with the rest of the hypnoanalgesic intervention. This can generally be achieved following four to six inductions.

Utilizing pain to induce hypnosis simply makes use of the fact that the patient is already absorbed. The patient is instructed to focus even more intently on the pain and to carefully notice some dimension of the pain (e.g., intensity, quality, temporality), to notice, for example, how the pain really is not constant but rather fluctuates, albeit ever so slightly, like the ebb and flow of the tides. It is suggested that the patient begin to highlight those fluctuations, first by intensifying the flow of the pain. Implicit is that if the pain can be increased volitionally, it can be decreased in intensity in a similar manner. Then, the patient begins to heighten the ebbing phase. Throughout the exercise the patient notes that with each flow and ebb of the pain a deeper level of relaxed hypnosis is attained. When the patient feels that the tide has subsided sufficiently, he/she can proceed with the hypnoanalgesic intervention.

MECHANISM OF HYPNOANALGESIA

The mechanism(s) of hypnoanalgesia and hypnoanesthesia remain unclear. The failure of naloxone to reduce hypnoanalgesia (93, 94) has led to the assertion that hypnoanalgesia occurs primarily at higher cortical levels (95). It has been reasoned that if hypnoanalgesia is mediated through a neurochemical mechanism involving the release of opioid peptides in the central nervous system (β-endorphins), then naloxone, an opioid antagonist, would reverse it. In contrast to this assertion, Stephenson (96) reported a single case of repeated reversal of hypnoanalgesia by naloxone, and Domangue and colleagues (90) found that mean plasma levels of β-endorphin were significantly higher following successful hypnoanalgesia in a group of arthritic pain patients. These seemingly conflicting results may reflect the fact that naloxone effects may not be comparable between clinical pain and laboratory-induced pain (97), and highlight the methodologic problems that need to be resolved before the mechanism(s) of hypnoanalgesia can be adequately investigated (98, 99).

CONCLUSIONS

Although there remains much to learn about the use of hypnosis in the relief of chronic pain, there clearly is sufficient scientific evidence substantiating its efficacy to warrant its clinical use. Equally important, the chronic pain patient is receptive to the use of hypnosis in the relief of pain and finds it very helpful (L.A. Gaupp, unpublished information). Of 145 chronic pain patients who completed a 6-week inpatient comprehensive pain management program, only 1 declined to attempt hypnoanalgesia. Further, when these patients were asked to indicate which of the 14 treatment elements that made up the program were most helpful in learning how to function more actively and productively in spite of pain, and in learning how to control and/or alter the perception of pain, hypnosis/self-hypnosis emerged as the treatment perceived as most helpful for both. This finding also supports the belief that hypnosis has the advantage of creating and promoting beneficial effects beyond the specific effect on pain (1, 93).

RELAXATION TRAINING

The induction of the psychophysiologic state of low arousal that has come to be known as the relaxation response (100) has gained widespread use in the management of chronic pain. The relaxation response has been characterized by a generalized decreased sympathetic nervous system activity and concomitant decreases in respiratory rate, oxygen consumption, heart rate, blood pressure, arterial blood lactate, and muscle tension, as well as increases in skin resistance, skeletal muscle blood flow, and electroencephalographic alpha activity (100). The amelioration of the chronic pain experience is presumed to result in part from the psychophysiologic changes attendant to the induction of the relaxation response (e.g., decreases in muscle tension believed to underlie musculoskeletal pain, such as muscle tension headache; decreases in cranial vasculature reactivity believed to underlie vascular headache). Although a variety of procedures have been devised to induce the relaxation response in the reduction of chronic pain, only the most commonly used procedures are reviewed here.

BIOFEEDBACK

Biofeedback has become a popular procedure for the treatment of chronic pain. This approach assumes that a maladaptive psychophysiologic response is of etiologic significance in chronic pain and that the normalization and/or control of the presumptive maladaptive response will attenuate the pain. These assumptions have led to the development of several frequently used biofeedback methods: (a) electromyographic (EMG) feedback to reduce muscle tension; (b) thermal feedback to increase finger temperature; and (c) cephalic blood volume pulse (BVP) feedback to reduce BVP of the cephalic temporal artery.

Numerous reports attesting to the efficacy of biofeedback in the reduction of chronic pain have appeared. Examples of these include the successful application of biofeedback in treating muscle tension headache (101–134), migraine headache (135–167), cluster headache (168–170), post-traumatic headache (171), low back pain (172–184), arthritis (185–187), temporomandibular joint pain (188–190), myofascial pain (191), phantom pain (192–194), benign chest pain (195), angina (196), dysmenorrhea (197), postherpetic neuralgia (198), causalgia (199), sickle cell disease (200), and burn pain (201).

Despite the fact that the support for the use of biofeedback in the reduction of chronic pain appears impressive in its magnitude, consistency, and diversity, the efficacy of application has yet to be firmly and scientifically established. Available reports are all too often methodologically weak, making unequivocal conclusions difficult. More troublesome, however, is the fact that the assumptions underlying biofeedback have been seriously questioned. For example, the belief that excessive muscle tension is the primary source of muscle tension headache has been challenged (102, 103, 108, 202–210), as have the belief that excessive cranial vasculature responsivity underlies migraine headache (211–213), and the belief that chronic low back pain reflects abnormal patterns of neuromuscular activity (214–217). Not surprisingly, then, numerous reports and reviews have dampened the enthusiastic claims of the efficacy of biofeedback in the reduction of chronic pain pending clarification of the relative contributions of the physiologic, physiologic self-control, psychological, social, and nonspecific factors involved (182, 218–248). Currently, it is fair to conclude that a scientific basis for the use of biofeedback in the reduction of chronic pain has yet to be established, and that there is only limited and qualified support for its efficacy in this regard, especially when it is used as the sole treatment intervention.

RELAXATION TRAINING

Like biofeedback, there are numerous reports attesting to the efficacy of various relaxation training procedures in the reduction of chronic pain. Examples of these reports include the successful application of such procedures to muscle tension headache (128, 134, 249–262), migraine headache (149, 153, 157, 161, 163, 167, 252, 260–265), post-traumatic headache (266), low back pain (267–269), temporomandibular joint pain (270–272), myofascial pain (273–276), arthritis (277), dysmenorrhea (278), cancer pain (279), phantom pain (280), abdominal pain (281), and chronic pain of mixed etiology (183, 184, 282–284).

In contrast to biofeedback, the efficacy of relaxation training is more firmly established (235, 285). In addition, it appears that biofeedback, which requires expensive equipment and technological support, is no more efficacious than relaxation training and, when successful, usually incorporates some form of home-based relaxation training. Finally, relaxation training can be taught more efficiently than biofeedback, and is more amenable to use as an active coping strategy.

Progressive muscle relaxation (286) is the most widely practiced method of relaxation training in the reduction of chronic pain. Although many variations of this approach are currently in practice (e.g., refs. 287, 288), all involve tensing a muscle group for several seconds, passive focusing of attention on how the tensed muscles feel, then releasing the tensed muscles with passive focusing of attention on how the muscles feel as the relaxation takes place. This sequence is systematically applied to the major muscle groups of the body, and highlights two skills that an individual must acquire if relaxation training is to be effective: recognition/discrimination and voluntary induction of the relaxation response. The patient must first learn to recognize the presence of muscle tension. Although this may seem a relatively easy matter, the chronic pain patient may adapt to a state of chronic muscle tension and thus exhibit a blunted awareness of its presence. Additionally, the patient must learn to recognize increasingly low levels of muscle tension because the pain experience may require only partial tightening of muscle fibers (289). Following this, the patient must first learn to discriminate the presence of muscle tension from the uniquely subjective feelings indicative of the state of relaxation (e.g., heaviness, warmth, calm). Finally, the patient must acquire the ability to induce the relaxation response without using the tensing-releasing procedures employed during training.

Several meditative approaches to relaxation training have demonstrated utility. One simple meditative approach calls for the patient to passively focus awareness on the breathing cycle and to silently repeat the word "one" with each exhalation (100). The patient is instructed to sit quietly in a comfortable position with eyes closed and to relax the muscles of the body, beginning with the feet and progressing up to the face and head. The patient is then instructed to passively focus awareness on the breathing cycle, to breathe easily and naturally through the nose, and to silently repeat the word "one" with each exhalation, for example, breathe in . . . out ("one"), in . . . out ("one"), and so on. Maintaining a passive attitude and permitting relaxation to occur at its own pace is emphasized. It is recommended that the technique be practiced once or twice daily for 10–20 min.

A more complex meditative approach to relaxation training is that of *autogenic training* (290). This approach relies on a series of self-directed formulas to induce the relaxation response. The patient is instructed to assume a relaxing position, to close the eyes, and to passively concentrate on a series of six standard autogenic formulas (e.g., "My right arm is heavy."). Standard formula one focuses on promoting the feeling of heaviness in the limbs, and formula two on promoting the sensation of warmth in the limbs. Formulas three and four focus on cardiac and respiratory regulation, respectively. Formula five focuses on promoting the sensation of warmth in the abdomen, and formula six on the feelings of coolness in the forehead. The patient is instructed to practice these formulas daily until such time that a voluntary shift to a state of wakeful low arousal is readily attained. In addition to the six standard formulas that focus on the psychophysiologic aspects of the relaxation response, there are a series of organ-specific formulas, intentional formulas, and meditative formulas.

Integrative Approach

Because a variety of relaxation training procedures and variations thereof have been used in the reduction of chronic pain, it is difficult to draw any conclusions regarding the effectiveness of any one relative to the others. Therefore, the practitioner should consider combining elements of the more commonly employed methods described above to form an integrative approach to relaxation training (e.g., the quieting response; ref. 291). One such approach is described below.

Phase 1: Progressive Muscle Relaxation This integrative approach begins with training in progressive muscle relaxation. Training is best conducted in a quiet, slightly darkened, and comfortably warm room with the patient in a posture conducive to relaxation. Most patients prefer to assume a supine position on a firm surface or recliner. The legs should be slightly apart and positioned so that the feet are inclined at a V-shaped angle; the heels should not touch each other. The trunk, shoulders, and head should be in a symmetric position. Particular care should be taken to determine the most relaxing position for the head, neck, and shoulders. The arms should lie relaxed and slightly bent beside the trunk. The fingers should remain slightly spread and flexed and not touch the trunk. If the patient presents with chronic low back pain, some support (e.g., folded blanket or pillows) under the knees will help to provide maximum postural relaxation of the back and both legs. Not everyone finds the supine or knees-raised training postures congenial; a sitting posture can be used (290). It is also advisable that the shoes be removed and clothing loosened, if necessary, to minimize any distracting stimulation. Finally, further reduction in unnecessary stimulation can be achieved by having the patient close the eyes.

Once the optimal relaxation training posture is assumed by the patient, the practitioner, speaking in a calm, melodic voice, instructs the patient to tense and release the gross muscle groups of the body, beginning with the dominant hand and forearm. For example, the practitioner may say: "Inhale slowly and make a fist, tensing the muscles of the right hand and forearm. . . . Tense until they slightly tremble . . . hold the tension (for 10 sec). . . . Notice how the tension in these muscles feels . . . become familiar with those sensations of tension so that you can recognize their presence even if they occur when you are not knowingly tensing. . . . Now . . . exhale slowly and relax . . . just letting go completely (3–5 sec) . . . allowing all the tension to drain from those muscles . . . just noticing how those muscles feel as the relaxation takes place . . . the comfortable feelings of heaviness . . . of warmth. . . . Passively focusing your awareness on these comfortable feelings and associated sense of inner peace and calm that is gradually coming over you. . . . As you do . . . allow the phrase, 'my right hand and arm are heavy and warm,' to gently settle into your mind . . ." and so forth, for 20–30 sec before repeating the sequence with the same muscle group for a second time. This sequence of breathing in and tensing, breath retention while focusing attention on the tension, breathing out and releasing, and normal breathing while passively focusing awareness on the relaxation is then systematically applied twice to the dominant upper arm, nondominant hand and forearm, nondominant upper arm, forehead, eyes and nose, cheeks and mouth, neck and throat, chest and back, abdomen, dominant upper leg, dominant calf, dominant foot, nondominant upper leg, nondominant calf, and nondominant foot.

The instruction to take a slow deep breath and to retain it until told to "relax" serves to enhance and maintain tension, facilitating its recognition. Conversely, the instruction to exhale slowly while releasing serves to enhance the feelings associated with relaxation, facilitating the discrimination process. When releasing the tensed muscles, the patient should take care not to release too rapidly or too slowly; 3–5 sec is about right for the release process. The 20–30 sec of practitioner-suggested feelings of relaxation (e.g., heaviness, warmth, comfort, calm) and the patient's passive concentration on the appropriate autogenic formula are designed to enhance the relaxation response. The patient is also cautioned to avoid retensing already relaxed muscle groups when tensing each new muscle group. This may take some practice but usually occurs readily.

Once all muscle groups have been relaxed, the patient is instructed to passively listen to the sound of breathing and to silently say the word "relax" with each exhalation. Pairing the word "relax" with the relaxation response allows the patient to develop a conditional cue for the eventual rapid induction of the relaxation response. This association also begins to prepare the patient for the second phase of relaxation training, training in proper breathing.

Training and practice sessions in progressive muscle relaxation usually last 20–30 min, and represent the focus of the first 2 weeks of relaxation training. The patient is instructed to practice at least once daily, twice if possible. Although tape-assisted practice is probably as effective as self-directed practice for inducing the relaxation response, self-directed practice is preferred because it is more likely to foster and/or restore the patient's sense of personal efficacy (292).

The patient is also asked to follow a number of guidelines in daily practice. Practice should take place in a quiet, slightly darkened and comfortably warm room. The relaxing posture employed during the training should be used during practice. Time(s) congenial to the patient's daily activities should be scheduled for practice so that practice becomes an integral part of the patient's daily routine. The patient should adopt a passive attitude while practicing and not be concerned about the level of success; differing levels of perceived success across practice sessions is natural. If the patient experiences the tendency to fall asleep during practice, he/she is instructed to silently repeat the phrase, "I stay free and fresh while practicing," while practicing. Finally, upon completion of practice, the patient should sit up slowly and remain seated for several minutes while gently moving the limbs before slowly standing up.

Phase 2: Proper Breathing The next phase of training involves training in proper breathing. Breathing rhythm, the sequence of inhalation and exhalation, is an important determinant of the level of arousal (293). In contrast to the rapid shallow breathing through the mouth indicative and facilitative of tension, proper breathing, characterized by slow and deep rhythmic breathing through the nose, promotes a low level of arousal.

Training in proper breathing begins with the patient assuming the relaxing posture used during the training and practice of progressive muscle relaxation. However, the hands are lightly placed over the abdomen just below the navel, with fingertips touching. The patient is instructed to inhale slowly and deeply through the nose, and at the same time to let the abdomen swell out, making a conscious but relaxed effort to distend the abdomen as if developing a "pot belly." The fingertips should move apart as the abdomen swells out. As the abdomen rises with inhalation, the diaphragm moves downward. As the breath continues, the lower part of the chest and finally the upper chest expands and slightly lifts and the inhalation is completed. The patient is instructed to retain the breath momentarily, and the process is then reversed. The breath is slowly released, the abdomen is drawn in, which lifts the diaphragm, the expanded chest relaxes, and exhalation is completed. The resultant emptiness is momentarily held and then the cycle repeated.

Thus described, training in proper breathing involves four distinct stages: (a) inhalation, (b) retention of breath, (c) exhalation, and (d) retention of emptiness. However, with practice this becomes one smooth continuous and effortless movement. Training in proper breathing may be facilitated by breathing to a count. Most patients find congenial a schedule of inhaling for a count of three or four (sec), holding for one count, and then exhaling and holding for the same count. In counting, then, a breathing cycle may sound like this: "(inhaling) one . . . two . . . three . . . hold . . . (exhaling) "relax" . . . two . . . three . . . hold." Beginning the exhalation count with the conditional cue "relax" facilitates the induction of the relaxation response by eliciting the feelings of relaxation previously associated with progressive muscle relaxation. Although the above count is appropriate for most patients, it may have to be shortened early in training for some. Whatever the count, it should be the same for both the inhalation and exhalation phase so that the breathing cycle is smooth and even.

Training and practice sessions in proper breathing usually last 10–20 min, and are the focus of the third week of training. The patient is instructed to practice proper breathing twice daily. The patient is also instructed to practice limited progressive muscle relaxation (i.e., one tensing-releasing sequence per muscle group) on every other day during this week of training.

For relaxation training to be maximally effective, the patient should use the skills acquired as an active coping strategy (235, 285). Thus, once the patient has begun to exhibit mastery of proper breathing, usually after 1 week of practice, the patient is instructed to practice the following applied breathing exercise roughly once every half hour while awake or each time the patient encounters a designated cue (e.g., small piece of tape on the time pieces in the patient's home and work environments). The patient is to first check the breathing rhythm. If it is proper breathing, the patient should smile and silently say, "What a nice thing to do for my body." If the breathing is rapid (shallow mouth breathing) the patient should silently say, "Proper breathing is better for my body." The patient then initiates proper breathing, allows the jaw to slightly lower and the body to relax, and recalls the feelings of deep relaxation (e.g., heaviness, warmth, calm). Once relaxed, usually after several minutes, the patient smiles and silently says, "What a nice thing to do for my body." The patient is also instructed to use the applied breathing exercise when encountering any annoyance or frustration, no matter how minor. On such occasions the patient is instructed to smile and say, "It's silly to get my body uptight and uncomfortable about this," complete the applied breathing exercise, and then smile and silently say, "It's healthier to keep my body relaxed no matter how disturbing things may seem."

Training and practice of the applied breathing exercise becomes the focus of the fourth week of training. The patient is also instructed to practice proper breathing once daily and limited progressive muscle relaxation on every other day during the fourth week.

Phase 3: Dissociative Visualization The final phase of this integrative approach to relaxation training involves dissociative visualization. Dissociative visualization is designed to induce "mental" relaxation as well as the relaxation response. It calls for the patient to master the ability of passive focusing on some personally meaningful, pleasing, relaxing, and absorbing memory or image. The patient is instructed to assume the relaxing posture used in the previous training phases, close the eyes, and use the applied breathing exercise to induce the relaxation response. Then, the patient is instructed to passively focus attention on the designated imagery and to allow complete absorption by the image and awareness of the sensory information inherent in the image (e.g., colors, sounds). Passive focusing is perhaps the most important element in relaxing at this point because distracting thoughts may occur, at least initially. The patient is informed that such intrusions may occur but that they do not mean the procedure is being performed incorrectly. Ideally, intrusions are best dealt with through the imagery rather than actively resisted. For example, the image may be one of a quiet beautiful lake nestled in a remote mountain valley. It reflects the brilliant warm sun by day and the distant stars by night. By day, distracting thoughts can become birds that fly from this peaceful sanctuary. By night, they become shooting stars that quickly disappear from the peaceful sky.

Training and practice sessions in dissociative visualization usually last 15–20 min, and are the focus of the fifth week of training. The patient is also instructed to continue practicing the applied breathing exercise daily and limited progressive muscle relaxation once every third day.

Week six of the training focuses on the practice of dissociative visualization as an active coping strategy either singly or in combination with the applied breathing exercise. The practice of limited progressive muscle relaxation once every third day is also prescribed. Thereafter, the patient may elect to adhere to the practice schedule of week 6, or focus on using the one or two procedures found to be most helpful. Regardless, periodic practice of each of the training procedures is strongly recommended so that the derived applied coping strategies do not lose their effectiveness.

Handling Adverse Patient Reactions

Relaxation training procedures designed to induce a low level of arousal may be aversive to some patients. When this occurs, care needs to be taken to determine if this is secondary to tension serving to defend against the florid expression of affectively laden material, for example, or if the tension and attendant pain represent internally augmented information that compensates for an extant and aversive state of low arousal (294). The latter is suspected if the patient has a history of seeking high-arousal activities and environments. In the former case, psychotherapy may be necessary before relaxation training can be initiated. If the latter is the case, relaxation training procedures should provide more adaptive ways to enhance arousal. High-arousal activities that are within any physical limitations posed by the patient's pain problem (e.g., games, dancing, jogging, bicycling, swimming, rowing) can be substituted for progressive muscle relaxation. Proper breathing can be modified such that the retention of breath is prolonged one count, which will serve to heighten arousal. Finally, dissociative visualization should employ high-arousal imagery (e.g., mountain climbing, sky diving).

Although relaxation training can be considered a benign treatment intervention, untoward reactions may occur. Most of these reactions are not cause for alarm (e.g., myoclonic jerks, cramping, muscle soreness, transient respiratory difficulties, dissociation), and usually reflect mild decompressive effects, high levels of tension, disuse effects, increased awareness of tension, or exposure to the unfamiliar state of low arousal. Although such occurrences may be unsettling for the patient, they readily resolve as training progresses or with reassurance that they will subside as the patient becomes familiar and comfortable with states of wakeful low arousal. Two untoward reactions, however, warrant the special attention of the practitioner and patient. Relaxation training may partially or completely restore physiologic dysfunction as a by-product of the general homeostasis facilitated by regular induction of the relaxation response. For example, patients taking antihypertensive medication, thyroid medication, and antidiabetic medication should be carefully monitored for possible symptoms of functional overdose. The hypertensive patient should be alert to hypotensive reactions marked by dizziness and/or light-headedness. The patient with hypothyroidism should be alert to heat intolerance, increased appetite, weight loss, increased nervousness or restlessness, increased activity or energy level, decreased need for sleep, and tremor. The diabetic should be alert to tremulousness, tachycardia, mental slowing, confusion, hypoglycemia, excessive thirst, excessive urination, excessive eating, intense itching, and weakness. Relaxation training should be temorarily discontinued with such occurrences and the prescribing physician consulted regarding medication adjustments.

Relaxation training may also precipitate an emotional decompression ranging from tearfulness to florid affective expression or abreaction. These expressions, usually of grief or anger or fear, occur when physiologic tension associated with psychological conflict is reduced. Although this is generally not cause for alarm, relaxation training may have to be temporarily discontinued in lieu of psychotherapy and/or continued within the context of psychotherapy.

CONCLUSIONS

Whereas conclusions regarding the efficacy of biofeedback in the reduction and/or management of chronic pain remain equivocal, sufficient scientific evidence has emerged substantiating the efficacy of relaxation training to warrant its use in the reduction of chronic pain. In addition, relaxation is cost-effective, found congenial by most chronic pain patients, and perceived by most patients as an effective treatment. In the study of chronic pain patients' perceived effectiveness of various treatment components of a comprehensive pain management program reported earlier (L.A. Gaupp, unpublished information), the integrative approach to relaxation training described above emerged as the second most helpful pain management strategy behind hypnosis/self-hypnosis. These authors would hold that for a chronic pain management strategy to be maximally effective it must: be congenial to the patient; restore and/or foster the often diminished sense of personal efficacy (292) exhibited by the chronic pain patient; be readily applied in vitro as an active coping strategy; offer a relatively immediate favorable impact on the perception of pain so that long-term in vitro utilization thereof is inherently reinforcing; and foster therapeutic benefit beyond the specific effect on pain. It is suggested that hypnosis/self-hypnosis and relaxation training not only meet these requirements but, when combined with operant strategies, which are more efficacious in increasing activity and decreasing medication usage than in the reduction of chronic pain (285), offer a reasonably comprehensive, efficacious, and cost-effective chronic pain management program.

ACUPUNCTURE

Acupuncture is one of the major therapeutic procedures of traditional Chinese medicine and, along with the use of herbs, has been in use for thousands of years. It had been standardized and was recorded in *The Yellow Emperor's Classic of Internal Medicine* 24 centuries ago (295). Its practice was consistent with Yin-Yang theory, the fundamental Chinese philosophy of active and passive principles of nature. Every entity was viewed as consisting of complimentary opposites, existing as parts of a whole, and inseparable from its relationship to other entities. Health was believed to result from a harmonious relationship of forces within the body and between the individual and nature. The major organs of the body, some of which were Yin and some Yang, were thought to be connected by 12 paired and 2 midline meridians or channels, which were named for the organs with which they were connected. In a state of health, vital energy (Qi or Chi) and four other fundamental substances flowed along these channels and harmonized the activity of the organs. Disease was believed to be associated with an imbalance of forces. It was corrected by inserting needles at appropriate points along the meridians at sites determined by the complex patterns of disharmony that were diagnosed (296, 297).

Acupuncture was first introduced to Western medicine in a book published in London in the latter part of the 17th century (298). It was used by a French physician in the early 19th century, and was condemned as reckless after an official investigation. There continued to be periodic references to its use in the medical literature, and a translation of a book on acupuncture published in France was available in the United States in 1825. In 1892 William Osler, in the first edition of his *Principles and Practice of Medicine*, recommended it as the most efficient treatment for acute lumbago, and commented that ordinary bonnet needles would do! However, acupuncture attracted little attention in American medicine until the early 1970s. Then, as a result of visits to China by western journalists and physicians, a widespread lay as well as medical interest developed in the phenomenon based on observations of surgery being performed under acupuncture anesthesia (299, 300).

USE OF ACUPUNCTURE FOR PAIN TREATMENT

Acupuncture involves inserting needles, usually stainless steel, 28–30 gauge, and approximately 1–10 cm in length, into selected anatomic points (297). Three hundred sixty-five points were recorded in the Yellow Emperor's treatise, but the number has differed subsequently. The depth of penetration varies, and a sensation of "take," described as tingling, numbness, and heaviness, is commonly experienced by the patient if the procedure is to be successful. The needle is twirled to facilitate the sensation of "take," and, once achieved, electrical stimulation may be applied.

Although acupuncture based on traditional concepts for the treatment of disease is practiced in the United States, particularly in areas with large Chinese populations, its major application has been for pain treatment. Classic acupuncture points as portrayed in ancient charts are commonly used. However, recent studies suggest that acupuncture need not be applied precisely at the classical points, and that stimulation close to the site of pain is generally more effective than stimulation at distant sites. Acupuncture analgesia has been attributed by some to a placebo effect, particularly after studies showed stimulation at nonacupuncture points was equally effective. However, it is likely that stimulation is effective within a large area. The production of analgesia in animals also suggests that the effect is not due to placebo alone. Further, it appears that needle puncture is not essential, and that an analgesic effect can be produced by various types of intense sensory stimulation (301). The relationship of acupuncture analgesia to afferent neural transmission is suggested by the demonstration that the analgesic effect is blocked by procaine infiltration of acupuncture points and by the observation that acupuncture points in hemiplegic limbs are ineffective unless sweating is present or there is other evidence that sympathetic nervous innervation is intact (297, 301).

The gate control theory as described by Melzak and Wall provided a possible physiologic mechanism to explain the relief of pain by acupuncture (302, 303). It now appears that this theory alone cannot account for this effect, since it was later shown that electrical stimulation of A fibers did not abolish the pain produced by C fiber stimulation (304). Melzak (303, 305) has subsequently postulated the existence of a central biasing mechanism at higher levels of the central nervous system that inhibits noxious stimulation when activated by intense somatic stimulation. A similar mechanism is thought to account for the pain relief produced by transcutaneous and dorsal column electrical stimulation. The existence of such a mechanism is suggested by the observation that stimulation of midbrain periaqueductal gray by electricity or opiates produces excitation of rostral medulla neurons and inhibits firing of trigeminal and spinal pain transmission neurons. As part of a negative feedback loop, the output of pain transmission neurons is an important factor in activating the pain suppression system (306). Some studies have suggested that the pain suppression mechanism may be mediated in part by endorphins. Pomerantz and Chiu (307) reduced the response to noxious heat stimulation in awake mice 54% by electroacupuncture, as measured by squeak response. Subcutaneous naloxone completely abolished this response. Mayer et al. (308) produced pain by electrostimulation of teeth in volunteers. Analgesia was produced by needling the Ho-Ku point on the hand. Significant analgesia was produced by acupuncture, compared to a no-treatment control group and a placebo group given saline injection. In a sample with a 20% increase in pain threshold, naloxone reduced the pain threshold to placebo levels, a significant difference compared to a saline-treated control group. Sjolund et al. (309) found a rise in an endorphin fraction in spinal fluid of patients with chronic pain who were being treated with acupuncture. Kiser et al. (310) studied endorphin levels in 20 patients treated by acupuncture for chronic pain syndromes. They found that symptom relief correlated with higher levels of met-enkephalin. However, other studies have not confirmed the reversal of acupuncture analgesia by naloxone. Chapman et al. (311) used acupuncture to reduce pain intensity, as measured by dental dolorimetry and smaller electroencephalograph evoked potential amplitude. Neither of these responses was reversed by naloxone. In a subsequent study Chapman et al. (312) were unable to demonstrate the reversal of dental acupuncture analgesia with a naloxone injection. Thus, the evidence linking endogenous opiates to acupuncture analgesia remains tentative.

Despite the metaphysical classical theory of acupuncture, and the conflicting results of attempts to understand its physiologic mechanism through scientific studies, a basic question of the clinician dealing with pain problems is—does it work? Although this question has been subject to serious investigation in the past 15 years, the answer is still unclear. Numerous anecdotal reports and clinical trials in both the Chinese and American literature have reported positive results (313, 314). However, in the absence of no-treatment or placebo control groups, no conclusions can be drawn. Millman (315), after a comprehensive review in 1977, took a rather skeptical stand, and while acknowledging reported pain relief in large, uncontrolled clinical studies in reputable institutions, concluded that suggestion and placebo effect have substantial roles. On the other hand, some early, controlled studies showed increased pain threshold and tolerance (308, 316, 317).

Some of the special problems encountered in research on the effect of acupuncture in pain have been described by Vincent and Richardson (318). Foremost of these it is the problem encountered in doing adequately controlled double-blind studies. In psychopharmacologic research, double-blind studies can be done with both the investigator and the patient unaware of whether an active or an inert substance is being given. In acupuncture studies, incorrect acupuncture points have been used as a control, but the acupuncturist is aware of the difference, and might transmit his expectations to the patient. Further, it appears that needle insertion even at incorrect points might produce some pain reduction. If so, the expectation that true acupuncture points should produce a significantly greater effect than bogus points would place an unrealistic expectation on demonstration of the effectiveness of acupuncture. On the other hand, bogus treatments such as taping needles to the skin have less credibility to the subject, and presumably less placebo power.

For these and other reasons, the overall quality of much acupuncture research has not been high. Richardson and Vincent (313) have recently done a thorough review of both controlled and uncontrolled studies of the use of acupuncture for the relief of pain. They evaluated a large number of uncontrolled studies that looked at the effects of acupuncture on mixed groups of pain patients. Although acknowledging that uncontrolled studies make a limited contribution to the evaluation of the effectiveness of acupuncture, they noted that most of these studies suggested that 50–70% of patients with chronic pain achieved clinically significant short-term pain relief, compared with the more commonly reported placebo response rate of 30–35%. Among controlled studies, they found headache and back pain to be the two most common pain disorders for which the effectiveness of acupuncture had been studied. In one study comparing acupuncture with a control condition, in which needles were inserted 1 cm from the correct point, true acupuncture reportedly had a significantly greater effect on tension headache than placebo acupuncture. In another study, comparing acupuncture with standard medical treatment for chronic headache, 58% of patients improved on acupuncture compared to 25% improvement on medical treatment. Thus there is evidence that acupuncture is an effective treatment for headache, although Richardson and Vincent believe there were methodologic problems in both studies that limited their validity. A carefully conducted study comparing acupuncture with placebo transcutaneous electrical nerve stimulation (TENS) revealed the commonly reported placebo response rate of 33% for the mock TENS, and at best an incremental response rate of 20% for acupuncture over placebo. Thus, Richardson and Vincent concluded that despite extensive claims for the effectiveness of acupuncture for the treatment of headache, the overall standard of research reports has generally been poor, and the result of the one adequately controlled study was not encouraging.

Richardson and Vincent's (313) review of controlled studies of acupuncture for low back pain included one study in which acupuncture was significantly more effective than spurious TENS, in which the skin electrodes were connected to a dummy electrical apparatus. In four of five studies they reviewed in which acupuncture was compared with needle insertion at incorrect sites, all but one of the studies reported substantial therapeutic effects of acupuncture. Although true acupuncture showed a tendency toward greater effectiveness than placebo, the difference was not significant. The one study that did not show substantial therapeutic effect was a carefully conducted study comparing locally anesthetized irrelevant acupuncture points with classical points. Using multidimensional evaluation and "blind" assessors, the overall success rate for acupuncture was reported to be 26%, compared to 20% for the control condition. Based on their review, Richardson and Vincent concluded that controlled studies suggest that a majority of back pain patients will derive clinically significant short-term benefits from acupuncture, with highly variable response rates ranging from 26 to 79%. Acupuncture shows no significant advantage over TENS, although the data show a trend in favor of acupuncture. Needling theoretically irrelevant sites showed no significant advantage over use of classical acupuncture points, although trends in the data marginally favored the latter.

From their exhaustive review, Richardson and Vincent (313) concluded that there is good evidence from controlled studies for the short-term effectiveness of acupuncture in relieving clinical pain. The reported success rate of 50–80% is greater than might be expected if the effects were mediated entirely by placebo response, which is generally in the 30–35% range. In studies comparing acupuncture with alternative treatment methods such as TENS and physiotherapy, the evidence is mixed, with the majority of studies finding no statistically significant advantage for acupuncture. Five studies comparing acupuncture at classical sites with needle insertion at random or theoretically irrelevant locations have found classical acupuncture to be significantly more effective, whereas six have found no significant difference in favor of acupuncture. Thus, Richardson and Vincent concluded that the significance of point location remains unclear.

USE OF ACUPUNCTURE ANALGESIA DURING SURGICAL PROCEDURES

Although many of the diseases treated with traditional acupuncture were associated with pain, it was not until the latter 1950s that the Chinese began using acupuncture anesthesia (or more accurately analgesia) for control of pain during surgical procedures (300). In the early use of acupuncture analgesia, multiple points were stimulated. Initially, for lung resection as many as 80 needles were used, but this was subsequently reduced and it is said that comparable results can be produced with one needle in the Nei-kuan point on the ventral forearm. One author described 29 acupuncture points as sufficient to produce analgesia for surgical procedures in any area of the body (297).

The impression of early visitors that most operations were successfully conducted under acupuncture analgesia was apparently inaccurate. Bonica (300) estimated that less than 10%, and perhaps no more than 1–2%, of the operations done in China during the 7 years prior to 1973 were conducted under acupuncture analgesia. Although reportedly effective in 90% of patients, the procedures rated as successful included patients who had obvious pain but for whom the operation could still be accomplished, as well as those in whom supplemental opiates and local anesthetic agents were used. The first American medical mission that visited China in 1974 believed that, using their own criteria, only 30–50% of the Chinese patients had pain relief that would be considered acceptable to American patients (300).

Acupuncture analgesia has not received wide acceptance in mainstream anesthesiology. In one standard text on anesthesiology its use in pain treatment is covered in one brief paragraph (319). It is said to apparently produce a relatively weak analgesia, through mechanisms similar to those in TENS, although less satisfactory because of the added expense and patient-therapist committment. In the chapter on obstetric anesthesia, it is mentioned as an example of various forms of psychological anesthesia such as hypnosis and natural childbirth, and dismissed as rarely used. Although the ability of acupuncture to alter pain perception can be accepted, the effect is not large, and apparently cannot alone account for the pain control observed in surgery. Psychological factors, not unlike those observed in natural childbirth, include careful selection of patients, explanations of what the patient can expect during the procedure, expectations that the patient will share responsibility for pain control, and contact with other patients who have undergone the procedure.

Few if any of the American anesthesiologists who have used acupuncture anesthesia on an experimental basis have seen fit to continue its application, presumably because of the high failure rate and unpredictable results, especially compared with the certainty of regional and general anesthesia (320). The Chinese are apparently more successful with the procedure because of intense preoperative counseling, their willingness to tolerate moderate to severe pain, the intense motivation provoked in the patient and the surgical team by shortage of anesthetic personnel and by political and ideologic factors, and the skill of Chinese surgeons and their willingness to accept less than optimal operating conditions. Other disadvantages of acupuncture include a 20–30-min waiting period before the onset of analgesia, the frequent need for needle placement close to the surgical field, the need for manipulation of needles by multiple acupuncturists, and the lack of muscle relaxation for abdominal procedures. Most of the patients receiving acupuncture anesthesia require supplemental analgesics or even anesthetic agents. For these reasons it seems unlikely that the use of acupuncture analgesia for surgical procedures will achieve any wide acceptance in the United States.

SUMMARY

Acupuncture is another treatment method that may be useful in some patients with pain complaints. Although sometimes used by inexperienced persons in an unscrupulous manner, it apparently can be useful when used ethically in appropriate settings. Although controlled studies have not yet fully resolved the questions of its efficacy, the preponderance of evidence seems to be that it is more effective than placebo. Like many other procedures such as TENS, hypnosis, and biofeedback, it apparently may provide relief for some patients for whom other methods have been unsuccessful. With the current intense research interest in pain mechanisms, and the increasing sophistication of treatment outcome studies, it can be anticipated that the role of acupuncture in the overall treatment of pain conditions will be further clarified.

PLACEBO ANALGESIA

Placebos may be defined as therapeutic substances or procedures that are deliberately given to have an effect on a system, syndrome, or disease, but that are without specific activity for the condition being treated (321). They can be viewed as medically doing something soothing when nothing curative can be accomplished (322). Substances given as placebos may be classified as to whether they are pharmacologically inert or whether they are pseudomedicaments, active medications that are ordinarily prescribed for a different condition or that are given in a subtherapeutic dose. Placebo effect may be defined as any effect attributable to a pill, potion, or procedure, but not to its pharmacodynamic or specific properties (322).

The use of placebos played an integral role in the practice of medicine for centuries, and in fact most of the therapies practitioners had at their disposal were actually placebos (322–325). Examples have included unicorn's horn, viper flesh, moss from the skull of a hanged criminal, eunuch fat, dried mummy, and oil of skinned puppy (323, 326). In ancient Egypt, according to the Ebers Papyrus in 1500 BC, patients were treated with such substances as lizard blood, crocodile dung, the teeth of an ass, putrid meat, and fly specs (323, 327). One scans the pages of Hippocrates in vain for any treatment of specific value (328).

The use of the quinine-containing cinchona bark, the introduction of which into Europe in the 17th century is attributed, perhaps erroneously, to the Countess of Chinchon, vicereine of Peru, is apparently the first example of a drug that was not a placebo. Sydenham, who demonstrated it was only effective for fever of malarial origin, contributed to the beginning of scientific medicine (329). Even after the introduction of effective drugs, many physicians recognized the limitations of their efforts and the role of factors other than their specific therapies. In 1859, Quimby stated that "Through a great many mistakes and the prescription of a great many useless drugs, I was led to re-examine the question, and came in the end to the position I now hold: the cure does not depend upon any drug, but simply in the patient's belief in the doctor or the medicine" (329). Oliver Wendell Holmes remarked that if all the drugs were sunk to the bottom of the sea it would be all the better for mankind and all the worse for the fish (330).

The use of the term *placebo* dates back to the 116th Psalm of the Hebrew Bible, which begins "I shall walk." Translated into Latin it became *placebo*, used in the 13th century in the sense of "I shall walk before" or "I shall please" (321, 322, 331, 332). The idea of doing something helpful in a difficult situation became associated with the meaning of the word "placebo." In 1787, Quincy's dictionary defined placebo as a "commonplace method or medicine" (321). In the 1951 *Dorland's Medical Dictionary*, it is defined as "an inactive substance or preparation, formerly given to please or gratify a patient, now also used in control studies to determine the efficacy of medical substance."

STUDIES OF PAIN RELIEF WITH PLACEBOS

Although prior to 1945 the word "placebo" had never appeared in the title of a medical article, there has since that time been an increasing interest, experimentally and clinically, in placebos (324, 329). Comparison of the effects of active analgesic drugs and placebo have been made in a variety of clinical settings. In a review of 15 clinical studies involving 1082 patients, the therapeutic effectiveness of placebo analgesia was determined (333). The patients suffered from a variety of conditions, including postsurgical wound pain, angina pectoris, and headache. About one-third of these patients received significant pain relief after ingesting placebos, a figure that is typical of most clinical studies. Placebo response has been reported for many types of pain, including postsurgical, labor, postpartum, angina pectoris, dental, cancer, arthritic, and peptic ulcer pain. Some clinicians probably underestimate the percentage of patients who will respond to placebo for pain control (324, 334). It is interesting to note that severe pain may be relieved by placebo in 35% of cases and that morphine may relieve pain in about 75% of cases (335). One might then speculate that about one-half of morphine's effectiveness is placebo effect.

The strength of the placebo response is exemplified by the many treatments that were miraculous when introduced, but proved to be no more effective than placebo when subjected to controlled trials. Benson and McCallie reviewed the use of medical and surgical treatments for angina pectoris that have subsequently been found to be ineffective (336). Between the 1930s and the early 1970s, the xanthenes, khellin, and vitamin E were introduced in turn. These were followed in the mid 1950s by internal mammary artery ligation and implantation. Before it was abandoned, 10,000–15,000 of the latter operations were done, with a mortality rate of about 5%. For all of these treatments uncontrolled trials indicated success rates in the 70–90% range, but controlled studies showed them to be no more effective than placebos. Internal mammary artery ligation was no more effective than a skin incision. The pattern was well recognized in the past. Armand Trosseau, an early 19th century physician, stated "you should treat as many patients as possible with the new drugs while they still have the power to heal" (327).

Experimental studies of the placebo effect have shown that placebo relief of pain is much less dramatic in experimental pain induced in the laboratory than in the clinical setting (331, 333). The former have shown an average pain relief of approximately 16%, compared to an average pain relief of 30–35% in the clinical setting. In studies of placebos and hypnosis in experimental pain, it has been found repeatedly that pain relief is related to the presence of anxiety (337). Apparently neither hypnosis nor placebo is as effective in producing pain relief unless some degree of anxiety is present (337, 338). In clinical pain, fear of its physical and economic implications, and its potential effect on important relationships to others introduce variables that increase the emotional suffering experience of pain. It is probably these components of the pain experience, which cannot be duplicated in the laboratory, that account for a significant part of the placebo effect.

THE PLACEBO RESPONSE

Not all studies show relief with placebo analgesia (339). It would be convenient to identify the situational and personality characteristics of placebo response. This is a complex area; however there are emerging data (340, 341). The patient's prior treatment experience is influential. Placebos were approximately twice as effective for patients for whom previous analgesics had been effective, compared to those who had had no previous analgesics or for whom they had been ineffective (342). Responsiveness was influenced by the nature of the pain, with pain of osteoarthritis more responsive than that due to rheumatoid arthritis. The classical observations of Beecher during World War II dramatically illustrated the importance of the meaning of the pain to the patient (343). He studied pain reports and the use of morphine in 215 soldiers who suffered major wounds in the European theatre during World War II. Only slightly more than 40% reported bad or moderate pain. Three-fourths of the total group of men wanted no morphine, even though they had received none for a matter of hours, and knew it was available for the asking. Beecher attributed the smaller need for morphine, compared to comparable civilian injuries, to the difference in the meaning of the wound. For the soldier it was a ticket to the hospital, and perhaps home, whereas for the civilian an accident is the beginning of a disaster. Other key elements related to predicting response to placebo analgesia seem to be related to the attitudes and expectations of the patient, attitude of the doctor, and the doctor-patient relationship (324). Patients who are treated by an individual who has a positive conviction about the treatment or drug potency seem to respond better (321). It has also been demonstrated that if the therapist conveys the concept of plausibility about a drug's potency there will be a better response (328, 341). Another potential predictor of placebo response is if the placebo is used for a pain syndrome that has previously responded to placebo analgesia in an experimental setting (344). The concomitant presence of distress or anxiety, as is often present in organic pain syndromes, has also correlated with placebo reactivity (322, 345). Other positive predictors may be the patient's faith in the treatment procedure with the expectation and anticipation of relief, previous positive experience with treatment, and the patient's acquiesence with the treatment (346).

The personality of the patient and his/her cultural attitudes about pain also play a part in the placebo response. Although some individuals are stronger placebo reactors than others, and seem to be characterized by enduring personality traits such as anxiety and social conformity, no typical placebo reactor personality has been consistently identified. One early study, using Rorschach data, suggested that the reactors were more anxious, dependent, emotionally labile, and preoccupied with their own internal processes (326). However, they were outwardly oriented and able to drain off their tension through talking with others. The placebo reactors were not "whiners" or "nuisances," not typically male or female, not typically young or old, and had the same average intelligence as nonreactors. In a preoperative period of stress, responders may behave in a more dependent yet outwardly responsive fashion and receive relief through attention from nurses and confidence in the effectiveness of drugs. A number of other investigators have analyzed the characteristics of placebo responses, with contradictory results. Some claim there is no predisposition to respond to placebos, whereas others find common denominators in responders. The most reasonable premise appears to be that there is no constellation of traits that will enable one to neatly pigeonhole people into responders and nonresponders. The placebo response will be determined by numerous factors, including the setting, the symptoms being treated, the specific medical figures involved, and the personality and past experience, anticipations, and fears of the individual (332).

The profile of nonresponders to placebo analgesia is not well delineated. In the past nonresponders have been characterized as being vague, nonspecific, rigid, hard to pin down, self-controlled, using denial, and not psychologically oriented (330, 346, 347). Unfortunately some medical personnel still regard the "placebo test" as a means of separating functional from organic pain (324, 348), and some practitioners have used placebos on "problem patients" about whom nursing staff had complained. In fact, the demanding, undesirable patients are reported to be the least likely to respond to placebos (324, 334).

MECHANISM OF ACTION OF PLACEBOS

The mechanism of action of placebos is not well understood and overlaps with the discussion of placebo responders. Potential mechanisms postulated include psychological, behavioral, and more recently, induction of the endogenous opioid system. From one perspective, placebos can be viewed as another active pharmacologic agent in their own right, whose analgesic effect can be independently evaluated using the same methods that would be used to test any other potent analgesic agent (321). Placebos can mimic certain characteristics of active drugs such as peak effects, cumulative effects, and carryover effects (349). Individuals receiving placebos have reported side effects such as nausea, thirst, headache, dizziness, insomnia, sleepiness, fatigue, depression, numbness, difficulty concentrating, hallucinations, feelings of cold or warmth, and itching (323, 337, 350, 351). It has also been suggested that tolerance to placebo analgesia may develop, as well as an abstinence-like syndrome when the substance is suddenly withdrawn (324). The above phenomena become particularly fascinating when considering a treatment modality that is not well understood from either a physiologic or psychological basis.

A review of the psychological and behavioral theories of action of placebos encompasses several topics. A regulatory effect produced by placebos has been proposed in that anxious and emotionally unstable individuals may well respond to placebo treatment (352). It has been proposed that such patients have a subjective reaction to illness, that a part of this reaction is anxiety, and that the role of the placebo in pain relief is primarily to relieve that anxiety (333, 353–355). Other authors have suggested the important role and powerful contribution of suggestion and the expectation that relief will be obtained (303, 356–359). The features of psychotherapy noted by Jerome Frank to be common to all psychotherapies, both primitive and contemporary, are similar to the factors that influence the effectiveness of placebos. These include a trusting relationship with a therapist in whom the patient has confidence, a setting that is identified as a sanctuary or place of healing (doctor's office or hospital), a plausible conceptual scheme accepted by the culture that enables the patient to explain and gain a sense of control over subjective distress, and a procedure based on the conceptual scheme that is believed to be effective (360). The effectiveness of the placebo will be influenced by its plausibility, and the intrisic character of the treatment. The latter would include such factors as taste, expense, and route of administration.

It has also been proposed that the placebo effect is a conditioned response that can be understood in terms of learning theory (359–361). For example, pills or injections of an active analgesic in the past have become associated with pain relief. Thus a similar stimulus, in this case an inert substance administered by mouth or by injection, will produce a conditioned analgesic response. It has been shown that both behavioral and physiologic responses can be conditioned in animals in this manner (321).

A proposed physiologic mechanism of action of placebos is related to the stimulation of endogenous opioids, although their role is still controversial (362). It has been suggested that placebo responders have increased levels of endorphins and that naloxone can reverse placebo-induced pain reduction (363). However, it appears that naloxone does not affect the placebo response in the absence of stress (362). The field is controversial and the data are not persuasive (332).

ETHICAL CONSIDERATIONS

Although the use of placebos is apparently not uncommon, most physicians would probably agree with the comments made by Richard Cabot, the eminent Harvard physician, 75 years ago (322), who expressed doubt that there "is a physician in this country who has not used them and used them pretty often," and deplored the fact that so many physicians believed it to be impossible to deal frankly and openly with patients. He argued against placebo use on the basis that the potential loss of trust in the physician by the patient and the community outweighed any short-term benefits. Although the deception might never be discovered, Cabot was of the opinion that it was not good for physicians to have their reputation rest on the expectation of not being found out. He countered the argument that patients will not be satisfied without medicine for every symptom by pointing out that the patient was not born with this expectation, but "learned it from an ignorant doctor."

On the other hand, many who recognize the ethical implications of placebo use believe that it may be justified in some situations, such as in temporary situations to placate the patient until a relationship can be established, in diseases for which placebos have proved efficacious experimentally, or in prolonged diagnostic testing during which the patient, if not placated, might not return for needed treatment. They also point out that there is a placebo component in almost every use of an active medication by a physician and that one should not withhold any remedy that affords some degree of relief (322, 330). However, the widespread use of placebos that some studies have revealed cannot be responsibly defended.

The *British Medical Journal* editorialized in 1952 that "a bottle of medicine is given as a placebo in about 40% of patients seen in general practice." In a 1952 analysis of 17,000 prescriptions in Great Britain, about one-third were considered to be placebos. This is close to Cabot's estimate in 1906 that placebos comprised 44% of prescriptions filled in Boston back bay drug stores (329). In a more recent study of placebo use by house staff and nurses, it was found that during a 6-month period nearly two-thirds of house staff had ordered placebos to see if a patient's pain was "real," 9 out of 10 had ordered placebos for patients they thought were asking for more pain medicine than the staff members thought necessary, and three-fourths had ordered placebos for patients the nurses were complaining about (334). Those who believe that placebos present an ethical dilemma would argue that this type of therapy is deceptive and risks the loss of patient trust. The possibility of nurturing unhealthy public attitudes also exists, in that people may become conditioned to expect medication for every symptom (322). Further, the practice does not take patient autonomy into consideration, nor does it honor the doctor-patient relationship or the right of informed consent.

CONCLUSION

Despite the remarkable technological advances made in medicine, there are many chronic conditions for which no cure is possible, and the most the physician can offer is symptomatic relief. For this group of patients particularly, the placebo effect can provide a significant benefit. This does not imply the intentional use of an ineffective or inert substance, but rather the conscious use of strategies that increase the expectiveness of any treatment.

Foremost of these is the doctor-patient relationship. Whatever increases the quality of this interaction will often facilitate treatment and contribute to the patient's comfort and symptom relief. A personal interest in the patient, demonstrated by a positive regard and nonjudgmental acceptance, are important ingredients of the relationship. A willingness to work with the patient to achieve the best possible result, to communicate through explanations and sharing responsibility for treatment decisions, and to provide plausible rationales for treatment modalities all potentially influence treatment response. One informative study compared the amount of morphine used by patients after undergoing abdominal surgery, who had received an explanation of the pain to be expected and instructions in relaxation techniques prior to surgery, with that used by a control group. The experimental group experienced significantly less pain and used significantly less morphine use (364).

Maximizing the placebo response to nonspecific therapies does not imply deception or an insincere and exaggerated assurance of benefits. Rather, it implies a manner that stimulates trust and inspires hope. In the context of a positive relationship, the placebo effect of modalities such as relaxation training, therapeutic exercise, diet, mild analgesics, and the like may be magnified, particularly if prescribed with a plausible rationale for their anticipated mental and physiologic effects. Within this type of relationship, placebos may even be openly prescribed. For example, if presented with an explanation as to the manner in which placebos can, through conditioning, have a genuine psychophysiologic effect, they can be introduced gradually into a patient's analgesic regimen on an unknown schedule with the concurrence of the patient. This strategy is often used in the behavioral component of pain treatment programs to facilitate reduction or discontinuation of narcotic-like analgesics. Used in these ways, within the context of positive doctor-patient relationships, the placebo response, which is actually inherent in and of greater or lesser importance to every therapeutic act, can be maximized and used as an integral part of the physician's healing armamentarium.

References

1. Hilgard ER, Hilgard JR: *Hypnosis in the Relief of Pain*. Los Altos, CA, William Kaufmann, 1975.
2. Ewin DM: Hypnosis in surgery and anesthesia. In Wester WC III, Smith AH Jr (eds): *Clinical Hypnosis: A Multidisciplinary Approach*. Philadelphia, JB Lippincott, 1984, p 210.
3. Shor RE: Explorations in hypnosis: a theoretical and experimental study. Doctoral dissertation, Brandeis University, 1959.
4. Hilgard ER: A quantitative study of pain and its reduction through hypnotic suggestion. *Proc Nat Acad Sci U.S.A.* 57:1581–1986, 1967.
5. Evans MB, Paul GL: Effects of hypnotically suggested analgesia on physiological and subjective responses to cold stress. *J Consult Clin Psychol* 35:362–371, 1970.
6. Hilgard ER, Ruch JC, Lange AF, et al: The psychophysics of cold pressor pain and its modification through hypnotic suggestion. *Am J Psychol* 87:17–31, 1974.
7. Knox VJ, Morgan AH, Hilgard ER: Pain and suffering in ischemia: the paradox of hypnotically suggested anesthesia as contradicted by reports from the "hidden observer". *Arch Gen Psychiatry* 30:840–847, 1974.
8. Shor RE: Physiological effects of painful stimulation during hypnotic analgesia under conditions designed to minimize anxiety. *Int J Clin Exp Hypn* 10:183–202, 1962.
9. Greene RJ, Reyher J: Pain tolerance in hypnotic analgesic and imagination states. *J Abnorm Psychol* 79:29–38, 1972.
10. Hilgard ER: Pain as a puzzle for psychology and physiology. *Am Psychol* 24:103–113, 1969.
11. Hilgard ER: Pain: its reduction and production under hypnosis. *Proc Am Philos Soc* 115:470–476, 1971.
12. McGlashan TH, Evans FJ, Orne MT: The nature of hypnotic analgesia and the placebo response to experimental pain. *Psychosom Med* 31:227–246, 1969.
13. Gottfredson DK: Hypnosis as an anesthetic in dentistry. *Dissert Abstr Int* 33(7-B):3303, 1973.
14. Wakeman RJ, Kaplan JZ: An experimental study of hypnosis in painful burns. *Am J Clin Hypn* 21:3–10, 1978.
15. Wolberg, LR: *Medical Hypnosis*. New York, Grune & Stratton, 1948.
16. Horan JS: Hypnosis and recorded suggestions in the treatment of migraine. *J Clin Exp Hypn* 1:7, 1953.
17. Blumenthal LS: Hypnotherapy of headaches. *Headache* 2:197, 1963.
18. Hanley FW: Hypnotherapy of migraine. *Can Psychiatr Assoc J* 9:254, 1964.
19. Harding CH: Hypnosis in the treatment of migraine. In Lassner J (ed): *Hypnosis and Psychosomatic Medicine*. New York, Springer-Verlag, 1967.
20. Greenleaf E: Defining hypnosis during hypnotherapy. *Int J Clin Exp Hypn* 22:120, 1974.
21. Anderson JAD, Basker MA, Dalton R: Migraine and hypnotherapy. *Int J Clin Exp Hypn* 23:48–58, 1975.
22. Andreychuk T, Skriver C: Hypnosis and biofeedback in the treatment of migraine headache. *Int J Clin Exp Hypn* 23:172, 1975.
23. Graham GW: Hypnotic treatment of migraine headache. *Int J Clin Exp Hypn* 23:165, 1975.
24. Maher LGP: Intensive hypno-autohypnosis in resistant psychosomatic disorders. *J Psychosom Res* 19:361–365, 1975.
25. Cedercreutz C, Lahteenmaki R, Tulikoura J: Hypnotic treatment of headache and vertigo in skull injured patients. *Int J Clin Exp Hypn* 24:195–200, 1976.
26. Daniels LK: The effects of automated hypnosis and hand warming on migraine: a pilot study. *Am J Clin Hypn* 19:91–94, 1976.
27. Daniels LK: Treatment of migraine headache by hypnosis and behavior therapy: a case study. *Am J Clin Hypn* 19:241–244, 1977.
28. Kroger WS, Fezler WD: *Hypnosis and Behavior Modification: Imagery Conditioning*. Philadelphia, JB Lippincott, 1976.
29. Kroger WS: *Clinical and Experimental Hypnosis*. Philadelphia, JB Lippincott, 1977.
30. Stambaugh EE, House AE: Multimodality treatment of migraine headache: a case study utilizing biofeedback, relaxation, autogenic and hypnotic treatments. *Am J Clin Hypn* 19:235–240, 1977.
31. De Piano FA, Salzberg HC: Clinical applications of hypnosis to three psychosomatic disorders. *Psychol Bull* 86:1223–1235, 1979.
32. Wain HJ: Pain control through use of hypnosis. *Am J Clin Hypn* 23:41–46, 1980.
33. Friedman H, Taub HA: An evaluation of hypnotic susceptibility and peripheral temperature elevation in the treatment of migraine. *Am J Clin Hypn* 24:172–182, 1982.
34. Howard L, Reardon JP, Tosi D: Modifying migraine headache through rational stage directed hypnotherapy: a cognitive-experiential perspective. *Int J Clin Exp Hypn* 30:257–269, 1982.
35. Milne G: Hypnobehavioral medicine in a university counselling centre. *Aust J Clin Exp Hypn* 10:13–26, 1982.
36. Milne G: Hypnotherapy with migraine. *Aust J Clin Exp Hypn* 11:23–32, 1983.
37. Toomey TC, Sanders S: Group hypnotherapy as an active control strategy in chronic pain. *Am J Clin Hypn* 26:20–25, 1983.
38. De Shazer S: The imaginary pill technique. *J Strat Syst Ther* 3:30–34, 1984.
39. Friedman H, Taub HA: Brief psychological training procedures in migraine treatment. *Am J Clin Hypn* 26:187–200, 1984.
40. Kapelis L: Hypnosis in a behaviour therapy framework for the treatment of migraine in children. *Aust J Clin Exp Hypn* 12:123–126, 1984.
41. Erickson MH: Special techniques of brief hypnotherapy. *J Clin Exp Hypn* 2:109, 1954.
42. Levit HI: Depression, back pain and hypnosis. *Am J Clin Hypn* 15:266, 1973.
43. Melzack R, Perry C: Self-regulation of pain: the use of alpha-feedback and hypnotic training for the control of chronic pain. *Exp Neurol* 46:452–469, 1975.

44. Crasilneck HB: Hypnosis in the control of chronic low back pain. *Am J Clin Hypn* 22:71–78, 1979.
45. Johnson LS, Wiese KF: Live versus tape-recorded assessments of hypnotic responsiveness in pain-control patients. *Int J Clin Exp Hypn* 27:74–84, 1979.
46. Lemmon KW: Chronic lower back pain differentiation of the real and imagined. *Med Hypnoanal* 4:17–30, 1983.
47. Michels PJ, Adams DB, McBride P: Chronic pain. *J Fam Prac* 17:591–610, 1983.
48. Butler B: The use of hypnosis in the care of the cancer patient. *Cancer* 7:1–14, 1954.
49. Butler B: The use of hypnosis in the care of the cancer patient. (Part I). *Br J Med Hypnot* 6(2):2–12, 1954.
50. Butler B: The use of hypnosis in the care of the cancer patient. (Part II). *Br J Med Hypnot* 6(3):2–12, 1955.
51. Butler B: The use of hypnosis in the care of the cancer patient. (Part III). *Br J Med Hypnot* 6(4):9–17, 1955.
52. Hedge AR: Hypnosis in cancer. *Br J Med Hypn* 12:2, 1960.
53. Lea P, Ware P, Monroe R: The hypnotic control of intractable pain. *Am J Clin Hypn* 3:3–8, 1960.
54. Cangello VW: The use of the hypnotic suggestion for relief in malignant disease. *Int J Clin Exp Hypn* 9:17–22, 1961.
55. Caricoppa JM: Hypnosis in terminal cancer. *Am J Clin Hypn* 5:205, 1963.
56. Cangello VW: Hypnosis for the patient with cancer. *Am J Clin Hypn* 4:215–226, 1962.
57. Sacerdote P: Additional contributions to the hypnotherapy of the advanced cancer patient. *Am J Clin Hypn* 7:308–319, 1965.
58. Sacerdote P: Theory and practice of pain control in malignancy and other protracted or recurring painful illnesses. *Int J Clin Exp Hypn* 18:160–180, 1970.
59. Sacerdote P: Some individualized psychotherapeutic techniques. *Int J Clin Exp Hypn* 20:1–14, 1972.
60. Sacerdote P: Convergence of expectations: an essential component of successful hypnotherapy. *Int J Clin Exp Hypn* 22:95–115, 1974.
61. Chong TM: The use of hypnosis in the management of patients with cancer. *Singapore Med J* 9:211–214, 1968.
62. LaBaw WL: Terminal hypnosis in lieu of terminal hospitalization: an effective alternative in fortunate cases. *Gerontol Clin* 11:312–320, 1969.
63. Crasilneck HB, Hall JA: Clinical hypnosis in problems of pain. *Am J Clin Hypn* 15:153–161, 1973.
64. Crasilneck HB, Hall JA: *Clinical Hypnosis: Principles and Applications*. New York, Grune & Stratton, 1975.
65. Willard RD: Perpetual trance as a means of controlling pain in the treatment of terminal cancer with hypnosis. *J Am Inst Hypn* 15:111–131, 1974.
66. Clawson TH: The hypnotic control of blood flow and pain and the potential use of hypnosis in the treatment of cancer. *Am J Clin Hypn* 17:160, 1975.
67. Margolis C: Hypnotic imagery with cancer patients. *Am J Clin Hypn* 25:128–134, 1982.
68. Araoz DL: Use of hypnotic techniques with oncology patients. *J Psychosoc Oncol* 1:47–54, 1983.
69. Davidson GP: Hypnotic augmentation of terminal care chemoanalgesia. *Aust J Clin Exp Hypn* 12:133–134, 1984.
70. Bachet M, Weiss C: Treatment of disorders of amputated subjects by hypnotic inhibition. *Br J Med Hypn* 4:15, 1952.
71. Dorcus RM: *Hypnosis and Its Therapeutic Applications*. New York, McGraw-Hill, 1956.
72. Papermaster AA, Doberneck RC, Bonello FJ, et al: Hypnosis in surgery: II. Pain. *Am J Clin Hypn* 2:220–224, 1960.
73. Chappell DT: Hypnosis and spasticity in paraplegia. *Am J Clin Hypn* 7:33, 1964.
74. Cedercreutz C, Uusitalo E: Hypnotic treatment of phantom sensations in 37 amputees. In Lassner J (ed): *Hypnosis and Psychosomatic Medicine*. New York, Springer-Verlag, 1967, pp 65–66.
75. Siegel EF: Control of phantom limb pain by hypnosis. *Am J Clin Hypn* 21:285–286, 1979.
76. Baker SR: Amelioration of phantom-organ pain with hypnosis and behavior modification: brief case report. *Psychol Rep* 55:847–850, 1984.
77. Swerdlow B: A rapid hypnotic technique in a case of atypical facial neuralgia. *Headache* 24:104–109, 1984.
78. Stam HJ, McGrath PA, Brooke RI, et al: Hypnotizability and the treatment of chronic facial pain. *Int J Clin Exp Hypn* 34:182–191, 1986.
79. Cheek DB: Therapy of persistent pain states: part 1, neck and shoulder pain of five years' duration. *Am J Clin Hypn* 8:281, 1966.
80. Williams JA: Ericksonian hypnotherapy of intractable shoulder pain. *Am J Clin Hypn* 26:26–29, 1983.
81. Elkins GR: Hypnosis in the treatment of myofibrositis and anxiety: a case report. *Am J Clin Hypn* 27:26–30, 1984.
82. Gould SS, Tissler DM: The use of hypnosis in the treatment of herpes simplex II. *Am J Clin Hypn* 26:171–174, 1984.
83. Smith SJ, Balaban AB: A multidimensional approach to pain relief: case report of a patient with systemic lupus erythematosus. *Int J Clin Exp Hypn* 31:72–81, 1983.
84. Zane MD: The hypnotic situation and change in ulcer pain. *Int J Clin Exp Hypn* 14:292–304, 1966.
85. Graham G: Hypnoanalysis in dental practice. *Am J Clin Hypn* 16:178–187, 1974.
86. Golan HP: Control of fear reaction in dental patients by hypnosis: three case reports. *Am J Clin Hypn* 13:279–284, 1971.
87. Schneck JM: Hypnotherapy for vaginismus. *Int J Clin Exp Hypn* 13:92, 1965.
88. Sachs LB, Feuerstein M, Vitale JH: Hypnotic self-regulation of chronic pain. *Am J Clin Hypn* 20:106–113, 1977.
89. Lehew JL: The use of hypnosis in the treatment of musculoskeletal disorders. *Am J Clin Hypn* 13:131–134, 1980.
90. Domangue BB, Margolis CG, Leiberman D, et al: Biochemical correlates of hypnoanalgesia in arthritic pain patients. *J Clin Psychiatry* 46:235–238, 1985.
91. Friedman H, Taub HA: Brief psychological training procedures in migraine treatment. *Am J Clin Hypn* 26:187–200, 1984.
92. Orne MT: Hypnotic control of pain: toward a clarification of the different psychological processes involved. *Res Publ Assoc Res Nerv Ment Dis* 58:155–172, 1980.
93. Goldstein A, Hilgard ER: Lack of influence of the morphine antagonist naloxone on hypnotic analgesia. *Proc Nat Acad Sci U.S.A.* 72:2041–2043, 1975.
94. Barber J, Mayer D: Evaluation of the efficacy and neural mechanism of a hypnotic analgesia procedure in experimental and clinical dental pain. *Pain* 4:41–48, 1977.
95. Hilgard ER: Hypnosis and pain. In Sternbach RA (ed): *The Psychology of Pain*. New York, Raven Press, 1980, p 219.
96. Stephenson JBP: Reversal of hypnosis-induced analgesia by naloxone. *Lancet* 2:991–992, 1978.
97. Terenius L, Wahlstrom A: Endorphins and clinical pain, an overview. *Adv Exp Med Biol* 116:262–277, 1979.
98. Frid M, Singer G: Hypnotic analgesia in conditions of stress

is partially reversed by naloxone. *Psychopharmacology* 63:211–215, 1979.
99. Sternbach RA: On strategies for identifying neurochemical correlates of hypnotic analgesia: a brief communication. *Int J Clin Exp Hypn* 30:251–256, 1982.
100. Benson H: *The Relaxation Response.* New York, WIlliam Morrow, 1975.
101. Budzynski TH, Stoyva JM, Adler CS, et al: EMG biofeedback and tension headache: a controlled outcome study. *Psychosom Med* 35:484–496, 1973.
102. Cox DJ, Fveundlich A, Meyer RG: Differential effectiveness of electromyograph feedback, verbal relaxation instructions, and medication placebo with tension headaches. *J Consult Clin Psychol* 43:892–898, 1975.
103. Haynes SN, Griffin P, Mooney D, et al: Electromyographic biofeedback and relaxation instructions in the treatment of muscle contraction headaches. *Behav Ther* 6:672–678, 1975.
104. Chesney MA, Shelton JL: A comparison of muscle relaxation and electromyogram biofeedback treatments for muscle contraction headaches. *J Behav Ther Exp Psychiatry* 7:221–225, 1976.
105. Hutchings DF, Reinkingy RH: Tension headaches: what form of therapy is most effective? *Biofeedback Self Regul* 1:183–190, 1976.
106. Reeves JL: EMG biofeedback reduction of tension headache. A cognitive skills training approach. *Biofeedback Self Regul* 1:217–225, 1976.
107. Kondo CY, Canter A: Time and false electromyographic feedback: effect on tension headache. *J Abnorm Psychol* 86:93–95, 1977.
108. Peck CL, Kraft GH: Electromyographic biofeedback for pain related to muscle tension: a study of tension headache, back, and jaw pain. *Arch Surg* 112:889–895, 1977.
109. Philips C: The modification of tension headache pain using EMG biofeedback. *Behav Res Ther* 15:119–129, 1977.
110. Budzynski T: Biofeedback in the treatment of muscle-contraction (tension) headache. *Biofeedback Self Regul* 3:409–434, 1978.
111. Tsushima WT, Hawk AB: EMG biofeedback treatment of traumatic headaches: a preliminary outcome study. *Am J Clin Biofeedback* 1:65–67, 1978.
112. Bruhn P, Olesen J, Melgaard B: Controlled trial of EMG feedback in muscle contraction headache. *Ann Neurol* 6:34–36, 1979.
113. Russ KL, Hammer RL, Adderton M: Clinical follow-up treatment and outcome of functional headache patients treated with biofeedback. *J Clin Psychol* 35:148–153, 1979.
114. Gray CL, Lyle RC, McGuire RJ, et al: Electrode placement, EMG feedback, and relaxation for tension headaches. *Behav Res Ther* 18:19–23, 1980.
115. Kumaraiah V: EMG biofeedback and progressive muscular relaxation in treatment of tension headache. *Ind J Clin Psychol* 7:1–5, 1980.
116. Schlutter LC, Golden CJ, Blume HG: A comparison of treatments for prefrontal muscle contraction headache. *Br J Med Psychol* 53:47–52, 1980.
117. Carrobles JA, Cardona A, Santacreu J: Shaping and generalization procedures in the EMG-biofeedback treatment of tension headaches. *Br J Clin Psychol* 20:49–56, 1981.
118. Philips C, Hunter M: The treatment of tension headache: I. Muscular abnormality and biofeedback. *Behav Res Ther* 19:485–498, 1981.
119. Satinsky D, Frerotte A: Biofeedback treatment for headache: a two-year follow-up study. *Am J Clin Biofeedback* 4:62–65, 1981.
120. Blanchard EB, Andrasik F, Neff DF, et al: Sequential comparisons of relaxation training and biofeedback in the treatment of three kinds of chronic headache or, the machines may be necessary some of the time. *Behav Res Ther* 20:469–481, 1982.
121. Blanchard EB, Andrasik F, Neff DF, et al: Biofeedback and relaxation training with three kinds of headache: treatment effects and their prediction. *J Consult Clin Psychol* 50:562–575, 1982.
122. Andrasik F, Blanchard EB, Edlund SR, et al: EMG biofeedback treatment of a child with muscle contraction headache. *Am J Clin Biofeedback* 6:96–102, 1983.
123. Bell NW, Abramowitz SI, Falkins CH, et al: Biofeedback, brief psychotherapy and tension headache. *Headache* 23:162–173, 1983.
124. Daly EJ, Donn PA, Galliher MJ, et al: Biofeedback applications of migraine and tension headaches: a double-blinded outcome study. *Biofeedback Self Regul* 8:135–152, 1983.
125. Janssen K: Differential effectiveness of EMG-feedback versus combined EMG-feedback and relaxation instructions in the treatment of tension headache. *J Psychosom Res* 27:243–253, 1983.
126. Onorato VA, Tsushima WT: EMG, MMPI, and treatment outcome in the biofeedback therapy of tension headache and posttraumatic pain. *Am J Clin Biofeedback* 6:71–81, 1983.
127. Ahles TA, King A, Martin JE: EMG biofeedback during dynamic movement as a treatment for tension headache. *Headache* 24:41–44, 1984.
128. Gada MT: A comparative study of efficacy of EMG biofeedback and progressive muscular relaxation in tension headache. *Ind J Psychiatry* 26:121–127, 1984.
129. Levine BA: Effects of depression and headache type on biofeedback for muscle-contraction headaches. *Behav Psychother* 12:300–307, 1984.
130. Werder DS, Sargent JD: A study of childhood headache using biofeedback as a treatment alternative. *Headache* 24:122–126, 1984.
131. Abramowitz SI, Bell NW: Biofeedback, self-control and tension headache. *J Psychosom Res* 29:95–99, 1985.
132. Daly EJ, Zimmerman JS, Donn PA, et al: Psychophysiological treatment of migraine and tension headaches: a 12-month follow-up. *Rehabil Psychol* 30:3–10, 1985.
133. Weranch HR, Keenan DM: Behavioral treatment of children with recurrent headaches. *J Behav Ther Exp Psychiatry* 16:31–38, 1985.
134. Lacroix JM, Clarke MA, Bock JC, et al: Muscle-contraction headaches in multiple pain patients: treatment under worsening baseline conditions. *Arch Phys Med Rehabil* 67:14–18, 1986.
135. Sargent JD, Green EE, Walters ED: The use of autogenic feedback training in a pilot study of migraine and tension headaches. *Headache* 12:120–124, 1972.
136. Sargent JD, Green EE, Walters ED: Preliminary report on the use of autogenic feedback training in the treatment of migraine and tension headaches. *Psychom Med* 35:129–135, 1973.
137. Johnson WG, Turin A: Biofeedback treatment of migraine headache: a systematic case study. *Behav Ther* 6:394–397, 1975.
138. Adler CS, Adler SM: Biofeedback therapy for the treatment of headaches: a five year follow-up. *Headache* 16:189–191, 1976.

139. Friar, LR, Beatty, J: Migraine: management by trained control of vasoconstriction. *J Consult Clin Psychol* 44:46–53, 1976.
140. Medtina JL, Diamond S, Franklin MA: Biofeedback therapy for migraine. *Headache* 16:115–118, 1976.
141. Mitch PS, McGrady A, Iannone A: Autogenic feedback training in migraine: a treatment report. *Headache* 15:267–270, 1976.
142. Reading C, Mohr PD: Biofeedback control of migraine: a pilot study. *Br J Soc Clin Psychol* 15:429–433, 1976.
143. Turin A, Johnson WG: Biofeedback therapy for migraine headaches. *Arch Gen Psychiatry* 33:517–519, 1976.
144. Feuerstein M, Adams HE: Cephalic vasomotor feedback in the modification of migraine headache. *Biofeedback Self Regul* 2:241–254, 1977.
145. Blanchard EB, Theobald DE, Williamson DA, et al: Temperature biofeedback in the treatment of migraine headaches: a controlled evaluation. *Arch Gen Psychiatry* 35:581–588, 1978.
146. Fahrion SL: Autogenic biofeedback for migraine. *Psychiatr Ann* 8:219–234, 1978.
147. Gainer JC: Temperature discrimination training in the biofeedback treatment of migraine headache. *J Behav Ther Exp Psychiatry* 9:185–187, 1978.
148. Sargent JD: Use of biofeedback in the treatment of headache problems. *Int Res Appl Psychol* 27:111–119, 1978.
149. Attfield M, Peck DF: Temperature self-regulation and relaxation with migraine patients and normals. *Behav Res Ther* 17:591–595, 1979.
150. Boller JD, Flom RP: Treatment of common migraine: systematic application of biofeedback and autogenic training. *Am J Clin Biofeedback* 2:63–69, 1979.
151. Drury RL, DeRisi WJ, Liberman RP: Temperature biofeedback treatment for migraine headache: a controlled multiple baseline study. *Headache* 19:278–284, 1979.
152. Lake A, Rainey J, Papsdorf JD: Biofeedback and rational-emotive therapy in the management of migraine headache. *J Appl Behav Anal* 12:127–140, 1979.
153. Silver BV, Blanchard EB, Williamson DA, et al: Temperature biofeedback and relaxation training in the treatment of migraine headaches: one-year follow-up. *Biofeedback Self Regul* 4:359–366, 1979.
154. Bild R, Adams HE: Modification of migraine headaches by cephalic blood volume pulse and EMG biofeedback. *J Consult Clin Psychol* 48:51–57, 1980.
155. Claghorn JL, Mathew RJ, Langen JW, et al: Directional effects of skin temperature self-regulation on regional cerebral blood flow in normal subjects and migraine patients. *Am J Psychiatry* 138:1182–1187, 1981.
156. Allen RA, Mills GK: The effects of unilateral plethysmographic feedback of temporal artery activity during migraine head pain. *J Psychosom Res* 26:133–140, 1982.
157. Houts AC: Relaxation and thermal feedback treatment of child migraine headache: a case study. *Am J Clin Biofeedback* 5:154–157, 1982.
158. Knapp TW: Treating migraine by training in temporal artery vasoconstriction and/or cognitive behavioral coping: a one-year follow-up. *J Psychosom Res* 26:551–557, 1982.
159. Gamble EH, Elder ST: Multimodal biofeedback in the treatment of migraine. *Biofeedback Self Regul* 8:383–392, 1983.
160. Gauthier J, Doyon J, Lacroix R, et al: Blood volume pulse biofeedback in the treatment of migraine headache: a controlled evaluation. *Biofeedback Self Regul* 8:427–442, 1983.
161. Jurish SE, Blanchard EB, Andrasik F, et al: Home versus clinic-based treatment of vascular headache. *J Consult Clin Psychol* 51:743–751, 1983.
162. Lahbe EE, Williamson DA: Temperature biofeedback in the treatment of children with migraine headaches. *J Pediatr Psychol* 8:317–326, 1983.
163. Lacroix JM, Clarke MA, Bock JC, et al: Biofeedback and relaxation in the treatment of migraine headaches: comparative effectiveness and physiological correlates. *J Neurol Neurosurg Psychiatry* 46:525–532, 1983.
164. Lichstein KL, Hoelscher TJ, Nickel R, et al: An integrated blood volume pulse biofeedback system for migraine treatment. *Biofeedback Self Regul* 8:127–134, 1983.
165. Marrazo MJ, Hickling EJ, Sison GF: The combined use of rational-emotive therapy and biofeedback in the treatment of childhood migraine. *J Rational-Emotive Ther* 2:27–31, 1984.
166. Reading C: Psychophysiological reactivity in migraine following biofeedback. *Headache* 24:70–74, 1984.
167. Fentress DW, Masek BJ, Mehegan JF, et al: Biofeedback and relaxation-response training in the treatment of pediatric migraine. *Dev Med Child Neurol* 28:139–146, 1986.
168. Blanchard EB, Andrasik F, Jurish SE, et al: The treatment of cluster headache with relaxation and thermal biofeedback. *Biofeedback Self Regul* 7:185–191, 1982.
169. Hoelscher TJ, Lichstein KL: Blood volume pulse biofeedback treatment of chronic cluster headache. *Biofeedback Self Regul* 8:533–541, 1983.
170. King AC, Arena JG: Behavioral treatment of chronic cluster headache in a geriatric patient. *Biofeedback Self Regul* 9:201–208, 1984.
171. McGrady AV, Bernal GA, Fine T, et al: Post traumatic head and neck pain, a multimodal treatment approach. *J Holist Med* 5:130–138, 1983.
172. Belar CD, Cohen JL: The use of EMG feedback and progressive relaxation in the treatment of a woman with chronic back pain. *Biofeedback Self Regul* 4:345–353, 1979.
173. Nouwen A, Solinger JW: The effectiveness of EMG biofeedback training in low back pain. *Biofeedback Self Regul* 4:103–111, 1979.
174. Freeman CW, Calsyn DA, Paige AB, et al: Biofeedback with low back pain patients. *Am J Clin Biofeedback* 3:118–122, 1980.
175. Jones AL, Wolf SL: Treating chronic low back pain: EMG biofeedback training during movement. *Phys Ther* 60:58–63, 1980.
176. Keefe FJ, Schapira B, Brown C, et al: EMG-assisted relaxation training in the management of chronic low back pain. *Am J Clin Biofeedback* 4:93–103, 1981.
177. Keefe FJ, Black AR, Williams RB Jr, et al: Behavioral treatment of chronic low back pain: clinical outcome and individual differences in pain relief. *Pain* 11:221–231, 1981.
178. Nigl AJ: A comparison of binary and analog EMG feedback techniques in the treatment of low back pain. *Am J Clin Biofeedback* 4:25–31, 1981.
179. Adams J, Pearson SC, Olson N: Innovative cross-modal technique of pain intensity assessment with lower back pain patients given biofeedback training. *Am J Clin Biofeedback* 5:25–30, 1982.
180. Wolf SL, Nacht M, Kelly JL: EMG feedback training during dynamic movement for low back pain patients. *Behav Ther* 13:395–406, 1982.
181. Flor H, Haag G, Turk DC, et al: Efficacy of EMG biofeedback, pseudotherapy, and conventional medical treatment for chronic rheumatic back pain. *Pain* 17:21–31, 1983.

182. Large RG, Lamb AM: Electromyographic (EMG) feedback in chronic musculoskeletal pain: a controlled trial. *Pain* 17:167–177, 1983.
183. Linton SJ, Melin L: Applied relaxation in the management of chronic pain. *Behav Psychother* 11:337–350, 1983.
184. Linton SJ, Götestam KG: A controlled study of the effects of applied relaxation and applied relaxation plus operant procedures in the regulation of chronic pain. *Br J Clin Psychol* 23:291–299, 1984.
185. Achterberg J, McGraw P, Lawlis GF: Rheumatoid arthritis: a study of relaxation and temperature biofeedback training as an adjunct therapy. *Biofeedback Self Regul* 6:207–223, 1981.
186. Bradley LA, Young LD, Anderson KO, et al: Psychological approaches to the management of arthritis pain. *Soc Sci Med* 19:1353–1360, 1984.
187. King AC, Ahles TA, Martin JE, et al: EMG biofeedback-controlled exercise in chronic arthritic knee pain. *Arch Phys Med Rehabil* 65:341–343, 1984.
188. Carlsson SG, Gale EN, Chman A: Treatment of temporomandibular joint syndrome in biofeedback training. *J Am Dent Ass* 91:602–605, 1975.
189. Carlsson SG, Gale EN: Biofeedback treatment for muscle pain associated with the temporomandibular joint. *J Behav Ther Exp Psychiatry* 7:383–835, 1976.
190. Funch DP, Gale EN: Biofeedback and relaxation therapy for chronic temporomandibular joint pain: predicting successful outcomes. *J Consult Clin Psychol* 52:928–935, 1984.
191. Stenn PG, Mothersill KJ, Brocke RK: Biofeedback and a cognitive behavioral approach to treatment of myofascial pain dysfunction syndrome. *Behav Ther* 10:29–36, 1979.
192. Sherman RA, Gall N, Gormly J: Treatment of phantom limb pain with muscular relaxation training to disrupt the pain-anxiety-tension cycle. *Pain* 6:47–55, 1979.
193. Dougherty J: Relief of phantom limb pain after EMG biofeedback-assisted relaxation: a case report. *Behav Res Ther* 18:355–357, 1980.
194. Tsushima WT: Treatment of phantom limb pain with EMG and temperature biofeedback: a case study. *Am J Clin Biofeedback* 5:150–153, 1982.
195. Schwartz DP, Large HS, DeGood DE, et al: A chronic emergency room visitor with chest pain: successful treatment by stress management training and biofeedback. *Pain* 18:315–319, 1984.
196. Hartman CH: Response of anginal pain to hand warming: a clinical note. *Biofeedback Self Regul* 4:355–357, 1979.
197. Bennink CD, Hulst LL, Benthem JA: The effects of EMG biofeedback and relaxation training on primary dysmenorrhea. *J Behav Med* 5:329–341, 1982.
198. Barth JT, Downs EJ: Post-herpetic neuralgia: a biofeedback case study. *Am J Clin Biofeedback* 4:104–106, 1981.
199. Blanchard GR: The use of temperature biofeedback in the treatment of chronic pain due to causalgia. *Biofeedback Self Regul* 4:183–188, 1979.
200. Thomas JE, Koshy M, Patterson L, et al: Management of pain in sickle cell disease using biofeedback therapy: a preliminary study. *Biofeedback Self Regul* 9:413–420, 1984.
201. Bird EI, Colborne GR: Rehabilitation of an electrical burn patient through thermal biofeedback. *Biofeedback Self Regul* 5:283–287, 1980.
202. Epstein LH, Abel GG: An analysis of biofeedback training effects for tension headache patients. *Behav Ther* 8:37–47, 1977.
203. Epstein LH, Abel GG, Colins F, et al: The relationship between frontal muscle activity and self-reports of headache pain. *Behav Res Ther* 16:153–160, 1978.
204. Beaty ET, Haynes SN: Behavioral intervention with muscle-contraction headache: a review. *Psychosom Med* 41:165–180, 1979.
205. Borgeat F: Some scientific feedback from biofeedback. *Acta Psychiatr Belg* 81:497–505, 1981.
206. Hart JD, Cichanski KA: A comparison of frontal EMG biofeedback and neck EMG biofeedback in the treatment of muscle-contraction headache. *Biofeedback Self Regul* 6:63–74, 1981.
207. Andrasik F, Holroyd KA: Specific and nonspecific effects in the biofeedback treatment of tension headache: 3-year follow-up. *J Consult Clin Psychol* 51:634–636, 1983.
208. Blanchard EB, Andrasik F, Neff DF, et al: Four process studies in behavioral treatment of chronic headache. *Behav Res Ther* 21:209–220, 1983.
209. Borgeat F, Gauthier B, Larouche LM: Muscle tension of patients with tension headaches during and between episodes of pain. *Acta Psychiatry Belg* 84:108–114, 1984.
210. Holroyd KA, Penzien DB, Hursey KG, et al: Change mechanisms in EMG biofeedback training: cognitive changes underlying improvements in tension headache. *J Consult Clin Psychol* 52:1039–1053, 1984.
211. Dalessio DJ, Kunzel M, Sternbach R, et al: Conditioned adaptation-relaxation reflex in migraine therapy. *JAMA* 242:2102–2104, 1979.
212. Gauthier J, Bois R, Allaire D, et al: Evaluation of skin temperature biofeedback training at two different sites for migraine. *J Behav Med* 4:407–419, 1981.
213. Gauthier J, Lacroix R, Coté A, et al: Biofeedback control of migraine headaches: a comparison of two approaches. *Biofeedback Self Regul* 10:139–159, 1985.
214. Biedermann HJ: Mechanisms of biofeedback in the treatment of chronic back pain: an hypothesis. *Psychol Res* 53:1103–1108, 1983.
215. Nouwevn A: EMG biofeedback used to reduce standing levels of paraspinal muscle tension in chronic low back pain. *Pain* 17:353–360, 1983.
216. Biedermann HJ: Comments on the reliability of muscle activity comparisons in EMG biofeedback research with back pain patients. *Biofeedback Self Regul* 9:451–458, 1984.
217. Bush C, Ditto B, Feuerstein M: A controlled evaluation of paraspinal EMG biofeedback in the treatment of chronic low back pain. *Health Psychol* 4:307–321, 1985.
218. McGeorge CM: Biofeedback and the headache. *NZ Psychol* 5:16–25, 1976.
219. Silver BV, Blanchard EB: Biofeedback and relaxation training in the treatment of psychophysiologic disorders: or are the machines really necessary? *J Behav Med* 1:217–239, 1978.
220. Belar CD: A comment on Silver and Blanchard's (1978) review of the treatment of tension headaches via EMG feedback and relaxation training. *J Behav Med* 2:215–220, 1979.
221. Blanchard EB, Ahles TA, Shaw ER: Behavioral treatment of headaches. In Eisler RM, Miller PM (eds): *Progress in Behavior Modification*. New York, Academic Press, 1979, vol 8, p 207.
222. Jessup BA, Neufeld RW, Merskey H: Biofeedback therapy for headache and other pain: an evaluative review. *Pain* 7:225–270, 1979.

223. Turk DC, Meichenbaum DH, Berman WH: Application of biofeedback for the regulation of pain: a critical review. *Psychol Bull* 86:1322–1338, 1979.
224. Adams HE, Feuerstein M, Fowler JL: Migraine headache: review of parameters, etiology, and intervention. *Psychol Bull* 87:217–237, 1980.
225. Cohen MJ, McArthur DL, Rickles WH: Comparison of four biofeedback treatments for migraine headache: psychological and headache variables. *Psychosom Med* 42:463–483, 1980.
226. Holroyd KA, Andrasik F, Noble J: A comparison of EMG biofeedback and a creditable pseudotherapy in treating tension headache. *J Behav Med* 3:29–39, 1980.
227. Kewman D, Roberts AH: Skin temperature biofeedback and migraine headaches: a double-blind study. *Biofeedback Self Regul* 5:327–345, 1980.
228. Nuechterlein KH, Holroyd JC: Biofeedback in the treatment of tension headache: current status. *Arch Gen Psychiatry* 37:866–873, 1980.
229. Sovak M, Dalessio DJ, Kunzel M, et al: Current investigations in headache. *Res Publ Assoc Res Nerv Ment Dis* 58:261–282, 1880.
230. Kremsdorf RB, Kochanowicz NA, Costell S: Cognitive skills training versus EMG biofeedback in the treatment of tension headaches. *Biofeedback Self Regul* 6:93–102, 1981.
231. Steiner SS, Dince WM: Biofeedback efficacy studies: a critique of critiques. *Biofeedback Self Regul* 6:275–288, 1981.
232. Ford MR: Biofeedback treatment for headaches, Raynaud's disease, essential hypertension, and irritable bowel syndrome: a review of the long-term follow-up literature. *Biofeedback Self Regul* 7:521–536, 1982.
233. Johansson J, Ost LG: Self-control procedures in biofeedback: a review of temperature biofeedback in the treatment of migraine. *Biofeedback Self Regul* 7:435–442, 1982.
234. Linton SF: A critical review of behavioral treatments for chronic benign pain other than headache. *Br J Clin Psychol* 2:321–337, 1982.
235. Turner JA, Chapman CR: Psychological interventions for chronic pain: a critical review. I. Relaxation training and biofeedback. *Pain* 12:1–21, 1982.
236. Barrios FX, Karoly P: Treatment expectancy and therapeutic change in treatment of migraine headache: are they related? *Psychol Rep* 52:59–68, 1983.
237. Haber JD, Thompson JK, Raczynski JM, et al: Physiological self-control and the biofeedback treatment of headache. *Headache* 23:174–178, 1983.
238. Holmes DS, Burish TG: Effectiveness of biofeedback for treating migraine and tension headaches: a review of the evidence. *J Psychosom Res* 27:515–532, 1983.
239. Kerns RD, Turk DC, Helzman AD: Psychological treatment for chronic pain: a selective review. *Clin Psychol Rev* 3:15–26, 1983.
240. Kewman DG, Roberts AH: An alternative perspective on biofeedback efficacy studies: a reply to Steiner and Dince. *Biofeedback Self Regul* 8:487–503, 1983.
241. Libo LM, Arnold GE: Does training to criterion influence improvement? A follow-up study of EMG and thermal biofeedback. *J Behav Med* 6:397–404, 1983.
242. Neff DF, Blanchard EB, Andrasik F: The relationship between capacity for absorption and chronic headache patients' response to relaxation and biofeedback treatment. *Biofeedback Self Regul* 8:177–183, 1983.
243. Thompson JK, Raczynski JM, Sturgis ET: The control issue in biofeedback training. *Biofeedback Self Regul* 8:153–164, 1983.
244. Diamond S, Montrose D: The value of biofeedback in the treatment of chronic headache: a four-year retrospective study. *Headache* 24:5–18, 1984.
245. Sorbi N, Tellegan B: Multimodal migraine treatment: does thermal feedback add to the outcome? *Headache* 24:249–255, 1984.
246. Spence ND: Relaxation training for chronic pain patients using EMG feedback: an analysis of process and outcome effects. *Aust NZ J Psychiatry* 18:263–272, 1984.
247. Trifiletti RJ: The psychological effectiveness of pain management procedures in the context of behavioral medicine and medical psychology. *Gen Psychol Monogr* 109:251–278, 1984.
248. Passchier J, van der Helm-Hylkema H, Orlekelke JF: Lack of concordance between changes in headache activity and in psychophysiological and personality variables following treatment. *Headache* 25:310–316, 1985.
249. Fichtler H, Zimmerman RR: Changes in reported pain from tension headaches. *Percept Mot Skills* 86:712, 1973.
250. Tasto DL, Hinkle JE: Muscle relaxation treatment for tension headaches. *Behav Res Ther* 11:347–349, 1973.
251. Warner G, Lance J: Relaxation therapy in migraine and chronic tension headache. *Med J Aust* 1:298–301, 1975.
252. Sallade JB: Group counseling with children who have migraine headaches. *Elem School Guid Counsel* 15:87–89, 1980.
253. Philips C, Hunter M: The treatment of tension headache: II. EMG "normality" and relaxation. *Behav Res Ther* 19:499–507, 1981.
254. DeBerry S: An evaluation of progressive muscle relaxation on stress related symptoms in a geriatric population. *Int J Aging Hum Dev* 14:255–269, 1981–1982.
255. Sherman RA: Home use of tape recorded relaxation exercises as initial treatment for stress related disorders. *Milit Med* 147:1062–1066, 1982.
256. Bhargava SC: Progressive muscular relaxation and assertive training in case of tension headache. *Ind J Clin Psychol* 10:23–25, 1983.
257. Jacob RG, Turner SM, Szekely BC, et al: Predicting outcome of relaxation therapy in headaches: the role of "depression". *Behav Res Ther* 14:457–465, 1983.
258. Hart JD: Predicting differential response to EMG biofeedback and relaxation training: the role of cognitive structure. *J Clin Psychol* 40:453–457, 1984.
259. Richter NC: The efficacy of relaxation training with children. *J Abnorm Child Psychol* 12:319–344, 1984.
260. Williamson DA, Monguillot JE, Jarrell MP, et al: Relaxation for the treatment of headache: controlled evaluation of two group programs. *Behav Mod* 8:407–424, 1984.
261. Blanchard EB, Andrasik F, Appelbaum KA, et al: The efficacy and cost-effectiveness of minimal-therapist-contact, non-drug treatment. *Headache* 24:214–220, 1985.
262. Janssen K, Neutgens J: Autogenic training and progressive relaxation in the treatment of three kinds of headache. *Behav Res Ther* 24:199–208, 1986.
263. Lutker ER: Treatment of migraine headache by conditioned relaxation: a case study. *Behav Ther* 2:592–593, 1971.
264. Hay KM, Maddens J: Migraine treated by relaxation therapy. *J R Coll Gen Pract* 21:664–669, 1971.
265. Andreychuk T, Skriver C: Hypnosis and biofeedback in the

treatment of migraine headache. *Int J Clin Exp Hyp* 23:172–183, 1977.
266. Smith TW, Denney DR: Relaxation training in the reduction of traumatic headaches: a case study. *Behav Psychother* 11:109–115, 1983.
267. Turner, JA: Comparison of group progressive-relaxation training and cognitive-behavioral group therapy for chronic low back pain. *J Consult Clin Psychol* 50:757–765, 1982.
268. Petty NE, Mastria MA: Management of compliance to progressive relaxation and orthopedic exercises in treatment of chronic back pain. *Psychol Rep* 52:35–38, 1983.
269. Sanders SH: Component analysis of a behavioral treatment program for chronic low-back pain. *Behav Ther* 14:697–705, 1983.
270. Newbury CR: Tension and relaxation in the individual. *Int Dent J* 29:173–182, 1979.
271. Stam HJ, McGrath PA, Brooke RI: The effects of a cognitive-behavioral treatment program on temporo-mandibular pain and dysfunction syndrome. *Psychosom Med* 46:534–545, 1984.
272. Stam HJ, McGrath PA, Brooke RI: The treatment of temporo-mandibular joint syndrome through control of anxiety. *J Behav Ther Exp Psychiatry* 15:41–45, 1984.
273. Gessel AH, Alderman M: Management of myofascial pain dysfunction syndrome of the temporomandibular joint by tension control training. *Psychosomatics* 12:302–309, 1971.
274. Raft D, Toomey T, Gregg JM: Behavior modification and haloperidol in chronic facial pain. *South Med J* 72:155–159, 1979.
275. Scott DS: Treatment of the myofascial pain-dysfunction syndrome: psychological aspects. *J Am Dent Assoc* 101:611–616, 1980.
276. Scott DS: Myofascial pain-dysfunction syndrome: a psychobiological perspective. *J Behav Med* 4:451–465, 1981.
277. Varni JW: Self-regulation techniques in the management of chronic arthritic pain in hemophilia. *Behav Ther* 12:185–194, 1981.
278. Quillen MA, Denney DR: Self-control of dysmenorrheic symptoms through pain management training. *J Behav Ther Exp Psychiatry* 13:123–130, 1982.
279. Dolan J, Allen H, Sawyer HW: Relaxation techniques in the reduction of pain, nausea and sleep disturbances for oncology patients: a primer for rehabilitation counselors. *J Appl Rehabil Counsel* 13:35–39, 1982.
280. Brena SF, Sammons EE: Phantom urinary bladder pain—case report. *Pain* 7:197–201, 1979.
281. Taylor CB, Zlutnick SI, Corley MJ, et al: The effects of detoxification, relaxation, and brief supportive therapy on chronic pain. *Pain* 8:319–329, 1980.
282. Kabat ZJ: An outpatient program in behavioral medicine for chronic pain patients based on the practice of mindfulness meditation: theoretical considerations and preliminary results. *Gen Hosp Psychiatry* 4:33–47, 1982.
283. Kabat ZJ, Lipworth L, Burney R: The clinical use of mindfulness meditation for the self-regulation of chronic pain. *J Behav Med* 8:163–190, 1985.
284. Linton SJ, Melin L, St Jernlof N: The effects of applied relaxation and operant activity training on chronic pain. *Behav Psychother* 13:87–100, 1985.
285. Linton SJ: Behavioral remediation of chronic pain: a status report. *Pain* 24:125–141, 1986.
286. Jacobson E: *Modern Treatment of Tension Patients*. Springfield, IL, Charles C Thomas, 1970.
287. Wolpe J: *The Practice of Behavior Therapy*. Elmsford, NY, Pergamon Press, 1969.
288. Bernstein DA, Borkovec TD: *Progressive Relaxation Training*. Champaign, IL, Research Press, 1973.
289. Brown BB: *Stress and the Art of Biofeedback*. New York, Harper & Row, 1977.
290. Schultz JH, Luthe W: *Autogenic Therapy: Autogenic Methods*. New York, Grune & Stratton, 1969, vol I.
291. Ford MR, Stroebel CF, Strong P, et al: Quieting response training: long-term evaluation of a clinical biofeedback practice. *Biofeedback Self Regul* 8:265–278, 1983.
292. Bandura A: Self-efficacy: toward a unifying theory of behavioral change. *Psychol Rev* 84:192–215, 1977.
293. Jencks B: Using the patient's breathing rhythm. In Wester WC II, Smith AH Jr (eds): *Clinical Hypnosis: A Multidisciplinary Approach*. Philadelphia, JB Lippincott, 1984, p 29.
294. de la Pena AM: *The Psychobiology of Cancer: Automatization Boredom in Health & Disease*. New York, Praeger, 1983.
295. Veith I: *Huang Ti Nei Ching Su Wen (The Yellow Emperor's Classic of Internal Medicine)*. Berkeley, University of California Press, 1966.
296. Kaptchuk T: *The Web That Has No Weaver*. New York, Congdon and Weed, 1983.
297. Lowe W: *Introduction to Acupuncture Anesthesia*. Flushing, NY, Medical Examination Publishing Co., 1973.
298. Quen J: Acupuncture and western medicine. *Bull Hist Med* 49:196–205, 1975.
299. Diamond E: Acupuncture, anesthesia, western medicine and traditional Chinese medicine. *JAMA* 218:1558–1563, 1971.
300. Bonica J: Anesthesiology in the Peoples' Republic of China. *Anesthesiology* 40:175–186, 1974.
301. Melzack R: Acupuncture and related forms of folk medicine In: Wall PD, Melzak R (eds): *Textbook of Pain*. Edinburgh, Churchill Livingstone, 1984, pp 691–699.
302. Melzack R, Wall P: Pain mechanisms: a new theory. *Science* 150:971–979, 1965.
303. Melzack R: *The Puzzle of Pain*. New York, Basic Books, 1973.
304. Nathan P, Rudge P: Testing the gate control theory of pain in man. *J Neurol Neurosurg Psychiatry* 37:1366–1372, 1974.
305. Melzack R: Prolonged relief of pain by brief intense transcutaneous somatic stimulation. *Pain* 1:357–374, 1975.
306. Basbaum A, Fields H: Endogenous pain control mechanisms: review and hypothesis. *Ann Neurol* 4:451–462, 1978.
307. Pomeranz B, Chiu D: Naloxone blocks acupuncture analgesia and causes hyperalgesia: endorphin is implicated. *Life Sci* 19:1757–1762, 1976.
308. Mayer D, Price D, Rafii A: Antagonism of acupuncture analgesia in man by the narcotic antagonist naloxone. *Brain Res* 121:368–372, 1977.
309. Sjolund B, Terenius L, Erikson M: Increased cerebrospinal fluid levels of endorphins after electro acupuncture. *Acta Physiol Scand* 100:382–384, 1977.
310. Kiser R, Khatami M, Gatchel R, et al: Acupuncture relief of chronic pain syndrome correlates with increased plasma met-enkephalin concentrations. *Lancet* 2:1394–1396, 1983.
311. Chapman C, Colpitts Y, Benedetti C, et al: Evoked potential assessment of acupunctural analgesia: attempted reversal with naloxone. *Pain* 9:183–197, 1980.
312. Chapman C, Benedetti C, Colpitts Y, et al: Naloxone fails to reverse pain threshold elevated by acupuncture: acupuncture analgesia reconsidered. *Pain* 16:13–31, 1983.

313. Richardson P, Vincent C: Acupuncture for the treatment of pain: a review of evaluative research. *Pain* 24:15–40, 1986.
314. Abstracts of the Second National Symposium on Acupuncture and Moxibustion and Acupuncture Anesthesia, Beijing, China, August, 1984.
315. Millman B: Acupuncture: context and critique. *Annu Rev Med* 28:223–234, 1977.
316. Anderson S, Erickson T, Holmgren E, et al: Electroacupuncture. Effect on pain threshold measured with electrical stimulation of the teeth. *Brain Res* 63:393–396, 1973.
317. Stewart D, Thompson J, Oswald I: Acupuncture analgesia: an experimental investigation. *Br Med J* 1:67–70, 1977.
318. Vincent C, Richardson P: The evaluation of therapeutic acupuncture: concepts and methods. *Pain* 24:1–13, 1986.
319. Miller R (ed): *Anesthesia*, ed 2. New York, Churchill Livingstone, 1986, vol 3, pp 1692, 2105.
320. Bonica J: Acupuncture analgesia and anesthesia. In: Eckenhoff JE (ed): *Controversy in Anesthesiology*. Philadelphia, WB Saunders, 1979, pp 185–200.
321. Jospe M: *The Placebo Effect in Healing*. Lexington, MA, DC Heath, 1978.
322. Brody H: *Placebos and the Philosophy of Medicine*. Chicago, IL, The University of Chicago Press, 1980.
323. Shapiro A: The placebo effect in the history of medical treatment: implications for psychiatry. *Am J Psychiatry* 116:298–304, 1959.
324. Reuler J, Girard D, Nardone D: The chronic pain syndrome: misconceptions and management. *Ann Intern Med* 93:588–596, 1980.
325. Critelli J, Neumann K: The placebo. *Am Psychol* 39:32–39, 1984.
326. Lasagna C, Mosteller F, VonFelsinger J, et al: A study of the placebo response. *Am J Med* 16:770–779, 1954.
327. Findley T: The placebo and the physician. *Med Clin North Am* 37:1821–1826, 1953.
328. Houston W: The doctor himself as therapeutic agent. *Ann Intern Med* 11:1416–1425, 1938.
329. Shapiro A: A contribution to the history of the placebo effect. *Behav Sci* 5:109–135, 1960.
330. Doongaji D, Vahia V, Bharveha M: On placebos, placebo responses and placebo responders (a review of psychological, psychopharmacological and psychophysiological factors). I: Psychological factors. *J Postgrad Med* 24:91, 1978.
331. Evans F: The placebo response. In Bonica J (ed): *Pain (Advances in Neurology 4)*. New York, Raven Press, 1974.
332. Lasagna L: The placebo effect. *J Allergy Clin Immunol* 78:161–165, 1986.
333. Beecher H: The powerful placebo. *JAMA* 159:1602–1606, 1955.
334. Goodwin J, Goodwin J, Vogel A: Knowledge and use of placebos by house officers and nurses. *Ann Intern Med* 91:106–110, 1979.
335. Beecher H: *Measurement of Subjective Responses: Quantitative Effects of Drugs*. New York, Oxford University Press, 1959.
336. Benson H, McCallie D: Angina pectoris and the placebo effect. *N Engl J Med* 300:1424–1429, 1979.
337. Sternbach R: *Pain: A Psychophysiological Analysis*. New York, Academic Press, 1968.
338. Thorn W: The placebo reactor. *Aust J Pharm* 43:1035–1037, 1962.
339. Khurmi N, Bowles J, Kohli R, et al: Does placebo improve indexes of effort-induced myocardial ischemia? An objective study in 150 patients with chronic stable angina pectoris. *Am J Cardiol* 57:907–911, 1986.
340. Woodforde J, Merskey H: Personality traits of patients with chronic pain. *J Psychosom Res* 16:167–172, 1972.
341. Liberman R: An analysis of the placebo phenomenon. *J Chronic Dis* 15:761–783, 1962.
342. Batterman R, Lower W: Placebo responsiveness—the influence of previous therapy. *Curr Ther Res* 10:136–143, 1968.
343. Beecher H: Pain in man wounded in battle. *Ann Surg* 123:96–105, 1946.
344. Bourne H: The placebo—a poorly understood and neglected therapeutic agent. *Rational Drug Ther* Nov, 1–6, 1971.
345. Merskey H: The status of pain. In Hill O (ed): *Modern Trends in Psychosomatic Medicine—3*. Boston, Butterworths, 1976.
346. Shapiro A: The placebo response. In Howells J (ed): *Modern Perspectives in World Psychiatry*. London, Oliver and Boyd, 1968, pp 596–613.
347. Fisher H, Olin B: The dynamics of placebo therapy—a clinical study. *Am J Med Sci* 232:504–512, 1956.
348. Hackett T: Chronic pain. In Sederer L (ed): *Inpatient Psychiatry: Diagnosis and Treatment*. Baltimore, Williams & Wilkins, 1983.
349. Lasagna L, Laties G, Dohan L: Further studies on the "pharmacology" of placebo administration. *J Clin Invest* 37:533–537, 1958.
350. Wolf S, Pinsky R: Effects of placebo administration and occurrence of toxic reactions. *JAMA* 155:339–341, 1954.
351. Haegerstam G: Placebo in clinical drug trials—a multidisciplinary review. *Methods Find Exp Clin Pharmacol* 4:261–278, 1982.
352. Medvedev V, Zavyalova E, Ovchinnikov B, et al: Functional structure of the placebo response. *Hum Physiol* 10:216–221, 1984.
353. Byerly H: Explaining and exploiting placebo effects. *Perspect Biol Med* 19:423–436, 1976.
354. Nash M, Zimring F: Prediction of reaction to placebo. *J Abnorm Psychol* 74:568–573, 1969.
355. Morris L, O'Neal E: Drug-name familiarity and the placebo effect. *J Clin Psychol* 30:280–282, 1974.
356. Wolf S: Effects of suggesting and conditioning on the action of chemical agents in human subjects—the pharmacology of placebos. *J Clin Invest* 29:100–109, 1950.
357. Petrie J, Hazleman B: Credibility of placebo transcutaneous nerve and acupuncture. *Clin Exp Rheumatol* 3:151–153, 1958.
358. Whitehorn J: Comment: psychiatric implications of the placebo effect. *Am J Psychiatry* 114:662–664, 1958.
359. Ullman L, Kraser F: Cognitions and behavior therapy. *Behavior Ther* 1:202–204, 1969.
360. Frank J: General psychotherapy: the restoration of morale. In Arieti S (ed): *American Handbook of Psychiatry*, ed 2. New York, Basic Books, 1975, vol 5, pp 124–125.
361. Voudouris N, Peck C, Coleman G: Conditioned placebo responses. *J Pers Soc Psychol* 148:47–53, 1985.
362. Ponser J, Burke A: The effects of naloxone on opiate and placebo analgesia in healthy volunteers. *Psychopharmacology* 87:468–472, 1985.
363. Levine J, Gordon N, Fields H: The mechanisms of placebo analgesia. *Lancet* 2:654–657, 1978.
364. Egbert L, Battit G, Welch C, et al: Reduction of postoperative pain by management and instruction of patients: a study of doctor-patient rapport. *N Engl J Med* 270:825–827, 1964.

chapter 16
Dysthymic Pain Disorder: The Treatment of Chronic Pain as a Variant of Depression

Dietrich Blumer, M.D.
Mary Heilbronn, Ph.D.

Pain is often the primary motivation for seeking the help of a physician, but is usually understood only as it relates to a somatic lesion. A substantial number of patients, however, challenge physicians with a persistent complaint of pain for which no physical origin can be found. Low back pain (1) and chronic headache (2, 3) are common examples, but the pain may be diffuse or of any location.

Physicians often become frustrated with such patients, and dismiss them as "crocks." Unfortunately, many physicians, including psychiatrists, are not aware that chronic pain not due to a physical lesion is now considered a distinct disease entity rather than a symptom of something else. A review of the literature indicates that chronic pain is a common clinical problem, but is poorly understood (4–11). Chronic pain may persist after transsection of nerves, rhizotomy, cordotomy, or even after total transsection of the spinal cord above the level of the painful region (12). No plausible neurologic theory has been proposed, yet the alternative concept of chronic pain as a psychiatric disorder has been little explored.

Our studies have led to the identification of a well-defined psychobiologic disorder, which we have termed the *dysthymic pain disorder* (13). Instead of an elusive somatic lesion, the variant of a very common disorder—of depression—tends to be implicated. Indeed, chronic pain can be viewed as the principal expression of a muted depressive state, that is, as a form of masked depression (5, 13–18).

Physicians must be wary not to consider the depression of these patients as merely a consequence of their constant pain. The bodily experienced suffering is part and parcel of a muted mental agony. Therefore, the search for a hidden physical cause must not be perpetuated.

Early recognition of the disorder is essential if disability is to be avoided. The drug treatment of dysthymic pain is identical to the treatment of depression. Drug therapy in combination with a behavior modification approach can be effective even for patients who have suffered for many years.

We had originally termed the dysthymic pain disorder "pain-prone disorder" in recognition of George Engel's pioneer studies (19). We subsequently adopted the term dysthymic pain disorder because it emphasizes the relationship to depression, the characteristic chronicity of the disorder, and the partly reduced symptom severity compared to that of major depression. The dysthymic pain disorder tends to be chronic, does not appear in bipolar form, and lacks psychotic features, but is characterized by a disabling degree of anergia.

PROFILE OF THE CHRONIC PAIN PATIENT

A general agreement on a link between chronic pain and depression is found in the literature (11), but little effort had been made to define it further. Our identification of the dysthymic pain disorder is based on the evaluation of approximately 2500 patients with chronic pain "of obscure origin." Over the years an increasingly comprehensive standardized psychiatric and psychologic evaluation of dysthymic pain patients was adopted. A remarkable homogeneity of traits among these patients has been observed (15–18), as summarized in Table 16.1. The characteristic psychiatric and psychological features of the entire group follow.

DEMOGRAPHICS

Men and women are equally affected by dysthymic pain. In a very few patients, onset of the chronic pain is dated as early as infancy and as late as the 70s; the mean age of onset is about 40 years, and the patients reach a pain clinic after their pain has persisted for an average of about 6 years. The average education completed by the patients is 12th grade. Although the entire spectrum of socioeconomic classes is affected, chronic pain is most prevalent among the lower middle class (blue-collar workers).

PREMORBID TRAITS

Patients with dysthymic pain disorder usually have a history of excessive work performance and generally relentless activity ("workaholism") prior to the onset of pain. This trait, which often takes the form of early work habits, has been termed "ergomania" (13, 17). Patients tend to come from families troubled by divorce, unfaithful parents, alcoholism, depression, or chronic pain (13).

Table 16.1
Characteristics of Dysthymic Pain Disorder

Family history	
Unipolar depression	
Alcoholism	
Chronic pain	
Crippled relative	
Premorbid traits	
Relentless activity	Ergomania
Overachievement	
Masochistic bonds	Masochism
Intolerance of success	
Clinical traits	
Continuous pain	Somatic presentation
Somatic preoccupation	
Anergia	
Anhedonia	Depressive features
Insomnia	
Depressive mood and despair	
Denial of conflicts	"Solid citizen"
Idealization of self and family relations	

They assumed precociously adult roles in support of the family and persist in viewing themselves as highly independent and more energetic than others. Their self-sacrifice in working for the well-being of the family is well motivated, but tends to be excessive. Self-sacrifice to the point of masochism is frequently evident in the past history of having submitted to an unfaithful, alcoholic, or physically abusive spouse for a prolonged period of time. The long-suffering patients display intolerance of success and, not so paradoxically, often develop chronic pain just when there is relief from the prolonged suffering of the abusive relationship. Frequently, a crippled next-of-kin is reported, serving perhaps as an object for unconscious identification with a victim (13).

In many patients, the listed premorbid traits are present in subtle form. The trend toward excessive physical activity and overachievement, however, is prevalent.

CLINICAL FEATURES

For the majority of patients who present with dysthymic pain, the suffering is continuous in nature—they wake up with the pain and go to sleep with it. Most display a more or less pronounced hypochondriacal preoccupation with the painful body parts. In many, a persistent desire for a surgical solution is evident. On an average, they undergo more than one surgical procedure for their pain, and the procedures provide little, if any, relief. Their entire misery is focused on the pain, and they desire to have it taken away by any means.

Most patients maintain an image of themselves as "solid citizens" in spite of years of disabling pain that often have rendered them dependent on relatives and the helping professions. They strongly deny difficulties in their interpersonal relationships, often describe their family relationships in idealized terms, still view themselves as independent, and resist a scrutiny of their personal lives. Many patients also suffer from clinical depression or alcoholism, preceding, alternating with, or concomitant with the chronic pain (5, 20, 21).

DEPRESSIVE FEATURES

Subsequent to the onset of pain, these patients tend to lose their initiative and zeal for work. The contrast between their frantic premorbid activity and their listlessness and helplessness after onset is striking. Their lack of energy (anergia) becomes associated with an increasing inability to enjoy social life, leisure time, and sexual relations (anhedonia). Premorbidly, with their relentless activity, they had already shown little ability to enjoy any leisure time or had preferred activity-oriented hobbies to more leisurely ones. The appetite is usually well maintained, but a sleep disorder often develops.

Anergia, anhedonia, and insomnia are highly characteristic traits of depressive disorders, but are almost invariably attributed to the pain by the patient. This is the prime reason why depression remains masked; the suffering is experienced more bodily than mentally. About one-third of the patients strongly deny being depressed and, although they may admit to feelings of despair, insist that it is because of the pain.

In his classic paper " 'Psychogenic' Pain and the Pain-prone Patient," Engel (19) discussed the theoretical and clinical problem of pain. He noted the common error made by physicians who assume that a patient is depressed because of the pain he experiences. On the contrary, Engel maintained that the experience of pain serves to attenuate the guilt and shame of the depression. Indeed, the pain not only masks the depressive mood, it may protect the patient from more intense depression and even suicide. Thus, pain comes to occupy a key position in the regulation of the entire psychic economy.

FAMILY HISTORY

We consider the genetic background a factor of great importance in the identification of chronic pain as a variant of depression. Every study has documented the high incidence of unipolar depression, alcoholism, and chronic pain among the families of patients with chronic pain, whereas bipolar disorders are rarely represented (13, 20–22). Thus, the evidence suggests that the dysthymic pain disorder may indeed belong to Winokur's depression spectrum disease (23). The recent finding that the patients themselves have a tendency toward clinical depression and alcoholism confirms the genetic relationships of the disorder (5, 13, 20, 21).

BIOLOGIC MARKERS

In recent years, it has become evident that patients with dysthymic pain share, to a significant extent, biologic markers found in patients suffering major depression. While abnormally shortened rapid eye movement sleep stage (REM) latency is found to a lesser degree in the dysthymic patient, abnormal sleep efficiency is at a very high level in both groups (13). Measurements of blood cortisol levels using the dexamethasone suppression test seem to correlate with the degree of depression found in the chronic pain patient (13, 24–27). Among the more depressed patients, one can expect a greater incidence of cortisol nonsuppression.

High levels of endorphins have been reported in both depression and chronic pain patients (28). Recently, the same researchers compared healthy volunteers with chronic pain patients and patients with definable neurogenic pain syndromes for depressive symptomatology, personality traits, and a series of biologic markers (29). Measuring 5-hydroxyindoleacetic acid and homovanillic acid in cerebrospinal fluid, platelet monamine oxidase activity, serum cortisol before and after dexamethasone suppression, and melatonin in serum and urine, it was possible to discriminate between the chronic pain patients and the other two groups.

PSYCHODYNAMIC FEATURES

In addition to rejecting any suggestion that their pain is a result of psychological factors, chronic pain patients have difficulty in expressing their feelings to other people (30). This indicates that the psychodynamics of patients with chronic pain are better understood if we consider the condition termed *alexithymia* (31, 32). A common finding in psychosomatic and addictive disorders, alexithymia is described by Stephanos (33) as a "psychosomatic phenomenon." The emotions tend to be undifferentiated and poorly verbalized and most are experienced in the somatic sphere; unawareness, blocking, and fear of affect prevail, and inability to mourn is marked. Individuals with alexithymia may appear very stoic, stone-faced, and stiff in posture; their thinking is oriented toward physical work and mechanical action, and they lack imagination and fantasy (34).

Such individuals make an overly compliant adjustment to reality and present with pseudonormality. The alexithymic individual tends to relate to others with apparent detachment, to care poorly for himself, and to relate to physicians with a child-like expectation to be cured. In our experience, the typical dysthymic pain patient presents all these characteristics for alexithymia, to a fault. They are, therefore, poor candidates for psychotherapy.

A summary of the psychodynamic issues characteristic of the dysthymic pain disorder, based on the sum of our clinical and test findings, is provided in Figure 16.1. The patients tend to show all the characteristics of alexithymia, as listed above. Beyond a detached attitude, a crucial set of core issues determines a dilemma: The patient has strong needs to be accepted, to depend on others, to receive affection, and to be cared for, yet he has never acknowledged these basic child-like needs. Guilt is easily provoked by anything socially unacceptable and is anxiously concealed and controlled; any hostile-aggressive trends are also denied. Anger and aggression, being overcontrolled, are turned inward against oneself (masochism). The inner insecurity and guilt may be soothed, and a certain degree of acceptance gained, by relentless activity and work performance, but the dilemma sooner or later becomes too painful. After a significant loss or disappointment, with or without the advent of a painful injury or ailment, a shift occurs that is drastic in its outward effect.

Alexithymia

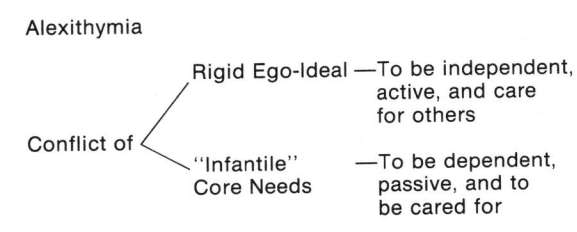

Conflict of ⟨ Rigid Ego-Ideal —To be independent, active, and care for others
"Infantile" Core Needs —To be dependent, passive, and to be cared for

Figure 16.1. Psychodynamic features of patients with dysthymic pain disorder.

This shift transforms the solid citizen into an invalid. The needs to depend, to be passive, and to be catered to, which have now asserted themselves, are still unacceptable, and the urge to be viewed as a strong and independent individual persists, causing the painful dilemma to intensify.

This explains the enormous need to maintain a physical problem as the culprit. With the failure of the solid citizen, the suffering becomes more evident. Both the frustration of the core needs and the failure of the ideal self represent prime sources of the depression. The lack of a secure inner core, the need to be accepted by a dominant other, and the conflict of guilt with concealed rage and aggression are indeed characteristic of depressive disorders.

A physical pain is viewed as honorable victimization, while a pain of mental origin is thought to be self-inflicted and proof of a weak mind. Thus the protest against having a mental problem serves to maintain self-esteem and the ideal view of oneself. "Nothing would be wrong if it weren't for the pain" is the common refrain.

A number of studies have found that groups selected for the presence of persistent pain show similar psychopathology, regardless of organicity (35, 37). These findings emphasize the trivial role of peripheral findings when it comes to chronic pain.

NOSOLOGIC CONSIDERATIONS

The criteria for the dysthymic pain disorder are compared to the DMS-III diagnostic criteria for major depressive episodes (13) in Table 16.2. Instead of the prominent and persistent dysphoric mood of the depressive episode, we list the prominent and persistent bodily pain of the dysthymic disorder as the leading symptom. A second major difference is the denial of emotional conflicts with sense of victimization and assumption of an invalid role, so prominent among the pain patients, which we list in place of the feelings of worthlessness, self-reproach, or guilt of the depressed patient.

Psychomotor agitation or retardation, as well as diminished ability to think or concentrate, are criteria of the major depressive episode virtually absent in the dysthymic pain disorder. Suicidal ideation is clearly less prominent in the dysthymic pain disorder, although it is not rare. Another difference is that weight loss is uncommon in the dysthymic pain disorder; in fact, patients often gain weight since they tend to maintain their appetite while lessening their activity. On the other hand, the major depressive traits of anhedonia, anergia, and insomnia tend to be equally present. Although the insomnia may be somewhat less prominent in the dysthymic pain disorder (patients characteristically have difficulty in falling and staying asleep but do not experience early morning awakening), the anhedonia and anergia of the chronic pain patient are almost invariably marked and tend to be devastating with their persistent impact on the ability to work and on family and social life. It is a critical error to subtract these traits when rating the chronic pain patient

Table 16.2
Diagnostic Criteria for Major Depressive Episode (DSM-III) and for Dysthymic Pain Disorder (Proposed)[a]

Major Depressive Episode	Dysthmic Pain Disorder
A. (One or both of the following) Dysphoric mood, prominent and persistent.	Bodily pain in the absence of any relevant lesion, prominent and persistent.
Loss of interest in all or almost all usual activities and pastimes.	
B. (At least four of the following)	
1. Poor appetite (or increased appetite)	Maintained appetite (or poor appetite)
2. Insomnia	
3. Psychomotor agitation or retardation.	—
4. Loss of interest or pleasure in usual activities, decrease in sexual drive (anhedonia).	
5. Loss of energy; fatigue (anergia).	
6. Feelings of worthlessness self-reproach or guilt.	Denial of emotional conflicts, sense of victimization, assumption of the invalid role.
7. Diminished ability to think or concentrate.	—
8. Recurrent thoughts of death, suicidal ideation.	(Suicidal ideation.)

[a] From Blumer D, Heilbronn M: Depression and chronic pain. In: Cameron O (ed): *Presentations of Depression: Depressive Symptoms in Medical and Other Psychiatric Disorders.* New York, John Wiley & Sons, 1987, pp 215–235.

for depression, as if they were due to a severe physical pain.

CONTROLLED STUDIES OF THE DYSTHYMIC PAIN DISORDER

Summaries of four of our representative studies follow. The first study compares patients with dysthymic pain disorder and patients with major depressive disease (13). The second study compares patients with dysthymic pain disorder and patients suffering rheumatoid arthritis, a well-defined chronic physical disease (5). The third study compares patients with chronic tension headaches and patients suffering noncephalic dysthymic pain of both single and multiple locations (2). Finally, a study is summarized of geriatric patients with chronic pain compared with patients with dysthymic pain of all ages (38). The first two studies were instrumental in establishing that dysthymic pain is a distinct disease entity. The latter two studies serve to illustrate that chronic pain is a treatable condition regardless of the pain location and regardless of the age of the afflicted.

COMPARISON BETWEEN PATIENTS WITH DYSTHYMIC PAIN DISORDER AND PATIENTS WITH MAJOR DEPRESSION

Patients with dysthymic pain disorder were 66 outpatients (41 females and 25 males, mean age 47.5 ± 14.8 years) referred to the Henry Ford Hospital Pain Clinic when no somatic cause for their pain could be determined by well-accepted clinical standards. Assessments were carried out during their initial two visits and prior to initiation of treatment. The 55 patients with major depressive disorder (37 females and 19 males, mean age 42.1 ± 15.5 years) were obtained from the Henry Ford Hospital psychiatric inpatient unit. All had been diagnosed as having unipolar endogenous depression by Research Diagnostic Criteria. The depressed control group underwent the evaluations after allowing time for adaptation for their inpatient stay, but prior to onset of treatment. The two groups did not significantly differ in age, sex, civil status, education, race, or occupation.

All patients underwent our standard workup for chronic pain, including completion of the Questionnaire for Pain Syndromes [QPS (15)], Hamilton Rating Scale for Depression [HDS (39)], dexamethasone suppression test [DST (40)], projective testing with the Szondi Experimental Diagnostic of Drives [SEDD (41)], and semi-structured interviews by both a psychologist and a psychiatrist. Additional data were obtained with the Family History—Research Diagnostic Criteria [FH-RDC (42)], and on other biologic measures (polysomnogram, urinary 3-methoxy-4-hydroxphenylglycol (MHPG), and urinary cortisol).

The data listed in Table 16.3 summarize the pertinent clinical findings. Both groups scored similarly high on the HDS. Although a majority of the depressed patients also complained of chronic pain, it was neither continuous nor disabling. Significantly more reports of poor appetite were present among the depressed patients, whereas both groups complained similarly of insomnia. The patients with dysthymic pain disorder stated significantly more often that their social life, sexual relations, and ability to work were impaired, a difference that apparently relates to the greater chronicity of the pain disorder. Anergia among dysthymic pain patients was found to be clearly more disabling.

Significant was the tendency of the pain patients to deny emotional and interpersonal problems. Suicidal ideation and attempts were significantly more frequent among the depressed patients. Analysis of the SEDD findings confirmed a preponderance of passive-submissive-masochistic trends and significant prevalence of dependency needs among dysthymic pain patients.

Table 16.4 shows a particularly high incidence of chronic pain (42%) among first-degree relatives of patients with the dysthymic pain disorder when compared with first-degree relatives of patients with major depression

Table 16.3
Comparison between Patients with Major Depressive Disorder and Dysthymic Pain Disorder (Clinical Findings)[a]

	Major Depressive Disorder (N=55)	Dysthymic Pain Disorder (N=66)	
Hamilton Depression Rating Scale	26.56±7.79	25.36±7.00	NS
Chronic pain	58%	100%	$p<.01$
(Mean duration of pain in years)	(3.81±4.67)	(8.29±11.79)	
Continuous pain	28%	86%	$p<.01$
Persistent depressed mood	84%	58%	$p<.01$
Poor appetite	36%	15%	$p<.01$
Insomnia	85%	79%	NS
Anhedonia			
Social life	47%	82%	$p<.01$
Sexual relations	45%	71%	$p<.01$
Leisure time	57%	67%	NS
Anergia			
Work disabled	9%	38%	$p<.01$
Decrease in activity	67%	75%	NS
Deny emotional problems			
Current	9%	49%	$p<.01$
Past	30%	62%	$p<.01$
Deny interpersonal conflicts	53%	82%	$p<.01$
Suicidal ideation	65%	27%	$p<.01$
Suicidal attempts	35%	9%	$p<.01$

[a] From Blumer D, Heilbronn M: Depression and chronic pain. In Cameron O (ed): *Presentations of Depression: Depressive Symptoms in Medical and Other Psychiatric Disorders.* New York, John Wiley & Sons, 1987, pp 215–235.

(25%). The first-degree familial incidence of alcoholism is likewise high (40%), and corresponds to the incidence of alcoholism in the first-degree family of patients with major depressive episodes (43%). Depressive patients show a significantly higher first-degree family incidence of affective illness (61%); however, the incidence of affective disorder among the relatives of chronic pain patients (42%) is also remarkably high. Three of the patients with major depressive disorder had first-degree relatives with histories of bipolar illness, and only one of the dysthymic pain patients had a family history of bipolar disorder. Only three of the patients with major depression and two of those with dysthymic pain disorder had a family history of chronic schizophrenia.

Urinary cortisol levels were abnormal among only 17% of the dysthymic pain patients, as compared with 82%

Table 16.4
Family History Comparison between Major Depressive Disorder and Dysthymic Pain Disorder[a]

	First-degree family history Number	First-degree family history Percentage	Multiple first-degree family history Number	Multiple first-degree family history Percentage	Range
Alcoholism[b]					
Major depressive disorder	21/49	43	6	12	2–6
Dysthymic pain disorder	26/65	40	7	11	2–4
Affective disorder[b]					
Major depressive disorder	30/49	61	8	16	2–4[d]
Dysthymic pain disorder	27/65	42	7	11	2–3[d]
Chronic Pain[c]					
Major depressive disorder	14/55	25	4	7	2–3
Dysthymic pain disorder	28/66	42	8	12	2–4
Handicapped-crippled[c]					
Major depressive disorder	10/55	18	1	2	3–3
Dysthymic pain disorder	21/66	32	3	5	2–3

[a] From Blumer D, Heilbronn M: Depression and chronic pain. In Cameron O (ed): *Presentations of Depression: Depressive Symptoms in Medical and Other Psychiatric Disorders.* New York, John Wiley & Sons, 1987, pp 215–235.
[b] Data obtained by FH-RDC method.
[c] Data obtained from the QPS.
[d] Significantly different at $p<.05$.

among the depressed patients. The urinary MHPG values, on the other hand, fell within the normal range for both the chronic pain and the depressed patients.

When we reported abnormal DST and shortened REM latency in a surprisingly high number (40% for both biologic markers) among a series of 20 patients with chronic pain (24), we pointed out that the patients had been selected for the significant insomnia and had to be considered more severely ill than the average chronic pain patient. Our later experience confirmed that a larger unselected group showed a lower incidence of these biologic markers (43). Here, only 10% of the chronic pain patients had an abnormally shortened REM latency, as compared with 44% among the depressed patients. Among the pain group, 70% had abnormal sleep efficiency, as compared with 94% among the depressed group. Prevalence of nonsuppression of dexamethasone was 24% among patients with dysthymic pain disorder compared with 57% among the group with major depression. It is no surprise that the presence of these markers is more pronounced among the more severely depressed chronic pain patients.

These data of significant similarities and differences between the two groups confirm our thesis that the syndrome termed dysthymic pain disorder is a specific variant of depression. Chronicity, lack of psychotic features, and a lesser incidence of biologic markers place the syndrome of chronic pain closer to the dysthymic disorder than to major depression.

COMPARISON BETWEEN PATIENTS WITH DYSTHYMIC PAIN DISORDER AND PATIENTS WITH RHEUMATOID ARTHRITIS

A sample of 129 patients (75 females and 54 males, mean age 46.4 ± 12.14) with chronic pain not related to somatic lesion (dysthymic pain disorder) underwent our standard evaluation. A control group of 36 patients (24 females and 12 males, mean age 55.1 ± 11.69) with classic rheumatoid arthritis receiving gold therapy treatment volunteered to complete the same evaluation.

The two groups showed significant differences in the duration, onset, and continuity of pain. The rheumatoid arthritis patients suffered pain twice as long as the dysthymic pain group, and the onset was mostly nontraumatic and gradual. The dysthymic pain patients showed mostly a sudden onset and more than half reported nontraumatic onsets. Only a few (12%) described an unquestionably severe trauma at the onset of their pain. Less than half of the patients with rheumatoid arthritis reported continuous pain, compared to 93% of the dysthymic pain patients.

Depressive traits were significantly more prevalent among the dysthymic pain patients. Impaired sleep, anhedonia, and anergia were clearly more prevalent, and the dysthymic pain patients were significantly more likely to admit frequent depressed mood.

When the historic traits of the two groups were compared, significantly more of the dysthymic pain patients were found to have suffered past physical abuse, chiefly at the hands of a former spouse. Although the prevalence of relatives with chronic pain did not vary significantly between the two groups, a significantly higher prevalence of crippled relatives was reported among the dysthymic pain disorder group. There was a significant prevalence of family history of manifest episodic mental disorders among dysthymic pain patients; none of the disorders were manic in nature, and they could best be classified as episodes of overt depression. Moreover, 12% of the dysthymic pain patients had a history of depression themselves, whereas none of the rheumatoid arthritis patients had such a history. The frequency of alcoholic relatives among dysthymic pain patients was considerably higher.

"Solid citizen traits" were not entirely different between the two groups. However, the tendency to idealize the relationship with the spouse, early work onset, chronic overtime work, and the failure to take annual vacations were traits prevalent among the dysthymic pain patients.

The somewhat younger age and lesser duration of illness of the dysthymic pain group hardly explains the prevalence of depressive traits among that group. Moreover, the finding of past personal and family history of depression among the dysthymic pain group favors the conclusion that the dysthymic pain disorder must be viewed as a variant of depressive disease.

COMPARISON OF PATIENTS WITH TENSION HEADACHES AND NONCEPHALIC PAIN

In a series of comparisons, we were unable to detect any significant differences among dysthymic pain patients grouped according to body parts affected, laterality, or peripheral versus central location of their chronic pain. We compared the psychobiologic profiles of patients whose pain was localized to the head with that of patients whose pain was localized to single and multiple areas elsewhere. Among 627 consecutive chronic pain patients referred to the Henry Ford Hospital Pain Clinic after no physical cause for their pain could be substantiated, there were 32 patients who complained of headache only. A total of 53 patients sampled complained of a single pain located elsewhere and this group served as a control group. A second control group of 53 patients with chronic pain of multiple (but not cephalic) location was randomly selected.

All of these 138 pain patients had undergone our standard evaluation for pain and all met our diagnostic criteria for the dysthymic pain disorder. Comparison of the two control groups indicated that the groups could be collapsed, averaged, and treated as a single control group.

Demographically, the headache patients did not differ significantly from the combined control group of noncephalic chronic pain with the exception that the headache patients were younger in age (37.2 versus 45.3 years). No significant differences appeared between the headache group and the control group across the premorbid traits, other biographic features, family histories, or psychodynamic traits. Importantly, no significant differences emerged between the groups in treatment response.

The headache patients differed significantly from the control patients on only three features: (a) fewer of the headache patients reported that their pain was continuous in nature (63% versus 88%); (b) a greater number of headache patients denied having any emotional problems (59% versus 30%); and (c) a significantly higher number of headache patients reported suicidal attempts or gestures (22% versus 8%), an interesting finding in view of their greater denial of emotional problems. The depressive traits characteristic for the dysthymic pain disorder are otherwise present in almost identical fashion among the headache and other pain patients. Of interest was a trend in our data for manual laborers to develop pain to body and limbs, whereas patients who chiefly use their head at work were more vulnerable to suffer headaches.

On the basis of these data we conclude that chronic headache generally referred to as tension or muscle contraction may best be understood as the chief symptom of masked depression, or more specifically, of a variant of depressive disease.

A STUDY OF 200 GERIATRIC PATIENTS WITH DYSTHYMIC PAIN DISORDER

Approximately 20% of the patient population of the Henry Ford Hospital Pain Clinic is comprised of individuals over the age of 60. The single criterion for referral to the Pain Clinic is the presence of a chief complaint of chronic pain in the absence of a plausibly related somatic disorder, as defined by accepted clinical standards. All referrals are accepted, regardless of the patients' age, motivation, mental status, or dependence on analgesics, and regardless of unresolved litigation.

In an effort to discern variances of the dysthymic pain disorder unique to geriatric chronic pain sufferers (age >60 years), we studied a random sample of 200 elderly patients evaluated and treated in our Pain Clinic. The sample consisted of 129 females and 71 males whose ages ranged from 60 to 86 years. Demographics and pertinent clinical traits, premorbid traits, and family histories of the geriatric sample were compared with a sample of chronic pain patients of all ages and the groups were not found to differ significantly. Of particular interest was the finding that at intake geriatric patients were taking from 0 to 12 medications, with an average of 2.6 medications. Ninety-five per cent of the medications were taken on a daily basis and the majority were classified as analgesics and minor tranquilizers.

A high degree of depressive symptomatology was reported by the patients and confirmed by the HDS mean average score of 24. A multiple regression analysis revealed that the HDS measures of hopelessness, decrease in work and/or activities, psychic anxiety, late insomnia, and hypochondriasis explained 86% of the variance of the total scale score.

The DST was taken by 41 of the patients prior to

commencement of treatment. Fourteen patients (34%) showed dexamethasone nonsuppression with values of greater than 5 μg/dl, one patient fell in the borderline range, and the remaining 26 patients showed normal suppression.

Among the total sample of 200 patients, there were 67 patients whose treatment response could be adequately assessed. Sixty patients (90%) responded favorably at least to a moderate degree, with 55% achieving considerable, near complete, or complete resolution of their pain and depression.

In short, it was found that elderly patients with chronic pain in the absence of pertinent somatic lesions do not depart significantly from the profile that has been documented among the dysthymic pain disorder sufferers of all ages. The higher prevalence of female patients, the less frequent complaint of loss of sexual interest, and the increased percentage of nonsuppression on the DST can all be explained by the characteristics of the advanced age. All of the traits of the variant of depression we have termed dysthymic pain disorder are present among the geriatric sample. It is apparent that individuals who derived their pride and self-esteem from their often extraordinary physical achievements will find it particularly difficult to adjust to the aging process and to retirement. They tend to become utterly preoccupied with their physical discomforts. Bodily ailments and depression secondary to physical disease are common fare of old age, but the role of physical ailments must not be overestimated. The common chronic pain secondary to depression can be recognized and treated.

TREATMENT

GENERAL PRINCIPLES

Pain in the absence of a significant somatic lesion should be recognized at its inception as the leading symptom of the dysthymic pain disorder, from day 1 if it began without any trauma, as is often the case. Once the condition has been diagnosed, the physician should explain the nature of the problem to the patient. The patient should be told that pain commonly occurs in the absence of mechanical factors. Although there is no hidden, undiscovered ailment, this type of pain is nevertheless very real. It is more related to a condition of the nervous system (a chemical imbalance) than to any injury. A depressive-tension state plays a role, and the condition can be treated.

Some patients may respond to simple reassurance. For others, one may need to prescribe exercises or physiotherapy in order to help them regain confidence in the use of their body parts. Prompt further treatment is indicated if a significant complaint of pain persists and a marked preoccupation with the pain becomes evident, together with other depressive symptoms such as anergia, anhedonia, and insomnia (all blamed on the pain by the patient). This is of great importance, since chronic pain tends to lead to early disability. Continuation or prompt resumption of work and regular activities need to be encouraged while treatment is carried out on an outpatient basis. However, the patients must learn to pace themselves and not be relentlessly active.

Based on our understanding of the dysthymic pain disorder, rational therapeutic approaches can be proposed. Treatment guidelines are summarized in Table 16.5. Effective treatment of chronic pain stresses avoidance of analgesics and benzodiazepines, deemphasis of the pain complaints, and gradual increase of activities (44–46). Systematic treatment with antidepressants, in accord with our view of chronic pain as a dysthymic disorder, needs to

Table 16.5
Treatment Guidelines for Dysthymic Pain Disorder[a]

1. Persistent pain not related to a somatic lesion is the warning signal for a depressive state: watch for excessive preoccupation with the pain, lack of energy and initiative (anergia), lack of ability to enjoy social life, sex, and leisure (anhedonia), as well as for insomnia and despair, as significant symptoms of a depressive state (dysthymic pain disorder).

2. Note that the patient typically will deny that he has any interpersonal problems, tends to idealize himself and his family relations, and will be unwilling to consider a psychiatric exploration. He will admit to being nervous or depressed only as a result of the pain. The pain is viewed as the one and only problem, as the cause of all the distress, and there is an intense plea to be relived.

3. Look for a premorbid history of relentless activity and overachievement (ergomania), past abuse at the hands of a spouse, presence of chronic pain or of a crippled individual in the kinship, and for a family and sometimes personal history of depression, alcoholism, or both.

4. Curb somatic investigations and avoid unnecessary procedures. Treat with antidepressants systematically. Do not treat minor incidental physical findings—the basic depressive disorder will persist: once the depression is improved, the patient's intense preoccupation with the body part in pain and his demand for relief will cease.

5. Antianxiety drugs (such as diazepam) and analgesics tend to worsen depression and are contraindicated. Analgesics can be withdrawn more easily once antidepressants are effective. Few patients with chronic pain are addicts. Involvement in litigation may intensify chronic pain but does not cause it and may make treatment more difficult but not necessarily ineffective.

6. Do not make light of the pain: there are cogent reasons for "non-somatic" pain, and it has to be dealt with as a real pain. You can instill hope that the pain may be brought under control.

[a] From Blumer D: Psychiatric aspects of chronic pain: nature, identification and treatment of the pain-prone disorder. In Rothman RH, Simeone FA (eds): *The Spine*, ed 2. Philadelphia, WB Saunders, 1982.

be carried out in conjunction with a firm and persistent effort at behavior modification. Although varying degrees of success, at least in the short run, are claimed for numerous procedures employed in many pain clinics, the combination of behavior modification and antidepressants is the most appropriate and effective treatment for dysthymic pain (47, 48).

BEHAVIOR MODIFICATION

Sound behavioral management of the chronic pain patient is based on the recognition that treatment must not be aimed at the alleged peripheral source of the pain. A rational, successful treatment for chronic pain in the absence of somatic findings, according to behavioral principles, was first developed by Fordyce (45).

Behavior modification is generally carried out in a well-staffed inpatient unit. Nonetheless, the principles of operant conditioning established by Fordyce (45, 46, 48), aimed at the unlearning of chronic pain, are applicable to office practice as well. If the patient is dependent on analgesics, they must not be prescribed on an as-needed basis, but at regular time intervals, in gradually decreasing doses. Activity needs to be prescribed in initially modest, well-tolerated quotas that are then gradually increased, with rest allowed after a set period of work rather than upon the occurrence of pain. The family must be instructed not to be solicitous of the pain but supportive of all attempts of the patient to become more active, although not to the previous excessive levels. The patients must be advised to ignore the pain as much as possible and to distract themselves by renewing their old interests or seeking new endeavors. The approach toward the patient in this regimen should be encouraging and somewhat forceful. While we emphasize the effectiveness of antidepressant drugs, we consider the application of behavioral principles essential.

SYSTEMATIC TREATMENT WITH ANTIDEPRESSANTS

Systematic treatment with antidepressant drugs can be very effective in the management of the dysthymic pain disorder (47, 49–51). This form of treatment is appropriate for a majority of patients and can be carried out by primary physicians on an outpatient basis. Referral to a psychiatrist is necessary when a depression becomes severe, or when a significant risk of suicide or other serious psychiatric complication develops.

Since patients with chronic pain resist the idea that their basic problem is of a depressive nature, it must be emphasized that antidepressant-type drugs, and not analgesics, are the drugs of choice *for their pain*. The medication should improve not only their pain, but their sleep, their mood, and their energy level. Full discussion of the nature of the dysthymic pain disorder is productive for a few patients only, but explaining the treatment to the spouse or next-of-kin can be very helpful.

Analgesics and antianxiety agents provide no sustained relief, are habituating, and may exacerbate the depression and the pain. Antidepressants are not habituating. They should be administered as in major depressions, patiently and systematically, by proper increases, with careful monitoring, to sufficient doses (as high as 150–300 mg daily for the major antidepressants). Substitution of another antidepressant drug may be needed if side effects occur. Whereas insomnia may improve promptly, pain and the other depressive traits tend to improve concomitantly from about 10 to as long as 30 days after institution of an effective antidepressant regimen. The patients must be alerted to this delayed effect of the drug. Table 16.6 provides the effective dose ranges for the antidepressant drugs.

We employ a more sedative type of antidepressant only if insomnia is a significant problem, and a nonsedative antidepressant if sleep has remained intact. Notwithstanding the myth that serotonergic drugs may be more effective for pain, we prefer the noradrenergic antidepressants (desipriamine, maprotiline), which have fewer anticholinergic side effects and less of a risk of weight gain. The drug is increased, if necessary, to a maximum dose. Thus, we may prescribe desipramine (25 mg, twice daily) initially, and increase the dose by 25 mg daily or every other day, until a dose of 50 mg three times a day is reached. Further stepwise increases to a maximum of 100 mg three times a day should be prescribed, if necessary, after 4

Table 16.6
Approximate Effective Dose Ranges of Antidepressant Drugs[a]

Generic Name	Trade Name(s)	Effective Dose Range (mg/day)
Tricyclics		
Imipramine	Tofranil	150–300
Amitriptyline	Elavil, Endep	150–300
Doxepin	Adapin, Sinequan	150–300
Desipramine	Norpramin, Pertofrane	150–250
Nortriptyline	Aventyl, Pamelor	50–100
Protriptyline	Vivactil	10–60
Trimipramine	Surmontil	150–300
Amoxapine	Asendin	200–400
Tetracyclic		
Maprotiline	Ludiomil	150–225
MAO inhibitors		
Phenelzine	Nardil	45–75
Tranylcypromine	Parnate	20–40

[a] From Blumer D: Psychiatric aspects of chronic pain: nature, identification and treatment of the pain-prone disorder. In Rothman RH, Simeone FA (eds): *The Spine*, ed 2. Philadelphia, WB Saunders, 1982.

weeks. The doses are smaller (by at least one-third) in patients past the age of 60, and are only cautiously increased. More sedative antidepressants (such as maprotiline) are best given as a once-daily bedtime prescription. Of course, it helps some anxious patients if they can take their medication distributed over the day.

Once an antidepressant has been tolerated at a maximum dose for 3 or 4 weeks yet the patient is not sufficiently improved, we proceed to combine a more modest dose of the drug with lithium carbonate or with a small amount of neuroleptic medication (e.g., 100–150 mg of desipramine with lithium carbonate at a modest therapeutic dose, or with 3–5 mg of trifluoperazine). Monoamine oxidase (MAO) inhibitors may also be effective for chronic pain.

We consider the noradrenergic antidepressant desipramine the drug of first choice for chronic pain; desipramine tends to have fewer side effects than other antidepressants and may be more effective for dysthymic pain because of the lack of excessive sedation. The key to success in the treatment of chronic pain, indeed, is the reactivation of the anergic patient. We tend to avoid both amitriptyline and doxepin, widely used in the treatment of chronic pain, for two reasons: they may be overly sedative, and they tend to be associated with weight gain. If a sedative effect is desirable because of persistent insomnia, we prefer the noradrenergic tetracyclic antidepressant maprotiline, given at bedtime.

Two points should be made clear to the patient at the very beginning of treatment: it may require patience before the correct dosage is established, and the first medication prescribed may have to be replaced because of side effects. Side effects may also require a slower introduction of the drug: they need to be promptly reported so that proper adjustments can be carried out. Table 16.7 contains a summary of possible side effects of the tricyclic antidepressant drugs.

The patient has to be prepared to continue the treatment for many months. Once the pain has subsided and the patient has found a more meaningful role in life, the medication can be slowly phased out. Many patients may require a maintenance treatment. Use of the behavior modification techniques, along with prompt employment of enhancement treatment with lithium carbonate or with low doses of a neuroleptic, undoubtedly has greatly improved our treatment results.

It is generally much easier to withdraw the analgesics from a patient once he is on an effective dose of an antidepressant. If a patient has a hard-core analgesic addiction, he will drop out of treatment as a strict withdrawal regimen of the particular analgesic drug is carried out. In our experience, however, only a small number of individuals among the chronic pain patients have a serious problem with addiction, and it is rare to find patients who are misleading the physician by their display of pain in order to get analgesic drugs.

Table 16.7
Side Effects of Tricyclic Antidepressants[a]

Sedative
    (Most with amitriptyline and doxepin; least with protriptyline and desipramine)
    Drowsiness, hypersomnia
Anticholinergic
    Dry mouth (very common), blurred vision, dizziness, constipation, epigastric disease, nausea, peculiar taste, palpitations, tachycardia, arrhythmia, postural hypotension, aggravation of narrow angle glaucoma, urinary hesitation (or retention)
Allergic
    Edema, skin rash, urticaria
Central Nervous System
    Tremor (fine, rapid), twitching, convulsions, dysarthria, paresthesias, ataxia, confusional state
Other
    Weight gain (or loss), decreased (or increased) sexual arousal, impotence, perspiration
ECG
    Flattened T waves, prolonged QT intervals, depressed S-T segments
Drug Interaction
    Intereference with therapeutic effects of guanethidine-type hypertensive agents; additive with sedatives, alcohol, and anticholinergics

[a] From Blumer D: Psychiatric aspects of chronic pain: nature, identification and treatment of the pain-prone disorder. In Rothman RH, Simeone FA (eds): *The Spine*, ed 2. Philadelphia, WB Saunders, 1982.

TREATMENT RESPONSE

Initially, our assessment of treatment effects was conducted through 1- and 2-year follow-up studies of dysthymic pain patients (49, 50). More recent studies have been carried out on a random sample of 1000 dysthymic pain patients evaluated and treated at the Henry Ford Hospital Pain Clinic (47).

The sample group of 1000 patients included 554 women and 446 men ranging in age from 16 to 84, with a mean age of 44.5 years. Mean duration of the pain complaint was 6.1 years. Of the patients, 760 were outpatient referrals, and 240 were referred when they were medical/surgical inpatients. Patients who maintained a significant improvement of pain and depressive symptoms for at least 3 months were judged to be responders.

Treatment compliance was the greatest problem, particularly among those who were initially seen as inpatients on the medical/surgical units. Because of the high dropout rate, treatment effects could only be assessed in 391 patients (196 women and 195 men).

The assessment showed that a preponderant majority of

the patients (89%) had positive treatment effects and were judged to be responders. Of the 349 responders, 202 (52%) showed moderate response, and 147 (37%) showed solid improvement, including 79 patients (20%) who showed either complete or near-complete resolution of their pain and depressive symptoms. Only 42 of the patients (11%) did not respond at all to treatment after a minimum trial of two antidepressants administered in optimal doses. The response data are summarized in Figure 16.2.

The sample revealed a significant sex difference, with a greater number of solid responders being women, whereas the number of men among nonresponders was disproportionately large. Few, if any, differences were found between the responders and nonresponders in age, pain duration, or number of clinic visits. However, complaints of drug side effects emerged as a variable, with complaints increasing dramatically from solid responders (15%) to moderate responders (50%) to nonresponders (100%). These complaints of side effects invite consideration of treatment compliance. A majority of the moderate responders were found to be intermittently noncompliant during the course of their treatment, whereas solid responders were generally complaint. Blood levels of the antidepressant drugs to establish compliance among nonresponders were not obtained.

An evaluation of nonresponders showed that 74% were blue-collar workers, compared to 61% among the solid responders. It is significant that 62% of the nonresponders were work disabled; all but two of the patients in this category was blue-collar workers. Among the 147 solid responders, 20 of the 56 work-disabled patients remained disabled after treatment. These findings show that relief from pain does not necessarily imply a return to work; many of the formerly hard-working patients, in fact, expressed a dread of returning to work after prolonged absence.

Over one-third of the 1000 patients sampled did not return for treatment at all after evaluation or returned for only one or two visits after evaluation. Among the sample group of patients whose treatment was assessed, 59% dropped out of treatment later on, with no significant differences between solid responders (52%), moderate responders (55%), or nonresponders (63%). The total combined dropout rate, both early and late, of 65% is an indication of the strong bias of dysthymic pain patients against treatment in a pain clinic affiliated with a psychiatric department. Even a number of patients who had shown remarkable improvement dropped out of treatment and did not resume it when their pain recurred.

Our assessment suggests that female patients tend to respond better and blue-collar workers respond less to antidepressants. Disabled blue-collar workers of the male sex tend to remain severely demoralized and predominate among the nonresponders; this emphasizes the need to recognize and treat their condition early, before they become unable to work.

REHABILITATION AT WORK

Chronic pain is the single most serious problem in the rehabilitation of workers (52). Among older workers, retirement on a disability pension may be unavoidable, but that is an inappropriate solution for individuals without significant impairment who are still in the midst of their best earning years.

The previously overachieving worker with chronic pain will find it increasingly difficult to function at work again, once he has been away from his job for a long time. Meanwhile, his position in the family as a breadwinner has been vitiated and much discontent has set in; diminished activities and social life have resulted in a monotony that further increases the mood of depression. The patient

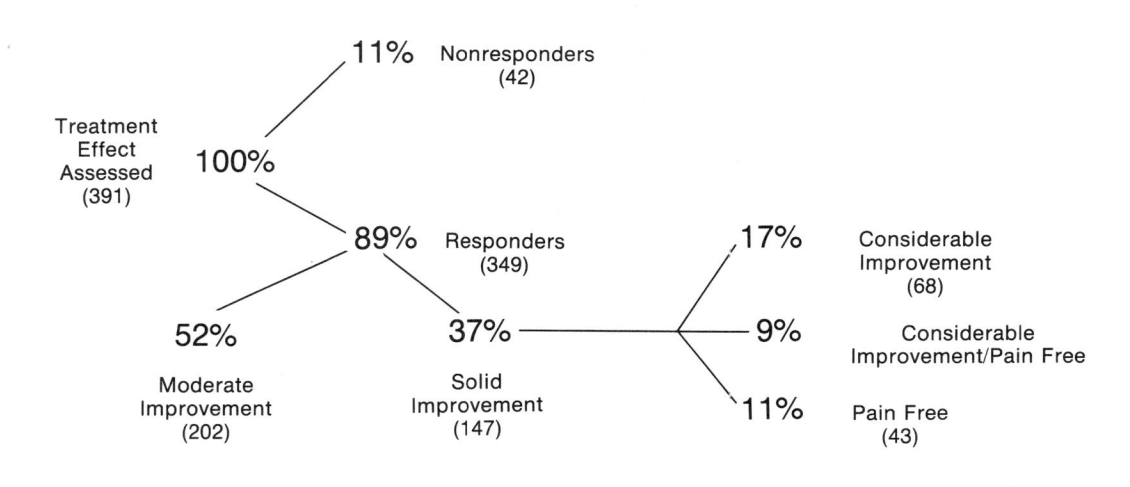

Figure 16.2. Treatment response of 1000 patients with dysthymic pain disorder.

often requires special consideration at his place of employment to be able to resume working again, or he may remain disabled even though the pain has improved. Thus the individual may become a permanent victim of work fatigue.

PROGNOSIS

Chronic pain appears to be less intractable than has been assumed. If the depressive disorder can be dealt with, the pain complaint may vanish. The basic conflicts, however, may turn out to be very persistent and difficult to confront. Many dysthymic pain patients will frustrate the best treatment efforts. This appears to be related to the masochistic or self-defeating tendency of such patients, who may even abandon the very treatment that has proved successful. Rather than continuing a required sustained treatment, many still prefer to shop around for the magical—but elusive—cure.

CONCLUSIONS

When compared with control groups of patients with major depression or with those whose pain can be related to a well-defined somatic disease, the dysthymic pain disorder proves to be a distinct entity with characteristic clinical, psychobiologic, biographic, and genetic traits. It meets rigorous criteria for identification as a psychobiologic disorder and warrants recognition as a specific variant of depressive disease. There is a clear suggestion of its kinship not only to unipolar depressions but also to alcoholism.

Early recognition and avoidance of the still customary physical mistreatments is of obvious importance. Once the disorder has been recognized and its origin understood, physical investigations should be curbed and futile surgical procedures avoided. The patients should be informed that pain such as theirs does occur commonly in the absence of a peripheral lesion, that a depressive-tension state plays a role, and that it can be treated. The combination of behavioral and antidepressant drug treatment has been proven as a rational and effective treatment for chronic pain.

References

1. Nachemson HL: Pathophysiology and treatment of back pain: a critical look at the different types of treatment. In Buerger AA, Tobias JS (eds): *Approaches to the Validation of Manipulation Therapy*. Springfield, IL, Charles C Thomas, 1977, pp 42–57.
2. Blumer D, Heilbronn M: Chronic muscle contraction headache and the pain-prone disorder. *Headache* 22:180–183, 1982.
3. Saper J: Chronic headache complex (CHC): the mixed syndrome. A new perspective. In Saper J (ed): *Headache Disorders, Current Concepts and Treatment Strategies*. Boston, John Wright PSG, 1983, pp 125–130.
4. Holden C: Pain, dying and the health care system. *Science* 203:984–985, 1979.
5. Blumer D, Heilbronn M: Chronic pain as a variant of depressive disease: the pain-prone disorder. *J Nerv Ment Dis* 170:381–406, 1982.
6. Bonica JJ (ed): *Advances in Neurology: International Symposium on Pain*. New York, Raven Press, 1974, vol 4.
7. Bonica JJ (ed): Pain. *Res Publ Assoc Res Nerv Ment Dis* 58, 1980.
8. Crue B (ed): *Chronic Pain. Further Observations from City of Hope National Medical Center*. New York, Spectrum Publications, 1979.
9. Lorenz KY, Bonica JJ (eds): *Developments in Neurology: Pain, Discomfort and Humanitarian Care*. New York, Elsevier, 1980, vol 4.
10. Melzack R: *The Puzzle of Pain*. New York, Basic Books, 1973.
11. Sternbach RA (ed): *The Psychology of Pain*. New York, Raven Press, 1978.
12. Melzack R, Loeser JD: Phantom body pain in paraplegics: evidence for central "pattern generating mechanism" for pain. *Pain* 4:195–210, 1978.
13. Blumer D, Heilbronn M: Depression and chronic pain. In Cameron O (ed): *Presentation of Depression*. New York, John Wiley & Sons, 1987, pp 215–235.
14. Blumer D: Psychiatric aspects of chronic pain: nature, identification and treatment of the pain-prone disorder. In Rothman RH, Simeone FA (eds): *The Spine*, ed 2. Philadelphia, WB Saunders, 1982, vol II, pp 1090–1117.
15. Blumer D: Psychiatric considerations in pain. In Rothman RH, Simeone JA (eds): *The Spine*. Philadelphia, WB Saunders, 1975, vol 2, pp 871–906.
16. Blumer D: A study of patients with "psychogenic" pain. Presented at the Annual Meeting of the American Psychosomatic Society, Philadelphia, 1965.
17. Blumer D, Heilbronn M: The pain-prone disorder: clinical and psychological profile. *Psychosomatics* 22:395–402, 1981.
18. Blumer D: Psychiatric and psychological aspects of chronic pain. In Keener EB (ed): *Clinical Neurosurgery*. Baltimore, Williams & Wilkins, 1978, vol 24, pp 276–283.
19. Engel G: "Psychogenic" pain and the pain-prone patient. *Am J Med* 26:899–918, 1959.
20. Schaffer CB, Donlon PT, Bittle RM: Chronic pain and depression: a clinical and family history. *Am J Psychiatry* 137:118–120, 1980.
21. Katon W, Egan K, Miller D: Chronic pain: lifetime psychiatric diagnosis and family history. *Am J Psychiatry* 142:1156–1160, 1985.
22. Krishnan KRR, France RD, Houpt JL: Chronic low back pain and depression. *Psychosomatics* 26:299–302, 1985.
23. Winokur G, Behar D, VanValkenburg MD, et al: Is a familial definition of depression both feasabile and valid? *J Nerv Ment Dis* 166:764–768, 1978.
24. Blumer D, Zorick F, Heilbronn M, et al: Biological markers for depression in chronic pain. *J Nerv Ment Dis* 170:425–428, 1982.
25. France RD, Krishnan KRR: The dexamethasone suppression test as a biological marker of depression in chronic pain. *Pain* 21:49–55, 1985.
26. Atkinson JH, Kremer EF, Risch SC, et al: Neuroendocrine function and endogenous opioid peptide synthesis in chronic pain. *Psychosomatics* 24:899–913, 1983.
27. Atkinson JH, Kremer, Risch SC, et al: Neuroendocrine responses in psychiatric and pain patients with major depression. *Biol Psychiatry* 21:612–620, 1986.
28. Almay BG, Johansson F, VonKnorring L, et al: Endorphins in

chronic pain. I. Differences in CSF endorphin levels between organic and psychogenic pain syndromes. *Pain* 5:153–162, 1978.
29. VonKnorring L, Almay BG, Haggendal J, et al: Discrimination of idiopathic pain syndromes and neurogenic pain syndromes and healthy volunteers by means of clinical rating, personality traits, monamine metabolites in CSF, cortisol in serum, MAO in platelets and melatonin in urine. *Eur Arch Psychiatry Neurol Sci* 236:131–138, 1986.
30. Pilowsky I, Spence ND: Illness behavior syndromes associated with intractable pain. *Pain* 2:61–71, 1976.
31. Krystal H: Alexithymia and psychotherapy. *Am J Psychother* 33:17–31, 1979.
32. Sifneos PE: Clinical observations on some patients suffering from a variety of psychosomatic diseases. In *Proceedings of the Seventh European Conference on Psychosomatic Research*. Basel, Karger, 1967.
33. Stephanos S: Das Koncept der "pensee operatoire" und "das psychosomatishe pahnomen." In von Eexkull T (ed): *Lehrbuch der Psychosomatischen Medizin*. Munich, Urban & Schwarzenberg, 1979, pp 217–219.
34. Marty P, deM'uzan M, David C: *L'Investigation Psychosomatique*. Paris, Presses Unversitaires, 1963.
35. Castelnuovo-Tedesco P, Krout BM: Psychosomatic aspects of chronic pelvic pain. *Int J Psychiatry Med* 31:109–126, 1970.
36. Sternbach RA, Wolf SR, Murphy RW, et al: Traits of pain patients: the low back "loser". *Psychosomatics* 14:226–229, 1973.
37. Woodforde JM, Merskey H: Personality traits of patients with chronic pain. *J Psychosom Res* 16:167–172, 1973.
38. Blumer D, Heilbronn M: Chronic pain and depressive illness in the elderly: a study of 200 geriatric pain-prone patients. In *Proceedings of The National Institutes of Mental Health Conference on Mental Health Aspects of Physical Disease in Late Life*. New York, University Press, in press.
39. Hamilton M: A rating scale for depression. *J Neurol Neurosurg Psychiatry* 23:56–62, 1960.
40. Carroll BJ, Feinberg M, Greden JF, et al: A specific laboratory test for the diagnosis of melancholia. Standardization, validation and clinical utility. *Arch Gen Psychiatry*, 38:15–22, 1980.
41. Szondi L: *Lehrbuch der Experimentellen Triebdiagnostic*, ed 3. Bern, Switzerland, Huber, 1972.
42. Andreasen NC, Endicott J, Spitzer RL, et al: The family history method using diagnostic criteria. *Arch Gen Psychiatry* 34:1229–1235, 1977.
43. Blumer D, Heilbronn M, Rosenbaum AH: Antidepressant treatment of the pain-prone disorder. *Psychopharmacol Bull* 20:531–535, 1984.
44. Black RG: The chronic pain syndromes. *Surg Clin North Am* 55:999–1011, 1975.
45. Fordyce WE: *Behavioral Methods for Chronic Pain and Illness*. St. Louis, CV Mosby, 1976.
46. Fordyce WE: The office management of pain. *Minn Med* 57:185–188, 1974.
47. Blumer D, Heilbronn M: Antidepressant treatment for chronic pain: treatment outcome of 1000 patients with pain-prone disorder. *Psychiatr Ann* 14:795–800, 1984.
48. Fordyce WE: Learning processes in pain. In Sternbach RA (ed): *The Psychology of Pain*. New York, Raven Press, 1978, pp 49–72.
49. Blumer D, Heilbronn M, Pedraza E, et al: Systematic treatment of chronic pain with antidepressants. *Henry Ford Hosp Med J* 28:15–21, 1980.
50. Blumer D, Heilbronn M: Second year follow-up study on systematic treatment of chronic pain with antidepressants. *Henry Ford Hosp Med J* 29:67–68, 1981.
51. Schatzberg A: Drug management of treatment resistant depression. *McLean Hosp J* 1:89–101, 1976.
52. Rowe ML: Low back pain in industry. *J Occup Med* 2:161–169, 1969.

chapter 17
Contingency Management in the Reduction of Overt Pain Behavior

Steven H. Sanders, Ph.D.

In keeping with the ever-expanding changes in our understanding of clinical pain, the application of behavioral principles and concepts to the area has resulted in major advancements in treatment practice (1–4). Although an array of behavioral methods has been increasingly utilized in both assessment and treatment of clinical pain (e.g., relaxation training, modeling, self-monitoring), the one with the longest history is contingency management (3, 5–7). Contingency management is a form of operant conditioning (8) and consists of increasing or decreasing the occurrence of overt behavior through the systematic application of consequences (positive or negative) contingent upon the behavior (cf. refs. 9, 10). As will be obvious from this chapter, overt pain behavior such as verbal pain complaints, activity level, and taking pain medication can be significantly influenced by operant conditioning effects (4, 11) and, thus, contingency management can be central to effecting therapeutic change.

Given the frequent importance of contingency management, this chapter is devoted to a discussion of its basic principles and application to overt clinical pain behavior. Although the focus is on reduction of overt pain behavior in chronic adult pain patients, consideration is given to its application with other pain conditions and patient populations (e.g., acute pain, cancer pain, pain in children and the elderly). The chapter concentrates on treatment; however, behavioral assessment principles necessary for proper application of contingency management are outlined. Other behavioral methods such as relaxation training, biofeedback, and social modeling, although often used in combination with contingency management, are not reviewed in this chapter. The reader is referred to other reviews (2, 4–7, 12–15) and chapters in the current text for more in-depth discussion of these behavioral methods.

The chapter has been divided into four main sections. The first offers some basic behavioral concepts and definitions for contingency management and clinical pain. With this background and understanding, the next section describes and discusses the application of contingency management principles to the specific reduction of overt pain behavior and reviews specific applications with commonly encountered behaviors. This includes guidelines for when, where, and how to use contingency management appropriately. The third section addresses issues inherent in contingency management with overt pain behavior and outlines research needs. The final section offers some conclusions regarding the use of contingency management and speculations regarding future trends.

BASIC CONCEPTS AND DEFINITIONS

Before discussing the specific application of contingency management to overt pain behavior, it is important to establish a conceptual and empirical basis for such an application. This section reviews the basic definition, principles, paradigms, and conditions for effective usage of contingency management, and offers a behavioral conceptualization and definition of clinical pain consistent with existing evidence.

CONTINGENCY MANAGEMENT
Definition

As noted in the introduction, contingency management can be defined as the control of overt behavior by application of positive or negative consequences. The technique is a form of operant conditioning and is substantiated by a rich body of knowledge. With this basic definition, let us now describe the primary contingency management paradigms typically used in behavior modification of human responses.

Positive Reinforcement

A positive reinforcement paradigm involves contingently following a specific overt behavior with a positive consequence (reinforcer), with the specific intent of maintaining or increasing the occurrence of the overt behavior. For example, a mother follows her child's use of the word "please" with praise. Soon, she sees an increase in its usage. This concept has been used extensively to effect changes in both child and adult behavior (10, 16). Positive reinforcers with children and adults have included food, social attention and praise, access to pleasurable activities, physical touch, music, and a host of other materials and experiences that individuals find enjoyable or pleasurable. Positive reinforcers are routinely identified by observing an individual's activity and by asking the person. Although there are common positive reinforcers that most individuals acknowledge (e.g., praise and money), important individual differences are quite frequent.

Negative Reinforcement

The second contingency management paradigm used to maintain or increase the rate of overt behavior is to follow the overt behavior with the removal of an unpleasant experience or aversive situation (negative reinforcer). This is also known as escape/avoidance conditioning (17), because it is assumed that the behavior is emitted to either escape or avoid an unpleasant experience. For example, consider the child who cries (overt behavior) whenever asked to clean up his room (aversive-unpleasant experience) and thus escapes or avoids having to clean the room. If you observe such a situation, you will typically see that crying becomes quite frequent where the threat or demand for cleaning up the room is present. Likewise, consider the adult who drives at 55 mph (overt behavior) to escape or avoid a traffic citation or automobile accident. It has clearly been established that overt behavior maintained or increased due to negative reinforcement (i.e., escape/avoidance conditioning) can be quite resistant to change and maintained even if the aversive experience is not actually present (e.g., our person driving at 55 mph even though a patrolman may not actually be in the area). As is described later, the negative reinforcement paradigm is often important in the development and maintenance of overt pain behavior.

Punishment

The third major paradigm included in contingency management involves the reduction of overt behavior through the application of an aversive-negative consequence or the removal of a positive experience. We are all familiar with this concept in child-rearing practices that might involve following behavior such as throwing food at the table (overt behavior) with a spanking (the aversive or unpleasant consequence) or sending the child to his room (removing pleasurable social interaction and access to activities and material outside of his room). As with reinforcers, aversive consequences or punishers are typically identified by observation and by questioning the individual. Common punishments include the experience of pain itself, social ridicule, interpersonal discord, job and school stress, loss of social attention-recognition, and loss of resources or valuables. By far the most prevalent and useful type of punishment in controlling and changing behavior involves the removal of pleasurable experiences contingent upon emission of a given overt behavior (cf. ref. 18).

Extinction

Another important paradigm within contingency management involves the reduction or termination of conditioning effects by elimination of the contingent relationship between an overt behavior and its positive or negative consequences. Such a removal of this contingent relationship is known as extinction, and typically results in a change in the target behavior. Removal of positive or negative reinforcers following an overt behavior routinely results in a reduction or elimination of that behavior, whereas removal of punishers may result in an increase in the behavior being punished. The rate of change in the target behavior varies once removal of contingencies has occurred and is typically not immediate.

An exception to the observed changes in overt behavior during extinction has been repeatedly observed for behavior maintained or increased by a negative reinforcement paradigm. As already noted, such learned escape/avoidance behavior appears to be remarkably resistant to the effects of extinction (17). Thus, it can persist indefinitely once established. This is particularly true if the target behavior actually avoids the occurrence of an unpleasant experience. Within this context, there is no opportunity for the negative experience to occur. As long as the individual perceives that she has successfully avoided it (e.g., getting a traffic ticket) this can be sufficient to sustain the behavior (e.g., driving 55 mph). Thus, the actual presence of an unpleasant experience is not needed once avoidance behavior has been established. Reduction or elimination often requires deliberate application of the unpleasant experience while preventing emission of the avoidance behavior (77), as well as discontinuing the contingency between occurrence of the behavior and removal (escape) of the unpleasant experience.

Discriminative Stimuli

Although contingency management is primarily concerned with the effects of consequences on overt behavior, it has also been repeatedly demonstrated that certain stimuli can acquire discriminative or cue-like qualities, thereby alerting the individual that a given behavior will result in a given consequence (19). For example, it is not unusual to see a child respond in one fashion when her mother is present and in another when her father is present. Such changes in behavior are many times a function of the child's learning that the father's presence will result in certain consequences for certain behavior that are different than those in the mother's presence. The mother and father are effectively serving as discriminative stimuli for various behaviors. Likewise, all of us have experienced a rather marked change in our driving behavior in the presence versus absence of a police officer. His presence is a definite discriminative stimulus that certain behavior such as reckless driving will result in certain consequences (e.g., being arrested or ticketed). The effect of discriminative stimuli on overt behavior is very important and can be quite potent. In fact, much of human behavior is directed by discriminative stimuli or cues in the environment that signal the presence (or potential for) a given consequence if an overt behavior is emitted.

Conditions for Effective Usage

The effective application of contingency management is dependent upon a number of basic conditions. These include clearly defining the overt behavior, applying consequences to the behavior as soon and consistently after its occurrence as possible, identifying truly positive-pleasurable and negative-aversive experiences or materials for a given individual, and the concept of shaping behavior. The concept of shaping applies primarily when one is trying to increase the occurrence of a behavior. It refers to gradually changing behavior and not expecting too much change too quickly. For example, in teaching someone to read you will get much farther if you positively reinforce and recognition and reading of letters, then words, then simple sentences, then more complex sentences. If you do not apply positive reinforcement until the individual has read a complex sentence, chances are reading will never occur. The basic notion here is to systematically reinforce successive approximations of the final overt behavior until the person is emitting the complete response (20). (Note: although the present chapter focuses on the reduction of overt pain behavior, as will be evident from subsequent sections, the concept of shaping is crucial to accomplishing this task.)

Although all of the preceding conditions are important for effective contingency management application, the requirement for immediate application of consequences with adults may not be as crucial as the other conditions. The primary requirement is an awareness that the consequences being applied are due to a specific overt behavior. Given our verbal and cognitive skills, this can be accomplished by reminding the individual why a certain consequence is being administered even if the overt behavior occurred sometime prior. However, it is preferable to administer consequences as soon after the occurrence of an overt behavior as possible.

It should be noted that, within contemporary behavioral interventions, contingency management is rarely if ever administered as the sole treatment technique. It is more often combined with other behavioral procedures (e.g., modeling, relaxation training, graduated exposure) that together produce the desired effects (cf. refs. 10, 11, 21). Nevertheless, contingency management is often an integral part of behavioral intervention. This section provides an overview of basic concepts and principles in contingency management. The reader is referred to other excellent sources (9, 10, 20–22) for a more in-depth review of this information. Let us now turn our attention to some important concepts and definitions in clinical pain.

A BEHAVIORAL CONCEPTUALIZATION OF CLINICAL PAIN

For the application of contingency management to have any credibility with clinical pain, it is mandatory that we establish a behavioral component within clinical pain and the existence of learning and conditioning effects upon these behaviors. This section establishes these points, thus laying the groundwork to apply contingency management to overt pain behavior. In light of a growing body of empirical knowledge over the past 20 years, it has become clear to most experts working with clinical pain that a great deal of the "pain experience" involves overt behavior. Fordyce (1, 3) is credited with establishing this initial point, which added to a basic shift in pain conceptualization. Building on Fordyce's concepts, the current author introduced the idea that clinical pain in its entirety be viewed as complex behavior (7, 11, 23, 24). Within this conceptual model pain can be defined as: "an interacting cluster of individualized overt, covert and neurophysiological responses capable of being produced by relevant tissue damage and irritation, as well as produced and maintained by other antecedent and consequence stimulus conditions" (11). At the neurophysiologic level, specific afferent, supraspinal, and efferent neurologic and muscular responses to tissue damage and irritation, as well as biochemical responses such as endorphin and enkephalin release, have been demonstrated (25). In addition, cognitive/subjective responses (e.g., thoughts of pain as horrible, visual images of being crippled, feeling states of discomfort and anxiety) have also been identified as part of the clinical pain experience (cf. ref. 26). Finally, overt, gross motor pain behaviors such as verbal pain complaints, moaning, taking pain medication, distorted gait, and lying down are a significant part of clinical pain (1, 11, 27, 28). Thus, it is not only reasonable but consistent with all we currently know about clinical pain that it be conceptualized as just noted.

The definition also denotes that pain responses can be maintained and influenced by a host of antecedent and consequence stimulus conditions in addition to tissue damage or irritation. This portion of the definition addresses the established effects of learning and conditioning on pain responses across the neurophysiologic, cognitive/subjective, and overt behavioral categories (cf. refs. 4, 11, 28, 29). Such stimulus conditions as stress, social reinforcement, reduction in distress, presence of others in pain, and administration of pain medication can significantly influence and maintain a host of pain responses. This appears particularly true as pain persists and develops into a chronic state.

Given the established presence of learning and conditioning effects in the development and maintenance of pain responses, it becomes a logical next step to consider using behavioral treatment procedures as part of managing and influencing these responses. Likewise, given that the most accessible pain responses occur in the overt behavioral category, these have been the most thoroughly investigated and frequently treated. The need for direct intervention to reduce or eliminate overt pain behavior becomes even more evident when we consider that most of it can be categorized as escape/avoidance behavior (11, 30). Although such behavior as lying down, taking pain medication, and verbal complaints of pain can be partially maintained by positive reinforcers, they are also very often partially maintained because they reduce or avoid the subjective feeling states of pain, distress, withdrawal, and the like. Thus, all the components for a negative reinforcement paradigm are in place. Given that behavior maintained by escape/avoidance conditioning is typically quite resistant to extinction, direct application of behavioral strategies such as contingency management are often required to effect any meaningful change. Likewise, in light of the frequent finding that pain responses in the chronic state are many times dominated by overt and cognitive/subjective responses, with pathophysiology and neurophysiologic responses not as predominant (cf. ref. 11), the potential utility of such strategies as contingency management becomes even greater.

With this outline of basic concepts in contingency management and a behavioral conceptual model of clinical pain, let us now focus on the specific application of contingency management as a method to reduce the occurrence of overt pain behavior.

REDUCTION OF OVERT PAIN BEHAVIOR WITH CONTINGENCY MANAGEMENT

This section reviews the application of contingency management to reduce overt pain behavior. The four most common categories of overt pain behavior are discussed. These include: (a) verbal pain behavior such as pain complaints, sighing, moaning, general conversations about pain, expressions of pain through verbally mediated intensity ratings, and general expressions of helplessness-hopelessness; (b) specific nonverbal motor pain behavior, including grimacing, bracing, limping, guarding, and rubbing; (c) activity level as seen by sitting, lying, standing, walking, exercising, working, and recreational behavior, or the lack of it; and (d) taking pain-related medication. The section first discusses when it is appropriate to consider using contingency management to effect changes in the overt behavior just described, and then how specific application strategies can be used. This is followed by considerations on where it is most appropriate to use contingency management methods, including some discussion regarding the types of patients (e.g., adult, pediatric, malignant and nonmalignant, low back pain) for which such methods might be most useful.

WHEN TO USE CONTINGENCY MANAGEMENT

Although the principles inherent in contingency management are rather straightforward, proper discrimination regarding under what circumstances contingency management should be considered is not. There are some rather obvious circumstances for contingency management to be of value in treatment. These include: (a) presence of overt pain behavior that appears to be at least partially maintained by learning-operant conditioning effects; (b) availability of effective and salient positive and negative reinforcers, as well as potential punishers; (c) presence of adequate environmental and stimulus control to effectively and contingently apply or withdraw appropriate consequences to specific behavior; (d) the absence of significant learning impairment (e.g., moderate-severe retardation or psychotic reaction); and (e) obtaining cooperation from the patient to allow sufficient application of contingency management methods (31, 32).

The following list outlines some rather basic conditions indicating that overt pain behavior is being influenced by learning-operant conditioning (cf. refs. 1, 6, 7, 11):

1. Overt pain behavior has persisted past the time for normal "healing" to occur.
2. Environmental stressors are present (e.g., marital discord, excessive work demands).
3. Overt pain behavior has a recognizable pattern of occurrence as a function of environment (more pain behavior noted in the physician's office versus home), situation, person (more pain behavior noted in the presence of the patient's spouse or physician versus when alone), or time (pain behavior occurs more frequently during the weekends).
4. Overt pain behavior is recognized and acknowledged by family and friends.
5. Reduction in activity and/or taking pain medication reportedly reduces pain perception.
6. Overt pain behavior appears to be in excess of that expected in light of current physical findings.
7. The patient is expressing concern and worry about increased pain with increased activity and/or return to work.
8. The patient is receiving economic compensation specifically for a medical condition (lumbar nerve root irritation) where pain is a predominate symptom.
9. In spite of significant pain behavior, the patient continues to engage in recreational, sexual, and adequate sleep activities.

Although clearly not definitive, the preceding list can be quite useful as a preliminary method of identifying patients in whom operant conditioning is present and, thus, contingency management strategies might be useful. Typically, one should identify at least three conditions on the list before drawing any assumptions regarding the presence of conditioning effects, with an increasing probability of such effects as the number of conditions increases. It should be noted that the presence of the preceding conditions does not exclude the real possibility that some or all of the overt pain behavior is also a function of underlying pathophysiology. Likewise, this checklist is not a substitute for a more thorough functional behavioral analysis performed by a qualified behavioral psychologist.

Even if conclusive data are not available establishing a specific causal relationship between certain aspects of overt pain behavior and learning-operant conditioning, contingency management principles are quite useful and applicable for increasing the occurrence of more adaptive "well" behavior (e.g., exercising, laughing-smiling, walking in a normal gait). As is outlined subsequently, this strategy is a very frequent approach to producing an actual reduction in overt pain behavior. Many well behaviors are, in fact, opposite to or incompatible with overt pain behavior. Thus, by systematically increasing and maintaining well behavior one automatically gets a reduction pain behavior.

In considering whether adequate control of environmental consequences is present, it is important to determine who is going to be monitoring and administering the consequences. Although historically contingency management has been externally mediated (i.e., behaviors are targeted, monitored, and contingently consequented by a health care professional), it is clear that at least with some overt pain behavior it might be possible for the patient herself to monitor and administer contingent consequences under the supervision of the heath care professional (more is discussed about this later). Thus, the need for exclusive control over the environment and relevant consequences becomes a function of the amount of instructional and self-control the patient is demonstrating. Practically speaking, it is typically best not to assume that the patient will be able to self-administer contingencies unless there is either a history of such behavior in other areas or initial demonstration by the patient of responsiveness to externally controlled contingencies.

The basic strategy utilized to establish the presence of those circumstances necessary to use contingency management involves an extended functional behavioral analysis (11, 33). During such an analysis, specific overt pain behavior and controlling stimuli (both antecedent and consequent) are identified, as well as the presence of adequate control, ability to learn, and cooperation. This information is typically obtained through a variety of assessment strategies, including patient self-report and self-observation via the use of interview, specific questionnaires, and self-monitoring, as well as direct observation by professional staff and significant others in the patient's environment. A thorough review and description of behavioral assessment techniques and tools is clearly beyond the scope of this chapter. The reader is referred to a variety of excellent resource materials (1, 6, 7, 34–38) and to Chapters 6 and 46 in the current text for in-depth descriptions of behavioral assessment techniques and tools. In general, it is recommended that whatever specific assessment techniques are utilized, they include both self- and direct observation of overt pain behavior in controlled and natural settings.

Now that we know when to use contingency management, let us provide a more detailed review of how to use contingency management across common overt pain behavior.

HOW TO USE CONTINGENCY MANAGEMENT

This section describes and offers guidelines for the application of contingency management to common overt pain behavior. For clarity, behaviors will be addressed separately, with contingency management methods demonstrated to be most useful for a given behavior outlined. As noted earlier, conditions for effective usage (e.g., identification of actual overt pain behavior and truly reinforcing or punishing consequences, consistent application) should always be established when applying contingency management.

Verbal Pain Behavior

Included in this category are such pain responses as verbal pain complaints, discussions about poor health, moaning, crying, sighing, and specific verbal expressions denoting the level of pain intensity (e.g., rating of pain intensity on a 0–100 or 0–5 scale). Although pain intensity ratings could also be categorized as cognitive/subjective responses, they are typically mediated by overt verbal behavior, and thus have been included here. The preceding list of verbal pain behaviors represents those routinely seen with chronic pain patients. Although their actual frequencies may vary, almost all patients will emit some verbal pain behaviors, with pain complaints and discussions about poor health and problems being the most obvious and frequently observed. Typically, these and other overt behaviors will show a recognizable pattern of occurrence and be associated with discriminative stimuli or cues (11, 39). For example, it is very common to observe an increase in verbal complaints and discussion of health problems when the patient is in the presence of a physician, nurse, or physical therapist. Furthermore, it has been demonstrated that the presence of a solicitous spouse can significantly increase the occurrence of such behavior (40). Likewise, research has demonstrated that increasing the occurrence of verbal pain complaints can consistently affect subsequent verbally mediated pain intensity ratings (28).

By far the most widely used contingency management methods to reduce verbal pain behavior have been the removal or withdrawal of pleasurable-positive experiences for the behavior through extinction or punishment, while systematically reinforcing verbal "well" behavior (e.g., statements of feeling better, pain is reduced, coping more effectively with problems). The most frequently used and readily available positive experience reinforcers withheld or withdrawn during extinction or punishment of verbal pain behavior and contingently applied to well behavior is social attention-praise. If the verbal pain behavior is also being maintained by other reinforcers such as administration of pain medications or escape from unpleasant home or work responsibilities, the contingent delivery of such consequences should be eliminated. The intent here is to minimize attention and gain or escape from unpleasant demands for verbal pain behavior, while systematically and contingently using positive and possibly negative reinforcers for the emissions of more adaptive verbal well behavior.

For example, take the patient who complains of having a terrible headache or back pain that is typically followed by expressions of concern and sympathy from the spouse and delivery of pain medication. Assuming the absence of serious pathophysiology, a contingency management program might include instructions to the spouse not to respond with sympathy toward pain behavior or application of medications, but rather to change the subject and discuss activity planning for the rest of the day. Likewise, whenever the patient made any verbal expressions about feeling better or marked reduction in pain intensity, the spouse could provide encouragement, praise, and affection. If this particular patient were being seen on an inpatient basis, the same basic strategies could be applied by the health care staff (with the exception of overt affection). With persistence and consistent application, the preceding contingency management strategy can result in significant reduction in verbal pain behavior and increase in more adaptive verbal behavior, particularly if administered in the context of a more general interdisciplinary pain rehabilitation treatment program.

Nonverbal Overt Pain Behavior

The other major overt behavioral category of pain responses involves nonvocal specific motor responses such as grimacing, limping, clutching, walking with a cane, and guarded posturing. (It should be noted that general activity level and taking pain medication are also nonverbal overt behaviors. However, given the need for more elaborate contingency management applications with these behaviors, they are discussed separately.) The same contingency management strategies discussed for overt verbal pain behavior are applicable to nonverbal behavior: specifically, the removal of any positive and negative reinforcers contingent upon these nonverbal behaviors and elimination of any negative reinforcers in concert with the systematic application of positive reinforcement for more adaptive nonverbal "well" behavior (e.g., walking in a relaxed gait, movement without the presence of grimacing or postural distortion). Likewise, the same kinds of positive and negative reinforcers are applicable by family and health care professionals. With regard to the pain behavior of walking with a cane or using a back brace, contingency management techniques should be incorporated with physical therapy. This might involve instructions with praise and the use of rest reinforcers to gradually "shape" walking without a cane or use of a brace by slowly increasing the amount of time, distance, or steps taken without the cane or brace aid. Again, the strategy is to stop reinforcing the pain behavior and systematically reinforce the more adaptive well behavior.

General Activity Level

Many chronic pain patients exhibit marked inactivity (behaviorally viewed as excessive sitting or lying down idle behavior). A major focus of many treatment programs is to increase the patient's overall activity level. Contingency management plays an important part in increasing activity level, primarily through the use of extinction, punishment, response prevention, and positive reinforcement for increased activity. These techniques are typically applied by behavioral specialists in concert with physical therapists. Specifically, the patient might be started on a series of limited exercises, with tolerance levels established. Gradually increasing quotas could then be set over days and weeks for completion of specific exercises (e.g., distance pedaled on an exercise bike) with social, rest, privilege (e.g., more leisure time if the patient is in the hospital), pleasurable activities, and physical or substance (e.g., deep muscle massage, cold or hot packs, special meals) reinforcers applied. Exercise quotas can be viewed not only as a positive reinforcement paradigm, but also as extinction whereby one is removing the contingency between stopping the behavior (exercise activity) and lying down, with the potential reduction in subjective pain experience and fatigue. Likewise, the quota system is a response prevention paradigm, where the act of stopping and lying down is prevented until a certain level of activity is reached.

Particularly for increasing activity, the response prevention aspect of intervention is important given that the pain behavior of sitting and lying down or stopping activity can be viewed as escape/avoidance responses. Thus, simply removing the contingency between the behavior and certain consequences is typically inadequate for change. You should also prevent the lying down/sitting/stopping activity pain behavior from occurring at will, so the individual can learn that the perceived negative consequences (i.e., more tissue damage or increase in pain) of engaging in the behavior do not necessarily occur over repeated trials. This provides the basis to effectively change the escape/avoidance response. Obviously, the concurrent reinforcement of more adaptive and often incompatible well behavior is also crucial. The literature has clearly demonstrated the efficacy of contingency management with chronic pain patients' activity level (1, 6, 41–47).

Medication Usage

The behavior of taking pain medication is one of the most common responses in the overt pain behavior constellation. Likewise, the reduction of this behavior for many patients is crucial to establishing and sustaining any long-term improvement in their condition. Fortunately, several very effective protocols combining medically safe detoxification schedules with contingency management principles have been developed to systematically reduce this overt pain response (1, 48; see Chapter 7). Based upon the assumption that requests for pain medication and its usage are primarily learned behaviors at least partially established and maintained because of positive-reinforcing consequences (e.g., reduction in subjective pain perception, euphoria-mood elevation, social attention, escape/avoidance of withdrawal symptoms) (1, 49, 50), the strategy involves eliminating the contingent relationship between the overt pain behavior and delivery of medication and the social attention it might bring. This is accomplished by administering medication on a "time-contingent" as opposed to a "pain-contingent" basis. Specifically, a baseline amount of medication usage is established under the supervision of a qualified physician. Then, medication is administered at fixed intervals and doses over time. Medication amounts can be systematically reduced within safe limits to avoid potential withdrawal symptoms and physiologic complications. The efficacy of this strategy has been widely demonstrated in the literature. Patients are routinely told that medications are being reduced, but not given specific information about the rate of reduction over time. The primary contingency management paradigms include extinction and response prevention. The patient is no longer given medication contingent upon requests and perceived pain level and is prevented from actually taking medication other than at certain times.

Part of a contingency management program for medication reduction involves the systematic reinforcement through praise and subjective reduction in pain of other nonpharmacologic pain control methods (e.g., relaxation, stretching exercises, transcutaneous electrical nerve stimulation, pacing of activities). Although these alternative pain control responses may not be incompatible with medication usage, they can reduce the stimulus situations of subjective pain perception and persistent tissue irritation, which set the occasion for medication usage behavior.

It should be noted that there are few data (46, 51) supporting the possibility that contingency management strategies within a detoxification schedule are not always necessary to reduce request and usage of medication. These studies have found that patients given proper instructions on reducing medication usage within a behavioral program were able to do so without contingency management. By far, however, the most widely accepted and utilized technique involves detoxification and contingency management as just described. The potential for patient-controlled medication reduction must await further empirical documentation.

Additional Guidelines

As a general rule, the contingency management techniques just described should be applied with the cooperation of the patient. Some have advocated the actual use of written behavioral contracts (42, 52) between the patient and health care professionals. Although no data are available demonstrating that such contracting procedures are necessary, some form of verbal or written understanding about the nature and intent of intervention is important. Likewise, the inclusion of family members in the application of contingency management is viewed as crucial. This typically takes the form of educating family members and obtaining their cooperation to systematically apply contingency management in the natural environment. Likewise, there is clear need to intervene on each pain and well behavior targeted. Current research suggests that effective change in one response (e.g., subjective pain intensity ratings) does not automatically correlate, or is not automatically consistent, with change in other pain responses (e.g., activity level) (cf. refs. 43, 46, 53, 54).

With regard to more broad-based economic consequences, it is also advisable to identify and hopefully reduce or eliminate any relevant contingencies between economic reinforcers (e.g., income supplement through workers' compensation) and overt pain or "illness" behavior. In addition, potential punishers (e.g., premature loss of health and income supplement payments prior to ability to return to work) for increasing more adaptive well behaviors should be removed whenever appropriate. Granted, many times such economic consequences are not controllable within the scope of clinical practice. The reader is referred to other sources for a more thorough review of this topic (55, 56).

Although by definition contingency management must be applied to an individual patient's behavior, it is possible to accomplish this within a group format for certain behaviors. For example, systematic reinforcement of exercise behavior to increase general activity level, and thus reduce lying down responses, could be effectively accomplished within the context of a group physical therapy exercise program. Likewise, extinction of verbal pain behavior and concurrent systematic reinforcement of more adaptive verbal well behavior could be partially accomplished during discussion and educational groups, using praise and attention of the group leader as an effective positive reinforcer. Although there are few empirical data specifically demonstrating such group application of contingency management methods, this format is seen in many pain treatment centers utilizing contingency management methods. Thus, it should not be overlooked as a potentially viable consideration.

When applying reinforcers to adaptive well behavior, it is also good clinical practice to begin by trying to reinforce every occurrence of the well behavior. The operating principle here is to maximize the amount of reinforcement given with the occurrence of target behavior. Once the behavior has been established and is occurring at a stable rate, it is wise to reduce or "thin" the schedule of reinforcement so not every occurrence is followed by reinforcement. It is usually a good idea to follow the behavior with reinforcement at least half of the time, using some form of random schedule of application with regard to which specific occurrence will result in a reinforcer. Such a strategy will maximize the maintenance of a given behavior once it has been established and is consistent with the observation that behavior that is reinforced only some of the time is more resistant to extinction than behavior reinforced all of the time (19, 20).

It is also quite important to administer the contingencies in the presence of as many discriminative stimuli or cues that are found to have influence on overt pain behavior as possible. For example, extinction of overt pain behavior via removal of the contingent consequences of social attention should occur both in the health care professional setting and at home in the presence of family members and friends. Likewise, any reinforcement for well behavior needs to be established across these environments and individuals, as well as possibly in the work environment if it is serving as a cue for increased pain behavior. This will enhance the potential for change in the behavior across these environments by changing the discriminative stimulus or cue values of settings and people. Without such a process, the potential for markedly different pain behavior patterns in one environment and around one group of people (e.g., in the physician's office or hospital room with a nurse) might well be expected. The more consistency there is in responding across environments, the more likely continuation of appropriate behavioral change will occur. Thus, association and establishment of discriminative stimuli or cues that set the occasion for engaging in adaptive overt well behavior is quite important. As noted, this can be done by changing the contingent application of reinforcement from the occurrence of overt pain behavior to well behavior in the presence of as many discriminative stimuli or cues that may have been associated with overt pain behavior as possible.

As with most treatment strategies for chronic pain patients, the maintenance of any improvements in overt behavior is partially a function of adequate follow-up. Although this will vary based upon need and patient availability, it is recommended that patients be followed on a biweekly to monthly basis during the first 6 months after initial intervention has been completed. This will allow the health care professional an opportunity to adjust contingencies, as well as the rate and level of reinforcers utilized to maintain more adaptive well behavior. The most common schedule involves following the patient biweekly during the first month after treatment, fading to once-a-month contact during the remaining 6 months after treatment. Obviously, variations of this schedule might be necessary depending upon the need for problem solving and changes in contingencies and consequences.

Having reviewed the important aspects of how to apply contingency management effectively with common overt pain behavior, let us now turn our attention to the question of where contingency management is most applicable.

WHERE TO USE CONTINGENCY MANAGEMENT

Historically, contingency management techniques were applied in well-controlled inpatient settings. Adult, non-malignant, chronic pain patients exhibiting overt pain behavior consistent with learning-operant conditioning effects were the main focus (1). More recently, the requirement of inpatient application has been reexamined (57, 58). In addition, because of a host of economic constraints, a growing number of pain centers that utilize contingency management techniques are offering more service on an outpatient basis. Unfortunately, there are no clear data to empirically direct decisions regarding inpatient versus outpatient application. Ideally, inpatient application would appear most appropriate given the need for environmental and contingency controls. However, this is still an empirical question. In practice, what is seen is a tendency to utilize inpatient environments for those patients exhibiting excessive pain medication usage behavior with the potential for physiologic dependency. Other patients not showing this behavior are considered for outpatient intervention. As a rule of thumb, it is advised that if contingency management techniques are the primary intervention strategy and the patient has exhibited excessive medication usage with evidence of physiologic dependency, initial intervention should be on an inpatient basis over 2–3 weeks. Obviously, this should be followed by outpatient work to ensure adequate stabilization and maintenance of improvements in the natural environment.

The problem with the preceding rule of thumb is that for the most part, pain treatment centers do not offer just contingency management techniques. Thus, we are left with the issue of excessive medication usage and potential physiologic dependency as a primary discriminator regarding inpatient versus outpatient application. Clearly, more research must be forthcoming to effectively examine the necessity of inpatient application of contingency management methods. Given anecdotal findings that it is quite possible to significantly change overt pain and well behavior on an outpatient basis within an interdisciplinary pain program that includes contingency management strategies, questions must be raised about the necessity of inpatient implementation. For now, no clear empirical guidelines are available with the exception of medication issues. Clinicians are left to their own judgment regarding the necessary setting to achieve desired effects using contingency management strategies.

With regard to the types of chronic pain patients for

whom contingency management techniques are most applicable, by far the vast majority have been low back pain patients (1, 11, 42, 46, 53). The next largest group includes cervical and headache chronic pain patients. Although these two groups constitute the majority of patients who have responded to contingency management methods alone or in concert with other strategies, the application of contingency management is not specific to site of discomfort. Given that overt pain behavior and the corresponding reduction of well behavior may be associated with injury or discomfort in any part of the body, contingency management techniques can be applicable regardless of pain type or location. Likewise, application of contingency management to overt pain behavior in children and the elderly has received at least limited empirical support (59–61). Although use of contingency management alone in the treatment of overt pain behavior in children and adults associated with malignant disease has yet to be adequately researched (62), its use in combination with other behavioral procedures (e.g., relaxation training) has at least some support from the literature on pediatric cancer patients (cf. ref. 63). Thus far, this intervention has focused on the reinforcement of "coping" behavior in children undergoing painful medical procedures such as bone marrow aspirations or lumbar punctures.

With the discussion of when, how, and where contingency management can be effectively applied to overt pain behavior, the next section highlights some important issues and needs that have been identified in this area.

ISSUES AND NEEDS IN CONTINGENCY MANAGEMENT WITH PAIN BEHAVIOR

Although contingency management with chronic pain patients has gained widespread acceptance and application in clinical practice, important issues and needs remain. These include cost, scope of application, generalization and maintenance of effects, and professional competence (3, 4, 28, 64, 65). The cost issue centers around the observed amount of economic and labor costs involved in the application of contingency management programs with chronic pain patients. Contingency management is a rather labor-intensive method, requiring time and energy on the part of health care professionals and family. Likewise, the incredible rise in hospital charges for inpatient delivery makes contingency management intervention rather expensive. This is a valid issue. Possible solutions include increased usage of outpatient settings, at least for part if not all of the treatment, and group application of contingency management principles. Likewise, the increased use of self-applied contingency management strategies for motivated patients appears quite reasonable (66). This would involve instructing the patient on appropriate application of contingencies to change pain and well behavior. A detailed review of such strategies is beyond the scope of this chapter. However, such self-management methods have exhibited widespread usage in behavior therapy and should be considered with chronic pain patients.

The second issue involves criticisms that contingency management is too narrow in scope and does not adequately address all aspects of the chronic pain syndrome. Particularly, repeated criticism has been made that contingency management does not typically reduce "subjective" pain (3). It is not clear that this is a truly valid criticism in that control studies have demonstrated effects on subjective pain reports as a function of contingency management (28, 42, 46). In addition, the fact that contingency management may not routinely produce significant changes in subjective pain experience does not detract from its very potent effects in modifying overt behavior. Included in this criticism of limited scope is the concern that contingency management techniques may be applicable to only a limited kind of chronic pain patient. Although it is clear that contingency management techniques may not be necessary for all chronic pain patients, at least that part of contingency management involved in the systematic reinforcement of more adaptive overt well behavior would appear quite applicable to most. Likewise, as already noted empirical support is growing for the utility of contingency management in treatment programs for pediatric and adult populations, as well as malignant and nonmalignant conditions. Obviously, much more research is still needed in this area.

Critics of contingency management strategies have also noted that the effects are not generalized to other environmental settings and are not maintained over time. Again, although there is some legitimacy to this criticism, follow-up in the natural environment through outpatient application and family involvement can significantly enhance generalization and maintenance.

A final important issue involves professional competency in applying contingency management techniques. Clearly, these are procedures that should be applied by someone thoroughly familiar with those principles and conditions for effective usage outlined at the beginning of the chapter. This routinely means that a behavioral psychologist should be involved in the design of any such contingency management program. Although such an individual might not be needed in the implementation of the program provided adequate training is given to other individuals (e.g., physical therapist, nurses, spouse), overall supervision of any contingency management program needs to be carried out by a well-trained behavioral psychologist.

There are a variety of clinical and research needs associated with contingency management of overt pain behavior. Clinically, there is an ongoing need to attempt systematic integration of contingency management methods with other behavioral procedures (e.g., relaxation training) and physical-medical interventions such as physical therapy, transcutaneous electrical nerve stimulation, and localized nerve blocks. This will typically allow application of contingency management across a broader range of chronic pain patients and facilitate overall effects. Contingency management should not be applied in isolation or in the absence of adequate data regarding the extent of pathophysiology.

There is also a significant need for more quality research in the area. Although a vast array of topics are worthy of more investigation, core areas include systematic research on the relative contribution, cost-effectiveness, and generalization of effects with contingency management; comparison studies of contingency management efficacy in inpatient, outpatient, individual, and group applications; and studies of comparative efficacy with other behavioral and nonbehavioral techniques. Likewise, further empirical tests of contingency management's utility with pediatric and geriatric chronic pain populations, malignant and nonmalignant progressive disorders (e.g., arthritis; cf. refs 67, 68), and more acute pain situations such as painful medical procedures, following surgery, or during childbirth are needed. In addition, continued studies to delineate individual differences and responses to contingency management and testing its limits of application within the chronic pain population are essential. Guided by the findings from such research, it should be possible to greatly enhance the current application of contingency management to maximize its utility in the treatment of overt pain behavior.

CONCLUSIONS AND FUTURE TRENDS

It is clear that contingency management is now well established as an important aspect of treatment with most chronic pain patients. It is also quite clear that contingency management is best utilized in concert with additional behavioral and medical strategies integrated in a uniform interdisciplinary treatment context. Given this, clinicians interested in seriously working with chronic pain patients must become familiar with contingency management concepts and applications if they are to succeed in delivering effective care. Given its demonstrated utility, contingency management should clearly continue to be a significant component in the future of chronic pain management.

Although future trends are often very difficult to predict, several directions appear to be emerging from current applications. One trend that has already started and would appear inevitable is the increasing use of contingency management techniques on an outpatient basis. Although possibly not ideal for environmental control, contingency management is currently being used effectively in concert with other methods on an outpatient basis in a growing number of interdisciplinary pain control programs. Given that such application is much more cost effective, ever-increasing application on an outpatient basis appears quite probable. Likewise, supported by those rather positive initial findings referenced in this chapter, the extension of contingency management techniques to other pain types and patient populations should also be forthcoming.

Again, quality research is the key to this expansion. Finally, the continued integration of contingency management techniques with other behavioral and medical strategies is quite evident. No longer are behavioral psychologists working in isolation when treating chronic pain patients. They have firmly established their presence and that of contingency management and other behavioral techniques as part of the interdisciplinary approach to chronic pain management.

References

1. Fordyce WE: *Behavioral Methods for Chronic Pain and Illness.* St. Louis, CV Mosby, 1976.
2. Keefe FJ, Gill KM: Recent advances in the behavioral assessment and treatment of chronic pain. *Ann Behav Med* 7:11–16, 1985.
3. Fordyce WE, Roberts KH, Sternbach RA: The behavioral management of chronic pain: response to critics. *Pain* 22:113–125, 1985.
4. Linton SJ: Behavioral remediation of chronic pain: a status report. *Pain* 24:125–141, 1986.
5. Linton SJ: A critical review of behavioral treatments for chronic benign pain other than headache. *Br J Clin Psychol* 21:321–337, 1982.
6. Linton SJ, Melin L, Gotestam KG: Behavioral analysis of chronic pain and its management. *Prog Behav Modif* 18:1–42, 1984.
7. Sanders SH: Behavioral assessment and treatment of clinical pain: appraisal and current status. *Prog Behav Modif* 8:249–291, 1979.
8. Skinner BF: *The Behavior of Organisms: An Experimental Analysis.* New York, Appleton-Century-Crofts, 1938.
9. Kanfer F, Phillips JS: *Learning Foundations of Behavior Therapy.* New York, John Wiley & Sons, 1970.
10. Goldfried MR, Davison GC: *Clinical Behavior Therapy.* New York, Holt, Rinehart & Winston, 1976.
11. Sanders SH: The role of learning in chronic pain states. In Brena SF, Chapman SL (eds): *Clinics in Anesthesiology: Chronic Pain Management and Principles.* London, WB Saunders, 1985, pp 57–73.
12. Turner JA, Chapman CR: Psychological interventions for chronic pain: a critical review. I and II. *Pain* 12:1–46, 1982.
13. Turk DC, Flor H: Etiological theories and treatments for chronic back pain: II. Psychological factors. *Pain* 19:209–233, 1984.
14. Chapman SL: Behavior modification for chronic pain states. In Brena SF, Chapman SL (eds): *Clinics in Anesthesiology: Chronic Pain Management and Principles.* London, WB Saunders, 1985, pp 111–142.
15. Chapman SL: A review and clinical perspective on the use of EMG and thermal biofeedback for chronic headaches. *Pain* 27:1–43, 1986.
16. Kazdin AE: *The Token Economy.* New York, Plenum Press, 1977.
17. Sidman M: Operant techniques. In Bachrach AJ (ed): *Experimental Foundations of Clinical Psychology.* New York, Basic Books, 1962, pp 170–210.
18. Kazdin AE: *Behavior Modification in Applied Settings.* Homewood, IL, Dorsey Press, 1975.
19. Skinner BF: *Science and Human Behavior.* New York, Macmillan, 1953.

20. Reynolds GS: *A Primer of Operant Conditioning*. Glenview, IL, Scott-Foresman, 1968.
21. Nay RW: *Behavioral Interventions: Contemporary Strategies*. New York, Gardner Press, 1976.
22. Staats A: Paradigmatic behaviorism, unified theory, construction methods, and the Zeitgeist of separationism. *Am Psychol* 36:239–256, 1981.
23. Sanders SH: Chronic pain: conceptualization and epidemiology. *Ann Behav Med* 7:3–5, 1985.
24. Sanders SH: A trimodal behavioral conceptualization of clinical pain. *Percept Mot Skills* 48:551–555, 1979.
25. Stimmel B: *Pain, Analgesia, and Addiction: Pharmacological Treatment of Pain*. New York, Raven Press, 1983.
26. Turk DC, Rudy TE: Assessment of cognitive factors in chronic pain: a worthwhile enterprise? *J Consult Clin Psychol* 54:760–768, 1986.
27. Keefe FJ, Gill KM: Behavioral concepts in the analysis of chronic pain syndromes. *J Consult Clin Psychol* 54:776–783, 1986.
28. White B, Sanders SH: The influence on patients' pain intensity rating of antecedent reinforcement of pain talk or well talk. *J Behav Ther Exp Psychiatry* 17:155–159, 1986.
29. Fordyce WE, Shelton JL, Dundore DE: The modification of avoidance learning pain behaviors. *J Behav Med* 5:405–414, 1982.
30. Foa EB, Steketee GS: Obsessive-compulsives: conceptual issues and treatment interventions. *Prog Behav Modif* 8:1–53, 1979.
31. Fordyce WE, Steiger JC: Chronic pain. In Pomerleau OF, Brady JP (eds): *Behavioral Medicine: Theory and Practice*. Baltimore, Williams & Wilkins, 1979, pp 125–153.
32. Roberts AH: The operant approach to the management of pain and excess disability. In Holzman AD, Turk DC (eds): *Pain Management: A Handbook of Psychological Treatment Approaches*. New York, Pergamon Press, 1986, pp 10–30.
33. Lake AE: Behavioral assessment considerations in the management of headache. *Headache* 21:170–178, 1981.
34. Keefe FJ, Brown C, Scott DS, Ziesat H: Behavioral assessment of chronic pain. In Keefe FJ, Blumenthal JA (eds): *Assessment Strategies in Behavioral Medicine*. New York, Grune & Stratton, 1982, pp 321–350.
35. Melzack R (ed): *Pain Measurement and Assessment*. New York, Raven Press, 1983.
36. Karoly P: The assessment of pain: concepts and procedures. In Karoly P (ed): *Measurement Strategies in Health Psychology*. New York, John Wiley & Sons, 1985, pp 461–515.
37. Keefe FJ, Crisson JE, Snipes MT: Observational methods for assessing pain: a practical guide. In Blumenthal JA, McKee DC (eds): *Applications in Behavioral Medicine Health Psychology: A Clinician's Sourcebook*. Saratoga, FL, Professional Resource Exchange, in press.
38. Brena SF, Chapman SL: Acute versus chronic pain states: "the learned pain syndrome". In Brena SF, Chapman SL (eds): *Clinics in Anesthesiology: Chronic Pain Management and Principles*. London, WB Saunders, 1985, pp 41–55.
39. Thelen MH, Fry RA: The effect of modeling and selective attention on pain tolerance. *J Behav Ther Exp Psychiatry* 12:225–229, 1981.
40. Block AR, Kremer EF, Gallor M: Behavioral treatment of chronic pain: the spouse as a discriminative cue for pain behavior. *Pain* 9:243–252, 1980.
41. Cairns D, Pasino J: Comparison of verbal reinforcement and feedback in the operant treatment of disability due to chronic low back pain. *Behav Ther* 8:621–630, 1977.
42. Roberts AH, Rinehart L: The behavioral management of chronic pain: long term follow up with comparison groups. *Pain* 8:151–162, 1980.
43. Fordyce WE, McMahon R, Rainwater G, Jackins S, Questad K, Murphy T, Delateur B: Pain complaint—exercise performance relationship in chronic pain. *Pain* 10:311–321, 1981.
44. Doleys DM, Crocker M, Patton D: Response of patients with chronic pain to exercise quotas. *Phys Ther* 62:1111–1114, 1982.
45. Cinciripini PM, Floreen A: An evaluation of a behavioral program for chronic pain. *J Behav Med* 5:375–389, 1982.
46. Sanders SH: Component analysis of a behavioral treatment program for low back pain. *Behav Ther* 14:697–705, 1983.
47. Dolce JJ, Crocker MF, Moletteire C, Doleys DM: Exercise quotas, anticipatory concern and self efficacy expectations in chronic pain: a preliminary report. *Pain* 24:365–372, 1986.
48. Hare BD, Milano RA: Chronic pain: perspective on physical assessment and treatment. *Ann Behav Med* 7:6–10, 1985.
49. White B, Sanders SH: Differential effects on pain and mood in chronic pain patients with time–versus pain-contingent medication delivery. *Behav Ther* 16:28–38, 1985.
50. Bertzen D, Gotestam KG: Effects of on-demand or fixed interval schedules in the treatment of chronic pain with analgesic compounds: an experimental comparison. *J Consult Clin Psychol* 55:213–218, 1987.
51. Keefe FJ, Bach AR, Williams RB, Surwit RS: Behavioral treatment of chronic pain: clinical outcome and individual differences in pain relief. *Pain* 11:221–231, 1981.
52. Sternbach R: *Pain Patients: Traits and Treatment*. New York, Academic Press, 1974.
53. Fordyce WE, Lansky D, Calsyn DA, Skelton JL, Stolov WC, Rock DL: Pain measurement and pain behavior. *Pain* 18:53–69, 1984.
54. Linton SJ: The relationship to an activity and chronic back pain. *Pain* 21:289–294, 1985.
55. Chapman SL, Brena SF: Pain and society. *Ann Behav Med* 7:21–24, 1985.
56. Brena SF, Chapman SL: Pain and litigation. In Wall PD, Melzack R (eds): *Textbook of Pain*. Edinburgh, Churchill-Livingstone (in press).
57. Follick MJ, Ahern DK, Attanasio V, Riley JF: Chronic pain programs: current aims, strategies, and needs. *Ann Behav Med* 7:17–20, 1985.
58. Kerns RD, Kirk DC, Holzman AD, Rudy TE: Comparison of cognitive-behavioral and behavioral approaches to the outpatient treatment of chronic pain. *Clin J Pain* 1:195–203, 1985.
59. Varni JW, Bessman CA, Russo DC, Cataldo MF: Behavioral management of chronic pain in children: case study. *Arch Phys Med Rehab* 61:375–379, 1980.
60. Miller C, LeLieuvre RB: A method to reduce chronic pain in elderly nursing home residents. *Gerontologist* 22:314–317, 1982.
61. Kelley ML, Jarvie GJ, Middlebrook JL, MacNeer MF, Drabman RS: Decreasing burned childrens' pain behavior: impacting the trauma of hydrotherapy. *J Appl Behav Anal* 17:147–158, 1984.
62. Jay SM, Elliot CH, Varni, JW: Acute and chronic pain in adults and children with cancer. *J Consult Clin Psychol* 54:601–607, 1986.
63. Jay SM, Elliot CH, Katz E, Siegel SE: Cognitive-behavioral and pharmacological interventions for childrens' distress during painful medical procedures: a treatment outcome study. *J Consult Clin Psychol* 55:860–865, 1987.
64. Latimer PD: External contingency management of chronic

pain: a critical review of the evidence. *Am J Psychiatry* 139:1308–1312, 1982.
65. Follick MJ, Zitter RE, Ahern DK: Failures in the operant treatment of chronic pain. In Foa EB, Emmelkamp P (eds): *Failures in Behavior Therapy*. New York, John Wiley & Sons, 1983, pp 311–334.
66. Stuart RB (ed): *Behavioral Self-Management: Strategies, Techniques and Outcome*. New York, Brunner/Mazel, 1977.
67. Bradley LA, Young LD, Anderson KO, McDaniel LK, Turner RA, Aqudelo CA: Psychological approaches to the management of arthritis pain. *Soc Sci Med* 19:1353–1360, 1984.
68. McDaniel LK, Anderson KO, Bradley LA, Young LD, Turner RA, Aqudelo CA, Keefe FJ: Development of an observational method for assessing pain behavior in rheumatoid arthritis patients. *Pain* 24:165–184, 1986.

chapter 18
A Cognitive-Behavioral Perspective on Chronic Pain: Beyond the Scalpel and Syringe

Dennis C. Turk, Ph.D.
Thomas E. Rudy, Ph.D.

Over the past two decades, numerous books and chapters have been written emphasizing the importance of viewing pain as more than simply a function of the extent of tissue damage. Authors have noted that pain is a much more complex, perceptual phenomenon that is comprised of a multitude of psychosocial factors as well as sensory stimulation. Chronic pain, in particular, extends over lengthy time periods and can be augmented, maintained, and even directly caused by cognitive, affective, and behavioral parameters (1).

Although historically the role of psychological factors was acknowledged, until recently the pendulum had swung to an extreme view of pain as solely sensory. This position evolved from the advent of sensory psychophysics and sensory physiology during the last half of the 19th century. Consideration of pain as a sensory phenomenon resulted in the efforts to measure pain per se, that is, as a sensory-physiologic phenomenon uncontaminated by psychological factors, and in the development of sophisticated surgical procedures to ablate the pain pathways from the periphery to the central nervous system and the synthesis of more and more potent analgesic agents. Unfortunately, these therapeutic advances have not always had the desired result of complete and permanent elimination of pain, nor is there agreement as to whether "pure" sensory pain can be isolated and measured. Dissatisfaction with the unidimensional sensory model was voiced by clinical practitioners who noted that patients with ostensibly the same degree of tissue damage reacted quite differently to identical therapeutic modalities and that patients with similar diagnoses responded quite differently to the syndrome or injury. Moreover, despite the advances in neuroanatomy and physiology, there continued to be many patients and many pain syndromes for which no intervention consistently and permanently eliminated complaints of pain.

The rather dramatic shift from pain as a purely sensory phenomenon to pain as a perceptual event was given the greatest impetus by developments in the mid-1960s, most notably by Melzack and his colleagues (2, 3) and Fordyce and coworkers (4). Melzack and his colleagues presented a multidimensional model of pain designed to deal with the inconsistencies manifest by different sensory models of pain, that is, the gate control model (3, 5). Melzack postulated that the experience of pain was the result of the integration of motivational-affective, cognitive-evaluative, and sensory-discriminative contributions. Note that this view differs greatly from sensory views that, when they consider psychological factors at all, relegate them to reactions to "pain" and, consequently, nuisance variables or at best epiphenomena. The gate control model did not give priority to sensory input nor did it treat the sensory input as isomorphic with pain. Rather, pain was postulated to be the result of the integration and interpretation of sensory and psychological processes, and, therefore, qualified as a perceptual process.

Coming from a very different orientation but at approximately the same time, Fordyce and his colleagues (6) emphasized the subjective aspect of pain. Rather than focusing on pain per se, Fordyce based his model on classical learning theory, specifically operant conditioning. From this perspective, the subjective experience of pain is irrelevant because it cannot be directly observed and reports and description of it are biased by a number of factors.

Forcye's (7) operant model focuses on behavioral expression of pain. These behavioral manifestations of pain or "pain behaviors" consist of overt sources of communication that convey to an observer that an individual is suffering (e.g., limping, grimacing, moaning, lying down). Once we begin speaking of observable behaviors, then we can consider the production and maintenance of those behaviors as being under environmental control through selective reinforcement. That is, significant others in the patient's environment, whether family, friends, or health care providers, respond to the patient's overt behavior. Significant others may positively reinforce these behavioral manifestations by providing attention or permitting the patient to avoid the performance of undesirable activities (e.g., physical activity), and thereby unwittingly contributing to the maintenance of these behaviors. Moreover, the insurance system may positively reinforce the expression of pain behaviors by providing financial incentives contingent upon the emission of pain behaviors. Thus, according to the operant conditioning model, pain behaviors may continue even in the absence of nociceptive stimulation. [Note that nociceptive stimuli are stimuli that are capable of being perceived as pain but are not conceptualized as pain stimuli (8). The analogy to potential energy is appropriate.]

The operant approach is particularly relevant when we consider chronic pain that extends over long periods of time. At an acute level, behavioral responses to injury and nociceptive stimulation may be appropriate and serve a protective function. However, extension of the performance of these behaviors over long periods of time may become detrimental and problems in their own right. [Recently, even the short-term production of such behaviors has been reported to be potentially detrimental to low back pain patients (9).] Extended performance of pain behaviors may directly influence the experience of pain because they lead to generalized deconditioning (reduction in muscle strength and flexibility and increased fatigue). Moreover, continuation of pain behavior may lead to reduction of previously enjoyed activities and increased affective distress. A vicious cycle may be initiated and perpetuated by the unwitting positive reinforcement of pain behaviors.

In the same way that the unidimensional sensory model suggests specific interventions (i.e., cutting or blocking pain pathways), the operant conditioning and gate control models each have important implications for treatment. The operant conditioning model emphasizes environmental manipulations whereby pain behaviors that were previously reinforced are extinguished and alternatively "well behaviors" are positively reinforced. Moreover, medications taken on an as-needed basis and exercise on a work-to-tolerance schedule are viewed as inappropriate. Rather, medication is changed to a time-contingent schedule and eventually eliminated and exercise is performed to quota, not until pain serves as a signal for termination. Treatment conceptualizations based on the gate control model lead to an increased emphasis on cognitive and affective factors. Both the operant and gate control formulations have contributed to a resurgence of interest in chronic pain treatment that extends beyond the scalpel and the syringe.

Although both the operant and gate control models provide important points of departure from sensory models and interventions, each provides a somewhat limited view and is inadequate in and of itself. The operant model fails to consider the contribution of cognitive appraisals of the patients as they affect patients' perceptions and responses to their physical problems. The gate control model seems more appropriate for acute pain in that it does not consider environmental influences as they extend over time. An alternative model that emphasizes both the importance of environmental factors underscored by the operant approach and the psychological contribution inherent in the gate control model has been formulated by Turk and his colleagues (10–12) and labeled a cognitive-behavioral perspective. A comprehensive intervention model based on the cognitive-behavioral conceptualization has been developed and employed with a diversity of pain syndromes [e.g., headaches (13), temporomandibular pain disorders (14), arthritis (15; K. Lorig, unpublished results), back pain (E.M. Altmaier and T.R. Lehmann, unpublished results), and heterogeneous pain syndromes (16, 17)]. In the remainder of this chapter we describe the cognitive-behavioral conceptualization and cognitive-behavioral approach to the treatment of chronic pain patients.

A COGNITIVE-BEHAVIORAL CONCEPTUALIZATION OF CHRONIC PAIN

To better understand the rationale for the advent of cognitive-behavioral conceptualizations it is worth considering the basic foundations of operant theory. The primary assumption of this approach is labeled the "law of effect" (18). Specifically, changes in response rates are postulated to occur in the presence or withdrawal of positive reinforcement and initiation or avoidance of negative reinforcement. We only consider the case of initiation of positive reinforcement to illustrate the operant model. An operant behavior has an initial level of occurrence in the absence of any reinforcement, which is referred to as the baseline level. The introduction of an external positive reinforcement increases the rate of responding, assuming the organism desires the reinforcement. When the positive reinforcement is terminated, the response rate increases markedly for a short time, then peaks and begins to subside, eventually returning to the baseline at the time the reinforcement was terminated. With prolonged withholding of the positive reinforcement, the response rate continues to decline until it reaches the baseline and then remains at that rate. At this point, extinction of the previously reinforced behavior has occurred.

From an operant perspective, therapy involves an attempt to increase the response rate of adaptive behaviors and the elimination of maladaptive ones. The use of positive reinforcement for desired behaviors can successfully accomplish this, and responding during positive reinforcement is reliably higher than baseline performance of the behavior. To provide a concrete example, Cairns and Pasino (19) demonstrated that the activity levels of pain patients could be increased as a function of attention (positive reinforcement) and that activity levels returned to baseline following elimination of the positive reinforcement (extinction). Although this study provides evidence to support the operant formulation, it also illustrates a major problem, the failure of the desired behavior to be maintained once the external reinforcement was withdrawn. This is a major problem for operant approaches because they have been plagued by the failure of treatment effects to be maintained and generalized beyond the therapeutic context (e.g., refs. 20, 21).

Cognitive-behavioral conceptualizations were originally developed in order to better understand how individuals function in general and not specifically in the area of pain. The impetus for the development of cognitive-behavioral models was the general dissatisfaction with what was perceived as the limited scope and consistent failure of the beneficial effects attributed to interventions based exclusively on operant conditioning to generalize and be maintained following treatment termination (e.g., refs. 22–24). It is our belief that attention to cognitive and affective factors that contribute to the pain experience can be integrated within a comprehensive treatment program that also gives attention to environmental sources of reinforcement and makes use of various behavioral techniques. We believe further than such a comprehensive approach has a greater likelihood of fostering maintenance of treatment benefits. The use of positive reinforcement for adaptive behaviors would play an important part in this approach; however, focus on intrinsic motivation should also play a major role because continued external reinforcement is unlikely to be maintained indefinitely. Some authors have suggested that cognitive and behavioral approaches and philosophies are "antithetical" and cannot be integrated (e.g., refs. 25, 26). We strongly disagree, and describe here how we have integrated cognitive and behavioral approaches within a comprehensive cognitive-behavioral approach.

ASSUMPTIONS OF THE COGNITIVE-BEHAVIORAL PERSPECTIVE

There are five general assumptions that characterize the cognitive-behavioral perspective. These are summarized in Table 18.1. The first assumption is that individuals are active processors of information rather than passive reactors. That is, individuals attempt to make sense of the stimuli that impinge upon them from the external environment by filtering information through organizing templates that have been derived through their prior learning histories and through the use of general strategies that guide the processing of information (e.g., refs. 27–29). Individuals' responses (overt as well as covert) are based on these appraisals and subsequent expectations rather than being contingent exclusively on the actual consequences of their behaviors (i.e., positive and negative reinforcements and punishments). Thus, from this perspective, the *anticipated* consequences are as important in the governing of behavior as the actual consequences.

A second assumption of the cognitive-behavioral perspective is that one's thoughts (e.g., appraisals, attributions, expectancies) can elicit or modulate affect and physiologic arousal, both of which may serve as impetuses for behavior. Conversely, affect, physiology, and behavior can instigate or influence one's thinking processes. Thus, the causal priority is dependent upon where in the cycle one chooses to begin. Causal priority may be less of a concern than the view of a transactional process that extends over time with the interaction of thoughts, feelings, physiology, and behavior (see ref. 30). Much energy has been devoted toward establishing the priority of thoughts, feelings, and behaviors. This approach seems to us to be futile and reminds us of a merry-go-round. Each champion has his or her favorite horse and thinks (feels,

Table 18.1
Assumptions of Cognitive-Behavioral Treatment

1. Individuals are active processors of information.
2. Thoughts can elicit or modulate affect and physiology and can serve as impetuses for behavior. Conversely, affect, physiology, and behavior can instigate or influence thoughts.
3. Behavior is reciprocally determined by the individual and the environment.
4. Clients or patients can learn more adaptive ways of thinking, feeling, and behaving.
5. Clients or patients are capable of and should be involved as active agents in change of their maladaptive thoughts, feelings, and behaviors.

behaves) as if he or she is leading the pack when in reality all are going around in circles with little progress but perhaps an exhilarating ride all the same.

Unlike the operant conditioning model that emphasizes the influence of the environment on behavior, the cognitive-behavioral perspective focuses on the reciprocal effects of the individual on the environment as well as the unidirectional influence of environment on behavior. That is, individuals elicit environmental responses by their behavior. The individual who acts in a hostile manner toward others is likely to elicit response in kind. In a sense, at least to some extent, individuals create their own environments. Thus, the third assumption of the cognitive-behavioral perspective is that behavior is reciprocally determined by both the environment and the individual (31).

If it is assumed, as it is from the cognitive-behavioral perspective, that individuals have learned maladaptive ways of thinking, feeling, and behaving, then successful interventions designed to change behavior should focus on each of these factors and not one to the exclusion of others with the expectancy that changing thoughts, feelings, or behaviors will necessarily result in the others following suit (for alternative views on this topic see refs. 25 and 32; the former gives priority to cognition and the latter to behavior). In a sense, then, the cognitive-behavioral perspective is one that is multidimensional, analogous to the integration of the operant and gate control models of pain described earlier. The possibility and feasibility of such an integration has been questioned by several authors (i.e., refs. 25, 26) and is discussed later in this chapter.

The final assumption of cognitive-behavioral models is that, in the same way as individuals are instrumental in the development and maintenance of maladaptive thoughts, feelings, and behaviors, they can, are, and should be considered as active agents of change of their own maladaptive modes of thinking, feeling, and behaving. Patients or clients, despite their initial conceptualization of their problems, are not helpless pawns of fate. They can and should be instrumental in learning and carrying out more effective modes of responding to their environment.

Unfortunately, most of us have learned to adhere to an acute model of illness; that is, there is a specific cause for any symptom, there is an appropriate treatment, there is a specific time course for resolution of the symptoms (usually days or weeks), and there are socially sanctioned healers who are virtually omnipotent and who will provide a cure. In this model, the "good" patient is the one who is passive, permits physicians to do things to him/her, asks few questions, complies with the physician's orders, and, consequently, gets better. Most patients with chronic illnesses, especially patients with chronic pain, are confronted with challenges to the acute illness model and, not surprisingly, are frustrating for physicians who, like their patients, ascribe to the acute illness model. Chronic pain patients often do not have sufficient objective evidence to account for their pain; many therapeutic interventions may have been tried with limited success, their pain extends over long periods of time and there is little encouraging information that there is an end to their suffering just over the horizon, and, despite the best efforts of physicians, the problem persists. Thus, it is hardly surprising that chronic pain patients become demoralized, and combating demoralization is the essential ingredient of any treatment (33).

OBJECTIVES OF COGNITIVE-BEHAVIORAL INTERVENTIONS

Given the description of the cognitive-behavioral perspective outlined above, we can now consider what the implications of this perspective are for developing interventions in general and then more specifically for use with chronic pain patients. There are a number of specific objectives for any cognitive-behavioral intervention. These are summarized in Table 18.2.

A primary objective, which is addressed repeatedly, is changing clients' or patients' views of their problem from overwhelming to manageable. That is, by the time patients or clients are seen for treatment of a chronic illness they have had sufficient time to become demoralized. They feel helpless and hopeless and the future appears bleak. After all, they have received multiple treatments by various health care providers and they are no better and possibly worse as a result of the potential iatrogenic consequences inherent in any somatic modality. A major component of any intervention, then, is to confront and overcome cli-

Table 18.2
Objectives of Cognitive-Behavioral Treatment

1. Reconceptualize clients' or patients' views of their problems from overwhelming to manageable. (Combat demoralization)
2. Convince clients or patients that skills necessary for responding to problems more adaptively will be included in treatment. (Enhance outcome efficacy)
3. Reconceptualize clients' or patients' views of themselves from passive, reactive, and helpless to active, resourceful, and competent. (Foster self-efficacy)
4. Ensure that client or patients learn how to monitor thoughts, feelings, and behaviors and learn the interrelationship among these. (Break up automatic, maladaptive patterns)
5. Teach clients or patients how to employ and when to execute the necessary overt and covert behaviors required for adaptive response to problems. (Skills training)
6. Encourage clients or patients to attribute success to their own efforts.
7. Anticipate problems and discuss these as well as ways to deal with them. (Facilitate maintenance and generalization)

ents' or patients' maladaptive conceptualizations because these conceptualizations contribute to and exacerbate the initial problem.

One way to bring about the change in patients' or clients' conceptualizations is to convince them that there are ways to address adequately their problems, and that the skills required by the patient to respond more effectively are included within the therapist's armamentarium and can be transferred to the patient. Unfortunately, convincing patients or clients that this is the case is not an easy task (if it was, there would not be a need to receive a lot of training to work with patients, nor would the high fees of treatment be warranted), and even if they believe in the efficacy of the proposed treatment regimen, they may not believe that they are competent to successfully learn and implement these skills as situations demand. Bandura (34) has emphasized the importance of enhancing clients' perceptions of self-control and self-efficacy. Convincing clients or patients of their ability is more likely to occur if they are successful and their own behavior then becomes a positive reinforcer than if one relies exclusively on logic and exhortation. Specific goals and paced mastery are primary strategies to employ in the fostering of patients' or clients' sense of competence. Only when they feel a sense of self-efficacy are they likely to try more difficult goals and to persist in their efforts in the face of difficulties.

Clients and patients need evidence that they can exert more control over their situation. It is all too easy to disregard successful behavior and goal attainment and to focus on failures. Moreover, unless individuals specifically attend to the impact of their thoughts, feelings, physiologic responses, and behavior on each other they are likely to see little interrelationship. To accomplish the levels of awareness of successful goal attainment and the relationship among thoughts, feelings, physiologic responses, and behaviors requires focused attention. Thus, cognitive-behavioral therapists emphasize self-observation and self-monitoring. Specific use of charts and diaries of goals and the antecedents and consequences of maladaptive thoughts, feelings, and behaviors are employed. Such self-monitoring can serve to bring maladaptive automatic modes of responding into conscious awareness and, consequently, can become the focus on voluntary control. Self-monitoring of overt behavior as well as some covert behaviors is an important component of many behavioral as well as cognitive-behavioral interventions. A difference is that the cognitive-behavioral approach is much more concerned about clients' or patients' self-monitoring of their own thinking as it relates to their appraisals, expectations, and dysfunctional modes of responding.

An additional objective of cognitive-behavioral interventions involves teaching clients and patients specific skills to employ that will foster more effective and adaptive modes of responding. A large number of specific skills may be employed but in general some of the most frequently used include problem-solving skills, rationale restructuring, communication skills, and muscular relaxation. Relaxation skills are generic and consist of a variety of different techniques (e.g., biofeedback, autogenic training) geared toward assisting patients to learn how to deal with stress in general and, in particular, how to reduce site-specific muscular hyperarousal. Cognitive-behavioral therapists not only focus on the performance of stress-management skills when the patient is aroused but also emphasize the use of problem-solving and communication skills to prevent the development of maladaptive stress responses. Problem solving consists of teaching patients to identify sources of distress as problems to be dealt with and then to generate and test various solutions. Rationale restructuring focuses on the identification and maladaptive appraisals and expectations and subsequent consideration of more appropriate modes of interpretation. Finally, communication skills relate to the client's or patient's mode of interacting with significant others, including health care providers, and more appropriate means to acquire attention and information. (For a discussion of these different clinical techniques and strategies see ref. 35.)

Teaching patients such skills is an important component of cognitive-behavioral interventions but, although skills training is viewed as necessary, it is not sufficient in and of itself. Clients and patients need to know not only how to perform specific skills but when to perform them as well. Most people can learn to relax when they are not upset, but it is more difficult to learn how to be aware of stress and automatic maladaptive responding and how to execute these skills within the natural environment. Moreover, factors that may interfere with the production of these skills needs to be addressed. Skills training may lead to a diminution in any skills deficiency, but cognitive-behavioral interventions also emphasize and address the importance of production deficiencies, that is, the factors that can inhibit the use of the skills acquired (e.g., insufficient motivation, automaticity of maladaptive responding, affective distress, maladaptive cognitions).

A final important objective of cognitive-behavioral interventions is the fostering of self-attribution of success. That is, much effort is given toward encouraging patients and clients to view themselves as the agents of change. To the extent that clients or patients attribute improvements to their own skills and efforts there is a greater likelihood that they will feel more competent and thus are more likely to expend greater efforts and to persist in the face of difficulties that evolve (34).

Before implementing any intervention with chronic pain patients, using cognitive-behavioral or other approaches, it is essential that a comprehensive assessment be conducted. The assessment of the chronic pain patient should evaluate and integrate psychosocial and behavioral information as well as organic and functional pathology (36). The treatment approach undertaken should be guided by the information provided by the through assessment of all relevant factors.

A COGNITIVE-BEHAVIORAL APPROACH TO THE ASSESSMENT OF CHRONIC PAIN PATIENTS

According to cognitive-behavoral theories of pain, it is the patient's perceptions that interact reciprocally with emotional factors, sensory phenomena, and behavioral responses. Moreover, the patient's behavior will elicit responses from significant others that can reinforce both adaptive and maladaptive modes of thinking, feeling, and behaving. Thus, a transactional model is proposed that does not include the linear causation postulated by unidimensional models such as sensory-physiologic models (see ref. 5), the cognitive model (25), or operant models (7, 32). Rather, the cognitive-behavioral, transactional model views pain as a complex, multidimensional perceptual phenomenon. Pain perception is not the end result of passive transmission and registration of impulses from physically defined stimuli. Instead, it is a dynamic, interpretive process. To better understand and treat pain, consideration must be given to the role of cognitions, emotions, and behavior as well as to sensory contributions in the formation of pain perception and as they evolve over time.

Three central questions guide assessment from a cognitive-behavioral perspective:

1. What is the extent of the patient's disease (physical impairment)?
2. What is the magnitude of the illness? That is, to what extent is the patient suffering, disabled, and unable to enjoy usual activities?
3. Is the illness behavior appropriate to the disease process or is there evidence of amplification of symptoms for any of a variety of psychological or social reasons or purposes ("abnormal illness behavior")?

We have recently proposed a model of pain assessment, labeled a Multiaxial Assessment of Pain (MAP), that incorporates each of these three questions. This MAP approach postulates that three axes, which parallel the questions listed above, are essential to appropriately assess chronic pain patients: medical-physical, psychosocial, and behavioral. From this perspective, each of these general domains must be assessed with psychometrically sound instruments and procedures *and* the results of the assessment of each axis must be combined into a meaningful taxonomy or classification system that will guide treatment decision making and planning. Table 18.3 lists the three axes and examples of the constructs that are incorporated within each.

The approach that we advocate is somewhat at variance with the recent taxonomy of chronic pain patients published by the International Association for the Study of pain (IASP) (37). The IASP taxonomy is based on inference starting with a priori syndromes or diagnoses and, subsequently, rating each diagnosis along each of five axes (i.e., body location, body system, temporal characteristics of pain, intensity and onset, and etiology). The end result of this process is the creation of a unique code for each of over 300 diagnoses. The MAP approach focuses on the empirical derivation of grouping of patients based on the statistical integration of medical-physical, psychosocial, and behavioral data. The suggested approach attempts to identify groups of patients based on their unique characteristics rather than assigning patients to a hypothesized set of diagnoses, as is the case with the IASP approach.

A cornucopia (or Pandorean box) of assessment instruments and procedures are available to operationalize the three MAP axes, and we do not review these here (see refs. 1, 38). What is described is our own attempts to operationalize each of these axes and to develop a taxonomy of chronic pain patients that is based on the integration of these results.

Table 18.3
Components of the Multiaxial Assessment of Pain

1. AXIS I: MEDICAL-PHYSICAL, quantification of:
   1.1. Laboratory and other diagnostic procedures
   1.2. Physical examination
   1.3. Functional mobility, strength, and flexibility
2. AXIS II: PSYCHOSOCIAL, including patients' perceptions of:
   2.1. Pain
   2.2. Affective distress
   2.3. Interference of pain with domains of life (e.g., social, vocational, marital, recreational, physical)
3. AXIS III: BEHAVIORAL-FUNCTIONAL, including:
   3.1. Observable communications of pain and distress
   3.2. Pain related use of health care system
   3.3. Medication
   3.4. Activity levels
   3.5. Responses of significant others

QUANTIFICATION OF MEDICAL-PHYSICAL FINDINGS

Difficulties in assessing the physical contributions to chronic pain are well recognized and there are no universal criteria for scoring the presence, absence, or importance of a particular sign (e.g., abnormal radiograph, distorted gait, limitation of spinal mobility), establishing the association of these findings to treatment success, or quantifying the degree of disability (39). Rather, interpretation of medical-physical findings has tended to rely on clinical judgments and medical consensus based on the physician's experience and occasionally quasi-standardized criteria (40, 41). As Brand and Lehmann (42) noted, "Most rating schemes provide only general guidelines from which a physician must develop his own standards" (p. 77).

A frequent source of confusion in the medical evaluation of chronic pain patients relates to what clinical and laboratory findings are useful and appropriate for chronic pain patients, how much importance should be given to each test result, and how to reliably assess physical pathology. For example, is determination of the amount of pathology based on radiographic and electromyographic findings equivalent to determining pathology based on physical examination? Should computed tomography (CT) scans be given more weight than a functionally oriented finding even though the structural finding may be less reliable than the functional finding? Does an abnormal radiograph predict a successful surgical outcome? Currently, there are no definitive answers to any of these questions.

Most assessments of physical pathology rely on a simple linear combination or summation of identified abnormalities, resulting in a total score (e.g., refs. 40, 41). This procedure is predicated on the assumption that the importance of all abnormalities, regardless of how they are assessed, is equivalent. It is possible if not probable, however, that some positive (abnormal) findings are more important than others and thus should be weighed more heavily in the total pathology or impairment score. Furthermore, some assessment procedures provide more reliable data than others.

To begin to address these questions, we conducted a study to establish the differential utility of the most commonly employed diagnostic procedures used by physicians specializing in the assessment and treatment of pain [i.e., members of the American Academy of Pain Medicine (AAPM), formerly, American Academy of Algology]. Eighty members of the AAPM were surveyed to establish the differential utility of 18 frequently used diagnostic test and examination procedures gleaned from the literature (e.g., electromyography, mobility of weight-bearing joints—see Table 18.4). These physicians displayed a high degree of agreement (Kendall's coefficient of concordance = .65, $p < .001$) regarding the relative importance of the different procedures included in the survey. The average individual physician's rank ordering of these procedures, from 1 (most useful) to 18 (least useful) in the evaluation of chronic pain patients is shown in Table 18.4.

The 80 AAPM members surveyed were also requested to list any additional procedures that would be included in medical assessment of chronic pain patients. Although psychological evaluation and testing were frequently listed, there were no consistent medical test or procedures suggested by those surveyed, and thus it appears that the content validity of the 18 medical tests and examination procedures is acceptable. Thus, if the information gained from these procedures can be reliably scored in the evaluation of chronic pain patients, the results will be of utility in developing a weighted scoring procedure for quantifying medical-physical findings.

A second study was conducted to assess the reliability of the medical-physical screening of the 18 procedures

Table 18.4
Rank-Ordering of 18 Medical Procedures Used in Chronic Pain Assessment

Rank Order Average	Medical Procedure
2.97	Neurologic examination
4.14	Observation of gait and posture
4.39	Assessment of spinal mobility
4.55	Examination of muscular function (tone, mass, strength)
5.94	Examination of soft tissues
6.35	Assessment of mobility of weight-bearing joints
7.95	Plain radiography
8.08	Assessment of mobility of joints other than spine or weight bearing
8.34	Computed tomography scan
9.61	Electromyography
10.42	Contrast radiography
11.69	Examination of internal organs (inspection, palpation, auscultation, percussion)
12.68	Nuclear medicine
13.45	Laboratory tests (other than blood count)
13.93	Thermography
14.00	Blood count
16.10	Electroencephalography
16.40	Electrocardiography

included in the survey of AAPM members. Two AAPM members performed chart reviews of 30 chronic pain patients using 3- or 4-point scales to rate each of the 18 procedures listed in Table 18.4, two AAPM members performed direct assessments on 30 chronic pain patients, and two AAPM members either reviewed the charts or directly examined the same 30 chronic pain patients. Although more complicated rating scales could have been devised, it would likely be more difficult to establish interjudge reliability for them and they would be less likely to be used in clinical settings.

Results from this study indicated that only one of the 18 procedures could not be reliably judged (i.e., assessment of mobility of joints other than spine or weight bearing); the remainder had an average kappa reliability coefficient of .64 ($p < .001$). The broad range in the linear utility weights computed for the 18 medical procedures (e.g., .394 for neurologic examination to .007 for electrocardiography) suggested that the development of assessment procedures that incorporate these medical findings should consider a weighted scoring system. For example, since neurologic examination findings were weighted over 56 times more useful than electrocardiographic findings in the evaluation of chronic pain patients, a scoring system that does not reflect these types of utility differences will likely lead to a skewed or biased scale that does not accurately reflect medical consensus. These results provide preliminary support for the appropriateness of assessing chronic pain patients using these basic quantification procedures and subsequently integrating the results of this examination with psychosocial and behavioral assessment data.

QUANTIFICATION OF PSYCHOSOCIAL AND BEHAVIORAL DATA

Recently, Kerns, Turk, and Rudy (43) developed a comprehensive assessment inventory, the West Haven–Yale Multidimensional Pain Inventory (MPI), that was designed to assess the impact of pain from the patient's perspective. That is, the MPI operationalizes psychological reactions to chronic pain, perceived responses of significant others, and activities interfered with because of pain. This inventory is comprised of three sections. The first section was specifically designed to evaluate chronic pain patients' (a) reports of pain severity and suffering; (b) perceptions of how pain interferes with their lives, including interference with family and marital functioning, work, and social-recreational activities; (c) dissatisfaction with present levels of functioning in family, marriage, work, and social life; (d) appraisals of support received from significant others; (e) perceived life control, incorporating perceived ability to solve problems and feelings of mastery and competence; and (f) affective distress, including ratings of depressed mood, irritability, and tension. The second section of the MPI assesses the patient's perspective as to how significant others within the environment respond when he/she is suffering (i.e., punishing, solicitious, or distracting responses). The last section evaluates the frequency of performing a set of common activities (e.g., cooking a meal). Thus, the first section of the MPI provides an operationalization of the psychosocial axis and the latter two sections the behavioral axis.

The MPI has demonstrated good internal consistency, test-retest reliability, and convergent and discriminant validity (43). Thus, the psychometric properties that are a prerequisite for the development of a classification system suggested by the MAP approach appear to have been met. The next step in the development of the MAP-based taxonomy consists of the integration of the medical-physical findings, based on the procedures described in the preceding section of this chapter, with the results of the psychosocial and behavioral data acquired on the MPI.

INTEGRATION OF ASSESSMENT FINDINGS: TOWARD A TAXONOMY OF CHRONIC PAIN PATIENTS

The MPI (43) and the medical-physical assessment described above were used in the initial phase of taxometric development. Utilizing recent statistical advances in clustering techniques that increase the accuracy of these methods (e.g., refs. 44, 45), cluster analyses and multivariate classification methods (46) were conducted on a heterogeneous group of 100 patients to determine whether there were different response patterns that could reliably classify patients into unique groups. The k-means clustering approach was used to discover more about the similarities and differences among chronic pain patients in order to identify subgroups or "homogeneous" samples of pain patients and to guard against the superimposing of an a priori but potentially invalid structure to the data.

Four distinct patient profiles were identified by means of this analysis:

1. "Disabled" patients who had higher than average medical-physical findings, who perceived the severity of their pain to be high, and who reported that pain interfered with much of their lives, a higher degree of psychological distress, and low activity levels.
2. "Dysfunctional" patients who had less severe levels of medical-physical findings than the disabled group but had high degrees of psychosocial and behavioral disability.
3. "Interpersonally Distressed" patients with a common perception that significant others were not very understanding or supportive of their pain problems.
4. "Adaptive Coper" patients who reported higher levels of social support, relatively low levels of pain and interference compared to the other three groups, and higher levels of behavioral activity.

The percentages of patients falling within each of the four clusters were 24, 24, 31, and 21, respectively.

Additional research is required to examine the incremental validity of behavioral observation of pain behaviors (e.g., ref. 47), coping resources (e.g., ref. 48), idiosyncratic cognitive styles (49), and more mathematically sound weighted scoring systems for medical-physical findings. The goal should be the development of a triarchic, MAP-based taxonomy that will enhance our understanding of pain, assist in evaluation and the prescription of specific therapeutic interventions, and further our ability to predict treatment outcome. The tendency has been to provide all patients with much the same intervention and to compare the treatment outcome to pretreatment measures or a no-treatment comparison group. The unfortunate result of this type of research is that, although patients with certain characteristics may benefit maximally from the intervention, others with a different set of characteristics may be inappropriate for the intervention. Combining both groups together in a single study is likely to lead to results of modest success at best and the subsequent wringing of hands about the inability of pain treatment programs to demonstrate their efficacy (e.g., ref. 50). Classification of patients into more homogeneous groups should permit the direct assessment of the relative effectiveness of different treatments for different patient groups on relevant characteristics and not just on the specific diagnosis as suggested by the IASP approach to classification (e.g., reflex sympathetic dystrophy of the arms, IASP classification code 203.91b) or heterogeneous groups comprised of generic "chronic pain syndrome."

The differential approach to treating pain patients does

not mean necessarily that the philosophy of treatment will change depending upon patient characteristics, but rather than specific interventions may be used to supplement treatment approaches that offer much that is consistent across patients. For example, the cognitive-behavioral philosophy may govern the treatment approach we use with all patients; however, patients with a profile that we have classified as "interpersonally distressed" might benefit from the inclusion of more active family involvement than patients who fall within the group we labeled "adaptive copers," who report that their social supports are more adequate.

COGNITIVE-BEHAVIORAL TREATMENT FOR CHRONIC PAIN

To understand the cognitive-behavioral approach to the treatment of chronic pain patients, it is important to understand that the techniques actually employed are viewed as significantly less important than the more general philosophy and orientation described in general above and more specifically to chronic pain in this section. These factors, which are often referred to somewhat disparagingly as the "nonspecifics" of treatment, are actually the most important component of successful treatment. Thus, we spend some time discussing these to emphasize their importance and to inoculate the reader against focusing on details, such as what method of relaxation to use, what are the specific images used to enhance distraction, where to place the biofeedback electrodes, what physical exercises are best for what types of patients, what is included in the homework assignments, and so forth. Although these technical minutiae are important, they will only contribute to treatment efficacy *if* they are embedded in a more general treatment framework (12, 33).

OVERVIEW

By the time patients come to a treatment program for chronic pain, they have received multiple evaluations and a range of treatment modalities, often beginning with suggestions for bed rest and nonnarcotic analgesic medication, progressing through therapeutic nerve blocks and passive physical therapy (e.g., hot pack, cold packs), and finally, when all else has failed, large dosages of psychotropic and/or narcotic analgesic medications and multiple surgical procedures. In addition to these conventional medical interventions, many patients have submitted to a host of alternative therapies (e.g., acupuncture, hypnosis, biofeedback, vitamin therapy). A common feature across all patients regardless of diagnosis is that the array of interventions have failed to adequately alleviate their suffering. Patients treated at the pain programs with which we have been affiliated have had a mean duration of pain of over 8 years. Thus, it is not surprising that by the time these patients are seen at a pain center they are quite demoralized and frustrated, and feel their situation is hopeless, yet still are seeking *THE* cure for the cause of their suffering. This, then, is the background against which any therapeutic regimen that will be offered must be viewed.

The general goal of a cognitive-behavioral pain treatment program is to assist patients to reconceptualize their view of their situation and their pain. Patients frequently come to pain clinics with a view of pain as a totally medical symptom that is all-encompassing and over which they have no control (fostered by the acute illness model describe earlier). The cognitive-behavioral approach is designed to be optimistic, emphasizing both the effectiveness of the rehabilitation approach *and* the patient's ability to alleviate much of his/her pain and suffering if he/she is willing to work *with* the treatment team. That is, the treatment methods that we will recommend will only be effective if the patient accepts responsibility for a large part of the treatment with the guidance, supervision, and support of all members of the treatment team. This view can be sharply contrasted with previous approaches that have been geared toward "doing something to the patient," with the patient assuming a passive "sick role."

Throughout the rehabilitation process, pain is reconceptualized so that the patient comes to view his/her situation as amenable to change by means of combined psychologically- and physically-based approaches. The treatment program is designed to teach the patient a range of physical and psychological coping skills and to assist him/her in dealing with maladaptive thoughts and feelings as well as noxious sensations that may facilitate or exacerbate suffering. The cognitive-behavioral treatment relies heavily on active patient participation and emphasizes a mutual problem-solving approach among the treatment team, the patient, and the significant others in the patient's environment.

The cognitive-behavioral approach is very much a collaborative endeavor that attempts to foster an increased sense of self-efficacy and intrinsic motivation. Even the most ideal treatment plan has little likelihood of success if the patient does not continue to engage in the prescribed behaviors once discharged from the treatment program. Thus the likelihood of the continued adherence to the self-care regimen is limited to the extent that the patient (*a*) does not have the necessary skills; (*b*) does not feel competent to perform the recommended overt and covert behaviors, particularly on an ad hoc basis; (*c*) permits other factors to interfere with the performance of the adaptive behaviors; and (*d*) experiences no external or intrinsic motivation to persevere with the performance of the behaviors (51). In one recent study surveying chronic pain patients 18 months to 10 years following treatment at a multidisciplinary pain center, adherence to various self-care behaviors was quite low, ranging from less that 10% for diet management and appropriate use of communication skills to 52% for following the recommended exercise regimen (52).

Kanfer and Karoly (53) suggested that for self-management to operate there must be a shift in the patient's repertoire from well-established, habitual, and automatic but ineffective responses toward systematic problem-solving and planning, long-term control of affect, and behavioral persistence. Cognitive and behavioral techniques are employed to teach the patient to recognize and alter the association between thoughts, feelings, behaviors, environmental factors, and pain. From the cognitive-behavioral perspective, therapeutic gain is enhanced and only maintained when the patient is actively involved, accepts responsibility for change, and is intrinsically motivated rather than externally manipulated (54). Improvement is thus a function of the clinic team, the patient, and other significant people in the patient's environment (e.g., family, lawyers, claims adjusters, and members of the health care system).

The cognitive-behavioral approach can be adapted for use with inpatients and outpatients, conducted on an individual or group basis, and can be used as a total program for treatment of chronic pain patients in a multidisciplinary setting or by a solo practitioner. Before describing the outline of treatment, we need to address briefly the composition and function of an interdisciplinary team, the involvement of significant others, and the disability/compensation morass.

INTERDISCIPLINARY TEAM

We use the term *interdisciplinary* rather than multidisciplinary to describe what we feel is the optimal treatment working relationship. Interdisciplinary implies a close working relationship among health care professionals rather than the distal involvement of many consultants with information integrated by the primary health care provider. The core of the team is comprised of members from medicine, nursing, psychology, and physical therapy disciplines. The specialty of the physician member of the team is less important than his/her dedication to working with pain patients and to a nonautocratic approach to participation on rather than command of a team. Each team member has specific areas of expertise, and their contribution to decision making and planning is essential and of equal importance in formulating the treatment.

Although we have listed the core professional team, it is important to realize that the patient and significant others are part of the interdisciplinary *team* as well. That is, patients and family members are not passive. They bring with them to the pain clinic thoughts, attitudes, and wishes that are important and must be incorporated or modified if treatment is to be successful. All too often health care providers forget to LISTEN to what patients and families are trying to tell them. We are not just referring to the "facts" of their injury but also to the impact on their lives. We could contrast the unidimensional health care provider as Sergeant Joe Friday (played by Jack Webb) in the 1950s detective show "Dragnet" with the cognitive-behaviorally oriented health care provider, Lieutenant Columbo (play by Peter Falk) in the late 1970s detective show "Columbo."[1] Sergeant Friday only wanted to "know the facts, nothing but the facts," whereas Lieutenant Columbo was probing, acknowledged confusion and lack of understanding, and readily asked for opinions and not "just the facts." (Perhaps that is why Joe Friday was never promoted from sergeant to lieutenant.)

Often there has been a tendency in the treatment of chronic pain patients to forget about the importance of the family (55). However, chronic pain, by virtue of extending over long periods of time, impacts on all aspects of the patient's life, including his/her family life. Failure to include family members is likely to contribute to the problems of maintenance of treatment gains. At a minimum, families need to be aware of the nature and logic for the treatment goals and modalities employed. Some families may require additional involvement or family counseling if there is to be any hope for success. We might speculate that patients who lie within the interpersonally distressed group described earlier might require extensive family counseling in addition to the basic family involvement required for all patients.

Important adjunctive members to the core professional team include vocational counselors, occupational therapists, and medical consultants, as well as a host of other health care professionals (e.g., dietitians, pharmacists), all of whom need to have a basic familiarity with the cognitive-behavioral orientation of the pain center. In specific cases, these adjunctive team members may assume a more central role and become part of the core disability management team. For example, when vocational issues are a primary concern, vocational counselors and occupational therapists trained in work capacity evaluation and work hardening become central team members.

Although not members of the core team, we should not loose sight of the important roles played by other clinic staff, receptionists, secretaries, and billing personnel. These individuals often have the first contact with the patient and referral sources and they can set the tone for much of the therapeutic milieu. Research suggests that the organizational structure and staff play an essential role in patient satisfaction and, consequently, continued clinic attendance and adherence to the therapeutic regimen (51).

There are three other groups who are essential to the maintenance of treatment gains, but they have been given much less attention—referring physicians, lawyers, and claims adjusters. Referring physicians provide the background set that patients acquire and carry with them to the clinic. Many patients are unsure why they are being referred ("Is this where I get more pills?"), others are angry

---

[1] We were unable to establish Lieutenant Columbo's first name. If any reader can provide this important bit of trivia, we would appreciate hearing from him/her.

("You're referring me there because you don't believe my pain is real."), and still others are given misinformation ("I was told to come here so that you could give a deposition indicating that I should receive complete disability from my worker compensation board."). Moreover, patients who are treated for chronic pain are going to return to referring or primary physicians for continued care. We have seen all too many patients who were successfully treated at other pain centers relapse shortly thereafter because, in part, the referring physician was not informed as to how best to follow through with the chronic pain patient, namely, positively reinforcing progress and avoiding rewards for abnormal illness behavior, including passivity and medication seeking. Thus, both prior to evaluation and treatment and subsequent to treatment termination, referring physicians play an essential role and need to be informed about the nature of the evaluation process and treatment program, what to tell patients who are being referred, and how to continue to care for patients following treatment at the pain center. Additionally, the referring physician should be provided with the evaluation results, a thorough description of the treatment plan, and how successful the patient was in accomplishing the treatment goals. Involvement and information sharing with referral agents is crucial to all phases of treatment and to facilitate maintenance of benefits.

Insurance companies have often had adversarial relationships with pain clinics. Part of the problems has been the failure of pain clinics to address the concerns of third-party payers while expecting them to continue to pay for the services provided (56). Health care providers have tended to take a "holier than thou" stance with insurance companies without understanding the needs of claims adjusters and thus contributed to the adversarial tension. Certain questions are essential from the standpoint of the insurance company, and these need to be addressed even if the answers are not what the insurance company would like to hear. Questions such as "Can this patient return to work?", "Can he or she be rehabilitated?", "Should he or she be awarded total and permanent disability?", "Could the car accident have exacerbated a previous pathological condition?", "What is this patients residual function capacity?", and "Is another surgery likely to permit us to close out this case?" are posed by insurance companies. Although health care providers need to be concerned primarily about the welfare of their patients, answers to these questions can be crucial in treatment planning and are important to address in order to assist third-party payers (56).

Personal injury lawyers and the legal system can hamper attempts to provide optimal rehabilitation. Often the litigation process extends over years and may make the task of rehabilitation much more difficult because the patient may be much more physically deconditioned and psychologically distressed following prolonged legal wrangling (57, 58). Pain centers have not done a very good job of education, and must be aware of these forces as they affect treatment and rehabilitation.

COMPONENTS OF COGNITIVE-BEHAVIORAL TREATMENT

With the background provided, we can now consider some of the specific components of the cognitive-behavioral treatment. Following assessment, although it should be noted that assessment is an ongoing process that should inform treatment, treatment is comprised of four interrelated components: (a) education (b) skills acquisition, (c) cognitive and behavioral rehearsal, and (d) generalization and maintenance.

EDUCATION

The educational component of treatment consists of the presentation of the cognitive-behavioral perspective on pain and the control of pain (i.e., role of cognitions, affect, behavior, environmental factors, and physical factors). At the outset of treatment and continuing throughout, we attempt to discuss pain and the impact on the patient's life in a manner that is most appropriate to each individual patient. We try to use patients' vocabularies, and start with their understanding of their situation and problems. We continue to this collaborative manner through the treatment (59). That is, we convey to the patient that we will not do anything to them but rather that we will work together to achieve the best possible outcome given the restraints imposed by any physical impairments. The collaborative approach can be contrasted with the more traditional autocratic medical approach inherent in many settings.

Many patients have unspoken fears about progression of their condition, injuring themselves by performing certain exercises ("I can't bend over too far or I might break my spinal fusion"), and that people think their pain is not real. In short, we begin by assuming the "Columbo" role and listen to the patient's "story," his/her fears and concerns. Many patients are reluctant to express such concerns or may not even be aware of them, even though these concerns influence their behavior. We often use the "imaginary patient" to help discuss sensitive issues. That is, we might say, "Some patients are concerned that they have limits on their physical activity due to their medical problem. Do you have any concerns about what activities might make your condition worse? Let me assure you that we will not recommend any exercises that would be detrimental to you." Or, we might ask, "Have any of the other physicians who have treated you suggested that you should not do certain things?" If the patient answers yes, we might ask "How long were you told you should not lift heavy objects and how heavy were the objects that you should not lift?" We have found the latter questions to be important because many patients misunderstand the information provided by previous health care providers. We saw one patient who continued to believe that he needed 6 hr of bed rest *2 years after a laminectomy* because his surgeon had told him upon leaving the hospital he should get this amount of bed rest. He did not tell the patient how long to follow this plan and the patient assumed it was permanent (we only wish our patients would adhere as well to our advice regarding the need to continue exercising). If significant others are present, we may turn to them and ask a similar set of questions to elicit their views, worries, and possible misconceptions. The important point is to not only reassure the patient and significant others but also to identify idiosyncratic beliefs and inaccurate understanding of information.

We then employ a more didactic approach, using the information obtained from the assessment, to clarify patients' medical conditions and explain to them what we have found and what is going on physically as well as psychosocially at a level that patients can understand. We prefer to do this with significant others present so that we can determine the misinformation they have acquired as well as educate them about any restrictions and provide them with appropriate reassurances. We review psychosocial and behavioral results acquired during the assessment and try to demonstrate to the patient how his/her situation may be influenced by these factors. We use this information to begin the process of reconceptualization. That is, pain interferes with different areas of peoples' lives, and people respond to them in different ways—how might these differential responses affect how they think, feel, and do, as well as influence how others respond to them?

The educational component continues throughout the treatment; all members of the treatment team use information and material that comes up during and between sessions to underscore the important interrelationships among thoughts, feelings, and behaviors. Specific homework tasks may be prescribed to help patients to identify situations in which thoughts, feelings, and behaviors exacerbated or inhibited their pain. Since homework is such a crucial element in cognitive-behavioral treatment, we devote a section to this topic later in this chapter.

SKILLS ACQUISITION

In all cases, it is important for patients to understand the rationale for the specific skills being taught and the behaviors they are being asked to perform. Again, unless patients understand the rationale for the treatment components and have an opportunity to raise issues and confusions, they are less likely to persevere in their efforts in the face of difficulty, to benefit from therapy, or to maintain any therapeutic gains. Cognitive and behavioral treatment techniques consist of a whole range of strategies and procedures designed to bring about alterations in patients' perceptions of their situation and thus their ability to control their condition (e.g., ref. 11).

Cognitive-behavioral therapists, regardless of speciality or discipline, serve as a teachers, coaches, collaborators, and at times "cheerleaders" helping patients learn new ways of behaving, feeling, and thinking. The health care provider, regardless of discipline, should encourage patients to become active contributors to their experience and not helpless victims. The responsibility for carrying out the program and maintaining any treatment gains rests ultimately with the patient.

Various strategies and techniques are available to the cognitive-behavioral team. As Holzman and his colleagues (54) noted, *"We have found no one treatment technique essential for all patients"* (p. 40, original emphasis). There is a need to individualize the treatment program for the specific patient. Although two patients both participate in a cognitive-behavioral pain management program, the specific details of their treatment or the treatment techniques that are employed may be very different. Therefore, commonalties among treatments may be obscured if only the techniques utilized are compared (33). Rather, the rationale for the techniques used and the overall plan of treatment are more important in this therapeutic approach. Techniques such as relaxation training, active physical therapy using paced mastery, problem-solving training, stress management, distraction skills training, rational restructuring, and communication skills training, to name only a few, have all been incorporated within the general cognitive-behavioral approach. Several recent publications have described in detail some specific techniques used, and the interested reader should consult these (i.e., refs. 10–12, 35, 54).

More important that the techniques is the goal of enhancing self-control and intrinsic motivation and the manner in which these skills are described, taught, and practiced. Once again, it is essential for therapists to keep in mind the patient's perspective and how he/she perceives each skill and assignment. The listening and observational skills of the therapist become quite important because they will influence subsequent strategies, revisions of goals and methods, and so forth. These clinical skills and the relationship that is established between therapists and patients become the oil that keep the gears of treatment moving forward; without these, treatment will come to a grinding halt (12).

COGNITIVE AND BEHAVIORAL REHEARSAL

In this component of the cognitive-behavioral treatment, the patient practices and further consolidates the skills that he/she has learned during the skills acquisition phase and learns to apply them to natural situations. The rehearsal techniques employed include rehearsal during mental imagery, during which time the patient imagines using the skills in different situation, difficulties encountered, and how these difficulties are handled and overcome. Role playing is also used. The patient interacts with the therapist as if he/she were in a specific situation and needed to employ specific skills (e.g., argument with spouse). Role reversal, where the patient and therapist switch roles and the patient "teaches" skills to the therapist, who has assumed the role of a new patient, is also employed. Specific details of these approaches are described in Holzman et al. (54) and Turk et al. (11).

HOMEWORK

An essential component of the cognitive-behavioral approach is the active involvement of the patient and significant others outside of the therapy sessions. Turk et al. (11) have outlined the purposes of the tasks to be conducted between sessions:

1. To assess various areas of the patient's and significant others' lives and how these influence and are affected by the pain problem.
2. To assess the typical responses of significant others and the patient to pain and pain behaviors.
3. To make the patient and significant others more aware of the factors that exacerbate and alleviate suffering.
4. To help the patient and significant others identify maladaptive responses to pain and pain behaviors.
5. To consolidate the use of coping procedures and physical exercises discussed during therapy sessions.
6. To increase physical activity levels.
7. To illustrate to the patient and significant others that progress can be made in living with pain but with less suffering.
8. To serve as reinforcers and as enhancers of self-efficacy as the patient achieves his/her goals.
9. To assist the therapist and patient in assessing progress and in modifying goals and treatment strategies.

Homework assignments are establish within the same consultative framework as all of the cognitive-behavioral therapy that we have described is conducted. Each homework assignment is geared toward observable and manageable tasks, starting with those that are most readily achievable and progressing to more difficult ones. The purpose of such graded tasks is to enhance the patient's sense of competence and to reinforce his/her continued efforts. The therapist uses the assessment results to establish short-, medium-, and long-term goals, and the accompanying tasks are designed to attain these goals. Goals and assignments are most effective when they are individually tailored to the particular condition, life-style, and whenever possible wishes of each patient. The emphasis on homework is consistent with operant approaches. This illustrates our point regarding the potential of integrating behavioral techniques within a cognitive-behavioral treatment regimen.

GENERALIZATION AND MAINTENANCE

In the final stage of treatment, discussion focuses on possible ways of predicting and avoiding or dealing with pain following treatment termination. We have found it helpful to assist patients to anticipate future stress or pain-eliciting events and to plan coping strategies and response strategies before they occur. Marlatt and Gordon (60) referred to this process as "relapse prevention."

It is important to note that all possible situations cannot be anticipated. Rather, our goal during this phase, as in the rest of the treatment, is to enable patients to develop a problem-solving perspective to coping where they believe that they have the skills and competencies within their repertoire to respond in an adaptive fashion. In this manner, the patient will learn to try to anticipate future difficulties, develop plans for coping, and adjust his/her behavior accordingly. Successful performance of these strategies should further serve to enhance self-efficacy and may help to form a "virtuous circle" in contrast to the "vicious circle" created and fostered by inactivity, passivity, physical deconditioning, helplessness, and hopelessness that characterize chronic pain patients.

The relapse prevention phase serves at least two purposes: first, it permits the patient to anticipate and plan for future events, and second, it focuses on the necessary conditions for long-term success. More specifically, relapse prevention provides the patient with the expectation that minor setbacks may in fact occur but that these setbacks do not signal total failure and should be viewed as cues to utilize in a more effective manner the coping skills already learned. It is important for the patient not to think of his/her work as ending at termination of treatment, but rather as entering into a different phase of maintenance.

During the final session, all aspects of the program are reviewed. A review with patients of what they have learned and how they have changed from the onset of treatment can encourage recognition of how patients' own efforts contributed to the positive changes. The goal is to help patients realize they have plans, skills, and abilities within their repertoire to cope with their situation without the need of direct contact with therapists. Thus, change has been achieved and can be maintained if the patient continues to take charge of his/her life.

CONCLUSIONS

Earlier we noted that some have suggested that cognitive and behavioral approaches are antithetical (25, 26). We disagree. From our perspective, the patient's attitudes and beliefs have an effect on motivation and behavior. We also believe that environmental contingencies can influence thoughts, feelings, and behaviors. Thus, we suggest employing both cognitive and behavioral techniques to bring about direct changes in behavior provided by environmental contingencies and indirect changes following changes in cognitive factors such as attitudes and beliefs. Behavioral techniques are essential at the beginning of treatment; however, unless significant changes in intrinsic motivation occur following from such direct behavioral techniques, it is our contention that treatment efficacy will not be obtained following the removal of direct environmental reinforcement. The literature on relapse following strict operant approaches for a diversity of problems lends support to our reservations regarding the long-term maintenance of treatment effects following exclusively operant approaches in the management of chronic pain (see refs. 19–21). Research, specifically in the area of chronic pain, needs to address the issue of maintenance.

Obviously in this chapter we have been unable to address all of the nuances of cognitive-behavioral treatments; however, we hope to have whetted the appetite of the reader to consider more carefully the nature of his/her treatment and mode of interacting with patients. As is obvious from any scanning of the literature, single-modality interventions imposed on passive patients seem of limited value for the complexity of problems inherent in chronic pain. The history of treatment of chronic pain is replete with technically elegant interventions that have proven to be failures (5, 61, 62). We do not mean to suggest that there is no place for conventional medical and surgical modalities in chronic pain; however, it seems apparent that optimal treatment for chronic pain patients must extend beyond the scalpel and syringe. We have attempted to describe one multidimensional approach to this major problem in health care. Research has begun to support the efficacy of this approach for a diversity of chronic pain syndromes (see refs. 11 and 63 for reviews). However, the hackneyed statement "more research is needed" is still relevant.

Acknowledgments Preparation of this manuscript was supported by grant #2 R01 DE07514-02 from the National Institute of Dental Research and #1 R01 ARNS 38698-01 from The National Institute of Arthritis and Musculoskeletal and Skin Diseases.

References

1. Turk DC, Rudy TE: Assessment of cognitive factors in chronic pain: a worthwhile enterprise? *J Consult Clin Psychol* 54:760–768, 1986.
2. Melzack R, Casey KL: Sensory, motivational and central control determinants of pain: a new conceptual model. In Kenshalo D (ed): *The Skin Sense*. Springfield, IL, Charles C Thomas, 1968.
3. Melzack R, Wall PD: Pain mechanisms: a new theory. *Science* 50:971–979, 1965.
4. Fordyce WE, Fowler RS, DeLateur B: An application of behavior modification technique to a problem of chronic pain. *Behav Res Ther* 6:105–107, 1968.
5. Melzack R, Wall PD: *The Challenge of Pain*. New York, Basic Books, 1983.
6. Fordyce WE, Fowler RS, Lehmann JF, DeLateur BJ, Sand PL, Trieschmann RB: Operant conditioning in the treatment of chronic pain. *Arch Phys Med Rehab* 54:399–408, 1973.
7. Fordyce WE: *Behavioral Methods for Chronic Pain and Illness*. St Louis, CV Mosby, 1976.
8. International Association for the Study of Pain: Pain terms: a list with definitions and notes on usage. *Pain* 6:249–252, 1979.
9. Deyo RA, Diehl AK, Rosenthal M: How many days of bed rest for acute low back pain? A randomized clinical trial. *N Engl J Med* 315:1064–1070, 1986.
10. Turk DC, Meichenbaum D: A cognitive-behavioral approach to pain management. In Wall PD, Melzack R (eds): *Textbook of Pain*. London, Churchill Livingstone, 1984.
11. Turk DC, Meichenbaum D, Genest M: *Pain and Behavioral Medicine: A Cognitive-Behavioral Perspective*. New York, Guilford Press, 1983.
12. Turk DC, Holzman AD, Kerns RD: Chronic pain. In Holroyd KA, Creer TL (eds): *Chronic Disease: A Handbook of Self-Management Approaches*. New York, Academic Press, 1985.
13. Holroyd KA, Andrasik F, Westbrook T: Cognitive control of tension headache. *Cogn Ther Res* 1:121–133, 1977.
14. Stenn PG, Mothersill KJ, Brooke RI: Biofeedback and a cognitive behavioral approach to treatment of myofascial pain dysfunction syndrome. *Behav Ther* 10:29–36, 1979.
15. Randich SR: Evaluation of a pain management program for rheumatoid arthritis patients. *Arthritis Rheum* 25(suppl):11 (abstr).
16. Kerns RD, Turk DC, Holzman AD, Rudy TE: Efficacy of an cognitive-behavioral approach for the treatment of chronic pain. *Clin J Pain* 1:195–203, 1986.
17. Moore JE, Chaney EF: Outpatient group treatment of chronic pain: effects of spouse involvement. *J Consult Clin Psychol* 53:326–334, 1985.
18. Thorndike EL: *The Psychology of Learning*. New York, Teachers College Press, 1913.
19. Cairns D, Pasino J: Comparison of verbal reinforcement and feedback in the operant treatment of disability due to chronic low back pain. *Behav Ther* 8:621–630, 1977.
20. Dolce JJ, Crocker MF, Moletteire C, Doleys DM: Exercise quotas, anticipatory concerns and self-efficacy expectations in chronic pain: a preliminary report. *Pain* 24:365–372, 1986.
21. Doleys DM, Crocker M, Patton D: Responses of patients with chronic pain to exercise quotas. *J Am Phys Ther Assoc* 62:1111–1114, 1982.
22. Bandura A: *Principles of Behavior Modification*. New York, Holt, Rinehart & Winston, 1969.
23. Keeley SM, Shemberg KM, Carbonell J: Operant clinical intervention: behavior management or beyond? Where are the data? *Behav Ther* 7:292–305, 1976.
24. Mahoney MJ: *Cognition and Behavior Modification*. Cambridge, MA, Ballinger, 1974.
25. Ciccone DS, Grzesiak RC: Cognitive dimensions of chronic pain. *Soc Sci Med* 19:1339–1346, 1984.
26. Sternbach RA: Behaviour therapy. In Wall PD, Melzack R (eds): *Textbook of Pain*. London, Churchill Livingstone, 1984.
27. Kahneman D, Slovic P, Tversky A: *Judgment under Uncertainty: Heuristics and Biases*. New York, Cambridge University Press, 1982.
28. Merluzzi TV, Rudy TE, Glass CR: The information processing paradigm: implications for clinical science. In Merluzzi TV, Glass CR, Genest M (eds): *Cognitive Assessment*. New York, Guilford Press, 1981.
29. Nisbett R, Ross L: *Human Inference: Strategies and Shortcomings of Social Judgment*. Englewood Cliffs, NJ, Prentice-Hall, 1980.
30. Lazarus RS, Folkman S: *Stress, Appraisal, and Coping*. New York, Springer-Verlag, 1984.
31. Bandura A: The self-system in reciprocal determinism. *Am Psychol* 3:344–359, 1978.
32. Rachlin H: Pain and behavior. *Behav Brain Sci* 8:43–53, 1985.
33. Turk DC, Holzman AD: Commonalities among psychological approaches in the treatment of chronic pain: specifying the metaconstructs. In Holzman AD, Turk DC (eds): *Pain Management: A Handbook of Psychological Treatment Approaches*. Elmsford, NY, Pergamon Press, 1986.
34. Bandura A: Self-efficacy: toward a unifying theory of behavior change. *Psychol Rev* 84:191–215, 1977.
35. Kanfer FH, Goldstein AP (eds): *Helping People Change: A Textbook of Methods*. Elmsford, NY, Pergamon Press, 1986.
36. Turk DC, Rudy TE: Assessment of chronic pain patients: toward a multiaxial system. *Behav Res Ther* 25:237–249, 1987.

37. International Association for the Study of Pain: Classification of chronic pain: descriptions of chronic pain syndromes and definitions of pain terms. *Pain Suppl* 3:S1–S225, 1986.
38. Bradley LA, Prokop CK, Gentry WD, Hopson LA, Prieto EJ: Assessment of chronic pain. In Prokop CK, Bradley LA (eds): *Medical Psychology: Contributions to Behavioral Medicine.* New York, Academic Press, 1981.
39. Brena SF, Turk DC: Vocational disability: a challenge to pain rehabilitation programs. In Aronoff G (ed): *Interdisciplinary Pain Clinics.* New York, Raven Press (in press).
40. Brena SF, Koch DL: A "pain estimate" model for quantification and classification of chronic pain states. *Anesthesiol Rev* 2:8–13, 1975.
41. Waddell G, McCulloch JA, Kummel E, Venner RM: Nonorganic physical signs in low-back pain. *Spine* 5:117–125, 1980.
42. Brand RA, Lehmann TR: Low-back impairment rating practices of orthopedic surgeons. *Spine* 8:75–83, 1983.
43. Kerns RD, Turk DC, Rudy TE: The West Haven–Yale Multidimensional Pain Inventory (WHYMPI) *Pain* 23:345–356, 1985.
44. Milligan GW, Cooper MC: An examination of procedures for determining the number of clusters in a data set. *Psychometrika* 50:159–179, 1985.
45. Scheibler D, Schneider W: Monte Carlo tests of the accuracy of cluster analysis algorithms: a comparison of hierarchical and nonhierarchical methods. *Multivariate Behav Res* 20:283–304, 1985.
46. Tatsuoka MM: *Multivariate Analysis.* New York, John Wiley & Sons, 1971.
47. Keefe FJ, Block AR: Development of an observation method for assessing pain behavior in chronic low back pain patients. *Behav Ther* 13:363–375, 1982.
48. Rosensteil AK, Keefe FJ: The use of cognitive coping strategies in chronic low back pain patients: relationship to patient characteristics and current adjustment. *Pain* 17:33–44, 1983.
49. Lefebvre MF: Cognitive distortion and cognitive errors in depressed psychiatric and low back pain patients. *J Consult Clin Psychol* 49:517–525, 1981.
50. Aronoff GM, Evans WO, Enders PL: A review of follow-up studies of multidisciplinary pain units. *Pain* 16:1–11, 1983.
51. Meichenbaum D, Turk DC: *Facilitating Treatment Adherence: A Practitioner's Guidebook.* New York, Plenum Press, 1987.
52. Meilman PW, Skultety FM, Guck TP, Sullivan K: Benign chronic pain: 18 month to ten-year follow-up of a multidisciplinary pain unit treatment program. *Clin J Pain* 1:131–137, 1985.
53. Kanfer FH, Karoly P: The psychology of self-management: abiding issues and tentative directions. In Karoly P, Kanfer FH (eds): *Self-management and Behavior Change.* Elmsford, NY, Pergamon Press, 1982.
54. Holzman AD, Turk DC, Kerns RD: The cognitive-behavioral approach in the management of chronic pain. In Holzman AD, Turk DC (eds): *Pain Management: A Handbook of Psychological Treatment Approaches.* Elmsford, NY, Pergamon Press, 1986.
55. Turk DC, Rudy TE, Flor H: Why a family perspective for pain? *Int J Fam Ther* 7:223–234, 1985.
56. Stieg RL, Turk DC: Chronic pain syndrome: the necessity of demonstrating the cost-benefit of treatment. *J Pain Management* (in press).
57. Beals RK: Compensation of recovery from injury. *West J Med* 140:232–237, 1984.
58. Brena SF, Turk DC: Chronic pain and disability: an overview for legal professionals. *Defense Counsel J* 54:122–130, 1987.
59. Hanlon R, Turk DC, Rudy TE: A collaborative approach in the treatment of chronic pain patients. *Br J Counsel Guidance* 15:37–49, 1987.
60. Marlatt GA, Gordon JR: Determinants of relapse: implications for the maintenance of behavior change. In Davidson PO, Davidson SM (eds): *Behavioral Medicine: Changing Health Life Styles.* New York, Brunner/Mazel, 1980.
61. Flor H, Turk DC: Etiological theories and treatments for chronic back pain: I. Somatic factors. *Pain* 19:105–121, 1984.
62. Turk DC, Flor H: Etiological theories and treatments for chronic back pain: II. Psychological factors. *Pain* 19:209–233, 1984.
63. Turner JA, Chapman CR: Psychological interventions for chronic pain: a critical review: II. Operant conditioning, hypnosis, and cognitive-behavior therapy. *Pain* 12:23–46, 1982.

pain management in selected disorders

section 3

part a
headaches

chapter 19
Differential Diagnosis of Headache Pain

Seymour Diamond, M.D.
Glen D. Solomon, M.D.
Frederick G. Freitag, D.O.

Headache has been termed the most common medical complaint of civilized people, and is the fifth most common reason for outpatient medical care (1). Headache may be intense whether its source is benign or malignant. Although the vast majority of headaches are unrelated to structural neurologic disease, headache can also be the presenting complaint in potentially life-threatening disorders such as meningitis, cerebral hemorrhage, and brain tumor.

In evaluating the diagnosis of headache, it is important to review the pain-sensitive structures of the head and their innervation (Table 19.1). These are the skin of the scalp and its blood supply and appendages, the head and neck muscles, aponeuroses, periosteum, spinal roots, joints, the great venous sinuses and their tributaries, parts of the dura mater at the base of the brain, the dural arteries, the intracerebral arteries, the fifth, sixth, and seventh cranial nerves, and the cervical nerves. The brain, cranium, the majority of the dura and pia mater, the ependymal lining of the ventricles, and the choroid plexus are not pain sensitive (2).

Pain pathways for structures of the anterior and middle fossae are contained in the ipsilateral trigeminal nerve. Pain from these structures is usually felt in the frontal, temporal, and parietal regions of the head. The posterior fossa is innervated by the ipsilateral upper three cervical roots with contributions from the glossopharyngeal and vagus nerves. Pain from these structures is usually felt in the occipital region (2).

HISTORY

Proper evaluation of a complete and detailed history will establish the diagnosis in most cases of chronic recurrent headache. A careful history is particularly important in the diagnosis of headache, because the majority of patients with headache will have normal neurologic and physical examinations.

The first inquiry in a headache history is a precise description of the headache. It is very common for patients to have two or more different types of head pain. For each separate type of head pain, the following data should be obtained.

1. Age at Onset, Length of Illness, Associated Life Events at Time of Onset The length of time that a patient has suffered from headache is the first guide to whether the symptom represents a malignant or progressive neurologic disorder that requires further evaluation. The sudden onset of severe headache, possibly with focal neurologic signs or decreased consciousness, suggests a serious illness such as subarachnoid hemorrhage or meningitis, whereas a recurrent course of headache over 30 to 40 years is likely to represent a form of vascular headache. The first attack of migraine may prove confusing to the physician,

Table 19.1
Pain Sensitivity of Cranial Tissues

	Pain Sensitive	Insensitive to Pain
Intracranial	Cranial sinuses and afferent veins Arteries of the dura mater Arteries of the base of the brain and their major branches Parts of the dura mater (in the vicinity of large vessels)	Parenchyma of the brain Ependyma, choroid plexus Pia mater, arachnoid membrane, parts of the dura mater
Extracranial	Skin, scalp, fascia, muscles Mucosa Arteries (veins: less sensitive)	Skull (Periosteum: slightly sensitive)
Nerves	Trigeminal, facial, vagal, glossopharyngeal Second and third cervical nerves	

unless it is preceded by a characteristic prodrome, and may suggest meningitis or intracerebral hemorrhage.

Headaches that have developed over weeks to months may be the most difficult to interpret. In these cases, the physician must consider sinusitis, occular disease, subdural hematoma, mass lesion, hydrocephalus, and, in the patient over 45 years old, temporal arteritis.

2. Time, Course, and Frequency of Headache The information should include the time of day when the headache begins, duration of headache, and relationship to menses, puberty, pregnancy, and menopause. Frequency and duration establish the temporal pattern that can be the key to the diagnosis of recurrent headache. Often, migraine will initially occur during puberty and may resolve after menopause. Migraine may recur irregularly for months or years, or may follow a pattern of occurring at the time of menses or 1–10 times per month. During the later months of pregnancy, migraines frequently improve. The duration of an acute migraine is usually from several hours to several days. It is usually preceded and followed by a headache-free interval.

Episodic cluster headache occurs in bouts lasting from 2 weeks to 3 months followed by episodes of quiesence ranging from months to years. The cluster periods tend to occur in the spring and fall months. During a cluster period, headaches recur one or more times per day, often at night, thus awakening the patient. The pain characteristically lasts from 10 min to 2 hr. This duration differentiates cluster headache from trigeminal neuralgia, which presents with transient, recurrent jabs of pain, lasting less than a second. Cluster variant headaches, such as chronic paroxysmal hemicrania, have pain patterns similar to cluster headache, although the attacks occur predominantly during the day.

Muscle contraction headache is characterized by the absence of periodicity or a headache-free interval. Most of these patients report a continuous, daily headache. The mixed headache syndrome is marked by intermittant paroxysms of severe, throbbing, sick headache superimposed on a background of constant, daily headache.

3. Location of Head Pain Muscle contraction headache is commonly bilateral. However, migraine occurs unilaterally in two-thirds of patients. Cluster headache and trigeminal neuralgia are always unilateral, as are headaches associated with local disease of the eye, nose, sinuses, or scalp. Headache due to subarachnoid hemorrhage and space-occupying masses may start as localized or unilateral pain, but will usually become bilateral. Migraine headache may alternate sides with different attacks buy may be localized to one side during an entire lifetime. Cluster headache invariably remains on one side during a series of attacks.

4. Severity and Pain Characteristics of Headache In differentiating migraine, the headache is either throbbing or pulsatile. A constant ache will suggest muscle contraction, whereas deep, boring, intense pain is descriptive of cluster headache. Shock-like intense jabs are typical of trigeminal neuralgia. Because the severity of pain is very subjective, its diagnostic value is limited. However, cluster headache and trigeminal neuralgia are consistently described as severe. The pain of cluster will generally make the patient unable to remain still. In contrast, the common response to migraine is to remain in a darkened, quiet room and limit activity.

5. Prodromal or Warning Symptoms and Signs The only type of headache with a recognizable prodrome is classic migraine. Visual (Table 19.2) or neurologic symptoms precede the onset of headache by 10–60 min. Premonitory symptoms commonly precede migraine by 12–24 hr and may include euphoria, fatigue, craving for sweets, or yawning.

6. Associated Symptoms Associated symptoms of migraine can include photophobia, gastrointestinal distur-

Table 19.2
Ocular Prodromata of Migraine

Positive	Teichopsia, or fortification spectra Zigzags Flashing lights and colors
Negative	Scotomata Hemianopsia
Metamorphopsia	Illusions of distorted size, shape, and location of fixed objects

bance, fluid retention, and focal neurologic signs. Cluster headache can be marked by partial Horner's syndrome, constricted pupils, injected conjunctiva, lacrimation, and rhinorrhea. Nasal congestion and rhinorrhea are also common in sinusitis. Stiff neck and other meningeal irritation signs can be seen with meningitis, encephalitis, and subarachnoid hemorrhage. Decreased level of consciousness can be observed in patients with mass lesions, hydrocephalus, or encephalitis. A colloid cyst blocking the flow of cerebrospinal fluid (CSF) in the third ventricle can cause positional headache and drop attacks. Seizures may reflect cortical irritation associated with mass lesions, or arteriovenous malformation. Fever and sweats may signal an acute infection.

7. **Precipitating Factors** Fatigue, specifically lack of sleep, can precipitate both migraine and muscle contraction headache. Stress is also a frequent trigger of muscle contraction headache, whereas migraine often occurs after a stressful period, weekends, or vacations. Patients with migraine often relate their headaches to menses, missing meals, and/or dietary indiscretion, particularly consumption of foods rich in tyramine (Table 19.3). Alcohol usually triggers an attack during a cluster series, but will have no effect during remission. Migraine can also be precipitated by alcohol, such as red wine. Weather changes can exacerbate sinusitis pain and can also trigger migraine.

8. **Emotional Factors and Other Evidence of Psychological Illness** Signs and symptoms of depression, including sleep and appetite disturbances, are frequent markers for muscle contraction headache and depression (Table 19.4).

9. **Relationship to Work and Occupational Exposure to Toxins, Chemicals, and Infectious Agents** Carbon monoxide poisoning will frequently be manifested by headache. Certain chemicals and toxins, such as nitrites, will induce withdrawal or reintroduction headache. It should be noted that exposure to infectious agents or AIDS may lead to encephalitis caused by fungi or microbacteria that may not produce fever or stiff neck (3).

10. **Family History of Migraine, Depression, Mental Illness, or Alcoholism** Migraine is a familial disorder, with positive family history noted in up to three-fourths of patients. Cluster headache is familial in only about 2% of patients.

11. **Medical and Surgical History** Head trauma suggests subdural hematoma or skull fractures. Lumbar puncture can be followed by a prolonged headache associated with CSF leakage. The headache is worse on arising and decreases with recumbancy. Immunocompromised patients (chemotherapy, cancer, steroids, AIDS) may be at risk for unusual types of meningitis and encephalitis, often without the sentinel signs of fever or stiff neck. Infectious disease, including syphilis or tuberculosis, may be manifested by headache. It is well to remember that fever, regardless of etiology, is the most common cause of infectious headache.

12. **Systems Review, Including Allergies** It has not been demonstrated that migraine and other types of head-

Table 19.3
Tyramine-Restricted Diet

Food	Types to Avoid
Meat, fish, poultry	Aged, canned, cured, or processed meats; canned or aged ham; pickled herring, salted dried fish; chicken liver; aged game; hot dogs, fermented sausage (no nitrates or nitrites): bologna, salami, pepperoni, summer sausage; peanut butter; any meat prepared with meat tenderizer, soy sauce, or yeast extracts
Dairy	Cultured dairy products, such as buttermilk, sour cream, chocolate milk
	Cheese: bleu, Boursault, brick, Brie types, Camembert types, cheddar, Swiss, gouda, roquefort, Stilton, mozzarella, parmesan, provolone, romano, Emmentaler
Breads and cereals	Hot, fresh homemade yeast breads; breads and crackers with cheese
	Fresh yeast coffee cake, doughnuts, sour dough breads
	Any containing chocolate or nuts
Vegetables	Pole or broad beans, lima or Italian beans, lentils, snow peas, fava beans, navy beans, pinto beans, pea pods; sauerkraut, garbanzo beans; onions except for flavoring; olives; pickles
Fruits	Avocados, banana (1/2 allowed per day), figs, raisins, papaya, passion fruit, red plums
	Nuts and seeds: peanut butter, sunflower, sesame, and pumpkin seeds; peanuts
Soups	Canned soups; soup cubes, bouillon cubes, soup bases with autolyzed yeast or MSG (read labels)
Desserts	Chocolate type: ice cream, pudding, cookies, cakes
	Mincemeat pies
Sweets	Chocolate candies, chocolate syrup, carob
Miscellaneous	Pizza; cheese sauce; soy sauce; monosodium glutamate (MSG) in excessive amounts; yeast, yeast extracts, Brewer's yeast; meat tenderizers, "Accent"; seasoned salt
	Mixed dishes: macaroni and cheese, beef stroganoff, cheese blintzes, lasagna, frozen TV dinners
	Nuts and seeds: peanut butter, pumpkins, sesame
	Some snack items are to be avoided; read all labels
	Any pickled, preserved, or marinated foods

Table 19.4
Patterns of Depression

	Incidence (%)
Physical complaints	
Sleep disturbances	97
Early awakening	87
Headache	84
Dyspnea	76
Constipation	76
Loss of weight	74
Trouble getting to sleep	73
Weakness and fatigue	70
Urinary frequency	70
"Spells"—dizziness	70
Appetite disturbances	70
Decreased libido	63
Cardiovascular disturbances	60
Sexual disturbances	60
Palpitations	59
Paresthesias	53
Nausea	48
Menstrual changes	41
Emotional complaints	
Blue, low spirits, sadness	90
Crying	80
Feelings of guilt, hopelessness, unworthiness, unreality	65
Anxious or irritable	65
Anxiety	60
Fear of insanity, physical disease, death; rumination over the past, present, future	50
Psychic complaints	
"Morning worst time of day"	95
Poor concentration	91
No interest; no ambition	75
Indecisiveness	75
Poor memory	71
Suicidal thoughts; death wishes	35

ache result from allergy (antibody-antigen reaction). The patient may confuse dietary triggers of headache for an allergic reaction. Patients with "triad asthma" (asthma, nasal polyps, and aspirin sensitivity) have a high incidence of migraine (4).

13. Previous Diagnostic Tests and Workup for Headache If a patient has recently had an adequate workup, and there are no neurologic or historic reasons to indicate further testing, it is prudent to not repeat tests.

14. Previous Treatments A past history of therapeutic successes and failures can serve as both a diagnostic aid and a guide to therapy. The dose and duration should be included if possible. Previous good response to ergotamine tartrate suggests the diagnosis of migraine, whereas acute cluster headache may respond well to oxygen inhalation as well as ergotamine.

15. Current Medications Migraine can be exacerbated by oral contraceptives, postmenopausal hormones, and vasodilators. Reserpine can promote both depression and migraine. Although indomethacin can be used in headache prophylaxis, it may trigger headache. The daily use of analgesics, especially those containing butalbital, caffeine, or narcotics, can eventually lead to rebound/withdrawal headaches, thus exacerbating a daily headache pattern. Overuse of ergot preparations can also cause rebound headaches.

The information obtained by each item in the headache history should contribute to the overall differential diagnosis of headache.

PHYSICAL AND NEUROLOGIC EXAMINATION

Every headache patient deserves a thorough physical and neurologic examination. The evaluation should include: mental status, examination of the head and skull, and palpation of both the temporomandibular joints and cervical spine to rule out tenderness and mobility. Neurologic examination should include tests of cerebellar, motor, and sensory function, testing of the cranial nerves, and careful inspection of the optic disks. Cardiopulmonary status should be evaluated, with measurement of vital signs. In most patients, the physical and neurologic examinations will reveal no abnormalities.

LABORATORY AND RADIOGRAPHIC STUDIES

As part of the initial evaluation of most headache patients, routine laboratory studies should be obtained in order to identify systemic causes of chronic recurrent headache, and to indicate potential hazards of certain medical therapies.

LABORATORY STUDIES

Laboratory studies should include complete blood count, chemistries, urinalysis, and, if clinically indicated, thyroid studies, serology, and prolactin measurement. In patients above the age of 45, erythrocyte sedimentation rate by Westergen method should be obtained to rule out temporal arteritis.

RADIOGRAPHIC STUDIES

Unless the headache history is clearly defined and the neurologic examination is essentially normal, radiographic studies, including skull x-rays and computed tomography (CT) scan of the head, are advised.

Skull Radiographs

Plain skull films can provide a large amount of clinical information, of both positive and negative importance, in the evaluation of the headache patient. This information may augment data from the CT scan, and has not been replaced by newer imaging techniques. The first step in evaluating skull x-rays is to ascertain satisfactory alignment of the films. On lateral views, the orbital plates and the mandibular rami should be superimposed. On the anteroposterior views, the distances from the orbital rim to the outer bony table should be equidistant. The examination should also include the outer and inner tables of the skull, the lines and sutures, the character and density of the bones, the shape and size of the sella turcica, pineal and unusual calcifications, the soft tissues of the skull, the craniocephalic index, and the general vault-to-base relationships. The basal angle should be calculated, and signs of basilar impression identified (5).

Abnormalities that may be identified include fractures, splitting of the sutures, pathologic vascular markings, shifts of the calcified pineal gland, abnormal sellar size or erosion of the sellar floor, metastatic disease, and increased digital markings suggesting increased intracranial pressure. Subgaleal hematoma, a benign cause of headache, can also be recognized on skull films.

Computed Tomography

Computed tomography is the most reliable method of identifying intracranial lesions in the headache patient, and probably represents the greatest diagnostic advance for these patients in the past several decades. This noninvasive technique, using a computer coupled with a special x-ray device, produces detailed cross-sectional images of the brain. It can detect variations in tissue density that assist in detection of pathologic lesions. The CT scan can identify most space-occupying lesions, and aid in discriminating between neoplasms, abscesses, and hematomas. It is useful in detecting hydrocephalus, cerebral edema, infarction, hemorrhage, and occasionally arteriovenous malformations. Computed tomography scanning is not particularly effective in detecting aneurysms. However, aneurysms rarely produce headaches unless they leak or rupture, on which occasion the bleed will be demonstrated by the scan. Some fourth-generation CT scans can visualize aneurysms (6).

The CT scan provides information on the brain and its appendages that previously could not be obtained, or required invasive techniques such as cerebral angiography, pneumoencephalography, or ventriculography. In addition, its accuracy in detecting supratentorial lesions far exceeds that of radioisotope scanning. The availability of CT scanning as an outpatient procedure, with its noninvasive technique and low radiation exposure, makes it the most cost-effective of diagnostic tests in headache evaluation.

The indications for the use of CT scan in patients with recurrent headache include:

Abnormal neurologic examination, especially if suspicious for intracranial mass lesion.

Recent onset of persistent headache, exertional headache, personality change, seizures, or loss of consciousness.
Change in the character of headache.

The CT scan can also be of great value in the detection of acoustic neuromas. Evaluation for these tumors requires special computer cuts and contrast dye enhancement. Routine CT scanning of the head to evaluate for supratentorial lesions, despite contrast enhancement, is inadequate to detect these tumors. If acoustic neuroma is suspected, CT scanning of the auditory canals should be obtained.

Magnetic Resonance Imaging

Magnetic resonance imaging (MRI), formerly called nuclear magnetic resonance (NMR), is the newest and probably the most revolutionary method of disclosing occult organic lesions that cause headache. Lesions of the posterior fossa not visualized by other techniques, including CT scan, can occasionally be found by MRI.

Magnetic resonance imaging works by magnetic induction of nuclei of hydrogen atoms, within tissues from random distribution, into a uniform array. Radiowaves transmitted into the tissues being imaged set the nuclei into resonant oscillating motion. When the radiowaves are stopped, the hydrogen nuclei return to their original positions, emitting their own weak radiowaves that are picked up by antennas in the magnet. These waves are then transformed into electrical impulses and processed into images by computer, similar to the method used in CT scanning (5).

Imaging can be done in frontal, sagittal, or axial projections. Although the images of MRI resemble those of CT scanning, there are important differences. The CT scan uses x-rays to measure densities of various tissues, and MRI measures the physiologic function of atoms within tissues. This enables the MRI to differentiate normal structures for pathologic tissues. Also, MRI demonstrates soft tissues with greater resolution than CT scanning, and may allow detection of tissue pathology at an earlier stage of disease.

Magnetic resonance imaging presents no known health hazards. Current FDA guidelines suggest that pregnant women in the first two trimesters of pregnancy should avoid MRI because the long-term effects of the magnetic field and radiowaves on the developing fetus are unknown. Additionally, patients with pacemakers or surgical steel clips from previous neurosurgery should not enter the MRI scanner.

Because of the lack of published studies specifically addressing the utility of MRI in headache patients, the clinical indications for MRI are uncertain. Brainstem and posterior fossa lesions, difficult to identify on CT scans because of bone artifacts, are well visualized on MRI scans. Soft tissue sensitivity is great enough to distinguish white and gray matter in the brain. Demyelinating lesions, such as those found in multiple sclerosis, can be detected. Brain tumors, infarcts, and hemorrhages are also easily delineated by MRI.

The high cost and lack of availability of MRI scanners limit their widespread use in the workup of the headache patient. With its great sensitivity, safety, and lack of both radiation exposure and need for contrast dye, MRI may in the future become the procedure of choice in the visualization of the central nervous system.

CLASSIFICATION OF HEADACHE

At present, there is no universally accepted classification scheme for headache. The classification used herein separates headache into three groups—vascular, muscle contraction, and traction and inflammatory (Table 19.5).

Included in the category of vascular headache, classic and common migraine are: hemiplegic and ophthalmoplegic migraine, cluster headache, toxic vascular headache, and hypertensive headache. The common pathway in these headaches is a tendency to vascular dilatation that provokes the headache phase.

Toxic vascular headache refers to systemic vasodilatation produced by fever, alcohol ingestion, poisons, carbon dioxide retention, and chemical vasodilators, such as the nitrates and nitrites. Hypertensive headache is associated with extreme elevations in systemic arterial pressure, such as hypertensive crisis of malignant hypertension. Cephalgia is rarely seen with mild or moderate hypertension, and the diastolic pressure must be 110 mm Hg or greater to produce symptoms.

The typical description of muscle contraction headache, sometimes called tension headache, is a dull, band-like, persistent pain. In the acute form, it is probably the most common form of headache, and is usually relieved by simple analgesics. These patients rarely seek professional help, except in the chronic form, when headache is frequently associated with depression or anxiety.

Traction and inflammatory headache are evoked by organic disease of the head, face, neck, brain, meninges, or vasculature. Mass lesions of the brain, including tumors, hematomas, abscesses, and cerebral edema, trigger traction headache. Traction and inflammatory headache can occur with subarachnoid hemorrhage, meningitis, arteritis, and disorders of the teeth, jaw, and neck. These disorders usually require specific therapy for the underlying disease.

VASCULAR HEADACHE

MIGRAINE HEADACHE

Migraine is a syndrome consisting of periodic headache associated with nausea and irritability, and, in many patients, photophobia and gastrointestinal dysfunction. In the 15–20% of migraine sufferers with classical migraine, attacks are preceded by scotoma, hemianopsia, unilateral paresthesia, or speech disorders.

The most frequent description of a migraine attack is a dull ache, progressively worsening into a throbbing pain. As it stabilizes, the headache may become constant and nonthrobbing. Migraine is unilateral about 70% of the time, usually affecting the frontal and temporal regions. Some patients will note generalized headache, or pain localized to the occipital areas. The intensity of pain may vary between attacks and between patients. For most patients, the pain will require alteration in normal activities. Attacks can occur from every few days to less than once per year. The duration usually lasts from 4 hr to 2 days, with severe episodes lasting up to 6 days. Between attacks, the patients are headache free.

Migraine is a common malady with a prevalence between 2% and 20% of the population, with women affected almost twice as often as men. In childhood, the incidence in males and females is equal.

Migraine may begin in childhood, with usual onset before age 40. It tends to decrease with advancing age, and up to three-fourths of female migraineurs note relief after

Table 19.5
Classification of Headache

Vascular Headache		Muscle Contraction Headache	Traction and Inflammatory Headache

Migraine
  Classic
  Common
  Hemiplegic
  Ophthalmoplegic
  Basilar artery
Cluster (histamine)
Toxic vascular
Hypertensive
	} complicated migraine	Depressive equivalents and conversion reactions
		Cervical osteoarthritis
		Chronic myositis
			Mass lesions (tumors, edema, hematomas, cerebral hemorrhage)
			Diseases of the eye, ear, nose, throat, teeth
			Arteritis, phlebitis, and cranial neuralgias
			Occlusive vascular disease
			Atypical facial pain
			Temporomandibular joint

menopause. About 70% of migraine sufferers have a positive family history for migraine.

Hormonal factors play a role in migraine, with 70% of female migraineurs relating migraine attacks to menstruation. Many women note dramatic improvement in migraine during the last two trimesters of pregnancy. Both oral contraceptives and postmenopausal hormones can aggravate migraine.

The hallmark of migraine is the association of headache with gastrointestinal complaints. The more common gastrointestinal symptoms include anorexia, nausea, and vomiting, with occasional abdominal bloating and diarrhea. Photophobia and phonophobia are frequent associated symptoms of migraine, often forcing the migraine sufferer to seek refuge in a dark, quiet room. Alterations in fluid balance can occur, with peripheral edema and fluid retention noted. Prior to the onset of head pain, the migraine patient may note oliguria, often followed by polyuria as the attack resolves. Other signs less commonly observed are pallor, sweating, chills, and cold extremities. Migraine has been linked to a number of other medical conditions, including Raynaud's phenomenon, systemic lupus erythematosus, mitral valve prolapse, vasospastic (Prinzmetal's) angina, and stroke.

The pathogenesis of migraine remains obscure. The prevailing vascular theory, based on the pioneering work of Wolff and Graham (7, 8), is that migraine represents a disorder of cerebrovascular regulation. In the classic migraine sequence, release of an as-yet-unidentified substance precipitates a cascade of events that includes platelet aggregation, release of platelet serotonin and thromboxane A_2, activation of prostaglandins and production of kinins, and the production of a localized sterile arteritis (9), causing symptomatic focal vasoconstriction. This is followed by reactive vasodilation, primarily in the extracranial cerebral circulation, stretching the pain-sensitive arterioles and producing the familiar throbbing headache of migraine.

Recent studies by Lance et al. (10), Olessen et al. (11), and Moskowitz et al. (12) have promoted the neurogenic theory of migraine. This work emphasizes the significance of central nervous system neurotransmitters (e.g., substance P) as the activators of intracerebral vasoconstriction and extracranial vasodilation.

Common (nonclassic) migraine is seen in 85% of all migraine sufferers. In this type of migraine, no neurologic aura precedes the headache attack. It is not unusual, however, for patients to experience disturbances of mood or appetite in the 1–3 days preceding the attack.

In *classic migraine*, distinct neurologic signs occur in the 15–30 min that precede the headache pain. Scotoma, or blind spots, are the most common aura symptom, but photopsia (flashes of light), teichopsia, or fortification spectra (bright borders resembling a wooden fort with a central blind spot) are also frequent. Other common visual aura include diplopia, micropsia, macropsia, and metamorphopsia. Nonvisual aura symptoms include paresthesias, olfactory hallucinations, and auditory hallucinations.

Complicated Migraine

Complicated migraine is defined by neurologic or visual symptoms that last beyond the head pain by more than 24 hr. The onset of the neurologic symptom may occur before the headache (aura) or during the pain phase. Complicated migraine can occur in any patient who suffers with migraine, just as classic and common migraine frequently occur in the same patient at different times. A small number of these patients suffer from residual neurologic deficit, and stroke (13).

Complicated migraine should be differentiated from *migraine accompagnee*, in which the neurologic symptoms begin during the pain phase and disappear before, or shortly after, the attack.

Basilar artery migraine, originally described by Bickerstaff in 1961, consists of bilateral, posterior, throbbing head pain preceded or accompanied by vertigo, tinnitus, hearing loss, ataxia, dysarthria, and occasionally bilateral sensory or motor symptoms (Table 19.6) (14). Also, basilar artery migraine is occasionally associated with drop attacks, cranial nerve affections, loss of consciousness, and transient global amnesia. These symptoms are thought to represent vascular disturbances within the vertebrobasilar circulation. This syndrome is usually observed in teenage

Table 19.6
Characteristics Useful in Distinguishing between Basilar Artery Migraine and Classic Migraine

	Basilar Artery Migraine	Classic Migraine
Age of onset	Childhood and early teens	Teens or early adult life
Frequency	Infrequent	Ranging through all degrees of frequency
Visual symptoms	Bilateral impairment or loss	Unilateral impairment or loss
Sensory symptoms	Bilateral, involving hands, feet, and mouth	Unilateral, involving hands, mouth, and tongue
Vertigo	Common	Rare
Ataxia (of gait)	Very common	Very rare
Speech disorder	Dysarthria	Dysphasia if on dominant side
Alteration of consciousness	Frequent	Very rare
Permanent sequelae	Very rare	Rare, but well recognized
Drop attacks	May occur	Do not occur
Origin	Posterior fossa lesions	Cerebral hemisphere lesions

females with previous migraine attacks, but may also be present in younger males. In this age group, the constellation of symptoms may suggest drug intoxication or encephalitis. Basilar artery migraine in adults must be differentiated from thrombosis of cerebral veins and sinuses, subarachnoid hemorrhage, space-occupying lesions in the brainstem, and transient ischemic attacks of the vertebrobasilar system. The differentiation of basilar artery migraine from vertebrobasilar transient ischemic attacks is based on patient age, family history of migraine, risk factors for occlusive arterial disease, and previous migraine symptomatology. Since cerebral infarction has been observed in patients with basilar artery migraine, invasive diagnostic workup, including four-vessel arteriography, may be required.

Hemiplegic migraine consists of unilateral motor and/or sensory deficits beginning before or during the migraine attack, but frequently not resolving for days to weeks. A positive family history for this type of migraine is often elicited, although it can occur sporadically in migraine sufferers.

Paresis of the extraocular muscles characterizes *ophthalmoplegic migraine*. The most common symptom is diplopia developing during the course of a headache and not as a symptom of an aura. Usually, the third cranial nerve is involved, but the fourth and sixth may also be involved. The ocular paresis may survive the headache by days or weeks, but will rarely become permanent. In order to differentiate this condition from compression of the third nerve by a space-occupying lesion or aneurysm, CT scan and/or angiography must be obtained. This procedure is also indicated in the differential diagnosis of hemiplegia migraine.

Benign Orgasmic Cephalgia

Benign orgasmic cephalgia is a type of exertional headache triggered by sexual intercourse. It is usually of brief duration and recurs with each episode of orgasm. The pain is usually throbbing, although muscular pain is often reported. If the onset occurs during exertion, subarachnoid hemorrhage is suggested. Unlike subarachnoid hemorrhage, benign orgasmic cephalgia has no accompanying hypertension or focal neurologic signs. Orgasmic cephalgia is extremely responsive to therapy with indomethacin.

CLUSTER HEADACHE

A variety of names are attributed to cluster headache, including histamine cephalgia, Horton's cephalgia, and migrainous neuralgia. Cluster is a form of headache that occurs in paroxysms of 2 weeks to 3 months, separated by long headache-free periods. Frequently, there is a seasonal incidence, with the cluster bouts occurring usually in spring and autumn. The individual attacks are severe, burning, and unilateral, usually localizing between or around the eye, and lasting from 10 min to 4 hr. During a paroxysm, attacks may occur from one to four times per day. Attacks frequently occur at night, awakening the patient from sleep. In contrast to migraine, there is no aura, and nausea and vomiting occur rarely.

Cluster headache is one of the most severe pains known to mankind. The pain may be so severe that the patient will contemplate suicide. It is usually described as constant and severe, and may be burning, tearing, or boring in quality. Cluster headache invariably occurs unilaterally, and usually affects the same side of the head in each bout. The pain may radiate ipsilaterally from the eye to the supraorbital region, temple, maxilla, and upper gum. Two-thirds of cluster patients will note simultaneous occipital/cervical pain with their attacks (15).

During an attack, patients may exhibit ptosis and miosis (partial Horner's syndrome), flushing or blanching of the face, injection of the conjunctiva, ipsilateral lacrimation, nasal congestion, and rhinorrhea. Focal neurologic signs, frequently seen in migraine, are rarely observed with cluster headache. Long-standing cluster sufferers are sometimes characterized by "leonine facies"—ruddy complexion, thick furrows across the forehead, telangiectasis, coarse cheek skin, and a square, thick chin.

Trigger factors for cluster are only implicated during the susceptible period. These include alcoholic beverages and other vasodilators, such as nitroglycerin. During the dormant periods, vasodilators are well tolerated.

In comparison with migraine (Table 19.7), cluster headache is uncommon, occurring in less than 2% of new patients in a headache clinic. Episodic cluster is predominantly a disease of young males, with a range of age at onset between 20 and 40 years, and an average of 25.5 years. Five to 10% of cluster sufferers are females. Over 70% of cluster patients are cigarette smokers, and peptic ulcer disease is reported in 20% of cluster patients (16). Coronary artery disease may also be more common in these patients.

The etiology of cluster headache remains uncertain. The sphenopalatine ganglion, when electrically stimulated, produces a syndrome similar to cluster headache. It is speculated that chronic irritation of the ganglion, possibly by cigarette smoke, may create unilateral hyperactivity. Nonspecific and repetitive stimuli of the ganglion may then induce attacks of cluster pain.

Vascular studies of cluster sufferers by Sakai and Meyer (17) demonstrated that, during a cluster attack, there is increased cerebral blood flow, primarily contralateral to the headache. The asymmetry of blood flow suggests autonomic dysfunction. They also found that during the headache, the vasodilator response to carbon dioxide was impaired, although the vasoconstrictor response to oxygen was increased. This may explain the therapeutic role of oxygen in acute cluster headache.

Hormonal abnormalities have also been recognized in cluster patients. Lower serum melatonin levels have been observed during cluster periods, as opposed to headache-free periods. Unexpectedly low levels of metenkephalin during the cluster attacks have also been observed, although the significance is unknown.

Chronic cluster headache is identical to episodic cluster

Table 19.7
Primary Distinguishing Features of Cluster and Migraine Headaches

Feature	Cluster	Migraine
Location of pain	Always unilateral, periorbital	Unilateral, occasionally bilateral
Age at onset	20–50 years	10–40 years
Sex incidence	90% male	65–70% female
Occurrence of attacks	Daily for several weeks to several months[a]	Intermittent, 2–8 times/month
Seasonal occurrence	More common in spring and fall	No variance
Number of attacks	1–6/day	1–8/month
Duration of pain	10 min to 3 hr	4–48 hr
Prodromes	Absent	25–30% of cases
Nausea and vomiting	2–5%	85%
Blurring of vision	Infrequent	Frequent
Lacrimation	Frequent	Infrequent
Nasal congestion	70%	Uncommon
Ptosis	30%	1–2%
Polyuria	2%	40%
Family history of vascular headaches	7%	90%
Miosis	50%	Absent
Chemical changes		
Decrease in plasma serotonin	None	80%
Rise in plasma histamine	90%	None
Rise in CSF acetylcholine	30%	None

[a] A small percentage of cluster headaches (2% to 3%) occur continuously and are refractory to all methods of treatment.

headache with regard to the individual attacks and patient demographics. However, headache-free intervals of 2 weeks or longer are not seen. These headaches are also identical to episodic cluster headaches in location, duration, and accompanying symptoms, resulting in the misnomer "chronic cluster" headache.

Two other syndromes are categorized as variants of cluster headache because of their unilaterality and the brief duration of individual attacks. *Chronic paroxysmal hemicrania* is a syndrome of strictly unilateral headache, never changing sides, without nausea or vomiting, with an attack frequency of 6–18/24 hr. Attacks can be triggered by neck flexion or rotation. These patients have a dramatic response to indomethacin.

Cluster headache variant, or *hemicrania continua*, occurs almost exclusively in women. The average age at onset is 35 years. Unlike cluster patients, peptic ulcer disease is rare in this group. Similar to chronic paroxysmal hemicrania, it is also noted for its dramatic response to indomethacin. The pain can occur in three patterns—atypical cluster headache, multiple stabs and jabs throughout the day, and unilateral throbbing headache that is chronic, continuous, and aggravated by exertion.

MUSCLE CONTRACTION HEADACHE

The muscle contraction headache group includes the syndromes of muscle contraction headache, cervical arthritis, and mixed headache. Muscle contraction headache can be acute, as in a typical, episodic "tension headache," related to contraction of the head and neck muscles. It is usually relieved by over-the-counter analgesics and may be associated with fatigue and temporary stress situations. Chronic muscle contraction headache is part of a symptom complex due in part to psychological problems and is particularly present in those persons subject to depression. Since acute muscle contraction headache responds well to simple analgesics, sufferers rarely consult a physician. Chronic muscle contraction headache usually manifests as a daily, or almost daily, headache, frequently lasting all day, and unresponsive to progressively larger amounts of analgesics.

Muscle contraction headache is described as a steady, nonthrobbing ache occurring bitemporally at the occiput, or in a "hatband" distribution. The muscles of the head, neck, jaw, or upper back may be contracted and tender, and may contain localized tender nodules on palpation.

Predominantly seen in women, muscle contraction headache does occur in men. These headaches may occur in families, and are considered in some a learned pattern derived from their parent's behavior.

It is crucial to recognize that chronic muscle contraction headache may conceal a *serious emotional disorder*, such as depression. For many patients, the physical symptom of headache is more socially acceptable as compared to the symptoms of anxiety or depression.

Some modern headache researchers have theorized that chronic muscle contraction headache results from disturbances of the monoaminergic, serotonergic, and endorphin functions, involving the hypothalamus, brainstem, and spinal cord. These disturbances may be due to referred or a central pain phenomena from the intermingling of major circuits of the brain and spinal cord.

Because muscle contraction headache is closely related to depression in a large percentage of patients, many associated symptoms of depression are observed. These include sleep disturbances, anorexia or excessive eating, decreased libido, and multiple somatic complaints. Biochemically, depression may be considered an illness involving depletion of biogenic amines and defects of neurotransmitters.

Cervical spine spondylosis may produce headache as a result of irritation of the structures of the spine, the adjacent musculature, and connective tissues. Pain is usually occipital, but may be anterior as a result of trigeminal nerve stimulation. Radiographs of the cervical spine will show osteoarthritic changes, with loss of the normal lordotic curve. Physical examination may reveal muscle spasm with increased tone and limited range of motion, and one or more tender areas on palpation of the posterior neck muscles.

The third major muscle contraction headache syndrome is the *mixed headache syndrome*. Patients with this type of headache pattern are the most frequently seen in a specialized headache clinic. It is comprised of the following symptomatology: (a) daily, continuous headache, (b) a sick headache (migraine) occurring 1–10 times monthly, and (c) easy susceptibility to habituation to over-the-counter or prescribed analgesics and/or ergotamine tartrate (18). Depression is also a common finding in this group of patients.

Once the diagnosis of mixed headache has been made, the use of sedatives, tranquilizers, habituating analgesics, and narcotics should be avoided in order to prevent addiction that would perpetuate the problem. The use of ergotamine should be limited to relief of the sick headache, and must not be repeated less than every fourth day. Ergotamine should never be prescribed on a daily basis for the mixed headache syndrome in order to avoid ergotamine rebound headaches.

TRACTION AND INFLAMMATORY HEADACHE

Headache from intracranial sources is usually produced by inflammation, traction, displacement, or distention of pain-sensitive structures, including susceptible blood vessels. Headache is the initial symptom of brain tumor in 25–35% of patients, and occurs in up to 80% of patients with brain tumors. The headache seen with brain tumors is not characteristic, but is often associated with signs or symptoms of increased intracranial pressure, including seizures, sudden loss of consciousness, weakness, or change in mental status.

The headache of *brain tumor* is often a deep, steady, dull, aching pain. It is intermittent in 90% of cases, does not interfere with sleep, may be worse in the early morning, and is aggravated by coughing or straining. The pain is not as intense as migraine or cluster, and is frequently relieved by minor analgesics. Nausea and vomiting are rare associated symptoms.

The headache of *brain abscess* is similar in quality to that of brain tumor. The presence of fever and leukocytosis with a brain abscess assists in the differential diagnosis.

Acute and chronic *subdural hematomas* frequently present with headache. Other common accompanying symptoms of subdural hematoma included altered consciousness, disorientation, drowsiness, and confusion. Although spontaneous subdural hematomas do occur, most cases are caused by head trauma, often minor injuries. The most susceptible groups to suffer subdural hematomas are the chronic alcoholics, the elderly, patients treated with anticoagulants, or those with bleeding disorders. Diagnosis can be confirmed by a skull x-ray showing a midline shift of the calcified pineal gland, or radionuclide brain scan, cerebral angiogram, or CT scan. Computed tomography scanning in chronic subdural hematoma may be negative during the second or third months, when the density of the hematoma is identical to that of surrounding brain tissue. During that period, radionuclide brain scan can be the most useful diagnostic test.

Post–lumbar puncture headache occurs after one-fourth of spinal taps. It usually begins a few hours to several days after lumbar puncture and lasts for days to weeks. The pain is a dull, deep ache, usually bifrontal and suboccipital. It is exacerbated by head movement and erect posture. This headache has been related to a loss of CSF, secondary to leakage from a dural hole.

Elevated CSF pressure, either from acute hydrocephalus (ventricular obstruction or shunt malformation) or pseudotumor cerebri, may cause headache. Pseudotumor cerebri is a syndrome of increased intracranial pressure and papilledema, without focal neurologic signs, and with normal CSF composition and normal- or small-sized cerebral ventricles. This condition usually occurs in children or obese young women with a history of headache for several weeks. Etiologies of pseudotumor include obstruction of cerebral venous drainage, rarely by slowly evolving tumors; endocrine and more commonly metabolic dysfunction, such as obesity or pregnancy; exposure to exogenous agents; and systemic illness, such as sarcoidosis or monoclonal gammopathy (19). Since papilledema usually occurs with this disorder, more serious pathology must be ruled out before a diagnosis of pseudotumor can be made.

Temporal arteritis frequently presents with a severe, throbbing, burning persistent headache. Often the involved artery is distended and tender. Associated symptoms may include jaw claudication, ocular symptoms including partial or complete loss of vision, depression, and polymyalgia rheumatica. This condition is primarily a disease of patients older than 50 years. Erythrocyte sedimentation rate is frequently elevated in temporal arteritis, but definitive diagnosis is made by temporal artery biopsy.

Cranial neuritides (Table 19.8), particularly trigeminal neuralgia, will present with episodic, recurrent unilateral pain. Trigeminal neuralgia (tic douloureux) causes unilateral facial pain in the distribution of the second or third division of the trigeminal nerve. Involvement of the first division occurs less frequently. This syndrome is most common in older patients, although it may be observed in younger patients, usually with multiple sclerosis, vascular anomalies, or fifth nerve tumors. The pain is usually described as a high-intensity jab lasting less than 30 sec, and is frequently triggered by trivial stimulation of the face

Table 19.8
Neuralgias: Signs and Symptoms

Trigeminal	Lancinating pain lasting seconds to minutes
	Maxillary-mandibular-ophthalmic divisions, in that order
	Older ages
	Trigger area unilateral
	Attacks often in October or March
Sphenopalatine ganglion	Sharp pain
	Lateral nose to frontotemporal area
	Older (40 years); females affected more often than males
	Often with lacrimation and rhinorrhea
	Unilateral
Glossopharyngeal	Deep, sharp pain
	Often ear-pharynx–roof of tongue
	Older patients (40 years)
	Unilateral
Geniculate ganglion	Sharp pain that is tic-like
	Tragus/external ear canal
	Unilateral
Gasserian ganglion	Postherpetic
	Unilateral
	Aching pain
	Often ophthalmic division of trigeminal
	Weeks to years duration
Dental	Short, throbbing pain
	Precipitated with thermal intraoral changes
Atypical pain	Pain does not follow anatomic distribution
	Constant with long duration, without trigger zones
	Younger patients

around the nose and mouth. This stimulation may include touching the face, washing, chewing, shaving, or even talking. The avoidance of facial stimulation by the patient helps the clinician differentiate trigeminal neuralgia from other facial pain syndromes. Glossopharyngeal neuralgia is similar to trigeminal neuralgia except that the pain is usually located in the pharynx, tonsil, or ear, and is usually triggered by swallowing, yawning, or eating. Postherpetic neuralgia frequently follows herpes zoster infection (shingles) in the elderly. The pain is described as an intense, aching and burning pain with dysesthesia and is unilateral. It is located in the trigeminal division that was previously infected with herpes zoster. Atypical facial neuralgias (or atypical facial pain syndrome) is the term used for facial pain syndromes that cannot otherwise be classified. The pain is usually a steady, diffuse, aching pain, lasting hours to days, without paroxysms or trigger zones. This condition is most commonly seen in 30–50-year-old women, and may be associated with depression. It may be differentiated from common migraine involving the face because of the lack of throbbing quality of the pain. These facial pain syndromes are covered in greater detail in Chapter 23.

Post-traumatic headaches occur in one-third to one-half of patients incurring head injury. The pathogenesis of post-traumatic headache suggests an organic basis, probably acceleration injury of the brain. The headaches may mimic any type of chronic recurrent headache syndrome, but predominantly fit into three groups: (a) headaches that mimic migraine, (b) headaches that mimic muscle contraction headache, and (c) headaches that mimic the mixed headache syndrome. In addition to the headache, symptoms may include lightheadedness, memory impairment, inability to concentrate, anxiety, and depression (Table 19.9). Workup for this type of headache will usually include a CT scan to rule out subdural hematoma, and a skull x-ray to evaluate for skull fracture.

Table 19.9
Symptoms Found in Post-traumatic Syndrome

Lightheadedness or true vertigo
Hyperacusis
Tinnitus
Impaired memory
Reduced attention span
Heightened distractibility
Inattentiveness
Decreased ability to concentrate
Forgetfulness
Difficulty in turning from one subject to another
Deterioration of synthetic thinking
Inability to grasp new or abstract concepts
Insomnia
Lack of spontaneity accompanied by apathy and loss of initiative
Easy fatigability
Reduced motivation
Decreased libido
Alcohol intolerance
Increased sensitivity to weather or temperature change
Irritability
Anger outbursts
Emotional callousness
Blunting or lability of emotional response
Mood swings
Anxiety, depression, and frustration
Syncope

Subarachnoid hemorrhage usually presents in a middle-aged individual, more frequently in females, with abrupt onset of an intense headache during exertion. The pain is generalized, and is associated with vomiting and, often, diarrhea, and usually with alteration of consciousness. The patient appears critically ill, with meningeal signs on examination. Lumbar puncture and CT scan will confirm the diagnosis. If the patient survives, the headache will remain severe for a few days, then slowly diminish over a 1–2-week period. Massive subarachnoid hemorrhage is usually due to either rupture of an intracranial aneurysm, bleeding from a cerebral angioma, or the extension of an intracerebral hemorrhage in a hypertensive patient. Congenital aneurysms present most frequently on the internal carotid artery, the middle cerebral artery, and at the junction of the anterior communicating and anterior cerebral arteries. Subarachnoid hemorrhage due to a cerebral angioma is much less common than one from a ruptured aneurysm [20].

The onset of subarachnoid hemorrhage from an intracranial aneurysm usually occurs without previous warning. However, aneuryms of the posterior communicating artery may present with headache in 20% of patients prior to hemorrhage. The pain is intermittent and boring in quality. As the aneurysm enlarges, an oculomotor palsy with a fixed, dilated pupil may result. Aneurysms of the internal carotid within the cavernous sinus may be associated with unilateral pain in or behind the eye. The pain may be increased by exertion and may be intermittent. Subarachnoid hemorrhage from a cerebral angioma is frequently preceded by symptoms of the cerebral lesion and focal neurologic signs.

The headache from subarachnoid hemorrhage is acute and persists for about a week. It is usually throbbing in character, is increased by head movement, and is frequently accompanied by meningeal signs, focal neurologic signs or altered consciousness, and arterial hypertension. Continuation or recurrence of the headache in the postbleeding period should raise the possibilities of recurrent bleeding usually occurring during the second week, cerebral edema, or acute hydrocephalus.

Ocular causes of headache are relatively rare, and include eyestrain (asthenopia), glaucoma, uveitis, and optic neuritis. A thorough history can easily differentiate these causes from the recurrent headache disorders. Painful ophthalmoplegia syndromes, including Tolosa-Hunt syndrome and Raeder's paratrigeminal syndrome, may be confused with ophthalmoplegia migraine or cluster headache.

Tolosa-Hunt syndrome is characterized by a boring, intense, sharp, or aching ocular pain followed in several days by ophthalmoplegia and diplopia. It may be associated with granulomatous lesions or arteritis within the orbit. Raeder's paratrigeminal syndrome is manifested by unilateral, deep throbbing pain around the eye, forehead, and cheek that may awaken the patient. A Horner's syndrome may also be present. This syndrome can easily be mistaken for cluster headache, except that the pain is usually constant. The pain is described an intense, sharp, and aching. Unequal pupil size and sensory loss may be noted. The etiologies for Raeder's paratrigeminal syndrome include tumors, injuries, and granulomatous lesions.

SUMMARY

Headache is a common symptom that, while usually benign, may be the presenting complaint in life-threatening conditions. Headache may be classified as vascular, muscle contraction, or traction and inflammatory. A careful history and examination will usually lead to the establishment of proper diagnosis.

References

1. Cypress BK: Patients' reasons for visiting physicians: National Ambulatory Medical Care Survey. United States, 1977–78. *Vital Health Stat* 13(56):1–128, 1981.
2. Diamond S, Dalessio DJ: *The Practicing Physician's Approach to Headache*, ed 4. Baltimore, Williams & Wilkins, 1986, p 36.
3. Goldstein J, Rose C: Headache in AIDS. In *Proceedings of the Fifth International Migraine Congress*. Basel, Karger, 1984, pp 138–143.
4. Grzelewskia-Rzymowska I, Bogucki A, Szmidt M, et al: Migraine in aspirin-sensitive asthmatics. *Allergol Immunopathol* 13:13–16, 1985.
5. Diamond S: Neuroimaging evaluation of patients with headaches. *Neurol Clin* 745–758, 1984.
6. Diamond S, Solomon G, Freitag F: Neuroimaging of the patient with headache. *J Mind Behav* (in press).
7. Graham JR, Wolff HG: Mechanism of migraine headache and action of ergotamine tartrate. *Arch Neurol Psychiatry* 39:737–740, 1938.
8. Dalessio DJ: *Wolff's Headache and Other Head Pain*, ed 4. New York, Oxford University Press, 1980.
9. Sandler M: Monoamines and migraine: a path through the woods. In Diamond S, Dalessio D, Graham J, et al (eds): *Vasoactive Substances Relevant to Migraine*. Springfield, IL, Charles C Thomas, 1975, pp 3–18.
10. Lance JW, Lambert GA, Goadsby PJ, et al: Brainstem influences in the cephalic circulation: experimental data from cats and monkeys of relevance to the mechanism of migraine. *Headache* 23:258–265, 1983.
11. Olesen J, Lauritzen M, Tfelt-Hansen P, et al: Spreading cerebral oligemia in classical and normal cerebral blood flow in common migraine. *Headache* 22:242–248, 1982.
12. Moskowitz M, Reinhard J, Romero J, et al: Neurotransmitters and the fifth cranial nerve: is there a relation to the headache phase of migraine? *Lancet* 2:883–885, 1979.
13. Spaccavento LJ, Solomon GD: Migraine as an etiology of stroke in young adults. *Headache* 24:19–22, 1984.
14. Bickerstaff E: Basilar artery migraine. *Lancet* 1:15–17, 1961.
15. Saper JR, Jones MJ: Simultaneous occipital/cervical pain in patients with cluster headache. *Headache* 26:315, 1986.
16. Diamond S, Solomon GD, Freitag FG, et al: Demographics of cluster headache patient attending an outpatient headache clinic. *Headache* 26:314, 1986.
17. Sakai F, Meyer JS: Regional cerebral hemodynamics during

migraine and cluster headache—measured by the Xe inhalation method. *Headache* 18:122–133, 1978.
18. Mathew NT, Stubits E, Nigam MP: Transformation of episodic migraine into daily headache: analysis of factors. *Headache* 22:66–68, 1982.
19. Powers MJ, Schnur JA, Baldree ME: Pseudotumor cerebri due to partial obstruction of the sigmoid sinus by a cholesteatoma. *Arch Neurol* 43:519–521, 1986.
20. Bannister R: *Brain's Clinical Neurology*, ed 5. New York, Oxford University Press, 1978, pp 270–274.

chapter 20
Medical Management of Headache Pain

Joel R. Saper, M.D., F.A.C.P.

In the previous chapter, the differential diagnosis of headache was reviewed with an emphasis upon the distinctive syndromes of migraine, muscle contraction headache, and cluster headache. This chapter provides the reader with an extensive survey of the medical management of headache as it pertains to the specific syndromes as well as to the transitional syndromes that are gaining increasing attention from headache specialists.

As our understanding of headaches changes, so too does our approach to treatment. In order to provide the proper perspective for the discussion that follows, it is important to provide this author's view of the changing attitudes toward headache pathogenesis as they influence the choices and development of treatment modalities.

In 1962, the Ad Hoc Committee on the Classification of Headache offered what was to become the standard classification for head pain disorders for the next 20 years (1). This report was based upon the premise of a clear distinction between migraine and tension headache, and focused on symptom-specific etiologies: vasculature in migraine and musculature in tension headache.

However, despite the many citations of the Ad Hoc Committee report and its traditional acceptance by researchers and clinicians alike, many authorities have been unable to reconcile the myriad of events and phenomena of migraine, tension headache, and cluster headache with the basic foundations of this classification (2). During the past several years, the emphasis on peripheral phenomena (blood vessels and muscles) and separateness between migraine and tension headache disorders has been challenged, and with this has come changing views on the treatment of this disorder.

Several authors (2-5) are now citing data that they believe support the view that migraine and tension headache are physiologically related entities, with a varied symptomatic expression reflecting a central disturbance of neuroreceptor function within the upper brainstem, limbic, and/or hypothalamic regions (2, 6).

The "central hypothesis" takes its support from the current understanding of brain mechanisms and the neurochemical and physiologic events that are purported to occur during headache (2, 5-8); the symptom overlap between migraine and tension headache (2-5, 8); the general acknowledgement that the clinical phenomena, including pain, cannot be satisfactorily or entirely explained by disturbances of the vascular or muscular structures alone (2-5, 8, 9); vascular flow studies that appear to challenge traditional views linking the preheadache and headache symptoms of migraine with specific changes in blood flow (10, 11); and therapeutic considerations that raise doubt as to the presumed mechanisms of well-known therapeutic agents (2, 12).

On this last point, drugs initially recognized to be useful for migraine or for muscle contraction headache may be of value in both disorders. Moreover, a large number of agents found useful in the treatment of tension headache, migraine, or both conditions do not demonstrate a consistent system (vascular or muscular) specificity sufficient to explain their effectiveness (2). In fact, the wide-ranging pharmacologic actions of drugs found useful in chronic headache disorders appear to share an influence on central brain mechanisms more than a specific vascular or muscular influence.

Thus, the perspectives on chronic headache are changing, and the villains of the past hundred years (the blood vessels and muscles) are now coming to be seen as possible victims, affected by chronic, intermittent, or continuous disturbances of central phenomena (2, 3, 6–8). Currently, the International Association for the Study of Headache is undertaking the first major attempt to reclassify headache since the Ad Hoc Committee report of 1963.

The following is an overview of the treatment of the primary headache conditions, including migraine, cluster headache, so-called tension headache, and chronic daily headache. Although the "separateness" concept still serves as the basis for treatment descriptions, the reader will soon note the substantial overlap of treatments between one headache entity and another, in part reflecting the transition period in understanding and terminology that currently exists.

GENERAL TREATMENT CONSIDERATIONS

In Chapter 21, the psychological therapies for headache are discussed. It is nonetheless critical to the success of any medical therapy for a proper physician/patient relationship to exist. Thus, the treatment of headache begins the moment the patient enters the office. Historically, patients claim that the medical profession reacts differently to the complaint of headache and chronic pain than to other similarly distressing illnesses. The merits of this claim aside, it is clear that helping such a patient is enhanced by conveying a sincere interest in their distress, understanding "the person" with the complaint, and establishing a worthwhile and frank communication forum.

A global recognition of the patient's life, emotional needs, and physiologic vulnerabilities is essential. Likewise, the physician's ability to enlist trust, allay anxiety and fear, and encourage cooperation are similarly important. In complex cases, the person, even more than the symptom, may require treatment, and the traditional focus of physicians on symptoms must make way for an emphasis on the individual first and the symptom second.

Although emotional factors are at times very important, in our need to explain that which is poorly understood, emotional phenomena may have been overemphasized as an etiologic basis for headache. Presumptions or premature emphasis on psychological elements early in the course of therapy is counterproductive and often clinically unfounded. Patients have come to feel defensive about these issues, because so many physicians are believed by patients to harbor preconceived notions as to the relevance of emotional considerations in the etiology of chronic headache.

The preventative as well as symptomatic treatment of chronic headache requires patience and innovativeness. Therapy in all cases must be modeled to meet individual differences in general health, psychological makeup, headache pattern, and patient compliance.

TREATMENT OF MIGRAINE

From its earliest recognition, migraine has defied a complete understanding of its pathophysiology, consistency of its diagnostic criteria, terminology, and reliability of treatment interventions. Although traditionally classified into *common* and *classic* forms, an expanded list of variants has evolved (3, 8, 9, 13). Also, differences of opinions exist as to whether classic migraine [forms with a preheadache (aura)], and *common* migraine (without a distinct, identifiable prodromal phase) are the same or different entities (14, 15).

Equally important is the growing recognition that many patients with migraine begin their headache years with acute intermittent "vascular"-type headache attacks, easily diagnosed as migraine by current criteria, but over the course of years evolve or "transform" into a chronic daily headache pattern that does not by current criteria fit the diagnosis of migraine (2, 8, 16, 17).

By traditional perspective, migraine is a common but periodic disorder, which undergoes natural remissions and spontaneous exacerbations. Prolonged uninterrupted use of preventative medications should be discouraged since remissions may not be appreciated when prolonged and successful therapy is continued indefinitely. Other nonpharmacologic treatments are of importance. Avoidance of migraine-provoking influences (3, 6, 8, 9), biofeedback, stress management, and adherence to life-style patterns that provide a regularity and sameness to the migraineur's daily activities may be important in many patients.

SYMPTOMATIC TREATMENT OF MIGRAINE

The pharmacologic symptomatic treatment of migraine should be considered when headaches occur infrequently and medications used for this approach are clinically acceptable (Table 20.1). The route of administration for symptomatic treatment may be as critical as the choice of medication. A delay of gastric absorption has been demonstrated in patients during both the acute phases of migraine and preheadache events, and can occur even in the absence of nausea and vomiting (6, 8). To abort a headache once begun, the use of one or more medications is usually required. The following are those noted to be of greatest value.

Ergotamine Tartrate and Other Alkaloids

Ergot alkaloids are estimated to be effective within the first 1–2 hr in up to 90% of cases when administered parenterally; in 80% of patients given the rectal form; and in up to 50% of the patients given the oral form (8). Historically, the effects of ergotamine have been con-

Table 20.1
Criteria for Symptomatic Versus Preventive Treatment of Migraine

Symptomatic Criteria
   Frequency less than 1–2 headaches/week
   General health does not contraindicate
      For ergot derivatives: coronary artery disease, severe hypertension, peripheral or cerebrovascular disease, etc.
      For analgesics containing aspirin: peptic ulcer disease, anticoagulant use, aspirin sensitive asthma, etc.
Preventive criteria
   Frequency greater than 1–2 headaches/week
   Medical contraindications for symptomatic therapies. Failure of symptomatic therapies. When attacks occur with reliable, predictable regularity, at or around menstrual period, etc. Known substance abuse tendencies

sidered to be via an arterial vasoconstrictive influence. More recently, a central (brain) effect has been considered (12).

Ergotamine possesses a smooth muscle–stimulating effect capable of producing vasoconstriction, a mild central sympatholytic effect in the medulla, and a peripheral adrenergic effect (18). Ergotamine may also delay gastric emptying by its direct action on stomach musculature, and may at high levels produces endothelial damage.

Ergotamine alkaloids [ergotamine tartrate and dihydroergotamine (D.H.E. 45)] are available in intravenous, intramuscular, subcutaneous, oral, rectal, inhalant, and sublingual forms. The oral and sublingual forms are not as effective as parenteral or rectal routes. The sublingual forms (Ergomar, Wigrettes, and Ergostat) contain 2.0 mg of ergotamine tartrate. The oral and rectal routes contain ergotamine tartrate in combination with caffeine with or without belladonna and barbiturate.

The dose required to alleviate an evolving migraine is variable and depends in part upon the method of delivery. Parenteral treatment with dihydroergotamine (1–2 ml intramuscularly or 0.5–1.0 ml intravenously) is usually effective. (D.H.E. 45 is currently the only available parenteral form of ergot alkaloids.)

In rectal form, a suppository containing 2 mg of ergotamine tartrate (Cafergot or Wigraine) can be administered initially with a repeat dose in 1 hr, and a maximum dose daily of 4.0 mg. The starting dose of one-third to one-half of a suppository is advisable because of the likely adverse effects if excessive or too rapid absorption occurs.

In tablet form (Cafergot or Wigraine), a 1.0-mg tablet is administered as two tablets initially, followed by one tablet every 30 min until relief is obtained or until 5 mg have been taken. Sublingual tablets (Ergomar, Ergostat, Wigrettes) contain 2.0 mg of ergotamine tartrate, and an inhalant form (Ergotamine Medihaler) can also be used. Although variability of the inhaled dose and concern over possible excessive pulmonary artery constriction has limited its usefulness, the inhalant form can be very effective.

Ergotamine and related alkaloids are contraindicated in patients with marked hypertension, peripheral vascular disease, ischemic heart disease, cardiac valvular abnormalities, collagen vascular disease, and thrombophlebitis, and in patients over the age of 60 (8). Caution must be exercised in patients with peptic ulcer disease, bradycardia, and renal and hepatic abnormalities. Current infection or fever may also promote excessive vasoconstriction. The use of these compounds must be avoided in pregnancy.

Among the minor untoward reactions are nausea and vomiting, muscle achiness, diarrhea, and difficulty swallowing (usually benign). Abdominal cramps, chest pain, vertigo, and paresthesiae of hands and feet are estimated to occur in 5–10% of patients. Symptoms lasting several hours or less are not generally considered contraindications to use.

The more serious consequences to ergotamine usage occur when excessive dosages are employed or when the drug is used in the presence of a contraindication. Severe reactions have been reported at acceptable dosages in otherwise healthy patients (8, 9). Ergotamine tartrate may cause bradycardia and should be used with considerable caution in patients with preexisting bradycardia, or with combined usage with β-blocking drugs or others that may slow the heart rate.

Ergotism is a serious and well-known consequence of ergotamine overusage (8, 12). Susceptibility to ergotism is variable. Recently, dependency on ergotamine tartrate has been reported in patients taking ergotamine as infrequently as three times per week, with the development of "rebound" or "ergotamine headache" as a consequence. Ergotamine tartrate should be used no more than 2 days per week, since greater frequency of usage can lead to dependency and increasing headaches (12).

Isometheptene Mucate

Isometheptene mucate is a sympathomimetic agent in a combined form (Midrin) that exerts a beneficial effect on the acute attack of migraine (8). Midrin is a combination of 65 mg of isometheptene mucate, 325 mg of acetaminophen, and 100 mg of dichloralphenazone (a tranquilizer). It produces less gastrointestinal distress than ergotamine preparations, and in one controlled study (19) was noted to be superior to ergotamine tartrate and caffeine preparations.

Midrin is an effective agent for the symptomatic treatment of mild to moderate migraine attacks, and is particularly useful in cases in which adverse effects to ergot medications exist. Although the general contraindications for the use of Midrin are the same as those for ergotamine, there exists a lesser likelihood of adverse responses. Mild sedation and gastrointestinal distress occur in some but not most patients. Generally the drug is well tolerated.

The dosage of Midrin is two capsules at the onset of an

attack, followed by one or two capsules 30 min and 1 hr later, up to a maximum of five capsules per attack. Simultaneous administration of two aspirin at the onset of an attack or a nonsteroidal anti-inflammatory drug (NSAID) may enhance effectiveness.

The drug should not be used more than two or three times per week in order to avoid "rebound" effects.

Nonsteroidal Anti-inflammatory Drugs

The NSAIDs have symptomatic as well as preventative value. A large number of agents are available (20). Naproxen sodium (Anaprox) has been most widely evaluated (21–23). The dose of naproxen is 275 mg (one to two tablets), to be taken at onset of headache. Other agents include meclofenamate sodium (Meclomen) at 100–200 mg, indomethacin (Indocin) at 25–50 mg, or ibuprofen (Motrin) at 400–800 mg, all taken at onset of the attack.

The NSAIDs have well known contraindications that generally include gastrointestinal or renal disease, or bleeding disturbances (20).

Analgesics

Although analgesics (narcotic and nonnarcotic) may benefit some patients during an acute migraine attack, the abuse potential for overuse is a sufficiently serious problem as to make the routine use of analgesics inappropriate for frequent headaches. This is particularly true of combination forms in which a narcotic or barbiturate ingredient is present. However, even the simple analgesics, when too frequently employed, can be troublesome.

Injectable narcotics are usually of greater value than oral medication, but the tendency for dependency must be emphasized. These drugs should not be employed as standard therapy for the acute migraine attack, unless other standard agents are of no value or are contraindicated, and the attacks are sufficiently infrequent as to justify this form of treatment. The physician must be alert to the somatic expression of psychological despair and drug-seeking behavior as manifested through the complaint of headache. Discouraging the employment of injectable narcotics for the treatment of headache is worthwhile. In selected cases, however, narcotics may represent the most appropriate and safest treatment.

Phenothiazines, Other Antiemetics, and Related Medications

The phenothiazines may be effective as antiemetics and may also have some pain-relieving benefit. These and related substances can be administered in conjunction with symptomatic drugs and are most effective by parenteral or suppository route.

The dose of chlorpromazine (Thorazine) is 25–50 mg intramuscularly, rectally, or in tablet form. Promethazine (Phenergan) is administered in a dose of 25 mg intramuscularly or rectally, or 50 mg orally. This author generally avoids employing prochlorperazine (Compazine) because of the higher incidence of acute dystonic reactions associated with its use when compared to other agents, such as chlorpromazine.

Reglan (metoclopramide hydrochloride) in dosages of 10 mg orally three times a day or in intravenous form can provide antiemetic effects and also may be of value in enhancing oral absorption. Hydroxyzine (Vistaril) in dosages of 50–100 mg orally or 75 mg intramuscularly may likewise be effective as an antiemetic and may enhance the benefit of other agents used to treat an attack. Hydroxyzine may also have primary analgesic effects (24).

The symptomatic usefulness of steroids should be noted (25). Prolonged refractory attacks may benefit from steroidal therapy. Prednisone in dosages of 40–60 mg administered orally for 3–5 days or 8–16 mg of dexamethasone by intramuscular administration may be used.

Recently, Raskin has recommended a treatment protocol using intravenous dihydroergotamine treatment for refractory migraine (26). This is discussed below under "Special Therapeutic Considerations and Situations."

Finally, many of the drugs useful for migraine prevention, including β-blockers, tricyclic antidepressants, and calcium channel blockers, may have a value in symptomatic protocols.

PREVENTIVE PHARMACOLOGIC AGENTS IN THE TREATMENT OF MIGRAINE

The preventive medical management of migraine employs the daily use of one or a combination of medications that are presumed to block the biologic events leading up to migraine. Such a program should be considered when the frequency of migraine attacks exceeds the safety limitations for the use of symptomatic medications or concurrent medical conditions contraindicate the use of medications employed to abort headaches. Generally, more than four major attacks per month justifies a preventative program. Preventative treatment should be employed at intervals of 3–6 months followed by a gradual reduction of medication, since natural remissions of headache may not be recognized when preventative medication therapy is maintained.

β-Blockers

The most widely used and important group of drugs for the prevention of migraine are the β-blockers. Among the β-blocking agents that are useful in the prevention of migraine are propranolol (Inderal) and nadolol (Corgard), which are nonselective blocking agents, imposing a competitive blockade in both β_1- and β_2-adrenergic receptors (3, 8, 27). Selective β-blockers, including metoprolol (Lopressor) and timolol (Tenormin), which selectively block β_1-adrenergic receptors, may be of equal value (8, 28), although the nonselective blockers have historically been considered more effective.

Because of their β-adrenergic blocking action, these drugs were initially presumed to affect migraine via a blocking of the peripheral vasodilatory receptors, thereby interfering with the presumed dilatory phase of migraine. Many clinicians now believe that other influences are responsible for the antimigraine effects of these agents, and an effect on the central nervous system is considered likely by some (8).

Therapy with the β-blocking drugs requires individual dose determination, and one agent may be more effective for a particular patient than another similar medicine. Inderal comes in two forms, the short-acting original form and the new Inderal LA. In the short-acting form, treatment may begin at dosages between 20 and 40 mg given three to four times a day and increased up to a total dose of 400 mg/day, in three or four divided doses. Inderal LA is best employed in a twice-per-day regimen, beginning at 80 mg once or twice per day, and increasing to 160 mg twice a day as tolerated.

Corgard (40-mg tablet) is begun at a dose of 20 mg twice a day and increased to the point of tolerance, often up to 120–160 mg twice a day (240–320 mg total dose). Corgard appears particularly reliable and can be effective in some patients in a once-a-day dose regimen. It seems considerably less likely to produce the frequently encountered "central" effects often seen with propranolol, and appears at least as effective, and perhaps more so, than propranolol.

High-dose regimens may be of value in some cases, but if efficacy is not demonstrated at moderate dosages, higher dosage regimens are usually of little value (29). However, exceptions exist.

Most individuals taking β-blocking agents will experience an initial lowering of blood pressure and pulse rate, and some patients have an unexpected sensitivity, resulting in rather dramatic hypotension and bradycardia even at low dosages. Caution and patient monitoring are essential. Other common side effects, including depression and mental changes, are well known and can be found in standard sources. Slowly discontinuing the medication over several weeks after prolonged usage is advisable. Approximately 24–48 hr are required for complete dissipation of its effect after final discontinuance (8).

Methysergide

Methysergide (Sansert) is an effective preventative medication for migraine (6–8), with a beneficial response demonstrated in up to 50–65% of patients. At one time, methysergide was the standard bearer for the preventive control of migraine headaches. The exact mode by which methysergide exerts its effect remains unknown, but it may occupy serotonin reuptake sites on the blood vessel walls, thereby stabilizing both vasoconstriction and vasodilation. Like many of the migraine agents, including ergotamine tartrate, methysergide may have its greatest influence on central aminergic physiology (2).

The usual dose of methysergide is 2.0 mg once or twice per day up to a maximum of 8.0 mg/day in four divided doses. It should not be used in patients with peripheral vascular disease, coronary artery disease, hypertension, serious gastrointestinal distress, and pregnancy. Activation of peptic ulcer disease is possibly related to its enhancement of gastric acid secretion (8).

Methysergide should not be administered for more than 5–6 months without interruption of therapy for at least 1 to 2 months because of the potential development of fibrosis in the retroperitoneal region, lungs, and heart valves. Although these changes tend to regress after discontinuance, they may not. A peripheral vascular occlusive reaction similar to Leriche's syndrome has been reported, and aggravation of preexisting angina pectoris is common. Intravenous pyelogram, chest x-ray, and cardiac exam are recommended after 6 months of therapy.

Adverse reactions of a mild to moderate degree occur frequently and thus limit methysergide's overall usefulness. The most common untoward reactions include transient muscle aching, abdominal distress, hallucinations, and a sense of swelling of face or throat. Frightening hallucinatory events after the first dose are not uncommon. Minor reactions are frequently transient, and continued use of the drug does not appear unsafe.

The use of methysergide should be limited to patients with migraine or related headaches who do not respond to other preventative medications, and when short-term prophylaxis is needed. It should not be given after the age of 50 or to persons at risk for vascular disease.

Calcium Antagonists (Calcium Channel Blockers)

Increasing attention has focused on calcium antagonists in treatment of various headache conditions. The mechanism of effectiveness is unknown but may not be directly related to effects on blood vessels, since central effects are present (30–33).

The three available calcium antagonists are verapamil (Isoptin, Calan), diltiazem (Cardizem), and nifedipine (Procardia). Isoptin is usually administered beginning at 80 mg two or three times a day and increased to approximately 160 mg three to four times per day. The starting dose of diltiazem is 30 mg two or three times a day, increased to 90 mg three times per day if tolerated. Procardia may be begun at 10 mg three times a day and increased to 60–90 mg three times a day.

The calcium antagonists are of special benefit in patients who suffer from migraine and simultaneous vasoconstrictive tendencies such as Raynaud's phenomena/disease or asthma. β-Blocking agents aggravate these conditions.

Among the side effects of calcium antagonists are headache (particularly with nifedipine), depression, vasomotor changes, tremor, gastrointestinal distress, dizziness, pedal edema, orthostatic hypotension, and bradycardia (particularly with verapamil and diltiazem). Numerous patients report an increase in headaches initially, with improvement occurring over several weeks. Periodic electrocardiographic evaluation is valuable, and special precautions in patients with bradycardia, hypotension, heart block, or vulnerability to heart failure are recommended.

The calcium channel blockers are generally considered safe and well tolerated. Their ultimate value in the prophylaxis of migraine remains to be determined.

Antidepressants

The tricyclic antidepressants (TCAs), particularly amitriptyline (Endep, Elavil), nortriptyline (Aventyl), doxepin (Sinequan, Adapin), and others, have been reported as effective in migraine prevention (3, 8), although their value in the treatment of daily chronic pain (tension headache) is better established (2, 34, 35). The usual dose of amitriptyline and doxepin ranges from 25 to 150 mg a day, often given in a single bedtime dose. Nortriptyline dosages range from 25 to 75 mg. Common side effects include sedation, dry mouth, urinary retention, constipation, blurred vision, intense dreaming with nightmares, weight gain, and hypotension. Contraindications include cardiac arrhythmias, narrow angle glaucoma, myocardial infarction, severe prostatism, and uncontrolled seizures.

The monoamine oxidase–inhibiting antidepressants (MAOIs), particularly phenelzine (Nardil), can be quite effective in the prevention of migraine (3, 6, 8, 9). MAOIs influence the intracellular metabolism of biogenic amines, and disturbances of this system have been proposed in migraine (6). The usual dose of phenelzine is 15 mg three to four times per day, usually given in divided dosages beginning with 15 mg/day for several days, with a gradual increase in dose until benefit is achieved or safety limitations reached.

The most common side effects of the MAOIs include insomnia, orthostatic hypotension, anticholinergic effects, weight gain, and loss of sexual desire and/or orgasm (8). Insomnia can sometimes be avoided by administering all doses prior to noon.

Traditional concern over the use of MAOIs has waned during the past several years since it has been recognized that their use may be much safer and less restrictive than historically believed (36, 37). Moreover, combinations of MAOI and amitriptyline have been reported efficacious in both pain and depression disorders. (For further discussion, see standard texts.)

Simultaneous use of MAOIs with β-blockers and calcium channel blockers must be carried out with extreme caution, since severe orthostatic hypotension with syncope is frequently encountered.

Nonsteroidal Anti-inflammatory Agents

The NSAIDs are useful in both the symptomatic and the preventative treatment of migraine (20–23). Naproxen sodium (Anaprox) has been most successfully established as an effective preventative agent. Indomethacin (Indocin) has shown its greatest value in the prevention of variants of cluster headache. The dose of naproxen sodium for migraine prevention is one or two 275-mg tablets twice a day. Gastrointestinal effects and long-term effects on renal function must be considered, and the drug should not be used in the presence of contraindications (20). The presumed mechanism is via an influence on prostaglandin and platelet metabolism.

The NSAIDs may be particularly valuable in the treatment of menstrual migraine (21).

Cyproheptadine

Although cyproheptadine (Periactin) has been used with minimal success alone in the prevention of migraine in adults, it is considered the treatment of choice for prevention of childhood migraine (8). Dosages range from 4 to 8 mg three to four times per day for adults and 4 mg two to three times per day in children.

Clonidine

Clonidine hydrochloride (Catapres) is an antihypertensive agent possessing α-adrenergic stimulating properties. Clonidine has been studied in several trials (8) and has been found useful in some but not in others. The recommended dose is 0.2 mg given two to three times per day. This drug may be worthy of trial in patients with migraine who are withdrawing from narcotic analgesics or in menopausal women experiencing headaches and vasomotor symptoms.

Bellergal/Anticonvulsants

Bellergal is a compound containing ergotamine tartrate, belladonna, and barbiturate. Bellergal-S is a sustained-release form of the same. The drug can be useful in some patients with migraine but should be used for only short-term intervention (such as around a menstrual period), since daily administration of ergotamine tartrate may result in dependency.

Occasionally, patients with intermittent migraine or mixed syndromes will appear to benefit from the anticonvulsants or antineuralgic agents, including carbamazapine (Tegretol), phenytoin (Dilantin), and baclofen (Lioresal). The mechanisms by which these agents help "nonneuralgic" syndromes is yet to be determined.

Long-term effectiveness of preventative therapy has been established in a report by Raskin and Schwartz (38).

TREATMENT OF CLUSTER HEADACHE

Perhaps the most sinister of the well-recognized headache disorders, cluster headache is a severely painful affliction primarily affecting men (3, 6, 8, 9, 39, 40). In this sense, a cluster headache is distinct from the other primary headache disorders (migraine, tension headache, and combined headaches), which by most surveys affect women in a ratio of 3:1. Few headaches more challenge the clinician's knowledge, compassion, and pharmacotherapeutic skills than the cluster headache condition.

Cluster headache can be divided into three major forms.

Episodic Cluster Headache This most well-known and common pattern is characterized by recurring bouts or clusters of headaches. During these cycles, typical headache attacks occur regularly and usually daily. Each cycle may last from weeks to months, and is then followed by a spontaneous remission, called the interim.

Chronic Cluster Headache Chronic cluster headache is divided into a *primary* form and a *secondary* form. In the absence of remission for 1 year or more, the term *chronic* is appropriate. Primary chronic cluster headache is characterized by recurring headache events for years without a remission. The *secondary* chronic cluster headache form is characterized by a pattern of typical recurring headache attacks that have become chronic but have evolved from an original episodic pattern.

Chronic Paroxysmal Hemicrania Chronic paroxysmal hernicrania is considered by many to be a true variant of cluster headache. It frequently affects children (8, 39). In 1974, Sjaastad and Dale (40) described this headache entity with striking similarity to cluster headaches. This disorder is quite similar to cluster headache despite some clinical differences. It primarily strikes young woman, although not exclusively. Although often indistinguishable from cluster headache, headache events of chronic paroxysmal hemicrania may be shorter than those of a typical headache, generally occur with greater frequency (usually during the day), and rarely awaken patients from sleep.

During cluster headache cycles, one or more attacks occur daily with an average frequency of one to three attacks every 24 hr, each lasting from 20 min to 2 hr with residual distress for several hours after the termination of the most intense pain. The clinical features of attacks are well described in standard texts (3, 6, 8, 9, 39).

Although cycles of headaches occur randomly in the episodic form, they appear most common at times of season change. Seasonal sensitivity may in part relate to adaptational changes of hypothalamic function, which may be the pathophysiologic locus of cluster headache (8, 39). Periodic depression may occur in conjunction with cluster headaches.

The actual mechanism of cluster headache is unknown, but disturbances within the circuits of cranial nerve V, nervus intermedius, and sphenopalatine ganglion have been considered. Dysfunction of the hypothalamus, involving chronobiologic abnormalities, may be of importance in cluster headache.

GENERAL TREATMENT CONSIDERATIONS

The treatment of cluster headache requires above all persistence, diligence, innovation, and compassion along with a commitment to a variety of tools available to curb the pain and desperation associated with this condition. As in other headache disorders, the choice must take into account the age and health of the patient, frequency of the attacks, the expected duration of a cluster cycle, previous therapies, and a patient's daily activities and habits.

Patients with cluster headache must discontinue all alcohol products and avoid daytime napping. Normalization of sleep cycles can be accomplished naturally by medication therapy, including tricyclic antidepressants. Awakening at the same time each day is very important since prolonged sleeping appears to provoke attacks (8). This author asks all patients to discontinue smoking and in those in whom this goal is accomplished, increased control seems apparent although not yet formally established.

SYMPTOMATIC TREATMENT

Inhalation of 100% oxygen is an effective means of symptomatically relieving the pain in many patients (8, 39, 41, 42). Patients must be given a mask and employ 100% oxygen at 7 liters/min for a period of 15 min or more. Between 65 and 75% of episodic cluster patients, and 50% of chronic headache patients, will experience improvement.

In addition to oxygen, effective symptomatic management generally requires the use of an ergotamine alkaloid, which, if administered and absorbed promptly, can reverse most attacks within minutes. Standard oral tablets are impractical. Although effective, ergot preparations must be used with great restraint because of the daily occurrence of attacks. Injectable narcotic analgesics are discouraged because of the obvious tendency for abuse with this headache pattern.

PREVENTIVE TREATMENT

The preventative therapy regimens are the most desirable treatment for cluster headache.

Prednisone

Prednisone is the most reliably effective drug for the immediate preventative control of cluster headache, and can dramatically prevent both chronic and episodic varieties within hours of first administration. Several regimens can be used. Kudrow (39) recommended a 3-week program starting with 40 mg for 5 days followed by a tapering course. This author employs a shorter regimen of 10 days beginning at 60 mg for four days and subsequently tapering (see Table 20.2) (8). Although some headache cycles can be terminated with such use, reemergence of headaches may occur as dosages fall to 15–20 mg/day. The risk from short-term usage in appropriate patients is small but the usual contraindications must be appreciated.

Steroid therapy is recommended in the following situations: to provide an immediate control, particularly in patients growing desperate from recurring attacks; to offer "insurance" treatment when patients are away from familiar medical care, such as when traveling; and during drug holidays from other medications.

Lithium Carbonate

Lithium carbonate (Eskalith, Lithobid, Lithane) can be effective in over 60% of cases (8, 39, 42–44). The usual starting dose is 300 mg administered two to four times per day. Therapeutic response does not necessarily correlate with blood levels, and serum levels exceeding 0.7 mEq/liter are rarely necessary for good results. Blood monitoring is appropriate to prevent toxicity. Lithium may have a direct effect on hypothalamic regulatory centers and may also influence enkephalinergic neuronal systems.

The adverse effects of lithium include nausea, vomiting,

Table 20.2
Protocols for Prednisone Treatment of Cluster Headache

10-Day Protocol[a]

Day	8:00 AM	4:00 PM	Bedtime	
1	20 mg	20 mg	20 mg	= 60 mg/day
2	20 mg	20 mg	20 mg	= 60 mg/day
3	20 mg	20 mg	20 mg	= 60 mg/day
4	20 mg	20 mg	20 mg	= 60 mg/day
5	20 mg	15 mg	15 mg	= 50 mg/day
6	15 mg	15 mg	10 mg	= 40 mg/day
7	10 mg	10 mg	10 mg	= 30 mg/day
8	5 mg	5 mg	5 mg	= 15 mg/day
9	5 mg	0	5 mg	= 10 mg/day
10	5 mg	(finished)		= 5 mg/day

7-Day Protocol[b]

Day	8:00 AM	4:00 PM	Bedtime	
1	20 mg	20 mg	20 mg	= 60 mg/day
2	20 mg	20 mg	20 mg	= 60 mg/day
3	20 mg	15 mg	15 mg	= 50 mg/day
4	15 mg	15 mg	10 mg	= 40 mg/day
5	10 mg	10 mg	10 mg	= 30 mg/day
6	10 mg	5 mg	5 mg	= 20 mg/day
7	10 mg	(finished)		= 10 mg/day

[a] 20 mg = 4 pills, 15 mg = 3 pills, 10 mg = 2 pills, 5 mg = 1 pill; total of 78 tablets needed.
[b] 20 mg = 4 pills, 15 mg = 3 pills, 10 mg = 2 pills, 5 mg = 1 pill; total of 54 tablets needed.

diarrhea, tremor, blurred vision, gait unsteadiness, and exacerbation of dermatologic conditions, including psoriasis. Hypothyroidism may occur with long-term use, particularly in women. Patients must avoid diuretics and salt-restrictive diets because of the increased risk of intoxication. Increased salt intake will reduce effectiveness.

During summer months, excessive salt loss through perspiration may result in lithium toxicity. Nephrotoxicity occurs in some patients even when lithium is maintained in the nontoxic range for short periods of time, although generally therapy is safe when given for short cycles. Other potentially nephrotoxic drugs such as NSAIDs should be used with caution during lithium treatment. Long-term, noninterrupted use in chronic headache patients should be discouraged. Frequent drug holidays and blood monitoring and alternate treatment programs are recommended.

Calcium Antagonists

The calcium antagonists can be of great value in cluster headache (30, 31). This author has found verapamil (Isoptin, Calan) particularly valuable (42). Many patients do not benefit until the upper levels of treatment are reached. Treatment effectiveness may require several weeks.

Diltiazem may be similarly effective and occasionally patients will report benefit from nifedipine, although worsening of pain to the point of intolerance is more likely with this latter drug.

Methysergide

Sansert is effective for many otherwise refractory patients with cluster headache, but the risks are well known. This ergot derivative is appropriate for a patient whose cluster periods last less than 3–4 months and who is refractory or cannot take other forms of therapy.

Chlorpromazine

Chlorpromazine (Thorazine) in dosages ranging from 75 to several hundred milligrams per day has been reported useful in cluster headache (45). A sustained benefit for up to 6–8 months was demonstrated on maintenance levels of 75 mg per day. Not all authorities believe this drug to be similarly effective. It can be used as an adjunctive therapy in refractory patients and may be particularly useful for nocturnal attacks. Risks and long-term side effects are well known and must be considered.

Cyproheptadine

Cyproheptadine (Periactin) has not been proven useful for most cluster headache patients; however, occasional benefits are recognized. Because of its overall safety, its use as an adjunctive agent in difficult cases is recommended.

Nonsteroidal Anti-inflammatory Agents

The NSAIDs may be effective for cluster headache (46), but appear to be most helpful for the variant called chronic paroxysmal hemicrania (CPH), which (by definition) is effectively treated with indomethacin (Indocin) at dosages of 25–50 mg three to four times per day. Whether other NSAIDs have similar benefits remains to be determined.

Other Therapies

Histamine desensitization to alleviate cluster headache was first described in 1939 by Horton et al. (47). Although recent attention to this form of therapy exists (48), most clinicians informally surveyed by this author fail to recognize a major contribution from this therapy. In severely intractable cases, however, this intervention could be considered.

Surgery and other ablative procedures on the sphenopalatine ganglion, nervus intermedius, or the other branches or ganglia of cranial nerve V may be effective and appropriate in some patients (49, 50). At this time, however, surgical treatment cannot be generally recommended except in the most severe and intractable cases, when all other traditional treatments, including inpatient care, have been tried.

Cluster headache and its variants are distressing disorders and, when uncontrolled, pose a serious threat to the patient's will to endure. Inpatient-level care has been used in numerous intractable cases and is to be recommended for difficult cases.

Cluster headache inflicts the most ravaging type of painful distress, and this is often accompanied by intense emotional despair. A relationship to cyclical depression is possible (8). Patients will frequently experience a personality change along with other constitutional, emotional, and physiologic changes during these cycles. Aggressive intervention and a committed involvement of the physician until control is established are essential, and bring profound satisfaction to the patient and physician alike.

TENSION, CHRONIC DAILY, AND COMBINED HEADACHES

Tension headache is defined by the Ad Hoc Committee (1) as:

> Ache or sensations of tightness, pressure, or constriction, widely varied in intensity, frequency, and duration; longlasting, and commonly suboccipital, associated with sustained contraction of skeletal muscles, usually as part of the individual's reaction during life-stress.

Combined headaches (vascular and muscle contraction) are:

> Combinations of vascular headache of the migraine type and muscle contraction headache prominently co-existing in an attack. (1)

Although historically clinicians have used the term *tension headache* to characterize a daily or almost daily chronic headache disorder without vascular-type features and that is likely but not necessarily associated with provocation by stress or emotional factors, traditionally migraine and muscle contraction headaches have been considered distinct entities (9).

So imprecise are the criteria for tension headache, and so casually has the diagnosis been rendered, that to many the diagnosis of tension headache or muscle contraction headache has become but a "wastebasket" diagnosis (2,8). In many instances, the diagnosis has been applied to any headache disorder that ostensibly is not vascular (migraine, cluster) nor associated with identifiable structural disease, and that occurs when elements of stress, anxiety, or depression are evident.

A serious reappraisal of attitudes on this headache entity is underway, as was mentioned earlier (2, 16, 17). Research studies over the course of the past several years have raised serious challenges to traditional positions. Attention to the transformation from intermittent migraine to daily chronic headache and to central elements purported to be involved in this process is growing in importance and is considered as the basis for the clinical events and for treatment approaches.

With this in mind, and recognizing that a transition in our understanding and classification of this disorder is currently underway, treatment regimens are described. The reader will quickly note that considerable overlapping between treatments of this condition and migraine exists, and that treatment frequently involves combinations of drugs.

SYMPTOMATIC TREATMENT FOR "ACUTE" TENSION HEADACHE

Acute tension headache may in fact be a separate and distinct entity from that of the chronic form. Acute tension headache is perhaps of muscular origin and results in occasional, intermittent headache, whereas chronic "tension headache" is prolonged, sustained, and more likely to be daily rather than intermittent. Acute tension headache can be brought on by stress, posture, or injury. The symptoms are usually generalized, with occipitofrontal tightness or "band-like" pain, and rarely does the pain reach sufficient level to cause limitations of function (8).

The treatment for acute tension headache consists of mild analgesics (aspirin, acetaminophen) or NSAIDs. Simple muscle relaxants may also be of value.

TREATMENT FOR CHRONIC DAILY HEADACHE (TENSION HEADACHE)

Symptomatic Treatment

From a therapeutic point of view, frequent, recurring headache patterns in which both muscular and vascular features coexist during a well-circumscribed attack are best treated with medications appropriate for the symptomatic alleviation of the predominant headache element. For acute muscular pain, simple analgesics, NSAIDs, or TCAs are useful. For acute migraine elements, ergotamine tartrate, Midrin, or other drugs mentioned in earlier sections are appropriate.

Preventive Treatment

Because most frequently chronic headache forms result in daily or almost daily headache, preventative treatment is advisable.

The TCAs (see "Preventive Pharmacologic Agents in the Treatment of Migraine," above) are used on a daily basis (3, 8, 51). In addition to their value in daily pain states, these medications are particularly valuable in controlling accompanying depression as well as sleep disturbance, which are both frequently encountered in this population (2, 8). Dosages range from 25 to 150 mg at bedtime if tolerated. Treatment response may have little to do with existing depression or its elimination.

Tricyclic antidepressants can be readily combined with β-blocking agents (51), and in this regard propranolol and nadolol have been found useful. Periodic acute attacks of migraine that are encountered commonly on a background of daily chronic headache should be treated in the standard fashion as described earlier. The addition of NSAIDs, benzodiazepine therapy, and other drugs mentioned earlier in the treatment of migraine may also be necessary.

This population of patients is very complex. Analgesic overuse, psychological distress, and family and other complicating problems frequently render even the most appropriate pharmacotherapeutic intervention ineffective. In this author's experience, a comprehensive treatment program including inpatient-level care, psychotherapy, family involvement in treatment programs, dietary control, biofeedback, and several other interventions are frequently necessary to bring about satisfactory control of this difficult headache process.

HEADACHES IN CHILDREN

Children, like adults, get headaches. Migraine, mixed element headaches, cluster headache, and others seen in adulthood can be encountered in childhood (8). Of some interest is that the female/male ratio among children with headaches is 1:1, whereas a 3:1 ratio in favor of women is characteristic of most adult chronic headaches, except cluster headache, which is predominantly an illness of men (8).

The pharmacologic treatment of headache in children does not differ appreciably from that of adults. Cyproheptadine (Periactin) may be the treatment of first choice for the prevention of childhood migraine. Children appear to tolerate both preventive and symptomatic agents quite well. Tricyclic antidepressants, β-blockers, NSAIDs (particularly for chronic paroxysmal hemicrania), and symptomatic medications are all appropriate. Nonmedical interventions including biofeedback, dietary restriction, avoidance of excessive "junk food" intake, regular eating patterns, stress management, and family counseling may all represent important elements in the treatment of childhood headaches.

POST-TRAUMATIC CEPHALGIA

The incidence of headache following closed head injury varies from 33 to 80% and may take one of several clinical forms. Often the headache is a component of the *posttraumatic* or *postconcussion* syndrome, which represents a constellation of symptoms that can follow even mild head or flexion/extension injury (3, 8, 9). Among the nonheadache symptoms that are generally considered common in this condition are vertigo or nonspecific dizziness, personality change (most notably depression and anxiety), impairment of memory, reduced attention span, insomnia, and reduced motivation. Prolonged neuropsychological impairment can be documented in many patients who exhibit little in the way of objective dysfunction (52).

The headache may take the form of one of several patterns. Among these are: a generalized throbbing and/or nonthrobbing cephalgia; unilateral intermittent or continuous throbbing pain (similar to migraine); localized occipitocervical pain with neuralgic qualities; and unilateral intense intermittent cephalgia in the anterior triangle of the neck or in the orbital area, and resembling episodic cluster headache (8, 9). Frequently, an intermingling of two or more of these forms is present. Occipitocervical soreness and myofascial-type complaints often accompany the more specific headache patterns.

TREATMENT OF POST-TRAUMATIC HEADACHE

Important nonpharmacologic interventions such as counseling, biofeedback, physical therapy, transcutaneous electrical nerve stimulation treatment, and others are appropriate. A variety of pharmacologic interventions should be considered. For prophylaxis, a TCA, β-blocker, or calcium antagonist can be efficacious alone or in combination. Nonsteroidal anti-inflammatory agents, intermittently or prophylactically, may be useful. Intermittent acute headache events can be treated in the manner described earlier for symptomatic treatment of migraine. Focal tenderness often responds to local anesthesia with or without steroids. Neuralgic symptoms may be controlled with carbamazepine (Tegretol), phenytoin (Dilantin), or baclofen (Lioresal). Local surgical procedures, including decompression or neurectomy, have been recommended in some patients.

Clinical experience, however, suggests that patients with post-trauma headache require a comprehensive treatment program. Lingering symptoms that are often refractory to simple intervention are common.

SPECIAL THERAPEUTIC CONSIDERATIONS AND SITUATIONS

SPECIAL DRUG TECHNIQUES

The pharmacologic treatment of patients with chronic headache must be individually determined. Persistent and innovative attempts to develop appropriate treatment protocols is frequently necessary to bring about recognizable improvement.

Raskin has recently described a program of intravenous administration of dihydroergotamine in dosages ranging from 0.5 to 1.0 mg every 8 hr over a period of 3–5 days (26). This treatment is purported to bring important control over even the most refractory cases of headache, including those due to substance withdrawal. Personal experience with this therapy supports Raskin's contention of efficacy, although the extent and applicability of this treatment remains to determined by the experience of others. Intravenous dihydroergotamine therapy is best carried out in an inpatient setting and should be reserved for those patients in whom standard interventions are of little value.

The MAOIs have proven useful in several of this author's most refractory cases. Although caution and special instructions to the patient are necessary, most patients can use these drugs without ill effects or undue risk.

In the symptomatic treatment of migraine, absorption from the gastrointestinal tract can prove to be the determining factor in establishing effectiveness. The use of metoclopramide (Reglan) 10 mg one to three times per day may be of value in enhancing the effectiveness of any of the oral tablets (8). Treatment with metoclopramide can precede the use of any of the oral agents by 10–15 min and can be helpful in avoiding some of the nausea that frequently occurs with the use of ergotamine tartrate or as part of the headache itself.

Inhalant forms of ergotamine tartrate or rectal forms are likewise useful in overcoming the gastrointestinal factors accompanying attacks.

Menstrual migraine represents a most difficult variation of migraine. Many women will experience their most severe headache at this time of the month and frequently it is superimposed upon other changes that occur as part of menses. Ergotamine tartrate is probably the most effective agent for the reversal of this headache, and preventive therapy that might include NSAIDs, Bellergal, β-blockers, and others may be necessary. Danazol (Danocrine) has been found useful anecdotally, but studies firmly establishing its efficacy are lacking.

It is particularly important when using combinations of medication to exercise appropriate caution, periodic educational review, and diagnostic monitoring. Laboratory reviews to monitor biochemical parameters, electrocardiographic evaluation to assess QRS intervals and conduction disturbances, and blood level assessments are strongly recommended (53).

Despite the apparent reliability of an individual patient, noncompliance either intentionally or inadvertently is common (54). Periodic review of treatment regimens and appropriate counseling are likewise worthwhile and add measurably to the likelihood of treatment efficacy.

TREATMENT OF MEDICATION OVERUSE AND DEPENDENCY IN HEADACHE PATIENTS

Physicians and other health care professionals treating patients with headache and other chronic pain syndromes must confront a serious medication overuse problem in a large number of their patients. The extent of this problem is difficult to assess. In our center, it is estimated that at least one-half of the patients seeking help for headaches indulge in excessive use of medications to relieve their distress, and it is not unusual for first-time patients to report the consumption of 10–30 simple analgesic tablets perday, 6–8 mg of ergotamine tartrate daily, or the regular ingestion of large amounts of tranquilizing, hypnotic, or narcotic analgesics.

Aside from the important health consequences of the daily use of many of these agents, recent interest has focused on the "rebound" phenomenon in which daily or almost daily use of symptomatic agents enhances and worsens headache frequency (8, 12, 55). Personal experience suggests that this problem represents the most important single factor contributing to treatment refractoriness in long-standing headache patients, and several reports have documented the importance of this problem (56).

The headache patient who overuses medication presents a special challenge to the clinician, frequently forcing hospitalization to establish meaningful treatment intervention. Although cynicism toward the patient is common, it must be emphasized that patients with legitimate chronic headache syndromes experience years of torment as a result of their unsuccessfully treated disorders. Many awaken each morning and retire each night with pain, and many have sought various medical as well as nonmedical avenues of help, ranging from qualified health care to nonqualified sources promising quick and simple explanations and therapies. Many have turned to symptomatic drugs simply to "get through the day." Marital, employment, and other relationships suffer. The quality of life deteriorates, and, if present, preexisting psychological disturbances are intensified.

In many ways, patients with headache are trapped. If patients resort to excessive analgesics, they come under assault for their "abuse." If they simply "take to bed" or accept their disabling illness by withdrawing from functional status, families, and other activities, they are identified as psychologically impaired, unmotivated, and achieving "secondary gain."

The treatment of patients with medication overuse and headache is difficult and tenuous. Detoxification and removal of the offending agents from the treatment regimen are essential. Patients frequently fear that elimination of analgesics prior to the development of a preventive treatment program will result in their having little in the way of reliable control over headaches, and will thus resist the removal of analgesics prior to efficacious prevention. Ironically, effective prevention is generally not forthcoming until detoxification and removal of analgesics have occurred, thus providing for a classic "catch-22" dilemma. We have found that open communication and instruction on this point, the use of reasonable and flexible timetables, and the use of a comprehensive inpatient treatment setting are the key elements to successful transition from use of analgesics to more acceptable prophylaxis. Psychological as well as physiologic dependency must be confronted, as must the practical considerations regarding the patient's need to remain functional and maintain some limited control over their own painful events. Patients with headache will resist and are frequently frightened of treatment efforts that remove entirely their own ability to manage pain, and cooperative treatment regimens with careful monitoring and instruction appear most effective.

INPATIENT UNITS

In 1979, this author and associates established the first inpatient program directed to the treatment of headache. Over the course of the past few years, several other units have developed. The patient treatment program provides a comprehensive intervention that includes detoxification from overuse of symptomatic medications, aggressive pharmacotherapy, milieu treatment, dietary manipulation, identification and restriction from aggravating influences, psychological and family intervention, and educational programs. Chronic illnesses such as headache frequently require this degree of intervention for treatment success. Recently, this inpatient unit has been awarded national accreditation from the Commission on Accreditation of Rehabilitation Facilities (CARF). This marks the first inpatient pain unit directed at headache management to achieve accreditation status, and initiates the establishment of standards for units treating headache.

FINAL THOUGHTS

Headache, like other painful syndromes, is a difficult condition to treat. Nonetheless, it is currently estimated that with proper technique upward of 75% of chronic recurring headache patients can achieve successful control. No universally effective solution to this complicated health problem currently exists. It is clear that most of the pharmacologic agents described in this presentation provide an indirect influence on the mechanism of headache. No therapy, despite its support in treatment studies, can be relied upon to be universally effective or always satisfactory. Indeed, one of the more frustrating phenomena encountered in the treatment of patients with headache is that from patient to patient with this condition, effective treatment requires individual consideration and treatment planning.

Many patients will benefit from programs described above, including the comprehensive and multidisciplinary approaches now available in specialty centers and inpatient units. Headache is a disabling condition, and medical science has not, until recently, begun to address it in a fashion consistent with its widespread impact. However, despite the limitations in our current understanding as well as the historic prejudice directed toward patients with this condition, our current understanding as well as the treatment approaches described above can provide hope and relief for most patients who suffer from these disorders.

Unfortunately, not all patients can be satisfactorily helped. For some, it is because their condition exceeds current knowledge. For others the need to be sick or fear to be well can defeat even the most committed effort. Nevertheless, persistence, patience, and compassion will bring recognizable and satisfying relief for most who suffer from recurring headaches. Although the chronic headache patient is prone to isolation and despair, knowing that someone cares, understands, and is willing to help is mightily useful in chronic, poorly understood illnesses such as headache.

Finally, while the use of multiple medication regimens is to be discouraged under most circumstances, this, like all other aspects of treatment for difficult-to-treat illness, must be considered in perspective. Neurologists commonly employ multiple treatment regimens for the control of Parkinson's disease and epilepsy. Multiple treatment regimens are frequently necessary in the control of hypertension, ischemic heart disease, congestive heart failure, and multisystem disease. That such efforts are sometimes appropriate in the treatment of the most refractory headache patients seems similarly justifiable. Attitudes that infer that similar efforts are excessive or inappropriate for this disabling disorder may be more a reflection of bias than a fair appraisal of treatment need.

References

1. Ad Hoc Committee on Classification of Headache: *Arch Neurol* 6:173–176, 1963.
2. Saper JR: Changing perspective on chronic headache. *Clin J Pain* 2:19–28, 1986.
3. Raskin NH, Appenzeller O: *Headache*. Philadelphia, WB Saunders 1980.
4. Featherstone HJ: Migraine and muscle contraction headaches: a continuum. *Headache* 25:194–198, 1984.
5. Cohen MJ: Psychophysiological studies of headache: is there a similarity between migraine and muscle contraction headache? *Headache* 18:189–196, 1978.
6. Lance JW: *Mechanism and Management of Headache*, ed 4. London, Butterworth Scientific, 1982.
7. Dalessio DJ, Camp WA, Goodell H, Wolff HG: Studies on headache. The mode of action of UML-491 and its relevance to the nature of vascular headache of the migraine type. *Arch Neurol* 4:235 1961.
8. Saper JR: *Headache Disorders: Current Concepts and Treatment Strategies*. Littleton, MA, Wright, PSG, 1983.
9. Dalessio DJ: *Wolff's Headache and Other Head Pain*, ed 4. New York, Oxford University Press, 1980.
10. Olesen J, Lauritzen M, Tfelt-Hansen P, et al: Spreading cerebral oligemia in classical and normal cerebral blood flow in common migraine. *Headache* 22:242–248, 1982.
11. Olesen J, Tfelt-Hansen P, Henricksen L, et al: The common migraine attack may not be initiated by cerebral ischemia. *Lancet* 2:438–440, 1981.
12. Saper JR, Jones JM: Ergotamine tartrate dependency: features and possible mechanisms. *Clin Neuropharmacol* 9:244–256, 1986.
13. Blau JN: Migraine prodrome separated from aura: "complete migraine." *Br Med J* 281:658–660, 1980.
14. Wilkinson M, Blau JN: Are classical and common migraine different entities? *Headache* 25:211–221, 1985.
15. Olesen J: Are classical and common migraine different entities? *Headache* 25:213, 1985.
16. Mathew NT, Stubits E, Nigam M: Transformation of migraine into daily headache: analysis of factors. *Headache* 22:66–68, 1982.
17. Saper JR, Johnson T, VanMeter M: "Mixed headache": a chronic headache complex. A study of 500 patients. *Headache* 23:143, 1983 (abstr).
18. Rall TW, Schliefer LS: Drugs affecting uterine motility. In Goodman LS, Gilman AG (eds): *Pharmacological Basis of Therapeutics*, ed 7. New York, Macmillan, 1985, pp 926–945.
19. Yuil GM, Swinburn WR, Liversedge LA: A double-blind crossover trial of isometheptane mucate compound and ergotamine in migraine. *Br J Clin Prac* 26:76–79, 1972.
20. Saper JR: Non-steroidal anti-inflammatory drugs. *Top Pain Manage* (newsletter) 1(3):9, 1985.

21. Saper JR: Naproxen sodium in the treatment of headache. *Top Pain Manage* (newsletter) 1(6):21–22, 1985.
22. Welch KMA, Ellis EJ, Keenan BA: Successful migraine prophylaxis with naproxen sodium. *Neurology* 35:1304–1310, 1985.
23. Pradalier A, Rancurl G, Dordain C, et al: Acute migraine attack therapy: comparison of naproxen sodium and ergotamine tartrate compound. *Cephalgia* 5:107–113, 1985.
24. Rumore MM, Schlichtine DA: Clinical efficacy of antihistaminics as analgesics. *Pain,* 25:7–22, 1986.
25. Gallagher RM: The emergency treatment of intractable migraine. *Headache* 26:74–75, 1986.
26. Raskin NH: Repetitive intravenous DHE as therapy for migraine. *Neurology* 36:995–997, 1986.
27. Sudilovsky A, Stern M, Mayer JH: Comparative efficacy of nadolol and propranolol in the prophylaxis of migraine. *J Headache* 26:311–312, 1986 (abstr).
28. Fanchamps A: Why do not all beta blockers prevent migraine? (Letter to the Editor). *Headache* 25:61–62, 1985.
29. Nadelmann JW, Phil M, Stevens J, Saper JR: Propranolol in the prophylaxis of migraine. *Headache* 26:175–186, 1986.
30. Meyers JS, Hardenberg J: Clinical effectiveness of calcium entry blockers in the prophylactic treatment of migraine and cluster headache. *Headache* 26:266–277, 1986.
31. Meyer JS, Nancy M, Walker M, et al: Migraine and cluster headache treatment with calcium antagonists supports a vascular pathogenesis. *Headache* 25:358–367, 1985.
32. Solomon GD, Steel JG, Spaccavento LJ: Verapamil prophylaxis of migraine. A double blind placebo-controlled study. *JAMA* 250:2500–2502, 1983.
33. Saper JR: Calcium channel blockers. *Top Pain Manage* (newsletter) 1(2):7, 1985.
34. *AMA Drug Evaluations,* ed 6. New York, American Medical Association, 1986, pp 239–252.
35. Saper JR: Treatment of chronic headaches. In Conn HF (ed): *Conn's Current Therapy.* Philadelphia, WB Saunders, 1983, pp 724–732.
36. White K, Simpson G: Combined MAOI-tricyclic antidepressant treatment: a re-evaluation. *J Clin Psychopharmacol* 1:264–282, 1981.
37. Pare CMB, Halstrom C, Kline M, et al: Will amitriptyline prevent the "cheese" reaction of monoamine oxidase inhibitors? *Lancet* 2:183–186, 1982.
38. Raskin NH, Schwartz RK: Interval therapy of migraine: long term results. *Headache* 20:336–340, 1980.
39. Kudrow L: *Cluster Headache.* New York, Oxford University Press, 1980.
40. Sjaastad O, Dale I: A new ? clinical entity: "chronic paroxysmal hemicrania." *Headache* 14:105–108, 1974.
41. Fogan L: Treatment of cluster headache: a double blind comparison of oxygen vs. air inhalation. *Arch Neurol* 42:362–363, 1985.
42. Saper JR: Cluster headache: diagnosis and treatment. *Pain and Analgesia* (in press).
43. Ekbom K: Lithium in the treatment of chronic cluster headache (editorial). *Headache* 17:39–40, 1977.
44. Mathew NT: Clinical subtypes of cluster headache and responses to lithium therapy. *Headache* 18:26–30, 1978.
45. Caviness VS Jr, O'Brien P: Cluster headache: response to chlorpromazine. *Headache* 20:128–131, 1980.
46. Mathew NT: Indomethacin responsive headache syndromes. *Headache* 21:147–150, 1981.
47. Horton BT, McLean AR, Craig WM: The use of histamine in the treatment of specific types of headache. *Proc Staff Meetings Mayo Clin* 14:247, 1939.
48. Diamond S, Freitag FG, Prager J: Treatment of intractable cluster. *Headache* 26:42–46, 1986.
49. Watson CP, Morley TP, Richards JC, et al: The surgical treatment of chronic cluster headache. *Headache* 23:289–295, 1983.
50. Onofrio BM, Campbell JK: Surgical treatment of chronic cluster headache. *Mayo Clin Proc* 6:537–544, 1986.
51. Mathew NT: Prophylaxis of migraine and mixed headache: a randomized control study. *Headache* 21:105–109, 1981.
52. Stuss DT, Ely P, Heugenholtz H, et al: Subtle neuropsychological deficits in patients with good recovery after closed head injury. *Neurosurgery* 17:41–47, 1985.
53. Boehnert MT, Lovejoy FH: The value of the QRS duration vs. the serum drug level in predicting seizures and ventricular arrhythmias after an acute overdose of tricyclic antidepressants. *N Engl J Med* 313:474–479, 1985.
54. Packard RC, O'Connell P: Medication compliance among headache patients. *Headache* 26:30, 1986 (abstr).
55. Rapoport A: Analgesic rebound. *Top Pain Manage* (newsletter) 1(8):29–32, 1986.
56. Rapoport A, Weeks RE, Sheftell FD, et al: The "analgesic washout period:" a critical variable in the evaluation of headache treatment of efficacy. *Neurology* 36(suppl):100–101, 1986.

chapter 21
Psychological Management of Headache Pain

Anthony Iezzi, M.S.
Henry E. Adams, Ph.D.
Robert N. Pilon, M.D.
Shepard S. Averitt, M.Ed.

Although headaches are usually not a life-threatening health problem, they are a major health problem when considered from an epidemiologic point of view. An estimated 35 million Americans apparently suffer from headaches (1). In terms of the frequency for which individuals seek outpatient medical care, headache was found to be one of the top 14 health problems (2). The social and economic costs of headaches also attest to the debilitating nature of this health problem. According to a recent national survey, the *Nuprin Pain Report*, 7% of a cross-sectional sample reported experiencing headaches at least 100 days or more over a 1-year period (3).

Even though the prevalence and significance of headache pain is readily apparent and the literature is substantial on the etiology and treatment of headache (4–6, 17), headache still remains an enigmatic health problem. The prevailing emphasis of this chapter is on the psychological management of headache pain. However, a brief review of the different headache types and their defining characteristics, the pathophysiology and etiology of the different headache types, and the assessment of headache is initially presented. The successful management of chronic headache is very dependent on a thorough assessment and accurate diagnosis of headache type and an understanding of the pathophysiology and etiology of headache type.

HEADACHE TYPES AND DEFINING CHARACTERISTICS

No useful information about etiology, mechanisms of pain, or treatment outcome can be generated without an adequate headache classification scheme. In 1960, the National Institute of Neurological Disease and Blindness formed the Ad Hoc Committee on the Classification of Headache (8). The Ad Hoc Committee outlined 15 types of headache that were commonly encountered in clinical practice. Although some controversy on the validity and the reliability of the committee's classification scheme has recently emerged (9), the classification scheme continues to be useful and helpful in guiding the differential diagnosis. Only four headache types are discussed here: (*a*) migraine; (*b*) muscle contraction; (*c*) combined vascular and muscle contraction; and (*d*) headache of delusional, conversion, or hypochondriacal states. These four headache types are discussed because they are seen most frequently in the clinical context and because psychological factors have been implicated in their etiology, exacerbation, and maintenance.

MIGRAINE HEADACHE

The following description of migraine headache is taken from the classification scheme proposed by the Ad Hoc Committee (8):

> Recurrent attacks of headache, widely varied in intensity, frequency, and duration. The attacks are commonly unilateral in onset; are usually associated with anorexia and, sometimes, with nausea and vomiting; in some are preceded by, or associated with, conspicuous sensory, motor, and mood disturbances; and are often familial. (p 378)

A migraine headache episode may occur at any time of the day, but is common upon awakening. Frequency of migraine headache can vary from several times per week to several times per year. Duration of an episode is usually from 30 min to several hours, but migraine can occur for several days at a time. A fully developed migraine episode will usually interfere with a patient's regular, daily activities.

Although the term *migraine* has often been used by the lay public as if it referred to a stereotypic pain phenomenon, migraine headache patients are really a heterogeneous group. The migraine headache category can be further divided into five subtypes (8): (*a*) classic migraine—sharply defined headache with sensory and/or motor prodromes; (*b*) common migraine—similar to classic migraine except without a clear-cut prodrome or aura; (*c*) cluster headache—unexpected bouts of severe headaches, usually in clusters of two or three 20–90-min headache episodes over several days; (*d*) hemiplegic and opthalmoplegic migraine—vascular headache with strong sensory and motor phenomena that persist during and after the headache; and (*e*) lower-half headache—headache centered primarily in the lower face. Of patients who report migraine, 85% tend to experience common migraine and 10% tend to experience classic migraine (10).

The pathophysiology of migraine headache involves the cranial and cerebral vascular systems and most likely involves the autonomic nervous system in some fashion (6, 7). The generally accepted pathophysiologic model of migraine, as suggested by Wolff (6), consists of a two-phase process. During the first phase, vasoconstriction of the cranial and cerebral arteries, with a subsequent reduction in blood supply to the brain, occurs. This initial phase is then followed by a vasodilation of cranial and cerebral arteries, including extracranial or scalp arteries. There then follows an inflamation of the arterial walls, vascular edema, and release of various local chemical and vasoactive substances. Actual head pain is believed to covary with the dilation of the extracranial arteries.

Although the pathophysiologic model of migraine headache has been fairly well established, the etiology remains somewhat equivocal. Exactly what initiates the two-phase pathophysiologic process is not known. Psychological (e.g., migraine personality), environmental (e.g., stress), neurovascular (e.g., platelet aggregation and amines), and hormonal (e.g., estrogen and progesterone) factors have been implicated in the etiology of migraine (4, 6, 7). It is unlikely that any one of these factors is singularly responsible or can account for the heterogeneity of migraine headache.

MUSCLE CONTRACTION HEADACHE

Muscle contraction headache, also known as tension headache, results from sustained contraction of the muscles of the shoulders, neck, and scalp (8). A description of sensation of tightness or pressure in a "hat band" distribution is commonly reported with this type of headache. Duration of a muscle contraction headache episode ranges from a few hours to several weeks, with varying degrees of intensity but usually not interfering with routine activities. Muscle contraction head pain is usually located bilaterally and described as a dull ache (as opposed to the commonly reported sensation of throbbing in migraine headache). Patients will usually report a worsening of head pain as the day progresses. Clearly defined prodromes in patients with muscle contraction headache are not common. The prevalence of muscle contraction headache varies, but it has been reported that as many as 80% of individuals experiencing headaches suffer from muscle contraction headaches (11).

As mentioned earlier, the pathophysiology of muscle contraction headache involves sustained elevations of muscle activity in several muscle groups of the head, face, and neck. These elevations in muscle activity are thought to occur in the absence of permanent structural change (8). Vascular changes have also been implicated in the pathophysiology of muscle contraction headache, but studies examining vascular changes have provided conflicting results (12). As is the case with migraine headache, exactly what initiates the pathophysiologic process of muscle contraction headache is unclear. Friedman (8) indicated that muscle contraction headache was due to an individual's reaction to life stress. Personality style and emotional lability have also been thought to be involved in the etiology of muscle contraction headache (13); however, this contention has met with little empirical support.

COMBINED VASCULAR AND MUSCLE CONTRACTION HEADACHE

Combined vascular and muscle contraction headache (also referred to in the headache literature as *mixed* headache) is characterized by the expression of vascular and muscular symptoms (8). Adams et al. (14) suggested that it may be more meaningful to think of patients with combined vascular and muscle contraction headache as individuals suffering from the two types of head pain independently. Very little is really known about this headache category because it has received little empirical study until recently. As one might expect, the pathophysiology and etiology of combined vascular and muscle contraction headache involve a combination of vascular and muscle changes, as discussed earlier.

HEADACHE OF DELUSIONAL, CONVERSION, OR HYPOCHONDRIACAL STATES

The Ad Hoc Committee defined headache of delusional, conversion, or hypochondriacal states as follows (8):

> Headaches of illnesses in which the prevailing clinical disorder is a delusional or a conversion reaction and a peripheral pain mechanism is nonexistent. Closely allied are the hypochondriacal reactions in which the peripheral disturbances relevant to headache are minimal. These also have been called "psychogenic" headaches. (p 379)

The term *psychogenic headache* will be used in place of headache of delusional, conversion, or hypochondriacal states for reasons of convenience, but also because psychogenic headache is similar to the pain disorder described in the *Diagnostic and Statistical Manual (DSM-III)* (15) as "psychogenic pain disorder."

A psychogenic headache tends to be relatively continuous in occurrence, with a waxing and waning quality; is often described as a dull pain; and is located frontally and posteriorly, although on occasion some patients report "it hurts all over my head, neck, and face." It is not unusual for patients to state that their pain travels; that is, the pain moves from one area of the head to another and often in a fashion that is not consistent with an anatomic distribution. Associated symptoms commonly include anxiety and depression (16, 17). The prevalence of psychogenic headache is unknown, but is probably much more frequent than most clinicians have acknowledged. This lack of recognition may have contributed to the confusing nature of the muscle contraction headache literature.

Given the definition of psychogenic headache, there is no pathophysiologic process that can adequately explain psychogenic headache. Although there appears to be an absence of a pathophysiologic process, the etiology of headache very likely involves the role of social learning and psychological factors (18). Through the environment, pain behavior is positively reinforced and "well" behavior is inadequately reinforced. Therefore, psychogenic headache can be viewed as a pain disorder reinforced by its consequences without the known peripheral pain mechanisms that are typical of migraine or muscle contraction headaches. The possible mechanism in the acquisition of psychogenic headache probably involves inappropriate positive reinforcement, modeling (e.g., family members who have headaches or other types of chronic pain), and/or avoidance conditioning (e.g., getting out of doing something aversive, such as school or work, by using pain). Although these etiologic hypotheses appear reasonable, ony further empirical research will determine their value and utility.

ASSESSMENT

Appropriate psychological management of headache pain is very much dependent on a thorough assessment. Table 21.1 presents a tripartite assessment model of head pain that has been used consistently for clinical and research purposes (14). The reader should find the table helpful in proceeding through this section on assessment.

A differential diagnosis of headache type involves the elimination of alternative medical (physical and physiologic) and psychological explanations of head pain. A comprehensive assessment requires collecting information from several sources (19): (a) an adequate medical examination, (b) a thorough interview with headache patient and significant other, (c) self-monitoring of head pain, and (d) performing a psychophysiologic assessment of the patient in headache and nonheadache states. A brief review of each assessment area is presented.

MEDICAL EXAMINATION

No treatment should ever be started on a headache patient who has not undergone a medical and neurologic workup. Although organic causes of headaches are somewhat uncommon, psychological treatment of a headache patient with an organic disorder would be ineffective, to say the least, and the consequences of choosing an inappropriate intervention can be very serious. The medical diagnosis of headache type is made on the basis of behavioral symptoms and positive/negative findings on a series of medical tests (20). A physical examination involves an evaluation of blood pressure, eye function, cranial nerve function, and general sensory and motor function. Also included in a thorough medical examination, if indicated, is the use of laboratory studies (e.g., blood and urine analysis, skull x-rays, computed tomography scan, angiogram, and electroencephalogram). Even when psychological intervention of headache is initiated, a careful record of symptoms and results should be monitored; if any unusual or unexpected symptoms are observed and do not fit the case formulation, then consultation with the referring physician is strongly recommended.

INITIAL INTERVIEW

Interview information obtained from a headache patient allows the clinician to make a correct diagnosis, to target psychological adjuncts to headache, establish rapport, and tailor a systematic treatment plan (19). Typically, a headache interview lasts anywhere from 1 to 1 1/2 hr and is usually conducted upon the initial visit. The critical areas to be covered in the interview include a detailed history of head pain, family history of head pain and other chronic pain disorders, possible treatments (medical and psycho-

Table 21.1
Tripartite Assessment of Head Pain[a]

Headache Type	Subjective	Behavioral	Physiologic
Migraine	Usually unilateral onset	Emergency room treatment	Cephalic vascular lability in headache and nonheadache states
	Prodomes	Bed rest required	
	Nausea	Avoidance of sound and light	
	Pulsating, throbbing pain	Vomiting and other signs of ANS distress	Response to vasoconstrictive and potent analgesic or sedative drugs
Muscle contraction	Dull, aching headband or neck pain	Only rarely requires cessation of ongoing activities or bed rest	Elevated muscle tension in facial and neck areas during headache episode and/or nonheadache states
	Pain attacks less severe; soreness of scalp and neck muscles	Pain elicited in stressful situations	Often responsive to mild analgesics
Conversion	Pain report typically not fitting pattern of migraine or muscle contraction	Presence of secondary gain (reinforcement)	Lack of physiologic basis for pain (e.g., no elevated EMG or vasomotor disorders)
	Iatrogenic effects	Presence of an initial precipitating event	
Combined	Characteristics of both muscle contraction and migraine, either coexisting in same attack or occurring in separate attacks	Disability as a function of type of headache	Physiology may vary as a function of type of pain
			When both types exist in same attack, physiologic changes may involve vascular and musculoskeletal components

[a] From Adams HE, Brantley PJ, Thompson K: Biofeedback and headache: methodological issues. In White L, Tursky B (eds): *Clinical Biofeedback: Efficacy and Mechanisms.* New York, Guilford Press, 1982, p 360.

logical) received for head pain and their success, an evaluation of the patient's psychological adjustment in order to construct a functional analysis of head pain and other psychological difficulties that may be present, and an evaluation of the reasons for seeking treatment.

An area often neglected in the interview process is the report of observations provided by significant others. Significant others can often provide useful information about the patient's pain behavior (e.g., localizing a patient's environmental stress, providing a check on the patient's self-report of head pain). Interviewing significant others will help establish rapport with them, which will also increase the probability of getting them to assist with the patient's treatment plan, and thereby increasing the possibility of positive therapeutic outcome.

A headache questionnaire can be administered to speed up the interview process. The critical areas assessed in a headache questionnaire are demographic information, headache history, current status and symptomatology of headache, and location of head pain. In addition, circumstances surrounding the onset of headache, modeling influences, and the antecedents and consequences of headache are vital data. A headache questionnaire is useful in that it saves some of the clinician's therapy time, it is easy for the patient to complete, and provides information that is more reliable than verbal report.

SELF-MONITORING

Self-monitoring or diary-keeping is a valuable component to the assessment and management of headache. On a daily basis, the patient is required to write the occurrence, intensity, degree of disability, duration, location, and associated symptoms of headache. Moreover, the type and amount of medications taken and other pain relief strategies used are reported. Possible triggers, stressors, or mood states that may be associated with the patient's headaches are also noted. The patient is usually required to keep a diary for 1 month before treatment, throughout the whole treatment process, and during follow-up. It is our experience that patients are very compliant with self-monitoring; in fact, if the patient has problems with diary-keeping, then the patient is likely to neglect other aspects of treatment.

There are several advantages to using a headache diary. The data obtained from the patient are more objective and reliable than global self-report. Diary-keeping facilitates the establishment of baseline levels of headache parameters and assesses for treatment effectiveness. Finally, functional relationship between antecedents and consequences of headache can be analyzed.

PSYCHOPHYSIOLOGY

The psychophysiologic evaluation is increasingly being used in the assessment and management of headache. This procedure essentially involves multichannel recording of multiple physiologic response systems. More specifically, physiologic activity (e.g., frontalis, trapezius, and splenius capitus electromyography, forehead and finger skin temperature, and cephalic blood-volume pulse) are assessed during baseline and in response to stress (e.g., "think of a typical day at work"). The most important aspect of the physiologic assessment is that the patient come in for an evaluation during nonheadache and headache states (two 1-hr sessions). As outlined in Table 21.1, this is the only way to differentiate some headache types. The clinician can also observe the behavioral presentation of the patient in these two states. For example, a migraine headache patient in a headache state will often exhibit obvious tearing of eyes, temporal artery distention, and pallor, whereas a muscle contraction headache patient should exhibit stiffness of movement, muscle tightness, and squinting or frowning expression.

SUMMARY

In sum, the essential point of an adequate assessment and understanding of relevant factors associated with head pain will yield information pertaining to the most logical and appropriate choice for the psychological intervention of headache pain.

PSYCHOLOGICAL MANAGEMENT OF HEADACHE PAIN

To date, there is no truly adequate treatment of chronic headache. Thus, "management" of headache is more accurate than "treatment" of headache, but as in the headache literature, in this chapter the two terms will be used interchangeably. Before discussing the different management strategies of headache, it should be pointed out that the clinician's choice of a particular intervention for a particular headache type needs to be made along several dimensions (21): (a) efficacy—Does treatment achieve the desired results? (b) relative efficacy—Is one treatment better than another? (c) generality—What proportion of a patient sample is able to derive benefit from treatment? (d) relative efficiency—Which treatment works faster? (e) convenience—What treatment is easier to give and which is easier for the patient? and (f) cost. Since many different treatment strategies seem to be equally effective in the treatment of headache, then it becomes important to consider the cost-effectiveness of a particular intervention.

Psychological management of headache pain has included a divergent range of approaches, including insight-oriented therapy, modification of pain perception, self-relaxation, desensitization to or modification of stressful environment, assertiveness training, control of peripheral hand temperature, self-regulation of temporal artery, and reduction of tonic and phasic levels of muscle activity. For our purposes, headache intervention strategies can be classified into three major groups: relaxation training, biofeedback training, and cognitive techniques. Even though there is not enough literature to warrant the categorization of operant pain control techniques as a major treatment approach of headache, these techniques are also reviewed. The following sections discuss each treatment approach, giving a description of procedure and appropriateness of procedure for headache type. It is beyond the scope of this chapter to provide a detailed review of the headache treatment literature; therefore, discussion of a few studies for illustration purposes are presented as necessary.

RELAXATION TRAINING

There are various forms of relaxation training, and the most commonly used technique is progressive muscular relaxation. This approach was originally developed by Jacobsen (22) and was popularized more recently by Bernstein and Borkovec (23). The rationale of this procedure involves the reduction of tonic states of muscular activity, learning to identify subtle differences in muscular tension, and a reduction of an overly active sympathetic nervous system. The ability to elicit the state of relaxation is ultimately implemented as an active skill to cope with situations that may trigger a stress response.

Relaxation training requires the individual to alternatively tense and relax a number of muscle groups throughout the whole body. The training sequence involves approximately 10 1-hr sessions. An individual's training progresses in turn from 16 muscle groups to 8 muscle groups to 4 muscle groups to 4 muscle groups through recall (no actual tensing, i.e., relaxation by remembering what it felt like when the muscle group had been previously relaxed), and cue-controlled relaxation (relaxation through recall and by counting backward from 10 to 1). Although the actual procedure becomes shorter as the training sequence progresses, by the end of the treatment regimen, the individual should be able to elicit a state of physical and mental relaxation that is equivalent to that achieved by practicing relaxation with 16 muscle groups. Twice-daily practice at home is recommended to the individual and is assisted by having the individual listen to audiotaped versions of the training sessions.

Another variation of relaxation, which is similar to transcendental meditation, was proposed by Benson (24). He advocated a passive relaxation response where the individual is required to sit quietly and to repeat "one" as a form of mantra. No actual tensing of muscles even occurs with this approach. The elicitation of the passive relaxation response is believed to result in physiologic changes that are thought to reflect an integrated hypothalamic response. Finally, Schultz and Luthe (25) proposed a passive suggestive type of relaxation using visual and auditory aids (e.g., beach scene) to induce mental, emotional, and somatic relaxation. This form of relaxation has come to be known as autogenic training.

Although relaxation training has been used to treat migraine, combined vascular and muscle contraction, and muscle contraction headache, the most appropriate target headache population for this form of treatment should be muscle contraction. Discussion regarding the efficacy and cost-effectiveness of relaxation training is deferred to the next section on biofeedback because of the considerable treatment literature comparing relaxation training and biofeedback.

BIOFEEDBACK TRAINING

Biofeedback training is an approach that involves the individual in a continuous interchange with a physiologic monitoring device (e.g., polygraph). The end goal of physiologic monitoring is the self-regulation of a target physiologic state that often results in an improved psychological state. More specifically, during biofeedback training the individual is provided with information about physiologic activity via an auditory signal or visual display that is proportional to the change in physiologic activity. The individual's task is to modify the target response in the desired direction, usually in a trial-and-error manner. Success in modifying a target response is indicated by the feedback provided (e.g., a decrease in the loudness of a tone). Clinicians will also often use cognitive aids (e.g., various mental images and blanking the mind) to achieve the desired physiologic change. The ultimate goal of biofeedback is to teach the individual to achieve the desired physiologic response without the aid of a feedback apparatus (i.e., voluntary control).

Several biofeedback training techniques have been used with headache patients. Biofeedback training techniques can essentially be grouped into three different forms: (a) electromyographic (EMG) biofeedback, (b) thermal biofeedback, and (c) cephalic vasomotor feedback. Electromyographic biofeedback came about through the pioneering work of Budzinski and coworkers (26). Basically, they attached three surface electrodes equidistant from each other on the midline of the forehead. In their original study, true feedback of frontalis muscle EMG in 15 subjects led to greater decreases in muscle activity than did pseudofeedback. This procedure was then applied to the treatment of muscle contraction headache subjects with substantial success (27). The rationale of EMG biofeedback is similar to that of relaxation training; EMG biofeedback is aimed at reducing elevated levels of muscle tension and at reducing sympathetic nervous system activity, albeit indirectly.

Thermal biofeedback consists of attaching a temperature-sensitive thermistor to a finger and requiring an individual to increase his finger temperature. Although skin temperature is an indirect measure of peripheral blood volume, the rationale for this procedure is that an increased peripheral blood flow (i.e., peripheral hand vasodilation) is associated with decreased sympathetic tone and increased relaxation. In addition, it is assumed that by increasing blood flow to the periphery, blood flow to the extracranial vasculature will be decreased (this treatment approach was originally designed to treat migraine headache). Clinical research work with thermal biofeedback was made popular by the Menninger Foundation Clinic (28, 29). With thermal biofeedback, these authors also included autogenic training (i.e., during thermal biofeedback training the individual repeats phrases such as: "I feel quite relaxed.", "I feel quiet.", "My arms and hands are heavy."). Of 62 patients, 74% of migraine headache suffers were considered "improved" in their original study (28).

Cephalic vasomotor response feedback requires the placement of a photoelectric transducer on the extracranial artery (usually the zygomaticofacial branch). The aim of cephalic vasomotor response feedback is to teach the patient to reduce the tonic pain associated with excessively high blood volume via the reduction of pulse amplitude. In other words, the patient is taught to constrict his temporal artery so as to avoid vasodilation and the associated pain that is concomitant with it. Although the first investigation on the utility of cephalic vasomotor feedback was not focused on the treatment of headaches per se, Koppman et al. (3) conducted an investigation examining whether patients who suffered from migraine headache could learn to control the temporal artery pulse with the aid of biofeedback. Of 9 patients who participated in 9–12 sessions (twice during each session), 7 patients were able to reliably demonstrate "bidirectional" control of temporal artery blood flow, thus indicating that the subjects had learned to control their temporal artery pulse.

As with the development of any new therapy, initial enthusiastic claims from the biofeedback literature subsequently were tempered by more realistic and cautious expectations. Many of the enthusiastic claims were based on anecdotal case reports, uncontrolled group studies, and studies with major methodologic flaws (accurate definition of headache type omitted, biased representativeness of samples used, poor outcome measures, etc.). Despite the plethora of problems in the headache literature, some statements about the treatment of headache can be made.

Much of what is known about the efficacy of headache treatment has been provided by the work of Blanchard and his associates (5, 31). Blanchard and his associates (31) used "meta-analysis" to evaluate treatment effect across research studies. In meta-analysis, mean changes in headache measures across research studies form the unit of analysis. An average percentage of improvement in headache density (product of intensity and duration of headache pain) from baseline was calculated. Only treatment studies with five or more subjects per group were included in the meta-analysis. Although the authors pointed to the consistency of results across studies as evidence for the reproducibility of their general findings, the authors also acknowledged that the utility of meta-analysis is somewhat compromised by the different dependent measures, sample sizes, treatment protocols, and methodologic quality of underlying studies. Many of the evaluative statements of the headache treatment outcome literature presented are based on the work of Blanchard and his associates.

The muscle contraction headache literature indicates that relaxation training and frontal EMG biofeedback appear to be equally efficacious (5). The average percentage of improvement in muscle contraction headache patients treated with relaxation training (nine studies) and frontal EMG biofeedback (12 studies) was 59.2% and 60.9%, respectively. Interestingly, the combination of relaxation training and frontal EMG biofeedback resulted in an average percentage of improvement of 58.8% (six studies); therefore, combining the two treatment approaches for muscle contraction headache did not lead to improved treatment outcome.

At this point in time, it is worth repeating the criteria in choosing the best treatment for a particular headache type. If relaxation training and frontal EMG biofeedback appears to be equally efficacious (i.e., which treatment works best) and equally generalizable (i.e., what proportion of a patient sample achieves significant benefit from treatment), then the choice of treatment for muscle contraction headache should be determined by the relative efficiency (i.e., which treatment works faster), convenience (i.e., which treatment is easier to administer and which is easier for the patient), and cost. Based on the literature and our own experience, the treatment of choice for muscle contraction headache is relaxation training. The results of a recent investigation suggested that muscle contraction headache patients should initially be treated with relaxation training, and those who do not improve should proceed sequentially with frontal EMG biofeedback (32). This appears to be an apropriate recommendation; however, if the patient also fails to derive any benefit from frontal EMG biofeedback, then the clinician should reconsider the case formulation and reevaluation for psychogenic headache, which would require treatment with operant pain control techniques. In another study, Teders and his coworkers (33) evaluated the comparative efficacy and cost-effectiveness of relaxation training for muscle contraction headache using a therapist-delivered relaxation treatment versus a procedure with minimal therapist-patient contact and based chiefly at home. Both procedures were highly effective and were equivalent in reducing headache complaints as assessed by measures of headache index, intensity, frequency, and medication consumption. Obviously, the minimal contact, home-based treatment was found to be more cost-effective when relating total amount of therapist contact to headache improvement. The home-based relaxation package appears promising for the treatment of muscle contraction headache, and further research with this approach is needed.

The number of studies investigating the treatment of migraine headache with relaxation training is relatively small (seven studies; ref. 5). Depending on which study one considers, relaxation training appears to be either ineffective or beneficial, but overall, across seven studies, the average rate of improvement was 47.9%, which was not significantly different from combined thermal biofeedback and autogenic training (64.9%; ref. 5). As far as combined vascular and muscle contraction headache, one study obtained a 22% average improvement rate when using relaxation training alone (32). However, when relaxation training was combined with thermal biofeedback, the overall improvement rate rose to 54%. One other study worth mentioning examined the utility of group relaxation training (34). The authors of this investigation found that 70% of 98 cases improved using this treatment approach. Two major weaknesses in this study were noted; the lack of a control group and the lack of any follow-up data. Although the relatively high success rate of this study is impressive and appears promising, it is interesting that this study has apparently not been followed up with another investigation. It would appear at this time that relaxation training is cost-effective in the treatment of a substantial number of migraine headache patients (probably best for the common migraine headache), and surely for those patients for whom it is not found to be helpful, there are other interventions that can be helpful.

Thermal biofeedback has been used rather extensively to manage migraine and combined vascular and muscle contraction headache. Thermal biofeedback alone does not appear to be helpful for either migraine or combined vascular and muscle contraction headache. The rate of improvement with thermal biofeedback (34.6%; seven studies) alone was significantly better than headache-monitoring alone (17.2%; six studies) and slightly but nonsignificantly better than psychological placebo (27.6%; five studies; ref. 5). Although Blanchard and Andrasik (5) concluded that thermal biofeedback combined with autogenic training and thermal biofeedback combined with relaxation training are the treatments of choice for migraine and for combined vascular and muscle contraction headache, respectively, other authors have questioned the utility and the mechanism of action in thermal biofeedback (35–37).

The use of cephalic vasomotor biofeedback in the treatment of migraine and combined vascular and muscle contraction headache has been found to be effective. Friar and Beatty (38) evaluated the therapeutic effects of eight sessions of cephalic vasomotor biofeedback training as compared to an attention control group. Post-training results indicated that the cephalic vasomotor biofeedback group demonstrated constriction of the extracranial arteries during a voluntary control assessment, whereas the attention-control group did not evidence vasoconstriction of the temporal artery. A significant reduction in the number of major headache attacks (over 3 hr) and total number of headaches per month in the treatment group was noted. Cephalic vasomotor biofeedback was also found to be superior to frontalis EMG feedback in reducing headache activity and medication intake in migraine headache patients (39). A number of experimental single-case studies evaluating cephalic vasomotor biofeedback have also been reported and indicate the clinical utility of this approach (40–42). Overall, the average rate of improvement in patients receiving cephalic vasomotor biofeedback was 42.3% (based on four studies), which was equal to relaxation training alone, thermal biofeedback alone, and psychological placebo, but significantly lower than thermal biofeedback combined with autogenic training (5). Which treatment of choice appears to be the best for migraine is uncertain. It would appear from a cost-effectiveness point of view that relaxation training should be the initial choice of treatment for migraine headache and any patient not improving should proceed to thermal biofeedback combined with autogenic training or cephalic vasomotor biofeedback. Although cephalic vasomotor biofeedback appears useful, one needs to consider that this kind of biofeedback training requires specialized equipment and a methodologic procedure that is still at the research state. In addition, for some migraine patients, voluntary control of the temporal artery may require an inordinate amount of training sessions (50–60; ref. 14).

COGNITIVE TECHNIQUES

The use of cognitive techniques in the treatment of headache is a fairly recent development. Much of the cognitive approach to treating headache borrows from the original work of Beck (43), Goldfried et al. (44), and Meichenbaum (45). Cognitive techniques have a much expanded focus and are aimed at providing the patient with a general set of problem-solving or coping skills that will be used with a wide range of situations or stressors that can give rise to headaches. The rationale for this type of treatment emphasizes that disturbed emotional and behavioral responses are a direct function of specific maladaptive cognitions (e.g., the belief that one should be a perfect manager or parent). A patient is encouraged to attribute the cause of his/her headaches to relatively specific cognitive aberrations rather than to external stimuli or complex inner dispositions. The therapist and patient focus on identifying cues that target tension and anxiety, how the patient responds when anxious, the patient's thoughts prior to becoming aware of tension, and how cognitions contribute to the patient's stress, tension, and emotional distress.

In reviewing the literature, it is difficult to evaluate studies using cognitive techniques because of the diversity in their approaches. Combinations of frontal and differential relaxation, self-desensitization, thought stopping, rational thinking, experiential focusing and flooding, cognitive reappraisal, and others have been used. With this comment in mind, the first controlled evaluation of cognitive therapy for headache was conduced by Holroyd et al. (46). Thirty-one muscle contraction headache subjects were randomly assigned to a waiting list control group, frontal EMG biofeedback, or cognitive stress coping training. Holroyd et al.'s treatment consisted of teaching subjects to identify and subsequently modify maladaptive cognitive responses assumed to mediate headache. When subjects were able to reliably identify their antecedent and consequent cognitions, subjects were then taught to use cognitive reappraisal, attention deployment, and fantasy as a way of modifying their cognitions. Results indicated that subjects receiving cognitive therapy evidenced significantly greater reduction in headache activity (89% improvement rate), which was also maintained at a 2-year follow-up (47).

Knapp and Florin (48) assigned 20 long-term migraine patients to one of four training conditions: (a) 10 sessions of cephalic vasomotor biofeedback, (b) 5 sessions of cephalic vasomotor biofeedback and 5 sessions of cognitive stress coping training, (c) 10 sessions of cognitive stress coping training, and (d) 5 sessions of cognitive stress coping training and 5 sessions of cephalic vasomotor biofeedback. The study also included a waiting list control group. The results indicated that all four treatment groups did equally well. In another study (49), migraine, muscle contraction, and combined vascular and muscle contraction headache groups received a cognitive-behavioral package (which was mostly based on Meichenbaum's work; see ref. 45). The results indicated that treatment gains were similar across all diagnostic groups. Finally, a more recent investigation compared home-based relaxation training alone, home-based cognitive stress coping training plus relaxation, and office-based cognitive stress coping training and relaxation (50). All three groups were equally effective and no significant differences in cost-effectiveness were noted.

Although it is still early, the use of cognitive techniques appears promising in the treatment of all headache types except for psychogenic headache. Cognitive techniques seem to be equally efficacious in the treatment of headache when compared to other treatment modalities.

OPERANT PAIN-CONTROL TECHNIQUES

Although operant pain-control techniques have frequently been used to treat chronic pain disorders (e.g., low back pain), they have received little attention in the headache literature. Operant pain control techniques are based on suggestions by Fordyce (18). Essentially, pain is an experience that is influenced by physical and psychological factors. As remarked by Fordyce, the issue is not whether the pain is real or organic but what factors are influencing pain. Although pain is a physiologic process, it can be controlled and maintained by learning factors. Therefore, if learning factors can influence the frequency, severity, and duration of pain, then it may be possible to extinguish learned components of pain, in this case, headache.

Following a functional analysis of headache and other pain behaviors, a clinician devises a pain control program and a behavioral contract (structured and formalized treatment goals and how to go about achieving them) is designed. The contract contains the following operant methods: (a) extinction procedures—the patient and significant other (S) will respond to pain behaviors with a neutral attitude; (b) reinforcement of nonpain behaviors—nonpain behaviors are to be reinforced with positive activities such as special meals, recreation, attention from significant others (S), and so on; (c) reinforcement of competing responses during pain behavior—patient will be encouraged to continue with ongoing activities even in the presence of pain; and (d) therapist reinforcement—therapist interaction is contingent on the decrease of pain behavior.

As of yet there are no control group outcome studies using operant pain-control techniques with headache. However, for illustration purposes, a case that was treated in our laboratory is presented (51). A 26-year-old female with a 13-year history of classic migraine headache was referred following hospitalization with severe head pain. Behavior assessment and analysis revealed that she received inordinant amounts of parental, social, and professional attention, as well as avoidance of school and work. The various treatments received by her included medication, acupuncture, chiropractic manipulation, psychotherapy, and even electroconvulsive shock. Following several trials of cephalic vasomotor feedback training, she was able to experience a decrease in headache, but treatment gains were lost following termination of each treatment program.

Self-monitoring data indicated that her headaches occurred five to seven times per week, lasted 8–12 hr per day, and were severely disabling. She avoided housework, meal preparation, working at her job as an L.P.N., socializing, and sexual activity. Domestic duties were completed by her parents and husband. Medications included, among others, as-needed injections of Demerol. Monitoring of the patient's pain behavior included verbal complaints, going to bed, cold compresses on her head, medication abuse, excuses from social obligations, and emergency room visits.

Her treatment consisted of having all the significant others completely ignore her pain behaviors, providing appropriate reinforcers by significant others for well behaviors, behavioral contracting that explicitly stated the above contingencies and expectations, with the cooperation of her physician and the patient's understanding that under no circumstances could she receive an injection of Demerol, muscle relaxation training as a procedure to handle daily stress or pain, and assertiveness training.

One month following treatment, the mean number of her daily pain behaviors went from 8 to below 1. Treatment results in the patient returning to work as an L.P.N. on a volunteer basis, maintaining an "A" average in a practical nursing program, walking 2 miles per day, and having been off all pain medication for slightly over a year. A 12-month follow-up, the client reported two headaches over the previous several months and her husband had reported that their marital and sexual relationship had greately improved. The results of this case study indicate the role of learning in migraine headache. This treatment approach has also been successfully used in the treatment of psychogenic headache in our laboratory. [For an excellent, detailed discussion on how to treat a psychogenic headache case, see Adams (52).] Obviously, it is too early to determine the efficacy of this treatment approach, but it does appear promising.

SUMMARY

To summarize the headache treatment literature, there is no treatment that is clearly more efficacious than another for any particular headache type. Relaxation training appears to be the most cost-effective treatment for headache. Home-based treatment also appears promising. If relaxation training does not work, there are certainly a number of viable management options. Frontal EMG biofeedback can be used in the treatment of muscle contraction headache, and migraine and combined vascular and muscle contraction headache can be further treated with combined thermal biofeedback and autogenic training and cephalic vasomotor biofeedback. Cognitive techniques also appear useful in the treatment of muscle contraction headache. In addition, the use of operant pain-control techniques appears to be beneficial in treating some migraine headache patients and surely is appropriate for psychogenic headache.

ISSUES IN THE PSYCHOLOGICAL MANAGEMENT OF HEADACHE PAIN

Despite the number of studies on the management of headache and that a substantial number of headache patients improve following psychological treatment, there are several issues that need to be addressed in the treatment literature. There is still little systematic research on predicting who responds to these treatments and who is more likely to relapse. Diamond and coworkers (53) conducted a 5-year retrospective study to examine the long-term effects of biofeedback (combined thermal and autogenic-training and frontal EMG biofeedback) on headache, and their results indicated that biofeedback training was significantly more effective in patients under age 18, patients of the female gender, and patients with no drug habituation problems; this is certainly not a representative example of most headache patients seen in clinical practice. More research is needed to elucidate these variables so that treatment could become more cost-effective.

Although biofeedback has received the most attention in the treatment literature, the clinical efficacy of biofeedback depends on the ability of the patient to demonstrate voluntary control (the ability to demonstrate bidirectional control of a physiologic response system). Clinicians usually include a voluntary control phase (e.g., patient is told to constrict his temporal artery) in their treatment, but very few studies ever evaluate or demonstrate true voluntary control. If no voluntary control can be demonstrated, then probably biofeedback at best has a nonspecific or placebo effect that has little to do with the hypothesized pain mechanisms of headache. Obviously, more research work investigating this issue of voluntary control is needed.

The treatment of headache will also become more successful as more is known about the mechanisms of headache pain and associated etiologic factors, which brings us back to the observation that the successful outcome of headache treatment is highly dependent upon the thorough assessment and accurate diagnosis of headache. More attention needs to be paid to providing clear descriptions and definitions of headache. The criteria to be used must also undergo tests of validity and reliability. The nature and the parameters of the intervention strategies used also need to be more clearly specified. The statement "more research of a controlled outcome nature is needed" is a cliche but very applicable to the headache treatment literature. Only with controlled outcome research will we be able to more clearly and effectively determine which are the treatments of choice for particular headache types.

References

1. Bonica JJ: Pain research and therapy: past and current status and future needs. In Ng L, Bonica JJ (eds): *Pain, Discomfort, and Humanitarian Care.* New York, Elsevier, 1980, p 1.
2. DeLozier JE, Gagnon RO: *National Ambulatory Medical Care Survey: 1973 Summary, United States, May 1973–April 1974* (DHEW Publication No. HRA 79-1772). Washington, DC, U.S. Government Printing Office, 1975.
3. Taylor H, Curran NM: *The Nuprin Pain Report.* New York, Louis Harris, 1985, p 233.
4. Adams HE, Feurstein M, Fowler JL: Migraine headache: review of parameters, etiology, and intervention. *Psychol Bull* 87:217–237, 1980.
5. Blanchard EB, Andrasik F: Psychological assessment and treatment of headache: recent developments and emerging issues. *J Consult Clin Psych* 50:859–879, 1982.
6. Dalessio DJ (ed): *Wolff's Headache and Other Head Pain,* ed 4. New York, Oxford University Press, 1980.
7. Lance JW: *Mechanism and Management of Headache,* ed 3. London, Butterworth, 1978.
8. Friedman AP: Ad Hoc Committee on the Classification of Headache. *Neurology* 12:378–380, 1962.
9. Thompson JK: Diagnosis of head pain: an idiographic approach to assessment and classification. *Headache* 22:221–232, 1982.
10. Friedman AP: *Chronic Recurring Headache: A Multimedia Learning System.* Basel, Switzerland, Sandoz Pharmaceuticals, 1973.
11. Philips C: The modification of tension headache pain using EMG biofeedback. *Behav Res Ther* 15:119–129, 1977.
12. Haynes SN, Cuevas J, Gannon LR: The psychophysiological etiology of muscle contraction headache. *Headache* 22:122–132, 1982.
13. Martin MJ: Muscle-contraction (tension) headache. *Psychosomatics* 24:319–324, 1983.
14. Adams HE, Brantley PJ, Thompson K: Biofeedback and headache: methodological issues. In White L, Tursky B (eds): *Clinical Biofeedback: Efficacy and Mechanisms.* New York, Guilford Press, 1982, p 358.
15. American Psychiatric Association: *Diagnostic and Statistical Manual of Mental Disorders,* ed 3. Washington, DC, Author, 1980, p 247.
16. Packard RC: Conversion headache. *Headache* 20:266–268, 1980.
17. Weatherhead AD: Psychogenic headache. *Headache* 20:47–54, 1980.
18. Fordyce W: *Behavioral Methods for Chronic Pain and Illness.* St. Louis, CV Mosby, 1976.
19. Sturgis ET, Adams HE, Brantley PJ: The parameters, etiology, and treatment of migraine headache. In Haynes SN, Gannon L (eds): *Psychosomatic Disorders: A Psychophysiological Approach to Etiology and Treatment.* New York, Praeger, 1981, p 485.
20. Ryan RE, Ryan RE: *Headache and Head Pain: Diagnosis and Treatment.* St. Louis, CV Mosby, 1978.
21. Blanchard EB, Ahles TA, Shaw ER: Behavioral treatment of headache. *Prog Behav Modif* 8:207–247, 1979.
22. Jacobsen E: *Progressive Relaxation.* Chicago, University of Chicago Press, 1938.
23. Bernstein DA, Borkovec TD: *Progressive Relaxation Training.* Champaign, IL, Research Press, 1973.
24. Benson H: *The Relaxation Response.* New York, William Morrow, 1975.
25. Schultz J, Luthe W: *Autogenic Therapy.* New York, Grune & Stratton, 1969.
26. Budzynski TH, Stoyva JM, Adler CS: Feedback-induced muscle relaxation: an appliation to tension headache. *J Behav Ther Exp Psychiatry* 1:205–211, 1970.
27. Budzynski TH, Stoyva JM, Adler CS, Mullaney DJ: EMG biofeedback and tension headache: a controlled outcome study. *Psychosom Med* 35:484–496, 1973.
28. Sargent JD, Green EE, Walters ED: The use of autogenic feedback training in a pilot study of migraine and tension headaches. *Headache* 12:120–124, 1972.
29. Sargent JD, Green EE, Walters ED: Preliminary report on the use of autogenic feedback training in the treatment of migraine and tension headaches. *Psychosom Med* 35:129–135, 1973.
30. Koppman JW, McDonald RD, Kunzel MG: Voluntary regulation of temporal artery diameter by migraine patients. *Headache* 14:133–138, 1974.
31. Blanchard EB, Andrasik F, Ahles TA, et al: Migraine and tension headaches: a meta-analytic review. *Behav Ther* 11:613–631, 1980.

32. Blanchard EB, Andrasik F, Neff DF, et al: Sequential comparisons of relaxation training and biofeedback in the treatment of three kinds of chronic headache or, the machines may be necessary some of the time. *Behav Res Ther* 20:469–481, 1982.
33. Teders SJ, Blanchard EB, Andrasik F, et al: Relaxation training for tension headache: comparative efficacy and cost-effectiveness of a minimal therapist contact versus a therapist-delivered procedure. *Behav Ther* 11:613–631, 1984.
34. Hay KM, Madders J: Migraine treated by relaxation therapy. *J R Coll Gen Pract* 21:449–464, 1971.
35. Holmes DS, Burish TG: Effectiveness of biofeedback for treating migraine and tension headaches: a review of the evidence. *J Psychosom Res* 27:515–532, 1983.
36. Kewman D, Roberts AH: Skin temperature biofeedback and migraine headaches. *Biofeedback Self-Reg* 5:327–345, 1980.
37. Mullinix JM, Norton BJ, Hack S, et al: Skin temperature biofeedback and migraine headache. *Headache* 17:242–244, 1978.
38. Friar LR, Beatty J: Management of migraines by trained control of vasoconstriction. *J Consult Clin Psychol* 44:46–53, 1976.
39. Bild R, Adams HE: Modification of migraine headaches by cephalic blood volume pulse and EMG biofeedback. *J Consult Clin Psychol* 48:51–57, 1980.
40. Feuerstein M, Adams HE: Cephalic vasomotor feedback in the modification of migraine headache. *Biofeedback Self-Reg* 2:241–254, 1977.
41. Feuerstein M, Adams HE, Beiman I: Cephalic vasomotor and electromyographic feedback in the treatment of combined muscle contraction and migraine headaches in a geriatric case. *Headache* 16:232–237, 1976.
42. Sturgis ET, Tollison CD, Adams HE: Modification of combined migraine muscle-contraction headaches using BVP and EMG feedback. *J Appl Behav Anal* 11:215–223, 1978.
43. Beck AT: *Cognitive Therapy and the Emotional Disorders.* New York, International University Press, 1976.
44. Goldfried MR, Decentecco ET, Weinberg L: Systematic rational restructuring as a self-control technique. *Behav Ther* 5:247–254, 1974.
45. Meichenbaum D: *Cognitive Behavior Modification: An Integrative Approach.* New York, Plenum Press, 1977.
46. Hoyroyd KA, Andrasik F, Westbrook T: Cognitive control of tension headache. *Cogn Ther Res* 1:121–133, 1977.
47. Holroyd KA, Andrasik F: Do the effects of cognitive therapy endure? A two year follow-up of tension headache sufferers treated with cognitive therapy or biofeedback. *Cogn Ther Res* 6:325–334, 1982.
48. Knap TW, Florin I: The treatment of migraine headache by training in vasoconstriction of the temporal artery and a cognitive stress-coping training. *Behav Anal Modif* 4:267–274, 1981.
49. Bakal DA, Demjen S, Kaganov JA: Cognitive behavioral treatment of chronic headache. *Headache* 21:81–86, 1981.
50. Attanasio V, Andrasik F, Blanchard EB: Cognitive therapy and relaxation training in muscle-contraction headache: efficacy and cost-effectiveness. *Headache* 27:254–260, 1987.
51. AuBuchon P, Haber JD, Adams HE: Can migraine headaches be modified by operant pain techniques? *J Behav Ther Exp Psychiatry* 16:261–263, 1985.
52. Adams HE: Case formulations of chronic headaches. In Turkat ID (ed): *Behavioral Case Formulation.* New York, Plenum Press, 1985, p 89.
53. Diamond S, Medina J, Diamon-Falk J, et al: The value of biofeedback in the treatment of chronic headache: a five-year retrospective study. *Headache* 19:90–96, 1979.

part b
facial pain

chapter 22
Differential Diagnosis of Orofacial Pain

Kim J. Burchiel, M.D.
Jeffrey A. Burgess, D.D.S., M.S.D.

In this chapter, we present a survey of the differential diagnosis of orofacial pain syndromes. No attempt has been made to produce an encylopedic litany of exceptionally rare syndromes. Rather, we discuss here the acute and chronic pain states that are seen with any frequency in a busy practice specializing in the treatment of orofacial pain problems. Where possible we have adhered to the Classification of Chronic Pain prepared by the International Association for the Study of Pain (IASP) Subcommittee on Taxonomy (1). Emphasis is placed on diagnosis; however, where appropriate, brief mention of relevant medical and surgical therapy is made. Specific discussions of therapy of orofacial pain can be found in Chapters 23 and 24. Primary headache syndromes and related disorders that produce craniofacial pain are not addressed in this chapter. For this the reader is directed to Chapters 19 to 21.

NEURALGIAS OF THE HEAD AND FACE

TRIGEMINAL NEURALGIA (TIC DOULOUREUX)

Trigeminal neuralgia, or tic douloureux, can be divided into three subcategories: so-called idiopathic trigeminal neuralgia, atypical trigeminal neuralgia, and symptomatic trigeminal neuralgia (in patients with multiple sclerosis). This discussion focuses primarily on idiopathic, or essential, trigeminal neuralgia, since the other two varieties are simply minor exceptions to the general criteria for diagnosis.

Idiopathic Trigeminal Neuralgia

The term *idiopathic* implies that no known etiology can be ascribed to this variety of trigeminal neuralgia. Although not yet universally accepted, considerable evidence from the surgical treatment of trigeminal neuralgia indicates that the pathophysiology of trigeminal neuralgia involves abnormal vascular cross-compression of the root entry zone of the trigeminal nerve (2). In the majority of patients who by most criteria would be considered to have a diagnosis of idiopathic trigeminal neuralgia, distortion of the nerve by a blood vessel can be demonstrated at the time of surgical exposure. Typically, an ectatic loop of the superior cerebellar artery or anterior inferior cerebellar artery impinges upon the nerve, and long-term pain relief can be obtained by surgical repositioning of the vessel, or padding of the neurovascular point of contact with a small prosthetic implant. Although hypotheses have been advanced to relate this vascular compression to the pathophysiologic mechanism of the genesis of the pain of trigeminal neuralgia (3), these remain speculative. If we accept the principle that most trigeminal neuralgia results from vascular compression, then the majority of these patients would more appropriately be classified as having "secondary" trigeminal neuralgia (see below). Nevertheless, this group of patients forms the largest subset of those individuals with trigeminal neuralgia, and they share historic characteristics, physical signs, and neuroradiologic features that, to some degree, distinguish them from patients with trigeminal neuralgia secondary to clearly defined central nervous system lesions. Thus, it seems prudent at this time, if only for semantic purposes, to discuss these patients under the rubric of "idiopathic."

The diagnosis of idiopathic trigeminal neuralgia can virtually always be made by a careful historic and physical examination of the patient. Trigeminal neuralgia is described as sudden, severe, agonizing, episodic but recurrent lacinating pains that are often "electric shock–like," in the distribution of one or more divisions of the fifth cranial nerve. Pain is felt superficially in the skin or buccal mucosa, and can often be triggered by light mechanical contact from a more or less restricted site, often in the perioral region. Duration of pain is usually brief, lasting only seconds, with repetition in bursts for several seconds to a minute or 2, followed by a refractory period of 30 sec or so up to a few minutes. Episodes may occur at intervals of several or many times daily, or in rare instances succeed one another almost continuously. Periodicity of the pain is characteristic, with episodes occurring as described for a few weeks to a month or 2, followed by pain-free intervals of months or years with recurrence of another bout of pain in exactly the same region. Occasionally a mild flush may be noted during the paroxysms of pain. Patients also sometimes report that some relief is obtained by firm pressure with the hands around but not touching the trigger point. The pain is strictly limited to the distribution of the fifth nerve, usually involves one or two divisions, and is slightly more common on the right side. Pains are virtually always confined to one side of the face, although occasionally treated patients or those in remission may experience contralateral typical neuralgic pain. Very rarely, bilateral trigeminal neuralgia can also be seen.

The prevalence of trigeminal neuralgia is relatively rare, with the incidence per year 2.7:100,000 for men, and 5.0:100,000 for women. Age of onset is usually after the fourth decade, with peak onset during the fifth and sixth decades. Onset of pain before age 40 is uncommon and should at least suggest the possibility of multiple sclerosis (MS).

In idiopathic trigeminal neuralgia, the neurologic examination is virtually always normal, although rarely some degree of trigeminal sensorimotor abnormality can be detected. Likewise, neuroradiologic studies [i.e., computed tomography (CT) or magnetic resonance imaging (MRI) scan] of the head are normal. Cerebral angiography should not be necessary, even preoperatively, unless the neuroradiologic studies suggest a vascular abnormality, such as an aneurysm, arteriovenous malformation, or tumor.

Atypical Trigeminal Neuralgia

Atypical trigeminal neuralgia differs from typical trigeminal neuralgia in that in addition to the episodic lancinating pain, there exists a component of a more persistent aching or burning pain (4). In this setting, careful consideration should be given to the presence of structural pathology in the nerve, or to an extrinsic compressive lesion such as a tumor or vascular malformation (5, 6). This is particularly true if sensory loss is detected on the face. Patients with atypical symptoms such as these should undergo CT or MRI scanning to rule out such pathology. If an etiology for the pain can be determined, the patient would then be classified as having a "secondary" neuralgia (see below), although a distinct pathologic lesion will not be demonstrable in all cases. Cases that have atypical features but lack structural pathology would then fall into this group [i.e., atypical (idiopathic) trigeminal neuralgia]. The significance of this subgroup is that in comparison to patients with more typical trigeminal neuralgia, these patients present somewhat different historic features and are generally more refractory to therapy (5).

Symptomatic Trigeminal Neuralgia

Patients with MS can also develop trigeminal neuralgia. The description of the pain is similar to that with idiopathic trigeminal neuralgia, although atypical features of a constant pain component and sensory loss are more common. The pathology in these cases appears to be demyelination either in the nerve or in the brainstem within the descending tract of the trigeminal system (7). In patients less than 40 years of age with trigeminal neuralgia not previously known to have MS, this diagnosis should at least be entertained, particularly if there is evidence of trigeminal sensorimotor dysfunction.

Treatment of Trigeminal Neuralgia

Approximately 70% of patients with trigeminal neuralgia will respond to pharmacologic therapy alone (8). Carbamazepine is the agent of choice and should be started at 100 mg (one-half tablet) orally twice a day, increasing the dose by 100–200 mg every 3–4 days until pain relief is achieved, or toxicity develops, to a final maximum dose in the range of 1000–1200 my/day. Because of its short serum half-life, carbamazepine administration should be spread out during the day in at least three or four doses. Rarely, carbamazepine may depress the peripheral leukocyte count, so a white blood cell count should be obtained prior to initiation of therapy, and then every few weeks for the first few months of treatment. Perhaps a less serious, but more insidious and pervasive, toxicity of carbamazepine is the mental dulling and mild to moderate gait ataxia that are frequent accompaniments of drug treatment. In some patients, no degree of cognitive impairment or ataxia is acceptable, and this argues for discontinuance of carbamazepine and consideration of other therapeutic options.

It is important to point out that a response to carbamazepine is virtually pathognomonic for trigeminal neuralgia, and thus it represents, in effect, a "diagnostic" test with high reliability. Not infrequently, patients may respond initially to carbamazepine therapy, only to become refractory, even at toxic doses, within the ensuing months or years. In these cases other medications can be substituted, but, in our experience, at this point it is not likely the pain will come under control by pharmacologic means alone.

Other drugs that should be considered are diphenylhydantoin and baclofen. Diphenylhydantoin can be given once a day and dosage ranges from 300 to 600 mg/day. Baclofen dose must be slowly increased, starting with 5 mg (one-half tablet) three times a day for 3 days, then 10 mg three times a day for 3 days, then 15 mg three times a day for 3 days, then 20 mg three times a day for 3 days, the usual dose being 40–80 mg/day. Both diphenylhydantoin and baclofen can cause mental slowing, ataxia, and, in the case of baclofen, frank weakness. Both drugs can be given in combination or with carbamazepine, although this is not usually necessary. All three drugs must be slowly tapered when discontinued to avoid complications of central nervous system hyperexcitability (i.e., seizures).

About 30% of patients with trigeminal neuralgia will not respond to pharmacologic therapy, will later become refractory to treatment, or will develop hypersensitivity reaction or other unacceptable toxic side effects of the drugs. These patients should then be considered for surgical treatment. Of the myriad surgical procedures available to patients with trigeminal neuralgia, perhaps three are currently the mainstays of surgical therapy: trigeminal gangliolysis, microvascular decompression of the trigeminal nerve, and peripheral trigeminal neurectomy.

Trigeminal gangliolysis can be performed by radiofrequency (RF) heating of a needle placed percutaneously through the foramen ovale into the ganglion, or by injection of glycerol into the cistern of Meckel's cave through a needle inserted by a similar route. Both are minor procedures, are performed with local or brief general anesthesia, have a very low incidence of morbidity or mortality, and, in about 80–90% of patients, provide years of pain relief (9–11). Both procedures appear to depend, in part, on the production of some degree of trigeminal sensory loss. These procedures appear to work as well for symptomatic trigeminal neuralgia as they do for the idiopathic type.

Microvascular decompression (MVD) of the trigeminal nerve attacks what is considered by some to be the underlying etiology of trigeminal neuralgia alluded to above, that is, cross-compression of the nerve by an ectatic posterior fossa blood vessel. This is a major operation performed under general anesthesia, with a small risk of mortality. In approximately 70–80% of individuals this procedure produces long-lasting or even permanent pain relief without sensory loss (2, 9).

Peripheral neurectomy of a branch of the trigeminal nerve, denervating the trigger area or the region in which pain is perceived, produces years of pain relief. Typically the supraorbital, infraorbital, or inferior alveolar (dental) nerves are avulsed for V_1, V_2, or V_3 pain, respectively. This procedure is particularly useful in patients who may be too debilitated to undergo prolonged general anesthesia and MVD, and are not sufficiently cooperative to tolerate a gangliolysis procedure (12).

There are many other surgical options for patients with trigeminal neuralgia, of which those noted above simply reflect the most commonly performed at present. The reader is directed to more thorough discussions of the surgical approach to this disorder, which are beyond the scope of this chapter (13, 14).

SECONDARY TRIGEMINAL NEURALGIA

Secondary trigeminal neuralgia, as noted above, constitutes a clinical syndrome of trigeminal neuralgia that is thought to be due to a definable structural pathologic lesion, such as tumor, aneurysm, or other vascular abnormality. These lesions are thought to produce a trigeminal neuropathy or neuritis by destruction, irritation, or demyelination of the nerve, and this in turn is responsible for the production of pain. It is much less common than idiopathic trigeminal neuralgia, representing only about 2% of trigeminal neuralgia. The age of onset corresponds to the appearance of the tumor or vascular abnormality, and may be somewhat lower than the idiopathic cases. Cases are equally distributed between males and females. The description of the pain is identical to that seen in primary trigeminal neuralgia, with the exception that nonparoxysmal pain of dull or more constant type may occur. The timing and progression of the pains mimic primary trigeminal neuralgia, and the severity is equal.

Structural lesions that may produce this syndrome include tumors in Meckel's cavity or in the cerebellopontine angle, which account for about 50% of cases. A partial list of associated conditions in given in Table 22.1. The likelihood of detecting one of these abnormalities is increased by documentation of hypesthesia in the trigeminal distribution, or depression of the corneal reflex (6). In these instances, a CT or MRI scan is mandatory.

Treatment in these cases is primarily directed at the offending structure or disorder, and pain relief frequently requires surgical intervention. However, drug therapy, as described above, can be effective, if a decision has been made to treat the neuralgia symptomatically and manage the patient conservatively.

SECONDARY TRIGEMINAL NEURALGIA FROM FACIAL TRAUMA

From 5 to 10% of patients will develop some degree of facial pain following facial fracture, or after reconstructive orthognathic surgery, and a further 1–5% of patients will develop such pain after removal of impacted teeth. The quality of the pain is sharp, with episodic triggered paroxysms and dull throbbing or burning background pain. Signs of this condition include tender palpable nodules over peripheral nerves, or neurotropic effects. The course of the disorder is characterized by progression over a period of 6 months or so, then stabilization of the pain

Table 22.1
Conditions Associated with Secondary Trigeminal Neuralgia

Tumors
Meningioma
Epidermoid tumor
Acoustic neurinoma
Nasopharyngeal carcinoma
Metastatic tumors
Brainstem glioma
Vascular lesions
Basilar artery or cavernous sinus aneurysm
Arteriovenous malformation
Tortuous basilar artery
Sarcoidosis
Connective tissue disease
Scleroderma
Syringobulbia
Pseudotumor cerebri
Paget's disease or acromegaly
Amyloidosis
Toxins
Syphilis
Déjérine-Sottas disease
Arnold-Chiari malformation

until treatment. The pathology is often vague, but may include neuromata or trigeminal deafferentation (15, 16).

This diagnosis overlaps to some extent with that of "atypical facial pain", a catch-all diagnosis that is not useful either from a taxonomic, diagnostic, or therapeutic standpoint (see "Pain of Psychological Origin in the Head and Face," below). The differential diagnosis of this type of pain is difficult since it lacks many of the characteristic attributes that signify primary or secondary (nontraumatic) trigeminal neuralgia. The differential diagnostic possibilities include idiopathic trigeminal neuralgia, secondary trigeminal neuralgia from intracranial lesions, postherpetic neuralgia, odontalgia, and musculoskeletal pain.

In general, the more these pains resemble typical trigeminal neuralgia, the more likely patients will respond to the anticonvulsant medications such as carbamazepine or diphenylhydantoin. If the pain has a constant or burning character, a tricyclic antidepressant such as amitriptyline in doses of 100–150 mg at bedtime in combination with fluphenazine 1–2.5 mg orally twice a day, represents a reasonable option. If a neuroma can be demonstrated, surgical excision can be recommended, but in our experience this is an unusual occurrence. Further trigeminal deafferentation by neurectomy, gangliolysis, or rhizotomy is notably unsuccessful in the management of this condition, and often worsens the pain state.

ACUTE HERPES ZOSTER (TRIGEMINAL)

Pain associated with an acute outbreak of herpetic lesions in the distribution of a branch or branches of the trigeminal nerve does not usually present a diagnostic dilemma. The etiologic agent is herpes zoster or varicella virus, which affects middle-aged and elderly individuals, males and females about equally. Pain is described as burning or tingling, with occasionally lancinating components felt in the skin. The pain usually precedes the onset of herpetic eruption by 1 or 2 days, or may develop coincident with the eruption. The pain is severe and usually lasts one to several weeks (17).

Associated symptoms include malaise, low fever, and headaches. Clusters of small vesicles, almost invariably located in the distribution of the ophthalmic division of the trigeminal nerve, appear. Herpetic eruptions are not uncommonly seen in patients undergoing treatment for systemic lymphoma, carcinomatous metastasis, or other conditions that predispose to immunosuppression. Elevated protein and pleocytosis of the spinal fluid are also observed. Corneal ulceration resulting from vesicles has been reported. The pathology of the lesions is small cell infiltrates in the affected skin and bullous cutaneous changes. Similar infiltrates in the trigeminal ganglion and root entry zone are also seen.

In the usual case spontaneous and permanent remission is the rule. However, in the older age group progression to chronic (postherpetic) neuralgia is not uncommon.

Acute herpetic neuralgia can be managed symptomatically with oral or parenteral narcotic pain medication. Because of the limited duration of the syndrome, tricyclic and anticonvulsant medications are probably not appropriate. Some evidence indicates that repeated sympathetic blockade (i.e., stellate block) may reduce the acute pain as well as the incidence of postherpetic neuralgia. Other agents that have been reported to be effective in the prevention of postherpetic neuralgia, when given in the acute phase, include corticosteroids, amantadine, levodopa and benserazide, vidarabine, and interferon-alpha (17).

POSTHERPETIC NEURALGIA

Chronic neuralgia that occurs in the distribution of one or more divisions of the fifth cranial nerve subsequent to an acute herpes zoster outbreak is described as postherpetic neuralgia. Pain of this type is usually associated with chronic skin trophic changes or scarring and most commonly occurs in the first (ophthalmic) division of cranial nerve V. It is a relatively infrequent disorder, predominantly seen in patients in their fifties or older, and is more common in males. The quality of the pain is described as burning, tearing, crawling, or itching dysesthesia in the affected area, and the pain is exacerbated by mechanical contact with the skin. The pain is moderate but present constantly, and may last for years, although spontaneous subsidence can occur. Because of the chronic and unremitting nature of the pain, depression and irritability are common associated symptoms.

On examination the skin of the painful region may show scarring, loss of normal pigmentation, hypesthesia or hyperesthesia, hypalgesia, or hyperpathia (allodynia). In the early phase of the disorder, pathologically there are chronic inflammatory changes in the trigeminal ganglion, and demyelination in the root entry zone. Later on, wallerian degeneration of the peripheral nerve fiber with fibrosis and a relative depletion of the large more than small myelinated and unmyelinated axons are seen (17).

Treatment of established postherpetic neuralgia is difficult. Fortunately, there is a tendency for the pain to diminish with time. Medications that are effective for trigeminal neuralgia are of little benefit in this disorder, although carbamazepine is useful in the treatment of any component of postherpetic neuralgia that is described as being paroxysmal and lancinating. For the more typical constant burning dysesthetic pain, tricyclic antidepressant medication alone or in combination with a neuroleptic agent is probably the most effective choice for pharmacologic treatment. Amitriptyline (75 mg given at bedtime) with fluphenazine (1 mg three times a day) is a commonly utilized regimen (17, 18).

In light of the natural history of postherpetic neuralgia, surgical therapy should be reserved for those patients with severe, unremitting pain that is refractory to medical management. Currently, stereotaxic trigeminal tractotomy is probably the only surgical procedure that has been shown, albeit in only a few cases, to be effective for the management of postherpetic trigeminal neuralgia (18).

GENICULATE NEURALGIA (SEVENTH CRANIAL NERVE)

The nervus intermedius is a component of the seventh (facial) cranial nerve that contains primary sensory afferent fibers whose somata are located in the geniculate ganglion. These fibers innervate part of the external canal and tympanic membrane, the skin of the angle between ear and mastoid process, the tonsillar region, and some other deep structures of the head and neck. Severe lancinating pain felt within the territory of the nervus intermedius (i.e., deeply within the external auditory canal, auditory meatus, concha, or retroauricular region) constitutes geniculate neuralgia.

The clinical syndrome of geniculate neuralgia, or intermedius neuralgia, occurs in young or middle-aged adults, predominantly in women. The pain can be described as sharp, shock-like, lancinating, and located in the external auditory meatus, with retroauricular radiation. Local tenderness in the pinna or external auditory canal may be present, and manifestations such as excessive salivation or nasal secretion, tinnitus, vertigo, or a bitter taste may accompany the pains.

This is an extremely rare entity, with only a few cases reported in the world's literature. Nevertheless, the syndrome is instructive since it demonstrates a pain syndrome due to involvement of the sensory component of the seventh cranial nerve, the nervus intermedius. Pain of this type must be differentiated from otic varieties of trigeminal and glossopharyngeal neuralgias (19, 20).

Geniculate neuralgia is not usually responsive to medical management, and a surgical procedure is therefore required. The most efficacious technique has been surgical division of the nervus intermedius, glossopharyngeal, and upper two strands of the vagus nerve in the posterior fossa. Ideally, this procedure should be performed under local anesthesia such that electrical stimulation of cranial nerves VII, VIII, IX, and X can be achieved. If under these circumstances pain can be reproduced by stimulation only of VII, IX, and the upper fibers of X, then rhizotomy of these nerves should be carried out. Otherwise, a medullary tractotomy is the procedure of choice (19).

GLOSSOPHARYNGEAL NEURALGIA (NINTH CRANIAL NERVE)

Glossopharyngeal, or more appropriately vagoglossopharyngeal, neuralgia is a rare syndrome that involves episodic bursts of pain in the sensory distribution of the ninth and tenth cranial nerves (21). The vagal and glossopharyngeal nerves are concerned with touch, pain, and temperature sensation in the posterior third of the tongue, tonsillar pillars and fossa, naso-, oro-, and laryngeal pharynx including pyriform recess, larynx, eustachian tube, middle ear, external auditory canal, part of the pinna, and a small cutaneous area anterior and posterior to the pinna. Pains in these regions can be mild to severe, and may be described as being sharp, stabbing, shock-like, hot, or burning. Other uncomfortable sensations, although not frankly painful, may occur in isolation or simply precede painful paroxysms. A dull aching or burning sensation may persist after an attack.

Swallowing, particularly of cold or acid fluids, often triggers the pain, and less commonly chewing, eating, talking, or other movements that involve the oropharyngeal musculature may also precipitate attacks. A discrete trigger point is commonly localizable on the fauces or tonsil, although this may be absent. Individual pains may last from seconds to minutes, and may occur from a few per year to dozens per day. Episodes may last for weeks to months and subside spontaneously, although commonly there is recurrence of the pain.

Bradycardia, tachycardia, syncope, hypotension, or seizures may accompany the painful paroxysms. The cardiovascular effects are thought to be mediated by the carotid sinus nerve or its central connections via the glossopharyngeal or vagus nerves.

The pathophysiology of glossopharyngeal neuralgia is unknown. However, vascular cross-compression by ectatic vessels in the region of the entry zones of the ninth and tenth cranial nerves, akin to what been observed in the fifth nerve in trigeminal neuralgia, has been suggested as a possible etiology.

A possible variant of this syndrome is neuralgia of the superior laryngeal nerve (vagus nerve neuralgia). In these cases paroxysms of unilateral lancinating pain radiate from the side of the thyroid cartilage or pyriform sinus to the angle of the jaw and occasionally to the ear. In all other aspects this syndrome is very similar to glossopharyngeal neuralgia. The differential diagnosis for pains in this area includes carotidynia, Eagle syndrome, or local lesions such as carcinoma.

Like trigeminal neuralgia, glossopharyngeal neuralgia typically does respond to anticonvulsant agents such as carbamazepine (22). If medical management fails to satisfactorily control the pain, the most promising approach has recently been to surgically explore the region of cranial nerves IX and X in the posterior fossa. Frequently, vascular loops impinging upon the nerve can be identified and repositioned. This results in pain remission in the majority of cases (21). If no vascular cross-compression is identified, the ninth and upper one-half of the tenth nerve are divided. Again, this rhizotomy is effective in relieving pain in most cases. If the syndrome is attributed to the superior laryngeal nerve, then temporary relief may be obtained from analgesic nerve block, alcohol nerve block, or nerve section.

OCCIPITAL NEURALGIA

In contradistinction to other cranial neuralgias, occipital neuralgia is quite common. Pain is usually deep, aching, or stabbing in the distribution of the second cervical dorsal root (i.e., unilaterally from the suboccipital area to the vertex), but may radiate toward the vertex, fronto-orbital area, or face. The temporal pattern of the pain is irregular, but it is usually worse later in the day, and may range from moderate to severe in intensity. A history of chronic recurring episodes is typical, although spontaneous cessation of the pain may also occur. Pains of this kind often occur after acceleration-deceleration injuries, and are more common in the third to fifth decades of life. Hyperesthesia of the scalp is a common complaint, and hypesthesia to pinprick in the C2 region of the scalp or tenderness of the great occipital nerve may be found. Local anesthetic block of the occipital nerve may produce effective temporary relief.

The pathophysiology of occipital neuralgia is unknown, although it may be secondary to trauma, including flexion-extension (whiplash) injuries. The mechanism may be related to increased muscle activity in the cervical region, or entrapment of the C2 root or dorsal root ganglion by paravertebral ligamentous structures (23, 24). The differential diagnosis of occipital neuralgia includes cluster headaches; posterior fossa, high cervical, or foramen magnum tumors; herniated cervical intervertebral disk; uncomplicated flexion-extension injury; and metastatic neoplasm at the base of the skull.

Since occipital neuralgia is merely a symptom of radicular or peripheral nerve pathology, treatment varies with the actual, or supposed, etiology. Treatment ranges from therapy directed at specific lesion of the C1–C2 region such as Arnold-Chiari malformation, gout, or neoplasm to generalized disorders such as diabetes. Often a specific etiology can only be postulated, and in these cases a wide variety of treatments have been advocated, such as rhizotomy, collar placement, massage, infrared heat, procaine and alcohol infiltrations, avulsion of the greater occipital nerve, traction, steroid injections, and excision or alcohol injection of all of the nerves in the back of the head (24). Recently, another mechanism has been proposed, that being entrapment of the second or third cervical root and dorsal root ganglion either by ligamentous or fascial structures in their respective neural foramina, or by osteoarthritis and spondylosis in these areas (23, 24). Surgical exploration of the C2 or C3 foramen may demonstrate neural compression, which when relieved may result in pain remission without the necessity for a neurodestructive procedure.

OTHER FACIAL NEURALGIAS

The following syndromes are unusual and are mentioned here only to complete the differential diagnostic possibilities in patients with paroxysmal facial pain secondary to presumed neuralgia.

Sphenopalatine Neuralgia

Sphenopalatine neuralgia (Sluder's syndrome or lower-half headache) consists of paroxysmal pains that begin on the medial side of the nose or medial canthus of the eye and radiate to the roof of the mouth, retro-orbitally, or rarely to the ipsilateral neck, shoulder, and upper extremity (25). Attacks occur many times a day and are often precipitated by sneezing or preceded by a sensation of nasal congestion. Unilateral lacrimation and conjunctival injection may accompany the attacks. Cocaine injection into the sphenopalatine ganglion affords temporary relief.

Vidian neuralgia, or Vail's syndrome, is a variant of sphenopalatine neuralgia. It is paroxysmal unilateral facial pain attributed to "irritation" of the vidian nerve, an afferent branch of the sphenopalatine ganglion. Pain may radiate backward into the ear, nape of the neck, and shoulder, and is occasionally associated with tinnitus and vertigo (25).

Raeder's Paratrigeminal Neuralgia

Raeder's syndrome, or "paratrigeminal" neuralgia, is characterized by frontotemporal pain and oculosympathetic paresis (incomplete Horner's syndrome). The syndrome may be due to the proximity of the ophthalmic division of the fifth nerve to the ocular sympathetic fibers that travel with the carotid artery in the region of the cavernous sinus (26). Two types of pain result: a migrainous variant with episodic and recurrent pains lasting hours or days, and a "symptomatic," more persistent type, often secondary to an aneurysm or tumor in the region of the middle fossa or cavernous sinus.

CRANIOFACIAL PAIN OF MUSCULOSKELETAL ORIGIN

Craniofacial pain of musculoskeletal origin may arise from the muscles of mastication or the temporomandibular joint (TMJ), depending on the sites of pathology, or be referred from the neck musculature (27). In this section we discuss chronic orofacial pain thought to originate specifically from the muscles of mastication or the TMJ. Information regarding head pain originating from the scalp muscles can be found in Chapters 19 to 21 and the neck musculature in Chapters 25 to 29.

Chronic orofacial pain of musculoskeletal origin can be divided into four major subcategories: (a) temporomandibular pain and dysfunction syndrome (28) (also called myofacial pain and dysfunction syndrome) (29); (b) specific myofascial disorders; (c) osteoarthritis of the temporomandibular joint; and (d) bone infections and tumors. Diagnosis in some cases may be confounded by the overlapping of conditions, pain referral from nonmasticatory muscles, lack of clear pathology, and psychosocial and behavioral factors contributing to symptom expression.

TEMPOROMANDIBULAR PAIN AND DYSFUNCTION SYNDROME

Temporomandibular pain and dysfunction syndrome has been equated by the IASP (1) with myofascial pain and dysfunction syndrome. In contrast, some workers consider these conditions to be distinctly different entities, with temporomandibular pain and dysfunction syndrome (TMPDS) by definition associated with altered TMJ physiology and myofascial pain and dysfunction syndrome primarily identified with sustained muscle activity (30). Practically, however, both conditions are characterized by the same triad of signs and symptoms: pain and tenderness of the masticatory muscles, joint sounds with jaw opening, and limited mandibular movement (31).

Diagnosis is based on the patient's history and clinical findings. In general, extensive radiographic evaluation is not necessary. However, radiographic analysis with panography or tomography may be required to rule out degenerative joint disease or other forms of joint pathology (32), and in some complex cases special procedures such as arthrography and CT scanning may be needed to define the nature of joint dysfunction or to rule out other forms of muscular disease such as myofibrositis. Unless the history or clinical findings are suggestive of systemic muscle pathology, rheumatoid arthritis, or lupus erythematosus, laboratory blood studies are not generally useful. Additional laboratory tests such as surface or needle electromyography or thermography have been recommended to assess TMPDS, but the significance of the data gathered from such testing is not presently understood. Since psychosocial stressors may be easily assessed by a detailed psychosocial interview, the use of more extensive psychometric testing is not generally necessary, unless to confirm or underscore a clinical impression.

Pain may be perceived on one or both sides of the face around the ear, in the cheek, jaw, or temple. Generally characterized as a dull, continuous, poorly localized ache of moderate intensity with a boring or gnawing quality, it may vary in degree of discomfort through the course of the day. Yawning, chewing, or moving the mandible will often result in stabs of severe pain and precipitate cramping of jaw locking. Long-term pain may also include cyclical periods of remission.

In addition to pain, patients frequently report symptoms such as jaw muscle fatigue with chewing, episodic jaw locking in either an open or closed position, and deviation with opening. Many patients note the presence of soft or hard clicking or popping joint sounds. If questioned, they may also relate grinding their teeth at night (bruxism) or keeping their teeth together during the day (clenching), or acknowledge other parafunctional habits (gum chewing or fingernail biting). There may be a history of trauma to the face or jaws and onset may often be associated with recent psychosocial stress. Other signs and symptoms that have been irregularly associated with TMPDS include: ear pain (33), headache (34), tinnitus and dizziness (35), malocclusion (36), and psychogenic pain.

TMPDS patients with chronic pain will display many of the psychological characteristics that have been observed for other chronic pain states, including anxiety, stress, depression, anger, and frustration. They may also demonstrate assorted illness behaviors, including increased treatment seeking and medication usage.

Examination will often reveal a limited mouth opening; whereas normal jaw opening is highly variable between individuals, an opening of less than 40 mm (or three finger-widths) is generally considered restricted (37). Reduced jaw opening may be the result of muscle dysfunction (e.g., spasm or splinting) (38); the result of meniscal displacement [e.g., failure of the condylar head to capture the meniscus (reduce) during opening]; or a combination of both conditions. Audible soft clicking or popping sounds resulting from meniscal reduction may occur at any point during jaw opening or closing and are not generally considered to be of significance. However, hard clicking consistently occurring late in opening (greater than 25 mm) coupled with periodic closed locking may indicate pathologic change in the meniscus or joint. In these rare cases arthrography may be useful in defining the nature of meniscus function and potential pathology. Palpation of the jaw-opening muscles, particularly the masseter, temporalis, and internal (lateral) pterygoid, will frequently elicit tenderness, but the pathophysiologic significance of such pain is presently unclear. Intraoral examination will sometimes demonstrate marked tooth attrition, cheek biting, or tongue indentations, findings associated with bruxism or clenching. In cases of dislocation of the meniscus there may be marked alteration in the occlusion.

The prevalence of TMPDS has been estimated to be between 10 and 15% of the population (39). It is a disease of the young (e.g., ages 15–45), with a three to five times greater incidence in females. Although TMPDS is generally acknowledged to be a psychophysiologic disease, its etiology remains unsettled. Fortunately, for approximately 80% of patients, the condition is self-limiting. Conditions that must be considered in the differential diagnosis of TMPDS are presented in Table 22.2.

The American Dental Association has recommended that until differences concerning the etiology, pathophysiology, and diagnosis of TMPDS are resolved, treatment strategies should be conservative and noninvasive (40). Interventions that address the muscular component of the problem include psychophysiologic (habit control, hypnotherapy, relaxation therapy, and biofeedback), psychological (counseling/stress management, communication/cognitive therapy, and behavioral modification), and pharmacologic (antidepressants, antianxiety agents, or muscle relaxants) modalities as well as massage, physical exercises, physiotherapy, splints, transcutaneous electrical neural stimulation (TENS), or myofunctional therapy. Relatively noninvasive strategies such as acupuncture and trigger point injections may also be useful. Aggressive intervention with orthodontics or dental reconstruction is very rarely necessary. In cases of severe TMJ dysfunction involving meniscus pathology, surgical therapy (e.g., disk repositioning and plication of the distal ligament, disk removal, or artificial meniscus implantation) may be indicated. The efficacy of the latter strategy, however, is increasingly being questioned because of premature breakdown and rejection. For greater detail about treatment methodologies the reader is referred to Chapter 23.

SPECIFIC OR DIFFUSE MYOFASCIAL PAIN SYNDROMES

The cardinal feature of what the IASP has described as "myofascial pain syndromes," upon which diagnosis is based, is the presence of latent or active myofascial "trigger points" (1). These are discrete nodular areas of hyperirritable muscle or fascial tissue that, when compressed, predictably produce what has been termed a "jump sign" and a reproducible pain referral pattern (41). Satellite tender points may be found within the area of pain reference of the initial trigger point. The presence of multiple "trigger points" distinguishes this pain disorder from pain of other muscle conditions (e.g., TMPDS).

Pain, described as deep, aching, or pressure-like, may be induced by passive stretch, functional movements, or strong voluntary contraction of shortened muscle, or by cold, damp weather, trauma, hyperactivity or inactivity, fatigue, and emotional distress. Activation of an initial trigger point may excite satellite points within the zone of reference and trigger points within synergistic muscles (42). If myospasm becomes a feature of trigger point activation, associated orofacial symptoms may include limited opening or joint clicking.

Evidence associating trigger points with specific or nonspecific pathologic features is limited (43) and there is virtually no experimental evidence supporting the presence of such discrete areas of pathophysiologic change within the muscles of mastication. Nonetheless, distinctive regions of tenderness described as trigger points have been reliably measured with a pressure algometer in the masseter and temporalis muscles (44). Laboratory procedures such as electromyography and thermography have not been thoroughly investigated in relation to masticatory trigger points and at present offer limited diagnostic utility. Blood studies are negative and not necessary, unless there is suspicion that the condition is secondary to systemic disease. Radiography with soft tissue imaging has not demonstrated abnormalities and is not recommended.

Although myofascial pain associated with the masticatory musculature appears to be quite common, its epidemiologic characteristics are unknown. In a recent study of 296 patients with complaints of head and neck pain, 55.4% were found to have a primary diagnosis of myofascial pain syndrome based on the presence of multiple trigger points (45).

Myofascial pain syndromes may occur within an indi-

Table 22.2
Differential Diagnosis of Temporomandibular Pain and Dysfunction Syndrome

Tumors
    Synovial chondromatosis
    Coronoid hyperplasia
    Sarcoma
Arthritis
    Infectious arthritis
    Traumatic arthritis
    Rheumatoid arthritis
    Osteoarthritis (degenerative joint disease)
    Psoriatic arthritis
    Juvenile rheumatoid arthritis
Connective tissue disease
    Systemic lupus erythematosus
    Dermatomyositis
Condylar agenesis
Myofascial disorders (myositis, fibrositis)
Myositis ossificans
Odontogenic or nonodontogenic infection
Otitis media
Parotitis
Reflex sympathetic dystrophy of the face
Elongated styloid process (Eagle's syndrome)
Pain of psychological origin in the face (psychogenic pain disorder)

vidual muscle (e.g., "specific" type) or involve several muscles (e.g., "diffuse" type). Synonyms for this condition include: fibrositis (syndrome), myalgia, tenomyositis, muscular rheumatism, and nonarticular rheumatism. Conditions from which myofascial pain syndromes should be differentiated are listed in Table 22.3.

Specific myofascial pain syndromes involving the masticatory muscles respond well to stretch-and-spray techniques, trigger point compression, massage, injection, or acupuncture. Low-dose amitriptyline (50–75 mg) may be helpful. The elimination of perpetuating postural or behavioral factors should be part of management strategy. Additional information concerning management of myofascial pain syndromes is found in Chapters 23 and 41.

OSTEOARTHRITIS OF THE TEMPOROMANDIBULAR JOINT

Pain is a fequent, but not consistent, finding in patients presenting with osteoarthritis of the TMJ. When present, it is often described as a deep ache within the ear or preauricular area of the face (with minimal radiation to surrounding regions) that increases in intensity from morning to evening and is exacerbated with use or cold weather. It may persist for months or years with cyclical periods of remission. Crepitus is the symptom most consistently related to osteoarthritis of the TMJ (46), but limitation of mandibular movement, presumably associated with muscle splinting, has also been reported (47). The sound of crepitus is distinctly different from clicking and has been described as a gristle, crackle, or soft-hard grating. It is assumed that damage to the soft tissue articulating components contributes to the noise, but the degree to which joint morphology, as opposed to degenerative change, contributes to the quality of sound is presently unknown. There is often a history of trauma. Patients with chronic osteoarthritis will appear to be less psychologically disturbed than those with myofascial conditions.

Diagnosis is based on history, the presence of crepitus revealed through stethoscopic evaluation, TMJ palpation pain (lateral and intrameatal), and radiographic interpretation. Change in occlusion may also be noted if joint degeneration has been rapid. Laboratory tests (e.g., blood or synovial fluid analysis) are not generally necessary, unless there is suspicion of infectious arthritis (bacterial, fungal, tubercular), connective tissue diseases (rheumatoid arthritis, systemic lupus erythematosus, dermatomyositis), or the rheumatoid variants (psoriatic arthritis, Reiter's syndrome, juvenile rheumatoid arthritis). Gross radiographic bone changes can be observed in panoramic and transcranial radiographs, but tomograms are currently considered the most accurate means of assessing the full extent of pathology. Osseous changes include: flattening of the condyle or eminence, osteophytes, marginal lipping of the anterior portion of the condyle, subarticular cystic changes or erosions in the lateral or superior portion of the condyle, sclerosis of marginal bone, and medullary distortions (48). Severe erosion of the TMJ is more indicative of connective tissue disease than osteoarthritis. Joint space narrowing has also been suggested as a sign of pathology, but this view remains controversial and unsupported. Other radiographic diagnostic techniques [e.g., MRI and single photon emission computed tomography (SPECT)] show promise for improving diagnostic capability.

Osteoarthritis of the TMJ is most likely to be observed in women past the age of 40 (49). However, it has been reported in young females (47). Epidemiologic studies suggest that between 4 and 14% of the population may have TMJ dengerative disease based on the presence of crepitus (50). Far fewer have pain or seek treatment. The histopathology of TMJ osteoarthritis is well documented, consisting of primary articular erosion and secondary joint space dystrophic calcification in the absence of inflammation (51). Histopathologic studies suggest that degenerative change may be correlated with articular disk perforations or deformations (52).

The etiology of TMJ osteoarthritis is unknown. The literature identifies a plethora of causes that include age, various forms of trauma (53), and functional or dysfunctional loading. The effects of genetic predisposition, systemic disease, metabolic-endocrine processes, and inflammation have not been thoroughly investigated. Recent evidence suggests that osteoarthritis may be related to condylar dysfunction, particularly chronic anterior meniscus displacement (52). However, the hypothesis that osteoarthritis may result from intermittent joint clicking remains speculative.

Conditions that should be considered in the differential diagnosis are listed in Table 22.4.

In general osteoarthritis of the temporomandibular joint follows a pattern similar to that in skeletal joints, with symptoms lasting 1–3 years and including bone remodeling. The condition may be conservatively managed with therapeutic strategies outlined above under "Temporomandibular Pain and Dysfunction Syndrome." In addition, anti-inflammatory medications and anesthetic injection into the joint may be helpful. Severe cases may require surgical management, and recurrence is likely.

Table 22.3
Differential Diagnosis of Myofascial Pain Syndromes

Temporomandibular pain and dysfunction syndrome
Myofascial pain and dysfunction syndrome
Connective tissue disease
    Systemic lupus erythematosus
    Dermatomyositis
Myositis ossificans
Odontogenic or nonodontogenic infection
The arthritides
Reflex sympathetic dystrophy of the face
Elongated styloid process
Pain of psychological origin in the face

Table 22.4
Differential Diagnosis of Osteoarthritis of the Temporomandibular Joint

Temporomandibular pain and dysfunction syndrome
Myofascial pain and dysfunction syndrome
Infectious arthritis (bacterial, fungal, tubercular)
Connective tissue diseases
    Rheumatoid arthritis
    Systemic lupus erythematosus
    Dermatomyositis
Rheumatoid variants
    Psoriatic arthritis
    Reiter's syndrome
    Juvenile rheumatoid arthritis
Traumatic arthritis

BONE INFECTIONS AND TUMORS

Orofacial pain resulting from infection and neoplasia is described as a constant, deep, aching sensation, sometimes localized to the teeth, but more often of a diffuse quality. Diagnosis is based on the patient's history, laboratory, radiographic, and clinical findings. In cases of nonpurulent infection (osteitis), radiography may reveal demineralization or remineralization of the bone. Signs and symptoms associated with chronic osteomyelitis include paresthesia (if the condition involves the mandibular nerve canal), low-grade fever, elevated white blood cell count and increased erythrocyte sedimentation rate values, sinus tract formation, limitation of opening, and occasionally exposed bone. Bone death and necrosis result in a distinctive radiographic presentation, with islands of bone, termed *sequestra*, surrounded by demineralization. The condition may result from periapical tooth abcess, fracture, or surgical contamination. Osteoradionecrosis, one form of osteomyelitis, may result from radiation treatment to the jaws or from radiation treatment that is followed by trauma (e.g., tooth extraction).

When neoplastic activity in the mandible (osteogenic sarcoma) is the source of the pain, there may be concurrent altered skin sensation (e.g., hypesthesia, dyesthesia, or paresthesia) over the chin or lower face. Chondrosarcoma, a relatively rare but exquisitely painful tumor, is most commonly found in the anterior maxilla. Diagnosis of neoplasm is straightforward and is based on history, clinical, laboratory, and radiographic findings.

LESIONS OF THE EAR, NOSE, AND ORAL CAVITY

OROFACIAL PAIN DUE TO SINUSITIS

Orofacial pain resulting from acute sinus infection can be mild to severe, and is often described as aching, throbbing, or as headache. Frontal or ethmoid sinus involvement generates bilateral forehead pain or pain felt between the eyes, whereas pain originating from the maxillary sinus is often experienced on one or both sides of the face in the upper cheek (zygoma) or the entire side of the face. Pain arising from chronic (as opposed to acute) maxillary sinusitis may be described as mild and continuous with a burning quality. Other associated symptoms may include a feeling of fullness in the face or, in cases of maxillary sinus involvement, tenderness of the maxillary premolar or molar teeth.

The diagnosis of chronic sinusitis is based on history, clinical, and radiographic findings. Forward bending or pressure applied over the affected sinus may intensify or exacerbate the pain in some cases. Examination may reveal hypertrophy or atrophy of the nasal mucosa and/or polyp formation. With maxillary involvement the upper teeth on the affected side will frequently be percussion sensitive. Cultures of the nose or nasal discharge, however, are often negative (54). In these cases the examiner should be alert to the possibility of allergy or a reaction to irritating dusts or toxic chemicals. Standard radiography may demonstrate a fluid level but may not be helpful in assessing mucosal changes. Computed tomography may be necessary to rule out neoplasm.

Acute sinusitis is quite prevalent in adults, with chronic sinusitis being less common. Males and females are equally affected. Inflammation of the sinus mucosal lining is considered to be the pathophysiologic mechanism responsible for facial pain genesis, and inflammation of elements of the superior alveolar nerve plexus the cause of tooth pain. Orofacial conditions that should be considered in the differential diagnosis include odontogenic infection and malignant disease.

Relief may be gained from antibiotics, decongestants, analgesics, moist heat, or lying down on the opposite side to promote drainage. Surgical lavage or drainage is necessary for intractable cases.

OROFACIAL PAIN OF ODONTOGENIC ORIGIN

Odontogenic pain or toothache, also termed *odontalgia*, is the most common source of orofacial discomfort. Highly variable in presentation, odontogenic pain may be intermittent or continuous, spontaneous or induced, and will often simulate other pain syndromes. It is most often described as a mild to unbearable aching or sometimes throbbing sensation with a dull or depressing quality. The IASP has chosen to differentiate five varieties of odontalgia: pain due to dentinoenamel defects; pain arising from the pulp (e.g., pulpitis); pain arising from the periodontal structures (e.g., periapical periodontitis and abscess); pain not associated with lesions (e.g., atypical odontalgia); and cracked tooth syndrome. With the exception of pain due to dentinoenamel defects, all of these conditions can be chronic in nature. Since atypical odontalgia is not associated with a known pathophysiologic mechanism, we have elected to describe this condition under the classification "Pain of Psychogenic Origin in the

Head and Face" (see below). A complete discussion of therapeutic considerations related to pain conditions of odontogenic origin is presented in Chapter 24.

Odontalgia: Toothache-Pulpitis

The term *pulpitis* implies that the etiology of this pain is only pulpal inflammation and not periapical infection. In these cases pain is very often poorly localized within the teeth, jaws, face, or head. It may occur spontaneously, or be activated (in severe cases exacerbated) by hot or cold stimuli. Pupal pain is often perceived as a sharp or dull ache of moderate or severe intensity.

Diagnosis is based on clinical signs and radiologic findings. Examination and radiography will often reveal deep dental caries, sometimes with erosion into the pulp chamber or root canal. Application of stimulants such as cold, heat, electric stimulation, and probing will induce pain. If inflammation progresses to infection and periodontal involvement, pain will be aggravated by percussion.

Differential diagnosis includes other forms of dental disease, trigeminal neuralgia, sinusitis, and migrainous headache syndromes.

Odontalgia: Toothache–Periapical Periodontitis and Abscess

Pain related to periodontal structures is similar in quality, occurrence, intensity, and duration to pain of pulpal origin. However, in contrast to pulpal pain, it is easily localized by the patient and diagnosis generally does not present difficulty. Pressure applied to the offending tooth will initiate or exacerbate tenderness. Associated symptoms may include localized redness, cellulitis, lymphadenitis, and drainage through the formation of a sinus tract. More severe complications can involve diffuse cellulitis and spread of the infection fo parapharyngeal spaces, with airway compromise; the central nervous system (CNS), with cerebral abscess; or the endocardium (55). Radiographic data are useful for initial diagnosis and for defining extensive fascial plane involvement. In cases involving diffuse cellulitis, hematologic, histopathologic, and microbiologic laboratory tests may be necessary to augment diagnosis or to provide baseline information should the infection not resopnd to initial treatment. Differential diagnosis includes other dental disease, nonodontogenic infections, and neoplasia.

Cracked Tooth Syndrome

Pain originating from a tooth with a fine crack can be acute or chronic and is described as sharp or shock-like and of brief duration, often produced by biting or chewing. Upon examination, percussion directed laterally toward the affected tooth cusp will usually exacerbate the pain. A visible crack may sometimes be apparent or the cusp may move with manipulation. Radiography is not beneficial. The differential diagnosis includes other forms of toothache associated with the dentine or pulp.

OROFACIAL PAIN OF MUCOSAL ORIGIN

Mucosal diseases produce pain that is intermittent in nature, although the patient may experience chronic discomfort. There are, however, a number of conditions that may produce persistent facial pain of an aching quality, including chronic periodontitis, benign mucous membrane pemphigoid, ulcerative lichen planus, major recurrent aphthous, Wegener's granulomatosis, and oral cancer with superimposed infection. Diagnosis in these cases is generally confirmed by history, examination, or laboratory findings (56).

One type of orofacial mucosal pain that may be encountered has been termed "burning mouth syndrome" (glossodynia). The typical patient is a postmenopausal woman. The onset of the disorder is often associated with a prior dental procedure. In these cases, pain, described as a persistent, severe, burning sensation, may occur in the tongue or other mucosal tissues within the mouth, often in association with other altered sensations (e.g., taste or dryness) (57). It may fluctuate during the day. The etiology and pathophysiology of this disorder remain unknown. The condition has been associated with local irritation (ill-fitting dentures), xerostomia, systemic disease, and nutritional deficiencies (especially of vitamin B_{12}, but also vitamins B_1, B_2, and B_6). Burning tongue has also been reported following the development of adenoid cystic carcinoma in the floor of the mouth. In addition, many workers consider burning mouth a psychogenic pain problem since symptoms are often associated with emotional upset in the absence of organic findings (see below).

PAIN OF PSYCHOLOGICAL ORIGIN IN THE HEAD AND FACE

The IASP has chosen to describe two general categories of "pain of psychological origin in the head and face": "delusional or hallucinatory pain" and "hysterial or hypochondriacal" pain (1). Classification of a pain condition as of psychological origin requires that there be no known physical cause or pathophysiologic mechanism; in addition, there must be proof of the presence of contributing psychological factors. As a result, these categories are roughly equivalent to what the American Psychiatric Association has described as "Psychogenic Pain Disorder" (58).

Historically, "atypical facial pain," or prosopalgia, has been the term most commonly used to describe diffuse, nonanatomic orofacial pain of unknown pathophysiology. In the authors' opinion, the diagnosis of "atypical facial pain" should be made only on the following basis: (*a*) when other etiologies for facial pain have been considered and evaluated where appropriate; (*b*) when objective evidence for most of the facial pain syndromes is lacking; and (*c*) when specific antecedent psychological or behavioral factors can be identified.

The predominant characteristic of psychologically induced pain is that it mimics pain of known pain syndromes. It is usually constant, is often bilateral, and is not confined to the trigeminal distribution. The description of the pain quality is often vague and variable, as is the location and precipitating factors. A constant aching or burning sensation is the dominant feature, paroxysmal pain being uncommon. Psychological features such as delusions, hallucinations, multiple physical complaints with classical conversion or pseudoneurologic symptoms, exaggerated symptom reporting, excessive concern or fear of the symptoms, depression, illness behaviors, and excessive treatment seeking or medication usage are common. The patient often appears morose, with evident suffering. A neurologic examination is usually normal except for some poorly localized tenderness and vague sensory loss in the painful region. Anticonvulsant medication is distinctly not helpful in these patients, and psychiatric evaluation with psychotherapy and antidepressant medication are perhaps the only reasonable courses (20).

References

1. International Association for the Study of Pain Subcommittee on Taxonomy: Classification of chronic pain: descriptions of chronic pain syndromes and definitions of chronic pain terms. *Pain* 3(Suppl):S1–S225, 1986.
2. Jannetta PJ: Treatment of trigeminal neuralgia by suboccipital and transtentorial cranial operations. *Clin Neurosurg* 24:538–549 1977.
3. Burchiel KJ: Abnormal impulse generation in focally demyelinated trigeminal roots. *J Neurosurg* 53:674–683, 1980.
4. Cusick JF: Atypical trigeminal neuralgia. *JAMA* 245:2328–2329, 1981.
5. Szapiro J Jr, Sindou M, Szapiro J: Prognostic factors in microvascular decompression for trigeminal neuralgia. *Neurosurgery* 17:920–929 1985.
6. Bullitt E, Tew JM, Boyd J: Intracranial tumors in patients with facial pain. *J Neurosurg* 64:865–871 1986.
7. Iragui VJ, Wiederholt WC, Romine JS: Evoked potentials in trigeminal neuralgia associated with multiple sclerosis. *Arch Neurol* 43:444–446 1986.
8. Crill WE: Carbamazepine. *Ann Intern Med* 79:844–847 1973.
9. Burchiel KJ, Steege TD, Howe JF, Loeser JD: Comparison of percutaneous radiofrequency gangliolysis and microvascular decompression of the trigeminal nerve for the surgical management of tic douloureux. *Neurosurgery* 9:111–119, 1981.
10. Sweet WH, Wepsic JG: Controlled thermocoagulation of trigeminal ganglion and rootlets for differential destruction of pain fibers: Part I. Trigeminal neuralgia. *J Neurosurg* 40:143–156, 1974.
11. Hakanson S: Tic douloureux treated by the injection of glycerol into the retrogasserian subarachnoid space; long term results. *Acta Neurochir Suppl* 33:471–472, 1984.
12. Quinn JH: Repetitive peripheral neuroectomies for neuralgia of second and third divisions of trigeminal neuralgia (tic douloureux). *Clin Neurosurg* 24:550–556, 1977.
13. Burchiel KJ: Surgical treatment of trigeminal neuralgia: minor operative procedures. In Fromm GH (ed): *The Medical and Surgical Management of Trigeminal Neuralgia*. Mount Kisco, NY, Futura, 1987, pp 71–99.
14. Burchiel KJ: Surgical treatment of trigeminal neuralgia: major operative procedures. In Fromm GH (ed): *The Medical and Surgical Management of Trigeminal Neuralgia*. Mount Kisco, NY, Futura, 1987, pp 101–120.
15. Goldstein NP, Gibilisco JA, Rushton JG: Trigeminal neuropathy and neuritis: a study of etiology with emphasis on dental causes. *JAMA* 184:458–462, 1963.
16. Thrush DC, Small M: How benign a symptom is face numbness? *Lancet* 2:851–853, 1970.
17. Loeser JD: Herpes zoster and postherpetic neuralgia. *Pain* 25:149–164, 1986.
18. Watson PN, Evans RJ: Postherpetic neuralgia; a review. *Arch Neurol* 43:836–840, 1986.
19. White JC, Sweet WH: *Pain and the Neurosurgeon*. Springfield, IL, Charles C Thomas, 1969, pp 264–265.
20. Hart RG, Easton JD: Trigeminal neuralgia and other facial pains. *Missouri Med* 11:683–693, 1981.
21. Laha RK, Jannetta PJ: Glossopharyngeal neuralgia. *J Neurosurg* 47:316–320, 1977.
22. Ekbom KA, Westerberg CE: Carbamazepine in glossopharyngeal neuralgia. *Arch Neurol* 14:595–596, 1966.
23. Poletti CE: Proposed operation for occipital neuralgia: C-2 and C-3 root decompression. *Neurosurgery* 12:221–224, 1983.
24. Ehni G, Benner B: Occipital neuralgia and the C1-2 arthrosis syndrome. *J Neurosurg* 61:961–965, 1984.
25. Aubry M, Pialoux P: Sluder's syndrome. In Vinken PJ, Bruyn GW (eds): *Handbook of Clinical Neurology*. Amsterdam, Elsevier North Holland, 1968, vol 5, pp 350–361.
26. Toussaint D: Raeder's syndrome. In Vinken PJ, Bruyn GW (eds): *Handbook of Clinical Neurology*. Amsterdam, Elsevier North Holland, 1968, vol 5, pp 333–336.
27. Travell J: Temporomandibular joint pain referred from muscles of the head and neck. *J Prosthet Dent* 10:745–763, 1960.
28. Schwartz L: *Disorders of the Temporomandibular Joint*. Philadelphia, WB Saunders, 1969.
29. Laskin D: Etiology of the pain-dysfunction syndrome. *J Am Dent Assoc* 70:147–153, 1969.
30. Moss RA, Garrett J: Temporomandibular joint dysfunction syndrome and myofascial pain dysfunction syndrome: a critical review. *J Oral Rehabil* 11:3–28, 1984.
31. Rugh JD, Solberg WK: Psychological implications in temporomandibular pain and dysfunction. *Oral Sci Rev* 7:3–30, 1976.
32. Laskin D, Block S: Diagnosis and treatment of myofascial pain-dysfunction (MPD) syndrome. *J Prosthet Dent* 56:75–84, 1986.
33. Dolowitz DA, Ward JW, Fingerle CO, Smith C: The role of muscular incoordination in the pathogenesis of the temporomandibular joint syndrome. *Laryngoscope* 74:790–801, 1964.
34. Magnusson T, Carlsson GE: A two and one half year follow-up of changes in headache and mandibular dysfunction after stomatognathic treatment. *J Prosthet Dent* 49:398–402, 1983.
35. Sharov Y, Tzukert A, Refaeli B, Israel J: Muscle pain index in relation to pain dysfunction, and dizziness associated with the myofacial pain dysfunction syndrome. *Oral Surg* 46:742–747, 1978.
36. Agerberg G, Carlsson G: Symptoms of functional disturbances of the masticatory system. *Acta Ondontol Scand* 33:183–190, 1975.
37. Bell W: *Clinical Management of Temporomandibular Disorders*. Chicago, Year Book Medical Publishers, 1982.
38. Griffin CT, Munro KK: Electromyography of the masseter and anterior temporalis muscles in patients with temporomandibular dysfunction. *Arch Oral Biol* 16:929–949, 1971.
39. Solberg W, Woo M, Houston J: Prevalence of mandibular

dysfunction in young adults. *J Am Dent Assoc* 98:25–34, 1979.
40. Griffiths RH: Report of the president's conference on the examination, diagnosis, and management of temporomandibular disorders. *J Am Dent Assoc* 106:75–77, 1983.
41. Travell J, Rinzler SH: The myofascial genesis of pain. *Postgrad Med* 11:425–434, 1952.
42. Travell JG, Simons DG: *Myofascial Pain and Dysfunction: The Trigger Point Manual.* Baltimore, Williams & Wilkins, 1983.
43. Awad EA: Interstitial myofibrositis: hypothesis of the mechanism. *Arch Phys Med Rehabil* 54:449–453, 1973.
44. Reeves JL, Jaeger B, Graff-Radford SB: Reliability of the pressure algometer as a measure of myofascial trigger point sensitivity. *Pain* 24:313–321, 1986.
45. Fricton JR, Kroening R, Haley D, Siegert R: Myofascial pain syndrome of the head and neck: a review of clinical characteristics of 164 patients. *J Oral Surg Oral Pathol Oral Medicine* 60:615–623, 1985.
46. Shira RB: Temporomandibular degenerative joint disease. *Oral Surg* 40:1651–1682, 1975.
47. Ogus H: Dengerative disease of the temporomandibular joint in young persons. *Br J Oral Surg* 17:17–26, 1979–80.
48. Wilkes DH: Structural and functional alterations of the temporomandibular joint. *Northwest Dent* 57:287–294, 1978.
49. Toller PA: Osteoarthrosis of the mandibular condyle. *Br Dent J* 134:223–231, 1973.
50. Gross A, Gale E: A prevalence study of the clinical signs associated with mandibular dysfunction. *J Am Dent Assoc* 107:932–936, 1983.
51. Moffett GC, Johnson LC, McCabe JB: Articular remodeling in the adult human temporomandibular joint. *Am J Anat* 115:119–142, 1964.
52. Wesstesson P-L, Rohlin M: Internal derangement of the temporomandibular joint: morphologic description with correlation to joint function. *J Oral Surg Oral Pathol Oral Med* 59:323–331, 1985.
53. Truelove E, Burgess J, Dworkin S, Lawton L, Sommers E, Schubert M: Incidence of trauma associated with temporomandibular disorders. *J Dent Res* 64:339, 1985, abstr 1482.
54. Weinstein L: Diseases of the upper respiratory tract. In Petersdorf R, Adams R, Braunwald A, Isselbacher J, Martin J, Wilson J (eds): *Harrison's Principles of Internal Medicine.* New York, McGraw-Hill, 1983, pp 1570–1571.
55. Hohl T, Whitacre R, Hooley J, Williams B: In Hooley J, Whitacre R (eds): *Diagnosis and treatment of odontogenic infections.* Seattle, Stoma Press, 1983, pp 50–106.
56. Wood NK, Goaz P (eds): *Differential Diagnosis of Oral Lesions.* St. Louis, CV Mosby, 1980.
57. Basker RM, Sturdee DW, Davenport JC: Patients with burning mouths—a clinical investigation of causative factors, including the climacteric and diabetes. *Br Dent J* 145:9–16, 1978.
58. American Psychiatric Association: *Quick Diagnostic and Statistical Manual (DSM-III).* Washington, DC, Author, 1980.

chapter 23
Medical/Neurosurgical Management of Orofacial Pain

Ronald Brisman, M.D.

Effective medical management of orofacial pain is dependent on appropriate diagnosis. Consultations from dental, otolaryngologic, and neurologic specialists are often necessary. Specific causes for the pain should be sought, because direct treatment may relieve the pain. Infection of dental or peridental structures or paranasal sinuses may be treated with antibiotics and occasional drainage. Temporomandibular joint degeneration, which may be caused by malocclusion of the teeth, requires dental correction. Tumors of the trigeminal nerve, a rare cause of facial pain, are usually associated with abnormalities of the trigeminal and other cranial nerves, and often require neurosurgical intervention.

In many instances of orofacial pain, a specific cause and definitive cure cannot be achieved, and medical or surgical management focuses on the relief of pain and suffering.

Most orofacial pains of nondental origin are either neuralgic (paroxysmal, episodic, unilateral, triggered by light touch about the mouth or face, and located in the distribution of the trigeminal or, rarely, the glossopharyngeal nerve) or atypical (continuous, burning, aching, or throbbing, often bilateral, and frequently distributed beyond the confines of one cranial nerve).

TRIGEMINAL NEURALGIA (TIC DOULOUREUX)

Episodic, triggered, severe, brief, lancinating paroxysms of pain, usually in the second and/or third divisions of the trigeminal nerve, without loss of sensation are characteristic of trigeminal neuralgia. At any one time, the condition is almost always unilateral, although 5–10% of patients will at some time in their lives have similar contralateral pain.

Multiple sclerosis should be suspected in younger patients with trigeminal neuralgia (those whose symptoms began before they were 45 years old) and those with bilateral symptoms (1). Other diagnostic tests for multiple sclerosis, such as cerebrospinal fluid (CSF) examination for α-globulin and oligoclonal bands, visual-evoked responses, and magnetic resonance imaging, should be pursued if multiple sclerosis is a possibility and microvascular decompression is being considered as treatment for the trigeminal neuralgia, because microvascular decompression is contraindicated in the presence of multiple sclerosis.

Only a few (1–5%) patients with trigeminal neuralgia will have a brain tumor, and many of these will have other neurologic abnormalities caused by the brain tumor (2). Rarely a patient with trigeminal neuralgia and no other signs or symptoms will have a brain tumor causing the trigeminal neuralgia. In those whose face pain symptoms are intractable enough to require a neurosurgical procedure, computed tomography should be done to exclude the possibility of a brain tumor, even though most patients will not have one.

MEDICAL MANAGEMENT

Carbamazepine (Tegretol) is so effective in treating trigeminal neuralgia (3, 4) that the diagnosis should be doubted if the patient does not show some response to this medication. Treatment is usually begun at a dose of 100 mg twice a day. The daily dose is increased by 100 or 200 mg until the patient gets relief. The usual maintenance dose is a total of 400–800 mg daily, which is given in divided doses from two to four times a day. It is rarely necessary to give more than 1200 mg daily. After the patient is free of pain for several weeks, attempts should be made to reduce the dose gradually to the minimum necessary.

Many unpleasant side effects may occur from carbamazepine. The most common are dizziness, drowsiness, unsteadiness, nausea, and vomiting, and they are most likely to develop when therapy is initiated or the dose is too high. They usually subside when the dose is lowered. Central nervous system toxicity is more likely to develop in the elderly (a group commonly afflicted with trigeminal neuralgia) and in those with multiple sclerosis. Carbamazepine is contraindicated in those with a known sensitivity to tricyclic compounds.

Other toxic effects may appear from the use of carbamazepine; these include skin rashes, bone marrow suppression, and liver or renal impairment. A complete blood count and liver and renal chemistries should be done as a baseline, after 2 weeks, and at approximately 6-week intervals. Substantial alterations require that the medication be stopped.

If satisfactory relief cannot be obtained from carbamazepine, then baclofen (Lioresal) should be tried alone or in combination with carbamazepine (if the patient does not have a toxic reaction to carbamazepine but it is no longer effective by itself) (5). The dose of baclofen is gradually titrated for each individual; an initial dose of 5 mg three times a day is given for 3 days, then increased every 3 days by a total daily dose of 15 mg until the optimal dose (usually 40–80 mg) is achieved. The most common adverse reactions are drowsiness, dizziness, and fatigue.

Although it is not effective in most patients, phenytoin (Dilantin) may be tried if treatment is not successful with carbamazepine and baclofen. The usual dose is 100 mg three times a day. Clonazepam (Klonopin) may also help; the initial dose is 0.5 mg three times a day, and may be increased every 3 days by a total daily increment of 0.5–1 mg. Chlorphenesin (Maolate) is used infrequently for trigeminal neuralgia, but has been reported to be effective in some patients. The dose ranged from 800 to 2400 mg/day (6).

NEUROSURGICAL MANAGEMENT

Neurosurgical procedures are recommended for those patients with trigeminal neuralgia who cannot obtain satisfactory relief from medications. Denervation of the sensory part of the trigeminal nerve can stop the pain of trigeminal neuralgia. Recurrent pain sometimes develops and is more likely if the denervation is peripheral to the gasserian ganglion or if it is partial. Denervation sometimes results in a new and unpleasant dysesthetic condition (anesthesia dolorosa), which occurs more frequently if the denervation is extensive. Fortunately, partial denervation also can relieve the pain of trigeminal neuralgia, and anesthesia dolorosa is much less likely to occur. Denervation of the cornea may result in keratitis, which if severe may cause impairment of vision. Selective denervation that spares the first division can usually be accomplished, and this significantly lessens the risk of keratitis.

Peripheral Denervation

Peripheral denervation can be done either by alcohol injection or neurectomy. The supraorbital, infraorbital, and mental nerves are readily accessible for such procedures. Pain usually recurs within 18 months, and repeating the procedure is more difficult, less likely to work, and associated with an even shorter remission. Because of these drawbacks and the development of newer and more effective surgical procedures, the peripheral denervations are infrequently recommended. They may still be useful in those patients with first division trigeminal neuralgia, because supraorbital denervation will not affect the cornea.

Radiofrequency Electrocoagulation

Controlled percutaneous radiofrequency electrocoagulation (RFE) is an important development in the neurosurgical treatment of trigeminal neuralgia, because it allows for partial and selective denervation in a proximal (gasserian and retrogasserian) location (7–9). If there is recurrence, the procedure can be repeated without added risk or difficulty and with a similar excellent chance of pain relief. Because of this, RFE is the procedure of choice for most patients with trigeminal neuralgia that is intractable in spite of appropriate medical treatment. This is especially the case for those with multiple sclerosis or the elderly.

The procedure is done percutaneously in an awake patient who is sedated using neuroleptanalgesia (2.5–5 mg of droperidol and 0.05–0.1 mg of fentanyl). Nasal oxygen is given, intravenous fluids are administered, and vital signs are monitored. After prepping the face with alcohol and draping with a sterile towel, the surgeon marks Hartel coordinates on the face with a sterile marking pen. These are a point just below the medial aspect of the pupil, a point on the zygoma 3 cm anterior to the tragus, and a point 2.5–3 cm lateral to the angle of the mouth. The cannula (Radionics), with 7 mm of uninsulated tip, is directed toward the foramen ovale.

Hartel coordinates and submentovertex and lateral skull x-rays are guides for cannula placement. Approximate target points are the midpoint of the foramen ovale as seen on the submentovertex x-ray and the clivus at its junction with the petrous bone as viewed on the lateral skull film (Figs. 23.1 and 23.2). Only when position is proper as verified by both x-ray projections is slumber induced with methohexital (Brevital) and the foramen ovale penetrated.

Final placement is between 5 mm anterior and 5 mm

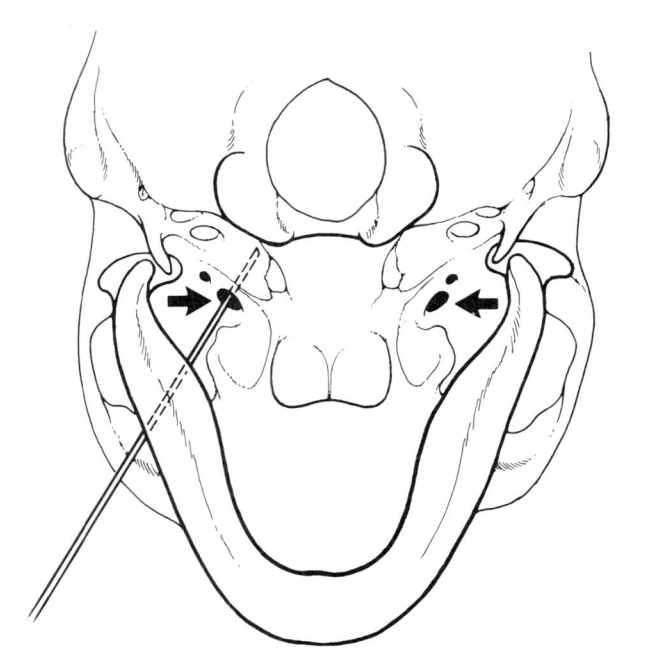

Figure 23.1. Radiofrequency electrocoagulation: Submentovertex skull x-ray shows the cannula through the foramen ovale (arrow).

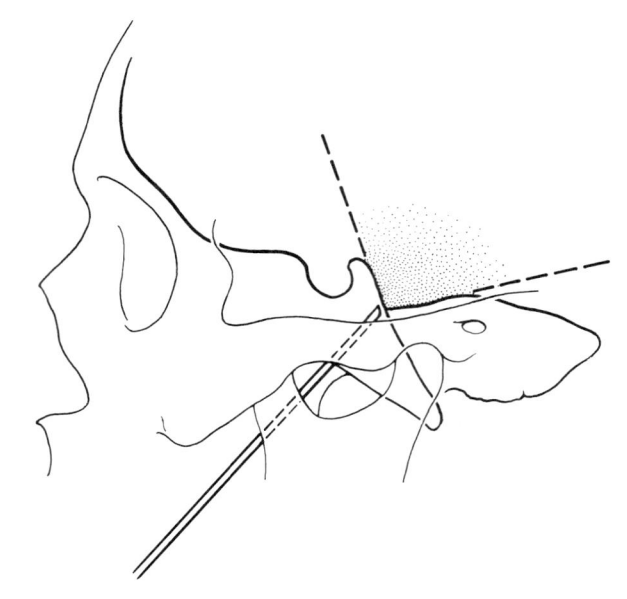

Figure 23.2. Radiofrequency electrocoagulation: Target on lateral x-ray is the angle between the petrous bone and clivus.

posterior to the clivus. First or second division lesions are easier to make if the cannula goes through the anteromedial half of the foramen ovale.

Precise localization of the specific trigeminal division desired is confirmed by very brief low-voltage stimulation at 50–100 cycles/sec in the awake patient. By advancing the cannula deeper, the surgeon can often move it from third to second or first division.

In the original descriptions of the procedure, small incremental lesions were made until analgesia developed in the division of the triggered pain (7). Since this may cause too much analgesia and hypoesthesia, with an added risk of anesthesia dolorosa, it is better to make a more modest lesion. Heating at 65°C for 60 sec will often relieve pain and will rarely cause anesthesia dolorosa or unwanted corneal anesthesia (10), although recurrence is more likely following such a denervation.

The hospital stay is usually less than 1 day. The procedure is very effective and well tolerated. Major complications with permanent morbidity are extremely rare and have not occurred at all in a consecutive series of 350 procedures done by this author.

RFE is not totally devoid of some risk of major complications. Infection may rarely occur, causing meningitis and, possibly, brain abscess. Early suspicion, diagnosis of meningitis by cerebrospinal fluid examination, and vigorous treatment with appropriate antibiotics will minimize and usually prevent permanent sequelae. A few intracerebral hemorrhages associated with hypertension have also been reported during RFE (11). Careful monitoring of blood pressure and early treatment with intravenous medication can lessen the likelihood of this unusual development.

Glycerol

Glycerol may be injected into the retrogasserian subarachnoic space with relief of trigeminal neuralgia pain (12, 13). The needle is placed in a manner similar to that used with RFE. Water-soluble contrast material may be given to identify the size of the gasserian cistern (12), or the response to electrical stimulation may help guide the final needle location (14). Although small doses of glycerol (0.15–0.25 ml) are rarely associated with profound analgesia or anesthesia dolorosa, larger doses may produce both of these.

By being prepared to use either RFE or glycerol or perhaps both, the surgeon may maximize the effectiveness of either method and minimize the risk of complications (15). If the response to electrical stimulation is in the desired division, a modest RFE (65°C for 45–60 sec) is made. If analgesia has not been produced, one more RFE at 70–75°C for 30–45 sec is performed, or instead, if there is free flow of CSF (a situation favorable for the use of glycerol), a small dose of glycerol may be injected. Sometimes the response to stimulation is not in the desired division (especially when a second division lesion is planned but only third division stimulation response is obtained even though the needle has been advanced deeper or attempts have been made to puncture the foramen ovale in a more medial location). If CSF is obtained from the cannula, 0.2–0.25 ml of glycerol may give a good result; a light RFE (60–65°C for 30–45 sec) may also be added.

When the cannula is posterior to the clivus or stimulation produces a second or first division sensation, extra caution is needed to prevent unwanted first division anesthesia. Smaller incremental lesions are indicated and the initial RFE should be at 55–60°C for 15–20 sec. Further denervation at the same electrode position should be made only after the awakened patient is tested and found not to be hypoalgesic in the first division.

Microvascular Decompression

Another important development in our understanding of trigeminal neuralgia is the recognition that a blood vessel may compress the trigeminal nerve close to its origin from the brainstem (16). This compression may cause trigeminal neuralgia, and pain relief may occur if the blood vessel can be decompressed away from the nerve (17).

There are several controversies associated with the above theory. The frequency with which such compression is found is disputed, and whereas some detect it in 100% of all patients with trigeminal neuralgia (who do not have a tumor or multiple sclerosis) (17), others find it in only 11% (18). The significance of the nerve–blood vessel relationship and the etiology of trigeminal neuralgia is also uncertain since such contacts are seen in many people who do not have trigeminal neuralgia (19). During microvascular decompression, denervation occurs in some patients, and it is not clear how much pain relief is due to denervation, decompression, or spontaneous remission—a factor that must be considered in evaluating any treatment for trigeminal neuralgia, no matter how intractable it initially appears to be.

The suboccipital craniectomy with direct exposure of the trigeminal nerve is a major neurosurgical procedure, which is done under general anesthesia with the use of the operating microscope. The lateral or three-quarter prone position is preferred. A vertical retromastoid incision is made and followed with a circular craniectomy that is 4 cm in diameter. It is important that the craniectomy extend superiorly to the transverse sinus and laterally to the sigmoid sinus. Mastoid air cells may be entered and should be waxed thoroughly. A cruciate dural incision is made.

If a three-quarter prone position was used initially, the table is now turned so that the head is lateral. This facilitates gentle retraction of the cerebellum, which is provided by a lightly applied self-retaining retractor. The initial exposure is at the superior lateral aspect of the cerebellum, which is retracted medially. The operating microscope with 275-mm objective is used.

The seventh and eighth nerves are often encountered first. The trigeminal nerve is more superior and deep, and a narrow brain retractor is required. The petrosal vein often has to be cauterized and divided. The arachnoid over the trigeminal nerve must be cut. Sometimes a blood vessel is found compressing the trigeminal nerve where it exits from the brainstem; this is usually a tortuous superior cerebellar artery. The trigeminal nerve may be surgically decompressed by placing a small prosthesis of either Ivalon foam sponge (Unipoint Industries, High Point, NC) or Telfa felt between the nerve and blood vessel. When compression is not found, the caudal third of the sensory part of the trigeminal nerve is divided close to the pons.

Although pain relief can be obtained in many patients from the suboccipital microsurgical procedure, the chance of a serious operative complication is higher than from the percutaneous techniques. Under the best of circumstances, the risk of death or severely disabling stroke from the suboccipital procedure is approximately 1–2%. Facial palsy and ipsilateral hearing loss occur more frequently. Because of this, the suboccipital operation should be reserved for those rare patients who have a posterior fossa tumor, or those few who persist with intractable trigeminal neuralgia in spite of appropriate management with medications and percutaneous procedures (radiofrequency and/or glycerol).

COMPARISON OF MANAGEMENT PROCEDURE EFFICACY

The relative value of different procedures for treatment of trigeminal neuralgia is difficult to assess because of the lack of valid concurrent controls. A number of factors will influence the apparent effectiveness of a given treatment. If recurrent pain is the measure of treatment failure, results will appear worse than if reoperation is used. Recurrent pain needs to be carefully standardized as to duration, frequency, and use of medication. The nature of the pain is also important, because patients with an atypical component to their trigeminal neuralgia may have a higher recurrence rate than those with pure trigeminal neuralgia (20). The degree of denervation (which is difficult to quantitate) must be compared in each treatment group, because patients with more denervation are less likely to develop recurrent pain. Most critical is the duration and thoroughness of follow-up; the likelihood of recurrence is increased as patients are followed for longer periods. One way to try to eliminate bias caused by losing patients from follow-up is to calculate Meier-Kaplan survival curves, which estimate probability of recurrence at specific intervals based on the actual numbers of patients available for follow-up at each interval (20–22).

ATYPICAL TRIGEMINAL NEURALGIA

Some patients with triggered, paroxysmal pain in the trigeminal distribution have the atypical feature of constant pain that persists in between the paroxysms. These patients are often helped by the medications used for trigeminal neuralgia (carbamazepine, baclofen, dilantin); if pain cannot be managed satisfactorily with medications, then RFE and/or glycerol will often help, although the results are not so reliable as with pure trigeminal neuralgia.

TRIGEMINAL NEUROPATHY

Patients with trigeminal neuropathy show signs of trigeminal nerve dysfunction, such as hypoalgesia or hypoesthesia or impairment of muscles of mastication and deviation of the opened jaw to the side of the lesion. There may also be pain in the distribution of one or more divisions of the trigeminal nerve; this pain may be paroxysmal and triggered by light touch, but sometimes is continuous and not triggered. Other nearby cranial nerves may also be involved and may cause impairment of extraocular movement, facial weakness, or eighth nerve dysfunction. Tumors, infection, granuloma, vascular abnormalities, demyelinating disease, or viral infections are sometimes responsible.

Direct neurosurgical intervention is helpful for removal of intracranial tumors involving the fifth nerve, which are often benign (epidermoid, meningioma, or neurinoma) and may be in the middle or posterior cranial fossae. Peripheral tumors that involve the trigeminal nerve at the base of the skull are usually malignant and are more likely to be associated with atypical facial pains (2). These can usually be biopsied via an otolaryngologic approach and are treated with radiotherapy.

GLOSSOPHARYNGEAL NEURALGIA

Patients with glossopharyngeal neuralgia have paroxysmal pain in the distribution of the glossopharyngeal and vagus nerves; the tonsillar pillars, base of the tongue, soft palate, and external auditory canal may also be involved (23, 24). Pain is triggered by swallowing or coughing, and temporary relief can be provided by spraying the throat with local anesthetics. Carbamazepine, baclofen, or dilantin may help.

Intractable cases are relieved by surgical denervation, which can be done via a percutaneous RFE technique (25). Denervation of the vagus nerve may produce difficulty swallowing or vocal cord paralysis. Stimulation of the vagus can cause bradycardia and hypotension. It is important to monitor the electrocardiogram and blood pressure continuously during the procedure to prevent excessive damage to the vagus nerve (26). Coagulation should be terminated at an early sign of vagal impairment; otherwise severe hypotension and even cardiac arrest could develop (27). If RFE is not successful, then intracranial section of the glossopharyngeal nerve (28) and upper rootlets of the vagus nerve (29) can be done. Some have advocated microvascular decompression (30).

GENICULATE NEURALGIA

Geniculate neuralgia has been described as pain in either the ear or the deeper structures of the face, orbit, or posterior nasal or palatal regions (31). Sometimes there is evidence of a herpetic rash in the auricle or external auditory canal, with possible facial palsy, hearing loss, vertigo, and tinnitus. Benefit from surgical section of the nervus intermedius has been reported (32, 33).

A reluctance to operate on this condition because of the uncertainty of the diagnosis and the possible damage to the seventh and eighth nerves during the surgical procedure (34) has been wisely advised. Even when the operating microscope was used, the nervus intermedius was identified as a separate nerve bundle in only one out of five cases (35).

Perhaps the best possible surgical candidates are those with paroxysmal intractable otalgia that is not satisfactorily managed with carbamazepine. Geniculate neuralgia must be differentiated from glossopharyngeal neuralgia, which can also cause otalgia, although local anesthetics in the pharynx and tonsillar area may temporarily relieve the pain of glossopharyngeal neuralgia. It has been recommended that posterior fossa surgery should be done under local anesthesia so that the nervus intermedius can be stimulated. If this reproduces the otalgia, then section of the nervus intermedius may relieve the pain (32).

It is difficult to operate in the posterior fossa under local anesthesia and maintain the patient in an alert enough state to respond reliably to electrical stimulation. An alternative that might be considered when treating a patient with intractable paroxysmal otalgia is stimulation of the ninth nerve via a percutaneous approach. If the otalgia is reproduced, then the nervus intermedius is not causing it. One could also temporarily block the ninth nerve at the same time with xylocaine or marcaine. If that relieved the pain, it would further suggest that the ninth nerve was responsible, and RFE of the ninth nerve could be carried out at the same time.

ATYPICAL FACIAL PAINS

Atypical facial pains are often continuous, not triggered, and not confined to the distribution of one cranial nerve. Depression is frequently present, and tricyclic antidepressants are appropriate. Usually there is no specific correctable underlying cause, and surgery is contraindicated because it is not likely to help and often makes the patient worse.

VASCULAR DYSFUNCTION

There are some conditions associated with face pain that are probably a result of vascular dysfunction and that respond to medications for migraine. These include cluster headache, lower-half face pain, and carotidynia. Ergotamine may abort an acute attack, and methysergide, lithium carbonate, prednisone, or propranolol may help prevent further episodes; indomethacin and calcium channel blockers may also be useful.

Cluster headache may involve the orbit and cheek as well as the head; men are usually afflicted. During an attack there are autonomic manifestations with conjunctival congestion, lacrimation, stuffiness in nasal passages and occasionally ptosis or myosis associated with facial sweating and ipsilateral erythema. During a cluster headache, patients often pace about. Pain lasts for 20 min to 2 hr and recurs for a varying number of times every day for several weeks, then disappears and returns months or years later. (Some have suggested that cluster headache is mediated by the nervus intermedius, is a form of geniculate neuralgia, and may be relieved by section of the nervus intermedius (31, 35). However, the data are not conclusive enough to make this a standard recommendation.)

Lower-half headache is more typical of migraine, except that the pain is in the face. Women are afflicted more often than men. The face pain is throbbing and unilateral and may be associated with nausea, vomiting, and photophobia. Menstruation and alcohol are frequent precipitating factors, and there is usually a family history of migraine.

Carotidynia is a syndrome of lateral neck pain with radiation to the side of the face and tenderness over the carotid artery in the neck (36, 37). The distribution of pain is not in the divisions of the trigeminal nerves, but rather along the branches of the external carotid artery. The pain is usually constant and dull, with episodes of throbbing exacerbations. Pain is aggravated by palpation of the carotid artery and sometimes by turning the neck or swallowing.

A painful condition of the internal carotid artery associated with oculosympathetic paralysis and anhidrosis of the forehead is the *"pericarotid syndrome"* (38). Pathogenetically associated conditions are migraine, cluster headache, infection, trauma, or dissecting internal carotid aneurysm; one of these is present in half the cases. In addition to treating the underlying condition when one is detected, symptomatic relief may result from the use of analgesics rather than vasoactive agents (38).

INFLAMMATORY VASCULAR DISEASES

Many patients with temporal arteritis will have pain and tenderness of the arteries of the scalp and face in addition to systemic disease, which may present with fever, malaise, anemia, or other protean manifestations (39). Vascular occlusion may cause blindness or infarction of the brain or facial structures. The elderly are affected, and the erythrocyte sedimentation rate is almost always elevated. The diagnosis is established by biopsy of the superficial temporal artery. A large segment of the artery (4–6 cm) should be obtained because pathologic abnormalities may be confined to short segments. A negative initial biopsy does not rule out the diagnosis, and contralateral biopsy is frequently positive. Corticosteroid therapy is beneficial.

Wegener's granulomatosis is associated with a systemic vasculitis but may cause pain of the paranasal sinuses, orbit, or palate (40). Cranial neuropathy, mononeuritis multiplex, and infarction or hemorrhage of the brain may occur. Immunosuppressive therapy with cyclophosphamide is often effective.

REFLEX SYMPATHETIC DYSTROPHY (14)

Facial reflex sympathetic dystrophy may follow trauma to the face. Most of these patients have a constant burning that is exacerbated by light touch. Treatment is directed at sympathetic denervation, which can be produced by oral medication (phenoxybenzamine), repeated local anesthetic blocks of the stellate ganglion, or, rarely, sympathectomy.

POSTHERPETIC NEURALGIA

As in other forms of trigeminal neuropathy, analgesia or hypoalgesia is usually present when patients have postherpetic neuralgia of the trigeminal nerve. The appearance of vesicles establishes the diagnosis. The first division of the trigeminal nerve is usually involved, and the pain is continuous and not triggered. Occasionally there is also a paroxysmal pain.

Amitriptyline provides good to excellent pain relief in 67% of patients, as demonstrated by a double-blind crossover study (42). The analgesia may be independent of the antidepressant effect. A single dose is given at bedtime, starting with 12.5–25 mg and increasing by one-half to one pill (25-mg size) every 2–5 days. Doses that are too high may sometimes result in increased pain, which is ameliorated after dose reduction.

Fluphenazine (Prolixin) (1 mg three times a day) is sometimes given in addition to amitriptyline, but the possibility of tardive dyskinesia, which may develop from the use of phenothiazines (such as fluphenazine), plus the uncertainty of the benefit of phenothiazines should temper their use.

Transcutaneous electrical nerve stimulation is a safe technique and has helped some of these patients (6); it is worth trying although it is frequently disappointing.

Neurosurgical procedures are rarely helpful but may be considered if there is a paroxysmal, triggered component in a patient who is not analgesic.

THALAMIC PAIN

Thalamic infarction can result in hemisensory dysfunction with agonizing, burning pain in the face as well as the rest of the body contralateral to the thalamic lesion. Tricyclic antidepressants and transcutaneous electrical nerve stimulation (6) sometimes help. The pain may persist in spite of all treatment.

EAGLE'S SYNDROME (ELONGATED STYLOID PROCESS)

Two clinical syndromes have been attributed to an elongated styloid process. The first "typical" form occurs after tonsillectomy and includes a sensation of a foreign body in the pharynx, pain in the ear, dysphagia, and a persistent sore throat (43). The second "atypical" syndrome is similar to that described for carotidynia (44). Tenderness in the distribution of the symptomatic pain is precipitated by palpation in the tonsillar fossa, and local anesthetics in this area abolish the pain temporarily. Panoramic radiographs demonstrate the elongated styloid process. Surgical reduction of the styloid process has been recommended if symptoms are severe (43, 44).

In a recent study (45), it was shown that the radiologic finding of elongated styloid process and/or ossification of the stylomandibular or stylohyoid ligaments occurred in about 30% of edentulous patients. There was a statistically significant relationship between facial pain and pain on turning the neck and radiologic evidence of anatomic aberrations in the styloid-stylohyoid complex. This relation existed only in women and could not be demonstrated for the other Eagle symptoms of pain on swallowing or tinnitus. The authors concluded that the finding of elongated styloid processes is of minor clinical importance.

SINUS DISEASE

Chronic sinus disease does not usually cause face pain, although an expanding mass can produce a dull aching sensation. Sinus disease is much more likely to cause pain when it is acute. The pain of acute sinusitis is usually in the overlying face, which is often tender, although it may be referred in acute maxillary sinusitis to the eye or teeth. Acute involvement of the frontal sinus causes pain in the forehead, and acute ethmoiditis causes pain in the bridge of the nose and between and behind the eyes. Infection requires treatment with appropriate antibiotics; surgical drainage is sometimes necessary.

TEMPOROMANDIBULAR JOINT DISEASE (46, 47)

Face pain and disturbance of mandibular movement are characteristic of myofascial pain dysfunction (MPD) and temporomandibular joint (TMJ) dysfunction. The pain is a unilateral aching in the jaw with radiation to the face, ear, temple, and occasionally the lateral cervical or retroorbital region. Tenderness may be in the muscles of mastication (MPD) or joint (TMJ). In only a few patients with pain, impaired mandibular movement, and tenderness are there organic abnormalities of the joint as demonstrated by imaging techniques; the term TMJ disease is restricted to these. TMJ disease may be caused by degenerative or rheumatoid arthritis, trauma, infection, or neoplasm; ankylosis or chronic dislocation may be present.

Treatment should usually be as conservative as possible. Excessive muscle contraction, if present, may be relieved by massage, moist heat, muscle-relaxing exercises, biofeedback, or psychological counseling. Obvious malocclusion should be corrected by dental maneuvers. Nonnarcotic analgesics, anti-inflammatory agents, antidepressants, muscle relaxants, and minor tranquilizers may be helpful. Some recommend local injections of trigger points in spastic muscles or intra-articular injections. Major surgical procedures on the joint may be required, but only for those rare patients with very advanced disease.

CARCINOMA

Malignant tumors of the face may cause pain that can usually be relieved by direct surgical excision and/or radiotherapy. Analgesics are appropriate, including narcotics, if nonnarcotic analgesics are not effective and life span is limited.

For patients with agonizing pain that cannot be satisfactorily relieved with medication, neurosurgical procedures can be considered. Ablative maneuvers to denervate the trigeminal nerve are appropriate if pain is confined to the distribution of the trigeminal nerve. Pain in the throat or pharynx may require denervation of the ninth and tenth cranial nerves, and pain in the auditory canal may possibly be helped by interruption of the nervus intermedius. When pain involves the neck, section of the appropriate cranial nerves may be combined with dorsal rhizotomies of C1–C4. Trigeminal tractotomy and thalamotomy have also been recommended. Deep brain stimulation (ventralis posteromedialis) combines the advantage of a small thalamotomy during passage of the stimulating electrode and the analgesic benefits of neuroaugmentation. Intraventricular infusion of small doses of morphine has also been reported to be effective in some of these patients (48).

SUMMARY

A careful multidisciplinary diagnostic evaluation of the patient with face pain may help direct attention to a specific condition such as infection, inflammation, malocclusion, or, rarely, neoplasm, for which precise treatment can be directed. It is helpful to recognize the paroxysmal, triggered, episodic, and usually trigeminal neuralgic pain that responds so exquisitely to carbamazepine and neurosurgical procedures, for those who cannot tolerate or are no longer helped by medication. Most other pains are called atypical (constant, burning or aching, not triggered, and frequently beyond the confines of one cranial nerve). These are often associated with depression, which should be treated, and are sometimes accompanied by myofascial or vascular dysfunction.

References

1. Rushton JG, Olafson RA: Trigeminal neuralgia associated with multiple sclerosis: report of 35 cases. *Arch Neurol* 13:383–386, 1965.

2. Bullitt E, Tew JM, Boyd J: Intracranial tumors in patients with facial pain. *J Neurosurg* 64:865–871, 1986.
3. Blom S: Trigeminal neuralgia: its treatment with a new anticonvulsant drug (G-32883). *Lancet* 1:839–840, 1962.
4. Rockliff BW, Davies EH: Controlled sequential trials of carbamazepine in trigeminal neuralgia. *Arch Neurol* 15:129–136, 1966.
5. Fromm GH, Terrence CF, Chattha AS: Baclofen in the treatment of trigeminal neuralgia: double-blind study and long-term follow-up. *Ann Neurol* 15:240–244, 1984.
6. Dalessio DJ: The major neuralgias, postinfectious neuritis, intractable pain, and atypical facial pain. In Dalessio DJ (ed): *Wolff's Headache and Other Head Pain*, ed 4. New York, Oxford University Press, 1980, pp 233–255.
7. Sweet WH, Wepsic JG: Controlled thermocoagulation of trigeminal ganglion and rootlets for differential destruction of pain fibers: Part 1. Trigeminal neuralgia. *J Neurosurg* 39:143–156, 1974.
8. Nugent GR, Berry B: Trigeminal neuralgia treated by differential percutaneous radiofrequency coagulation of the Gasserian ganglion. *J Neurosurg* 40:517–523, 1974.
9. Tew JM, Tobler WD: Percutaneous rhizotomy in the treatment of intractable facial pain (trigeminal, glossopharyngeal, and vagal nerves). In Schmidek HH, Sweet WH (eds): *Operative Neurosurgical Techniques* New York, Grune & Stratton, 1982, vol 2, pp 1083–1106.
10. Salar G, Mingrino S, Iob I: Alterations of facial sensitivity induced by percutaneous thermocoagulation for trigeminal neuralgia. *Surg Neurol* 19:126–130, 1983.
11. Sweet WH, Poletti CE, Roberts JT: Dangerous rises in blood pressure upon heating of trigeminal rootlets; increased bleeding times in patients with trigeminal neuralgia. *Neurosurgery* 17:843–844, 1985.
12. Hakanson S: Trigeminal neuralgia treated by the injection of glycerol into the trigeminal cistern. *Neurosurgery* 9:638–646, 1981.
13. Lunsford LD, Bennett MH: Percutaneous retrogasserian glycerol rhizotomy for tic douloureux: Part 1. Technique and results in 112 patients. *Neurosurgery* 14:424–430, 1984.
14. Sweet WH, Poletti CE, Macon JB: Treatment of trigeminal neuralgia and other facial pains by retrogasserian injection of glycerol. *Neurosurgery* 9:647–653, 1981.
15. Brisman R: Treatment of trigeminal neuralgia: radiofrequency electrocoagulation with/without glycerol. *Contemp Neurosurg* 8(3):1–5, 1986.
16. Dandy WE: Concerning the cause of trigeminal neuralgia. *Am J Surg* 24:447–455, 1934.
17. Janetta PJ: Microsurgical approach to the trigeminal nerve for tic douloureux. *Prog Neurol Surg* 7:180–200, 1976.
18. Adams CB, Kaye AH, Teddy PJ: The treatment of trigeminal neuralgia by posterior fossa microsurgery. *J Neurol Neurosurg Psychiatry* 45:1020–1026, 1982.
19. Hardy DG, Rhoton AL Jr: Microsurgical relationships of the superior cerebellar artery and the trigeminal nerve. *J Neurosurg* 49:669–678, 1978.
20. Latchaw JP, Hardy RW, Forsythe SB, Cook AF: Trigeminal neuralgia treated by radiofrequency coagulation. *J Neurosurg* 59:479–484, 1983.
21. Lee ET: *Statistical Methods for Survival Data Analysis.* Belmont, CA, Lifetime Learning Publications, 1980, pp 75–156.
22. Piatt JH Jr, Wilkins RH: Treatment of tic douloureux and hemifacial spasm by posterior fossa exploration: therapeutic implications of various neurovascular relationships. *Neurosurgery* 14:462–471, 1984.
23. Weisenburg TH: Cerebello-pontile tumor diagnosed for six years as tic douloureux. The symptoms of irritation of the ninth and twelfth cranial nerves. *JAMA* 54:1600–1604, 1910.
24. Harris W: Persistent pain in lesions of the peripheral and central nervous system. *Brain* 44:557–571, 1921.
25. Lazorthes Y, Verdie JC: Radiofrequency coagulation of the petrous ganglion in glossopharyngeal neuralgia. *Neurosurgery* 4:512–516, 1979.
26. Isamat F, Ferran E, Acebes JJ: Selective percutaneous thermocoagulation rhizotomy in essential glossopharyngeal neuralgia. *J Neurosurg* 23:575–580, 1981.
27. Ori C, Salar G, Giron G: Percutaneous glossopharyngeal thermocoagulation complicated by syncope and seizures. *Neurosurgery* 13:427–429, 1983.
28. Dandy WE: Glossopharyngeal neuralgia (tic douloureux). Its diagnosis and treatment. *Arch Surg* 15:198–214, 1927.
29. Robson JT, Bonica J: The vagus nerve in surgical consideration of glossopharyngeal neuralgia. *J Neurosurg* 7:482–484, 1950.
30. Laha RK, Jannetta PJ: Glossopharyngeal neuralgia. *J Neurosurg* 47:316–320, 1977.
31. Hunt JR: Geniculate neuralgia (neuralgia of the nervus facialis); a further contribution to the sensory system of the facial nerve and its neuralgic conditions. *Arch Neurol Psychiatry* 37:253–285, 1937.
32. Furlow LT: Tic douloureux of the nervus intermedius (so-called idiopathic geniculate neuralgia). *JAMA* 119:255–259, 1942.
33. Wilson AA: Geniculate neuralgia; report of a case relieved by intracranial section of the nerve of Wrisberg. *J Neurosurg* 7:473–481, 1950.
34. Stookey B, Ransohoff J: Geniculate ganglion neuralgia. In *Trigeminal Neuralgia: Its History and Treatment.* Springfield, IL, Charles C Thomas, 1959, pp 111–119.
35. Solomon S, Apfelbaum RI: Surgical decompression of the facial nerve in the treatment of chronic cluster headache. *Arch Neurol* 43:479–481, 1986.
36. Fay T: Atypical facial neuralgia, a syndrome of vascular pain. *Ann Otol Rhinol Laryngol* 41:1030–1062, 1932.
37. Orfei R, Meienberg O: Carotidynia: report of eight cases and prospective evaluation of therapy. *J Neurol* 230:65–72, 1983.
38. Vijayan N, Watson C: Pericarotid syndrome. *Headache* 18:244–254, 1978.
39. Goodman BW: Temporal arteritis. *Am J Med* 67:839–852, 1979.
40. Wolff SM, Fauci AS, Horn RG, Dale DC: Wegener's granulomatosis. *An Intern Med* 81:513–525, 1974.
41. Jaeger B, Singer E, Kroening R: Reflex sympathetic dystrophy of the face. Report of two cases and a review of the literature. *Arch Neurol* 43:693–695, 1986.
42. Watson CP, Evans RJ, Reed K, et al: Amitriptyline versus placebo in postherpetic neuralgia. *Neurology* 32:671–673, 1982.
43. Eagle WW: Elongated styloid process: report of two cases. *Arch Otolaryngol* 25:584–587, 1937.
44. Eagle WW: Elongated styloid process: further observations and a new syndrome. *Arch Otolaryngol* 47:630–640, 1948.
45. Keur JJ, Campbell JPS, McCarthy JF, Ralph WJ: The clinical significance of the elongated styloid process. *Oral Surg* 61:399–404, 1986.
46. Booth DF, Hagens GA, Altshuler JL: Facial pain. In Aronoff

GM (ed): *Evaluation and Treatment of Chronic Pain.* Baltimore, Urban & Schwarzenberg, 1985, pp 131–147.

47. Guralnick W, Kaban LB, Merrill RG: Temporomandibular-joint afflictions. Medical progress. *N Engl J Med* 299:123–129, 1978.

48. Lenzi A, Galli G, Gandolfini M, Marini G: Intraventricular morphine in paraneoplastic painful syndrome of the cervico-facil region: experience in thirty-eight cases. *Neurosurgery* 17:6–11, 1985.

chapter 24
Dental Management of Orofacial Pain

Jerome D. Buxbaum, D.D.S., F.A.D.G.
Norbert R. Myslinski, Ph.D.
Daniel E. Myers, D.D., M.S.

Traditionally, discussions of nociception and pain as applied to the orofacial area have been fragmented and to a degree confusing. Part of the problem stems from the fact that some pathologic entities have, over the years, been given several different names. The more significant part of the problem is due to the inability of the professions to compartmentalize the vast array of pathologies that may produce similar symptomatologies. As this is written, well over 100 pathologic and psychological entities have manifestations of orofacial discomfort (1). One of the aims of the authors is to attempt to organize this material in a logical and cogent manner so that the physician and dentist can easily utilize it to the betterment of their patients. To accomplish this purpose the chapter is divided into four sections: (a) basic information, (b) temporomandibular dysfunction (TMD), (c) other orofacial pathologies, and (d) systemic pathologies that may produce orofacial pain.

It may seem simplistic to say so, but the single most important factor in the management of the orofacial pain patient is proper diagnosis. Yet the authors' clinical experience has shown, and the literature supports the fact, that most orofacial patients have consulted multiple health specialists and have been treated without benefit of a reasonable workup and diagnosis (2). It is not within the scope of this chapter to discuss diagnostic procedures in detail. It is appropriate to state that most orofacial chronic pain is multifactorial and requires the expertise of a team of health specialists to reach an accurate diagnosis and appropriate treatment plan. This chapter focuses on the dentist's role in chronic orofacial pain. It emphasizes the importance of cooperation and interaction between the dentist and other medical specialists in the diagnosis and management of the chronic orofacial pain patient.

On the basis of the above statements, it is not surprising that a significant percentage of these patients have been subjected to nociceptive and/or pain sensations for extended periods of time. Patients with pain of longer than 6 months' duration become classified as "chronic pain" patients. The autonomic, psychological, and therapeutic responses of these patients are markedly different from those of the acute pain patient. Even the nerve fiber pathway for acute nociception is different from the pathway for chronic pain. Indeed, the chronic pain symptoms may persist long after the alleviation of the etiologic pathology (3). Hendler et al. have classified the characteristic differences between the acute and chronic pain patient, and Table 24.1 is a summary of these differences (3).

It is reasonable at this point for the authors to briefly state their definitions of nociception and pain. Mersky (4) defined pain as

> an unpleasant sensory and emotional experience associated with actual or potential tissue damage, or described in terms of such damage. Pain is always subjective. Each individual learns the application of the word through experiences related to injury in early life. It is unquestionably a sensation in a part of the body, but it is also always unpleasant and, therefore, also an emotional experience.

Table 24.1
Characteristics of Acute and Chronic Pain

Characteristic	Acute	Chronic
Onset	Current	Continuous or intermittent
Duration	Less than 6 months	6 months or more
Autonomic responses	Increased heart rate Increased stroke volume Increased blood pressure Pupillary dilation Increased muscle tension Decreased gut motility Decreased salivary flow Flight-or-fight response	Habituation of autonomic responses
Psychological aspects	Anxiety modified by cortical response; screening tests normal	Increased irritability Associated depression Somatic preoccupation Withdrawn from outside interests Decreased strength of relationships Occupational disability
Other changes	Screening tests are normal	Decreased sleep Decreased libido Appetite changes Screening tests abnormal
Responsive to analgesic medication	Responsive	Not responsive

There have been several theories proposed over the years in an effort to explain the many clinically observed aspects of "pain." One of these, the specificity theory, proposes that a pattern of specific pain receptors in the body tissues project to a brain center devoted to the sensation of pain. If we say that a specific sensory receptor responds to liminal noxious stimulation, it is a physiologic statement. To term this receptor a "pain" receptor is a psychological assumption. The former statement carries the concept that there is a direct connection from the receptor to a cortical area where pain is perceived. It further implies that stimulation of the receptor must always elicit the sensation of pain and only pain. At present there is no substantive evidence to support the position that there is a special class of receptor-fiber units that are exclusively devoted to the detection and transmission of a "pain" modality. Burgess and Perl have discovered a small class of A-delta fibers that are specific for nociception (5). However, this small fiber group could not begin to account for the overall pain response.

There are, however, a broad spectrum of receptor-fiber units that are capable of responding to tissue injury. These receptors can physiologically be termed nociceptors, and their associated fibers nociceptive fibers. We therefore have nociceptive receptors but not pain receptors. If nociception is a response to tissue injury, what is pain? Pain is always a psychological event. The impulses in the nociceptive fibers are no more "pain" than the visual impulses from the retina are the perceptual impression of color and pattern that present to us when we have our eyes open. Pain is, in part, the psychological response to nociceptive perception. However, pain can exist without any demonstrable tissue injury (6, 7).

Epidemiologic studies of orofacial pain in a number of countries of the world have shown striking agreement. These studies indicate that approximately 50% of the population displays one or more of the symptoms associated with orofacial pathology (8). The problem of chronic orofacial pain is therefore significant in scope and challenging to solution.

PHYSIOLOGIC BACKGROUND FOR OROFACIAL PAIN TREATMENT

OROFACIAL PERIPHERAL NERVES

The orofacial nociceptor fibers are found mainly in the trigeminal (fifth) nerve. However, other cranial nerves contribute to the orofacial nociceptive spectrum. These include the facial (seventh) nerve, with receptors in the deep face; the glossopharyngeal (ninth) nerve, with receptors in the middle ear and pharynx; and the vagus (tenth) nerve, with receptors in the external auditory meatus.

The trigeminal nerve consists of three divisions: the ophthalmic, the maxillary, and the mandibular, each with many important branches (Fig. 24.1). The ophthalmic nerve is the smallest of the three divisions and has three main branches: the lacrimal, nasociliary, and frontal nerves. The branches of the maxillary nerve are the palatine, zygomatic, infraorbital, and superior dental nerves. After giving off the nervus spinosus the mandibular nerve separates into anterior and posterior parts. The anterior part gives off the masseteric, deep temporal, lateral pterygoid, and buccal nerves. The posterior part gives off the auriculotemporal, lingual, inferior dental, incisor, and mental nerves.

Figure 24.1. Trigeminal innervation.

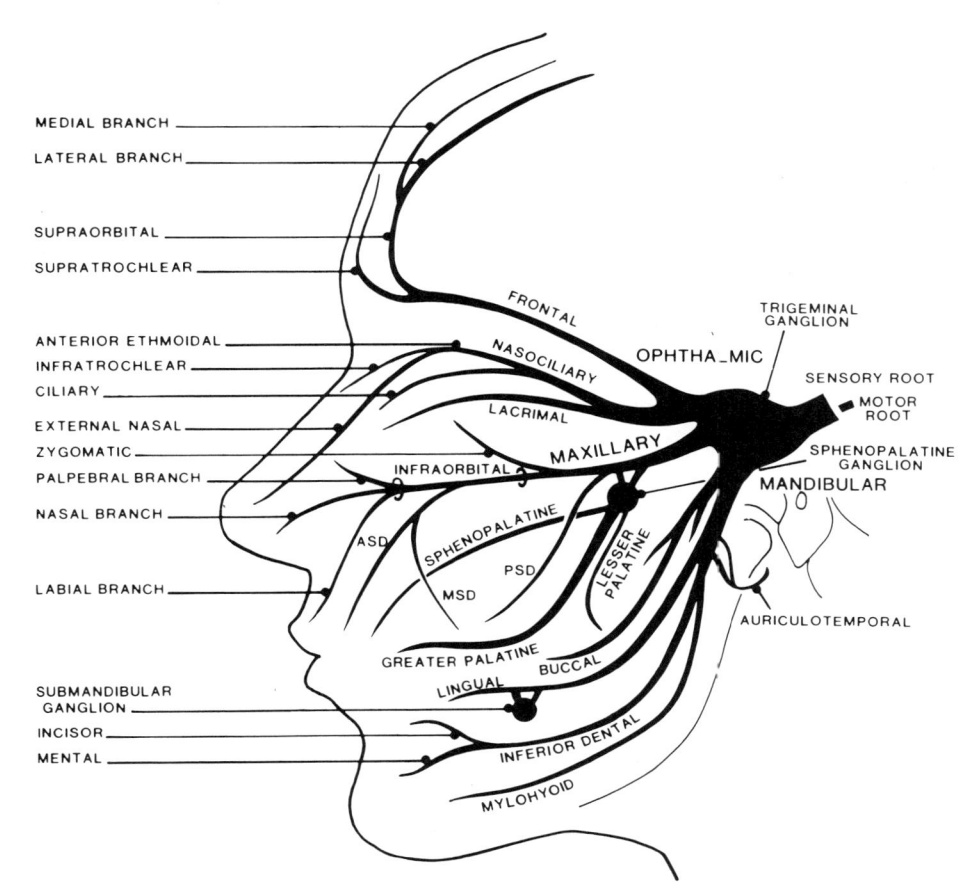

OROFACIAL CENTRAL PATHWAYS (FIG. 24.2)
First-Order Neurons

There are many similarities between the orofacial nociceptive system and that already described for the rest of the body. The primary afferents of the orofacial region have nonmyelinated (C fiber range) and thinly myelinated (A-delta fiber range) peripheral processes that function as dendrites. The C fibers are polymodal nociceptive afferents, whereas the A-deltas are divided into two groups: the high-threshold mechanoreceptive afferents and the heat-nociceptive afferents.

The trigeminal nerve differs from the spinal nerves in a number of respects. It has a higher ratio of myelinated to unmyelinated fibers, a higher density of nociceptors (especially around the mouth and nose), and shorter conduction distances. The last point leads to differences in the temporal dispersion of afferent activity reaching the central nervous system, which probably accounts for the absence of human reports of first and second pain sensations on the face (9).

The cell bodies of the first-order neurons are small and medium-sized pseudounipolar cells. They are located in the semilunar (gasserian) ganglion of the trigeminal nerve, which lies in a depression on the petrous portion of the temporal bone where it is situated lateral to the internal carotid artery and the posterior end of the cavernous venous sinus. These cell bodies are also located in the geniculate ganglion of the facial nerve, the superior ganglion of the glossopharyngeal nerve, and the superior ganglion of the vagus nerve.

The central or proximal processes enter the brainstem and bend inferiorly to form a distinct bundle, the spinal tract of the trigeminal nerve. This tract descends ipsilaterally through the pons and medulla to end in the third or fourth cervical segment. As it descends, its fibers pass to the spinal nucleus (or descending nucleus), which lies medial to it. Here they synapse in the substantia gelatinosa (laminae II and III) and the more superficial marginal layer (lamina I).

The spinal nucleus is divided into the subnucleus oralis (or rostralis), subnucleus interpolaris, and subnucleus

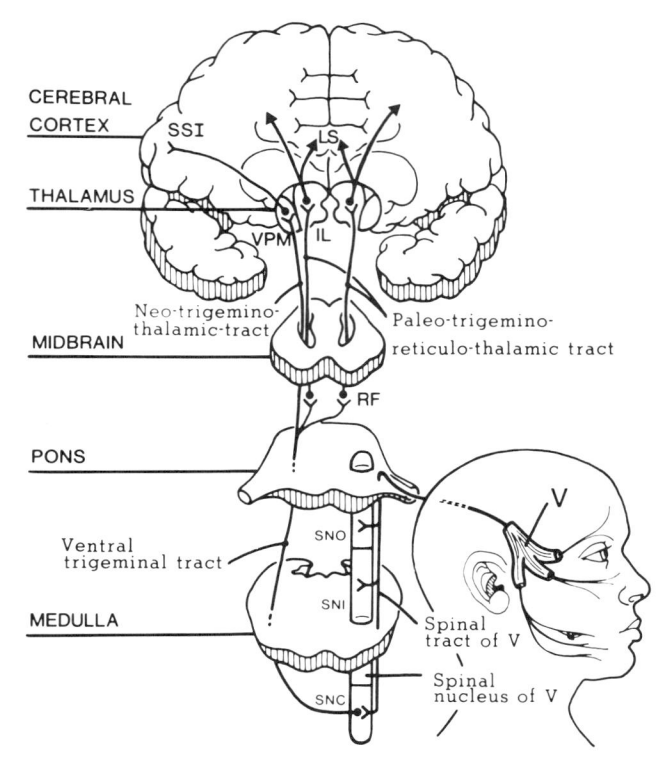

Figure 24.2. Central nervous system pain pathways. SNC = subnucleus caudalis, SNI = subnucleus interpolaris, SNO = subnucleus oralis, RF = reticular formation, VPM = ventral posteromedial nucleus, IL = intralaminar nucleus, LS = limbic system, SSI = somatosensory cortex I.

caudalis. The subnucleus caudalis extends into the spinal cord and merges with the dorsal horn. Nociception is primarily relayed in the subnucleus caudalis, whereas tactile sensibility is primarily relayed in the more rostral subnucleus oralis and main sensory nuclei. Anatomic studies show that the superficial laminae of the subnucleus caudalis almost exclusively receive the small-diameter afferent fibers that can be stimulated by noxious orofacial stimuli. This anatomic arrangement is the basis for the trigeminal tractotomy operation, which is used for the relief of trigeminal neuralgia (10). The operation selectively interrupts the smaller fibers that extend caudal to the subnucleus caudalis but leaves intact the larger fibers that leave the spinal tract earlier to synapse in the more rostral sections of the trigeminal sensory complex. This produces an almost complete loss of orofacial pain sensibility but a less dramatic loss of touch. In the spinal tract the nerve fibers derived from the mandibular division of the trigeminal nerve run posteromedially, fibers from the opthalmic division run laterally, and the maxillary division fibers run in between (11). This arrangement is constant, and allows for selective cutting during tractotomies.

Tooth pulp afferent fibers are different in that they project to all levels of the trigeminal spinal nucleus (12, 13). Whereas relay through the subnucleus caudalis is important for the transmission of nociception to higher centers, the importance of the relay through the subnucleus oralis and the main sensory nucleus is controversial and much less clear. Tooth pulp afferent fibers may be involved in the localization and discrimination of pulpal stimuli in referred pain mechanisms, or in reflex responses to pulpal stimuli. They may also be involved in nonnociceptive input, or "prepain," since it is now known that pain is not the only sensation experienced in stimulating human teeth, as was once thought. This is especially reasonable since Hu and Sessle (14) found that the larger tooth pulp fibers go to the main sensory nucleus and the subnucleus oralis.

Second-Order Neurons

There are two general types of nociceptive neurons in the subnucleus caudalis. One type consist of nociceptive-specific neurons that respond exclusively to noxious mechanical and thermal stimuli. The second type are the wide dynamic range neurons that respond to nonnoxious as well as noxious stimuli. Tooth pulp stimuli can activate not only both types of nociceptive neurons, but also the low-threshold mechanoreceptive neurons, which otherwise are only responsive to light touch, pressure, or facial hair movement.

These two types of nociceptive neurons are excellent candidates for the transmission cells described in the gate control theory of Melzack and Wall (15). They receive input from the nociceptive and nonnociceptive afferents, and mechanisms of convergence, central summation, inhibition, and descending control determine what sensory messages are relayed by these neurons.

These nociceptive neurons exist particularly in the superficial (layers I to III) and deep (layer V) parts of the subnucleus caudalis and in the adjacent reticular formation. From these locations some of the neurons connect with cranial nerve motor nuclei or other subnuclei of the sensory complex. Others make up two major secondary pathways that cross ventromedial to the contralateral side and ascend to higher centers in the trigeminal lemniscus. These two trigeminothalamic pathways are analogous to the neo- and paleospinothalamic pathways that originate from the lower centers.

The neotrigeminothalamic pathway is epicritic in nature. It transmits information concerning sharp, pricking pain that is highly discriminative and localizable. It conveys this information in a point-to-point fashion to the medial part of the ventroposterior thalamic nucleus.

The paleotrigeminoreticulothalamic pathway is protopathic in nature. Its messages are consciously translated as poorly localized sensations usually described as aching or burning pain. It is this pathway that is most involved in chronic pain of the orofacial region. Some of this information goes directly to the intralaminar nuclei of the thalamus. The rest goes to two different zones of the reticular formation. The first zone is the lateral reticular formation lying immediately subjacent to the subnucleus caudalis. The second is the medial reticular formation, which receives convergent high-intensity input from all over the body and is responsible for the alerting response. This processed information is in turn transmitted to the intralaminar nuclei of the thalamus. The fact that input to this area is widely spread is of tremendous importance in the treatment of chronic pain. It means that impulses mediating pain can find a way around any localized destruction that the surgeon might produce.

Third-Order Neurons

The cell bodies of the thalamus and their ascending axons make up third-order neurons. The axons from the ventroposterior thalamic nucleus pass through the internal limb of the internal capsule and corona radiata to terminate in the inferior portion (face area) of the postcentral gyrus of the parietal lobe (areas 3, 2, and 1). The orofacial region has a disproportionately large area of neuronal representation in the somatosensory cortex, thus producing a high level of sensory discrimination for this region. The intralaminar thalamic nuclei are at the origin of the diffuse thalamocortical projection system, which serves to activate (desynchronize) the whole cortex, except the primary sensory and motor areas.

There are research data on nonhuman mammals to indicate a tooth pulp projection area within the face area of the primary somatosensory cortex. These neurons activated by pulp stimulation are located in deep cortex in the base of the central sulcus, and are of three types: those activated from one pulp alone, those activated from more than one pulp, and those activated from one pulp and its adjacent soft tissue (16, 17).

However, electrical stimulation of the cortex in conscious humans does not often lead to a feeling of pain (18). Penfield and Boldrey (19) found that out of more than 800 responses to direct electrical stimulation of the cortex only 11 were described as pain and none were of pain in the jaws or teeth. It is not yet possible to say at what anatomic level impulses from nociceptive stimuli reach consciousness and become pain. What happens in the cortex is complex and not well understood, but probably pain is localized and interpreted here, and evaluated in terms of past experiences.

Orofacial nociceptive information is also transmitted to the limbic system, mainly by way of the reticular formation. This system is largely responsible for the affective components of pain, including fear and aversion.

TOOTH INNERVATION (FIG. 24.3)

The teeth are innervated primarily by the maxillary and mandibular branches of the trigeminal nerve. Muscle nerves such as the mylohyoid may be involved, and may be responsible for the incomplete anesthesia of the inferior dental and buccal nerves. Anatomic observations of the pulp have indicated unmyelinated as well as myelinated fibers. The myelinated fibers are mainly A-deltas, but A-betas have also been found. As for the unmyelinated fibers, there is still no physiologic evidence that they are nociceptive afferents. They may be autonomic efferent fibers that regulate the pulpal vasculature, or the unmyelinated pulpal component of the nerve fibers that are myelinated outside the pulp.

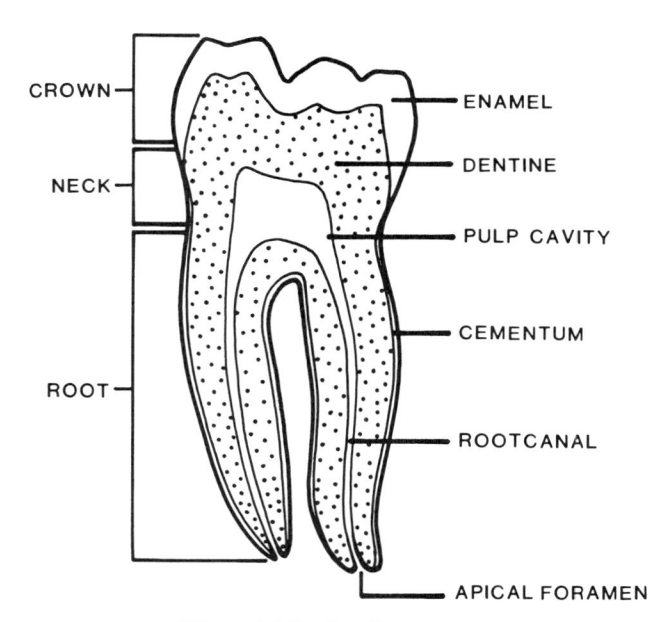

Figure 24.3. Tooth anatomy.

Both the deciduous and permanent teeth have similar innervation densities; however, their numbers are not constant throughout life. A marked decrease in numbers of nerve fibers occurs during root resorption in deciduous teeth, and with age in permanent teeth. Pulp nerve degeneration is also associated with caries and poor dental restorations.

Although most tooth pain is acute, chronic pain can occur in both the pulp and dentine with such conditions as chronic pulpitis or cracked tooth syndrome.

TOOTH PULP

Nerve fibers enter the tooth via the apical foramen. They form a common pulpal nerve and proceed coronally through the radicular pulp, dividing several times. Some fibers terminate in the pulp proper, but many spread out toward the roof and walls of the coronal pulp and branch repeatedly on approaching the cell-free zone of Weil. Many fibers continue into the odontoblastic layer, and some may even proceed into the predentine and dentine.

Electrophysiologic recordings from the inferior dental nerve, the trigeminal ganglion, and the tooth itself have revealed that pulpal nerve fibers can be excited by a number of stimuli, including thermal, osmotic, electric, and chemical (20). It is still not clear whether the response of single pulpal afferents is nonspecific or specific for one form of stimulation.

The response of pulpal nerve fibers to thermal stimulation can be quite effective and is sometimes of a rhythmic nature, very similar to the throbbing seen with many types of toothaches. If a heat stimulus is repeated a number of times prolonged afferent neural discharges can occur, which may suggest sensitization or damage to the pulp.

Like most other neural afferents in the body, the pulp afferents are sensitive to the chemical serotonin (5-hydroxytryptamine). However, unlike the others the pulp afferents are relatively insensitive to such endogenous chemicals as histamine, bradykinin, and substance P. Electrical stimulation is used clinically in pulp vitality testers. Unfortunately, many pulp testers do not deliver reproducible stimuli. The stimuli may also go beyond the pulpal tissue and produce pain by stimulating the periodontium. Nonvital teeth could therefore respond falsely to the pulp tester. There also does not seem to be any correlation between electrical stimuli thresholds and the extent of pathology in the tooth. Bipolar, constant-current stimulators have been shown to produce less spread of excitation to extrapulpal tissues than the monopolar, constant-voltage stimulators (21).

TOOTH DENTINE

In the past it has been very difficult to histologically preserve and identify neural elements of the tooth. Distinguishing them from connective tissue and odontoblastic processes has also been difficult. For these reasons there has been a prolonged controversy as to whether or not nerve fibers enter the dentine. Based on transsection/degeneration experiments and retrograde transport of radioactive material, it is now accepted that they enter the inner layer of the dentine. There is still doubt, however, about how far they extend beyond that. Also, it is possible that some of these intradental nerve fibers are autonomic efferents that serve neurotrophic or metabolic support functions, and not afferents at all. Gap junctions have been identified in the odontoblastic zone that may involve neural elements or odontoblasts or both. The existence of coupled nerve fibers is supported by the finding that sending a nerve impulse into the tooth antidromically may result in an orthodromic impulse in another nerve fiber (22).

Another controversy that has not yet been resolved concerns the basis for dentinal sensation. The neural theory, the odontoblastic transduction theory, and the hydrodynamic theory are all important attempts at explaining the mechanism of dentinal sensitivity (Fig. 24.4). The neural theory assumes that the intradentinal nerve fibers are in fact afferent fibers and that they are the morphologic substrate for dentinal sensitivity to enamel or dentinal stimuli. This is supported by electrophysiologic recordings of dentinal activity that disappears after transsection of the inferior alveolar nerve (23). Contrary evidence includes the lack of intradental nerve fibers in deciduous teeth and the enamel-dentine junction, which are both nonetheless clinically sensitive. Also, a number of substances that normally either block or activate nociceptors have no effect when applied to the dentine. The odontoblast transduction theory attributes an active role to the odontoblast, which transmits its own excitation to adjacent nerve fibers. The neural chest origin of the odontoblast and its apparent tight gap relationship with nerve fibers are supporting evidence.

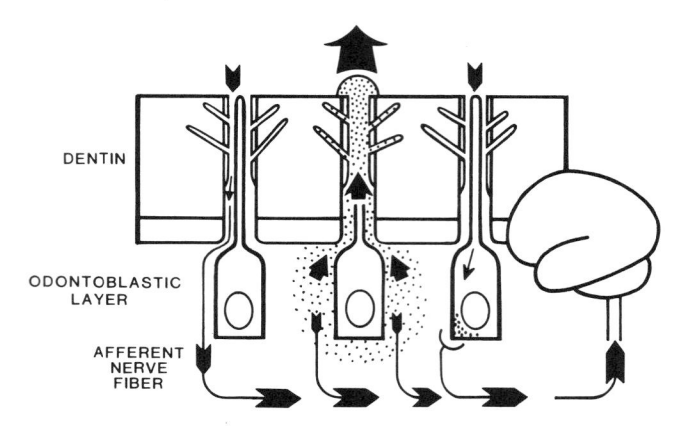

Figure 24.4. Three main theories of dentinal sensitivity.

Probably the most accepted theory is the hydrodynamic theory (24). It is based on in vitro findings regarding pressure changes produced in the pulp and on fluid flow through capillary tubes sealed in the pulps of recently extracted teeth. The theory states that stimuli to the enamel or dentine cause an outward or inward flow of dentinal tubular contents. This perturbation is transmitted to the pulp, causing a mechanical displacement that excites the pulpal nerve fibers. Most painful stimuli, whether drilling, air, temperature changes, osmotic changes, or the like, cause a change in flow. However, the amount of flow change is not always correlated with the pain, and certain substances that do not cause pain cause changes in flow. Clearly the controversy is not resolved, and possibly parts of all these theories could be true.

OROFACIAL ANALGESIC SYSTEMS (FIG. 24.5)

As with other parts of the body, the brain's own pain-suppressing systems, whether they be sensory interaction or descending central control, are also effective on orofacial pain (25). Activation of large nonnociceptive fibers can suppress responses of trigeminal brainstem neurons to noxious stimuli. The trigeminal nociceptive neurons can also be suppressed by stimulation of certain brain sites, especially the periaqueductal gray matter in the midbrain

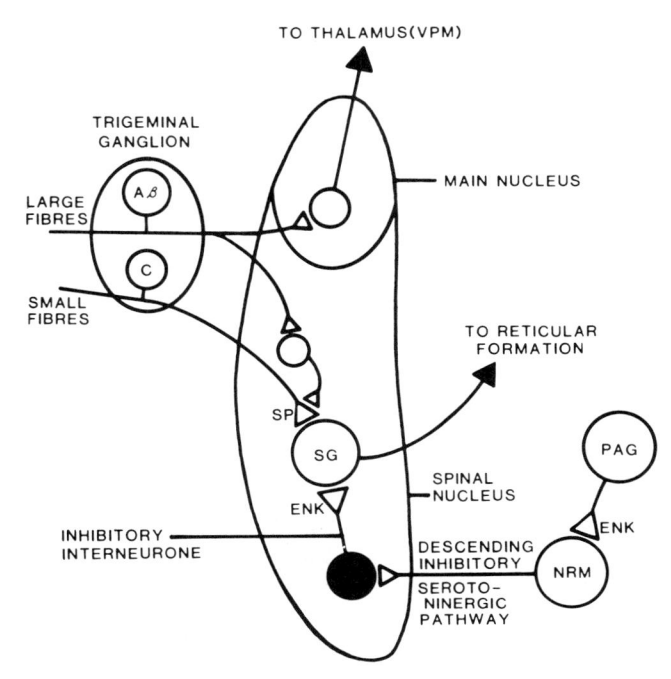

Figure 24.5. Orofacial pain inhibitory pathways. VPM = ventral posteriomedial nucleus, SP = substance P, SG = substantia gelatinosa, ENK = enkephalius, PAG = periaqueductal gray, NRM = nucleus raphe magnus.

and the nucleus raphe magnus in the medulla. The response of nociceptive neurons in the subnucleus caudalis can also be suppressed by local application of enkephalin, which is one of the neurotransmitters involved in descending pain suppression. Many important therapeutic procedures, such as narcotic analgesia, may exert their therapeutic effects by utilizing this natural pain-suppressing system. It is also suggested that dysfunction of this system may be a cause of chronic orofacial pain.

PAIN, REFERRED PROJECTED PAIN, AND NEUROMAS

REFERRED PAIN

Pain that is perceived as occurring at a site distant from the source of tissue damage is known as referred pain. Well-known clinical examples include the left arm pain of angina pectoris and the left-sided chest pain and back pain of cholelithiasis. Referred pain also occurs in the orofacial region and is all the more significant because of the large number of anatomically discrete structures in this area (not the least of which are the 32 teeth).

Although the physiologic mechanism for referred pain is not completely understood, there is some anatomic and physiologic information relevant to this phenomenon. The most widely accepted concept is that there is central convergence of multiple afferent inputs with receptive fields covering a wide area of tissue. Evidence supporting this concept comes from a study in the cat (26) that demonstrated that nociceptor-specific neurons of the trigeminal spinal nucleus receive multisynaptic input from high-threshold cervical afferents. This convergence of peripheral nociceptive input could provide a dilemma for the cortex in identifying the source of a pain. The pain may be perceived as coming from one source, the other source, or both sources.

Regardless of the mechanism, pain referred to and from dental structures is a common clinical situation, and efforts have been made to identify the locations to which pain may commonly be referred in the orofacial region. Wolff (27) electrically stimulated the teeth of volunteers in an effort to identify the sites to which pain from specific teeth may be referred. He found that stimulation of the lower posterior teeth produced a sensation of pain extending from the ipsilateral chin to the ipsilateral ear, including the posterior portion of the ipsilateral maxilla. Stimulation of the posterior maxillary teeth produced pain that was perceived in the ear, maxillary teeth and sinus, and temporal region. These results are in basic agreement with clinical experience, but there are situations in which pain may be referred to even more distant sites than those seen experimentally by Wolff. The most common clinical management problem caused by referred dental pain is in the localization of the offending tooth or other dental structure in the chronic facial pain patient. Standard endodontic tests such as percussion, palpation, thermal and electrical testing, and selective local anesthesia are extremely effective in identifying painful teeth. It is critical that teeth not be extracted without clearly identifying an irreversible pathologic condition. Although a patient may feel certain about the source of his pain he may be mistaken. Extraction of noninvolved teeth may exacerbate the problem by leading to a condition known as the phantom tooth syndrome. Occasionally, pain emanating from a pulpally involved tooth will produce a pain perceived by the patient as an "earache" or "headache" rather than a "toothache." It is therefore incumbent upon the practitioner who manages facial pain to either become familiar with the diagnosis of dental pain or call upon a dentist for assistance in facial pain of unclear origin. This may save the patient from unnecessary pain and medical procedures.

Just as pain may be referred from the teeth to other structures, pain from other sources may be perceived as a toothache. Clinical examples of this are sinusitis, cluster headache, TMD, and periodontal disease. Countless healthy teeth have been extracted because of pain produced in these nearby structures.

Although the pain of angina pectoris may be referred to the left mandible and ear, there is generally associated chest pain. Thus very few patients mistake angina for toothache, yet this may occur (28).

After the teeth, the most common source of referred

maxillofacial pain is the temporomandibular joint with its associated structures. Although pain from the joint proper is generally perceived as being preauricular, many patients, either because of referred pain or through lack of knowledge of the existence or location of the temporomandibular joint (TMJ) believe they have an "earache" and initially seek medical attention.

PROJECTED PAIN

Pain is most often initiated by noxious stimulation in which nonneural tissue damage is present or threatened. This nonneural tissue damage, through mechanisms yet undefined, causes stimulation of the free nerve ending of the nociceptor, thus initiating the neural signal that travels to various regions of the pain pathway. The pain is perceived (with the exception of referred pain) as originating from the site of noxious stimulation. However, a very different situation may occur when peripheral nerves are damaged.

When a nerve involved in a pain pathway is injured in any way, including cutting, crushing, ischemia, or burns, one possible consequence is the development of pain that may become chronic. Although the neural damage may occur anywhere within the pain pathway, the pain is perceived as originating in the dermatome supplied by the injured nerve. For example, injury to the cell body (in the trigeminal ganglion) of a neuron supplying the posterior mandibular teeth will produce a "toothache" in the patient's perception, regardless of the health or even presence of the tooth in question. This is known as projected pain.

An example of projected trigeminal pain occurs in tic douloureux, where pathology in the region of the trigeminal ganglion may produce pain perceived as a toothache.

There are several possible mechanisms of projected pain, including neuroma formation, deafferentation, and development of epileptogenic foci.

Neuromas

When a nerve trunk is cut the proximal end begins regrowth in an attempt at reinnervation. To be successful the regenerating axons must find the proper neurilemma tubes and follow them to the original receptive field. If they do not they may randomly overgrow into disorganized bundle of intertwined intraneural and extraneural tissue and Schwann cells. These are called neuromas. The neurogenic pain that results is thought to be partly due to the ephaptic transfer of neural impulses generated by pressing or stretching the nerve tissue mass. This neurogenic pain in many cases is exacerbated by norepinephrine or sympathetic activity, in which case it is called causalgia.

Traumatic neuromas formed in scar tissue usually produce no discomfort except when a certain mandibular movement stretches the affected scar tissue. The nociceptive response is greater in intensity than would be expected from the applied stimulus, and is quite faithful in incidence and duration. There are usually no accompanying sensory or motor symptoms indicative of a neural deficit. There is usually no visible or palpable mass. The pain can be temporarily arrested by a small injection of an anesthetic at the pain site. Sympathetic blockade is sometimes helpful in attenuating the pain, or if accessible, the traumatic neuroma can be surgically removed.

The placement of pressure on a neuroma produces pain projected to the dermatome supplied by the nerve in which it forms. Thus, neuroma formation in the infraorbital or alveolar nerves may produce pain perceived as a toothache. It is important to note that there may be spontaneous or evoked pain in a nerve regenerating properly. This pain generally may be expected to have a duration of up to 6 months.

Deafferentation

There is evidence that demonstrates that extracranial trigeminal nerve sectioning can produce retrograde degeneration of nervous tissue in the trigeminal ganglion and spinal nucleus (29–32). This degeneration includes cell necrosis and glial scarring. It is most prominent in the chief sensory nucleus and the rostral portions of the spinal nucleus and occurs from 3 to 20 weeks after the injury.

Gregg has hypothesized that this central degeneration of neural elements produces an imbalance in the ratio of large sensory fibers to smaller (nociceptive) fibers (30). Therefore, according to the gate control theory, pain may be produced by an increase of the activity of small fibers in comparison to large fibers.

Development of Epileptogenic Foci

Another theory that can be applied to explain the occurrence of projected pain is based on the concept that long-lasting pain signals may be initiated spontaneously or by brief light touch. This has led to some authors to believe that reverberating circuits or epileptogenic foci are sometimes established following nerve injury. Although the exact mechanism by which this takes place is not known, it is believed that the efficacy of certain anticonvulsant drugs (i.e., phenytoin and carbamazepine) is based on their ability to reduce this neural reverberation. It has been shown that anticonvulsants reduce post-tetanic facilitation in the trigeminal ganglion, and this may account for their effectiveness in the control of tic douloureux and other trigeminal neuralgias (33).

A different theory that may explain the phenomenon of pain evoked by light touch is that of neural crosstalk. It is postulated that following damage to a peripheral nerve one of two things may occur. One possibility is that the proximal end of a severed small fiber may regenerate and connect with the distal end of a larger fiber, thus producing pain evoked by light touch (33). Another possibility is that, following nerve damage, activity in the axon of a large fiber may induce activity in a small fiber axon as a result of the neural crosstalk phenomenon (33).

TEMPOROMANDIBULAR DYSFUNCTION AS A CAUSE OF OROFACIAL PAIN

DIFFERENTIAL DIAGNOSIS AND TREATMENT

The stomatognathic system is a closed system consisting of four parts: the TMJ, its associated neuromusculature, the dentition, and the periodontium including its sensorineural components (Fig. 24.6). Although the parts are not of equal importance, if present, they must all function within the physiologic tolerances of the patient in order to maintain orofacial health. Any change in one component of the system will have an immediate effect on one or more of the other components. These changes may or may not be of a magnitude to produce clinical symptoms.

Temporomandibular dysfunction syndrome is, at present, an ill-defined psychopathologic entity. Over 100 different pathologies may have the typical TMD symptoms of reduced mandibular range of motion, joint noises, myospasm, and pain. In order to organize this material in a cogent fashion it is logical to categorize these entities in a continuum (see Fig. 24.7).

The pathologies to the left and right of the vertical lines in Figure 24.7 are discussed in other sections of this chapter. In this section we discuss those pathologies that affect the TMJ and its associated structures. The area at the left side of the continuum within the vertical lines represents pathologies of the articulating elements of the TMJ. Many authors use the term *temporomandibular joint disease* (TMJ disease) to describe these disabilities. Although

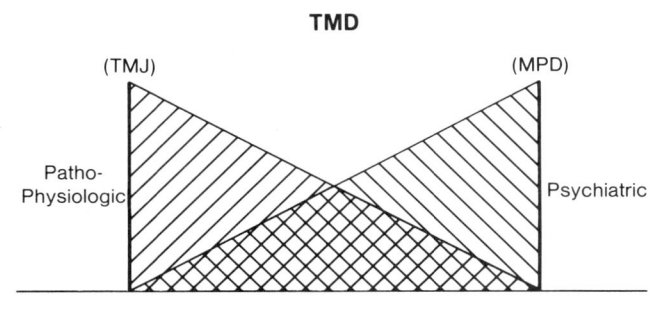

Figure 24.7. Continuum of pathologies with typical TMD symptoms.

most of these pathologies may be treated nonsurgically, some require surgical intervention. However, almost all of these joint disabilities will, over time, produce sequelae that result in disease on the right side of the continuum. The right side of the continuum represents neuromuscular-psychological pathologies. Moving from left to right, the pathophysiologic aspect decreases and the psychological aspect increases. In the literature, the term *myofacial pain dysfunction* (MPD) is used to categorize these items. However, just as articulating structure pathologies can affect the neuromusculature, long-standing neuromuscular pathologies can produce disease in the articulating elements. I believe that the continuum represents a more logical way to visualize all of these interrelated disease entities, and the term TMD is a more comprehensive title for this syndrome.

The TMJ is a ginglymoarthrodial (rotating and translating) synovial joint. The articulating components are the condyle, the meniscus or articular disk, and the articular eminence of the temporal bone. The TMJ is a single joint with a bilateral articulation. Therefore, sensory input from receptors in the joint must be centrally integrated in a fashion similar to that of the vestibular sense. Unlike other synovial joints, the osseous parts of the TMJ are both convex. This means that the biconcave disk is essential for normal joint movement. The articulating bones are covered with fibrocartilage, which is usually found only in relatively immobile joints. Its purpose in the TMJ is to aid in preserving the condyle-disk-eminentia relationship (fibrocartilage is deformable).

Under normal function the disk position is maintained by medial and lateral collateral ligaments that bind the disk tightly to the condyle. In addition, under loading, the osseous aspects of the joint deform the disk, producing a mechanical anulus that also contributes to preserving the integrity of the disk-bone relationship. Although the superior belly of the lateral pterygoid muscle attaches to the disk, it does not pull the disk forward in translation. Its function is to resist the pull of elastin fibers when the mandible closes. Therefore, there is no muscle system that is involved in disk movement. The disk itself is divided into an anterior, thin intermediate, posterior, and bilam-

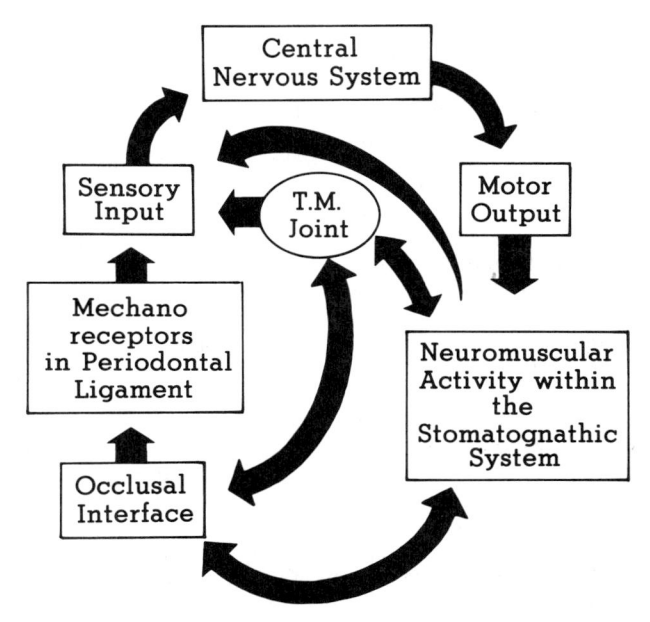

Figure 24.6. Factors in temporomandibular joint problems. (Adapted from Solberg WK, Clark GT: *Temporomandibular Joint Problems.* Chicago, Quintessence, 1980.)

inar zone. The disk is thicker posteriorly than anteriorly and medially more than laterally. The functional area is the thin intermediate zone. In function the anterior, then the anterior superior, then the posterior superior aspect of the condyle rotates against this thin intermediate zone as the mandible is depressed. The sequence is reversed in closure. This functional area of the disk is both avascular and aneural.

INTERNAL DERANGEMENTS

Internal derangements of the TMJ are a frequently encountered pathology. The term implies a dyscoordination between the disk, condyle, and eminentia as described above. The disk tends to prolapse anteriorly or anteriomedially. Internal derangements may be self-reducing or nonreducing. In the self-reducing derangement the disk is located anterior to the condyle in the closed mouth position. During opening an audible "click" represents the disk reducing into its normal position. There is almost always a reciprocal "click" on closure that corresponds to the disk relapsing into its anterior state. The closure click is usually less audible than the opening sound.

The signs and symptoms of patients with internal drangements are usually similar to those of TMD patients in general. These are a reduction in the range of mandibular motion, earache (more precisely pain and tenderness in the preauricular area), joint noises, myospasm, and headache. Some patients complain of a feeling of fullness in the ear.

Headache is a common symptom in TMD patients. According to Farrar and McCarty retro-orbital headache is also the most common symptom of internal derangements (34). The above statement notwithstanding, headache is such a common symptom that it should not, without other joint signs and symptoms, be a major indicator of internal derangements.

Preauricular pain, often mistakenly reported by the patient as otic pain, is a frequent sign. In fact most TMD patients present initially to their physician believing they have otic involvement. It is essential that otic involvement be eliminated as a cause of the patient's symptomatology. The TMJ on the affected side is tender to palpation both directly and intermediately. In addition, there are usually multiple myospastic areas in the musculature associated with mandibular movement.

Since one of the cardinal symptoms of a reducing derangement is the reciprocal "click," both sides of the TMJ should be auscultated to ascertain if "clicks" are present. Usually the earlier the "click" appears in the opening movement of the mandible the more amenable it is to nonsurgical management. Joint sounds may now be visualized by means of TMJ sonograms, which have the capability of both locating the derangement in the opening and closing cycles as well as performing a diagnostically significant power spectrum analysis on all joint sounds. If a "click" is demonstrated, the clinician should have the patient protrude the mandible and repeat the opening and closing movements. In most reducible derangements the "click" will disappear. This indicates that the derangement has reduced itself. In internal derangements the opening and closing "clicks" do not appear at the same point in the opening and closing cycle. If the "click" should appear at the same position in both opening and closing it is indicative of an anatomic abnormality rather than an internal derangement (35). It has been demonstrated both arthrographically and surgically that the opening "click" is the condyle slipping over the posterior zone of the disk onto the thin intermediate zone. The fainter sounding closing "click" is the condyle slipping posterior to the posterior zone of the disk.

The normal range of mandibular motion is approximately 50 mm vertically, 9 mm laterally, and at least 6 mm protrusively. The mandible should open without deviation. In the reducible internal derangement the degree of reduction in these parameters is variable. It is usually dependent on the extent of associated myospastic activity. The mandible may deviate toward the affected side until the disk prolapses into place and then complete the opening movement in a normal fashion.

Intermittent "clicks" in the absence of any other clinical finding (pain, myospasm, reduced range of motion, etc.) should not be treated.

In a percentage of patients who have reducing derangements and are not treated, the derangements will cease to reduce. The history would reveal the presence of a "click" that has now disappeared. There is almost always an increase in pain and a reduction in the mandibular range of motion. The mandible will deviate toward the affected side. This condition is known as a closed lock.

The treatment for a reducible internal derangement consists of the fabrication of an orthopedic repositioning appliance that maintains the mandible in a protruded position. Care must be exercised to be certain that there is no movement of the dentition during the period of joint therapy. A number of appliances are acceptable and the reader is referred to any of the texts on TMD management for the details of appliance construction. The myospastic areas are treated with trigger point injections of local anesthesia without vasoconstrictor and the external use of refrigerant sprays such as Fluori-Methane. Muscle relaxants and diazepam-type drugs are of little value. However, nonsteroidal anti-inflammatory agents have proven helpful in providing symptomatologic relief in association with the regimen outlined above. If reduction does occur, an effort should be made to evaluate the stomatognathic system to determine any correctable pathology that may have served as an etiologic base for the derangement.

If there is no symptomatologic improvement within 3–4 months of nonsurgical therapy, the patient should undergo arthrographic studies to determine if the conservative measures should be continued or if surgical intervention is required. In the case of the closed lock patient, arthrographic studies should be obtained immediately. On the basis of the results of these tests either a surgical or nonsurgical treatment plan should be formulated. At the time this text is written, magnetic resonance imaging appears to offer promise as a noninvasive, reasonably accurate alternative to arthrography. However, at present there is no alternative to arthrography as the definitive diagnostic evaluator of internal derangements.

ARTHRITIDES

A traditional definition of arthritis is a disease entity that exists within the joint itself (36). A listing of arthritides that may affect the TMJ would include: (a) osteoarthritis (arthrosis), (b) rheumatoid arthritis, (c) polyarthritis (e.g., gout, lupus erythematosus, Reiter's syndrome), (d) rheumatoid variants (e.g., psoriatic, juvenile), and (e) traumatic arthritis (37). Many authors equate the term *synovitis* with arthritis. This amalgamation of semantics fails when applied to the TMJ. One of the major signs of synovitis is swelling, and this symptom is not commonly associated with this joint (38). In the confirmed arthritic, the dentist's role is confined to restoring and maintaining the stomatognathic system in its optimal state of function.

Osteoarthritis

Osteoarthritis is also known as hypertrophic arthritis or degenerative joint disease (DJD). It is the most common form of joint disease affecting the TMJ (39). In clinical practice, osteoarthritic patients fall into one of two classes even though there may be only one pathohistologic profile of the disease.

In one group the patients are relatively asymptomatic, with the diagnosis of DJD being made rather serendipitously from routine radiographs. The condyle may show lipping or flattening and Ely's cysts may be present. On auscultation, crepitus is discernible. The disease is more often unilateral than bilateral. It is a relatively common finding after the fifth decade.

The other group of osteoarthritic patients present with a variety of TMD symptoms. These include pain and tenderness over the TMJs, pain in the joint area on mastication, reduced range of mandibular opening, luxation and subluxation, bruxism, otic symptomatology, dizziness, headache, deviation of the mandible toward the affected side, and pain and stiffness in the neck and shoulder areas.

The diagnostic workup should include a complete examination by an otolaryngologist and appropriate blood studies. Cephalometrically corrected tomograms are especially revealing for this type of pathology. Whenever possible nonsurgical regimens should be tried as initial therapy. These regimens include eliminating any discrepancies between the mandibular closure position (dictated by the dentition) and the physiologic position (determined by the joint and its associated neuromusculature); orthopedic repositioning appliances to interdict any bruxing or clenching habits; and nonsteroidal anti-inflammatory medications. Surgical intervention should only be considered if these noninvasive procedures have proven to be ineffectual.

Rheumatoid Arthritis

The role of the dentist in rheumatoid arthritis is rather limited. The principal clinician obviously should be the rheumatologist. Rheumatoid arthritis patients may display limited range of mandibular movement and pain in the preauricular area. The clinician should be aware of patients who have developed an "open bite" in the anterior area. This sign can indicate the presence of rheumatoid arthritis in the TMJ. Open bites should not be corrected either surgically or by occlusal equilibration until rheumatoid arthritis has been completely eliminated as an etiologic possibility.

Traumatic Arthritis

Traumatic injury to the facial area may cause a chipping of the condyle without fracture. This condition produces chronic preauricular discomfort often accompanied with a reduction in the range of mandibular motion and some evidence of myospasm. Although a thorough history will usually reveal a moderate trauma to the jaw, some patients cannot recall a precipitating event. The diagnosis is confirmed by means of transcranial and tomographic radiographs.

TUMORS

Although malignant tumors of the TMJ have been reported, most lesions of this joint are benign (40). Osteochondroma is the lesion most often encountered. The growth of the tumor produces an asymmetric condyle, and if the lesion is rapidly growing there may develop an ipsilateral posterior open bite. These patients complain of preauricular pain on the affected side as well as a reduction in the range of mandibular motion and associated myospasms. When the preauricular area is palpated there is no rebound felt when a tumor is involved. This is opposite to the rebound that is associated with pain of myospastic origin. Diagnosis is confirmed radiographically. The patient should be referred immediately for a surgical consultation.

FRACTURES

Most fractures are of an acute nature and are therefore beyond the scope of this text. However, an undetected and untreated condylar fracture that heals in an abnormal position will place a strain on the remaining components of the stomatognathic system. Although the neuromusculature is capable of adaptation, this capability is not infinite. It will vary from individual to individual and in the same person during their lifetime. The reported symptoms are typical of TMD and include pain in the TMJ area, restricted mandibular movement, headache, and myospasms. Nonsurgical therapy to alleviate the strain on the system should always be attempted initially. Only when these nonsurgical measures have proven ineffective should surgical intervention be considered. The nonsurgical treatment plan should include physical therapy, mild stretching exercises, trigger point injections with a local anesthetic without any vasoconstrictor, refrigerant spray (e.g., Fluori-Methane), and the construction of an orthopedic repositioning appliance. It is important in these patients that any imbalance between the dentally dictated closure position and the neuromuscular closure position be eliminated.

NEUROMUSCULAR PATHOLOGIES

If the skeletal, traumatic, neoplastic, internal derangement, and infectious causes of orofacial pain are eliminated, there still remain 70–80% of the patients presenting with typical TMD symptoms (41). These are the patients with active myospastic areas, demonstrable trigger points, referred pain, occlusal disharmonies, parafunctional occlusal habits, emotional stress patterns, and a reduced range of mandibular movement.

The diagnosis and treatment of these TMD patients requires clinicians to use their full range of biologic and clinical knowledge and experience. It is essential to remember that, although a variety of therapeutic regimens may prove to be effective, there can only be one accurate diagnosis. The etiology of these patients' symptoms is usually multifactorial. The authors also believe that no definitive treatment should be initiated until the clinician has completed the diagnostic workup and a presumptive diagnosis has been determined. The above statement notwithstanding, it is often necessary to initiate some emergency therapy to assist the acutely distressed patient. Even if the emergency measures alleviate the acute symptoms, they do not remove the responsibility of the clinician to discover the etiologies of the problem and seek their remediation. It must always be rememberd that many TMD patients are psychologically labile. It is often necessary to obtain counseling support (conducted by an appropriate specialist) coincident with the physical treatment of the stomatognathic system. The chronicity of "pain" in these patients is an important factor. Many of these patients' complaints originate as part of the "chronic pain pattern" and are not related to actual TMD pathology. These symptoms may continue to be manifested after all pathology in the stomatognathic system has been eliminated. The authors also emphatically believe that reversible treatments, when indicated, should be the initial treatment modes of choice. Irreversible procedures should be initiated usually only after all reversible techniques have been attempted without alleviating the patient's discomfort.

Etiologic Theories

The etiology of TMD of neuromuscular origin is unresolved at present. However, several etiologic theories have evolved and most TMD specialists will be devotees of one of these major schools of thought. Deboever has categorized these theories into five groups: mechanical displacement theory, muscle theory, neuromuscular theory, and the psychological and psychophysiologic theories (42).

Mechanical Displacement Theory (Costen's Theory) The mechanical displacement theory is based on the observation that some TMD patients have overclosure of the mandible. This may be caused by the loss of or improper eruption of the posterior dentition. The overclosure of the mandible is thought to place undue pressure on the auriculotemporal and chorda tympani nerves and the eustachian tube. Adherents of this theory place great emphasis on the visualization of equal anterior and posterior joint spaces on roentgenographic examination. The theory has been challenged on anatomic grounds.

Muscle Theory The basis of the muscle theory is muscle hyperactivity. The hyperactivity serves as an initiator of myospasm, which then spreads to its primary and secondary referred pain sites. Although there is no basis for refutation of this theory, the authors believe this theory is narrow and restrictive. It does not take into account other viable causes of the TMD problem.

Neuromuscular Theory The neuromuscular theory is based on a functional disharmony between the occlusal interface and a physiologic joint-muscle position. The incompatibility leads to parafunctional habits such as grinding and clenching of the dentition (bruxism). The grinding and clenching may occur during the waking hours but are most often manifested during sleep. The bruxing habit leads to abnormal contractile states and, hence, myospastic activity. The theory covers many of the clinical TMD problems that are commonly seen and, indeed, may be the most popular theory. Its major weakness is that it does not explain why many patients with abnormalities in the occlusal interface do not have TMD problems.

Psychological and Psychophysiologic Theories The basis of the psychological and psychophysiologic theories is that patients under stress have increased tension and activity in the masticatory and associated musculature. Supporters of the psychological school believe that the syndrome is purely psychogenic and should be treated from a psychoanalytic point of view. Laskin (42) has evolved a psychophysiologic approach to TMD problems. This theory states that myospastic activity is the primary cause of TMD symptomatology. It is further believed that fatigue caused by tension-related oral habits is the major cause of the abnormal myospastic activity. The theory does take into account the necessity for physiologic harmony between the components of the stomatognathic system as well as the obvious influence that psychological factors have in the TMD syndrome. At present there are too few data to unequivocably support this theory. However, the authors believe that its multifactorial base is far more rational than the other existing theories of TMD dysfunction.

It can be stated that the myofacial aspect of the syndrome is multifactorial, and there can be little doubt that the emotional status of the patient is one of the most important of these factors. However, for any lasting improvement in the patient's symptoms, all of the components of the stomatognathic system must also be functioning within the physiologic parameters of the patient. TMD has both a physical and an emotional aspect. Both must be accurately diagnosed and both must be treated.

The Myospastic Cycle

Although there is a multiplicity of theories, the one common denominator in all of them is the presence of myospastic areas. The origin of muscle spasm is prolonged or abnormal muscle contraction. This abnormal muscle reaction is a response to one or more of three variables: alterations in skeletal muscle length, protective neuromuscular responses associated with occlusal relationships, and emotional stress. The two major effects of this abnormal muscle contraction are ATP depletion and vasoconstriction. The cycle is diagramed in detail in Figure 24.8.

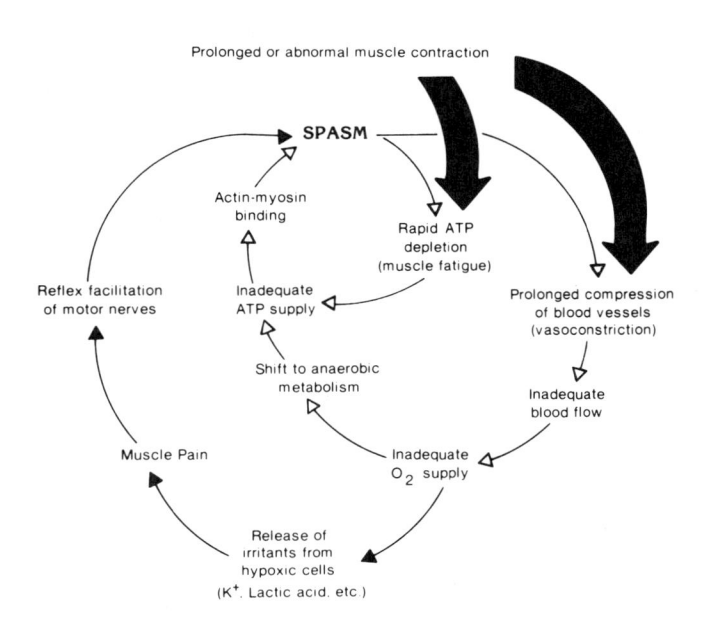

The cycle once started tends to perpetuate itself. In addition, once a muscle has been subjected to a myospastic episode it tends, for reasons not yet understood, to become more susceptible to future episodes. The nociceptive area may be in the muscle itself or it may be referred to other orofacial areas. These referred pain sites have been meticulously mapped by Dr. Janet Travell, and the reader is referred to her text for exact referred site locations (43).

There are several techniques currently employed to break the cycle. These are refrigerant sprays (e.g., Fluori-Methane), trigger point injections using local anesthetics without any vasoconstrictor, mild stretching exercises, and ultrasound. It is incumbent on the clinician to discover and treat the cause of the myospasm even if the above-noted measures temporarily break the cycle. Refrigerant sprays combined with mild stretching exercises are often effective in breaking the myospastic cycle. The technique employs sprays such as Fluori-Methane (Gebauer). The bottle is held about 6 inches from the affected area and the spray is applied in unidirectional parallel lines from insertion to origin. The skin should not be blanched. After spraying, the muscles are gently stretched by use of graduated rubber stoppers or tongue blades. The spray is then repeated. The stretch part of the exercise is then used for about 10 additional minutes. The entire process is repeated four or five times per day.

Trigger point injection of anesthetic without vasoconstrictor is also an excellent technique for breaking myospasm. An aspirating syringe and 30-gauge needle is the usual delivery system. Care must be exercised to make certain not to deposit the solution into the vascular system.

The TMD Workup

The diagnostic procedures involved in a TMD workup are both numerous and complex. They include a thorough systems review and history, an examination of the oral and perioral hard and soft tissues, a study of the occlusal relationships, measurement of the mandibular range of motion, patterns of mandibular movement, auscultation of the TMJ, palpation of the adnexal musculature of the joint, radiographs, deprogrammed occlusal analysis, electromyographic studies, sonograms, and laboratory tests. It is beyond the range of this work to discuss each of these entities in detail. For additional information the reader is referred to any one of a number of texts devoted to the diagnosis and treatment of temporomandibular pathologies. However, it is appropriate to elaborate on several basic diagnostic entities.

The mandibular range of motion can easily be measured by any clinician. Vertical movement is determined by first measuring the number of millimeters an upper central incisor overlaps its lower counterpart. The patient is then asked to open as far as possible and the interincisal dimension is recorded. The vertical range is the sum of these two parameters. Lateral excursions are the number of millimeters that the lower center incisors move either left or right from their central position. Protrusive excursion is the number of millimeters that the lower central incisors can move directly forward from their normal closure position. The normal values for these movements are as follows: left and right lateral, 9.1 mm; protrusive, at least 6.1 mm; and vertical, 50.3 ± 6.9 mm (44).

Joint auscultation is performed by placement of a stethoscope over the preauricular areas and asking the patient to open, close, move left, move right, and protrude the mandible. Note should be made of the presence of any "clicks" or crepitus and where the sounds are detected in the opening and closing movements of the mandible. During opening and closing, the mandible should be observed to detect any deviation from the midline.

Figure 24.8. The myospastic cycle.

If TMD is suspected from the examination, the patient should be referred to an appropriate specialist. Muscle relaxants, tranquilizers, and narcotics are of little value in support of these patients. Symptoms can temporarily best be handled medically by use of nonsteroidal anti-inflammatory drugs and tricyclic antidepressants.

OROFACIAL PATHOLOGIES EXCLUDING THE TEMPOROMANDIBULAR JOINT AND ITS ADNEXAL STRUCTURES

Although the single most common group of disorders that produce chronic facial pain are the musculoskeletal conditions collectively known as TMD, many other conditions are best treated by medical/surgical means and are not within the purview of the dentist or maxillofacial surgeon. On the other hand, there are some conditions that may best be managed by a combination of dental, medical, and psychological means.

Perhaps the best example of this multidisciplinary approach can be found in the neurogenic pain disorders (neuralgias). These include tic douloureux, post-traumatic trigeminal neuralgia, postherpetic neuralgia, glossopharyngeal neuralgia, and multiple sclerosis neuralgia. Dental and maxillofacial surgical aspects of the treatment of these conditions are described using post-traumatic neuralgia as an example. This condition responds best to these approaches. There are also atypical neuralgias.

POST-TRAUMATIC (POSTSURGICAL) NEURALGIAS

One common source of facial pain is produced by damage to the dental branches of the trigeminal nerve. Although this pain may be caused by infection, sports injuries, automobile accidents, or other accidental trauma, the majority of such injuries are brought on by dental extractions (45) and, to a lesser extent, other oral and maxillofacial surgical procedures (46) (e.g., implants and orthognathic surgery) and root canal therapy (47). The inferior and superior alveolar nerves travel precariously close to the surface in an area where infection, fractures, and traumatic injuries are common (48). These nerves are also subjected to the trauma of local anesthetic injections, which will, on rare occasion, produce a chronic pain condition. Furthermore, third molar impactions often put pressure on the inferior alveolar nerve, causing some level of trauma. The psychological significance of the orofacial region and the symbolic importance of tooth extraction further complicate the management of post-traumatic neuralgias (49).

The pain of post-traumatic neuralgia may be severe at times. Generally, there is a persistent, nearly continuous low level of baseline pain with episodic bouts of severe pain brought about by the application of moderate to intense pressure to the site of injury. The baseline pain is often described as deep, boring, and sometimes burning. Such daily activities as eating and wearing of dentures may be extremely difficult. This severe pain is usually described as being sharp. Complicating the pain of post-traumatic neuralgia are paresthesias and dysesthesias, which may also occur. In the event that the lingual nerve is damaged, usually from mandibular third molar extraction, taste sensation may be impaired ipsilaterally.

Timing is a critical factor in the management of post-traumatic neuralgia, and the prognosis for this type of pain is highly dependent upon the duration of the problem at the time of presentation. Acute post-traumatic neuralgias are quite common, and a certain degree of neurogenic pain probably accompanies most oral surgery and endodontic procedures without chronic sequellae. In contrast, chronic post-traumatic neuralgias may persist for decades, and the prognosis for satisfactory recovery from this condition deteriorates after 2 years' duration.

As described in the section on nerve regeneration following injury, several months may be required for complete recovery from peripheral nerve trauma under normal circumstances. Therefore, this kind of pain cannot be considered to be chronic until it extends beyond the expected healing period, generally held to be 6 months.

The first step in the management of postsurgical neuralgia actually occurs before the surgical procedure is performed. This involves making a definitive diagnosis before planning surgery and informing the patient that nerve damage involving pain may be a risk of the procedure. Those procedures that involve surgery near major nerve branches or extraction of deeply impacted teeth might be expected to produce more neuralgic pain than other procedures, but any oral and maxillofacial surgical procedure can cause this problem. By informing a patient that he may expect the possibility (although not a common one) that pain or paresthesia may last for several months following surgery, anxiety is reduced in the event nerve damage does occur.

It is well known that acute pain follows tooth extraction and other surgical procedures. In general, the treatment for this focuses on the use of analgesics, including the use of low doses of narcotics, such as codeine or other narcotic agents. However, following the acute phase, pain may persist, especially if significant nerve damage took place. This pain is often combined with paresthesias that increase in severity as the nerve heals properly. At this time reassurance and nonnarcotic analgesics are the best management techniques. If the pain and paresthesias do not improve or become more severe as the 6-month mark is reached, the pain may be considered to be chronic and appropriate management as described below should be initiated.

The introduction of the long-duration local anesthetic agent bupivacaine (Marcaine) has added a new dimension to the treatment of post-traumatic trigeminal neuralgias (50). Bupivacaine is an amide-type local anesthetic that is chemically similar to mepivacaine. The concentration best used in the management of chronic trigeminal pain is 0.5%

with epinephrine 1:200,000. Bupivacaine is available in either the cartridge or vial form. Generally one cartridge (1.8 ml) is sufficient to produce the desired anesthetic effect, but because of its low toxicity, up to 10 cartridges of bupivacaine may be safely administered at one time. However, because of the possibility of intravascular injection higher concentrations should not be used.

In many cases, serial nerve blocks with bupivacaine are sufficient to satisfactorily manage post-traumatic trigeminal neuralgias (51). The following text describes the use of serial local anesthetic blocks of the branches of the trigeminal nerve. During the initial block, anesthesia may be difficult to obtain and additional injections may be required. Along similar lines, the duration of anesthesia and analgesia may be relatively short.

The onset of anesthesia may also be somewhat delayed so that in emergency pain situations, lidocaine should be injected before bupivacaine. The duration of anesthetic action varies widely among individuals, but it generally lasts between 5 and 8 hr. However, the relief from neuralgic pain usually outlasts the anesthesia, with a duration of 12–24 hr being common. A diary is kept by the patient to document the duration of pain relief and the general intensity of pain during the following week.

At the next appointment (approximately 1 week later), the injection is repeated. This time the duration of neuralgia analgesia is somewhat greater. The injections are then continued in a series of increased intervals between blocks until the injections are required only once every several months.

In some cases, nerve blocks provide only partial relief for trigeminal neuralgias (this is especially true in cases of tic douloureux). Blocks then may serve as adjunctive therapy when combined with anticonvulsant medications (51). Since anticonvulsants may produce severe side effects, which are dose dependent, the advantage of combined therapy is the reduction of anticonvulsant dosage required to achieve a therapeutic effect.

Furthermore, some patients do not benefit sufficiently from anesthetic blocks, anticonvulsants, or their combination. For these patients, a variety of surgical procedures are available. These procedures can be categorized as being either intracranial (i.e., at the level of the trigeminal ganglion or centrad) or extracranial (i.e., in the peripheral branches of the trigeminal nerve). The intracranial procedures are described in Chapter 23.

Gregg has pioneered the development of extracranial surgical procedures for trigeminal neuralgias (45, 48). There are two basic procedures available on a limited basis at this time: peripheral thermoneurolysis and neural decompression. The extracranial approach has several advantages over the intracranial one. Most importantly, there is no possibility of damaging intracranial contents, especially cranial nerves. There is also the advantage of easier access to the nerve and less discomfort during the procedure.

In this procedure a radiofrequency lesion is made in the mental nerve, inferior alveolar nerve, lingual nerves, or infraorbital nerve (48). These thermal lesions selectively destroy the nociceptive fibers while primarily sparing the larger fibers. The technique involves the localization of the damaged nerve by electrical stimulation of the needle probe. The probe is then heated to a controlled temperature (60–70°C) for 30 sec. This procedure may then be repeated. Radiofrequency lesions are highly effective in relieving pain without producing significant paresthesia. However, there is often recurrence of pain and the procedures must be repeated every several years for continued relief in many cases.

Another type of oral surgery operation that may prove to be effective in those cases where neuroma formation is a major problem is the neural decompression procedure (48). Such cases may be identified by the development of pain and paresthesia projected distally when pressure is placed over the site of the neuroma (Tinel's sign). In essence, the operation involves (a) exposure of the operative site, (b) removal of any tissue such as bony sequestra that may entrap the nerve, (c) removal of connective scar tissue, and (d) microsurgical repair of the nerve. As more cases are treated in this way, success rates, complications, and recurrences will be determined.

VASCULAR AND OTOLARYNGOLOGIC ETIOLOGIES

There are a number painful vascular conditions of the face that either produce pain referred to the teeth or may on occasion affect oral vasculature, thus producing a perception of toothaches or TMD pain. These include facial migraine, cluster headache, angina pectoris, and temporal arteritis. These conditions must be recognized and treated and unnecessary tooth extraction prevented.

Likewise there are otolaryngologic diseases such as sinusitis, otitis, and tonsillitis that may be confused with tooth and jaw pain. Of special concern is the linkage, especially in the lay press, of TMD with auditory and vestibular dysfunction. Although treatment of TMD may relieve some ear symptoms, such as feelings of pain and fullness, others, such as tinnitus or hearing loss, are unlikely to improve.

PHANTOM TOOTH SYNDROME

Just as when a limb is amputated, the extraction of a tooth may produce the perception that the missing tooth is still present and perhaps painful (52, 53). The mechanism of this phantom tooth pain is similar to that of other projected pains, involving neuroma formation, deafferentation, and epileptogenic foci. However, one aspect that may be unique to the pain associated with phantom body parts (including teeth) is the psychological one. This is due to the sense of loss associated with a missing body part as well as perceived changes in body image.

In the phantom tooth syndrome there is either persistent pain in a tooth treated endodontically or toothache-like

Figure 24.9. Panorex x-ray at the time of presentation of a patient suffering from phantom tooth syndrome. The patient complained of pain in the left maxillary molar region that was not relieved by root canal therapy, apicoectomies, or extractions. In the past similar conditions existed on the right side of the maxilla and mandible.

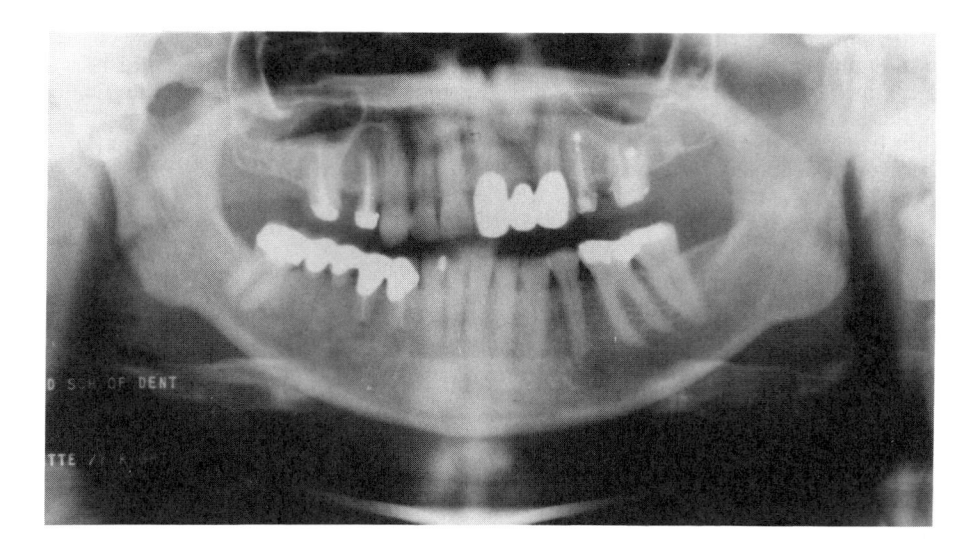

pain in the area of a previous extraction. Because there are potentially 32 teeth all in close proximity, it is natural for a patient to think that the pain of a phantom tooth actually is caused by an adjacent tooth. The dentist must evaluate this possibility and at the same time recognize the fact that dental pain may be refered from dental and nondental structures. In some cases many teeth receive root canal therapy or extraction if the syndrome is not recognized (Fig. 24.9). There are several features of phantom tooth pain as defined by Marbach et al. (54). First, the likelihood of phantom pain developing is greater if the tooth was painful before root canal treatment or extraction. This fact makes it essential to determine when the onset of any pain in the tooth in question occurred. Chronicity may be determined using this onset time as a guide. Second, the pain must persist after proper healing is expected (i.e., the pain must be chronic). Third, there must be pain on palpation of the area. Fourth, there is often a lack of response to generally reliable therapy such as nerve blocks and analgesics. It is estimated that between 3 and 6% of the population undergoing endodontic or oral surgery procedures suffer from this problem.

Although it is correct to consider the phantom tooth syndrome as a type of postsurgical neuralgia, its unique features warrant its designation as a discreet entity with management considerations of its own. One consideration of crucial importance is that a moratorium on further extractions or endodontic procedures should be placed on the patient until the nature of the problem can be addressed. The only exception are teeth in which there is a compelling need for such work based on radiographic or clinical information (not on the basis of subjective pain complaints alone). Because of the unusual nature of phantom tooth pain this condition may be considered to be an atypical facial neuralgia (54). Clinical experience suggests that psychological depression is often found in atypical facial pain patients (49). Thus, the management of this problem involves the skillful balance of nerve blocks, anticonvulsant medication, psychological counseling, and antidepressant medication (51). Surgery is not recommended until a thorough psychological evaluation has been undertaken.

Although the dentist is not a psychotherapist, he should be a sympathetic listener with whom a patient may develop a relationship based on trust. From a psychosocial history he should be able to broadly identify the nature and severity of a psychiatric problem and assist the therapist in management of the patient (49).

Phantom phenomena occur in orofacial regions other than the teeth. Phantom tongue has been described (55), and the authors have seen phantom pain following the removal of a salivary gland and a phantom mandible following hemimandibulectomy. However, the most commonly seen phantom situations occur following tooth extraction and root canal therapy.

One type of dental pain that may be particularly baffling is due to a fracture of the tooth and is known as the cracked tooth syndrome (56). The diagnosis is made primarily by symptomatology and may be supported by clinical detection of a fracture. Sometimes disclosing solutions may help to identify a crack. The tooth is painful when heavy pressure is placed on it as during mastication of hard foods (57, 58). In every other respect the tooth responds normally to all tests. The pain is of the sharp, shooting type (57, 58). The specific treatment is dependent upon the extent of fracture. However, the goal of treatment is to prevent separation of the tooth segments by masticatory forces and is often best accomplished by the fabrication of a cast metal crown (57, 58).

PAIN FROM THE SALIVARY GLANDS

Deep pain of the facial area may be caused by pathologic inflammation of the salivary glands, or sialadenitis. It most often originates in the excretory duct, and is caused by mechanical irritation of the duct followed by infection. Less frequently the inflammation results from the spread of infection from the oral cavity or the tonsils. The pain can be localized quite well by manual palpation and the presence of other signs of inflammation.

One of the most common causes of sialadenitis is the obstruction of the duct by calculi, or sialothiasis. Salivary stones occur most often in the submandibular duct and gland. When a salivary stone obstructs a duct, eating or other forms of salivary stimulation can increase pressure in the gland until salivary colic results. The pain may radiate to the ear and neck regions. Distention, compression, and mastication can accentuate the pain, and therefore may be mistaken for masticatory pain. If left untreated the stone may occasionally be shed. Some fibrosis may result together with a reduction in salivation. Surgical treatment may be required to remove the calculus.

Other causes of salivary gland pain may be cystic degeneration, tumor formation, infectious mononucleosis, or neoplasia. With chronic inflammation the gland is permanently enlarged as a result of the exudate and proliferative changes in the stromal connective tissue. Compression interferes with the formation of saliva, and pressure from the fibrosing stroma produces atrophy of the acini.

GLOSSODYNIA (BURNING MOUTH AND BURNING TONGUE)

Superficial, steady, and continuous are characteristics given to the somatic pain of the common oral complaint of glossodynia, or burning mouth and burning tongue. The immediate cause is the abrasive effect of the tissues rubbing against themselves, teeth, or ill-fitting dentures, bridges, or crowns. The location of the pain depends on which tissues are being rubbed and where, and this usually corresponds to the areas of greatest movement. The oral examination often reveals a clean hygienic mouth. Sometimes hyperemia, inflammation, and ulceration are seen. Infection of the irritated tissues may also complicate the condition.

Sometimes the complaint is cyclic in nature based on its inhibitory effect on movements. This inhibition permits some improvement of the tissue and decrease in pain. This in turn leads to an increase in rubbing and return of the pain.

Some causes are emotional tension, oral consciousness, dental appliances, and habits such as bruxism and tongue thrusting. One of the most common causes is xerostomia, which is an inadequate quantity or quality of saliva. Many modern medicines such as some diuretics, tranquilizers, muscle relaxants, antihypertensive agents, antihistamines, or other anticholinergic agents can alter and depress salivation. Radiation and the aging process can also depress salivation. Dietary influences and systemic conditions can also affect salivary functioning. An early sign of vitamin B_{12}, folic acid, or iron deficiency can be a pain and burning sensation in the tongue. The tip and margins of the tongue become smooth and red in these deficiencies.

All oral irritants can exacerbate the condition. Acidic juices, spices, hot liquids, strong coffee, and certain mouth washes can all increase the irritation.

This condition can be diagnosed by the application of a topical anesthetic, which should promptly and effectively arrest the pain. Deep or referred pains should not be affected.

Treatment includes the removal of any sharp cusps or sharp edges of the teeth that may cause irritation. It is only necessary to grind away small amounts of tissue to restore comfort. Sources of irritation from bridges, crowns, partial dentures, and denture clasps should also be removed. Dentures may have to be adjusted, or new dentures may have to be made. Sliding pressures should be avoided and clasps placed carefully so as to avoid inviting the tongue to play with them. All oral irritants should be avoided.

Possible dietary causes should be considered, and any nutritional deficiencies rectified. Iron deficiency can be treated with 200 mg of ferrous sulfate twice daily, or folic acid deficiency with 5 mg of folic acid once a day. Artificial saliva or sialogogues can be used to reduce xerostomia. Psychological problems should be considered, and stressful situations avoided or reduced. The patient should be reassured that the tongue symptoms do not indicate cancer. Despite all treatment, however, sometimes the pain persists. Fortunately, a relatively large percentage of these patients eventually exhibit spontaneous recovery.

HERPES SIMPLEX

The herpes simplex viruses are usually divided into type 1 and type 2 viruses. The distinction between the infections caused by these two types of viruses, however, are not exact. There is overlap regarding the anatomic sites and clinical features.

Mucocutaneous lesions of the mouth and face are usually caused by herpes simplex type 1. The virus is virtually ubiquitous in the general population and most individuals have prior exposure and some partial immunity. A primary infection called acute herpetic stomatitis may occur early in life. There is malaise, raised temperature, and submandibular lymphadenitis. Vesicles occur and break down to form ulcers. The condition resolves itself in about 10 days. Primary infections can also be subclinical, but in both cases the individual continues to harbor the virus for life. Any patient debilitation can lead to outbreaks of herpes in the form of cold sores or fever blisters, usually on or near the lips. The first sign is a slight prodromal burning or tingling sensation followed by the formation of vesicles. These break down and become crusted over. Although the surface heals it can break down again because of the movement of the lips.

For the treatment of *primary* infections due to herpes simplex, acyclovir, an antiviral agent, appears to be significantly beneficial. Local therapy to ameliorate symptoms may include topical anesthetics such as viscous zylocaine or protective emollient mixtures such as Orabase. Bed rest, maintenance of adequate fluid intake, and a soft diet supplemented by proteins are recommended. Acetaminophen may also be used.

In the treatment of *secondary* or recurrent oral-labial herpetic lesions no existing antiviral agents are effective. There are nevertheless other forms of treatment that can be recommended. Symptomatically, bland emollient creams or ointments such as Herpecin-L or Blistex are recommended. The sooner and more often applied the better the results. During the prodrome or if the lesion has already developed, the emollient should be applied liberally as often as convenient or about every hour. Benzoin tincture or 70–90% topical alcohol can also be used. Where secondary infection is evident or likely, administration of antibiotic creams or ointments containing bacitracin, neomycin, or a combination of the two is recommended. Topical anesthetics applied to the oral lesions are helpful, especially prior to meals to alleviate pain while eating. Caustic or escharotic agents, such as phenol or silver nitrate, and topical corticosteroids are contraindicated in secondary herpes.

Type 1 herpes simplex infections are usually more severe in patients with impaired cellular immune functions. A simple blister of the lip may progress to an invasive oral-pharyngeal necrotizing lesion, esophagitis, pneumonia, or diseminated disease. Such patients should be referred for medical treatment.

OTHER SYSTEMIC PATHOLOGIES THAT MAY PRODUCE OROFACIAL NOCICEPTION

Although there are a number of systemic diseases that fall into this category, the authors have selected some of the more commonly encountered entities. These may be grossly classified into diseases of musculoskeletal origin and collagen disorders.

MUSCULOSKELETAL DISORDERS
Thoracic Outlet Syndrome

Thoracic outlet syndrome represents an abnormal compression of the brachial plexus produced by either a cervical rib or an abnormally tight anterior scalene muscle. At one time it was believed that the syndrome was ficticious. However, it has now been validated and is seen in some post-traumatic patients. The symptoms include tingling in the fingers, diffuse pain, and myospasm in the shoulder and neck area that may be referred to the orofacial region. If thoracic outlet syndrome is suspected the patient should be checked for Adsen's sign. This is the absence of a pulse when the arm of the affected side is elevated above the head and the head rotated in the contralateral direction. If a positive Adsen's sign is found the patient should be referred to an orthopedist or neurosurgeon for further evaluation.

Cervical Spondylosis

Spondylosis in its simplest form is defined as degenerative changes in the spine. These changes usually involve the cervical and lumbar regions (27). Although most individuals past the fifth decade will have demonstrable degenerative changes in the spinal cord, most of these subjects are asymptomatic. The predisposing factor for pain appears to be the size of the spinal canal. Narrower canals are predisposed to produce pain in the presence of spondylosis. The pain is produced on neck movement and may be referred to the orofacial area. Diagnosis is made by x-ray or magnetic resonance imaging, and the patient should be referred to an orthopedist or neurosurgeon.

Hyperextensive Trauma

As discussed in an earlier section of the chapter, the anterior aspect of the TMJ is its weakest section. Almost all hyperextensive-type injuries, such as whiplash, will produce symptom-producing injury to the joint or its adnexal structures. This injury is frequently overlooked by the physician because of the concentration on the coexistent pain in the neck, shoulder, and back area. It is suggested that all patients involved in whiplash-type traumas be evaluated for TMD as quickly as practical.

Spastic Torticollis

Abnormal head posture associated with dyskinetic movements of the musculature of the neck are the distinguishing symptoms of this disorder. The etiology is unknown. It has been associated with psychiatric, kinesthetic, ocular, and neurologic disorders. The myospastic activity in the neck produces a profound response in the TMJ and its associated neuromusculature. The patient requires simultaneous treatment by the dentist, psychiatrist, internist, and other appropriate medical specialists.

COLLAGEN DISORDERS

The proliferative collagen disorders lupus erythematosus and systemic sclerosis may produce facial pain and mandibular dysfunction or complicate the management of the facial pain patient. Temporomandibular joint inflammation similar to that found in rheumatoid arthritis may be a manifestation of the polyarthritis found in lupus and systemic sclerosis. A polymositis involving the head and neck muscles may also be present. In addition, the skin tightness of systemic sclerosis can cause difficulties in all dental and oral surgical procedures.

Ehlers-Danlos syndrome is a disorder of collagen formation that produces joint hypermobility (among other problems). This syndrome may produce TMJ hypermobility with clicking and popping (59). Such patients are treated in basically the same way as others with TMJ disorders. However, the prognosis is not as favorable and therapy must be continued beyond the time required by TMJ problems of other etiologies. Furthermore, excessive strain on the TMJ and other joints must be avoided. TMJ surgery is contraindicated because of excessive scar formation and poor healing (59).

RARE OROFACIAL PAINS

Damage to the auriculotemporal nerve produces the auriculotemporal, or Frey's, syndrome. This involves a

Table 24.2
Dental Management of Orofacial Pain Patients

Treatment Modalities	Indications
Analgesic blocking—the use of local anesthetics to arrest pain input, interrupt cycling, resolve trigger point activity, or produce sympathetic blockade.	Pain of muscle origin Vascular pains Other visceral pains Neurogenic pains
Sensory stimulation—stimulating nonnociceptive afferents to produce pain-inhibiting effects. This includes cutaneous (vibration, counterirritation, hydrotherapy, vapocoolant therapy), and transcutaneous (TENS, electroacupuncture) stimulation.	Pains of dental origin Pains of muscle origin TMJ pains Other musculoskeletal pains Vascular pains Neurogenic pains
Physiotherapy—this includes cutaneous and deep massage, exercise, deep heat therapy, and trigger point therapy.	Pain of muscle origin TMJ pains Other musculoskeletal pains Other visceral pains
Medicinal therapy—this includes analgesics, anti-inflammatory agents, analgesic balms, antibiotics, antiherpes agents, local anesthetics, anticonvulsants, neuroactive drugs, antianxiety drugs, muscle relaxants, antidepressant drugs, and vasoactive agents.	Cutaneous pains Mucogingival pains Pains of dental origin TMJ pains Other musculoskeletal pains Vascular pains Other visceral pains Neurogenic pains
Surgery—this includes TMJ surgeries such as eminectomies, condylectomies, condylotomies, disk repair and disk plication; and neurosurgeries such as peripheral thermoneurolysis and neural decompression.	TMJ pains Neurogenic pains

[a] TENS = transcutaneous electrical nerve stimulation, SCNS = subcutaneous central nervous system.

paradoxical gustatory reflex with parazyms or unilateral burning pain in the temple or the temporomandibular joint area, associated with flushing and sweating when the patient eats. The skin may be hyperesthetic between attacks.

Eagle's syndrome induces a sensation of persistent raw throat, pain and difficulty in swallowing, pain referred to the auricular area, and limited neck movement. This syndrome is caused by an elongation of the styloid process or calcification of the stylohyoid ligament. Encroachment of the elongated styloid process on the carotid artery may produce carotid arteritis and carotidynia. Pain is sometimes referred through the face to the ophthalmic area. This encroachment on the carotid artery can also produce syncope when the head is turned from side to side.

These, plus other rare syndromes, such as Raeder's syndrome, are best treated by the physician and not the dentist.

SUMMARY

Although the subject of chronic orofacial pain is diverse and complex, the author has attempted to present a rational, in depth, organized discussion of the subject. In closing, Table 24.2 is presented to summarize much of the material in this chapter.

References

1. McNeill C: Craniomandibular disorders: the state of the art. *J Prosthet Dent* 49:393–395, 1983.
2. Morgan DH, House LR, Hall WP, et al: *Diseases of the Temporomandibular Apparatus.* St. Louis, CV Mosby, 1982, p 73.
3. Hendler NH, Long DM, Wise TN: *Diagnosis and Treatment of Chronic Pain.* Boston, John Wright PSG, 1982, pp 1–20.
4. Merskey H: Pain terms: a list with definitions and notes on usage. Recommended by the IASP Subcommittee on Taxonomy. *Pain* 6:249–252, 1979.
5. Burgess PR, Perl ER: Myelinated afferent fibers responding specifically to noxious stimulation of the skin. *J Physiol (London)* 190:541–562, 1967.
6. Weisenberg M (ed): *Pain, Clinical and Experimental Perspectives.* St. Louis, CV Mosby, 1975, p 132.
7. Buxbaum JD, Myslinski NR, Myers DE: *The Physiology, Pathophysiology, Diagnosis and Treatment of Temporomandibular Dysfunction and Related Pain.* Baltimore, University of Maryland, 1986.
8. Solberg WK, Clark GT: *Temporomandibular Joint Problems.* Chicago, Quintessence, 1980, p 17.
9. Dubner R, Sessle BJ, Storey AT: *The Neural Basis of Oral and Facial Function.* New York, Plenum Press, 1978, pp 9–55.
10. Dubner R, Gobel S, Price DD: Peripheral and central trigeminal "pain" pathways. In Bonica JJ, Albe-Fessard D (eds): *Advances in Pain Research and Therapy.* New York, Raven, 1976, pp 137–148.
11. Kunc Z: Significance of fresh anatomic data on spinal trigeminal tract for possibility of selective tractotomies. In Knighton RS, Dumke PR (eds): *Pain.* London, Churchill Livingstone, 1966, pp 351–363.
12. Greenwood F: An electrophysiological study of the central connections of primary afferent nerve fibers from the dental pulp in the cat. *Arch Oral Biol* 18:771–785, 1973.
13. Vyklicky L, Keller O, Jastreboff P, et al: Spinal trigeminal tractotomy and nociceptive reactions evoked by tooth pulp stimulation in the cat. *J Physiol (Paris)* 73:379–386, 1977.
14. Hu JW, Sessle BJ: Trigeminal nociceptive and nonnociceptive neurons: brain stem intranuclear projections and

modulation by orofacial, periaqueductal gray and nucleus raphe magnus stimuli. *Brain Res* 170:547–552, 1979.
15. Melzack R, Wall PD: Pain mechanisms: a new theory. *Science* 150:971–979, 1965.
16. Anderson SA, Keller O, Roos A, et al: Cortical projection of tooth pulp afferents in the cat. In Anderson DJ, Matthews B (eds): *Pain in the Trigeminal Region*. Amsterdam, Elsevier/North Holland, 1977, pp 355–364.
17. Biedenbach MA, Van Hassel HJ, Brown AC: Tooth pulp-driven neurons in the somatosensory cortex of primates: role in pain mechanisms including a review of the literature. *Pain* 7:31–50, 1979.
18. Albe-Fessard D: Central nervous mechanisms involved in pain and analgesia. In Lim RKS, Armstrong D, Pardo EG (eds): *Pharmacology of Pain*. Oxford, Pergamon Press, 1968, pp 131–168.
19. Penfield W, Boldrey R: Somatic motor and sensory representation in the cerebral cortex of man as studied by electrical stimulation. *Brain* 60:389–443, 1937.
20. Matthews B: Responses of intradental nerves to electrical and thermal stimulation of teeth in dogs. *J Physiol (Lond)* 264:641–664, 1977.
21. Matthews B, Searle BN: Some observations on pulp testers. *Br Dent J* 137:307–312, 1974.
22. Matthews B, Holland GR: Couplings between nerves in teeth. *Brain Res* 98:354–358, 1975.
23. Scott D Jr: The arousal and suppression of pain in the tooth. *Int Dent J* 22:30–32, 1972.
24. Brannstrom M, Astrom A: The hydrodynamics of dentine: its possible relationship to dentinal pain. *Int Dent J* 22:219–227, 1972.
25. Sessle BJ, Hu JW, Dubner R, Lucier GE: Functional properties of neurons trigeminal subnucleus caudalis of the cat. II. Modulation of responses to noxious and non-noxious stimuli by periaqueductal grey, nucleus raphe magnus, cerebral cortex and afferent influences, and effect of naloxone. *J Neurophysiol* 45:193–207, 1981.
26. Sessle BJ, Hu JW, Zhong G, Amano N: Responsiveness of trigeminal (V) brainstem neurons to cervical afferent stimulation. *J Dent Res* 64(spec issue):284, 1985.
27. Dalessio D (ed): *Wolff's Headache and Other Head Pain*. New York, Oxford University Press, 1972, pp 463–476.
28. Tzukert A, Hasin Y, Sharar Y: Oro-facial pain of cardiac origin. *Oral Surg* 51:484–486, 1981.
29. Tyndall DA, Gregg JM, Hawker JS: Evaluation of peripheral nerve regeneration following crushing or transection injuries. *J Oral Maxillofac Surg* 42:314–318, 1984.
30. Gregg JM: Post-traumatic pain: experimental trigeminal neuropathy. *J Oral Surg* 29:260–267, 1971.
31. Gobel S, Binck JM: Degenerative changes in primary trigeminal axons and in neurons in nucleus caudalis following tooth pulp extirpation in the cat. *Brain Res* 132:347–354, 1977.
32. Westrum LE, Canfield RC, Black RG: Transganglionic degeneration in the spinal trigeminal nucleus following removal of tooth pulps in adult cats. *Brain Res* 101:137–140, 1976.
33. Gardner WJ: Trigeminal neuralgia. In Hassler R, Walker AE (eds): *Trigeminal Neuralgia: Pathogenesis and Pathophysiology*. Philadelphia, WB Saunders, 1967, pp 153–174.
34. Farrar WB, McCarty WL Jr: The TMJ dilemma. *J Ala Dent Assoc* 63:19, 1979.
35. Helms CA, Katzberg RW, Dolwick MF: *Internal Derangements of the Temporomandibular Joint*. San Francisco, Radiology Research and Educational Foundation, Radiological Institute, 1983, p 34.
36. *Dorland's Illustrated Medical Dictionary*, ed 26. Philadelphia, WB Saunders, 1981.
37. Gibilisco JA: Temporomandibular joint dysfunction and treatment. *Dent Clin North Am* 27(3):459, 1983.
38. Gibilisco JA: Temporomandibular joint dysfunction and treatment. *Dent Clin North Am* 27(3):461, 1983.
39. Solberg WK, Clark GT: *Temporomandibular Joint Problems*. Chicago, Quintessence, 1980, p 123.
40. Solberg WK, Clark GT: *Temporomandibular Joint Problems*. Chicago, Quintessence, 1980, p 115.
41. Greene CS: The temporomandibular joint syndrome. *JAMA* 224:622, 1973.
42. Deboever J: Functional disturbances of the temporomandibular joint. *Oral Sci Rev* 2:140, 1973.
43. Travell JG, Simons DG: *Myofascial Pain and Dysfunction: The Trigger Point Manual*. Baltimore, Williams & Wilkins, 1983.
44. Clark GT, Lynn P: Horizontal plane movements in controls and clinic patients with TMD. *J Prosthet Dent* 155:730–735, 1986.
45. Gregg JM: Post-traumatic trigeminal neuralgia: response to physiologic, surgical and pharmacologic therapies. *Int Dent J* 23:43, 1978.
46. Rasmussen OC: Painful traumatic neuromas in the oral cavity. *Oral Surg* 49:191–195, 1980.
47. Siegel MA, Van Hassel H: Traumatic neuroma subsequent to endodontic therapy. *J Endodont* 11:179–180, 1985.
48. Gregg JM: Neurological disorders of the maxillofacial region. In Kruger GO (ed): *Textbook of Oral and Maxillofacial Surgery*. St. Louis, CV Mosby, 1979, pp 666–710.
49. Baile W, Myers DE: Psychological and behavioral dynamics in chronic atypical facial pain. *Anesthesia Prog* 1986 (in press).
50. Moore PA: Bupivicaine: a long-lasting local anesthetic for dentistry. *Oral Surg* 58:369–374, 1984.
51. Myslinski NR, Myers DE: Drugs used in the treatment of facial pain. In Holroyd SV, Wynn RL (eds): *Clinical Pharmacology in Dental Practice*, ed 4. St. Louis, CV Mosby, 1987 (in press).
52. Myers DE: Illustrative case of neurogenic toothache. *Headache* 25:173–174, 1985.
53. Marbach JJ: Phantom tooth pain. *J Endodont* 4:409–419, 1971.
54. Marbach JJ, Hulbrock J, Hohn C, Segal AG: Incidence of phantom tooth pain: an atypical facial neuralgia. *Oral Surg* 53:190–193, 1982.
55. Hanowell ST, Kennedy SF: Phantom tongue pain and causalgia: report of a case. *Anesth Analg* 58:436–438, 1979.
56. Cameron CE: Cracked tooth syndrome. *J Am Dent Assoc* 68:405, 1964.
57. Gibbs JW: Cuspal fracture odontalgia. *Dent Diagn* 60:156–160, 1954.
58. Silvestri AR: The undiagnosed split-root syndrome. *J Am Dent Assoc* 92:930–935, 1976.
59. Myers DE: Ehlers Danlos syndrome as a cause of TMJ disorders. *Anesthesia Prog* 33:23–24, 1985.

part c
back and spinal pain

chapter 25
Spinal Surgery

Clark Watts, M.D.

Surgery upon the spine for the management of pain is conducted for pain arising from spinal and extraspinal locations. It is performed for pain of neoplastic origin and also for pain of chronic nonneoplastic origins. The surgery is of two types. First, there are procedures designed to correct the cause of the pain. An example would be a spinal fusion for pain secondary to chronic instability, or decompressive laminectomy for the pain of neurogenic claudication secondary to spinal stenosis. The second type of surgery is directed primarily to affect pain itself rather than the cause of the pain. The patient with a chronic "failed back" syndrome or widespread metastatic carcinoma has an uncorrectable "lesion" requiring the surgeon to, in some way, modify the sensation of pain.

Techniques for pain modification are varied depending upon the location of the pain and the neurologic status of the patient. The implantation of a dorsal column stimulator results in no change in the neurologic status of the patient, whereas a cordotomy or a lesion placed in the dorsal root entry zone may result in neurologic changes, both sensory and motor. All of these issues are dealt with in greater detail by other authors in Chapters 11 and 26 to 29. The purpose of this chapter is to give a thoughtful, some might even say philosophical, analysis of the issues that should be considered by physician and patient alike in spinal surgery for pain management.

Surgeons who operate for pain management function constantly under the shadow cast by the dictum "if one operates for pain, pain is what one gets." This underscores the realization by these surgeons that patients who undergo surgery for the management of pain require a great deal of perioperative support, both medical and psychological. Often these patients are medical and psychological cripples by the time surgery is considered. More than one program of nonsurgical pain management has failed. They are often drug dependent and also have experienced more than one personal failure, whether it be loss of the support of family or a negatively altered doctor-patient relationship.

The support that is required in the perioperative period is not unique to the perioperative state. In fact, if the support that is required at this time for successful management of the patient's pain had been available earlier in the patient's management, it is possible the patient would not have suffered the failures bringing him to the surgeon in the first place. These concepts can be illustrated using as an example the experience of the patient with the chronic "failed back" syndrome.

This patient initially experiences an episode of back pain that does not respond to self-treatment with a period of sedentary activity. The patient is then seen by a physician with a nonspecific, but to the patient disabling, back pain, which is not very intellectually challenging to the busy physician. After a cursory examination that reveals little in the way of positive findings, the physician instructs the patient to return to sedentary activity with some medication and no appointment to return for reexamination, but the suggestion that if the patient has not improved in a few days to call or return for another examination.

The patient at this time feels somewhat guilty for taking the physician's time but also feels some anger because at further cost to himself he has acquired little in the way of additional understanding of his problems. The interactions of these complex emotions along with lack of acceptance on the part of the patient's family, and possibly employer, result in poor compliance. The patient does not improve.

After a few days the patient returns still complaining of the low backache, which has now become interpreted by the patient as suffering. The physician at this point, finding nothing in the way of objective evidence of disease, must deal with his own emotional complexities. He is perturbed that his patient is not improving from what he considers to be a minor problem. There may be a sense of frustration that is transmitted to the patient in one way or another. The physician handles this problem, however, by proceeding to the next step, which is to obtain a battery of studies including a blood test (possibly an erythrocyte sedimentation rate), some x-rays, perhaps even a computed tomography (CT) scan, despite finding nothing on the physical examination that would suggest that these studies have a high degree of probability of providing useful information.

If in fact little information is gained from further studies, the physician takes one of several avenues, all but one guaranteeing a continuation of the patient's relentless trip to the pain surgeon. The physician may tell the patient there is nothing wrong, even suggesting that the pain is simply "in the mind" of the patient, and dismiss him (whereupon the patient will seek some other health care provider, where the above scenario will be repeated). Alternatively, the patient may be referred to a back surgeon, either a neurosurgeon or an orthopaedic surgeon (more on this below).

It is hoped, but unfortunately this is infrequent, that the physician recognizes that he has more than a set of somatic complaints in this patient. He has a patient who needs education and direction. If this is the physician's approach to the patient, he will properly educate the patient about the biomechanics of the back and the interrelationships between those mechanics and the pain the patient is suffering. The physician will explain carefully, tactfully, and with a great deal of sensitivity the chronic effect that pain may have on the mind, and on the patient's outlook on life. A careful analysis of the sociodynamics of the patient's life at home, at work, and at play will be conducted. The physician will develop a management protocol, skillfully incorporating into that protocol activities that the patient will understand and accept as useful to him but also, just as important, as instructions from a knowing and caring physician. It is the resultant harmony in the doctor-patient relationship that will, as much as attention to the physical needs of the healing backache, guarantee success.

I noted above that one of the avenues the physician may take is to refer the patient to another physician for further evaluation, perhaps even a back surgeon. This is a critical step. In this referral it is important the physician not suggest, by the referral, rejection of the patient, but rather communicate an understandable desire to seek what is in the patient's best interest. The back surgeon, receiving the patient who has failed medical management from a physician perceived as being insensitive or not knowledgeable, will face a number of pressures both from within and without the doctor-patient relationship that too often result in the first of a number of surgical procedures not indicated, leading to the chronic "failed back" syndrome. The net result of these pressures is to bring into conflict noninterventional therapy, which I will call inactive, and interventional therapy, which I will call active. The simplest way to analyze these pressures is to look at each one, and the contributors, individually.

The first contributor is the back surgeon himself. If he recommends no surgery but rather a continuation of the noninterventional or inactive management protocol that has already failed the patient, the surgeon has to admit the inability of his skills to be effective. This admission is hard for most physicians, especially surgeons, because of the general view that surgery is so definitive. The surgeon feels professionally impotent. This drives the surgeon to be less than objective about the "soft" signs that accompany the patient's story. The inconsequential findings on x-ray, CT scan, or myelography carry more weight in the deliberative process. Questionable additional studies such as epidural venography, diskography, and the like are interpreted in the favor of intervention. Once the surgeon becomes committed, he proceeds aggressively, with his talents and skills, to apply the definitive management, intervention.

It is the failure of ill-advised surgery that has driven the search for simpler, less invasive, techniques for the management of these patients, such as epidural and intradiskal steroids, chemonucleolysis, and the currently developing percutaneous nuclectomy. Although each of these techniques is effective in a narrowly defined group of patients, their simplicity and the pressures on the surgeon to intervene have resulted in their use in a wider group of patients, guaranteeing a higher degree of failure. It is this escalating failure coupled with, in some cases, serious complications that has resulted in rapid disenchantment with the procedures by both medical professionals and lay people alike, and the acquisition by these procedures of poor reputations that may have been undeserved.

The conflict of inactive versus active therapy is contributed to by employers and third-party payers. They perceive the patient undergoing inactive treatment as receiving less than definitive management. They perceive the diagnosis to be uncertain. They are unable to accurately calculate, actuarially, their costs and to know with any acceptable (to them) degree of certainty when they will close the case file. On the other hand, they understand that if the patient has some form of intervention, they can calculate, based upon past rates of success of the surgeon and the return to work rate of the patients, their costs and work load scheduling responsibilities. They prefer the latter, apparently more precise degree of certainty. It was, for example, the support of this group when told of the promises of chemonucleolysis that permitted the rather brief but astonishing degree of incorporation of this procedure into the standard surgical armamentarium of back surgeons. It is thought by some that the uncritical acceptance of chemonucleolysis on the part of employers and insurance companies, with its promise of more rapid return to work even without promise of significant cost reduction, led, as much as any other influence, to its rapid widespread use.

A third group that contributes to the conflict between active and inactive therapy for the patient with back pain is comprised of the families and friends of the patient. The back surgeon who prescribes inactive treatment may be perceived by the family as noncaring, and as senselessly prolonging the agony of the patient, whereas the surgeon who decides to intervene is perceived as just the opposite. In addition, the family may look upon the patient who accepts additional inactive treatment by the back surgeon as being duped, or worse, wishing to "punish" the family by requiring of them additional attention. Once again, the unknowing family, when presented with the option of active treatment, feels just the opposite about the patient.

Finally, what of the patient himself? The patient is suffering from pain. This is the reason he accepts the advice of the initially treating physician to see the back surgeon. If he learns nothing new about himself, if he receives no detailed treatment protocols by the surgeon, he feels additionally frustrated. He believes health care professionals generally, and the surgeon specifically, really do not care. This attitude is readily transmitted to the surgeon. On the other hand, if the patient is offered surgery, he believes he is moving toward certain success. He is apprehensive about the additional risks of intervention, an increase in pain, and additional costs he will undertake, but the apprehension itself can lead to a curious reversal of priorities, enhancing the desire for more aggressive, more active treatment. This desire, for example, along with the suggestion that chemonucleolysis was simpler and might get the patient back to work earlier with few risks, contributed to the acceptance by the public of this form of treatment.

Once the ill-advised intervention has occurred, failure is almost certain. This leads to additional interventions, and eventually the patient becomes one for whom intervention is being undertaken not to alleviate the cause of pain, but to alleviate the pain itself.

Do the ideas and concepts discussed above apply at this point? Yes, they do. Pain and suffering on the part of the patient will tend to push the patient and the physician to more active forms of therapy, to intervention for the pain itself. The same pressures, often more intense, come into play. The large number of pain management techniques and protocols underscore the disappointment felt by most who participate in these interventions, whether patient or physician. This disappointment drives the constant search for new means of management, such as complex pain programs with biofeedback (nonsurgical) and chronically implanted central nervous system–stimulating electrodes (surgical).

The thesis of this essay is not that spinal surgery for pain management is not appropriate. Rather, it is that this surgery should be considered, in most cases, as intervention of a "last resort." In some cases, it may be the most humane management technique. The patient with widespread cancer and only a few months left to live will certainly benefit the less she must use mind-dulling medication. On the other hand, large numbers of patients who fail surgery for chronic non-life-threatening pain speak to the need for extreme care and sensitivity on the part of the pain management team in recommending such surgery, especially in view of risks of additional neurologic deficits brought on by surgery.

It is with this in mind that the reader should critically review techniques of spine surgery for pain presented in this book by extremely well respected, experienced, and thoughtful surgeons.

chapter 26
Differential Diagnosis and Management of Cervical Spine Pain

John Aryanpur, M.D.
Thomas B. Ducker, M.D.

"Pain in the neck" is such a common complaint and is so universally understood that the expression alone is used to describe certain people, situations, and experiences. Within any given month approximately 10% of the population will experience pain in the neck, with or without radicular pain into the arms (1). More than one-third of the population can recall a significant episode of severe neck pain, often with radicular components (1). In epidemiologic studies, a history of significant stiff neck with or without arm pain has been found in one-half to three-quarters of all individuals (2–4). Often these people will see their physician with this complaint. The scope of this problem is therefore tremendous.

Fortunately, 70% of people with the complaint of new-onset neck pain who visit a doctor are well or improving within 1 month (2), and a majority of the remaining 30% obtain symptomatic relief with time and appropriate therapeutic interventions. Thus, only a small proportion of patients with acute neck pain go on to develop more chronic pain problems.

The human neck is evolutionarily an extremely complex structure with multiple bony, ligamentous, muscular, vascular, and neural components, all of which are capable of generating "neck pain." As such a structure, the neck can be affected by such processes as degenerative osteoarthritis, inflammatory diseases of muscle and ligament, vascular insufficiency, and neural compression syndromes, to mention only a few. Dermatomal, myotomal, and sclerotomal pain patterns may be distinguished.

More importantly, in a social sense the neck acts as a fulcrum from which our eyes, ears, nose, and mouth function to interact with our environment. Neck mobility is essential for the full aprpeciation of the world around us. More than we realize, the neck is active in common activities—nodding, turning, smiling, and shaking hands. Any disruption of its normal function may quickly be appreciated as uncomfortable, and even painful.

To complicate the situation, pathologic processes in other areas, such as the shoulder, the diaphragm, the heart, or the jaw, may cause pain that is referred to the neck—thus the complaint of "neck pain" in patients with acromioclavicular joint disease, diaphragmatic irritation, hypertension and myocardial infarction, or temporomandibular joint syndromes. Disease of the apical lung and pleura also may impinge upon the brachial plexus to give pain in a C8 or T1 distribution.

Finally, even the most minor discomfort in the neck may be colored by certain psychosocial and psychoneurotic factors, in which case the complaint of "pain in the neck" is in reality but a physical outlet for a variety of personal and psychological problems.

The differential diagnosis of cervical spine pain is therefore quite large and it is often only with repeated office visits and multiple investigations and therapies that the proper diagnosis is made.

In the next few pages we review some basic aspects of cervical anatomy and biomechanics as well as bony and neurologic pathology and specific referred pain syndromes. Following that diagnostic studies are outlined. From a synthesis of the above a list of differential diagnoses can in most cases be made, with the ultimate goals of focusing in upon the most appropriate diagnosis and treatment for each patient.

ANATOMY AND BIOMECHANICS

The neck is the most mobile region of the spine. Over 50% of all neck motion occurs at the atlanto-occipital and atlantoaxial joints, and the remaining 50% of neck motion is equally distributed through the C3–C7 segments. In quadriped animals the motion allowed at the atlanto-occipital and atlantoaxial joints is even greater than it is in humans.

Mechanically there are many places where the system may cause pain. In the seven cervical vertebrae there are 14 zygoapophyseal joints (usually referred to as facet joints) as well as five Luschka's joints (referred to as uncinate processes), and a muscular and ligamentous apparatus that is innervated not only by the eleventh cranial nerve but also by all of the eight cranial nerves on both sides. Muscle and ligamentous tears and sprains are by far the most common causes for neck pain, but other pathologies may exist as well. The facet joints and joints of Luschka are lined with synovial membrane, and are subject to the same inflammatory pain-producing pathologies as synovial joints elsewhere. The normal intervertebral disk absorbs axial loading pressures on the spine, serving as a "shock absorber." Disk rupture or degeneration or anulus tear can produce severe focal pain that may be difficult to diagnose and treat. Bony structures themselves may degenerate secondary to osteoporosis or metabolic or infiltrative processes, leading to pathologic fractures and pain. Finally, the neural tissues themselves may be a source of pain when compressed or irritated. These pathologic mechanisms are discussed in more detail below.

THE CERVICAL SPINE

The anatomy and relevant biomechanics of the cervical spine are most pertinent to clinical disorders if considered segmentally. Thus, the occiput–C1 region (comprising the occiput and C1 vertebrae, the joints between them, the muscles and ligaments affecting movement at these joints, and the spinal cord and nerve roots exiting at that level) may be considered an independent segment, and so on for the C1–C2, C2–C3, and remaining regions down to C7–T1.

The seven small cervical vertebrae balance the 15-pound weight of the head and its contents. The center of weight of the skull is slightly anterior to the midaxis of the spine, and naturally causes the head to fall forward. For this reason there is constant tension on the posterior cervical musculature to hold the head in the upright position. Relaxation and contraction of this posterior musculature, aided by the upper one-third of the trapezius, allows cervical flexion and extension. The vast majority of this flexion and extension occurs at the atlanto-occipital joint, and this joint is commonly referred to as the "yes" joint. Conversion of the emotion of "yes" into the "yes" nodding motion of the head is mediated by branches of the eleventh cranial nerve supplying the trapezius and sternocleidomastoid muscles, as well as by all eight cervical roots, including the C1 motor root, which exists at this level. There is no C1 sensory root.

Beneath this atlanto-occipital joint the neural anatomy is terribly complex. Within the spinal cord at that level there is the decussation of the long motor tracts as well as the descending spinal tract of the fifth cranial nerve, which is responsible for pain and temperature sensation over the face. The lower cranial nerve nuclei are also vulnerable at this location. Compression of the cord at this level can cause a variety of signs and symptoms (neck pain, limitation of flexion and extension, headaches, "onionskin" facial numbness, lower cranial nerve palsies, upper extremity weakness, and lower extremity spasticity) that may be diffuse enough to confuse even the best trained clinician. Suffice it to say that a patient presenting with complaints and physical findings as listed above should be suspected of having pathology at the occiput–C1 level.

Movement at the C1–C2 level is greatly influenced by the dens, which acts as a stable pin about which rotation may occur. The rotary movement of the atlantoaxial joint has led to its being refered to as the "no" joint. Again, motion through a cervical joint is controlled by one's emotions! Extremes of rotation, up to 80–100°, are possible at this joint.

The actual turning of the neck to produce a "no" movement is primarily a function of the sternocleidomastoid muscle. This muscle, with its attachments on the mastoid process at the base of the skull, clearly provides the major fulcrum for turning of the atlantoaxial joint. Posteriorly, the smaller capitis musculature, with attachments onto the spinous process of C2 extending up to the skull, acts primarily as a stabilizer and servo-mechanism balance system to maintain the head in proper alignment with the motions initiated by the stronger sternocleidomastoid muscle. Other posterior muscle groups, including the trapezius, complement this stabilizing action. Motor innervation for the sternocleidomastoid occurs primarily through the eleventh cranial nerve, supplemented by small fibers from C2 and C3 to the lower half of the muscle. At the C1–C2 segment a sensory nerve component is present in the form of large C2 sensory nerve roots. These divide peripherally into several branches, the largest of which on each side is the greater occipital nerve. This nerve provides sensory innervation of the superior aspect of the neck and the entire posterior half of the hemicranium, including the occiput and superior parietal areas of the skull and scalp. The greater occipital nerve may be trapped peripherally as it passes through the thick fascial attachments of the posterior neck musculature over the occipital region. This can be a source of pain and tenderness on the posterior aspect of the head. Prolonged contraction of the posterior cervical musculature, due to stress or fatigue, can cause compression of both greater occipital nerves, contributing to the tension headache syndromes.

The C2–C3 segment is in a sense a transitional segment between the hypermobile occiput–C2 area and the remaining cervical segments. The C2–C3 joint has multiple components: the intervertebral disk, the vertebral joints, and the zygoapophyseal joints. These limit the degrees of freedom at that segment, but also provide a degree of stability not present at higher levels. This joint will allow approximately 10° of motion in flexion and extension and 5–6° in rotation or lateral flexion. It is rarely involved in the degenerative arthritic changes that are so common at lower cervical levels.

The C3 vertebra has the C3 nerve root above and the C4 nerve root below. The motor innervation of the diaphragm, and of the accessory muscles of respiration in the neck, basically comes from these two nerve roots. (Occasionally the C5 roots make several smaller contributions to this innervation.) These motor roots also contribute to the innervation of the intrinsic neck muscles, as do all motor roots in the cervical region. The sensory component of the C3 root supplies the superior half of the neck anteriorly, and can extend up to the angle of the jaw and ear. Below, the C4 dermatome covers the lower half of the neck, and will extend over the clavicles. C5 through C8 dermatomal patterns are carried primarily out through the brachial plexus into the upper extremities.

From the C3–C4 segment caudally the motion of each vertebra upon its adjacent vertebra is basically the same. All are associated with approximately 10° of rotation and/or lateral flexion. All have intervertebral disks and uncovertebral and zygoapophyseal joints. Although disease within any of these vertebrae, adjacent ligaments, or joint structures can cause focal pain, more commonly the pathologic process is associated with a prominent component of local nerve root irritation and a strong radicular element is apparent. Pathology in the C4–T1 segments, therefore, commonly produces varying degrees of upper extremity pain and neurologic deficit. For this reason, the discussion of the caudal cervical segments simplifies to a neuroanatomic discussion of each of the individual cervical nerve roots that lead to the brachial plexus. Although the specific organization of the brachial plexus is complex, individual nerve root patterns are well recognized and easy to distinguish.

The C5 nerve root, which exits between the fourth and fifth cervical vertebrae, supplies the major innervation of the deltoid muscle. It also contributes to the biceps, the supra- and infraspinatus, serratus anterior, and levator scapulae. All are muscles involved in stabilizing the shoulder, and in abduction of the arm. The biceps reflex can be associated with the C5 nerve root, although in fact the C6 root may make a significant contribution. The sensory innervation of the C5 root is fairly specific, covering the shoulder and down the radial aspect of the arm to middistal forearm.

The motor component of the C6 nerve root, which exits between the C5 and C6 vertebrae, is responsible for the innervation of the brachioradialis and biceps muscles, as well as the extensors of the wrist. Clinically, the brachioradialis reflex is linked with the C6 root—in truth the C5 root is also involved. The C6 dermatomal pattern is very specific and definitely involves the dorsal radial aspect of the hand, the entire thumb, and sometimes part of the dorsal surface of the index finger.

The C7 nerve root makes an important contribution to the posterior aspect of the brachial plexus, which leads directly into the radial nerve. For that reason is strongly influences the triceps musculature, as well as the extensors of the wrist and the intrinsic muscles of the hand. Its sensory dermatomal pattern always involves the middle finger, but can involve the index finger as well. The triceps reflex is subserved by this nerve root.

The C8 nerve root, which comes off beneath the seventh cervical vertebra just above the first thoracic vertebra and the first rib, contributes heavily to the inferior cord of the brachial plexus and the medial cord. Its primary myotome includes the flexors of the hand—it is responsible for grip. The sensory innervation of this root covers the ulnar aspect of the forearm and the dorsal and palmar ulnar aspects of the hand extending up over the fourth and fifth fingers. This differs from the sensory distribution of the ulnar nerve in that the latter covers only the ulnar half of the fourth finger and does not extend proximally beyond the palmar crease.

Although it exits outside the cervical spine at the T1–T2 region, the T1 nerve root obviously contributes to the brachial plexus and the intrinsic muscles of the hand. Its sensory contributions are into the axilla and down the medial aspect of the upper arm. There is no specific reflex associated with this nerve root.

THE SPINAL CORD

The relationship between the spinal cord and nerve roots at the C3–T1 levels is clinically important and is constant in the mid- and lower cervical spine. The spinal cord lies within the vertebral canal, with nerve roots exiting via foramina at each level. The neural foramen at each level is bounded dorsolaterally by the facet joint capsule, anteromedially by the disk space and uncovertebral joints, and superiorly and inferiorly by the arches of the vertebra above and below. Each foramen can therefore be impinged upon in many ways. Degenerative changes leading to hypertrophy of the facet joint and/or the uncovertebral joints can often cause foraminal stenosis. The nucleus pulposis of the intervertebral disk is usually held in place by strong posterior longitudinal ligaments. However, under certain extremes of pressure and stress the disk material can herniate posteriorly or posterolaterally to impinge upon the spinal cord or nerve root. The neural foramina are slightly larger at C2–C3 and become progressively smaller down to C6–C7. Generally speaking the foramina have an average vertical diameter of 10 mm and a transverse diameter of 5 mm. The nerve roots lie near the upper vertebral pedicle, and as they exit further they descend slightly toward the intervertebral joint space itself. Since the nerve roots themselves occupy only one-third of the cross-sectional area of the foraminal space the actual shape of the foramen may be the most important consideration in determining its adequacy. A decrease in foraminal height is not as critical as a decrease in foraminal width. Consequently foraminal stenosis may be fairly advanced before the patient becomes symptomatic.

Cross-sectionally the normal spinal cord has a diameter in the lateral dimension of 12–13 mm throughout most of the cervical regions. In the anteroposterior (AP) dimension this diameter is generally less, from 8 to 9 mm. The spinal canal is largest in the high cervical region, and tapers progressively from there down. Assuming a normal AP diameter of 8–9 mm and allowing for 1 mm thickness of cerebrospinal fluid and 1 mm thickness of dural coverings surrounding the cord anteriorly and posteriorly, a minimum spinal canal diameter of 12–13 mm is required to allow for a healthy, noncompressed spinal cord. Clinically, the AP diameter of the spinal canal is easily obtainable from plain films or computed tomography, thus allowing quick estimates of the adequacy of the spinal canal. In practice, an AP diameter of 14 mm is considered to be normal, and anything less than that indicates a degree of central spinal stenosis with narrowing of the canal that could adversely affect the spinal cord.

VASCULAR SUPPLY

The vertebral artery travels through the transverse foramina of the C6–C1 vertebrae, making a tight arch over the atlas as it pierces the dura between the atlas and occiput. The spinal cord and nerve roots derive their blood supply bilaterally from myeloradicular arteries that branch from each vertebral artery and accompany specific nerve roots toward the cord substance itself. In the neck there are often three or four of these arteries, the largest of which usually accompanies the C6 or C7 root and is usually larger on the left than the right. This is commonly termed the artery of the cervical enlargement. This supply feeds into bilateral contributions from the intracranial vertebral artery, which joins at the midline to form the anterior spinal artery. A system of parallel posterior spinal arteries also exists. Although anastomoses between anterior and posterior spinal arteries are numerous, in general the anterior spinal artery supplies blood to the anterior two-thirds of the cord (including the anterior and lateral funiculi and gray matter of the cord). The posterior spinal artery system supplies the posterior columns exclusively. In rare individuals the anterior spinal artery may be vestigial, and a single large myeloradicular artery may supply most of the cervical spinal cord. Embolic or thrombotic events, or occlusion of major spinal arteries or veins during surgical interventions or by trauma, can lead to spinal cord ischemia, and ultimately spinal infarction.

PATHOLOGY

Pathology within the cervical spine can involve the central nervous system and its adjacent nerve roots, the vertebral joints, or the bones themselves. When initially attempting to ascertain where the pathology lies the first major division is between involvement of the nervous system itself and involvement of bony and soft tissue structures. In many cases both go hand in hand, and consequently may be difficult to tease apart. For discussion's sake we will begin centrally with problems of the spinal cord itself, and then proceed peripherally to quickly review pathology of the bones, joints, and muscles.

Clinically, the prototypical intrinsic spinal pathology is an expansile mass of the cord, and the simplest of central spinal masses is the syrinx. These can develop idiopathically or as a long-term sequela of spinal trauma, and may be initially associated with arm and facial pain and discomfort, especially at night. This latter is thought to be secondary to changes in differential pressure between syrinx and subarachnoid space that occur during recumbency. The pain then becomes less prominent as the neurologic deficit becomes more pronounced. There can be focal sensory loss on the face as well as over the trunk and limbs as a consequence of compression of the anterior white commissure and lateral spinothalamic tracts. Clumsy, wasted hands and a stiff gait reflect a combination of upper and lower motor neuron deficits in the upper extremities and pure upper motor neuron deficits in the lower extremities. Bowel and bladder problems may occur as well.

On occasion, a spinal cord cyst is associated with a tumor, such as an ependymoma. More frequently the tumor itself can develop cystic degeneration, as in astrocytomas of the cord.

Other degenerative processes besides intrinsic compressive cord lesions may lead to neurologic deficit and pain. Anterior motor horn cell loss, as in amyotrophic lateral sclerosis and polio, or ischemic processes of the cord may result in clinical syndromes that are difficult to distinguish from those of the more common spinal cord compressive syndromes.

Rather than being in the spinal cord itself, the mass may be centered along the meninges or adjacent nerve roots. These are locations at which meningiomas and neurofibromas are commonly found. Even though these tumors may initially develop on one root alone, they progress so slowly that the true root pathology may not be fully appreciated. Again, the common initial symptomatology is often pain, but it is often only when spinal cord compression has reached the point of upper extremity weakness, myelopathy, or gait disturbance that the clinical syndrome is recognized.

Extradural processes as well may cause a syndrome identical to the above. By far the most common source of extradural compression is degenerative joint disease of the intervertebral joints. Normal degenerative joint changes lead, over time, to reactive pannus and bony spur formation that when severe can cause spinal cord or nerve root compression. These degenerative processes can be accelerated by coexistent disease, such as rheumatoid arthritis, which characteristically attacks predominantly the atlanto-occipital and atlantoaxial regions of the spine, leading to ligamentous laxity and spinal column instability as well as cord and nerve root compression. In contrast, ankylosing spondylitis causes calcification of joints and longitudinal spinal ligaments, leading to spinal fusion and abnormal bone formation that once again may compress neural tissues.

Other epidural masses such as metastatic tumors (usually from the breast or lung) and benign and malignant primary bone tumors may cause cord or root compression as above and can therefore be included in this category of extradural compressive masses.

Intervertebral disk herniation typically affects only a single nerve root. However, the herniation may be directly posterior into the canal to cause acute spinal cord compression and symptomatology similar to that of other extradural lesions. In addition, joint and ligamentous pathology may cause pain independent of a compressive effect on neural tissue. Joints that are inflamed or unstable may produce focal, mechanical pain quite different from that of neural compression. Thus, a common clinical presentation is that of the patient with severe degenerative changes of the cervical spine who has both mechanical (joint and ligamentous) and radicular (neural compressive) pain components.

Intrinsic pathology of the bone, such as with osteoporotic fractures, bony tumors, or Paget's disease of the spine, may produce focal pain. This pain may be exacerbated by neck movement, as is pain originating from the joints, but more commonly is not. Palpation of the involved vertebra, however, almost invariably reproduces the pain. The pain from bony lesions is characteristically described as dull or aching.

Finally, all the above pathologies may contribute to the development of cervical muscle spasm and irritation, making this a nearly universal accompaniment of all complaints of neck pain. Pain on movement and superficial palpation, and muscle tightness are characteristic.

MEDICAL HISTORY

In evaluating a patient with cervical pain, as with any patient, the physician has the responsibility of directing the interview process. If this is skillfully done, in 70–80% of patients a reasonable initial diagnosis can be made even without a physical examination or further diagnostic studies. As always, open-ended questions yield the greatest information.

The interview begins as the patient enters the room, and his or her habitus, posture, and gait should be observed. Age, sex, and occupation are all readily ascertained. Next, a description of the pain is needed.

Pain always has at least three characteristics—onset, course, and severity. These need to be described in terms of location, exacerbating and relieving factors, quality, and severity. It is essential to have the patient begin by pointing to the painful area of the neck or arm. One must literally have the patient stand up and show the examiner where he/she hurts. This will allow the examiner to sidestep any confusion the patient may have with anatomic description or terms.

Leading questions about particular activities (i.e., twisting the neck, running, doing sports, working, etc.) are useful. If the patient does not spontaneously provide descriptions of the type and severity of the pain then questions such as how sharp or dull, aching or burning, throbbing or cramping the pain is may be employed. Although it is important not to put words in the patients mouth, certain general types of pain may indicate certain pathologies. For example, pain deep within the bone is usually described as dull and nagging, whereas fracture pain is sharp, severe, and immediately associated with muscle spasm. Pain that is worse at night can suggest a spinal cord tumor or mass. Pain that radiates sharply is usually radicular in origin.

Finally, patients may have initiated treatments on their own or sought advice elsewhere prior to being seen. Responses to over-the-counter drugs such as aspirin, Motrin, Tylenol, and the like are important. Some patient have seen physical therapists or chiropractors, and a knowledge of the response to such manipulations is always beneficial. As always, how the patient reacts to his/her disease psychologically is of paramount importance. If there is obvious secondary gain or malingering involved the examiner may do better to direct treatment toward these psychological factors.

It is also important to be cognizant of the many patterns of referred pain. As discussed earlier, numerous noncervical pathologies may cause various types of neck pain. Consequently, in difficult cases where no conspicuous cervical pathology can be held accountable for the patient's pain, consultation with colleagues in other specialties should be the rule rather than the exception.

CLINICAL EXAMINATION

In dealing with patients with neck pain the physical examination must have two basic components. The first component must involve an examination of the anatomy and mechanics of the neck itself. The second component must include an accurate assessment of the patient's neurologic status.

ANATOMY AND MECHANICS OF THE NECK

In evaluating the mechanics of the neck it must be appreciated that, as described above, 50% of cervical motion occurs at the occipital C1 and C2 joints alone. Thus the "yes" and "no" motions may be intact in the face of many a severe cervical disorder. The first three cervical vertebrae are anatomically located behind the face and are covered by the jaw at the base of the skull. C4 through C7 are centrally placed, and are the vertebrae that make up the neck as we view it from the surface.

Grossly the neck should have a gentle lordotic curve, as in the lumbar region. Most patients should be able to easily extend their neck to look at the ceiling, and to flex their neck to look at the floor. A neck that is fixed and lacks motion has either mechanical or pain-evoked limitations to a full range of motion.

The head compression, or Spurling's, test (5) is a valuable aid in localizing the level of the pathology. This maneuver causes compression of the vertebral bodies on one another and narrows the neural foramina. If this maneuver produces radicular pain a nerve root pathology is probable. However, if only local neck pain is elicited, joint or ligamentous disease is more likely. The reverse of compression (i.e., distraction) is often helpful as well. The radicular pain of a soft disk herniation or formainal stenosis may be relieved by the opening of the foramina caused by cervical distraction. If pain is from joint disease, distraction will simply accentuate the pain as much as compression.

In cervical nerve root disorders due to either soft disk disease or osteophytes, extending the neck and turning the head to the side of the pain commonly reproduces the radicular pain symptoms. Patients will often volunteer that they will not turn or extend their neck because of this discomfort.

In addition to testing the range of motion of the neck the range of motion of the shoulder and upper extremity must be evaluated as well. In many cases, it is very difficult to distinguish between shoulder joint disorders and certain nerve root compression syndromes. Furthermore, with certain neck disorders weakness within the deltoid or biceps leads to shoulder stiffness and tightness, so the patient may in actuality have both problems. Nonetheless, if the patient has pain in the neck that radiates down the arm it is useful for the patient and examiner to demonstrate that passive movement of the wrist, elbow, or shoulder will not reproduce the pain, thereby confirming that the upper extremity pain is not caused by pathology in the limb itself. If this is followed by measures that do reproduce the upper extremity pain (i.e., compression, extension, and rotation of the neck), ordering x-rays and other diagnostic studies of the neck will seem logical to the patient as well as reassuring to the physician.

NEUROLOGIC STATUS

The neurologic examination should be performed in a systematic way. The patient can be sitting on an examining table, although it may be found helpful to have the patient sitting in a chair. This way the examiner can walk around the patient to observe at many angles. A motor, sensory, and reflex examination can be done in a matter of a few minutes. The examiner begins by walking behind the patient and observing as he/she raises the arms above the head and lowers them back down. By looking at how the neck is held and at the mechanics of the neck and shoulders throughout this movement one has already learned a good deal of information. Palpation of neck muscles and individual spinous processes may also yield valuable information regarding the origin of neck pain.

Next the patient is instructed to flex the arms at the elbows and abduct at the shoulder, and to maintain this position. By exerting counterpressure the strength of the deltoid muscles may be tested simultaneously. This is essential because, although absolute strength is important, it is more crucial to detect an asymmetry in strength from side to side. The patient now lowers the arms to his/her side, keeping them flexed at the elbow. In this position biceps strength can be assessed. Again, one is looking above all for asymmetry. Moving behind the patient, the patient's fist is then placed inside the examiner's hands with instructions to extend the arms, thus utilizing the triceps muscle. If the arm is only minimally flexed to begin with the mechanical advantage will be with the examiner, and no patient will be able to overcome the examiner. A false impression of weakness might thus be given. It is therefore always crucial to examine individual muscles in positions that allow the patient maximal mechanical advantage. The triceps musculature has widespread innervation (C6–C8) so that asymmetry of the strength of this muscle is often a very sensitive indicator in patients with neurologic dysfunction. Finally the examiner faces the patient and has him/her extend the wrist, spread the fingers, and squeeze down tightly, all as a measure of the strength of the wrist extensors and intrinsic hand musculature. Although more sophisticated motor examinations are possible, these simple maneuvers can be rapidly performed and will pick up the majority of upper extremity dysfunctions. The lower extremities can be tested in a similar fashion.

The sensory examination is best done with a safety pin. This will not cause bleeding, can be used to test the patient's ability to distinguish between sharp and dull, and can be discarded after each examination. Comparing dermatomal patterns from side to side is usually the best way to appreciate a subtle hypoalgesia. As discussed above, a simple way to remember dermatomal patterns is to think of C5 as covering the shoulder, C6 covering the thumb, C7 involving the index and middle fingers, and C8 the ring and little fingers. Often testing down onto the chest wall is helpful, and it is important to remember that the C4 dermatomal pattern comes over the clavicle and is adjacent to the T2 dermatomal pattern on the anterior chest wall. Thus, a change in the sensation just below the clavicle may reflect a C4 sensory level deficit. Often, assessment of lower extremity proprioception is useful.

When cervical problems are suspected the reflex examination should include the upper and lower extremities as well as a comparison between the two. The biceps, triceps, and brachioradial reflexes are the significant deep tendon reflexes in the upper extremities. Inversion of the upper extremity reflexes or a positive Hoffmann's sign are evidence of hyperreflexia. Subsequent to this, lower extremity reflexes should be evaluated, especially at the knees. If the reflexes are perfectly normal in the upper extremities and at the knees, assessment of ankle and Babinski's reflexes are unlikely to yield much new information, and may be omitted in the interest of time. However, if any pathologic reflexes are noted then full lower extremity reflex assessment, including Babinski's reflex, is mandatory. The examination may be concluded by watching the patient walk from the examining room.

DIAGNOSTIC STUDIES

The investigation of any complaint of neck pain must first begin with plain films of the cervical spine. Oftentimes the plain films alone will show pathology such as bony erosion or degenerative osteoarthritis with osteophyte formation, which will guide further investigations and diagnostic decisions. Flexion and extension views of the cervical spine are indispensible in evaluating spinal stability radiographically. Oblique views allow visualization of the neural foramina. Other views may be tailored to the specific area being investigated.

With the plain film information in hand, further radiologic, electrophysiologic, or laboratory investigations may be ordered.

Unenhanced computed tomography remains the procedure of choice if detailed visualization of the bony anatomy is desired. Fractures, destructive processes, or osteophytes are all well visualized. Unfortunately, soft tissue and neural tissue visualization, although possible, is not optimal.

In instances in which a more detailed view of the spinal cord or nerve roots is desired several options exist. Classically the best way to obtain information regarding spinal cord and roots has been via myelography. This is still appropriate in many cases. Recently, however, both intrathecally enhanced computed tomography (CT) and magnetic resonance imaging (MRI) techniques have allowed myelography to be bypassed in selected cases. Thus, the patient in whom a syrinx or spinal cord tumor is suspected clinically could be studied by either intrathecally enhanced CT or MRI rather than traditional myelography. Indeed, the imaging study of choice for certain cervical disorders such as spinal syrinxes and Arnold-Chiari malformations is now the MRI scan. It should always be recognized, however, that if visualization of fine bony detail is required, supplementation of MRI with CT scanning will be needed. Many patients who are reluctant to undergo the invasive myelogram study can be evaluated adequately in this way.

Nuclear medicine studies, such as gallium and leukocyte-tagged scans, are not capable of providing detailed anatomic information. They are useful, however, when infectious etiologies are suspected as a cause of neck pain. It is always necessary to remember that these are fairly nonspecific tests, and may be positive for several months after surgery or other interventions.

Electrophysiologic testing utilizing electromyography (EMG) and nerve conduction velocity (NCV) testing techniques is indicated when evidence exists of damage to neural tissue. Decrease in motor potential in muscle groups and/or slowing of conduction velocities along nerves are among the many pathologic responses detected by these tests. In particular, EMG/NCV tests are useful in delineating the level and extent of neurologic injury. Nerve conduction velocities may be decreased relatively quickly after injury to the involved nerve, whereas electromyographic changes may take weeks to become apparent. For this reason the NCV is a more sensitive test early in the disease course.

Laboratory investigations will supplement all the above tests. Determination of the complete blood count and differential, the serum protein electrophoresis, the erythrocyte sedimentation rate, the rheumatoid factor, or the serum calcium may be crucial to arriving at the final diagnosis. Obviously, individual tests will be ordered depending upon the details of the history, physical examination, and radiographic studies.

SPECIFIC CERVICAL PAIN SYNDROMES

Based upon the history and physical examination, it should be possible to arrive at a tentative diagnosis. Diagnostic studies can bolster or refute these initial impressions. Certain disorders are common and should be familiar to every clinician. These are listed in Table 26.1, and are discussed individually. This table is in no way meant to be all-inclusive. Creating a huge differential diagnosis is not helpful in the day-to-day practice of treating cervical pain syndromes. Once again the key differential here is to determine whether the disease syndrome is primarily neurologic or bony in nature. Deciding this will allow a narrowing of the differential

Table 26.1
Common Disorders of the Cervical Spinal Area Causing Neck and Upper Extremity Pain

Spinal cord compression due to tumor or syrinx
Intrinsic motor and sensory disorders of the cord (including torticollis, toxins, and viral, vascular, and metabolic diseases)
Extrinsic spinal cord neoplasms
Osteoarthritis
Nerve root irritations (soft and hard disk protrusions)
Traumatic injury to the cervical spine
Rheumatoid arthritis
Ankylosing spondylitis and diffuse idiopathic skeletal hyperostosis
Infections

diagnosis list into manageable subclasses, and will direct further studies that will allow the final diagnosis to be reached. Obviously there are other esoteric diseases that may cause pain in the neck and upper extremities. A full discussion of these disorders is beyond the scope of this chapter. For this the reader is referred to a more comprehensive text (6).

SPINAL CORD COMPRESSION

Compression of the spinal cord can occur from mass lesions either extrinsic or intrinsic to the cord itself. The most common intra-axial spinal mass lesions are syrinxes, and the most common primary spinal tumors are spinal ependymomas and spinal gliomas, respectively accounting for 60 and 30% of all primary spinal tumors (7).

The ependymoma literally starts from the central spinal canal, taking origin from vestigial ependymal cells lining this cavity. The tumor expands slowly to compress the spinal cord between it and the confines of the spinal canal.

Spinal gliomas arise from malignant transformation of astrocytes or other glial elements. These tumors are more infiltrative than ependymomas and are consequently much more difficult to deal with surgically.

The pain from such lesions is usually insidious in onset and is poorly localized. It is often worse at night or in the early morning, for reasons discussed above. It may occasionally be exacerbated by activity, leading to the speculation that increased blood supply to the tumor during exercise may aggravate any ongoing compression.

The key to arriving at the proper diagnosis is in recognizing that this pain is invariably associated with a defined but sometimes subtle neurologic deficit. There may be slight lower extremity hyperreflexia, or subtle weakness of the upper extremities. Often, a cape-like distribution of sensory deficit over the shoulders and upper arms is the first appreciable evidence of neurologic problems. These deficits rapidly progress, however, to become more readily apparent. Soon there is loss of motor function and coordination in the hands. Invariably at some point in the progression of the syndrome lower extremity hyperreflexia will develop, as will stiffness of gait and other signs of myelopathy.

There are often intradural tumors that may be associated, initially at least, predominantly with unilateral symptoms. These are tumors that usually lie within the dura but are extramedullary, the classic examples being neurofibromas and meningiomas. Here again, the history of night pain is common. These tumors may grow to totally envelop a single nerve root with no appreciable neurologic deficit on exam. Often, the patient presents with unilateral radicular pain and numbness only. Once again, as the mass grows and the spinal cord is compressed, signs and symptoms of myelopathy point the way to the correct diagnosis.

Once the tentative diagnosis of intrinsic spinal cord compression is reached the diagnosis may be confirmed by radiologic studies. Intrathecally enhanced CT and MRI scans are most commonly available, and should be the radiologic studies of choice following the plain x-ray. Treatment of these lesions is surgical and, in the case of tumors, is often supplemented by local radiation.

INTRINSIC MOTOR AND SENSORY DISORDERS

There are many primary neurologic disorders that can disrupt spinal cord function. When the disorder primarily involves the motor system it may disrupt spinal cord circuitry and cause a lack of balance between agonist and antagonist motor functions. This may cause constant paradoxical muscle spasms, or torticollis. This disorder can quickly be recognized by the patient's posturing. In severe torticollis there is almost constant head jerking to one side or the other and the patient soon develops osteoarthritic changes in the facet and uncinate joints that may be a source of additional pain. Unfortunately, there is no good treatment for spontaneous idiopathic torticollis. Cutting the various motor roots that innervate the involved muscles can indeed reduce the constant and abnormal motor movement; however, this comes at the price of muscle denervation and associated atrophy. Such treatment is justified only in extreme cases. Other experimental procedures are being tested that may have more promise.

Toxins can affect the nervous system and give severe burning pain as well as neurologic deficit. In our highly industrialized society the chance of significant exposure to potential neurotoxins is always present. The heavy metals lead and mercury as well as more complex organic compounds are in this group.

There are natural factors as well that have been implicated in neurologic disease. Recent reports of linkage between plants and amyotrophic lateral sclerosis (8) and the long-standing suspicions of a viral/infectious etiology for multiple sclerosis are prominent examples. Certain coral elements in the Caribbean, when eaten by fish and then by humans in the food cycle, may cause severe cervical pain. This is called ciguatera. Treatment of such conditions is directed toward ending exposure to the offending agent and providing supportive and curative care as needed.

On rare occasions, vascular insufficiency to the spinal cord can itself cause pain. This may occur as a result of surgery or trauma or preexistent cardiovascular disease. Characteristically the early stages of spinal cord ischemia will give truncal pain that is poorly localized. Within a matter of hours, if not sooner, spinal infarction may occur guaranteeing a devastating neurologic deficit and poor ultimate progress. Unfortunately we do not know a great deal about how these various metabolic, toxic, or infectious disorders bring about disease on a cellular level. Further advances will be required for rapid and more effective treatment and diagnosis of such disorders.

EXTRINSIC SPINAL CORD NEOPLASMS

Extra-axial neoplastic lesions of the cervical spine may cause mechanical symptoms and localized pain or may lead to neurologic deficit depending upon the site of origin of the process. Bony tumors may be divided into benign primary tumors of bone, malignant primary tumors of bone, and metastatic tumor to bone. Malignant tumor metastases to bone are far and away most common. A list of various tumor types is presented in Table 26.2.

Primary malignant bony tumors such as chordomas, osteosarcomas, and chondrosarcomas may occur in the cervical region. Unfortunately the bones of the cervical spine can also be involved by metastatic tumor processes. Hematologic malignancies such as multiple myeloma or lymphoma very commonly involve the axial skeleton, causing bony destruction and neurologic deficit.

It is obvious that with such an extensive list of pathologic processes it would be impossible to formulate a "typical" clinical presentation. However, some typical clinical features exist that would allow the clinician a hint as to the presence of one of the diseases.

Pain deep within the bone itself is the most common clinical presentation of all of the above-listed processes. This complaint in any patient with previously diagnosed malignancy should trigger a full diagnostic workup aimed at detection of possible bony metastases. The pain is initially mechanical in nature, and may be worse with motion. In addition there is often an element of night pain. The patient typically falls asleep only to be awakened in the middle of the night with a deep underlying gnawing pain, possibly due to tumor expansion. As the pain increases in severity a radicular component usually develops. If the tumor irritates adjacent nerve roots a radiculopathy with definite motor and sensory loss becomes apparent. As the tumor expands into the spinal canal a cervical myelopathy will readily occur. Usually, however, the neurologic symptoms occur well after the onset of pain.

Fortunately the radiologic appearance of these diseases is fairly specific. Cervical spine films with obliques followed by CT scanning will reveal osteolytic lesions, pathologic fractures, and abnormal soft tissue masses in the majority of cases. Definitive diagnosis requires tissue biopsy, either from the cervical lesion itself or, as is sometimes possible in metastatic lesions, from the primary tumor site itself. Multiple myeloma produces "punched out" osteolytic lesions of the spine as well as a severe generalized osteoporosis, and pathologic fractures may ensue. Appropriate hematologic evaluations will usually clinch the diagnosis in these cases.

In all cases in which the cervical spine is involved by tumor there are two important treatment considerations. Assuring the stability of the spine and maintaining neurologic function are of paramount importance in planning treatment. Nonsurgical interventions such as radiation or chermotherapy and bracing are appropriate first-line treatments in many cases if a tissue diagnosis is already available. These may eliminate the need for surgical intervention. Close follow-up with radiologic studies and serial neurologic exams is necessary to detect progression of disease. If spinal stability or neurologic function are at risk, further consultation is required with specialists who are honestly interested in spinal surgical problems, be they neurologic or orthopedic surgeons. A variety of new techniques are now available to stabilize and decompress the spine, even in the most advanced or disease states. Patients with reasonable life expectancies (usually greater than 6 months) who are in medical condition to tolerate extensive operative procedures are candidates for these techniques. Unfortunately, in patients with a very limited prognosis as a result of extensive tumor spread or general poor health, simple bracing, supportive care, and radiation or chemotherapy are often all that is possible.

OSTEOARTHRITIS

In the vertebral column osteoarthritic changes are usually associated with intervertebral disk dgeneration. Disk degeneration, resulting from trauma or advanced age, reduces the shock absorber effect of a well-hydrated intervertebral disk and causes abnormal stresses to be applied

Table 26.2
Tumors of the Cervical Spine

Primary tumors
  Giant cell tumor
  Osteoblastoma
  Osteochondroma
  Eosinophilic granuloma
  Plasmacytoma
  Chondromyxoid fibroma
  Desmoid tumor
  Hemangioma
  Osteocartilaginous exostosis
  Rheumatoid pannus
Malignant tumors of the cervical spine
  Chordoma
  Chondrosarcoma
  Osteosarcoma
  Ewing's sarcoma
  Aggressive solitary plasmacytoma
  Hemangiopericytoma
Metastatic from solitary organs
  Breast
  Prostate
  Renal
  Gastrointestinal
  Thyroid
  Lung
  Nasopharyngeal
Hematogenous metastatic process
  Multiple myeloma
  Hodgkin's disease
  Lymphoma

to the vertebral body, the adjacent uncinate process (joint of Luschka), and the posterior facet areas. Over a period of time reactive osteophyte formation occurs along the joint interfaces. The buildup of these bony spurs may extend directly posteriorly toward the spinal canal and cause cord compression and myelopathy. More commonly spur formation occurs at the uncinate process and facet joints, resulting thereby in neural foraminal stenosis. The most common sites of degenerative osteophytes are the C5–C6 and C6–C7 joint spaces.

Pure cervical osteoarthritis in itself (when not involving the nervous system) is not usually associated with a great number of symptoms. On occasion the patient may describe mechanical neck pain with radiation suggestive of but not corresponding to a radicular distribution. This may be associated with a variety of symptoms—headaches, shoulder pains, clicking sounds—that seem to be exacerbated by purely mechanical factors. For unclear reasons high cervical disk degeneration with joint collapse and osteoarthritic changes is commonly associated with a headache that at times is impossible to separate from a tension headache. Periodically the patient may suffer acute attacks with increased neck discomfort and severe muscle pains resembling acute torticollis. These episodes are often triggered by activity and physical exertion, and peak after a 2–3-day period with total recovery within 7–10 days.

When the cervical osteoarthritis has progressed to cause nerve root compression, radicular pain and symptoms are common. Lesions of this type are often referred to as "hard" disks (to be discussed below). When the cervical osteoarthritis extends posteriorly and causes central canal stenosis, cord compression and cervical spondylotic myelopathy occur. The common term for this myelopathy is cervical spondylosis, and the classic references describing this disorder were written in 1967 and 1971 (9, 10). The combination of neck pain, increased lower extremity reflexes, stiff gait, and plain spine films showing osteophytic spurs is sufficient to make the presumptive diagnosis. The diagnostic study of choice under these circumstances remains at present time the intrathecally enhanced CT scan. MRI will allow good visualization of the cord itself, but is generally not optimal for visualizing bony and osteophytic anatomy. In all types of osteoarthritic disease, nonsteroidal anti-inflammatory medications often speed recovery from mechanical symptoms (such as local pain and muscle spasm) and are helpful in keeping the patient active. Once the osteoarthritic changes have progressed to cause problems related to compression of neural tissue, remission of the symptomatology is rare. Anti-inflammatory medications and mechanical stabilization in bracing devices may prevent progression of symptoms for a long period of time; however, in the majority of cases well-planned operative decompressions will afford relief of symptoms and ensure that further neural tissue compression does not occur.

NERVE ROOT IRRITATIONS

The spinal cord is the conduit for carrying information to and from the brain. At the segmental level nerve roots gather information from the periphery and deliver motor messages to the trunk and limbs. Each of these nerve roots exits through a foramen, and can be compressed by disk protrusion or osteophytes. Such compression will lead to pain in the distribution of the nerve root, and often locally as well. In explaining the problem to the patient it is often helpful to use the analogy of a telephone wire being rubbed on by a tree, which in turn produces static on the line.

Cervical radiculitis is a term applied when a nerve root is irritated and inflamed. The extension of this term, cervical radiculopathy, implies that damage to the root has produced a clinically appreciable motor or sensory neurologic deficit in the distribution of the root. Typically, patients with cervical root pain syndromes have neck pain made worse by extension and turning to the painful side. In addition, they will have pain that radiates either into the lower neck and shoulder (C4–C5 roots) or well down into the upper extremity (C6–T1 roots). C6 and C7 nerve root irritation in particular causes significant arm pain. These patterns are described in the anatomic section of this chapter. Unfortunately, differentiation between these patterns can sometimes be difficult in a clinical setting. For example, differentiation between C6 and C7 root involvement may be difficult at times. In both of these syndromes biceps and triceps strength is affected and the patterns of sensation loss are similar—C6 involvement causes sensation loss on the thumb and C7 on the middle finger. Either of these syndromes can cause sensation loss on the index finger, although the C7 syndrome does so more frequently.

The predominantly radicular nature of these patients' symptoms and complaints is the key element of the history and physical. Although the roots as they exit from the spinal canal can be compressed by numerous factors, by far the most common source of such irritation is either an acute disk herniation and/or a degenerative disk that in turn has caused focal osteoarthritic changes with foraminal stenosis. We commonly refer to these as soft and hard disk disease, respectively. The soft disk disorders tend to occur in patients under the age of 50. The hard disk/osoteoarthritis spur formation tends to occur in the older population, although obviously there are no absolutes.

After obtaining a medical history and physical examination, diagnostic studies will often pinpoint which root is involved. Neurophysiologic studies such as EMG/NCV are helpful in pinpointing the level involved; however, diagnostic imaging is essential to making the correct diagnosis and in formulating treatment. In addition, in some patients (particularly those who have ill-defined neck and shoulder pain that is not clearly radicular in nature) plain shoulder films may be useful to rule out glenohumeral joint disease.

The first and most basic diagnostic study, however, should be the plain cervical spine film with oblique views. In younger patients and in those who have normal-appearing plain x-rays, the next diagnostic study of choice is MRI, which will usually show the soft disks better than other diagnostic modalities. In older patients and in those who have evidence of degenerative disk disease and spurs on plain films, the preferable next study is an intrathecally enhanced CT scan, which will allow better visualization of bony anatomy than MRI.

Treatment of these lesions requires decompression of the affected root. In selected cases cervical bracing and traction or physical therapy may be of long-term benefit; however, in the vast majority this decompression is best accomplished surgically.

GOUT, MULTIPLE SCLEROSIS, AMYOTROPHIC LATERAL SCLEROSIS, SYRINGOMYELIA, KLIPPEL-FEIL SYNDROME

Gouty arthritis is associated with elevation of uric acid level and deposits within various joints. Although the disease commonly affects such joints as the big toe, it definitely can influence the spinal axis, including the cervical spine. Patients with known gouty arthritis have an increased incidence of degenerative changes in the cervical spine. The x-ray appearance is identical to that of osteoarthritis. The symptomatology cannot be differentiated from the cervical myeloradiculopathies, and the treatment is basically the same. In the acute episode of the presentation, confirmation of the uric acid levels and use of uricosuric agents is appropriate as well.

Multiple sclerosis can occur in conjunction with osteoarthritic changes in the cervical spine. It is true that the two diseases together can accentuate an existing myelopathy. Decompressive procedures are only half as successful in this condition as they are in the routine setting, and the chance of symptomatic relief after surgery is less than 50%. Consequently, operating in these settings, only 50% of the patients truly benefit from any type of decompressive laminectomy, foraminotomy, anterior cervical diskectomy, or the like. It appears that when a fusion is done with an anterior diskectomy, the spine is slightly more stabilized and there are better results in the relief of not only the pain but the intrinsic neurologic problem. This probably is related to immobilization of the spinal cord, which is already diseased.

Amyotrophic lateral sclerosis can be present in patients with some pain caused by the associated arthritic changes that occur in the spine. The neurologic disease itself is painless. However, because of the imbalances along the spine caused by muscular weakness arthritic changes can occur with some discomfort to the patients. Symptomatic treatment is all that is required. Rarely do any of these cases need operative care.

Syringomyelia was always thought to be a painless disease. In specific, patients experienced numbness in a cape-like distribution over the shoulders and arms, with muscle weakness primarily in the hands. Often they would have a myelopathy as well. However, as revealed by information obtained from MRI studies, syringomyelia usually presents initially as pain, often in a root fashion. This pain accompanies the initial development of the syrinx. As the syrinx enlarges, the pain fibers are destroyed and the patient has less pain. It is most beneficial to treat these patients early, with correction of the syrinx itself. This can be done by correcting the Arnold-Chiari malformation at the base of the skull if that exists and/or draining the syrinx into either the pleural or peritoneal cavity. If the syrinx is adequately drained, patients will have less pain. Even with the most successful procedure, rarely is all the patient's discomfort obliterated.

When a patient has congenital blocked vertebrae, as in Klippel-Feil syndrome, there is an increased instance of osteoarthritic changes at an adjacent level, usually cephalad and rarely caudally. With an immobile joint in the cervical spine, the next superior joint often has accelerated degenerative changes with osteophyte formation. This can lead to a radiculitis and/or myelopathy. If the usual measures of physical therapy, proper exercises, and anti-inflammatory medications fail, then the patients often do require decompressive procedures on the nerve roots. If there is marked compression anteriorly, then an anterior operation can be done. Rarely do patients require more extensive fusions posteriorly.

CERVICAL TRAUMA

Cervical spine trauma is almost invariably diagnosed on the historic facts alone. In taking a history, details of the traumatic event should be recorded succinctly and accurately, because this may prove germane to further events in our current litigious society. The trauma itself may be divided into its neurologic, bony and ligamentous, and muscular components, and each may give rise to significant pain. The most frequent cervical spine traumatic event that causes pain is muscle sprain or strain—more commonly referred to as whiplash injury. Under normal conditions of wear and tear the cervical muscles modulate many of the forces being transmitted to the cervical spine via balanced contraction and relaxation. Rapid, large changes in motion or force, as occur in cervical spine injury, may exceed the capacity of the cervical musculature to compensate, leading to muscle strain and tears. Larger disruptive forces may cause bony and ligamentous damage in addition to the muscular injury. Classically the pain associated with muscle strain develops to a maximum after about 2–3 days and then resolves slowly over 2–3 weeks. In the setting of trauma local neck pain with spasm and stiffness of cervical muscles, normal neurologic examination, and normal diagnostic studies (if performed at all; usually plain x-rays only) are the criteria that must be met before this diagnosis can be confidently made. If any one of these criteria is not met then other cervical spine injury beyond muscle spasm must be suspected, and further diagnostic workup is appropriate and necessary.

Similarly, traumatic neck pain that persists for more than 2–3 weeks after injury should raise a red flag, and should be considered of bony or ligamentous origin until proven otherwise.

Treatment of mild cases of cervical sprain is usually best done with mild nonnarcotic analgesics and application of heat packs. In more severe cases, decreasing cervical mobility with a bracing device such as a soft collar and the judicious use of antispasm medications such as Flexeril or Diazepam may be required.

Trauma with bony or ligamentous disruption is caused by extreme abnormal movements or compressive forces in the neck. Although the head itself only weighs from 10 to 15 pounds, that weight alone is in extreme flexion and extension sufficient to damage bones. Furthermore, although protected from extremes of movement in flexion and extension by muscle and ligament, the cervical vertebrae are very vulnerable to axial compressive forces. These forces are commonly generated in diving and automobile accidents, thus accounting for the high percentage of cervical spine injury in such cases. The injury from such forces is variable, and may result in ligamentous tear, bony fracture, or dislocation and malalignment depending upon the location and force vectors involved.

In general, bony and ligamentous cervical spine injuries can usually be classified into flexion-, compression-, or extension-type injuries. On rare occasions distraction injuries may occur, especially in the upper cervical and occipital areas. The pain associated with bony and ligamentous trauma is mechanical, sharp, and exacerbated by even the slightest cervical motion. In the absence of damage to neural structures radicular or dysesthetic pain should not be present. Significant paraspinous muscle spasm and tenderness is almost always present.

In the setting of trauma and neck pain, plain cervical spine films (particularly the lateral view) are essential. All seven cervical vertebrae must be visualized, as must be the occiput–C1 and C7–T1 junctions. Additional views such as obliques are often helpful. Cooperative patients may have flexion and extension films (with careful monitoring of neurologic function at each position, of course) to further document the degree of instability. Generally the more abnormal the first lateral cervical spine x-ray the less the necessity for further films. If the films initially appear normal and bony pathology is still suspected, then additional views such as oblique or flexion/extension should be attempted. If following adequate films any uncertainty remains regarding bony anatomy, CT scan becomes mandatory.

Trauma may leave the patient neurologically intact and with x-rays that are unimpressive. In these cases ligamentous and or joint capsular tearing is usually the source of pain. In most cases the patients can localize the discomfort accurately to the level of the lesion. Local injection of damaged facets or ligaments with anesthetic agents is both diagnostic and therapeutic in this case.

In the neck with unstable bony disruption or significant malalignment secondary to trauma, skeletal tong traction must be initiated early to achieve stability. The only exceptions to this rule are disruption injuries causing distraction of the occiput from C1 or C1 from C2. In these cases the application of traction can worsen the distraction and literally "pull the head off." In all other instances, however, bony alignment with judicious use of traction, multiple sequential lateral cervical spine films, and close monitoring of neurologic status, is the appropriate course of action, and should be carried out as rapidly as feasible.

Finally, cervical spine trauma may result in injury to the nervous tissue itself. Although this most commonly occurs in the setting of cervical spine fractures, damage to neural structures may also occur independently of this, as in traumatic anterior spinal artery or central cord syndromes. Focal pain at the site of injury and the presence of neurologic deficit are presumptive evidence of traumatic cord/root injury. The classic picture is of flaccid plegia or paresis during the spinal shock phase that eventually gives way to spasticity and upper extremity lower motor neuron deficits. Proximal motor function may be preserved, but the fine motor control needed for adequate hand function is invariably lost. Numbness, clumsiness, and even complete paralysis of the hands is the rule rather than the exception in these situations, and hand dysfunction may even exceed lower extremity dysfunction. This is particularly true with central cord syndromes, where upper extremity lower motor neuron lesions figure prominently.

When there is neurologic deficit in the presence of spinal trauma adequate visualization of the spinal cord/thecal sac is essential for planning further treatment. Bony fragments, herniated disks, and epidural hematomas may all cause persistent cord compression and significant cord compression independent of that caused by the initial traumatic blow itself. Intrathecally enhanced CT or MRI scanning is therefore required.

Treatment centers around the dual needs to stabilize the spinal column and to alleviate ongoing neural compression. The institution of skeletal traction is a valuable first step toward stabilizing the spinal column, and may alleviate neural compression as well. Thus, judicious use of skeletal traction is the first treatment choice. Surgery, either to relieve ongoing neural compression or to internalize a stabilization, should be considered rapidly thereafter if the patient's clinical status will allow. This will be followed with 6 weeks to 3 months in a rigid cervical orthosis until the surgical fusion is stable.

RHEUMATOID ARTHRITIS

Rheumatoid arthritis is a chronic inflammatory disease of probable, although undefined, infectious etiology. Subsequent to the presumed infection, a broad immunologic response is generated that after prolonged periods of time leads to characteristic changes in many joints of the body. The prevalence of this disorder in the United States is roughly 1% of the population. Although juvenile forms exist, more frequently it is the elderly patient with rheumatoid arthritis who develops cervical spine pain and arthritic changes. The cervical spine is commonly involved, especially in the C1–C2 area. Inflammatory processes in this region cause exuberant pannus formation, bony destruction, and ligamentous laxity. Atlantooccipital subluxation, basilar invagination, and atlantoaxial subluxation are frequent end results.

Mechanical neck pain is the initial presenting symptomatology. Occipital headache and muscle spasm can also occur. Extremes of bony and ligamentous instability may allow cord compression, resulting in lower cranial nerve palsies, myelopathy, and facial numbness. Trivial trauma in the presence of this instability may cause acute, devastating neurologic deficit. More commonly, the patient presents with simple neck pain and as followed over time develops a gait disturbance with myelopathy and associated changes.

The diagnosis of rheumatoid arthritis is often made on physical examination alone because the findings in patients with rheumatoid arthritis are multiple and characteristic. Confirmatory laboratory evidence is obtained by elevated erythrocyte sedimentation rate and rheumatoid factor screen. Radiologic evidence of rheumatoid arthritis is best obtained on plain spine films. Tomograms will also disclose the loss of bony tissue with further appreciation of atlantoaxial subluxation. More recently, with MRI, the actual pannus buildup in and around the dens can be seen. Treatment of the mechanical pain of cervical spine rheumatoid arthritis relies upon steroidal and nonsteroidal anti-inflammatory agents. The development of significant (usually greater than 1 cm) subluxation at C1–C2, spinal instability, or neurologic deficit warrants serious consideration of surgical decompressive/stabilization procedures. Such a procedure is a major operation for many of the senior patients involved, and the morbidity of the postsurgical bracing devices (i.e., the halo brace) is not insignificant in this population. Nonetheless, such treatment is warranted since the natural history of this disease in a patient with symptomatic neural compression is indeed most bleak.

ANKYLOSING SPONDYLITIS

Ankylosing spondylitis is an inflammatory joint disorder with a striking predilection for the cartilaginous joints of the axial skeleton. The main pathologic features involve abnormal deposition of calcium and spontaneous fusion of the ligamentous and facet structures. Although ankylosing spondylitis is commonly associated with the lumbosacral spine, it may also advance to involve the neck. It is initially associated with gradual onset of pain and aching in the lower back and buttocks. Morning stiffness is often present; this tends to improve with exercise during the day. There may be an associated mild peripheral arthritis. Mechanical spine pain and restriction of mobility go hand in hand. Compression of neural structures is rare, and radicular and myelopathic pain patterns are therefore rarely present. The abnormally fused spine becomes brittle and is therefore fractured easily even with minor trauma. This may cause acute onset of neurologic complaints.

Diagnosis may be made on the basis of plain spine films. The high association of this disease with the HLA-B27 antigen type warrants this type of testing as well.

Often confused with ankylosing spondylitis is a hyperostotic disorder that primarily affects the anterior longitudinal ligament of the spine. This is referred to as the diffuse idiopathic skeletal hyperostosis (DISH) syndrome. It has also been termed Forrestier's disease (11). Fortunately this unusual form of ankylosing hyperostosis does not require specific therapy outside of occasional nonsteroidal anti-inflammatory medications and continuous physical therapy modalities.

INFECTIONS

Although infections of the cervical spine are rare, the consequences of failure to make a proper diagnosis and initiate therapy in a timely fashion are so devastating that discussion is appropriate.

Whereas neoplastic processes usually begin in the bone and spare the disk space, infection is just the opposite; it usually begins in the disk space with bony destruction occurring only later. The most common offending organisms are staphylococcal and streptococcal species, usually introduced into the area by iatrogenic means or by hematogenous spread from other foci. Other infectious organisms, such as tuberculosis, brucellosis, anaerobic bacteria, and fungi, are rare in this country except in specific host populations. Younger patients especially are susceptible to streptococcal infections, which may spread to the nasopharyngeal and tonsillar area and into the retropharyngeal space and on rare occasions become localized in a disk space. In the young adult the most common infection is usually staphylococcal. In the older person or in immunosuppressed individuals tuberculosis and other more indolent infections may be seen. Finally, select patients with severe immunosuppressions may develop fungal infections of the spine.

When the infections occur within the spine there is relatively little systemic and/or immunologic response initially. Fever, sweats, and constitutional symptoms are common but not universal. Neck pain, with radiation to the shoulders and back of the head, is a predominant symptom of cervical spine infection. Invariably patients will have restricted range of motion of their neck and rather striking muscle spasms. These nonspecific complaints are often present for several weeks to months before the diagnosis is even entertained. If the infection tracks into the prevertebral space, dysphagia, dysphasia, and hoarseness may occur. Myelopathy is a late and ominous sign, indicative of epidural compression and possible epidural abscess.

Unfortunately, radiographic bony changes usually take 3–6 weeks to develop; thus the diagnosis of earlier, potentially more easily curable infections is difficult. Bone scanning with gallium or technetium or labeled white cells has become an important diagnostic adjuvant in these disorders. Elevated systemic white count as well as high erythrocyte sedimentation rate will point to possible infectious processes as well.

Making the proper microbiologic diagnosis may require aspiration or open biopsy and drainage. More recently more aggressive care has been widely recommended. This protocol includes biopsy, drainage, curettage, and concomitant bony fusion occurring as the initial surgical procedure, and it has been very successful. The organism is identified and appropriate antimicrobial coverage is continued for at least 6 weeks. After the cervical stabilization procedure, external immobilization with a rigid orthosis is commonly required.

CLINICAL CONCLUSIONS

The study of neck pain in cervical spine disorders is almost a specialty within itself, with rheumatologists, neurologists, orthopedic surgeons, and neurosurgeons all very interested in and committed to understanding these disorders. With a complaint so common as neck pain it is obvious that every patient cannot and should not see a specialist. Therefore some general guidelines should be outlined for the initiation of treatment of these patients.

Patients with pain in the neck with or without cord or root complaints will need to be seen on several occasions in order to make the proper diagnosis and assess treatment. The interval between these visits may vary, but in general should be proportionate to how ill the patient is. If the patient is suspected of harboring a serious neoplastic process or infection, or has suffered severe trauma, with neurologic deficit, then hospitalization and more than two or three visits a day may be appropriate. The majority of patients with new-onset cervical pain will do well with a 2–3-week interval between office visits. On the other hand, if the patient has a long-term complaint without impressive physical or radiographic findings, then the interval between visits can be 3–4 weeks if not longer. The fundamental steps in managing the patient at each visit are basically the same, and are outlined below.

VISIT 1

Visit 1 includes the initial history and physical examination. Initial diagnostic testing, such as plain spine films, is often carried out at this time, although in most cases of simple neck pain from muscle sprain this is not indicated. It is also wise at this time for the physician to give the patient an initial impression of what he/she believes the patient is suffering from. Treatment can be based upon diagnostic impressions, and oftentimes will be symptomatic only, such as with nonsteroidal anti-inflammatory medications. The neck may be immobilized with some type of collar or brace, with instructions to evaluate response to immobilization. The majority of patients will not require more than a single office visit.

VISIT 2

If the patient's neck pain has not improved after a sufficient (usually 2–3-week) period of initial treatment, several options exist. It is mandatory first, however, to reexamine the patient for evolution in signs and symptoms. If the patient is clinically stable at this point, medications could be changed to either another nonsteroidal anti-inflammatory medication or to stronger pain medications. Utilization of such modalities as exercise and physical therapy also may be appropriate at this time. At this second visit complete cervical spine films with flexion, extension, and oblique views should be obtained regardless of diagnostic impressions. This study remains the single most important diagnostic study available to us. While the cervical spine x-rays are being done, screening hematologic evaluation, including complete blood count, rheumatoid factor, or erythrocyte sedimentation rate, could also be obtained.

VISIT 3

If the patient has not responded to the second line of treatments after a reasonable time and all the studies obtained during the second office visit are normal, again repeat physical examination is warranted, and the differential diagnosis should be mentally reviewed. If the patient is clinically stable, medications should again be changed and additional studies ordered as below. In younger patients and those with normal cervical spine films MRI is the next most important diagnostic study. This will point out soft tissue defects and herniated disks as well as visualize the neural elements. On the other hand if there are significant arthritic changes, bony destruction, or malalignment on plain films, then the CT scan with or without intrathecal contrast is the study of choice.

VISIT 4

In some patients an acceptable diagnosis will still not have been reached even after repeat physical examination, plain films, CT scan, and/or MRI. At this time looking for clinical oddities is warranted. Patients who have had MRI studies should have CT studies next, and vice versa. Other testing, such as EMG/NCV and bone scans, may be appropriate in specific situations. Additional blood work is also done.

VISIT 5

If the patient is continuing to suffer from cervical spine pain at this point, now usually 2–3 months after initial presentation, then consultation and further diagnostic tests/procedures should be carried out. A more sophisticated mechanical examination of the neck by orthopedists or rheumatologists is warranted. A more detailed neurologic exam by neurologists or neurosurgeons is often appropriate as well. Further diagnostic studies also should be carried out, such as bone scanning, complete myelography, and lumbar puncture if indicated. Obviously, decisions need to be made on an individual basis. With each visit, if the patient is still failing to improve medication changes should be considered. There are over a dozen nonsteroidal anti-inflammatory medications, and it is important to try many, for patients may vary greatly in their response.

SUBSEQUENT PATIENT MANAGEMENT

Visits subsequent to the fifth one should be to either a competent rheumatologist or orthopedic or neurosurgeon, because the patient will probably not get well quickly and further consultation and advice is needed. This is frequently the beginning of the chronic neck pain syndrome. It may be that nothing more can be done for the individual. It may also be that secondary gain or conversion disorders may be operative, especially in cases involving litigation and workers' compensation. In this case psychological evaluation should be seriously considered.

In any case, by following this guideline a logical and fairly complete evaluation of the patient with cervical spine pain will have been performed. In the vast majority of cases an appropriate diagnosis is obtained and appropriate treatments started, with excellent relief of symptoms.

References

1. Lawrence J: Disc degeneration, its frequency and relationship to symptoms. *Ann Rheum Dis* 28:121, 1969.
2. British Association of Physical Medicine: Pain in the neck and arm. *Br Med J* 1:253, 1966.
3. Hult L: Cervical, dorsal and lumbar spinal syndromes. *Acta Orthop Scand [Suppl]* 17:1, 1954.
4. Hult L: The Munkford Investigation. *Acta Orthop Scand [Suppl]* 16:1, 1954.
5. Spurling RG, Scoville WB: Lateral rupture of the cervical intervertebral discs. *Surg Gynecol Obstet* 78:350, 1944.
6. Bland J: *Disorders of the Cervical Spine*. Philadelphia, WB Saunders, 1987, p 40.
7. Wilkins R, Regachary SP: *Neurosurgery*. New York, McGraw-Hill, 1985.
8. Spencer P, Nunn P, Hugan J, et al: Guam amyotropic lateral sclerosis–parkinsonism–dementia linked to a plant excitant neurotoxin. *Science* 237:517–522, 1987.
9. Brain W: *Cervical Spondylosis*. Philadelphia, WB Saunders, 1967.
10. Wilkonson M: *Cervical Spondylosis: Its Early Diagnosis and Treatment*. Philadelphia, WB Saunders, 1971.
11. Resnick D, Niwayama G: Radiographic and pathological features of spinal involvement in diffuse idiopathic skeletal hyperostosis (DISH). *Radiology* 119:559, 1976.

chapter 27
Differential Diagnosis of Low Back Pain

John A. McCulloch, M.D., F.R.C.S.(C)

This question is frequently asked by doctors at various stages of training and practice experience: "How can I assess and treat a patient with back pain when the diagnosis is so elusive?" It is hard on the ego to assess a patient and fail to arrive at a concrete diagnosis on which to base a treatment program. All too often, a treatment program for low back pain is based more on hope than science. This should not be so. In today's medical world, our clinical skills and our investigative tools are such that we should be able to arrive at the correct diagnosis for most patients with "lumbago or sciatica." This chapter outlines the simple steps needed to assess a patient who presents with a complaint of low back pain.

ASSESSMENT METHOD

Do not initiate your assessment with a long list of time-consuming differential diagnoses on your menu. In family practice, this presents an overwhelming burden to the multitude of chief complaints heard during a day. Instead, adopt a simple, methodical approach. Your goal is to sort those patients who have mechanical or structural problems in the low back from those who have not. In a family practice setting, perhaps 20–25% of patients presenting with low back pain will have a source outside of the back as the cause of their symptoms. This fact presents many pitfalls for the unwary. For this reason, accurate evaluation requires a logical, step-by-step method. The foundation of this method is the clinical assessment, the good old-fashioned history and physical examination. Investigations such as computed tomography (CT) scanning and myelography should play a secondary role to clinical assessment. Today, our investigative tools are so sophisticated that one can find pathology in almost every patient whether or not the patient is sick (1, 2). Moreover, minor insignificant pathology can become the red herring that causes you to miss the symptom-producing lesion.

In assessing a patient with a low back complaint, ask yourself five questions:

1. Is this a true physical disability or is there a setting and a pattern on history and physical examination to suggest a nonphysical or nonorganic problem?
2. Is this clinical presentation a diagnostic trap?
3. Is this a mechanical low back pain condition, and if so, what is the syndrome?
4. Are there clues to an antomic level on history and physical examination?
5. After reviewing the results of investigation, what is the structural lesion and does it fit with the clinical syndrome?

Although these questions may not be answered sequentially during the history and physical examination, they ultimately must be answered sequentially before arriving at a diagnosis and prescribing a treatment program. That is to say, do not answer question 5 and plan a treatment program until you have satisfactory answers to each preceding question. Probably the biggest pitfall is to answer question 3 before you have satisfactorily answered questions 1 and 2. The answers to questions 1 and 2 should routinely be made outside the hospital, and before

CT, myelography, magnetic resonance imaging (MRI), and other sophisticated investigative modalities are used. The classic trap is to ignore questions 1 and 2 and admit a patient with a complaint of low back pain to the hospital, seek pathology with sophisticated investigative tools, and then prescribe a treatment plan based on false-positive findings.

QUESTION 1

Is this a true physical disability or is there a setting and a pattern of history and physical examination to suggest a nonphysical or nonorganic problem?

That medicine should concern itself with the whole person is often stated but frequently ignored. The hallmark of a good clinician is the ability not only to diagnose disease but also to assess the "whole patient." No test of the art of medicine is more demanding than the identification of the patient with a nonorganic or emotional component to a back disability.

To start, recognize the disability equation:

$$\text{Disability} = A + B + C$$

where:

A = the physical component (disease).
B = the patient's emotional reaction.
C = the situation the patient is at the time of disability (e.g., compensation claim, motor vehicle accident).

Each patient presenting with a back disability may have some component of each of these entities entwined in their disability. For example, a patient presenting a collection of symptoms, with no physical disability evident on examination, should lead one to think of the other aspects of the equation and look for emotional disability or situational reactions.

A classification of nonorganic spinal pain is outlined in Table 27.1. The term *nonorganic* has been chosen over other terms such as nonphysical, functional, emotional, and psychogenic. The following definitions are used for the classification in Table 27.1.

Table 27.1
Nonorganic Spinal Pain

1. Psychosomatic spinal pain
   a. Tension syndrome (fibrositis)
2. Psychogenic spinal pain
   a. Psychogenic spinal pain
   b. Psychogenic modification of organic spinal pain
3. Situational spinal pain
   a. Litigation reaction
   b. Exaggeration reaction

1. Psychosomatic Spinal Pain Psychosomatic spinal pain is defined as symptomatic physical change in tissues of the spine that has as its cause anxiety. The expression of anxiety is mediated as a prolonged and exaggerated state that eventually leads to structural change (spasm) in the muscles of the neck or low back.

2.A. Psychogenic Spinal Pain Psychogenic spinal pain is defined as the conversion or somatization of anxiety into pain referred to the neck or back, unaccompanied by physical change in the tissues of these regions. The pain is variously known in the literature as conversion hysteria, psychogenic regional pain, traumatic or accident neurosis, and hypochondriasis.

The emotional upset brings pains to the back just as it may bring tears to the eyes. The reason for the conversion is found in complex psychodynamic mechanisms beyond the scope of this chapter. The reaction represents a sincere unconscious emotional illness that offers the patient the primary gain of solving inner conflicts, fears, and anxieties. Inherent in the conversion reaction is the concept of suggestion and hypnosis, the importance of which will become apparent later in this chapter.

2.B. Psychogenic Modification of Organic Spinal Pain Psychogenic modification of spinal pain is a sincere emotional reaction that modifies the appreciation of an organic pain. Usually, the organic pain by itself would not be disabling, but with the psychogenic modification a significant disability ensues. No associated physical change occurs as a result of anxiety, and a conversion reaction may or may not coexist (3).

An example is the patient burdened with life situational pressures (mortgage payments, car payments) who, because of his physical illness, believes he cannot sustain the effort necessary to meet these demands. A resulting depression may occur, and the symptoms of fatigue, loss of appetite, insomnia, impotence, constipation, and the like so dominate the history that the underlying physical condition is missed. Other examples are patients with passive-dependent personality, drug or alcohol dependence, or psychosis who, in the face of a minor physical problem, use their illness to step out of the demands of the real world.

Some obsessive-compulsive patients cannot adjust to a minor physical problem, and this personality trait leads them to believe they have a significant disability.

3. Situational Spinal Pain Situational spinal pain is a reaction whereby a patient, through a collection of symptoms, maintains a situation (with potential secondary gain) through overconcern or conscious effort.

3.A. Litigation Reaction The litigation or compensation reaction is defined as overconcern by the patient for present and future health, arising out of a litigious or compensable event that initially affected health. The reaction manifests itself in patient's complaint of continuing neck or back pain coupled with a concern that, upon formal severence from his claim to compensation, deterioration in health may occur. The patient with this reaction is neither physically nor emotionally ill.

This reaction is not to be confused with the ambiguous terms *litigation neurosis* or *compensation neurosis*. Like "whiplash," these terms have no medical or legal value and should be dropped from our vocabulary. If a patient has a true neurosis arising out of a litigious or compensable event (accident), then those terms listed under "Psychogenic Spinal Pain" (2.A) should be used for diagnostic purposes (e.g., traumatic neurosis or accident neurosis). If the patient's disability appears to be based more on his awareness of the commercial value of his symptoms, his reaction should not be legitimized by the use of the term *neurosis* in conjunction with the words "litigation" or "compensation" (thus litigation reaction).

3.B. Exaggeration Reaction Exaggeration reactions are attempts by the patient to appear ill or to magnify an existent illness. *Malingering* is a term frequently applied to the reaction, and is defined as "the conscious alteration of health for gain."

As is described below, it is possible for the physician to detect efforts to magnify, but it is not proper for him to assign motives (gain) to the patient. The lawyer involved is in a reversed role. He may raise doubts about the plaintiff's motives (gain), but he is in no position to clinically detect effort to magnify or exaggerate. The choice of the word "malingering" implies proficiency in two professions, an uncommon occurrence. For this reason, the terms *malingering* and *conscious effort* are best not used by the physician when discussing nonorganic spinal pain.

Alteration of health in order to deceive, to evade responsibility, or to derive gain does occur. Those who would deny its occurrence deny the existence of human nature. The patient who tries to alter or reproduce symptoms or signs of a spinal problem may do so in a number of ways:

1. *Pretension*: No physical illness exists and the patient willfully fabricates symptoms and signs. Occurring infrequently in the military during wartime, it is a rare civilian event.
2. *Exaggeration*: Symptoms and signs of a spinal disability are magnified to represent more than they really are.
3. *Perseveration*: As a manifestation of back disability, perseveration is a continuing complaint by the patient after the physical cause of the disability has ceased to exist.
4. *Allegation*: Genuine disability is present, but the patient fraudulently ascribes these to some cause, associated with gain, knowing that, in fact, his condition is of different origin.

Civilian nonorganic situational spinal pain is usually the exaggeration or perseveration type. Pretension and allegation are uncommon forms of gainful alteration of health in civilian practice. Like the patient with the litigation reaction, these patients are neither emotionally nor physically ill. However, they differ from patients with the litigation reaction in that they are attempting to demonstrate physical illness through the effort of exaggeration or perseveration. The reason for this effort is usually, but not always, found in secondary financial gain.

Clinical Description

Before describing each of these entities, it is important to emphasize a few points. First, the above classification is a simplistic one that is useful only to the family practitioner or the spinal surgeon. It does not allow for the more complex assessments done by psychologists, psychiatrists, and the like, but it does allow for a foundation on which to build clinical recognition of these entities so that the patient can be referred to others more skilled in the field. Second, one cannot rigidly define disability, because there are gray areas. However, there is a tendency for a nonorganic disability to fall largely into one category.

Third, it is most important to determine if one of the following setting exists for nonorganic disabilities:

1. A patient who has had previous emotional problems is prone to have an emotional component to a disability. Symptoms such as fatigue, sleeplessness, agitation, gastrointestinal upset, and excessive sweating should signal that an emotional component is likely present.
2. A patient who is in a secondary gain situation such as a motor vehicle accident claim has the potential for these nonorganic reactions. It is important to establish the presence of such circumstances early in the patient encounter. If a patient states that low back pain started suddenly with an incident, it is important to document whether or not the incident is a claim type of accident and whether or not insurance and legal factors are involved. Conversely, if there is no secondary gain detected on history, it is unusual to arrive at a secondary gain diagnosis such as litigation reaction or exaggeration reaction.
3. A vague and confusing history, a baffling physical examination, and an elusive diagnosis signal a possible nonorganic diagnosis. Reflect on this before taking the expensive step of hospital admission and sohisticated testing.
4. A patient who quickly establishes an abnormal doctor-patient relationship has a potential nonorganic component to his disability. These abnormal doctor-patient relationships include a hostile or effusively complimentary patient, a patient who has had many other doctors involved in care prior to your assessment, a patient who fails to respond to standard conservative treatment measures, and a patient who is critical of other doctors.

Psychosomatic Spinal Pain The psychosomatic phenomenon of muscle spasm arising out of tension states usually affects the neck, but may affect the low back. It should be known as the "orthopedic ulcer," but more often is given the label of fibrositis. The patient with this problem is overtly strained and tense, as evidenced by facial expression. They are fidgety and restless and may sit on the edge of the chair while they wring their hands. Some of these patients will place their hands on their neck or back during the history and literally wring the area while describing the pain. They have a general feeling of restlessness and a specific feeling of a tightness in their neck with associated sensations of cracking and a constant feeling of the need to stretch out the neck and shoulder muscles. The pain is not specifically mechanical but does tend to accumulate with the day's activity, especially when that activity is carried out in the tension-producing environment (e.g., work).

The pain typically responds to chiropractic or physiotherapeutic intervention, but relief is usually temporary, a fact that makes the patient tend to seek prolonged care.

Physical examination reveals a good range of movement in the back, with a complaint of pain only if movement is done too quickly or carried to extremes. The significant physical finding is the presence of firm, tender muscles when the affected part is examined in a position of rest. The patient may be able to demonstrate the "cracking" to the touch or auditory perception of the examiner.

No evidence of nerve root involvement exists in the lower extremities. Skin tenderness, the significance of which is explained below, is not a usual finding.

Psychogenic Spinal Pain The patient with psychogenic spinal pain is emotionally ill. These patients often have a history of past illnesses replete with emotional problems. It follows that the history of the present illness contains a preponderance of emotional symptoms and the description of the pain will not be typical of any organic condition. The patient is convinced that he is ill, and that conviction extends to the frequent demand for consultations with numerous doctors. Considerable financial hardship and aggravation will occur in some cases when these consultations take the patient great distances to and from major clinics or spas throughout the world. Throughout their constant demand for care, these patients notice times when their symptoms do improve. This is due to the institution of some new form of treatment that affects the patient through suggestion or hypnosis, a fact that makes placebo trial of little value in the evaluation of these problems.

It follows that because these patients are emotionally ill, no causative organic problem will be found on physical examination. The conversion reaction is associated with an upset body image appreciation such that a topographic unit (the back and leg), indifferent to matters of innervation or anatomic relationship, will contain physical findings of skin tenderness and dulled sensory appreciation (3). The somatization infrequently reaches the stage of weakness with wasting and depression of all the reflexes in the contiguous part (e.g., an arm or leg).

However, the important observation on physical examination of this patient is the paucity of physical findings, which separates him from the magnifier and exaggerator, who by definition have many "physical" findings.

Psychogenic Modification of Organic Spinal Pain Of all the nonorganic causes of spinal pain, the patient who psychogenically modifies organic pain presents the most difficult diagnostic and therapeutic challenge. Sometimes, but not always, the organic problem by itself would not be disabling. Thus, the historic and physical component of the disability related to the organicity is not significant. Those findings indicative of a physical illness will be appropriate and a quantitative guide to the extent of physical illness. However, the life situational pressures or the personality of the patient modifies the disability to a significant point. Also, the psychogenic reaction interferes with response to treatment and leads to persistence of the disability. In a surgical practice, this failure to respond to conservative treatment is the classic indication for operative intervention. If the surgeon fails to recognize that the failure to respond to treatment is due in this instance to a psychogenic disability, he will gradually build a practice containing a number of spinal surgery failures. Psychogenic modifications are commonly seen in the patient with an inadequate personality. By definition, the patient's personality may limit advancement up the social, educational, and occupational ladder and confine him to the unskilled worker classification. Some of these patients can be found in the Workers' Compensation Board population and may be one of the reasons for poorer results of treatment sometimes obtained in the "Comp" patient.

These patients are seen with a minor physical problem (e.g., back strain), yet have a total disability. All attempts at treatment fail to return the patient to the work force. Frequent office visits reinforce the disability for the patient. If the doctor fails to recognize this maladaptive reaction and reinforcement, he may add a scar to or stick a needle into the back, which will not help the patient in any way.

Other psychogenic modifications come about through drug addiction and alcohol dependence. Occasionally, psychotic behavior will convert a minor physical problem into a prolonged disability. Physical examination will reveal the nature and extent of the physical impairment. Usually the physical impairment by itself would not be significantly disabling. The loss of movement in the back is minor, the limitation of straight leg raising is minimal, and the neurologic changes are of questionable significance. In the face of repeated assessments and a continuing statement of disability, the patient's minor physical problem may become magnified in the mind of the clinician who does not assess personality and life situational factors.

Situational Spinal Pain—Litigation Reaction The litigation reaction patient is neither physically nor emotionally ill. Thus, few emotional symptoms will be present on historic examination. The patient is in the process of litigation or under the care of the Worker's Compensation

Board. These patients often state that they do not care about the litigious or compensation issue, yet they also state that they are afraid to settle or return to work for fear that further illness will develop. Their continuing complaints are rather vague and would not normally be incapacitating. If they are on treatment, they are not improving. Physically, there may be an increased awareness of the part as manifested by skin tenderness in the affected area, but no organic illness is detectable, and there is no attempt to exaggerate or magnify a disability.

Situational Spinal Pain—Exaggeration Reaction Some or most of the following historic characteristics will be obtained from the exaggeration reaction patient. The most obvious historic point is the secondary gain situation, which usually involves the fault of someone else and/or payment of financial compensation. Other secondary gain situations can occur. The initiating event is usually a trivial or minor incident. There may be a latent period of hours or days between the incident and the onset of symptoms, during which time the patient speaks to friends and relatives and learns the commercial value of the injury.

The patient describes the pain with some degree of indifference as evidence by a smile or a laugh when describing his severe disability. He is vague in describing and localizing the pain, giving the examiner the impression of someone struggling to remember a dream. Specificity and elaboration require memory for repetition, a quality not present to a significant degree in this type of patient. The individual wishes you to believe this pain is unique and severe. This attempt to have you believe in the pain is often accompanied by a salesman-like attitude with many examples of the disability spontaneously listed. Inability to engage in sex is frequently mentioned.

In spite of the trivial initiating event, the disability may have been present for a long time. Three types of treatment patterns occur:

1. The patient follows a "straight line" course of treatment; he does not respond to the standard treatment nor to the suggestion and hypnosis of treatment (i.e., he does not improve or he gets worse).
2. The patient is not on treatment because he is "allergic" to all medications prescribed, he "suffocates" in the neck or back braces, or he becomes ill in a physiotherapy setting.
3. The patient is not on treatment because he has not sought treatment.

Certain behavioral patterns become apparent after seeing a number of these patients. Some never appear for appointments in spite of weeks of notification. Others appear late for the appointment and do not apologize or state indifferently that the traffic was heavy. There may be an attempt to manipulate your feelings with a compliment about your reputation or your office. There may be an effort to play one doctor against another by making false statements about the other doctor. Finally, hostility may appear during the assessment. A patient truly ill will not be aware or afraid of exposure and will not be hostile unless provoked. A patient exaggerating a disability is suspicious. He may start out hostile, but the usual pattern is one of developing hostility as discrepancies in the history and physical examination are exposed. Examiners are advised, for obvious reasons, not to precipitate this final behavioral pattern.

The patient who is magnifying or exaggerating a disability can be exposed only through an adequate physical examination. Those physicians who do not physically examine patients will not recognize this reaction, which may explain the reluctance of the psychiatric community to accept this clinical entity.

The physical findings of exaggeration reaction are classified into those that demonstrate acting behavior, those that indicate anticipatory behavior, and those that fail to support the patient's claim to illness.

Acting Behavior Exaggerating a disability requires acting by the patient. This acting may be general in nature, such as the Academy Award performances put on by some patients as they moan and groan through the examination, walk around the examining room with their eyes closed, and either reach for objects to support themselves or reach for their painful areas. The incongruity of this acting behavior may be evident when the patient mounts the examining table with considerable ease and/or dresses within minutes of the examination and smiles and waves goodbye as he leaves the office.

Specific examples of acting behavior are the rigid back, a condition that disappears on the examining table, the reduction of straight leg raising (SLR) in supine (Fig. 27.1A) that disappears in the sitting position (Fig. 27.1B), tender skin, and the paralyzed insensitive extremity. That these findings are a result of acting can be demonstrated through the use of distraction testing (Table 27.2). Using nonpainful, nonemotional, and nonsurprising examination techniques, it is possible not only to change the acting behavior but also to demonstrate normal physical function. It is the author's opinion that proper distraction

Table 27.2
Demonstration of Acting Behavior

Condition	Response
Physical finding (acting behavior)	Reduction in straight leg raising
Distraction test (e.g., Flip test): nonpainful, nonemotional, nonsurprising	Normal straight leg raising (normal physical function)

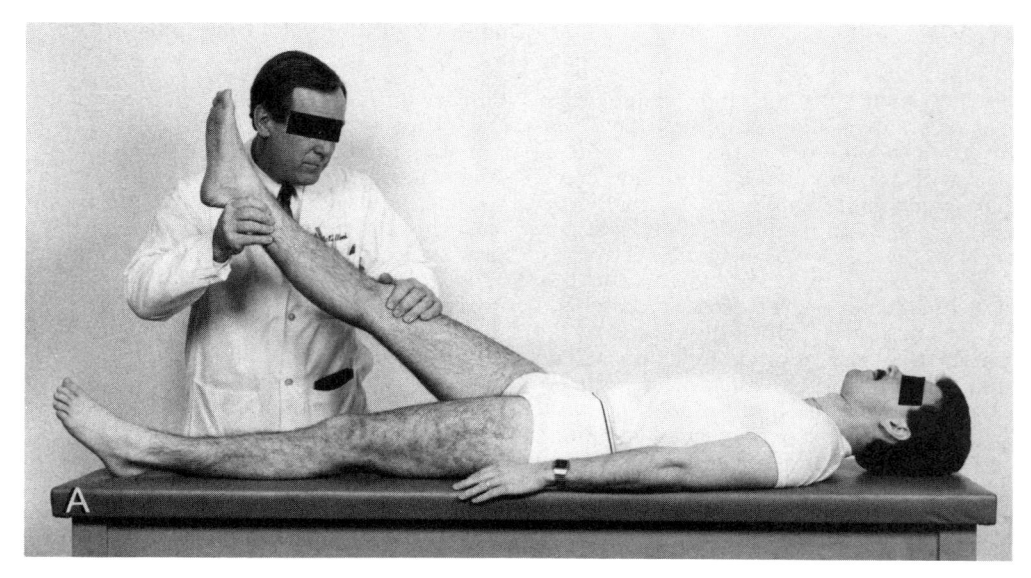

Figure 27.1A. Patient demonstrating significant SLR reduction in supine position.

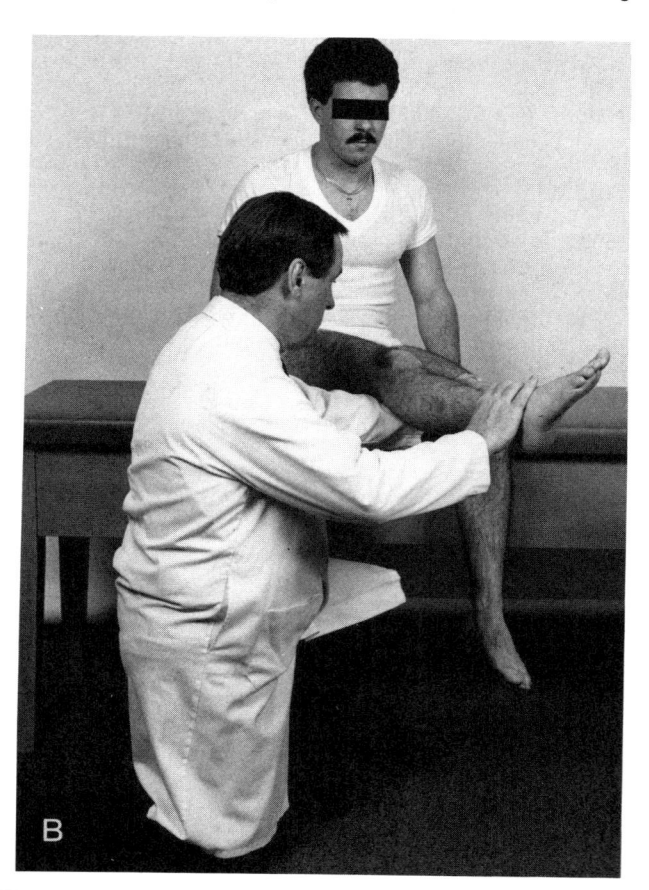

Figure 27.1B. SLR ability in sitting position is 90°—a difference from Figure 27.1A that cannot be explained by root involvement, but rather represents magnification/exaggeration effort by the patient.

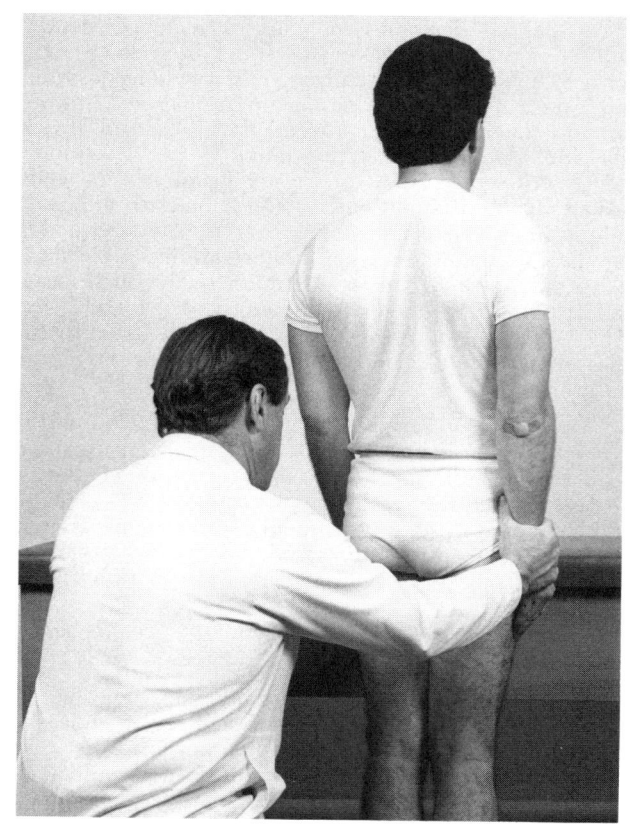

Figure 27.2. Simulated movement testing. Holding the patient's arms fixed to the pelvis allows for rotation through the hip joints without moving the back. If the patient complains of back pain, this is considered anticipatory behavior, one of the many indications of nonorganic pain.

testing that abolishes an acted physical finding and demonstrates normal physical function is a method of demonstrating exaggeration behavior. The best distraction test is simple observation of the patient as he gets undressed and moves about the examining room.

Varying degrees of acting behavior occur in different patients. In general, the more sophisticated the patient, the more sophisticated the acting behavior, and the more sophisticated the examiner must be.

Anticipatory Behavior The second group of physical findings in this reaction represent anticipation on the part of the patient to the test situations. This anticipatory behavior leads to an appropriate response by the patient in an attempt to indicate illness. An example of this test is illustrated in Figure 27.2.

Contradictory Clinical Evidence Statements by the patient to the effect that he is unable to work may not be supported by clinical observations. Some patients will say they are unable to drive, yet will have driven by themselves great distances to get to the examination. Some patients will say that they require frequent medication, yet will arrive from great distances without their medication. The patient who claims to be continuously wearing a collar or a brace should show signs of this wear on his body and the appliance. Patients with callouses on their hands and knees contradict their story of a prolonged inability to work. Other evidence of work may be in the form of paint stains or a particular distribution to their sunburn. Patients with nicotine stains on a grossly paralyzed limb should start to demonstrate similar stains on the opposite hand. Finally, those patients who demonstrate a prolonged and profound weakness in an extremity will not have associated wasting of that extremity.

It is important to stress that one swallow does not make a spring! The fact that a patient has one of these findings does not mean the patient should be classified as a exaggerator or litigant reactor. It is important to stress that a collection of symptoms and signs should be present with the appropriate clinical setting to make the diagnosis of exaggeration behavior. Waddell et al. (3) have documented the significant symptoms and signs that, when collected together, suggest that a nonorganic component to a disability is present. These symptoms and signs have been scientifically documented as valid and reproducible. As a screening mechanism, they are an excellent substitute for pain drawings and psychological testing (Table 27.3).

Conclusion

Every human attends the school of survival. Sometimes the lessons lead patients to modify or magnify a physical disability at a conscious or unconscious level. One word of caution—the presence of one of these nonorganic reactions does not preclude an organic condition such as a herniated nucleus pulposus. The art of medicine is truly tested by a patient with a physical low back pain who modifies the disability with a nonorganic reaction of tension, hysteria, depression, or emotional factors.

Table 27.3
Symptoms and Signs Suggesting a Nonorganic Component to Disability

Symptoms
1. Pain is multifocal in distribution and nonmechanical (present at rest)
2. Entire extremity is painful, numb and/or weak
3. Extremity gives way (as a result the patient carries a cane)
4. Treatment response:
    A. No response
    B. "Allergic" to treatment
    C. Not on treatment
5. Multiple crises, multiple hospital admissions/investigations, multiple doctors

Signs
1. Tenderness is superficial (skin) or nonanatomic (e.g., over body of sacrum)
2. Simulated movement tests positive
3. Distraction tests positive
4. Whole leg weak or numb
5. Academy Award performance

QUESTION 2

Is this clinical presentation a diagnostic trap?

It is to easy, when trying to arrive at a mechanical diagnosis, to fall into the many traps in the differential diagnosis of low back pain. An example is the young man in the early stages of ankylosing spondylitis who presents with vague sacroiliac joint pain and mild buttock and thigh discomfort who is thought to have a disk herniation. The patient with a retroperitoneal tumor invading the sacrum or sacral plexus may present with classic sciatica and also be diagnosed as having a disk herniation. It is not uncommon that patients with pathology within the peritoneal cavity will refer pain to the back. To avoid missing these various diagnostic pitfalls, always ask yourself the second question: Is this clinical presentation a trap?

Two broad categories of disease are included in this question:

1. Back pain referred from outside the spine may come from within the peritoneal cavity (e.g., gastrointestinal tumors or ulcers) or from the retroperitoneal space (genitourinary conditions, abdominal aortic conditions, or primary or secondary tumors of the retroperitoneal space). These patients can be recognized clinically on the basis of two historic points. First, the pain is often nonmechanical in nature and troubles the patient just as much at rest as it does with activity. Second, the pain in the back often has the characteristics of the pain associated with the primary pathology.
2. Painful conditions arising from within the spinal column, including its neurologic content. This group is subdivided into the differential diagnosis of low back

pain or lumbago (Table 27.4) and the differential diagnosis of radicular pain or sciatica (Table 27.5).

These patients have nonmechanical back pain or a pain more characteristic for the primary pathology. Radiating extremity pain is not common unless neurologic territory has been invaded by the disease process, which usually occurs late in the disease. Unfortunately, many of these conditions are not obvious on history and physical examination and are often missed on reviewing plain x-rays. The following diagnostic tests are useful as a screening mechanism:

1. Hemoglobin, hematocrit, white blood count, differential, and erythrocyte sedimentation rate.
2. Serum chemistries, especially calcium, acid and alkaline phosphatase, and serum protein electrophoresis.
3. Bone scan.

These three screening tests can be completed outside of the hospital and almost routinely identify these conditions. Magnetic resonance imaging (MRI) will start to play a bigger role in the diagnosis of these various nonmechanical conditions.

Although the most common cause of leg pain in a radicular distribution is a structural lesion in the lumbosacral region, there are many other causes of radiating leg discomfort that must be considered. Missing these conditions is probably the most common error made in a spine surgical practice. For example, the high sensitivity of today's investigative modalities is capable of showing a minor and insignificant herniated nucleus pulposus when in fact the patient has a conus tumor higher in the spinal canal. This situation is being abetted by the tendency to do a computed tomography (CT) scan and skip myelography in an attempt to arrive at a structural diagnosis for mechanical low back pain. This may seem a good idea to avoid the complications of myelography, but it will present problems unless you adhere to the following rule: *An equivocal CT scan requires completion of myelography.* As more MRI is done, the issue is going to be resolved. Soon, all patients with low back pain who do not respond to usual conservative treatment measures will automatically have an outpatient hematologic and serum screen, a bone scan, a CT scan, and MRI. (Is it far down the road that one day robots will deal with the structural lesion?)

Table 27.4
Differential Diagnosis of Nonmechanical Low Back Pain

1. Referred pain (e.g., from the abdomen or retroperitoneal space)
2. Infection—bone, disk, epidural space
3. Neoplasm
   A. Primary (multiple myeloma, osteoid osteoma, etc.)
   B. Secondary
4. Inflammation—arthritides such as ankylosing spondylitis
5. Miscellaneous metabolic and vascular disorders such as osteopenias and Paget's disease

Table 27.5
Differential Diagnosis of Sciatica

1. Intraspinal causes
   A. Proximal to disk—conus and cauda equina lesions (e.g., neurofibroma, epindymoma)
   B. Disk level
      Herniated nucleus pulposus
      Stenosis (canal or recess)
      Infection—osteomyelitis or diskitis (with nerve root pressure)
      Inflammation—arachnoiditis
      Neoplasm—benign or malignant with nerve root pressure
2. Extraspinal causes
   A. Pelvis
      Cardiovascular conditions (e.g., peripheral vascular disease)
      Gynecologic conditions
      Orthopedic conditions (e.g., osteoarthritis of hip)
      Sacroiliac joint disease
      Neoplasms
   B. Peripheral nerve lesions
      Neuropathy (diabetic, tumor, alcohol)
      Local sciatic nerve conditions (trauma, tumor)
      Inflammation (herpes zoster)

Etiology of Radiating Leg Pain

Space does not permit discussion of all the differential diagnoses of radiating leg pain, but three common conditions must be recognized: (a) cardiovascular conditions (peripheral vascular disease), (b) hip pathology, and (c) neuropathies.

Cardiovascular Conditions Cardiovascular disorders in the form of peripheral vascular disease can cause leg discomfort that is easily confused with nerve root compression. Since these conditions tend to occur in the older patient population, they may coexist. Table 27.6 is an attempt to separate vascular claudication from neurogenic claudication.

Hip Pathology Usually it is easy to diagnose conditions of the hip because they so commonly cause pain around the hip and specifically pain in the groin. In addition, walking causes a limp, and physical examination reveals a loss of internal rotation early in the disease. Occasionally, however, a patient with hip pathology will have no pain around the hip and will have only referred pain in the distal thigh. In these patients, it is easy to miss hip pathology unless one specifically examines the hip for

Table 27.6
Differential Diagnosis of Claudicant Leg Pain

Findings	Vascular Claudication	Neurogenic Claudication
Pain		
Type	Sharp, cramping	Vague and variously described as radicular, heavyness, cramping
Location	Exercised muscles	Either typical radicular or extremely diffuse
Radiation	Rare after onset	Common after onset, usually proximal to distal
Aggravation	Walking	Only 50% aggravated by walking, can be aggravated by standing
Relief	Stoping muscular activity even in the standing position	Walking in the forward flexed position more comfortable; once pain occurs, relief comes only with lying down
Time to relief	Quick (minutes)	Slow (many minutes)
Neurologic symptoms	Not present	Commonly present
Straight leg raising tests	Negative	Mildly positive or negative
Neurologic examination	Negative	Mildly positive or negative
Vascular examination	Absent pulses	Pulses present

loss of internal rotation. If there is any doubt, an x-ray of the pelvis must be taken.

Neuropathies The most easily missed diagnosis is diabetic mononeuropathy. Although it more commonly occurs in poorly controlled diabetes mellitus, it may occur in an undiagnosed late-onset diabetic. It is thought to be due to an ischemic episode affecting the peripheral nerve, and is characteristically manifested by acute onset with pain in a typical radicular distribution easily mimicking a disk herniation. If the peripheral neuropathy of diabetes is a mononeuropathy multiplex, a symmetrical polyneuropathy, or an autonomic neuropathy, the diagnosis is more readily apparent. The distinguishing features of diabetic mononeuropathy are as follows:

1. It occurs in the older patient with or without known diabetes.
2. There will be a history of the sudden onset of radicular pain with no back pain.
3. The patient will describe nonmechanical leg pain; the patient is extremely uncomfortable at rest.
4. The pain is usually more severe than the pain associated with lateral recess stenosis or spinal stenosis, and of equal severity to the leg pain associated with a herniated nucleus pulposus.
5. The paresthetic discomfort often has a burning or numbing characteristic to it.
6. Although the sensory symptoms predominate, it is the author's experience that mononeuropathy affecting the femoral or the lumbosacral nerve roots has a more significant motor and reflex component on examination.

The diagnosis is supported with abnormal blood sugars and electrical studies showing slower nerve conduction velocities and the presence of fibrillation potentials, positive waves at rest, and a decrease in the number of motor unit potentials on electromyography (EMG).

Conclusion

Although there are many other causes of extremity *symptoms* not listed in this table, it is important to recognize that the table includes most causes of lower extremity *pain*. Extremity symptoms such as numbness and weakness, in the absence of pain, should suggest very strongly that a primary neurologic disorder is possible rather than a mechanical low back condition.

QUESTION 3

Is this a mechanical low back pain condition, and if so, what is the syndrome?

The two important words are "mechanical" and "syndrome." Mechanical pain is pain aggravated by activity such as bending and lifting, and relieved by rest. There may be specific complaints relative to household chores or specific work efforts. These mechanical pains are usually relieved by rest. Although these statements seem straightforward, clinical assessment is not always easy. A poor historian may not be able to relate a history of mechanical aggravation or relief. In addition, if significant leg pain is present, implying a significant inflammatory response around the nerve root, then much rest will be needed before the patient describes a relief of leg pain. Significant mechanical back pain may sometimes be aggravated by simply rolling over in bed. To the unsophisticated historian, this may have the appearance of nonmechanical back pain. However, if one takes a careful history, and if a patient is a good historian it is possible to determine that mechanical back pain is pain aggravated by activity and relieved by rest.

The second important word is "syndrome." It is much safer to make a syndrome diagnosis for mechanical low back pain and then, after investigation, try matching a structural lesion with the clinical syndrome. There are two reasons for taking this approach:

1. Today's investigative techniques are so sophisticated that it is possible to find abnormalities whether a patient has symptoms or not.
2. A patient may have an obvious structural lesion such as spondylolisthesis, yet may have an acute radicular syndrome due to a disk herniation at a level other than that of the spondylolisthesis. In fact, a patient with spondylolisthesis may have any one of the potential diagnoses discussed in this chapter. To focus on the structural lesion of spondylolisthesis shown on x-ray and ignore the history and physical examination will lead to errors in diagnosis and treatment.

There are basically two syndromes in mechanical low back pain (Table 27.7): (a) lumbago (mechanical instability), and (b) sciatica (radicular syndrome). Before enlarging on these syndromes, it is well to take a moment to reflect on the concept of "referred pain." Many state that leg pain that does not go below the knee and is associated with good SLR ability is likely referred leg pain. This idea is further entrenched if there is an absence of neurologic symptoms or signs. The gate control theory of pain is one of the theories used to explain referred pain. The phenomenon is thought to occur when painful stimuli are reflexly shifted around at the cord level. This shunting results in pain being felt in a myotomal or dermatomal distribution away from the origin of the pain, such as in the leg. The concept is altogether too simplistic and needs to be reworked in light of new investigative techniques such as CT scanning and MRI. I predict that referred leg pain will be a lot less common than originally thought. It is more likely that patients labeled as having referred pain for their leg radiations have various degrees of radicular pain due to nerve root encroachment by either bone or chronic disk herniations.

The diagnosis of referred leg pain should be reserved for the patient who has the following clinical presentation:

1. There is significant mechanical back pain present as the source of referral.
2. The leg pain affects both legs, is vague in its distribution, and has no radicular component.
3. The degree of referred leg discomfort varies directly with the back pain. When the back pain increases in severity, the referred leg pain occurs or increases in severity. Conversely, a decrease in back pain results in a decrease in the referral of pain. Referred pain is less likely to radiate below the knee.
4. There are no neurologic symptoms or signs in concert with the complaint of refered leg pain.

It is safer to assume that any patient with radiating leg pain, especially unilateral leg pain, has a radicular syndrome until proven otherwise.

Lumbago–Mechanical Instability

The lumbago–mechanical instability syndrome is easy to recognize. These patients present exclusively with lumbosacral backache aggravated by activities such as bending, lifting, and sitting. The pain may radiate toward either iliac crest, but does not radiate down into the buttock or legs. The pain is almost always relieved by various forms of rest, for example, reduced activity, weight reduction, corset support, or bedrest. Most patients have no trouble describing these relieving efforts.

Most importantly, there are no associated leg symptoms or signs.

Unilateral Acute Radicular Syndrome

Before describing the unilateral acute radicular syndrome syndrome, it is important to note that the leg includes the buttock and sacroiliac joint areas proximally (Fig. 27.3). In fact, the younger patient may lateralize discomfort off the midline as high as the top of the sacroiliac joint or iliac crest region. Even this is considered leg pain in the young patient. Obviously, any pain below the buttock crease is to be considered leg pain. A radicular distribution to leg pain is just what it implies—not a diffuse, but a specific distribution to the pain that follows a radical distribution.

History Approximately half the patients will attribute the onset of their acute radicular syndrome to some traumatic experience. This may be retrograde rationalization on the part of the patient. Experimental studies and careful statistical analysis of case histories do not support the concept that direct trauma or sudden weight loading of the spine are routinely the causal agents of disk rupture, although they may aggravate a preexisting lesion. This

Table 27.7
Syndromes in Mechanical Low Back Pain

1. Lumbago–mechanical instability
2. Sciatica–radicular pain
   A. Unilateral acute radicular syndrome
   B. Bilateral acute radicular syndrome
   C. Unilateral chronic radicular syndrome
   D. Bilateral chronic radicular syndrome

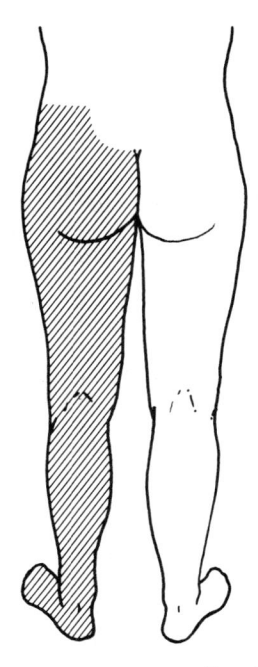

Figure 27.3. When a spine surgeon talks of leg pain, he also includes any pain located in the buttock.

aspect in the history becomes important when litigation or compensation is involved.

The younger the patient, the more likely sciatica is the only symptom. When asked specifically, many patients may state they noted numbness in the calf or foot before the pain developed. This is a stage of root compression before the inflammatory radiculitis begins. The majority of patients, however, develop back pain that subsequently radiates to the buttock and then down the leg. Most patients report that as the sciatic pain increases, the back pain decreases in severity. The history of pain is spondylogenic in character. That is to say, the pain is aggravated by general and specific activities and is relieved by rest. Bending, stooping, lifting, coughing, sneezing, and straining at stool will intensify the pain. Infrequently, referral patterns of pain occur such as perineal or testicular discomfort (pain or paresthesia) and lower abdominal discomfort. The former symptoms are likely due to irritation of lower sacral roots laterally or at the midline, and the latter may be due to muscular splinting of the pelvis.

Patients with acute radicular syndrome may complain of a dermatomal distribution to the paresthetic discomfort. It is interesting to note that although pain occurs in the buttock, thigh, and calf, the symptom in the foot is almost exclusively paresthesia.

Physical Examination

The Back The posture is characteristic. The lumbar spine is flattened and slightly flexed. The patient often leans away from the side of his pain and this sciatic scoliosis becomes more obvious on bending forward. The patient is more comfortable standing with the affected hip and knee slightly flexed, a manner accentuated by asking the patient to flex forward (Fig. 27.4). He walks in obvious discomfort, sometimes holding his loin with his hands. The gait is slow and deliberate and is designed to avoid any unnecessary movement of the spine. With gross tension on the nerve root, the patient may not be able to put his heel on the ground, and walks slowly and painfully on tiptoe.

Forward flexion may be permitted, so the hands reach the knees by virtue of flexion of the hip and knee joint. If the examiner keeps his fingertips on the spinous processes, it is observed that the lumbar spine is splinted and nonmobile. Limitation of flexion in such instances is therefore the result of root tension. The degree of flexion should be recorded by measuring the distance between the fingertips and the floor.

Extension is also limited, although to a lesser degree than flexion. The complaint on extension is usually back pain but at times the patient may feel buttock pain.

Lateral flexion may be full and free, but in the presence of a sciatic scoliosis, lateral flexion toward the concavity of the curve (side of sciatica) is limited.

The phenomenon of sciatic scoliosis and the relief of

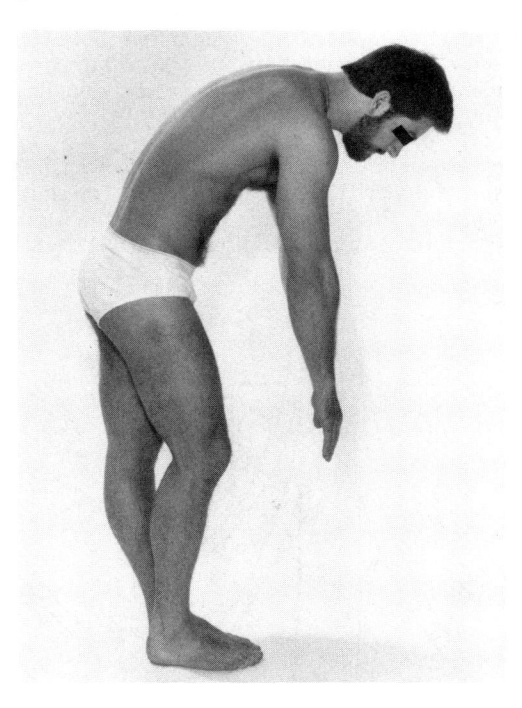

Figure 27.4. Typical posture assumed by patient with herniated nucleus pulposus when forward flexion is attempted—flexion of knee on affected side and forward rotation of pelvis to affected side.

aggravation of pain on lateral flexion have been attributed to the position of the protrusion in relation to the nerve root (Fig. 27.5). However, this may be a simplistic explanation in view of the fact that the sciatic scoliosis disappears on recumbency. This observation, the loss of lateral curvature of the lumbar spine on recumbency, differentiates the sciatic list from a structural scoliosis. On further assessment of the degree of root involvement present, it is imperative to test the extremities specifically for root tension, root irritation, and impairment of root conduction. These are the cardinal signs of lumbar root compromise.

Back Tenderness and Muscle Spasm In the standing position, especially in the presence of scoliosis, muscle spasm can be observed. At rest, however, the spasm often subsides and there is little tenderness to be found in the back musculature. Selectively palpating and applying a lateral thrust to the spinous process may cause some back pain, and on rare occasions may produce leg pain. By and large, when the patient with an acute radicular syndrome is at rest on the examining table, there is little to find in the back. The patient's major complaint is leg pain and the majority of physical findings are in the extremity.

The Extremities in the Unilateral Acute Radicular Syndrome

Root Tension and Irritation The term *root tension* denotes distortion of the emerging nerve root by an extradural lesion. The three most useful tests for the presence of root tension are limitation of SLR, crossover pain, and the bowstring sign, the latter also arising in part from root irritation.

When testing SLR, it is important not to hurt the patient. Never suddenly jerk the leg up in the air. The standard for SLR testing is a fully extended knee with the hip in slight internal rotation and adduction. Figure 27.1A demonstrates a good way of doing the SLR test. A positive SLR test is present when the test reproduces pain in the buttock or leg, which limits SLR ability to something less than normal.

Two additional maneuvers are useful to support the finding of limitation of SLR:

1. Aggravation of pain by forced dorsiflexion of the ankle at the limit of SLR.
2. Relief of pain by flexion of the knee and hip.

Physiogenic sciatic pain due to nerve root compromise is always relieved by flexion of the knee and hip. Continuing to flex the patient's hip with the knee bent does not reproduce and aggravate sciatic pain. This phenomenon is seen only in the emotionally destroyed patient.

If SLR is permissible to 70° before leg pain is produced, the finding is equivocal for the acute radicular syndrome. Below this level the reproduction of leg pain on SLR, aggravated by dorsiflexion of the ankle and relieved by flexion of the knee, is strongly suggestive of the tension on the L5 or S1 nerve roots. Reproduction of the sciatic pain in the affected extremity by raising the unaffected leg is irrefutable evidence of root tension in the acute radicular syndrome. This is known as contralateral or crossed SLR pain.

False-Positive SLR Test Hamstring tightness may cloud the assessment of the SLR test. These patients generally have a tight body build (e.g., inability to fully extend the elbow). Their hamstring tightness limiting SLR is bilateral and the discomfort the patient feels is distal in the thigh in the region of the hamstring tendons. Hamstring tightness does not produce pain radiating below the knee. Finally, other physical findings of root tension, irritation, and compression are absent when hamstring tightness is the sole cause of decreased SLR ability.

False-Negative SLR Test On occasion you will en-

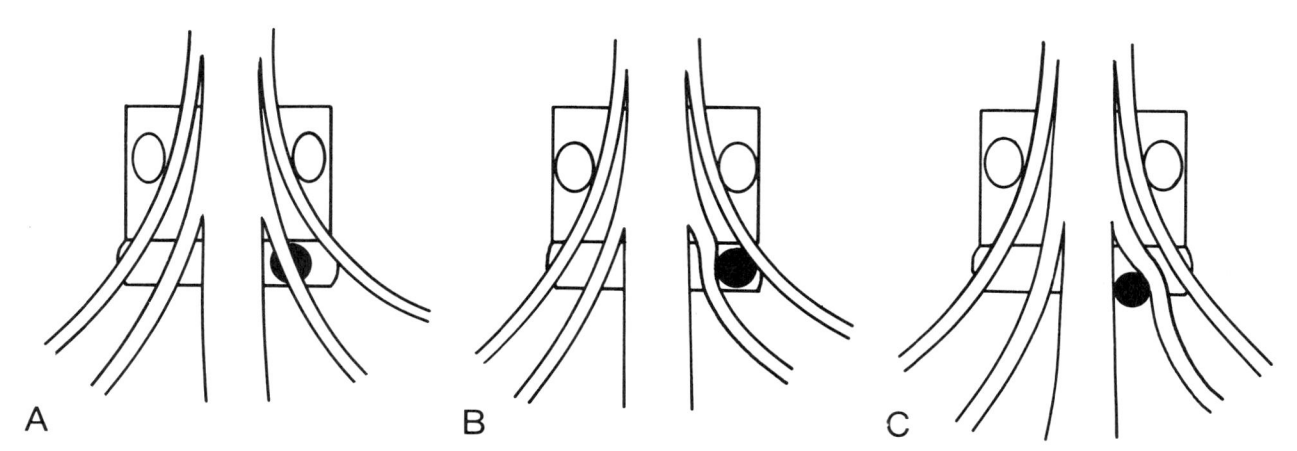

Figure 27.5. *A,* Usual relationship of herniated nucleus pulposus (HNP) ventral (anterior) to nerve root. *B,* Rare location of HNP lateral to nerve root such that flexion to affected side increases pain. *C,* Not unusual location of HNP in axilla of nerve root such that flexion to opposite side increases pain.

counter a loose-jointed individual with sciatica due to an herniated nucleus pulposus. On SLR testing you may not be impressed with the degree of impaired SLR ability until you examine the unaffected leg and see the patient's ability to straight leg raise well beyond 90°.

The Bowstring Sign The bowstring sign is an important indication of root tension and irritation. To perform the test the examiner carries out SLR to the point at which the patient experiences some discomfort in the distribution of the sciatic nerve. At this level, the knee is allowed to flex and the patient's foot is allowed to rest on the examiner's shoulder (Fig. 27.6). The test demands sudden, firm pressure applied to the tibial nerve in the popliteal fossa. Do the test in the following stages. Apply firm pressure to the hamstrings: this will not hurt. Then, move your thumbs over to the tibial nerve. Apply sudden, firm pressure with your thumb over the nerve. A positive bowstring test is reproduction of radiating leg discomfort. Most commonly the radiating discomfort is pain felt proximally in the thigh and even into the back. Less commonly, radiating discomfort will travel distally, and this discomfort is more often paresthetic in nature than being painful. It is important to emphasize that if the test only produces local pain in the popliteal fossa, then it is of no significance. This demonstration of root irritation is probably the single most important sign in the diagnosis of tension and irritation of a nerve root by a ruptured intervertebral disk; unfortunately it is not alway present in patients with herniated nucleus pulposus.

Tests to Verify SLR Reduction When the patient sits with the legs dangling over the side of the bed, the hip and knee are both flexed to 90°. If the knee is now extended fully, the position assumed by the leg is equivalent to 90° of SLR. If the patient is suffering from root compromise, this will cause sudden, severe pain and the patient will lean backward to avoid tension on the nerve (Fig. 27.7). This is commonly referred to as the "positive flip test." With the psychogenic regional pain syndrome, the patient will permit the examiner to extend the knee of the painful leg without showing any response.

Sometimes crossover pain can be demonstrated only in the sitting position. If one crosses over pain from the asymptomatic leg to the symptomatic leg in the sitting position, this is also considered a positive crossover sign and almost certainly indicative of an acute radicular syndrome.

Patients with acute radicular syndrome may also have tenderness over the sacroiliac joint and down the course of the sciatic nerve. This tenderness has led to the erroneous diagnosis of sacroiliac joint strain. It is very unusual in these patients to see any clinical or radiologic evidence of damage to the sacroiliac joint.

Femoral Nerve Stretch With higher lumbar disk herniations and acute radicular syndromes, the SLR test may be negative, but the femoral stretch test will be positive. Figure 27.8 shows the femoral nerve stretch test. It is not nearly as satisfactory as an SLR test, but if this test reproduces radiating thigh pain, aggravated by knee flexion, then the test is considered to be positive.

Summary Table 27.8 summarizes the historic and physical foundation on which to build the diagnosis of an acute radicular syndrome.

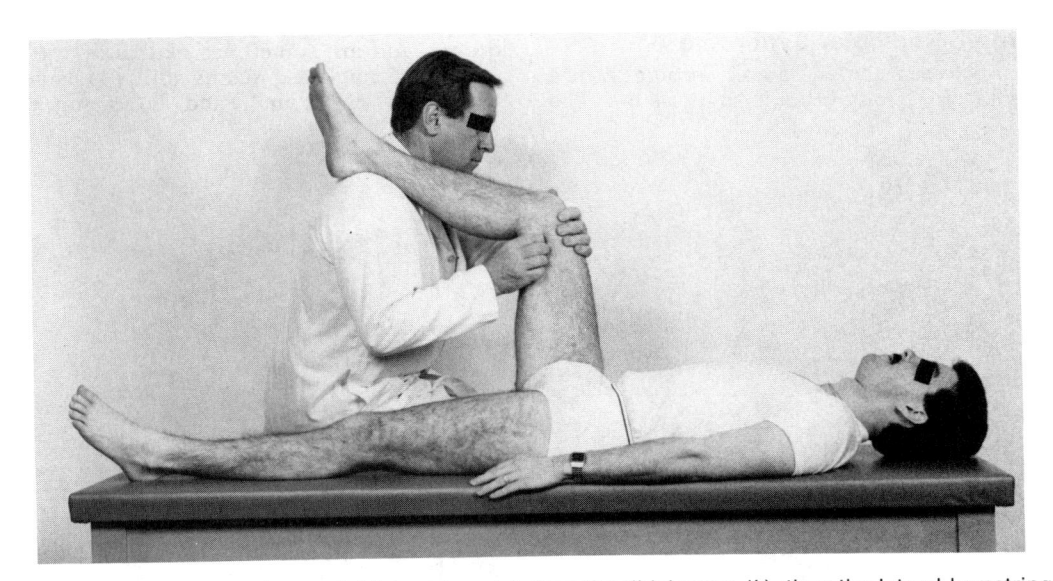

Figure 27.6. Bowstring test. First do the medial hamstrings (*a*), then the tibial nerve (*b*), then the lateral hamstrings (*c*), then the lateral popliteal nerve (*d*). A positive response at (*b*) and (*d*) equates with organic root irritation. A negative response at all four test sites is a negative test. A positive test at (*a*) and (*c*) is indicative of nonorganic reaction.

Figure 27.7. A positive flip test. Because of root tension, an attempt to straight leg raise in the sitting position causes buttock or leg pain and the patient flips back on the examining table to relieve the increased tension.

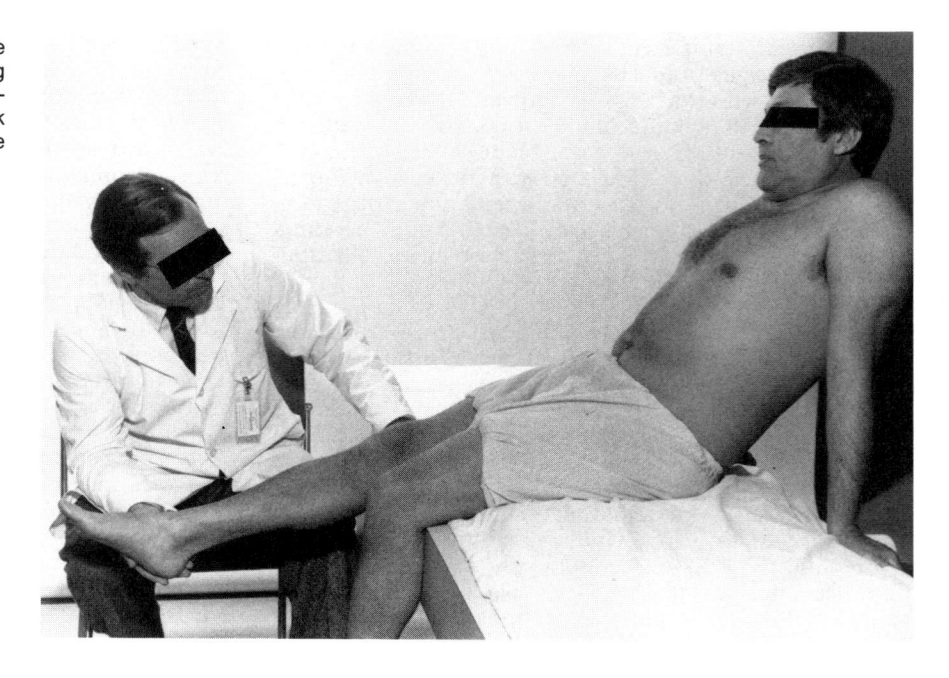

Bilateral Acute Radicular Syndrome

Fortunately, the bilateral acute radicular syndrome is rare. It is usually due to a massive midline sequestered disk. The syndrome is manifested by the sudden onset of bilateral leg pain usually accompanied by bladder and bowel impairment. It is obviously an emergency and is a diagnosis that is rarely missed.

Unilateral Chronic Radicular Syndrome

The difference between acuteness and chronicity in a radicular syndrome is often difficult to measure. The severity and the duration of the syndrome usually combine to distinguish acute from chronic radicular pain. Chronic unilateral radicular pain is usually a complaint for many months or more. It follows a typical radicular distribution, including pain below the knee, and is usually associated with much in the way of mechanical back pain. Both pains are usually aggravated by walking. Neurologic symptoms are less prevalent than in acute radicular syndrome, and are sometimes extremely diffuse and nonlocalizing. Straight leg raising ability is usually much better than 50% of normal, and bowstring discomfort and

Figure 27.8. Method of doing femoral stretch.

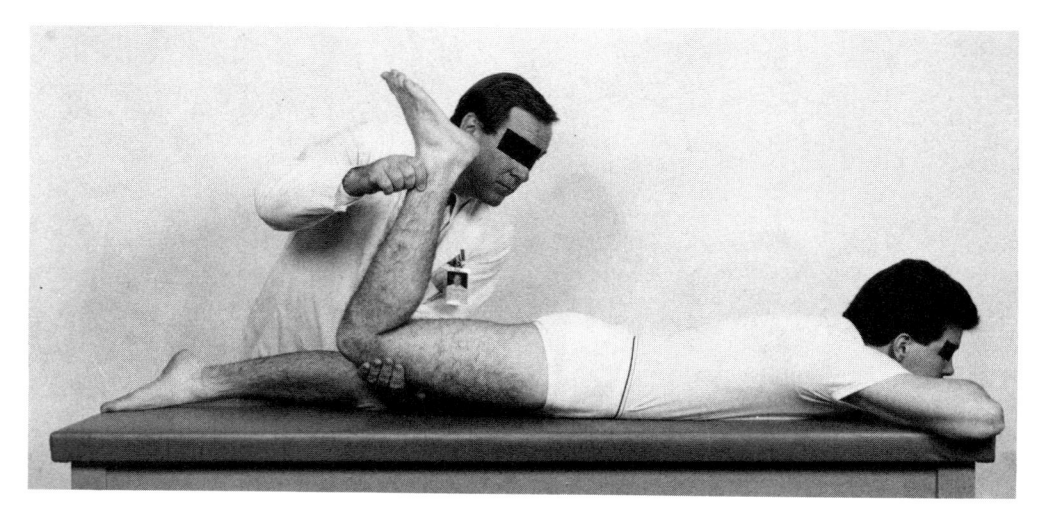

Table 27.8
Criteria for the Diagnosis of Acute Radicular Syndrome[a]

1. Leg pain (including buttock) is the dominant complaint when compared to back pain.
2. Neurologic symptoms that are specific (e.g., paresthesia in a typical dermatomal distribution).
3. Significant SLR changes (any one or a combination of these)
   A. SLR less than 50% of normal
   B. Bowstring discomfort
   C. Crossover pain
4. Neurologic signs (see section on anatomic level

[a] Three or four of these criteria must be present, the only exception being the young patients who are very resistant to the effects of nerve root compression and thus may not have neurologic symptoms (criterion 2) or signs (criterion 4).

crossover pain are not seen in this syndrome. Neurologic findings are very few and usually not helpful in localizing the degree of nerve root involvement.

Bilateral Chronic Radicular Syndrome

To many, the bilateral chronic radicular syndrome is known as neurogenic claudication. However, bilateral leg symptoms specifically aggravated by walking are present in only 50% of patients with chronic bilateral radicular syndrome. For this reason, the term *chronic bilateral radicular syndrome* is preferred. This syndrome differs from the unilateral radicular syndrome in two ways:

1. Both legs are affected rather than one leg.
2. The pain of the bilateral radicular syndrome may not be a typical radicular-type pain. Some patients describe typical claudicant leg pain in a radicular distribution. Other patients describe a diffuse type of claudicant leg discomfort that cannot be localized to a radicular distribution.

Many other symptoms are present in this syndrome, including weakness, "heaviness," and "rubberiness" in the legs. Numbness is also prevalent in this syndrome and is often of no value in localizing which nerve roots are compromised. There is a typical march phenomenon with the chronic bilateral radicular syndrome. Symptoms get much worse with prolonged walking, radiate further down the leg, and ultimately interfere with the ability of the patient to ambulate. Some patients may report noticing that if they attach themselves to a shopping cart and walk in the flexed position, they can get more distance before their leg symptoms appear. Characteristically, physical examination in chronic bilateral radicular syndrome reveals little. Straight leg raising is usually very good, and if the syndrome is due entirely to canal narrowing rather than lateral recess narrowing, there are limited neurologic findings except where the syndrome has significantly progressed.

QUESTION 4

Are there clues to an anatomic level on history and physical examination?

Is there an anatomic level clinically? There is an important intermediate question to consider between a syndrome diagnosis and a structural diagnosis. If it is possible to determine an atomic level clinically, then any structural lesion has to be at the appropriate level. Otherwise it cannot be considered a significant defect. A patient who has an anatomic level of S1 root involvement rarely should have a structural diagnosis localized to the L3–L4 interspace!

There are three ways to determine an anatomic level: distribution of leg pain, neurologic symptoms, and neurologic signs.

Distribution of Leg Pain

Pain in the posterior thigh and posterior calf distribution incriminates the fifth lumbar root or the first sacral root. Whether this pain is posterior or posterolateral in the thigh and calf is of little use in separating fifth lumbar root lesions from first sacral root lesions. However, pain down the anterior thigh almost certainly incriminates the fourth lumbar nerve root or higher lumbar nerve roots, and excludes involvement of the fifth lumbar or first sacral roots.

Neurologic Symptoms

A paresthetic discomfort with a dermatomal distribution is the most helpful historic feature in localizing an anatomic level. Paresthetic discomfort along the lateral edge of the foot incriminates the first sacral nerve root, paresthetic discomfort over the dorsum of the foot and the lateral calf incriminates the fifth lumbar nerve root, and paresthetic discomfort down the medial shin incriminates the fourth lumbar nerve root.

Neurologic Signs

The diagnosis of acute radicular syndrome is in no way totally dependent on the demonstration of root impairment as reflected by signs of motor weakness or changes in sensory appreciation or reflex activity. However, the presence of such changes reinforces the diagnosis. The common neurologic changes are summarized in Table 27.9.

Changes in Reflex Activity The ankle jerk may be diminished or absent with an S1 lesion. This is tested with the patient kneeling on a chair or sitting comfortably. (If a patient's sciatica is so severe he cannot sit comfortably, then testing of the reflexes in the sitting position is invalid, because the guarding and posturing will depress the reflexes.) This explains the occasional depressed knee reflex seen in the presence of sciatica due to an L5–S1 disk protrusion. If the patient has suffered a previous attack of

Table 27.9
Common Neurologic Changes in Acute Radicular Syndrome

Change	Root L4	Root L5	Root S1
Motor weakness	Knee extension	Ankle dorsiflexion	Ankle plantar flexion
Sensory loss	Medial shin to knee	Dorsum of foot and lateral calf	Lateral border of foot and posterior calf
Reflex depression	Knee	Tibialis posterior	Ankle
Wasting	Thigh (no calf)	Calf (minimal thigh)	Calf (minimal thigh)

sciatic pain, with compression of the first sacral nerve sufficient enough to obliterate the ankle jerk, this may not return to normal. The absence of the ankle reflex therefore may be merely a remnant of a previous episode of disk rupture, and the present attack may be due to a disk rupture at another level.

With an L5 root compression, the tibialis posterior reflex (obtained by striking the tendon of the tibialis posterior near its point of insertion) may be absent. Diminution of the lateral hamstring jerk is also seen on occasion with an L5 root compromise, but multiple innervation of this muscle group make this an unreliable reflex.

With L4 and L3 lesions, the knee jerk may be diminished.

Wasting Muscle wasting is rarely seen unless the symptoms have been present for more than 3 weeks. Very marked wasting is more suggestive of an extradural tumor than of a disk rupture.

Always measure the girth of the thigh and the girth of the calf. This is a useful baseline from which to assess the progress of the lesion. Remember, if there is gross weakness of the gastrocnemii, the main venous pump of the affected extremity is no longer working and these patients may even show some measure of ankle edema. The combination of calf tenderness due to S1 root irritation and the observation of a swollen ankle may give rise to the erroneous diagnosis of thrombophlebitis.

Motor Loss The weakness of the gastrocnemii is best demonstrated by getting the patient to rise on tiptoe five or six times. The patient is then asked if it requires more effort do this on the affected extremity. If the quadriceps is weak, the physician must be aware of this before ascribing the difficulty of tiptoe rising to weakness of the calf muscles; also, if sciatic pain is severe, the test cannot be performed by the patient.

The power of ankle dorsiflexion is best tested by applying full body weight to the dorsiflexed ankle. Testing the dorsiflexors by asking the patient to walk on his heels will only demonstrate marked weakness in this muscle group. Weakness of the flexor hallucis longus (S1) or weakness of the extensor hallucis longus (L5) is often the first evidence of motor involvement. The evertors of the foot may be weak with an L5 lesion. The gluteus maximus may become weak with lesions involving the first sacral nerve root and may be demonstrated by the sagging of one buttock crease when the patient stands. Weakness of the gluteus medium is seen with an L5 lesion and occasionally is marked enough to produce a Trendelenberg lurch, particularly noticeable when the patient is tired. When the gluteus medius is involved, there is frequently marked tenderness on pressure over the muscle near its point of insertion, and this may be confused with a trochanteric bursitis or with gluteal tendonitis.

Quadriceps weakness is seen with an L4 lesion and can be assessed by the examiner placing his arm under the patient's knee and asking the patient to extend the knee against the resistance of the examiner's hand.

Sensory Impairment The regions of sensory loss are reasonably constant. Within the sensory dermatomes, there appear to be areas more vulnerable to sensory loss than others. Loss of appreciation of pinprick is first noted in an S1 lesion below and behind the lateral malleolus and in an L5 lesion in the cleft between the first and second toes. Sensory appreciation is a subjective response and, as such, may sometimes be difficult to assess. Certain precautions must be followed. Sensory perception varies in different parts of the limb. Identical areas in each limb must be tested consecutively. The examination must be carried out as expeditiously as is compatible with accuracy, because the patient will soon tire of this form of examination and his answers may not be accurate. When the skin is pricked with a pin, the physiologic principle of recruitment is present. Thus, the overall sensory appreciation depends not only on the action of the pinprick, but also on the number of pinpricks experienced.

A sensory examination is only interpreted as positive when the sensory loss approximates one dermatomal distribution, and when the loss is not present in the adjacent dermatomes or the same contralateral dermatome.

QUESTION 5

After reviewing the results of investigation, what is the structural lesion and does it fit with the clinical syndrome?

The potential structural lesion diagnoses are listed in Table 27.10. This table covers only degenerative conditions of the spine; it omits postoperative scarring of arachnoid or nerve roots and fractures and dislocations. It is important to stress here that it is possible to have multiple syndromes related to a single structural lesion. For example, a dengerative spondylolisthesis can cause both mechanical instability (back pain) and bilateral claudicant leg pain as a result of encroachment on the spinal canal. Table 27.11 links syndromes with structural lesions.

Conclusion

It is important to make a clear-cut syndrome diagnosis on the basis of a history and physical examination, and match it to a clear-cut bonafide structural lesion on investigation. Failure to do this leads to wrong diagnoses and futile treatment interventions.

METHODS USED TO DOCUMENT THE STRUCTURAL LESION

Steps to document the presence of a structural lesion in mechanical low back pain should be taken only after a satisfactory answer has been obtained for questions 1, 2, and 3 above. Seeking a structural lesion in a patient with an unrecognized nonorganic problem is usually a waste of time and money, and is a danger to the patient.

False-positive investigative findings are easy to come by with today's sophisticated techniques. Before discussing each of these possible investigative procedures, it is assumed that a thorough history, physical examination, and other necessary investigations have satisfactorily answered questions 1 and 2.

PLAIN X-RAYS

It may not be necessary on the first assessment to do lumbar spine films, but if a patient does not quickly respond to treatment, anteroposterior, lateral, and oblique films should be obtained. Plain x-rays may demonstrate a narrowed disk space, facet joint disease, or a spondylolisthesis, but one must not assume that one of these is the causative structural lesion.

In reading plain x-rays, look at the nonskeletal areas first. Review the retroperitoneal area in specific regard to the kidneys and ureters, and the abdominal aorta. Be sure that the psoas shadows are intact. After reviewing the nonskeleton part of a lumbar spine x-ray, consider the skeleton. Look at the sacroiliac joints, survey the pedicles and vertebra bodies for erosions, and finally consider the structural defects that may have a potential for causing the patient's syndrome. Such things as narrowing of the disk space and translation of vertebral bodies are important to note. Various measurements of plain x-rays are not helpful in assessment of canal or recess narrowing.

MYELOGRAPHY

Myelography should be considered only when adequate conservative treatment has failed, and surgery is contemplated. Myelography has three purposes:

1. To rule out higher spine pathology.
2. To localize the exact level of root involvement.
3. To determine if any migration of disk material has occurred.

It is not the purpose of this text to discuss in detail the radiologic changes that may be seen on myelography, but some general principles regarding interpretation of myelograms are described.

Myelography was introduced in 1921 by Sicard (4) using iodized poppyseed oil injected into the epidural space. This is a logical place to put radiopaque material because the lesion is, indeed, an epidural lesion and should be demonstrated more easily by a radiopaque substance introduced into the epidural space. However, difficulty in aspirating the radiopaque material at the

Table 27.10
Structural Lesions in Mechanical Low Back Pain

1. Instability
   A. Intrinsic to disk—degenerative disk disease (DDD)
   B. Extrinsic to disk
      Facet joint disease (FJD)
      Spondylolisthesis
2. Soft tissue lesions—muscle spasm, ligamentous strain
3. Herniated nucleus pulposus (HNP)
4. Narrowing of spinal canal
   A. Spinal canal stenosis (SCS)
   B. Lateral recess stenosis (LRS)

Table 27.11
Relationship of Syndromes and Structural Lesions

1.	Lumbago	DDD
		FJD
		Spondylolysis/ spondylolisthesis
		Soft tissue
2.	Unilateral acute radicular	HNP
		HNP + LRS
3.	Unilateral chronic radicular	LRS
		HNP
4.	Bilateral acute radicular	Central HNP
5.	Bilateral chronic radicular	SCS

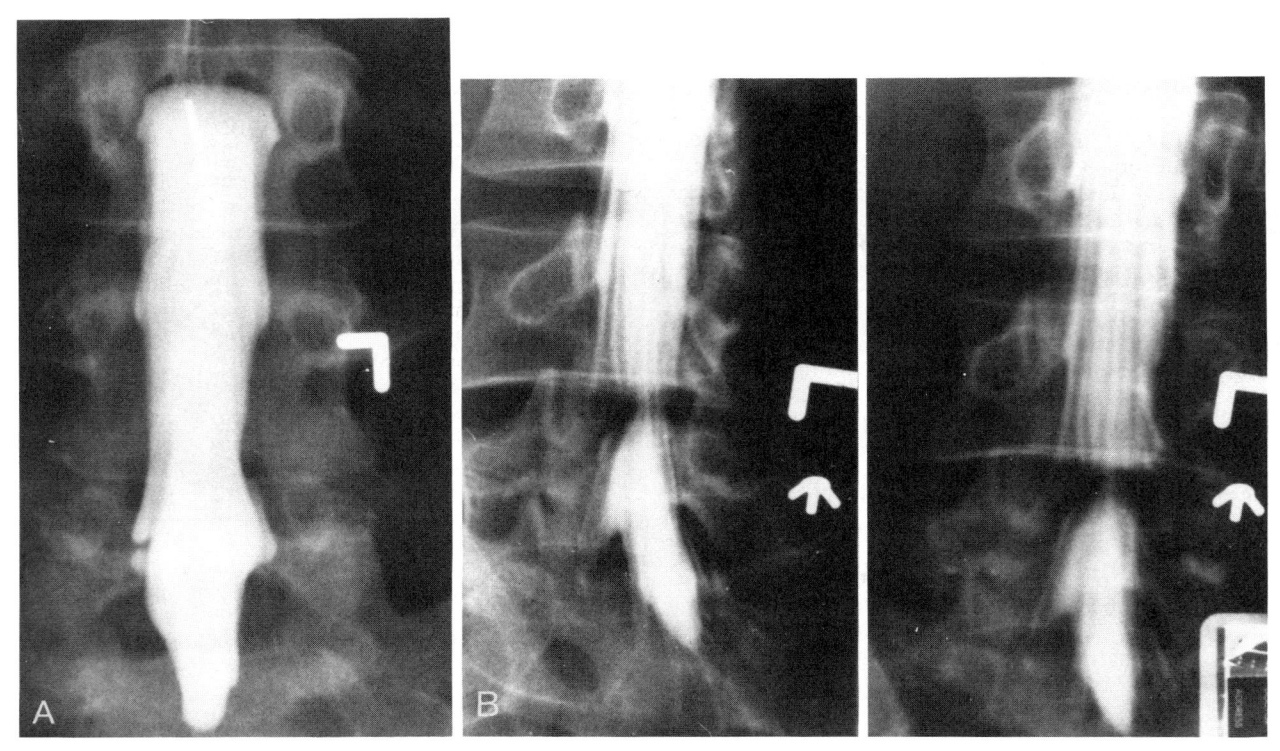

Figure 27.9. *A*, Oil-soluble contrast myelography showing defect in contrast column at L4–L5 left. Notice the lack of filling of nerve roots that made interpretation of apparent defect of L5–S1 left difficult (ultimately found to be not significant). *B*, Water-soluble contrast myelography showing large HNP central and left L4–L5. Notice how well nerve roots fill.

conclusion of the epidural myelography and the suggestion that this might give rise to root irritation at a later date persuaded surgeons to use the intrathecal injection of oil-soluble radiopaque compounds. Because these compounds are emulsified with the cerebrospinal fluid, it is not possible in the majority of instances to aspirate all of the dye injected.

Although many surgeons ordered oil myelograms, few themselves would undergo the procedure because of its difficulty and the postmyelographic complications. However, with the advent of water-soluble opaque materials and their refinement, myelography has become a much safer procedure.

The most popular water-soluble contrast material was metrizamide, but more recently this has been replaced by iohexol and iopamidol. These water-soluble compounds have several advantages over oil-soluble myelography in that the water-soluble contrast material is easier to inject and flows more readily through the nerve root sheaths. Obviously, it has a higher degree of sensitivity in documenting extradural lesions. Figure 27.9 is an example of oil- and water-soluble myelography.

Some neuroradiologists have popularized dynamic myelography. This entails flexion and extension of the patient on the fluoroscopic table with pictures being taken in these positions. Flexion supposedly opens up the spinal canal and reduces the degree of spinal stenosis encroachment on the contrast column. Conversely, extension decreases the dimensions of the spinal canal and if a spinal stenotic lesion is present, then more constriction of the contrast column will be evident on extension x-rays.

Myelography is still accompanied by some complications such as headache, nausea, and vomiting. More severe complications such as convulsions and infections have also been reported after myelography.

COMPUTED TOMOGRAPHY SCANNING

Presently, CT scanning of the lumbar spine is the single most popular investigative step. In fact, some doctors are so enamored with the CT scan that they order it before plain x-rays or before treatment intervention. I have even known doctors to order a CT scan before examining the patient. This abuse of the CT scan is leading to many erroneous diagnoses, especially when the doctor looks exclusively to the CT scan for guidance, and ignores an adequate history and physical examination. Bell and others have published excellent articles on the overuse and pitfalls of routine CT scanning (1).

Axial images are the most valuable and should be cut

from L3 to the midportion of the sacrum. Therefore any lesion above or below these levels will not be documented by the CT scan. Many neuroradiologists believe that reconstructions are of value, but the author is not convinced. Crude measurements from the CT scan can also give some impression as to the integrity of the spinal canal and the lateral recesses. Figure 27.10 demonstrates a narrowed spinal canal.

CT scanning is so simple, so readily available, and so nice to look at that many pitfalls await the unwary. Before embarking on treatment, especially surgery, be sure that the patient's clinical syndrome fits the structural lesion on CT scan. If there is any doubt, then a myelogram must be combined with the CT scan to further document the structural lesion.

MAGNETIC RESONANCE IMAGING

Magnetic resonance imaging will become the test of choice in the near future. The procedure requires no x-ray radiation and with the recent development of surface coils, the technique of MRI has improved to the point where it has become extremely sensitive in demonstrating soft tissue abnormalities in the lumbar spine. The major drawbacks to MRI are its cost, its time, and the claustrophobic effect it causes to patients lying in the chamber for imaging purposes. However, these drawbacks will be overcome and MRI will have a profound effect on the investigation of a patient with mechanical low back pain. Figure 27.11 is an MRI scan demonstrating a cervical disk herniation. MRI is limited in its outline of bony detail, a handicap not encountered with the CT scan. In the future a patient who has a mechanical low back pain syndrome, failing to

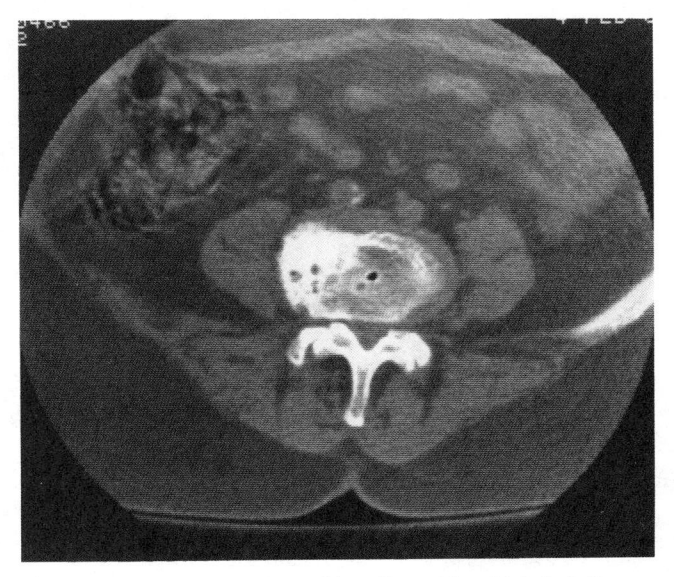

Figure 27.10. CT showing subluxation of facet joints (left more than right) and canal stenosis.

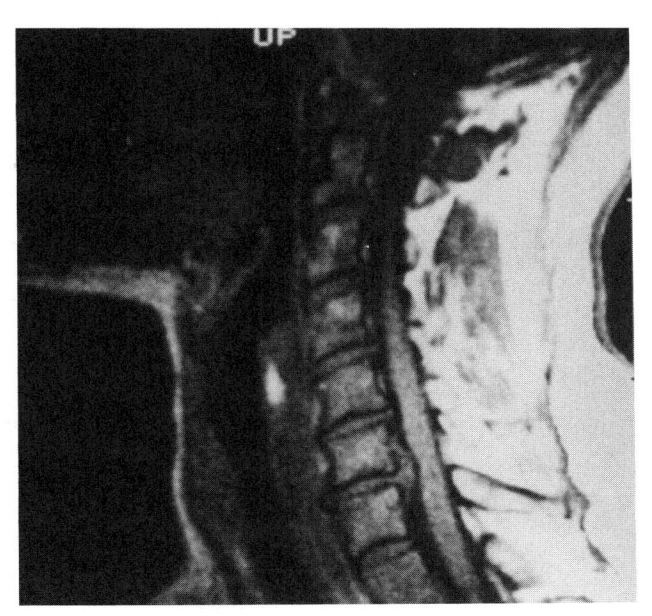

Figure 27.11. An MRI demonstrating a cervical disk herniation.

respond to conservative treatment, will be investigated with a CT and an MRI scan. Myelography will be less commonly ordered.

NERVE ROOT INFILTRATION

Nerve root infiltration is an investigative procedure that invovles blocking the anterior primary ramus of a single nerve root. It is usually the fifth lumbar or first sacral nerve roots that are blocked, but any root can be blocked. It is an investigative procedure that is useful only when one is sure that a radicular syndrome is present, but unsure of which nerve root is affected. It is of no value in trying to separate referred pain from radicular pain, or a herniated nucleus pulposus from lateral recess stenosis. Most often the procedure is used in chronic unilateral radicular syndrome (due to lateral recess stenosis) when structural recess stenosis lesions are noted at the level of the fifth lumbar and first sacral nerve roots and there are no clinical clues as to the anatomic level. The second indication for a nerve root infiltration is in the presence of scarring or arachnoiditis when trying to decide which root is most symptomatic.

The technique is accomplished in the prone position under image intensifier control. A paraspinal approach is used to the fifth lumbar nerve root, catching it just as it exits under the pedicle of L5. The S1 nerve root is blocked through the posterior first sacral foramen. Under image intensifier control, a long needle is slowly advanced toward the nerve root. When the nerve root is encountered, radiating discomfort down the leg will result. Usually this radiating discomfort is typical enough that the block can then be accomplished with 3 ml of 0.5 or 0.75% Marcaine, a long-acting anesthetic agent. On occasion, the radiating discomfort will not be striking, and water-soluble contrast material must be injected to be sure of needle placement.

Although x-ray is used to assist in accomplishing a nerve root infiltration, the procedure is not an x-ray evaluation procedure. The first principle of nerve root infiltration is to obtain a good root block. That is to say, if a fifth lumbar nerve root is blocked, the patient should have a drop foot and numbness over the dorsum of the foot when the procedure is finished. Similarly, if the first sacral root is blocked, then the patient should have numbness to pinprick sensation along the alteral border of the foot and weakness of plantar flexion. Once a good nerve root block is obtained, the patient is then asked to participate in the activity that was most aggravating to him. Usually, the patient needs a cane for support because of the profound nature of the root block. Long-acting anesthetic agents last 4–6 hr, and at the end of that time the patient should record his impressions of relief or lack of relief of his symptoms with the root block. If you suspected the fifth lumbar nerve root as the culprit, and a good fifth lumbar nerve root block relieves the patient's pain, then the procedure has satisfactorily pinpointed the fifth lumbar nerve root as the source of symptoms. The appropriate surgical procedure can then be carried out with confidence.

FACET JOINT BLOCK

A facet joint block is a local anesthetic procedure to temporarily denervate the facet joint. This is accomplished by blocking the facet joint itself and the posterior primary ramus supply to the facet joint. Facet joint innervation from the posterior primary ramus is from multiple segments and thus multiple blocks have to be done. It is routine to block the facet joint and posterior primary ramus at L3–L4, L4–L5, and L5–S1, and also block the ascending posterior primary ramus branch coming out of the S1 foramen. Also, the procedure is done bilaterally.

Again, an image intensifier is used to guide needle placement. There is little in the way of radiating discomfort to help localize the block, and thus anatomic placement of the needle is important. Figure 27.12 shows such needle placement at the junction of the lateral edge of the superior facet and the superior edge of the transverse process. Here, the posterior primary ramus comes through a ligamentous tunnel to supply the facet joint at that level and send branches to adjacent levels. Next, a needle should be placed within the facet joint itself so that the joint can be blocked. Long-acting anesthetic agents are also used for this procedure. After a satisfactory block is obtained, the patient is asked to participate in the activities that aggravated his pain and, at the end of 4–6 hr, to sit down and record his impressions of the effect of the procedure. If a patient has mechanical low back pain prior to the procedure that is abolished by the procedure, this

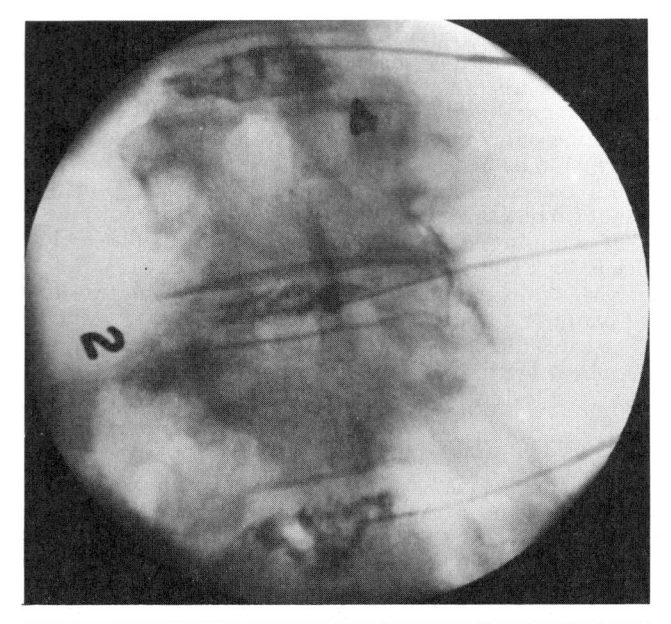

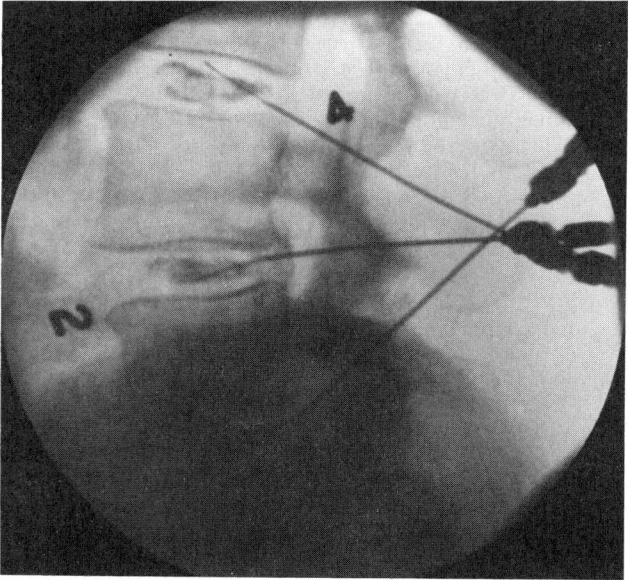

Figure 27.12. Intraoperative x-rays showing good needle tip position. *Top*, anteroposterior; *bottom*, lateral.

suggests that the facet joints are the source of symptoms, and appropriate procedures can be prescribed.

Both nerve root infiltration and facet joint blocks are procedures that depend on patient response for evaluation. Obviously, if the patient is an abnormal responder (e.g., a patient with nonorganic pain), these two procedures are useless. Both will misguide you if you have missed the diagnosis of a nonorganic syndrome.

ELECTRODIAGNOSIS

There are three electrodiagnostic procedures that are used in the investigation of a patient with lumbar disk disease: electromyography (EMG), nerve conduction tests (NCTs), and evoked potentials.

Electromyography

The EMG is a motor unit examination. Any disruption in the anterior horn, the nerve fiber, or the muscle fiber has the potential of producing an abnormal EMG. Thus, an abnormal EMG is indicative of lower motor dysfunction. Electromyographic examination for a lumbar spine abnormality includes needle electrode placements in the paraspinal muscles and specific extremity muscles. Electrical activity is recorded on insertion, at rest, and with voluntary contraction or stimulation. Normally, there is unsustained electrical discharge on insertion of the needle and no signal discharge (a silent EMG) at rest. With voluntary contraction, biphasic or triphasic forms of action potentials are seen. Theoretically, with lower motor nerve root dysfunction, insertional activity is abnormal in that more positive sharp waves appear; at rest, there are fibrillation potentials and positive sharp waves; and with stimulation, the quantity of motor units recorded decreases and multiple polyphasic waves are seen. Extending the theory further, in a herniated nucleus pulposus with single root involvement, the EMG findings will be localized to a single root. With spinal stenosis (multiple root involvement), there will be multiple root findings on EMG. In fact, EMG has a very low sensitivity and specificity in evaluating patients with lumbar disk disease. More blinded studies are required to determine the value of EMG in diagnosing lumbar disk disease. At present, there is overreliance on EMGs when, instead, a good clinical history and physical examination can be more helpful.

Nerve Conduction Tests

Nerve conduction tests measure the speed at which nerve fibers conduct. They are useful in separating peripheral neuropathy from a radiculopathy (trying to answer question 2). In radiculopathy one should see normal NCT velocities, whereas in peripheral neuropathy NCT velocities are often slowed.

Evoked Potentials

With the failure of EMG to play a significant role in the evaluation of lumbar disk disease, a search began for new electrodiagnostic fields. Probably the most interesting to date is somatosensory-evoked potentials, which focus on the sensory side of the nerve fiber. These highly sophisticated evaluations have been used for some time in scoliosis and major spine reconstructive surgery. The spinal evoked potential is transmitted through the dorsal column and is detectible with receptors in the spine or on the skull. Theoretically, lesions of peripheral nerves will prolong the latency response of the sensory input, and root and cord lesions cause change in the wave form. Conflicting evaluations of this technique have appeared in the literature (5). At this stage, it is considered experimental, and represents a very sophisticated technique. However, some authors see great promise in this approach to the evaluation of patients with lumbar disk disease.

OTHER TESTS OF LIMITED OR NO VALUE

There are three tests that I place in this classification: epidural venography, thermography, and ultrasound.

Epidural Venography

In the early 1970s, epidural venography enjoyed a brief popularity. It represented an attempt at a more accurate diagnosis of disk lesions at the L5–S1 level, where an oil-based myelogram had at least a 25% false-negative rate. A secondary reason was the false-positive rate of oil-based myelography at the L4–L5 level. However, epidural venography turned out to be a difficult technical exercise and also stressful for the patient. Limitations resulting from previous surgery also detracted from its value. Eventually, epidural venography was displaced by the advent of water-soluble myelographic compound and CT scanning.

Thermography

Many doctors have promoted and popularized thermography as a test of nerve root physiology. In theory, it states that pathology causing nerve root irritation will result in changes in skin temperature that can be detected with liquid cholesterol crystals or infrared photography. Although the principle is simple and attractive, there are limited blinded studies to support the claims of thermographers. In fact, a number of very good blinded studies have appeared that seriously question the clinical value of thermography (6, 7). Until thermography is submitted to more blinded studies on specificity and sensitivity, its use should be limited to experimental medicine only. Unfortunately, thermography has found its way into the courts and is being used extensively by judges and juries to determine financial awards. This is an unfortunate occurrence and one that should be halted until further blinded studies are completed.

Ultrasound

In spite of excellent scientific efforts by Porter in England (8), the use of ultrasound for the evaluation of patients with mechanical low back pain has severe limitations. The technique is exacting and difficult because the bony cover of the spinal canal interferes with visualization of its soft tissue contents. It has become a useful tool during spine surgery for spine trauma in detecting residual fragments anterior to the dura. However, at this point, it is not a useful investigative tool for the ambulatory patient with mechanical low back pain.

CONCLUSION

The assessment of a patient with a low back disability does not need to be difficult. By keeping a simple system in mind, it is possible to arrive at a good clinical impression by asking yourself the five questions listed below and committing yourself, eventually, to sequential answers.

1. Is this a true physical disability or is there a setting and a pattern in the history and physical examination to suggest a nonphysical or nonorganic problem?
2. Is this clinical presentation a diagnostic trap?
3. Is this a mechanical low back pain condition, and if so, what is the syndrome?
4. Are there clues to an anatomic level on history and physical examination?
5. After reviewing the results of investigation, what is the structural lesion and does it fit with the clinical syndrome?

Do not commit yourself to any major investigative step until questions 1 and 2 have been adequately answered. Then, if you are satisfied that you have a mechanical low back pain problem, dissect it into a syndrome first, an anatomic level second, and a structural lesion third. The structural lesion diagnosis should fully support the clinical syndrome and the anatomic level. If not, take one step back and repeat the history and physical examination. Listening to the patient's story, doing a thorough physical examination, and supporting your diagnosis with investigation is the best way to avoid erroneous diagnoses and ill-fated surgery.

References

1. Bell GR, Rothman RH, Booth RE, et al: A study of computer-assisted tomography. *Spine* 9:552–556, 1984.
2. Hitselberger W, Witten R: Abnormal myelograms in asymptomatic patients. *J Neurosurg* 28:204–206, 1968.
3. Waddell G, McCulloch JA, Kummel EG, et al: Nonorganic physical signs in low back pain. *Spine* 5:117–125, 1980.
4. Sicard JL: Roentgenologic exploration of the central nervous system with iodized oil (Lipiodol). *Arch Neurol Psychiatry* 16:420–426, 1926.
5. Aminoff MJ, et al: Dermatomal somatosensory evoked potentials in unilateral lymbosacral radiculopathy. *Ann Neurol* 17:171–176, 1985.
6. Mahoney L, McCulloch JA, Czima A: Thermography as a diagnostic aid in sciatica. *J Am Acad Thermol* 1:51–54, 1985.
7. Mills GH, Davies GK, Getty CJM, Conay J: The evaluation of liquid crystal thermography in the investigation of nerve root compression due to lumbosacral lateral spinal stenosis. *Spine* 11:420–432, 1986.
8. Porter RW, Hubbert CS, Wicks M: The spinal canal in symptomatic lumbar disc lesions. *J Bone Joint Surg* 60B:485–487, 1978.

chapter 28
Painful Arthropathies

J. Leonard Goldner, M.D.
James Nitka, M.D.
Patricia Howson, M.D.
Bruce Tobey, M.D.

SPINAL COLUMN AND SACROILIAC JOINTS

Pain arising from the spine may be related to the spinal joints, including the intervertebral disk complex; the facet joints, which have synovial coverings; the ligaments surrounding the vertebral bodies and the adjacent joints; the neural elements that are adjacent to the spine, protected by the posterior elements; and the pain receptors (nociceptors) that exist in the supporting ligaments. Many other extraneous factors that influence the severity and duration of pain are included in any discussion of painful joints, but the intent of this material is to describe the reasons for and the conditions that are known to produce pain.

A logical way to determine the cause of the complaints of the patient who describes back pain in any region of the spine is to gather data in a clear, concise, and knowledgeable way, perform a detailed and accurate physical examination, and order and interpret certain essential laboratory studies in order to assist in differentiating mechanical, inflammatory, neoplastic, metabolic, and vascular lesions from each other. In this way, a reasonable diagnosis is established and appropriate treatment initiated. This analysis includes a knowledge of the physiology of the pain and the alterations that occur when a pathologic lesion exists. Furthermore, the emotional, social, and the administrative aspects of pain cannot be eliminated from the methods of management, but these aspects of the patients' complaints, along with their personality profile, are placed in proper perspective.

PATHOPHYSIOLOGY OF SPINAL JOINT PAIN

Pain related to vertebral disease is divided into two general categories: (a) pain associated with compression of or impingement on neural tissue that results in local or radicular sensations, and (b) pain related to stimulation of nociceptors of ligaments and muscle fascia causing referred pain in a myotome or sclerotome pattern.

The innervation of vertebral ligaments attached to the vertebral body is by a plexus of nerve fibers associated with the external and internal venous plexuses of the spine. Also, pain is conducted through the sinuvertebral nerve to innervate the posterior longitudinal ligament and the posterior aspect of the anulus fibrosis, and the ventral aspect of the dural sac. These nerve fibers travel with the vertebral veins into the vertebral bodies and innervate at least the posterior aspect of these structures. Each sinuvertebral nerve is composed of a somatic root from the ventral ramus and an autonomic root from the gray ramus communicans. This nerve supplies the adjacent vertebra and one or two levels above the origin of the nerve.

The anterolateral aspect of the anulus fibrosis and the anterior longitudinal ligament are innervated by a series of nerve fibers from the ventral rami and from the sympathetic nerve chains. Also, free nerve endings have been described within the interspinous ligaments and the zygoapophyseal joints of the lumbar spine. These receptors are thought to represent type IV pain fibers. Very few of these have actually been found within the ligamentum flavum or the lumbodorsal fascia of the back. However, the muscles of the back contain abundant type IV nociceptor free nerve endings.

The assumption is that certain kinds of back pain originate with the nociceptor input, are conducted to the spinal cord, and are referred back to a dermatome distribution that coincides with a particular level of nociceptor nerve supply. Or, the fibers may conduct through the posterior sensory ganglion and be recognized as myotome or sclerotome sensations.

The origin of this stimulus is usually mechanical and is associated with abnormal activity or stress of the ligamentous and muscular structures around the disk complex that are attached to the vertebral elements opposite the intervetebral disk joint. Furthermore, pain arising from the fascia and ligaments in the thoracolumbar region may be referred to the lumbosacral region through the L4–5 or S1 nerve root distribution (1).

Injection of hypertonic saline into the thoracolumbar fascia results in referred pain to the L4–S1 anatomic areas of the spine. Upper cervical sensory root irritation may result in headache, occipital numbness, and autonomic nervous system symptoms.

Radiculopathy is due to compression of a mixed nerve root by adjacent structures. The causes of nerve compression or disruption of soft tissue vary with each region of the spine and with each pathologic syndrome causing the root irritation. These lesions may cause a dermatome pattern as well as a sclerotome sensation. The latter is dull, deep, and aching, whereas the former is more likely hypesthesia, paresthesia, or hyperpathia.

CERVICAL SPINE ARTHROPATHY PAIN

Osteophytes

Cervical spine pain varies from chronic, intermittent, aching pain, as in cervical spondylosis, to sharp, lancinating pain with increased muscle tension and radicular distribution, noted in cervical osteoarthritis and degenerative intervertebral disk disease.

C1–C2 Instability (Congenital, Traumatic, or Rheumatoid Disease) Atlantoaxial instability may initially present with occipital headache, upper neck pain (dull or sharp), and occasional cranial nerve involvement if the occipital compression is significant. Lower extremity paresthesias and dysesthesias as well as upper extremity paresthesias may also occur in an asymmetric manner. Paresthesias in all four extremities require careful review of the occipital cervical region. Electrical shocks may be associated with forceful flexion of the neck or percussion of the head with the neck in a neutral or a flexed position. This suggests instability of the atlas on the axis or possible stenosis. Pain receptors in the loose synovium, the interspinous ligaments, and the intervertebral disk complex cause unpleasant sensations, and cervical or occipital stenosis may cause spinal cord or cerebellar compression symptoms.

The position of the head and neck that causes pain depends on the location and severity of the pathologic lesion. Posterior compression is due to laminal arches, radicular canal stenosis, compression by the ligamentum flavum, or combinations of these conditions causing compression. Extension of the head and neck may result in anterior compression by anterior osteophytes from the anulus or indentation from the posterior overgrowth of the zygoapophyseal joints and the anular ligaments (2).

With the head and neck in extension, posterior indentation occurs and anterior subluxation is diminished. With the head in flexion, anterior indentation occurs and posterior structures cause compression if the vertebral body displaces anteriorly.

Cervical Spine Stiffness and Neck Pain Degenerative disease of the cervical interspaces results in narrowing, incongruity of the articulations, and irregularity of the articular facets and the synovial apophyseal joints (Fig. 28.1). The range of motion diminishes and pain may increase at the extremes of movement. The deep dull aching sensation is caused by abnormal stress on the nonelastic ligaments, by irritation of the synovial linings, and by instability and incongruity of the vertebral bodies and the facet joints. Very reactive hypertrophic osteophytes occur because of the narrowed intervertebral disk space and facet joints. The formation of osteophytes is associated with either instability or incongruity.

If encroachment on the spinal canal or the short radicular canals occurs, the classic findings of a degenerative cervical intervertebral disk syndrome result, with localized neck pain, decreased range of motion with or without radicular dermatome pain, and muscle weakness.

The severity of the neck and extremity pain is related to the patient's age and the rapidity of onset of the pathologic condition. The extent of the adaptation of the involved joints depends on the influence of other factors such as congenital synostosis of the cervical region, the hormonal and biochemical factors that influence the nerve receptors, and the coalition of the mucopolysaccharides and the proteoglycans that make up the nucleus and anulus of the cervical joints.

As the biochemical make up of the degenerating disk complex changes, the pain complaints become both mechanical and inflammatory. The mechanical and inflammatory irritation of the nociceptors in the anulus and the ligaments and the stimulation of the sinuvertebral nerves and the sensory roots cause varying degrees of pain that usually respond initially to anti-inflammatory medications and to intermittent periods of rest. Most patients with degenerative arthrosis of the cervical spine adapt to limited activity, use anti-inflammatories, and accommodate to the gradual onset of the condition. If the wear and de-

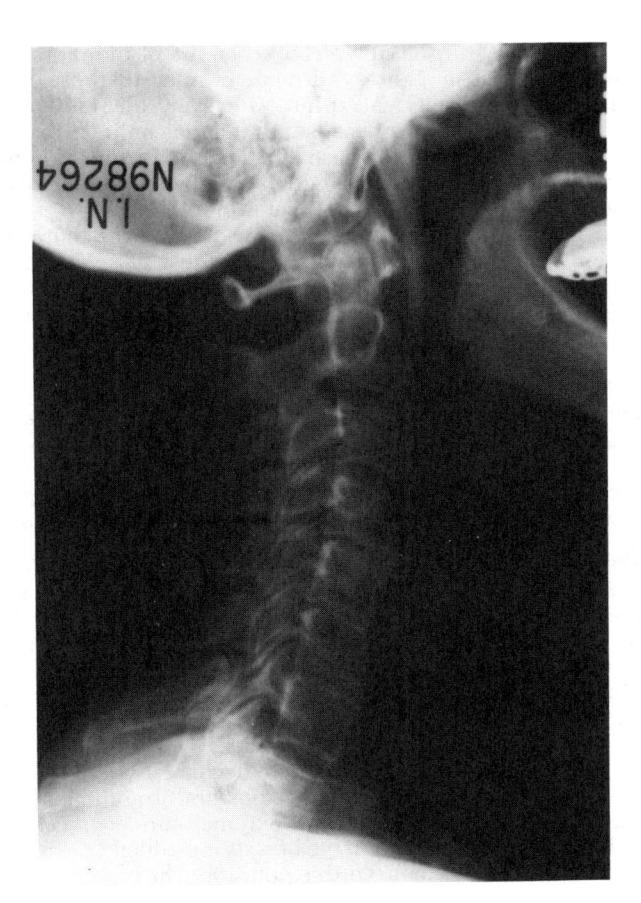

Figure 28.1. Cervical spine of a 50-year-old female showing degenerative arthrosis of C4–C5. Nonoperative treatment did not relieve the neck symptoms or the radiculopathy. Anterior spine diskectomy and iliac bone arthrodesis resulted in reestablishment of the height of the nerve root foramina and fusion of the vertebral body interspaces.

generative changes occur relatively slowly, the healing and accommodation response is rapid enough to allow the patient to become relatively asymptomatic in a reasonable period of time.

Inflammatory disease of the cervical spine, such as rheumatoid arthritis, ankylosing spondylitis, or other collagen conditions, causes inflammatory reaction with pain that is eventually also associated with mechanical changes. The destructive lesions of rheumatoid disease may lead to encroachment on the spinal cord and the upper or lower cervical roots. Atlantoxial instability may require external support if the condition is mild or surgical stabilization if the condition is severe and progressive (3, 4).

Ankylosing spondylitis, on the other hand, results in spontaneous stabilization of the vertebral bodies and limited rotation of the head and neck. Once the spontaneous fusion occurs and the inflammatory condition subsides or goes into remission, the patient is comfortable but neck motion is limited. If the position of spontaneous fusion is in acute flexion, then corrective osteotomy and restabilization are necessary.

Benign or Malignant Lesions of the Cervical Spine

Benign or malignant cervical spine lesions are characterized by intermittent or continuous pain regardless of neck position or the time of day. The pain may be related to increased or constant pressure on nociceptors within the intervertebral disk bond or the osseous tissue; or radicular pain occurs as a result of encroachment on nerve roots or on the spinal cord.

Osteoid osteoma of the vertebral body or posterior spinal elements, for example, is usually associated with persistent or continuous or varying degrees of pain and may be partially or completely relieved by salicylates. A *giant cell tumor* of the cervical spine will be associated with intermittent pain, the range of motion will be diminished, and the pathologic lesion is progressive.

A *metastatic tumor* to the vertebral body and sparing the interspace may eventually involve the disk bond because of mechanical alterations. A *bacterial septicemia* may affect the interspace initially and the vertebral body secondarily and cause severe constant pain and limited motion.

Acute Neck Trauma

Traumatic cervical injuries may include acute herniation of the nucleus pulposus and be associated with intense paravertebral muscle tension, radicular dermatome changes with peripheral motor weakness, and dermatome deficiencies. If the spinal cord is involved by trauma or a central herniation of the disk, upper and lower extremity dysesthesias, paresthesias, and muscle weakness may be present.

Acute hyperextension of the cervical spine after a fall may cause hyperpathia along the C5–C8 dermatomes without evidence of fracture and without evidence of ruptured disk. This is particularly true in patients who have osteoarthrosis, small nerve root foramina, and limited elasticity of the neural tissue. This primary traumatic causalgia usually responds to limited activity and rest, but may require several months, and as much as a year, before the hypersensitivity reaches a point of equilibrium.

Management of Cervical Spine Arthropathies

Neck pain caused by mild degenerative arthrosis and facet joint involvement is managed by:

1. Regular active and relaxation exercises of the cervical spine.
2. Alteration of head and neck positions during work, recreational activities, and sleep. This may be done

with contour pillow, feather pillow, and rearrangement of working habits. (5)

Before exercise is initiated, slow warm-up motion should be performed. Relaxation techniques should be acquired from a physical therapist so muscle tension associated with pain is relieved by massage and gentle activity and muscle tension associated with anxiety and stress is improved by behavioral modification.

Accessory methods are used to support the head and neck, maintain protection from intermittent cool and damp air, and provide protection of the neck during automobile riding. The soft molded neck collars are used to unload the neck, to provide moderate warmth, and to provide support and prevent sudden forceful flexion or extension when the patient is in an automobile.

Cervical spine traction for several hours at a time when the patient is in bed or intermittently with special arrangement of the apparatus using graduated weights, may be helpful. The bed traction apparatus should be arranged so that the pull is on the occiput, the strap under the chin is only supportive, the direction of pull is in slight flexion, and the head of the bed is elevated about 6 inches. A 6-pound weight is sufficient to provide the necessary traction and relaxation. Intermittment cervical traction is performed with greater weight, and the patient is usually in the sitting or standing position.

Intervertebral disk degeneration and pain and interbody pain may respond to methods already described and anti-inflammatory medications. However, if pain persists for several months, and if the condition is progressive and the range of motion is limited, then localized intervertebral disk excision and arthrodesis should be considered.

If neck pain and cervical radiculopathy are present, and if the condition does not respond to limited activity, traction, nonsteroidal anti-inflammatories, and observation for a reasonable period of time, then the necessary diagnostic studies are performed in order to determine if there is localized nerve root irritation. If the lesion is localized by imaging and electrical studies, and if the condition does not respond to traction, limited activities and pharmacologic agents, then anterior diskectomy and iliac bone graft to the interspace will eliminate the pain and provide a stable neck (6).

Referred Pain in the Cervical Region

Suboccipital headache may be associated with upper cervical disk degeneration or facet joint arthrosis. Primary shoulder disease may cause proximal tapezius pain that is confused with cervical lesion. Pulmonary and cardiac lesions may be referred to the supraclavicular or lateral neck area and suggest the occurrence of a cervical syndrome. A Parsonage-Turner neuronitis may be associated with severe neck and shoulder girdle pain and resemble a cervical arthropathy.

THORACIC SPINE ARTHROPATHY

Lesions affecting the intervertebral disks, the facet joints, or the soft tissue structures around the intervertebral spaces and the nerve root foramina of the thoracic spine may cause pain syndromes similar to those described for the cervical spine. However, the radicular pattern is less obvious because it remains confined to the chest wall, except in the case of a severe thoracic radiculopathy after herpes zoster, which may be readily defined and may remain painful for several months.

Degeneration of the intervertebral disks in the thoracic region may be associated with dermatome or sclerotome pain and with narrow interspaces on the radiograph.

The melted candle effect of ankylosing spondylitis may not be evident for several years after the origin of vague back pain.

Calcification of the intervertebral disks is noted in chondrocalcinosis and may be associated with acute pain followed by dull aching discomfort for many months.

The pain syndromes affecting the joints of the thoracic spine follow the same pattern in their pathologic changes as do those that have been described for the cervical spine.

Management of Thoracic Spine Arthropathy

The method of treatment depends upon the final diagnosis. Thoracic spine pain associated with osteopenia is managed by external corset support and an antiosteopenic medication program that includes Premarin, Provera, calcium, vitamin D, and limited exercise. The specific doses and the duration of treatment depend on the individual problem and the patient's complaints.

Thoracic pain associated with degenerative arthrosis may be improved by exercise, postural training, anti-inflammatory medications, and external support. Weight reduction and support of large breasts are added considerations in order to manage this condition in certain individuals.

If ankylosis spondylitis is the cause of the thoracic pain, the appropriate anti-inflammatory medication may be helpful; the three-point brace may diminish pain moderately. This condition is usually self-limiting, although several years may pass before the pain is readily tolerated by the patient.

LUMBAR AND LUMBOSACRAL SPINE ARTHROPATHY

The lesions affecting the intervertebral disks account for the greatest proportion of pain complaints referable to the low back. Intervertebral disks degeneration, facet joint arthrosis, radicular canal stenosis, and laminal arch and facet encroachment on the cauda equina are the major causes of progressive lumbar arthropathy.

The diagnosis of single or multiple intervertebral disk or facet joint disease in the lumbar or lumbosacral region follows the same pattern as already described for the cervical region. Careful history, a detailed physical and neurologic examination, specific laboratory tests, and the proper imaging studies will usually result in an accurate diagnosis. In the absence of any specific findings other than subjective complaints, the assumption is usually correct that the condition has to do with ligament attachment pain, early subtle intervertebral disk disease, or overuse syndromes that may be muscular-ligamentous in their origin (7).

Intervertebral disk disease varies according to the location of the pathologic lesion. An acute rupture of an intervertebral disk may cause nerve root irritation and not only back pain but also extremity pain. Neurologic changes indicate that the involved nerve root is being seriously compressed.

Management of Lumbar Spine Arthropathy

Options for treatment depend on the severity of the onset, the presence or absence of bowel or bladder involvement, and the degree of neurologic deficit.

If there is no bowel or bladder involvement, and if the neurologic deficit is not severe, then a program of nonoperative management is usually adequate. Limited bedrest, anti-inflammatory medications, and avoidance of stress on the spine, including torque, flexion, and extension, will usually result in remission of the condition. However, if the neurologic findings progress, and if pain persists to the point where the patient is not able to function, then disk excision with or without spine fusion should be considered. The diskectomy alone is the usual method of management if there is no instability or incongruity of the interspace. However, if the disk bond is badly disrupted and damaged, then posterior and posterolateral spine fusion may be indicated (8).

If the first diskectomy fails and several months have elapsed since treatment, then an anterior diskectomy and fusion should be considered (9) (Fig. 28.2).

SACROILIAC JOINT ARTHROPATHY

Involvement of the sacroiliac joints by pathologic processes is relatively uncommon. Ankylosing spondylitis (Marie-Strumpell arthritis) is the most common specific condition affecting these joints. The onset of that syndrome is relatively slow and subtle, with vague complaints and a delayed diagnosis.

The history of early morning pain, limited chest expansion compared to the population average, radiograph showing sclerosis of the subchondral bone on either side of the sacroiliac joint, partial narrowing of the joints, and a positive HLA-B27 are the findings that will establish the diagnosis after the process has been present for several months or even years. Many patients who are affected by this condition have numerous diagnostic studies, particularly myelography, or currently computed tomography scan inspecting the nerve roots of the cauda equina, before a definite diagnosis is established.

The treatment is use of Indocin and other anti-inflammatories, a regular exercise program to attempt to maintain chest expansion, and occasionally a three-point brace to avoid the development of a kyphosis.

HIP JOINT ARTHROPATHIES

The hip joints are a major cause of painful arthropathy.

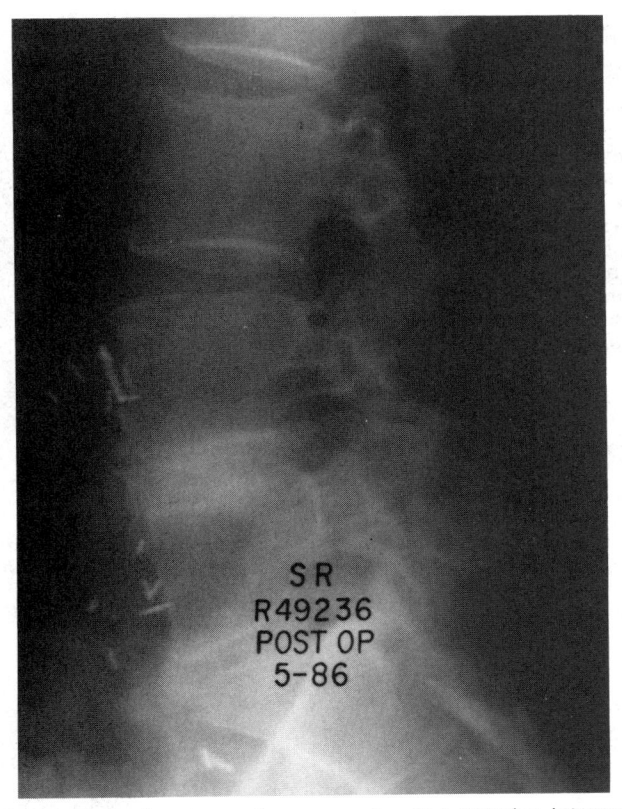

Figure 28.2. Lumbar spine x-ray showing anterior intervertebral body arthrodesis for painful arthropathy at L4–L5 and L5–S1. This adult patient had two prior diskectomies at both interspaces. Extremity pain was improved but back pain persisted. Anterior diskectomy and iliac bone graft arthrodesis immobilizes the spine at this level, diminishes nerve root irritation, and eliminates interbody pain.

HIP JOINT PATHOLOGY

The most common cause of persistent hip pain is osteoarthrosis or degenerative arthrosis of the hip joint. The onset is usually subtle, but the symptoms gradually increase with time. The differential diagnosis early in the course of the disease includes trochanteric bursitis, synovitis from trauma, pseudogout, iliopsoas bursitis, or pain at the insertion of the adductor tendons.

Other conditions, such as pain originating in the symphysis pubis, ischial tuberosity bursitis, or stress fracture associated with osteopenia, simulate the painful hip.

CLINICAL EXAMINATION

Limited rotation of the hip joint is the earliest clinical finding associated with osteoarthrosis or other pathology of the hip. A hip limp that consists of a shift of the trunk to the involved side and pain on contraction of the gluteus medius are constant findings.

Figure 28.3. *A*, Preoperative degenerative arthrosis of both hips, probably associated with acetabular dysplasia, in a 55-year-old female. Pain was severe on the left, moderate on the right. The condition had been controlled with ibuprofen, but eventually the distorted gait and the fatigue associated with excessive energy expenditure in walking required a porous coated total hip replacement. *B*, Both hip joints have been replaced with porous coated total hip joints. The acetabulum is high-density polyethylene with metal-backed porous coated cobalt-chromium alloy. The femoral component is a cobalt-chromium-molybdenum alloy.

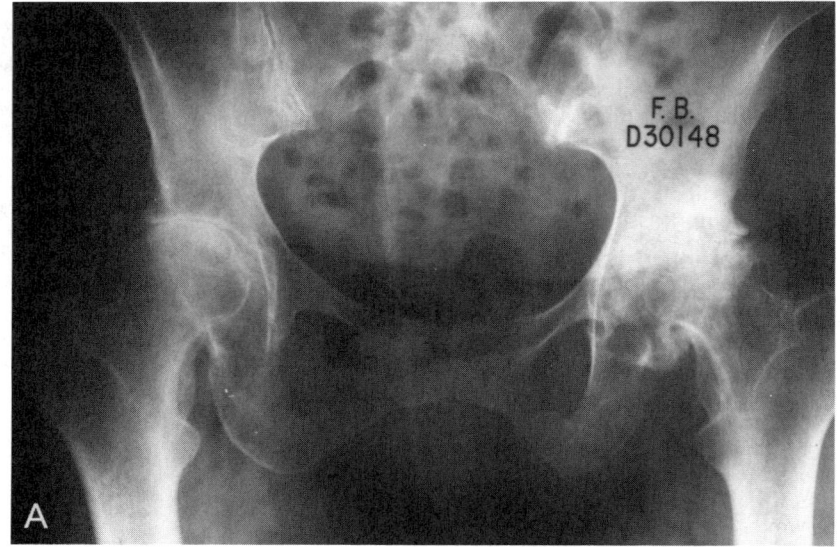

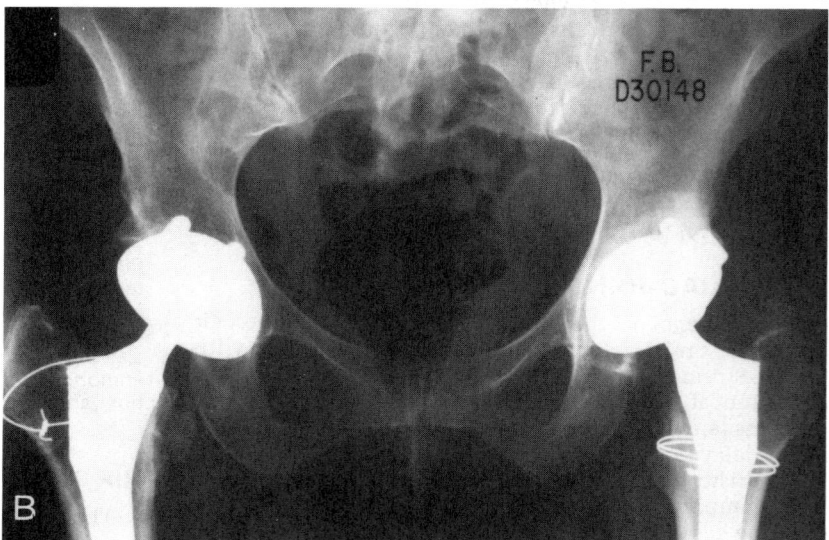

DIAGNOSTIC STUDIES

Radiographs demonstrate subchondral cyst formation either on the acetabular or the femoral side of the joint. Areas of increased density in the subchondral bone may occur, and osteophytes signifying narrowing of the articular cartilage are eventually obvious. Acetabular dysplasia, detected by a wide "teardrop" of the acetabulum, accounts for many changes in the hip joint that are not apparent in a younger individual. The pathologic changes may be superior or medial in relationship to the congruity of the femoral head and the acetabulum. Superior changes are more noticeable than medial alterations.

Additional diagnostic studies include aspiration of the hip joint for crystals, serologic studies with reference to possible rheumatoid disease, technetium-99 bone scan, tomography, magnetic resonance imaging, and computed tomography. These studies will usually allow a diagnosis and influence the ultimate treatment.

TREATMENT OF HIP JOINT ARTHROPATHY

If the condition is caused by a specific disease such as gout, psoriasis, ankylosing spondylitis, or rheumatoid disease, the primary disease should be treated.

The hip joint is unloaded by use of a cane in the opposite hand, and anti-inflammatories are helpful. Weight reduction, exercise activity to improve muscle

Chapter 28/Painful Arthropathies 363

tone, limited physical stress on the hip joint, and appropriate medication may protect the hip joint for many years.
More aggressive forms of therapy are:

1. Osteotomy of the femur and/or acetabulum.
2. Removal of osteochondral loose bodies if the condition is osteochondromatosis.
3. Excision of osteochondritis dessicans and drilling of the subchondral bone.
4. Prosthetic hip replacement.

Hip Arthroplasty

There are gradations of hip arthroplasty depending on the patient's age, the primary pathology involved in the hip joint, and the patient's general health.

Prosthetic Replacement of the Proximal End of the Femur This procedure is performed by replacing the upper end of the femur with a stainless steel or alloy prosthesis. The A.T. Moore prosthesis has been used successfully for about 40 years. Its usual period of pain relief is about 15 years. The acetabular cartilage wears and additional surgical revision is necessary (see below).

Total Hip Replacement without Methacrylate Using Porous Coated Acetabulum and Femoral Component This prosthesis has been developed during the past 10 years and has been inserted in a large number of patients during the past 5 years. Currently the success rate is high but the patients may requires as long as a year before thigh pain is diminished and stable ingrowth of tissue into the prosthesis has occurred. The final information concerning longevity and need for revision is not known.

Total Hip Replacement with Methacrylate This procedure has been performed since 1968. The average length of time that the patient with strong bone and no systemic disease can expect satisfactory performance from this prosthesis is 12–15 years; thus, the procedure should be saved for those individuals over age 65 or those who have systemic problems such as renal disease or rheumatoid arthritis.

Figure 28.3A shows the preoperative condition of the hip joints in a 55-year-old female with severe involvement on one side and a lesser amount on the other. Porous coat total joint hip replacements, including an acetabular cup

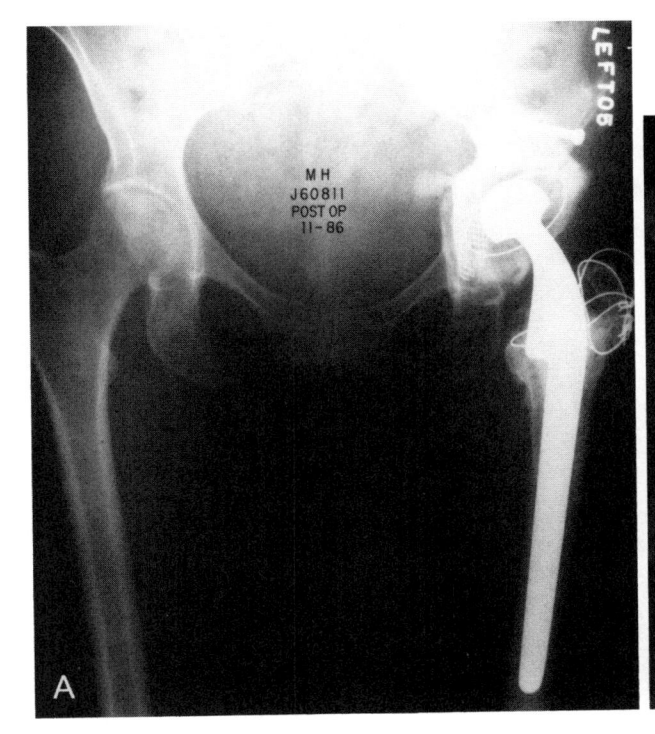

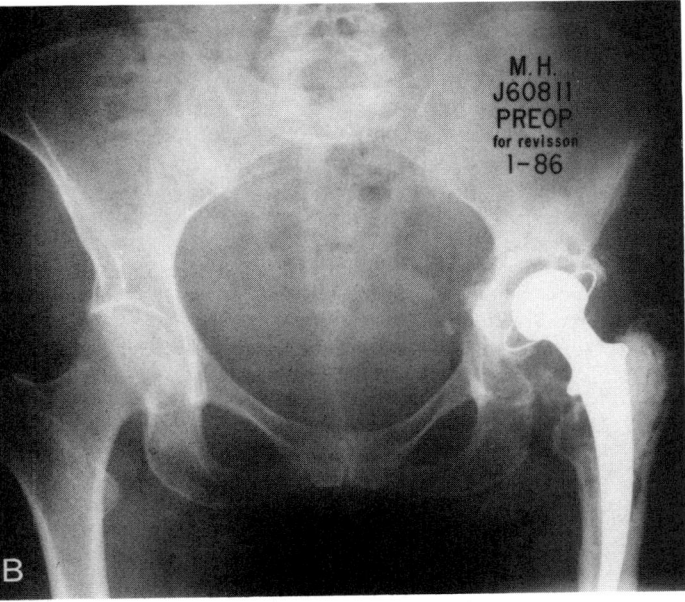

Figure 28.4. This patient had degenerative arthrosis of the left hip, that was severely incapacitating in 1970. A total hip replacement was performed at that time. A, Preoperative x-ray showing migration of the acetabulum superiorly and loosening of the femoral component in 1985. Bone absorption had resulted in both the acetabulum and the femur. B, A new prosthesis was inserted with iliac bone graft to the superior acetabulum. The bone graft is held by a screw. Additional bone was placed in the base of the acetabulum, and a large high-density polyethylene prosthesis was inserted over the reinforced bone graft with Gelfoam, vitallium mesh, and methacrylate. The femoral component replaced the absorbed neck and trochanteric region. The patient is pain free, has a stable hip, and walks with minimal limp but is required to use a cane in the right hand to unload the left hip joint.

and femoral component on both sides (Fig. 28.3B), have resulted in complete relief of pain, elimination of limp, and return of the patient to full activity, excluding axial loading such as running and jumping.

Total Hip Revision

The length of time that a high-density polyethylene–stainless steel–methacrylate fixed total hip joint will be painless and useful varies from patient to patient. Once the prosthesis shows evidence of loosening, settling, or methacrylate fracture, replacement is necessary.

Early replacement with a noncemented prosthesis or with a methacrylate-bonded prosthesis with supplementary bone graft and additional techniques for better bonding of the methacrylate will diminish the likelihood of rapid bone erosion in the future (Fig. 28.4).

References

1. Depalma A, Rothman R: *The Intervertebral Disc.* Philadelphia, WB Saunders, 1970.
2. Ferlic DC, Clayton ML, Leidholt JD, et al: Surgical treatment of the symptomatic unstable cervical spine in rheumatoid arthritis. *J Bone Joint Surg* 57A:349, 1975.
3. Bland JH, Davis BH, London MG, et al: Rheumatoid arthritis of the cervical spine. *Arch Intern Med* 112:130–136, 1963.
4. Fielding JW, Hensinger RN: The cervical spine. In Cruess RL, Rennier J (eds): *Adult Orthopaedics.* New York, Churchill Livingstone, 1984, pp 747–765.
5. Gibson JW: Cervical syndromes: use of a comfortable cervical collar as an adjunct in their management. *South Med J* 67:205–208, 1974.
6. Robinson RA, Smith GW: The treatment of certain cervical-spine disorders by anterior removal of the intervertebral disc and interbody fusion. *J Bone Joint Surg* 40A:607, 1958.
7. Nachemson A, Bigos SJ: In Cruess RL, Rennier J (eds): *Adult Orthopaedics.* Churchill Livingstone, 1984, vol 2, pp 843–937.
8. Goldner JL: The role of spine fusion in management of low back pain. *Spine* 6:293–303, 1981, pp 293–303.
9. Goldner JL, Wood K, Urbaniak J: Anterior lumbar discectomy and interbody fusion: indications and technique. In Schmidek ED, Sweet (eds): *Operative Neurosurgical Technique.* New York, Grune & Stratton, 1982, vol II, pp 1373–1379.

chapter 29
Painful Neuropathies and Nerve Root Lesions and Syndromes

Benjamin L. Crue, Jr., M.D., F.A.C.S.

The task of writing this chapter is exceedingly difficult for the present author, as it has long been my contention that neuropathies are seldom, if ever, painful. Furthermore, it is my belief that therapy for the entrapment syndromes, usually involving cervical and lumbar nerve roots, as well as the carpal and tarsal tunnel syndromes, does not, in my opinion, belong in a book about *chronic* pain.

The above introductory paragraph is obviously written with tongue in cheek, as the writer (and, I am certain, the reader) is well aware that the basic problem in communication lies usually in the definitions of the terms used. Just what do we mean by the terms *neuropathy* and *chronic pain*? The problem of the taxonomy and classification of pain syndromes, and the difference between acute and chronic pain, has been tackled on numerous occasions by man, including the present author, and reported almost ad nauseam (1–9). There remains considerable controversy over the "centralist" versus the "peripheralist" concept of chronic pain (2). The present author is a centralist and believes that to use the term *chronic pain* correctly is to imply a lack of clinical or experimental evidence of continued somatic or visceral peripheral nociceptive afferent input to the central nervous system. This is stated with the understanding that, in many chronic pain conditions, pain severity can be made worse (and the pains of neuralgia can be triggered) by several forms of "nonnociceptive" peripheral afferent input, which have usually been considered as central "perversions" of the normal patterns of sensory input. If this concept of chronic pain requiring a central underlying pain mechanism within the brain itself is accepted, then it can be logically stated that *all* "chronic pain" is *always all* basically psychosomatic (10). That is, the brain contains both the underlying central generator mechanism producing the chronic pain and also the apparatus necessary for the chronic pain patient's conscious perception of the pain and the continued suffering that follows. It thus logically also follows that any therapeutic approach aimed at stopping any imaginary peripheral nociceptive input in patients with chronic pain can logically bring about a therapeutic improvement only through what we know as the "placebo" response. This is true of peripheral nerve blocks as well as such neurosurgical interventions as rhizotomy, chordotomy, and tractotomy.

The statement that all chronic pain is always all psychosomatic at first sounds like a fanatical statement. However, it must be understood that it is merely a classification. That is, if it is not central pain, it should not be called chronic pain, no matter how long the pain has existed clinically. Our temporal classification of pain (outlined in Table 29.1) has been presented many times. Acute pain, subacute pain, recurrent pain (at times with underlying chronic ongoing pathology), and ongoing acute cancer pain are all believed to be related to nociceptive input, but the term *chronic pain* is reserved for those states that have no continued nociceptive input and hence are centrally generated and by definition psychosomatic.

The fact that the present writer may well be in the minority in his view of chronic pain is well known, but the controversy continues, and I refer interested readers to a recent article by Brena, Crue, and Stieg that attempts

Table 29.1
Temporal Classification of Pain Complaints

1. *Acute:* up to a few days in duration, mild or severe with cause known or unknown, presumed nociceptive input (the "fix me" medical model)
2. *Subacute:* a few days to a few months in duration (although no longer an emergency, in most ways treat like acute pain)
3. *Recurrent acute:* recurrent or continued nociceptive input from underlying chronic pathologic process, i.e., arthritis (either rheumatoid or osteoarthritis)
4. *Ongoing acute:* due to uncontrolled malignant neoplastic disease, with continued nociceptive input
5. *Chronic:* benign, nonneoplastic, usually more than 6 months, no known nociceptive peripheral input, but pain often made more severe by any type of subsequent sensory input; basically a "central" pain, but with seemingly adequate coping by the patient.
6. *Chronic intractable benign pain syndrome (CIBPS):* chronic pain with poor patient coping; pain becomes central focus of the patient's existence (no known nociceptive peripheral input)

to elucidate further this problem of definition of chronic pain (10).

For the purposes of a definition of neuropathy in the present chapter, we must discuss the meanings of the precise use of the words *neuritis, neuropathy,* and *neuralgia* (11). In 1958 Wartenberg offered a book entitled *Neuritis, Sensory Neuritis and Neuralgia* (12). Since then much has changed in our thinking about mechanisms underlying chronic pain (1, 13–19). However, the author has been unable to find a more recent reference that deals specifically with this subject. Let us examine in terms of human pain the three suffixes attached to the stem *neuro:* -itis, -opathy, and -algia.

NEURITIS

Derived from the Greek, the suffix *-itis* denoted inflammation, not just infection. In a given peripheral neuritis inflammation of a nerve can be due to bacterial infection, but it appears that, when pain is involved, a disproportionate number of cases are due to other causes. For example, the herpes zoster virus in a person with shingles leads to pain in almost all cases. Inflammation can also accompany toxicity, and painful inflammation of the nerves, presumably the sensory portion, can be due to a whole host of toxins. It must be remembered that inflammation supposedly accompanies any type of injury or trauma, including compression such as that in the carpal tunnel syndrome with acute flare-up of pain in the median nerve at the wrist, or radiculoneuritis from nerve root compression from a herniated nucleus pulposus. This type of pain can be considered to be on a neuritic basis. This neuritis or radiculoneuritis has been the object of many presently accepted therapeutic endeavors to decrease the inflammatory element of the painful syndrome. Specifically, the term *neuritis* means peripheral neuritis. Nerve root inflammation is radiculoneuritis or radiculitis, and inflammation with the spinal cord itself is myelitis, and that within the cranial cavity is encephalitis or cerebritis. It is generally recognized that any sensory nerve can emit pain when it becomes inflamed, regardless of the cause. It becomes edematous, undergoes an infiltration of polynuclear leukocytes and, later, of lymphocytes and other monocytic cells, and so forth.

There are two points to raise here. First, when we talk about an inflamed peripheral nerve, we are generally referring to an acute process. Although it may indeed be accompanied by a severe and, for a time, seemingly intractable pain, this classification of neuritis probably should be kept entirely for consideration of the etiologic agent and the mechanism underlying acute pain syndromes. There really is no evidence that neuritis plays any role in human chronic pain and suffering. Chronic pain due to continued nociceptive input probably does not exist, although it is a widely held *myth* within medicine. Second, in spite of our recent tremendous scientific advances in the use of neurophysiologic microelectrodes, electron microscopes, and special staining or isotope techniques, we still know very little as to how the inflammation in the nerve itself contributes to the increased barrage of nociceptive sensory input information that is apparently the underlying neurophysiologic mechanism leading to the acute pain. Even under the circumstances of neuritis, the awareness of pain when it is acute is still to be considered perception, and it must be remembered that even acute pain is not really limited to a primary sensory modality or sensation (14, 15).

Much work has been done to improve our understanding of some aspects of the neurochemical and neuropharmacologic activity resulting from acute trauma of peripheral tissues that give rise to severe acute clinical pain. In recent years studies of that old standby, aspirin, have been carried out in the periphery. Studies with histamine, then bradykinin, and more recently with the prostaglandins have led to an ever-increasing understanding of the whole arachidonic acid cascade and to the newer nonsteroidal anti-inflammatory analgesic agents that act in a number of ways to block the chain reaction in the periphery involving the prostaglandins and the leukotrienes. Yet, much is still unknown concerning how neurochemistry and neuropharmacology relate to inflammation of neural tissue itself. This fuzzy area must include the finer peripheral elements, which are referred to as the chemoreceptor portion of the nociceptor apparatus. Just how they relate to the clinical syndromes of peripheral neuritis, which many clinicians almost automatically visualize as somehow having to do with larger sensory nerves, remains unidentified, even when we talk about this most common aspect of acute pain.

Over the last decade much new information has emerged about neural transmission as it relates to the endorphins, enkephalins, and other short peptide chains (20). The connection to the feedback loop descending to the region of the dorsal horn that modulates and apparently turns off subsequent nociceptive input has also received much attention (13). However, the endorphin system plays as yet no proven role whatsoever in neuropathy and neuralgia (to be discussed below).

Activation of the acute pain-blocking feedback endorphin system to treat acute pain of great severity due to presumed afferent nociceptive input, regardless of the cause, is one of the possible and permissible uses of narcotics. Thus opiates and many of the newer synthetic narcotic-like compounds are certainly indicated in acute pain of clinical severity. Nevertheless, it has been well recognized that physicians often tend to undertreat the pain aspects and to be too conservative in the use of narcotics for patients in the recovery room after surgery, in the emergency room after injury, and in pain due to acute inflammation with neuritis, such as acute herpes zoster and the cutaneous lesions of shingles. Not only is there sound neuropharmacologic evidence that narcotics are effective with a central blocking mechanism, but also the accompanying sedation and euphoria can be helpful adjuncts in the treatments of severe acute clinical pain with presumed nociceptive input. Although it must always be stated that narcotic use should not be prolonged in nonterminal conditions, the fear of producing addiction generally has been stressed to a point that the frequent result is administration of the wrong narcotic in inadequate doses over too long a time interval on a symptom-contingent rather than a time-contingent basis. Many physicians today unfortunately do not understand the optimal use of narcotics, even in acute pain associated with somatic or visceral tissue abnormalities with its neuritic component. This argument is being advanced as forcefully as possible, because I will later state that narcotics should have *no* role in either neuropathy or neuralgia.

Despite all the work that has been done on peripheral prostaglandins and central endorphins, the treatment of the inflamed nerve itself is still a confused issue. This is true for all of the therapeutic modalities that physical therapists can now provide, including diathermy, ultrasound, and microwave. In general, for inflammation both of peripheral nerves (neuritis) and of joints (arthritis), it is still preferable to rest the afflicted part, and then to apply cold during the first few hours, and heat thereafter; or, whatever sequence gives the most subject relief on an empirical basis. For arthritis or synovitis, if the foregoing does not work after a reasonable length of time, injections of cortisone can be added. The inflamed nerves themselves in neuritis, however, should not be the site of injection.

Pain of an ongoing nature seen with the invasion of malignant neoplasms into either peripheral nerves or frequently the brachial or the lumbosacral plexus should properly be included under neuritis rather than neuropathy. Although the mechanisms of pain from distended viscera, involvement of the periosteum, bony metastases or direct pressure on major nerve trunks have all been clearly demonstrated as causes of acute as well as continuing pain in terminal cancer, they probably always cause some type of inflammation in the nerve structures so affected. This is especially true when cancer of the lung or breast involves the brachial plexus and the perineurium is invaded, when carcinoma of the cervix involves the lumbosacral plexus, and when carcinoma of the rectum and sigmoid involves the presacral neural structures (21). Thus, such pain due to neoplasm should be classified as an acute pain problem, not only because of the hypothesized ongoing nociceptive input, but because the ongoing pain seen in cancer indicates some degree of neuritis in the sensory nerves involved.

It has always been interesting just how quickly even this fearsome pain can at times be turned off. For example, after hormonal manipulation through hypophysectomy (22, 23) in a hormone-sensitive metastatic tumor of the breast, the severe pain may be gone by the time the patient awakens from general anesthesia. The prompt cessation of pain after the injection into the pituitary gland under local anesthesia of larger amounts of alcohol than the sella turcica can be expected to hold gives rise to the hypothesis that at times this inflammation may be under the control of the hypothalamic structures rather than the pituitary gland itself. Be that as it may, neuritis comprises acute pain, subacute pain, recurrent acute pain, and the ongoing pain of malignancy (24).

NEUROPATHY

The suffix *-opathy* refers only to pathology, and neuropathy is usually used clinically in the sense of damaged nerve with no evidence of neuritis or inflammation. Neuropathy also has myriad causes, usually bringing to mind initially the concept of injury, such as post-traumatic neuropathy. However, the process may also be the end stage of neuritis, when the inflammation subsides; and, if the sensory nerves or their coverings have sustained permanent damage, then a form of neuropathy becomes a secondary stage that follows the neuritis. For instance, the end stage of herpes zoster or shingles after neuritis is usually a postherpetic neuropathy. Because a number of patients with shingles proceed to a specific, painful syndrome known as postherpetic neuralgia, we sometimes forget that most get over their acute neuritic pain and are left only with areas of temporary numbness and underlying neuropathy. Many patients suffering from difficult, chronic, postherpetic neuralgic pain are very elderly and have severe underlying contributing emotional factors, concomitant diabetes, or a depressed immunosuppressive system from treatment of, for example, a preexisting lymphoma. Nonetheless, most patients with herpes zoster neuritis end up with a neuropathy, and postherpetic neuralgia does not develop to any great severity or for a long duration in the majority.

Some syndromes designated neuropathies are probably

types of neuritis when they are painful. For example, diabetic neuropathy is well known and is usually painless, but when the sensory nerves are involved (usually in patients with juvenile diabetes, although persons with adult-onset diabetes can be so affected as well), it is often cited as the cause of the resultant pain. In all probability, these patients have a neuritis. Some patients also may have a known diabetic neuropathy as well as a new episode of neuritis with pain; then, with clinically continued pain, they end up with chronic pain and a diabetic neuralgia, a seldom-heard term.

Such a differentiation between neuritis, neuropathy, and neuralgia is necessary, in my opinion, because neuropathy is never painful. In fact, even in some neuritis patients a neuropathy develops without their ever having had pain associated with the original neuritis, provided that onset is slow enough or the virulence of the causal bacterial infection is low grade. Three examples illustrate this possibility:

1. Many elderly people with cervical osteoarthritis may have never had any severe radicular pain from traumatic radiculoneuritis or radiculopathy and experience numbness of the hands from sensory nerve involvement, as well as the atrophy from motor involvement.
2. In Hansen's disease, especially before the advent of newer treatments with chemotherapeutic agents, the bacillus is of such low-grade virulence in its inflammatory response that profound numbness would often develop and body parts would even be lost as part of the slowly progressive neuritis leading to neuropathy without the patient's reporting any significant pain syndrome.
3. Most cases of tardy ulnar nerve palsy are of a nonpainful nature; repeated minor trauma at the elbow can often lead, without pain, to severe motor or sensory changes in the ulnar distribution in the hand. In fact, most experienced neurosurgeons will not perform an ulnar transplant at the elbow if there is much clinical pain, unless the motor or sensory deficits are also very severe. The painful component frequently is not relieved for long, and the surgeon may be left postoperatively with a complaining patient in whom the central emotional factors potentiating the pain have been recognized too late.

Some researchers believe that it is possible to have pain on the basis of a peripheral generator after nerves have undergone pathologic changes. However, this just does not make sense clinically, even after limb amputation. The phantom limb syndrome occurs almost universally, but only a small percentage of patients have a painful phantom. There is no good clinical evidence that, when phantom pain occurs, it is related to peripheral nociceptive input; in contrast, there is a tremendous amount of clinical evidence that it is related to central factors. Some neurophysiologists do not differentiate between the clinical entity of phantom limb pain and peripheral neuroma stump pain (especially when the patient attempts to wear a prosthesis), which may involve inflammation and nociceptive input generated by repeated trauma to the peripheral traumatic neuroma.

It must be admitted, however, that in some cases of neuropathy with damaged peripheral nerves, "cross-talk" may take place and may well contribute initially to the formation of a central "causalgia" syndrome (25).

There is no question but that the central mechanisms that we have been discussing in the establishment of central pain (to be discussed under neuralgia, rather than neuropathy) may relate to organic peripheral and/or organic central factors, and not merely be due to centrally preprogrammed environmental factors. Thus, the pain seen in central syndromes in some cases clinically appears to be much more organic than in other syndromes. For example, trigeminal neuralgia, and perhaps acute recurrent pain of migraine, may well be related to some form of sensory epileptiform discharge and may respond to the anticonvulsants, and is certainly "organic." Although the chronic intractable benign pain syndrome with poor patient coping may be entirely central as well, it is usually considered as "functional overlay" with no known continued peripheral pathophysiology or known continued nociceptive input, but where both early nurturance and then later postinjury reactive factors might play a role from a psychogenic standpoint (see Table 29.2). However, we are digressing from neuropathy and getting into the next subject of central pain and neuralgia.

If pathologic findings in a nerve per se are not a source of pain, we must revise our attitudes toward treatment of some of the clinical entities presently believed to be due to such changes. Our current state of medical knowledge sometimes leads to rather heroic therapeutic interventions, including surgery. For example, most cases of

Table 29.2
Predisposing Central Factors to Chronic Pain

1. Organic lesion with CNS involvement
    a. Pathologic (e.g., following stroke)
    b. Physiologic from abnormal peripheral input (e.g., causalgia)
    c. Mixture of pathologic and physiologic (possible example, tic douloureux)
2. Possible "genetic" inherited defects, or, at least, individual differences
3. "Functional" environmental factors from physiologicaly normal but psychologically often "abnormal" peripheral input from external milieu
    a. Past input into memory storage including early nurturance ("psychosomatic")
    b. Reactive factors to acute pain (as often the etiologic trigger) ("somatopsychic")
    c. Mixture of the two (the CIBPS syndrome)

postlaminectomy or postmyelography "arachnoiditis" are, in fact, "arachnoidopathy." Although inflammation can occur initially, and although rare cases of progressive arachnoiditis from various etiologic agents may occur, most persons in whom arachnoiditis is diagnosed are the "failed back" patients who have undergone previous surgical intervention. After a while, the proper diagnosis almost certainly becomes arachnoidopathy with damage to the nerve roots within and without the canal, not arachnoiditis. These patients usually do not demonstrate nociceptive input from the condition. Many are being operated on inappropriately on the basis of modern scientific diagnostic techniques, such as computed tomographic scans of the spine showing spinal or lateral recess "stenosis" that may or may not accompany the clumping of fibers on subsequent metrizamide myelography. Furthermore, positive thermographic results should not be taken as an indication for repeat laminectomy, especially in the absence of electromyographically demonstrated denervation fibrillations. The overwhelming evidence suggests that these patients have centrally generated chronic pain with underlying unresolved emotional conflicts. In any case of chronic pain, actively treating any neuropathy in the belief that one is treating the source of continuing nociceptive input is medically inappropriate.

NEURALGIA

According to *Dorland's Illustrated Medical Dictionary*, *-algia* comes from the Greek *algos*, meaning pain, and *ia*, meaning condition; the word, therefore, suggests a painful condition. It goes on to define neuralgia as "paroxysmal pain which extends along the course of one or more nerves" and describes many varieties, distinguishing them by the anatomic part affected, the distribution of the nerve involved, and (even more unconvincingly) the etiology.

There are a number of things wrong with this definition. First, not all neuralgic pain is "paroxysmal"; in some cases if may be constant. Second, when one talks about the cause of any given case of neuralgia, it must be kept in mind that, although *etiology* and underlying neurophysiologic *mechanisms* are related sequentially, they are two different aspects of the problem and must never be confused. Third, defining neuralgia as pain of unknown origin in the distribution of a peripheral or cranial nerve implies that the cause of the pain may be within that cranial or peripheral sensory nerve and that, through biopsy, electron microscopy, or other yet-to-be-invented techniques, one might find pathologic changes to explain the pain felt subjectively in the distribution of that sensory dermatome.

A quote from Wartenberg regarding neuralgia still illustrates the present state of confusion regarding the use of the term:

> One is struck by the indiscriminate use of the term "neuralgia". It clearly illustrates the rampant confusion regarding this so extensively used term. This usage tacitly implies that any term which includes the word "neuralgia" or ends in "algia" signifies a definite morbid condition, and not merely pain in a certain area.
>
> The indiscriminate use of the term neuralgia to designate almost every undeterminable, and often not neurogenic [*sic*] painful affection is a menace to exact medical diagnosis. As a result, it is well nigh impossible to get a firm hold on the true meaning of the term. It covers so much that it has become almost useless for precise application. (12)

I would like to suggest a different concept: *All neuralgia* is *centrally generated pain* that is *referred* to the *periphery*, at some part of the body image; thus neuralgia, of however short duration, is central and is a form of chronic pain. Furthermore, as a centralist (who believes that the term *chronic pain* should not be used for a condition with continued nociceptive input), It would like to suggest conversely that all chronic pain is not only psychosomatic, but also basically a form of neuralgia.

This concept is not far from the schema proposed three decades ago by Ramzy and Wallerstein (26) (see Fig. 29.1). In an attempt to give a hypothetical taxonomy to purely psychogenic (mental) and bodily pain, they subdivided the latter into somatic and neurotic categories. The somatic category included both peripheral (somatic) and internal (visceral) pain, which is equivalent to pain from continued nociceptive input and, per the temporal classification outlined in Table 29.1, comprises acute, subacute, recurrent acute, and ongoing cancer pain. Neuritis falls into this category for the purpose of this presentation. Ramzy and Wallerstein also delineated a second type, "neurotic bodily pain," involving memory. This can be considered to be "real" pain from a prior injury (or neuritis) that originally entailed nociceptive input, but for which no presently continuing underlying organic pathophysiologic process justifies the assumption that a "discernible stimulus to the body" provides continuing nociceptive input. This concept fits well with the definition by Pinsky of the chronic intractable benign pain syndrome, where it is suggested that there is no ongoing pathophysiology in the here and now; that is, no continued nociceptive input (27) (see Table 29.3). Long ago, I suggested that this central mechanism of "neurotic bodily pain" could be relabeled neuralgia (28–30). This classification includes not only the few patients with hypochondriacal or hysterical features, or phantom limb pain, but also *all* patients with chronic pain.

In some forms of central neuralgia with a presently unknown etiology, such as idiopathic primary trigeminal neuralgia, the *cause* may be presumed to be peripheral. In secondary trigeminal neuralgia, acoustic tumors, entry zone multiple sclerosis, the carotid artery's beating under the trigeminal ganglion in the region of the foramen lacerum, and even pulsation of a smaller artery against the trigeminal root near the pons have all been listed as

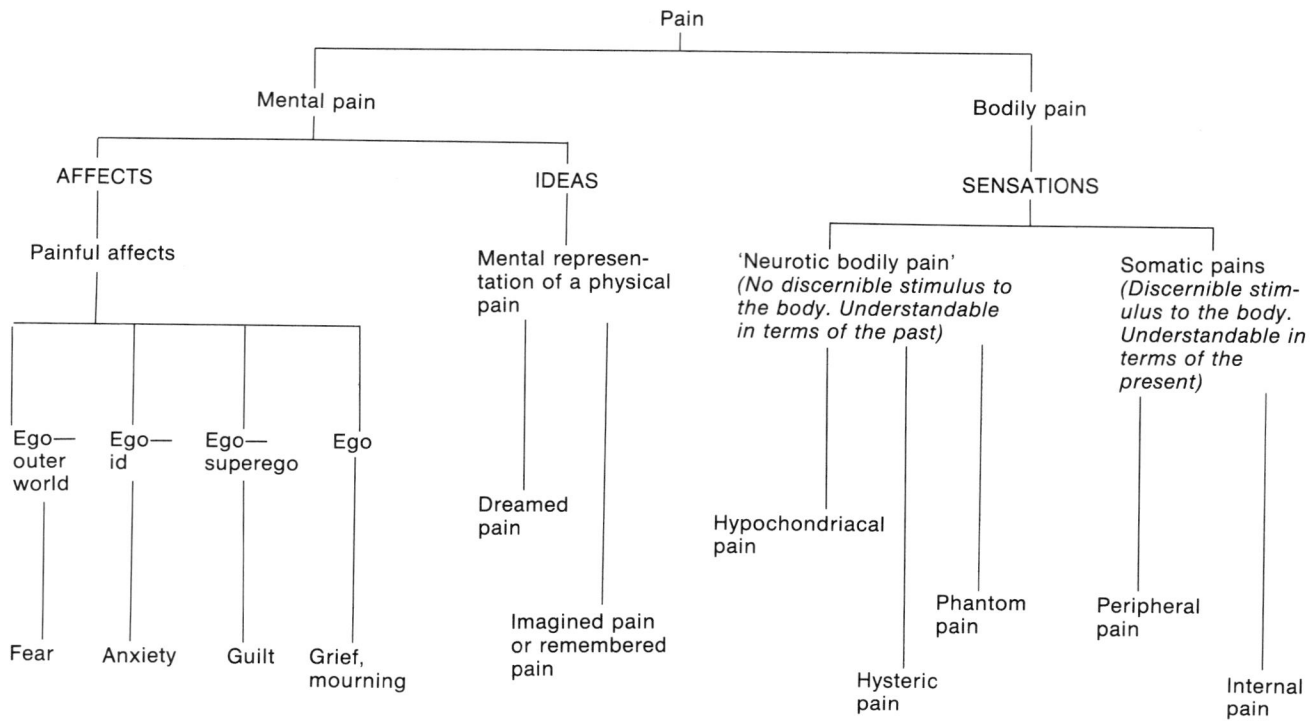

Figure 29.1. Psychoanalytic schematization of pain. (From Ramzy I, Wallerstein RS: Pain, fear, anxiety. A study in their inter-relationships. *Psychoanal Study Child* 13:147, 1958.)

etiologic agents. However, in all neuralgia, the mechanism is central. We have postulated that trigeminal neuralgia is a form of sensory epilepsy (repetitive, uncontrolled, epileptiform neuron firing) within the trigeminal nucleus in the brainstem (31–35). Hence, it is the drugs with anticonvulsant properties that have proved effective in treatment; first phenytoin (36), then mephanesin carbamate (37) (no longer available), then carbamazepine, and now recently baclofen. The anticonvulsants also seem to help in the paroxysmal jabs of pain after spinal cord injury, the lightning pains of tabes dorsalis, and postherpetic neuralgia as well. However, they do not affect the constant pain of many chronic syndromes, especially the deafferentation hypersensitivity states, which often leads to the diagnoses of causalgia and reflex sympathetic dystrophy. For this type of constant "dysesthetic" chronic pain, often seen in postherpetic neuralgia, the antidepressants amtriptyline and doxepin have given partial relief, presumably by a central analgesic action. Fortunately, the vast majority of neuralgic pain syndromes are of short duration, usually self-limiting (in spite of attempted therapy), and do not become intractable. Consequently, therapeutic success has been attributed to virtually everything: nerve block, rhizotomy, transcutaneous electrical nerve stimulation, hypnosis, transcendental meditation, biofeedback, acupuncture, moxibustion, and even wearing a string of garlic. The last certainly is to be preferred to electroconvulsive therapy and depth electrode placement for stimulation, cingulotomy, or even prefrontal lobotomy, which are still being done in this country without adequate trial of the pain team–oriented method of intensive treatment (38). Some patients and many physicians seem to be unable to accept that psychologically based treatment is indicated. The confluence of attitudes agrees with the rationale "if there is something wrong in my head, fix it there," an approach that can lead to the use of essentially unproved chemical and surgical central nervous system treatments.

CONCLUSION

It is time that we in medicine, especially we surgeons, live up to the dictum that we all learned in medical school: "First do no harm!" When it comes to treating patients with chronic pain or the neuralgia syndromes of unknown etiology, we should always use the simpler, noninvasive, and nondestructive methods first (39), rather than try the newest therapeutic medication or operation available or even resort to them as a last desperate measure without adequately determining what we are trying to accomplish.

If the pain syndrome is chronic, then psychotherapy

Table 29.3
Chronic Intractable Benign Pain Syndrome (CIBPS)[a]

General characteristics of pain
1. Cannot be shown to be causally related to the here-and-now with any active pathophysiologic or pathoanatomic process
2. Has an antecedent history of generally ineffective medical and surgical intervention in the pain problem
3. Has come to be accompanied by disturbed psychosocial function that includes the pain complaint and the epiphenomena that accompany it

Epiphenomena
1. Substance use disorders of varying severity with their attendant CNS side effects
2. Multiple surgical procedures or pharmacologic treatments with their own morbid side effects separate from those related to above
3. Escalated decrease in physical functioning related to accompanying pain and/or fear that this pain is a signal of increased bodily harm and damage
4. Escalated hopelessness and helplessness as persistent or increased dysphoria does not give way in the face of mounting numbers of "newer" or different treatment interventions
5. Emotional conflicts with medical care delivery personnel (doctors, nurses, therapists, technicians), which result in therapeutic goal interference
6. Interpersonal emotional conflicts with significant others
7. Lasting, unpleasant mood and affect changes
8. Decrease in feelings of self-esteem, self-worth, and self-confidence
9. Escalated withdrawal and loss of gratifications from psychosocial activity
10. Decreased ability to obtain pleasure from the life process, reflected in the presence of profound demoralization and, at times, significant depression

[a] From Crue BL: The centralist concept of chronic pain. *Semin Neurol* 3:331–339, 1984.

(40), however it may function as a therapeutic tool, is the best we presently have to offer (41). If physicians are not able to accept this concept, regardless of therapeutic outcome, patients who seek their advice will not have much chance of staying away from eventually harmful treatments. Group psychotherapy, usually by a trained pain team in the milieu of a multidisciplinary, interdisciplinary, comprehensive pain center, offers the best therapy presently available for these chronic pain syndromes.

Thus, one can see the difficulty in carrying out the assignment of talking about the management of painful neuropathies and entrapment syndromes, if one believes the neuropathies are not painful. We are instead usually either talking about acute neuritis or, in the chronic syndromes, the central neuralgic painful syndromes. It is obvious how complicated this can be, since we do not have agreed-on definitions within the field of neurology and neurosurgery. It continues to lead to confusion. I ask the interested reader to look through the recently published second edition of Dyck et al.'s two-volume set *Peripheral Neuropathy* (42). It is obvious at once that under the rubric of neuropathy are included many of the syndromes that the present author would refer to as neuritic or neuralgic. It must be admitted that there are esoteric causes of peripheral nerve damage that can on occasion be painful where it has not been proven that there is inflammation or a central mechanism. However, the present writer contends that the division of "neuropathy" into the concepts of neuritis, neuropathy, and neuralgia presented above make a very useful clinical framework on which to consider treatment rationale in any given case with intractable pain. Perhaps one of the best examples of how confused we still are about this can be seen in a recent book, *Evaluation and Treatment of Chronic Pain*, edited by my good friend Gerald Aronoff (43). The present author wrote the foreword, in which I discussed the problem between the central and peripheral concept of chronic pain; then neurologist Dave Agnew, in Chapter 4, carried this on, and appears to agree with the present author, when under the diagnosis of painful neurologic disorders, he discussed the usual lack of pain in the truly neuropathic syndromes (44). Yet the editor himself joined with coauthor Walter Panies in Chapter 5 of the same book when, under the title of "Painful Peripheral Neuropathies," he talked about pain in neuropathy, but *included* the "entrapment syndromes" and the "neuralgic syndromes" (45). No wonder students of human pain syndromes remain confused!

References

1. Crue BL: A physiological view of the psychology of pain. *Bull LA Neurol Soc* 44:1, 1979.
2. Crue BL: The centralist concept of chronic pain. *Semin Neurol* 3:331–339, 1983.
3. Crue BL: Defining the chronic pain syndrome. In Long DM (ed): *Current Therapy in Neurosurgery*. Toronto, Ontario, BC Decker Co, 1985, pp 205–208.
4. Crue BL, Pinsky JJ: Chronic pain syndrome—four aspects of the problem: New Hope Pain Center and Pain Research Foundation. In *New Approaches to Treatment of Chronic Pain*. Research #36, Monograph Series. Rockville, MD, National Institute on Drug Abuse, 1981, pp 137–168.
5. Crue BL: Multidisciplinary pain treatment programs—current status. *J Clin Pain* 1:31–38, 1985.
6. Crue BL: Foreword. In Aronoff GM (ed): *Evaluation and Treatment of Chronic Pain*. Baltimore, Urban & Schwarzenberg, 1985, pp xv–xxi.
7. Crue BL: Foreword. In Aronoff G (ed): *Pain Centers in the U.S.A.: A Revolution In Health Care*. (In press).
8. Crue BL: Historical perspectives. In Ghia JN (ed): *Organization of Pain Clinics and Function of Personnel*. (in press).
9. Crue BL: Outpatient management of acute and chronic pain.

In Wolcott MW (ed): *Ambulatory Surgery*. Philadelphia, JB Lippincott, 1988.
10. Brena S, Crue B, Stieg R: Comments on the classification of chronic pain; its clinical significance. *Bull Clin Neurosci* 49:67–81, 1984.
11. Crue BL: Neuritis, neuropathy, and neuralgia. *Curr Concepts Pain* 1:3–10, 1983.
12. Wartenberg R: *Neuritis, Sensory Neuritis, Neuralgia*. New York, Oxford University Press, 1958.
13. Crue BL, Carregal EJA: Pain begins in the dorsal horn—with a proposed classification of the primary senses. In Crue BL (ed): *Pain Research and Treatment*. New York, Academic Press, 1975, pp 35–68.
14. Crue BL, Kenton B, Carregal EJA: Speculation concerning the possibility of a unitary peripheral cutaneous input system for pressure, hot-cold, and tissue damage: discussion of relationship to pain. *Bull LA Neurol Soc* 41:13–42, 1976.
15. Crue BL, Kenton B, Carregal EJA: Review article—neurophysiology of pain—peripheral aspects. In Crue BL (ed): *Chronic Pain*. New York, Spectrum Publications, 1979, pp 59–96.
16. Crue BL, Kenton B, Carregal EJA, Pinsky JJ: The continuing crisis in pain research. In Crue BL (ed): *Chronic Pain*. New York, Spectrum Publications, 1979, Chapt 44.
17. Crue BL, Saltzberg B: Dynamic pain. *Bull LA Neurol Soc* 44:127, 1979.
18. Crue BL: Neurophysiology and taxonomy of pain. In Brena S, Chapman S (eds): *Management of Patients with Chronic Pain*. New York, Spectrum Publications, 1983, pp 21–36.
19. List CF: Cranial neuralgia—introduction, definitions, anatomic and pathologic aspects. In Vinken PJ, Bruyn LW (eds): *Handbook of Neurology*. Amsterdam, North Holland Publishing Co, 1968, vol 5, pp 281–295.
20. Crue BL: Comments on recent neurochemical brain stem aspects of pain. In Crue BL (ed): *Chronic Pain*. New York, Spectrum Publications, 1979, pp 193–209.
21. Crue BL, Todd EM: A simplified technique of sacral rhizotomy for pelvic pain. *J Neurosurg* 21:835–837, 1964.
22. Freshwater DB, Crue BL, Shelden CH, Pudenz RH: A technique for hypophysectomy. *Calif Med* 84:229–233, 1956.
23. Freshwater DB, Crue BL, Shelden CH, Pudenz RH: Further experience with a technique of total extracapsular hypophysectomy. *Cancer* 10:105–110, 1957.
24. Crue BL: Treatment of patients with pain due to cancer. In Gross SC, Garb S (eds): *Cancer Treatment and Research in Humanistic Perspective*. New York, Springer-Verlag, 1985, pp 118–133.
25. Crue BL: Causalgia and the deafferentiation syndromes. In Brena S, Chapman S (eds): *Management of Patients with Chronic Pain*. New York, Spectrum Publications, 1983, pp 73–83
26. Ramzy I, Wallerstein RS: Pain, fear, anxiety. A study in their inter-relationships. *Psychoanal Study Child* 13:147, 1958.
27. Pinsky JJ, Crue BL: Intensive group psychotherapy. In wall PD, Melzack R (eds): *Textbook of Pain*. New York, Churchill Livingstone, 1984, pp 823–831.
28. Crue BL, Todd EM: Neuralgia: consideration of central mechanisms. *Bull LA Neurol Soc* 29:107–132, 1964.
29. Crue BL, Todd EM, Carregal EJA: Cranial neuralgia—neurophysiological considerations. In Vinken PJ, Bruyn GW (eds): *Handbook of Neurology*. Amsterdam, North-Holland, 1968, vol 5, pp 281–295.
30. Crue BL, Todd EM: Vagal neuralgia. In Vinken PJ, Bruyn GW (eds): *Handbook of Neurology*. Amsterdam, North-Holland, 1968, vol 5, pp 362–367.
31. Carregal E, Crue BL, Todd EM: Further observations of trigeminal antidromic potentials. *J Neurosurg* 20:277–288, 1963.
32. Crue BL, Shelden CH, Pudenz RH, Freshwater DB: Observations on the pain and trigger mechanism in trigeminal neuralgia. *Neurology* 6:196–207, 1956.
33. Crue BL, Sutin J: Delayed action potentials in the trigeminal system of cats. *J Neurosurg* 16:477–502, 1959.
34. Crue BL, Kilham OW, Carregal EJA, Todd EM: Peripheral trigeminal potentials. *Bull LA Neurol Soc* 32:17–29, 1967.
35. Crue BL, Carregal EJA: Postsynaptic repetitive neuron discharge in chronic neuralgia pain. *Adv Neurol* 4:643–649, 1974.
36. Crue BL, Todd EM, Carregal EJA: Observations on the present status of the compression procedure in trigeminal neuralgia. In Crue BL (ed): *Pain and Suffering—Selected Aspects*. Springfield, IL, Charles C Thomas, 1970, pp 47–63.
37. Crue BL, Todd EM, Loew AG: Clinical use of mephensin carbamate (Tolseram) in trigeminal neuralgia. *Bull LA Neurol Soc* 30:212–215, 1965.
38. Pinsky JJ, Crue BL: Comments on psychosurgery for pain. In Crue BL (ed): *Chronic Pain*. New York, Spectrum Publications, 1979, pp 535–542.
39. Todd EM, Crue BL, Vergadamo M: Conservative treatment of post herpetic neuralgia. *Bull LA Neurol Soc* 30:148–152, 1965.
40. Crue BL, Pinsky JJ: An approach to chronic pain of nonmalignant origin. *Postgrad Med J* 60:30–36, 1984.
41. Lee J: Lemons from a shady dealer. *Time* 23 May 1983, p 60.
42. Dyck PT, Thomas PK, Lambert EH, Bunge R: *Peripheral Neuropathy*, ed 2. Philadelphia, WB Saunders, 1984.
43. Aronoff GM (ed): *Evaluation and Treatment of Chronic Pain*. Baltimore, Urban & Schwarzenberg, 1985.
44. Agnew DC: Painful neurological disorders. In Aronoff GM (ed): *Evaluation and Treatment of Chronic Pain*. Baltimore, Urban & Schwarenberg, 1985, pp 61–73.
45. Panis W, Aronoff GM: Painful peripheral neuropathies. In Aronoff GM (ed): *Evaluation and Treatment of Chronic Pain*. Baltimore, Urban & Schwarzenberg, 1985, pp 75–82.

part d
genitourinary pain

chapter 30
Gynecologic Pain

J. Greg Johnson, M.D.

Pelvic pain in the female patient is a very common occurrence leading the woman to seek gynecologic consultation. Symptoms of pelvic pain along with vaginal bleeding are the two most common reasons for a woman to seek gynecologic consultation. Pelvic pain can be a disabling problem accounting for many lost work days, and having severe impact on psychosocial interrelationships of the female patient. I attempt here to describe and delineate a practical approach to the recognition and management of gynecologic or pelvic pain.

Because the pelvis contains all of the female genital organs and also includes portions of the urinary tract and gastrointestinal tract, it is sometimes quite difficult to differentiate in a clinical setting the origin of pelvic pain. Possible etiologies of nongynecologic pelvic pain include diseases of the gastrointestinal tract, including appendicitis, diverticulitis, ulcerative colitis, and other inflammatory bowel diseases, and functional disturbances, or the so-called spastic colon. One must also differentiate pain that originates from the urinary tract. This may include ureteral stones, urinary tract infections, and trigonitis. The urinary tract infection is easily diagnosed by urinalysis and culture, whereas the other disorders may need further radiographic and cystoscopic evaluation. This discussion does not include the workup and management of urologic conditions.

Pain arising in the female genital tract may be of multiple origins. It may vary from an early intrauterine pregnancy to an ectopic pregnancy to infectious or inflammatory disease of the uterus, tubes, and ovaries to neoplasia or various endocrinologic abnormalities. Included also in this discussion is pelvic pain for which one cannot find a readily identifiable cause. Pelvic pain without obvious pathology is a significant problem requiring a multidisciplinary solution.

The women presenting with pelvic pain can usually be categorized as those with acute, severe onset of pain versus those whose pain is of a more chronic, nagging nature. Those with acute, severe pain usually have had the onset of the pain within the last few hours or days and it has become so severe that it is incapacitating. In these patients, one must consider the possibility of an ectopic pregnancy, an ovarian cyst with torsion or rupture, and acute pelvic inflammatory disease. The patient with chronic pelvic pain is more likely to have endometriosis, a neoplasia, or chronic pelvic inflammatory disease, or to fall into the category of pelvic pain without obvious pathology.

DIAGNOSTIC TOOLS IN GYNECOLOGY

Two of the more useful tools available to us are ultrasound and laparoscopy. With the development and progression of these two tools, visualizing the pelvis, both noninvasively and invasively, has become an easier task.

Ultrasound is defined as mechanical radiant energy with a frequency rate above the audible range. The use of ultrasound as a diagnostic tool is a major advancement in the investigation of pelvic abnormalities and disease. With the development of real-time ultrasound, the image is very much like watching a TV in black and white. Ultrasound has the ability to visualize tissue interfaces, which x-ray is incapable of doing. This provides us with an anatomic picture of an object within the body cavity. Ultrasound has greatly enhanced our diagnostic capabilities in gynecology and in general is superior to standard radiographic procedures, including computed tomography (CT) scan, in imaging the pelvic organs.

Laparoscopy, although an invasive procedure, is relatively safe and, in experienced hands, simple. With the use of fiberoptics, one is allowed to directly visualize the pelvis to delineate and diagnose conditions that may present a similar clinical picture. With the progression of technique in laparoscopy, it is even possible to do more and more operative procedures through the laparoscope, thus sparing the patient the major trauma of laparotomy. In diagnosis, the development of laparoscopy has greatly enhanced our early diagnosis of such conditions as pelvic inflammatory disease, ectopic pregnancy, and pelvic endometriosis. One may also delineate between functional and pathologic ovarian growths or cysts. The laparoscope is also useful in the management of malignant neoplasms of the pelvis.

These two procedures are referred to frequently in the following discussion because they are both very helpful in diagnosing the causes of pelvic pain.

ECTOPIC PREGNANCY

Implantation of the fertilized ovum outside of the uterine cavity is known as an ectopic pregnancy. Although the vast majority of these will occur in the fallopian tube, ectopic pregnancies can also occur in the ovary, pelvis, and other parts of the abdominal cavity. Ectopic pregnancy is definitely on the rise, with the overall incidence exceeding 1%. The increase that is seen in pelvic infections and pelvic inflammatory disease, the use of intrauterine devices, and the increasing rate of tubal surgery have all led to the increased incidence of ectopic pregnancy.

The patient with an ectopic pregnancy may have a variety of symptoms that can be confused with an early intrauterine pregnancy, spontaneous abortion, or pelvic inflammatory disease. It is imperative to recognize the possibility of an ectopic pregnancy early, because if one can diagnose it in the unruptured state, the fallopian tube can be preserved for future fertility. Commonly, the patient will present with a history of a missed period, vaginal bleeding, and abdominal pain. The pain may be variable. If it is early in the pregnancy, the pain may be of a mild nagging nature. However, if it is later and impending rupture is occurring, the pain will be very severe. On examination in the unruptured state, the patient will have adnexal tenderness, usually on the side of the ectopic pregnancy, but this tenderness may be bilateral. There is frequently tenderness upon motion of the cervix also. If the ectopic pregnancy has ruptured, this may be accompanied by hypotension and shock and signs of intraabdominal hemorrhage. These signs include weakness, dizziness, abdominal distention, hypotension, and tachycardia. If the bleeding has been profuse, there may be shoulder pain, which is an ominous sign.

Newer diagnostic techniques, including ultrasound, quantitative human chorionic gonadotropin (HCG) assays, and laparoscopy, are very helpful in the early diagnosis of an ectopic pregnancy. If one is presented with a woman who has a history of a missed period, a positive pregnancy test, and abdominal pain, it is useful to obtain ultrasound examination. Six weeks after the last menstrual period, one should see the gestational sac and early development of a fetus. By eight weeks since the last menstrual period, one should see definite fetal cardiac activity if there is an intrauterine pregnancy. If the gestational sac and embryo are not seen at ultrasound at the appropriate times, it is helpful to obtain a quantitative HCG assay. An HCG titer of greater than 6500 MIU/ml with absence of an intrauterine pregnancy on ultrasound should lead one to the diagnosis of ectopic pregnancy (1, 2). With these diagnostic tools, when one suspects an ectopic pregnancy, it is usually beneficial to proceed with laparoscopy prior to laparotomy to definitely establish the diagnosis. With the laparoscope, one can directly visualize the uterus, tubes, and ovaries to determine, without major surgery, the correctness of one's diagnosis. If an ectopic pregnancy is found, it is then necessary to proceed with definitive surgery to remove it. In the unruptured state, this may be done by a linear salpingostomy with removal of only the ectopic pregnancy from the fallopian tube. If the fallopian tube has ruptured, however, it is usually necessary to remove at least that portion of the fallopian tube that is involved with the ectopic pregnancy. With modern reconstructive surgery, it is preferable to be conservative and save as much of the fallopian tube as possible, because it may lend itself to repair at a future date.

Ovarian and abdominal pregnancies are rare, but many present as a surgical emergency with an acute abdomen and massive internal hemorrhage. Diagnosis preoperatively may be difficult, and it is necessary to proceed with laparotomy based on the patient's signs and symptoms.

UTERINE CAUSES OF GYNECOLOGIC PAIN

Dysmenorrhea is that pain that occurs with the menstrual period. This usually includes lower abdominal pain and low back pain associated with menstruation. In the past, this has been divided into primary and secondary dysmenorrhea, with primary dysmenorrhea being that for which no etiology could be found and secondary dysmenorrhea the painful menstruation associated with a variety of pathologic conditions. In a patient with primary dysmenorrhea, the pain begins near or at the onset of menstrual flow and will usually become increasingly worse during the first or second day of the menstrual period and then gradually diminishing as the menstrual flow diminishes. Women with dysmenorrhea have been documented to have increased levels of prostaglandins in their endometrium and menstrual discharge (3). This information is important because of the development of prostaglandin synthetase inhibitors that can block the production of prostaglandins. These substances not only reduce the level of prostaglandin but also have some analgesic effect of their own in most cases. In the office experience, it is useful to give a trial of the various prostaglandin synthetase inhibitors to find one to which the individual will respond. It is unusual with primary dysmenorrhea to find a patient who does not respond to one of the variety of prostaglandin synthetase inhibitors that are available. Use of oral contraceptives in the patient with dysmenorrhea may additionally benefit her with pain relief by reducing the amount of menstrual discharge and relieving intrauterine pressure.

Benign tumors of the uterus may produce secondary dysmenorrhea that initially will present with a painful nature similar to that of primary dysmenorrhea. Usually on pelvic examination these tumors are palpable, but in the early stages they may not be readily apparent. The most common of these tumors are leiomyoma and adenomyosis. Other less common tumors will produce a similar picture. Adenomyosis, also known as internal endometriosis, is a condition in which the glands grow into the myometrium or muscle layer of the uterus, producing swelling and inflammation within the wall of the uterus. Since this is endometrial tissue, it is under the control of the hormonal cycle and will initially cause pain at the time of menses. As the condition progresses, the pain may occur at other times during the menstrual cycle. There is also usually associated increased flow at the time of menstruation. On pelvic exam, one may find an enlarged, boggy, tender uterus that is symmetrical and globular in shape. Adenomyosis usually occurs in the patient at the upper end of her reproductive years, in the late thirties and early forties. The definitive treatment for this condition, and the only definite way to make the diagnosis, is hysterectomy and pathologic examination.

Leiomyoma of the uterus may occur at any time during the reproductive years, but is more common as women age. This is probably the most common benign disease in women. Twenty percent of women at age 40 will have developed uterine leiomyomas. The vast majority of these are asymptomatic and require no therapy; if the woman reaches menopause, then these tumors will decrease in size after removal of the influence of estrogen. The most common sign of a problem with leiomyoma is that of increasing and irregular menstrual flow. At times this flow can be very heavy, producing an associated anemia. If the leiomyomas increase in size rapidly, they can produce sudden, sharp pain, particularly if there is degeneration within the center of an enlarging fibroid. More commonly, the patient will complain of a painful pressure sensation in the pelvis that is of a nagging nature. As the fibroids become larger, they are more easily palpable on pelvic examination. Surgical management is indicated when the leiomyomas are producing significant pain or significant abnormal uterine bleeding or when they become so large that they are greater than the size of a 12-week pregnancy. At this time, ureteral compression can occur. It is also difficult to differentiate between a tumor originating in the ovary and a tumor originating in the uterus when these tumors become this large. In the young woman who desires further childbearing, a myomectomy may be preferable to hysterectomy. Leiomyomas are very rarely malignant.

Malignant tumors of the uterus usually do not present with pain as a significant symptom. Cancer of the endometrium will initially present with abnormal uterine bleeding and only late in its course will pain be a significant symptom. Other malignant tumors of the uterus are very rare, and it can also be stated that only late in their course would pelvic pain be a significant problem.

OVARIAN CAUSES OF GYNECOLOGIC PAIN

This section considers those conditions that are unique to the ovary, not including inflammatory or infectious causes of ovarian pain. One may have a nonneoplastic ovarian cyst, including the follicular cyst, corpus luteum cyst, and theca-lutein cyst. Usually these are of no clinical significance, but must be included in the differential diagnosis in ruling out neoplastic ovarian tumors. A neoplasia may be either benign or malignant. Most benign ovarian tumors occur in women in their reproductive years, but they may occur at any age. Malignancy is most common in the postmenopausal women, but can be seen in young women in their teens and twenties, and must be included in the differential diagnosis of ovarian tumors.

Follicular cysts occur when the ovarian follicle does not rupture at the time of ovulation and there is a subsequent accumulation of fluid within the follicle. Follicular cysts are usually small and rarely become larger than 5 cms. They are confined to one ovary and will usually not cause any symptoms. The patient, however, may complain of fullness and occasionally a sharp pain in the area of the involved ovary. If these cysts are found at the time of pelvic examination, there may be tenderness present that is of a mild to moderate nature. Following this cyst through one to two menstrual cycles will usually result in spontaneous resolution of the cyst. Occasionally, spontaneous rupture will occur, producing a sharp pain that may last several hours. Typically, these patients present with a history of a sharp, stabbing pain that is now somewhat better, and on pelvic examination the findings are essentially normal. On rare occasions, the cyst may be involved in torsion of the adnexa, leading to a picture similar to that of an acute abdomen. It may be accompanied by fever, chills, severe abdominal pain, an elevated white blood cell count, and an extremely tender unilateral pelvic mass. When this occurs, emergency surgical treatment is necessary, with removal of the involved adnexa because of the thrombosis that occurs in the ovarian vessels.

A patient may also develop a corpus luteum cyst after ovulation. After release of the egg, the corpus luteum remains and, for reasons unknown, may produce an excessive amount of fluid within the corpus luteum. This may lead to cyst formation, usually in the 5-cm or less range, with symptoms similar to those of the follicular cyst. Rarely, rupture of a corpus luteum cyst may produce severe intra-abdominal hemorrhage that requires immediate surgical attention. A patient may also have a persistent corpus luteum cyst, known as Halban's syndrome, that is characterized by amenorrhea followed by irregular uterine bleeding, pelvic pain, and a tender adnexal mass. In this case, a pregnancy test is negative. The corpus luteum may occur within the menstrual cycle or early in pregnancy and it is at this time that it can be confused with an ectopic pregnancy. Following the cyst through one to two menstrual cycles or through early pregnancy will result in resolution.

A theca-lutein cyst develops in the absence of ovulation and is more commonly bilateral. These occur as a result of elevations of the gonadotropin level. Similarly to follicular cysts, the theca-lutein cyst will usually regress spontaneously.

Ovarian neoplasia, as previously stated, may occur in any age group, with benign tumors occurring more frequently in women in their reproductive years. Fortunately, the vast majority of ovarian tumors are benign. Unfortunately, there are no specific symptoms related to ovarian malignancy. The patient with an ovarian neoplasia will usually present with a dull, chronic discomfort that produces fullness and pressure in the pelvis without severe pain. In the younger woman, the findings of an adnexal mass do not clearly establish the diagnosis of ovarian neoplasia, as can be seen from the previous discussion. In the postmenopausal woman, however, the finding of a mass in the pelvis warrants immediate surgical attention for pathologic diagnosis. If one sees a young woman in her reproductive years with an adnexal mass that is producing a mild to moderate degree of discomfort, one may choose to follow her through one to two menstrual cycles to see if it will regress spontaneously. A mass of greater than 6 cm, however, is usually an ovarian neoplasia and may be handled by laparoscopic examination and further surgical intervention as necessary.

Ovarian malignancies, unfortunately, produce few specific symptoms in their early stages. This makes early detection and thus improved outcome very difficult. A woman with an ovarian malignancy may present complaining only of a vague pelvic discomfort and gastrointestinal distress with nausea, dyspepsia, and vague lower abdominal discomfort. It is not until later in the progression of ovarian cancer that the patient will have increasingly severe abdominal and pelvic pain, which, by that time, is usually accompanied by ascites and abdominal distention. Severe pain in the early stages of ovarian cancer usually is related to a complication of torsion or rupture of the cystic structure. A thorough discussion of the types of ovarian neoplasia is left for a gynecology textbook.

Associated with the ovary are paraovarian cysts. These result from incomplete resolution of embryologic structures related to the mesonephros and metanephros. These cysts are usually asymptomatic and small but may distend, producing a large, painful mass in the adnexa. Ultrasound examination may be helpful in differentiating the simple-type cyst, that is, the follicular or corpus luteum cyst, from the more complex ovarian neoplasm, which may have a more echogenic appearance. One may also be able to distinguish areas of calcification within the ovary that indicate an ovarian neoplasia is present. The ultrasound cannot, however, distinguish a benign from a malignant mass. Radiographic examination may be very helpful in distinguishing the nature of an ovarian or pelvic mass. Computed tomography, in the author's experience, has not been helpful in delineating the type of pelvic tumor present, but may demonstrate metastatic disease.

Occasionally at laparoscopy done for pelvic pain, one will see an ovary that has a thickened capsule and is filled with multiple small cysts. This patient's pain may be due to the distention of the ovarian capsule by functional cysts. These patients may have a variation of the polycystic ovarian syndrome, which results from tonic elevations of luteinizing hormone. These patients respond well to oral contraceptives by suppression of ovarian function or diminished gonadotropin output secondary to the oral contraceptive.

ENDOMETRIOSIS

Endometriosis is one of the more intriguing causes of pelvic pain. It occurs when the endometrium locates in areas outside the uterine cavity. Endometriosis is a very common finding during gynecologic surgery. The incidence is difficult to establish because women with endometriosis may be asymptomatic. This may occur anywhere within the body, but is most frequent in the pelvic organs. The most common pelvic location of endometriosis is the ovary, but it may be found on any of the peritoneal surfaces covering the bladder and the cul-de-sac, particularly along the uterosacral ligaments, the fallopian tubes, the round ligaments, and the broad ligaments. Commonly, one may find endometriotic lesions in the appendix, cecum, and small intestine. The umbilicus, bladder, and ureter, previous laparotomy scars, and the vagina, vulva, and cervix may also be included. Interestingly, endometriosis has been described in the lung, pleura, kidney, spleen, gallbladder, and brain.

Typically, these lesions appear as powder burn areas with dark brown or black pigmentation that may have a hemosiderin-laden fluid within the lesion and are surrounded by fibrosis. Lesions may vary from a few millimeters to much larger lesions in the centimeter size, and may turn into endometriomas within the ovary, producing large cystic structures with old blood that has been broken down into a chocolate-like material.

The most common symptom of endometriosis is pelvic pain and dsymenorrhea. Also common is dyspareunia.

Most women have some degree of pelvic pain; however, it is interesting that one may have a woman with extensive disease with few or no symptoms and another with minimal disease may have severe pelvic pain. Also associated is a history of infertility and abnormal uterine bleeding. Frequently one will see a patient whose pain initially began with her menstrual period, but instead of having the onset and diminution synchronously with the menstrual period the dysmenorrhea will become progressively worse as the menstrual period continues and may take several days beyond the menstrual period to diminish. As the endometriosis spreads and progresses within the pelvis, the pelvic pain will increase and become dissociated with the menstrual period. As previously stated, the nature and severity of the pain associated with endometriosis is quite variable. Pain with intercourse may occur as the disease involves the cul-de-sac and uterosacral ligaments and produces pelvic adhesions and scarring within the pelvis.

In approximately one-third of women, abnormal uterine bleeding will occur, primarily characterized by premenstrual spotting. Infertility is quite common and may occur in as much as 40% of these patients (4).

On physical examination, one may find tenderness in the uterus, cul-de-sac, or adnexa. There may be some thickening and nodularity along the uterosacral ligaments posterior to the uterus. If there is scarring and adhesion formation, there may be fixation of the uterus and adnexa. If endometriomas are present, these will present as a tender cystic mass. In other cases, however, physical findings will be that of a normal pelvis. There can be significant pain without significant physical findings.

The only definitive way to diagnose endometriosis is by direct visualization either by laparoscopy or laparotomy. Ultrasound and laboratory evaluation are of no value in diagnosing endometriosis with absence of physical findings.

The management of endometriosis depends on several factors, including the woman's age and desire for childbearing and the extent or severity of the endometriosis. In the young, infertile woman with mild endometriosis, an expectant therapy approach is appropriate. One must correct other causes of infertility during this time and then, if no pregnancy occurs, medical or surgical alternatives may be instituted.

Medical therapy initially included androgens and estrogens and then progestins and eventually progressed to estrogen-progestin combination therapy (pseudopregnancy). The symptomatology improved in over half the cases and pregnancy rates were 40–50%. With the addition of danazol to the medical therapeutic regimen of endometriosis, use of the pseudopregnancy therapy has decreased. In young women who are not desirous of childbearing, low-dose contraceptive therapy will usually relieve the pain.

The most common medical therapy today is danazol. This drug produces its effect by reducing the production of gonadotropins from the pituitary, which then produces atrophy in the normal endometrium and endometriotic implants. Common side effects from danazol are related to its menopausal-type effect. The average duration of therapy is 6 months, with improvement in women with mild to moderate disease in the 72–100% range and improvement of disease by laparoscopy in the 85–95% range. Pregnancy rates following danazol therapy vary from 28 to 60% (5). In a patient who is having significant pain but does not desire pregnancy in the near future, a 6-month course of danazol followed by a low-dose oral contraceptive may be very effective.

Conservative surgical therapy of severe endometriosis is indicated when there is the presence of an adnexal mass or symptoms that are not responding to medical therapy in a patient who desires pregnancy. At surgery, one should attempt to resect endometriomas and remove as much endometriosis, either by excision or cauterization, as can be done safely without injury to bowel, bladder, or ureters. Any disease in the cul-de-sac should be carefully removed.

In the patient who has completed her reproductive function, definitive surgical therapy is warranted. Abdominal hysterectomy with bilateral salpingo-oophorectomy can be done in women for whom childbearing is not a consideration. Also, in those women without children who have progressive severe disease that has been refractory to medical or conservative surgical therapy, definitive surgery should be considered.

Some gynecologists consider central pelvic pain to be a clear indication for presacral neurectomy. This procedure has decreased in use in recent years, but may still be of value at the time of conservative surgery for endometriosis. Along the same lines, a number of surgeons believe that uterine suspension is desirable in the patient who has had surgery for pelvic endometriosis.

INFECTIOUS CAUSES FOR GYNECOLOGIC PAIN

Thanks to the sexual revolution, we are in the midst of an epidemic of sexually transmitted diseases. Although there are several that can cause clinical problems, most of these are localized problems within the lower genital tract and do not produce significant pain other than the local irritation and inflammation within the vagina or vulva. Included in these, but not exclusively limited to these, are trichomoniasis and herpetic infections. These can be recognized either by microscopic examination of a vaginal discharge or visualization of vulvar or vaginal lesions characteristic of herpes simplex II. The two most common agents producing pelvic inflammatory disease are gonorrhea and *Chlamydia*. The term *pelvic inflammatory disease* refers to an infection in the endometrium, ovary, or fallopian tube. Previously gonorrhea was the most common organism producing pelvic inflammatory disease; however, in the past decade *Chlamydia* infections have become more common than gonococcal infections. It is currently estimated by the Centers for Disease Control that there are 3–4 million *Chlamydia* infections annually in the United States. Either of these organisms may produce the classic signs and symptoms of pelvic inflammatory disease, which may then lead to chronic pelvic pain.

The patient with gonococcal or chlamydial infection varies from being asymptomatic to developing severe pelvic inflammatory disease and pelvic abscess formation. To prevent the sequelae of pelvic inflammatory disease with destruction of the fallopian tube, it is imperative to diagnose this entity early in its course.

Unfortunately, it may be easy to confuse acute salpingitis with acute appendicitis, ectopic pregnancy, or pelvic endometriosis. Typically, the patient with acute salpingitis will have bilateral lower abdominal tenderness that usually begins shortly after a menstrual period. The pain becomes progressively worse over several days to the point where the patient is having severe pelvic pain at the time of presentation. Although patients with pelvic inflammatory disease at any stage may be asymptomatic and afebrile and have a normal white blood cell count, in the acute phase typically the patient will have an elevated temperature that may be quite high, in the 102–104° range. At this point, the white blood cell count is usually elevated. As the infection progresses further, the patient may develop an ileus with nausea and vomiting and may develop the Fitz-Hugh and Curtis syndrome with right upper quadrant pain from perihepatitis. On examination, the patient will usually have bilateral lower abdominal tenderness with guarding and rebound present depending on the degree of pelvic peritonitis. On pelvic exam, there will be a profuse yellow discharge and a great deal of tenderness with motion of the cervix. The adnexa may feel thickened and will be very tender on both sides, but it may be difficult to delineate a mass because of the patient's guarding and tenderness.

In contrast, in the patient with acute appendicitis, the abdominal pain is usually migratory in nature and will localize in the right lower quadrant. The classic pain of pelvic inflammatory disease is bilateral. Bowel symptoms occur late in the course of the disease of acute salpingitis, only after severe peritonitis has developed. Tenderness upon motion of the cervix may be present in acute appendicitis, particularly if the appendix is low in the abdomen or in the pelvis, or in ectopic pregnancy.

In women with pelvic inflammatory disease, the laboratory may not be particularly helpful, as has been previously mentioned. A significant number of patients with acute salpingitis will have normal white blood cell counts. Cultures of the endocervix are useful, but take several days to report and, in particular, the chlamydial culture takes very careful handling to be valid. Laparoscopy is very useful in the patient with a confusing picture, in that one may visualize the fallopian tubes and may see erythema and a purulent discharge from the fibria and rule out an ectopic pregnancy or endometriosis. One may also visualize the appendix and rule out appendicitis at the same time.

Appropriate medical therapy should be instituted as soon as one makes the diagnosis of pelvic inflammatory disease. Antibiotic therapy for gynecoccal and chlamydial infection may be found by referring to the latest recommendations of the Centers for Disease Control.

The patient with chronic pelvic inflammatory disease will usually have exacerbation of her symptoms after each menstrual period, which then gradually abate into her cycle. These patients should initially be tried on a course of antibiotics with each menstrual period, but if they fail to respond after two to three cycles, it may be necessary to surgically correct their problem. This may be done by laparoscopy or laparotomy, depending on the severity of the pelvic adhesions. In more extreme cases with the formation of pelvic abscess, appropriate surgical intervention is necessary in a timely fashion. This may necessitate the drainage of the abscess or, in more severe cases, definitive surgery with total abdominal hysterectomy and bilateral salpingo-oophorectomy.

UNEXPLAINED CAUSES FOR PELVIC PAIN

After careful and thorough evaluation to eliminate the possibility of organic causes of pelvic pain, one will still be left with a group of patients in whom the etiology of the pain is not readily apparent. These patients will have been carefully screened with appropriate radiographic, ultrasonographic, and laparoscopic procedures, but no organic cause for the pain can be found. This leads one to conclude that there is an underlying psychological cause for this pain. However, this may not necessarily be the case. As our knowledge of physiology progresses, the syndrome of primary dysmenorrhea, for example, which was once thought to be a psychosomatic problem, has been found to be related to the excess secretion of prostaglandins.

Typically, patients in this category are in their twenties and thirties, married or in this day and age probably divorced, with children, and have a number of psychosomatic complaints along with their pelvic pain. Generally they will also complain of nervous tension, fatigue, constipation, diarrhea, and bowel irritability. Dyspareunia is also a common complaint. In this author's experience, although tenderness may be elicited upon initial examination of the uterus and adnexa, if one is able to distract the patient with conversation, this tenderness may diminish or dissipate.

Numerous authors have attempted to attribute chronic pelvic pain without obvious pathology to a vascular or autonomic nervous system disorder (6, 7). Renaer (8), in a comprehensive review article in 1980, concluded that although a good percentage of patients with chronic pelvic pain without obvious pathology present radiographic signs of passive pelvic congestion, there are a certain percentage who do not present these signs. He also concluded that many persons who do not complain of pain may also have radiographic signs of passive pelvic congestion (8).

The psychological aspects of chronic pelvic pain certainly cannot be underplayed. In women who have undergone laparoscopy and no pathology has been demonstrated, there is a definite difference in response to psychological questionnaires. Women who have chronic pelvic pain and are laparoscopically negative are significantly less positive about themselves and their male partners; they feel less sexually attractive, less physically attractive, and are more anxious. They tend to have fewer orgasms than women who are in a control group. These women also have a poorer relationship with their families (9). I find that these women are generally under a great deal of stress either because of an unhappy marriage, divorce, stressful job situations, or overwhelming demands of motherhood.

With these factors in mind, it is important for the physician to maintain an open attitude toward these patients. One must be prepared to take the symptoms seriously but not alarm the patient, thereby producing a "cancer mentality." A thorough evaluation must be done, but when one cannot find an organic cause for the pain syndrome, one must be prepared to take a multidisciplinary approach to helping these patients. Even in this modern era, psychiatric evaluation is considered to be taboo by some. The gynecologist should gently probe the patient's life-style and sexual history looking for situational problems that might be producing the chronic pain syndrome. It is helpful to have a psychologist or psychiatrist with whom the patient will feel comfortable in exploring these possibilities. As part of this, it may be necessary to look for personality disorders through the standard testing mechanisms. Frequently one will find associated depression and anxiety. Availability of a chronic pain center is of great benefit in helping these patients to deal with their pain, and to accept therapeutic modalities that improve their response to stressful situations and enable them to better live their lives with this entity of chronic pelvic pain without obvious pathology.

SUMMARY

I have explored the possible etiologies of pelvic pain. The majority of women entering the gynecologist's office with a complaint of pelvic pain will have an organic reason for this pain. One must thoroughly evaluate cases of pelvic pain. Medical trial with oral contraceptives, prostaglandin synthetase inhibitors, and antibiotics are appropriate. However, if these fail to improve the pain, a thorough evaluation including laparoscopic examination is warranted. Any organic findings should then be corrected in the appropriate manner. In patients with chronic pelvic pain without obvious pathology, one should look very carefully for environmental causes.

References

1. Kadar N, Devore G, Pomero R: Discriminatory HCG zone: its use in the sonographic evaluation for ectopic pregnancy. *Obstet Gynecol* 58:156, 1981.
2. Kadar N, Caldwell BV, Romero R: A method for screening for ectopic pregnancy and its indications. *Obstet Gynecol* 58:162, 1981.
3. Picles VR, Hall WJ, Best FA, et al: Prostaglandins in endometrium and menstrual flow from normal and dysmenorrheic subjects. *J Obstet Gynaecol B Commonw* 72:185, 1965.
4. Kitchin JD: Endometriosis. In Sciarra JJ, Droegenueller W (eds): *Gynecology and Obstetrics*. Philadelphia, Harper & Row, 1985, vol 1, p. 10.
5. Butler L, Wilson E, Belisle S, et al: Collaborative study of pregnancy rates following danazol therapy of stage I endometriosis. *Fertil Steril* 41:373, 1984.
6. Taylor HC: The problem of pelvic pain. In Meigs JV (ed): *Problems in Gynecology*. New York, Grune & Stratton, 1957, vol III, pp 191–207.
7. Hobbs JT: The Pelvic Congestion Syndrome. *Practioner* 216:529–540, 1976.
8. Renaer M: Chronic pelvic pain without obvious pathology in women—personal observations and a review of the problem. *Eur J Obstet Gynecol Reprod Biol* 10:415–463, 1980.
9. Beard RW, Belsey EM, Lieberman BA, et al: Pelvic pain in women. *Am J Obstet Gynecol* 128:556, 1977.

chapter 31
Pain in the Male Genitalia

Terrence R. Malloy, M.D.
Charles Witten, M.D.

In assessing pain in the male genitalia, the physician must be aware of the many areas from which pain can be referred to this anatomic region. Because of the anatomy and nerve supply, pain is often felt in the genitalia that originates at some distance. It is not uncommon, for example, for men to complain of pain in the glans penis. This pain, however, is very rarely caused by a lesion in the glans; rather, it is referred pain that may come from such diffuse organs as the ureter, bladder, trigone, or prostate.

Therefore, in assessing the management of pain in the male genitalia the physician must utilize all of the classic investigative modalities to truly identify the cause of the discomfort. It is essential that a complete history be taken, and a thorough physical examination and then laboratory and radiographic studies performed in many instances prior to delineating the exact cause of the patient's discomfort. In dealing with this problem, the anatomy of the male genitalia must be carefully considered.

ANATOMY

KIDNEY, RENAL PELVIS, AND URETER

The kidney, renal pelvis, and ureter are retroperitoneal organs lying beneath the diaphragm, traversing caudally to the area of the bladder and prostate. The renal pelvis tapers to become the ureter, which crosses the pelvic inlet anterior to the bifurcation of the common iliac artery (1). The ureter descends to the level of the ischial spine, where it proceeds anteriorally and medially to enter the bladder at its lateral border. Proximal to the area where the ureter enters the bladder it is crossed by the vas deferens. The ureter traverses the bladder muscle to open in the region of the bladder neck at the trigone.

URINARY BLADDER

The urinary bladder is a pelvic organ that is posterior to the pubic bones and anterior to the sacrum (2). Its lateral attachments are the arteries coming from the internal iliac artery. Distally the bladder neck joins into the prostate to become the prostatic urethra. The urethra is anchored at this area by the urogenital diaphragm. The puboprostatic ligaments secure the prostate to the symphysis pubic. The bladder and prostate are separated from the rectum posteriorly by Denonvilliers' fascia. In this area lies the vas deferens and the seminal vesicles. Anteriorly the dome of the bladder is covered with parietal peritoneum, which is in direct contact with small and large bowel.

The efferent nerve supply to the bladder originates from the vesical plexus, which arises from the inferior hypogastric plexus. Multiple branches accompany the vesical artery to the bladder, delivering further branches to the seminal vesicles. Sympathetic fibers that arise from the lower two thoracic and upper two lumbar segments of the cord synapse in the bladder wall to provide motor fibers to the smooth muscles of the sphincters at the bladder neck and inhibition fibers to the detrusor muscle of the bladder. Parasympathetic efferent fibers arise from the second through the fourth sacral segments. They produce the pelvic splanchnic nerves, which provide excitory synapses to the detrusor muscle and inhibit the smooth muscle sphincter. The majority of afferent sensory fibers from the baldder and proximal urethra pass via the pelvic splanchnic nerves. However, some afferent nerves travel with the sympathetic supply via the hypogastric plexus and enter the first and second lumbar segments of the spinal cord. Bladder pain fibers can be stimulated by distention or spasm of the bladder wall, ureteral obstruction, inflammation, or malignant growth. Because of the dual afferent supply, simple division of the appropriate sympathetic nerves or division of the superior hypogastric plexus does not materially alter bladder pain. Additionally, while bilateral anterior cordotomy may transect pain fibers in the anterolateral columns, those afferents that sense filling of the bladder travel in the posterior fasciculus gracilis and allow the patient to be aware of filling and the need to micturate.

PROSTATE GLAND

The prostate gland is a pear-shaped organ in the adult male that can vary in size from 10 to 100 g (2). It is a fibromuscular and glandular structure that surrounds the prostatic urethra and is bounded superiorly by the bladder neck and inferiorly by the urogenital diaphragm. The prostate is surrounded by a fibrous capsule as well as an outer fibrous sheath. Anteriorly the prostate is attached to the pubic symphysis by the puboprostatic ligaments. Posteriorly the prostate is separated from the rectal ampulla by the rectovesical septum, called Denonvilliers' fascia. Laterally the prostate is suspended by the anterior fibers of the levator ani muscles. The prostate is divided into a central zone and a much larger peripheral zone that constitutes 95% of the glandular structure. The remaining 5% forms the transition zone, which lies superior to the verumontanum and is the site of origin of benign prostatic hyperplasia.

The arterial blood supply to the prostate is from branches of the inferior vesical and middle rectal arteries. Veins from the prostatic venous complex situated between the capsule and the fibrous sheath traverse with the arteries. This venous complex receives the deep dorsal vein of the penis and numerous vesical veins, which eventually drain to the internal iliac vein or the vertebral veins, called Batson's plexus.

The efferent nerve supply to the prostate forms a prostatic plexus that arises from the inferior hypogastric plexus. Large nerves enter the base and sides of the prostate, with branches distributed to the prostate, seminal vesicles, prostatic urethra, ejaculatory ducts, corpora cavernosa, corpus spongiosum, and membranous and penile urethra. Sympathetic fibers provide the glandular elements with secretory function. They also innervate the prostatic capsule. Parasympathetic nerves arise via the pelvic splanchnics and supply most of the muscular stroma of the prostate.

URETHRA

The male urethra, unlike the female, both serves as a urinary conduit and participates in sexual activity. It extends from the bladder outlet to the meatus within the glans penis. It is divided into three main components: prostatic urethra, membranous urethra, and penile urethra (3).

The prostatic urethra is a wide, distensible organ averaging 3 cm in length. A median longitudinal ridge arises posteriorly at the bladder neck. The verumontanum is found at the distal portion of the prostatic urethra. The utricle has a slit-like orifice through which ejaculatory ducts open into the prostatic urethra. Prostatic sinuses are found on either side of the crista urethralis, with additional prostatic ducts on the floor of the prostatic urethra.

The membranous urethra passes through the genitourinary diaphragm. It is enveloped in skeletal smooth muscle components, the skeletal muscle components forming the external or voluntary urinary sphincter. This area is approximately 2 cm in length, extending from the apex of the prostate to the bulbous portion of the urethra.

The longest portion of the urethra, the penile urethra, is contained within the corpus spongiosum and averages 15 cm in length. Proximally a fusiform segment is called the bulbous urethra. Terminally the urethra traverses the glans penis, where it is called the fossa navicularis, and then tapers to the external urinary meatus.

Muscular elements of the prostatomembranous urethra receive innervation from autonomic and somatic nervous systems. Parasympathetic and sympathetic fibers are found through the entire length of the urethra. Somatic fibers derive branches mainly from the pudendal nerve supply and its branches, including muscular branches from the perineal nerve. The afferent supply to the urethra is similar to that of the bladder and proximal urethra.

PENIS

The penis arises embryologically from paired genital tubercles that form the paired corpora cavernosa and their crura. The root of the penis is situated in the superficial perineal pouch and provides fixation stability to the penis. The body of the penis is composed of two corpora cavernosa and the corpora spongiosum urethra. The glans penis is the distal extension of corpus spongiosum. The corpora cavernosa traverses the penis on the dorsal side, with the corpus spnogiosum urethra being on the ventral surface of the penis. These structures are surrounded by dense connective tissue labeled Buck's fascia. The corpora cavernosa diverge proximally to form the crura, which attach to the pubic arch at each ischial tuberosity. In this area they are surrounded by fibers of the ischiocavernosus muscle.

The skin of the penis is easily distensible and is based on loose fascial connections to the glans penis and to the Buck's fascia. At the distal end the skin folds on itself to be the foreskin, which overlaps the glans penis.

Arterial supply to the penis is derived from the internal pudendal arteries branching from the right and left internal iliac arteries. Three main branches constitute the deep penile arteries, the urethral artery, and the bulbal artery.

There is also a branch of the deep dorsal artery of the penis that runs on the dorsal surface of the copora cavernosa with the dorsal veins and nerve supply. This structure is called the neurovascular bundle. Venous drainage for the penis is via the cavernosa veins, the deep dorsal veins, and the superficial dorsal vein. The deep dorsal vein empties into the prostatic plexus while the superficial veins enter the external pudendal vein.

The nerve supply of the penis is derived from the pelvic plexus, made up of sacral parasympathetics and sympathetic fibers from the hypogastric plexuses via the pudendal nerve. These fibers form the perineal nerve, which supplies muscular branches to the perineum and sensory nerves to the posterior scrotum. The pudendal nerve also has a dorsal component that innervates the penis. The ilioinguinal nerve also contributes sensory innervation to the skin of the proximal penis and scrotum.

SPERMATIC CORD STRUCTURES

The spermatic cord structures consist of the artery and vein to the testicle, the vas deferens, and the artery and vein to the vas. These structures arise from the testicle, traversing the scrotum to enter the external inguinal ring. The ilioinguinal nerve tranverses the inguinal canal along the floor, separated from the structures by loose areolar tissue. The inguinal canal extends from the internal to the external inguinal ring. The transversalis fascia forms the internal spermatic fascia, the internal oblique fibers create a continuum with the cremasteric muscle fibers that surround the cord structures, and the aponeurosis of the external oblique is continued into the cord structures as the external spermatic fascia that arises at the external ring.

Deep to these layers the lining of parietal peritoneum that descended with the testicle through the inguinal canal forms the tunica vaginalis. The arterial supply to the spermatic cord structures is the testicular, the cremasteric, and the vasal. Testicular veins form the pampiniform plexus. Lymphatic vessels ascend to the lumbar lymphatics. Nerves include the genital branch of the genitofemoral nerve and the testicular plexus, which is composed of fibers from the renal and aorta plexus as well as the superior and inferior hypogastric plexuses.

SCROTUM

The scrotum is partitioned into two compartments by a medial septum, with each half containing a testicle, epididymis, and lower portions of the spermatic cord structures. Beneath the skin of the scrotum is the dartos muscle, which replaces the superficial fat and Colles' fascia. The external spermatic fascia, cremasteric muscle fibers, and internal spermatic fascia are the next layers encountered in dissecting the scrotum. The tunica vaginalis is deep to all these structures surrounding the testicle. This is normally sealed from the peritoneum shortly after the testicles descend in utero. The scrotal blood supply is derived from branches of the external pudendal artery that perfuse the anterior scrotum. The posterior scrotum is perfused by branches of the internal pudendal artery. Additional vascular supply comes from the cremasteric and testicular branches that traverse the spermatic cord. Lymphatic drainage from the testicle is to the superficial inguinal nodes. The nerve supply to the scrotum is provided by the ilioinguinal and genital branches of the genitofemoral nerve supply. The perineal division of the pudendal nerve supplies the cutaneous branches to the posterior scrotal wall. Additionally, the posterior femoral cutaneous nerve has fibers to the posterior scrotal skin.

TESTICLE AND EPIDIDYMIS

The testicle is an egg-like structure approximately 5 cm by 3 cm by 3 cm in size (2). The tunica vaginalis covers the testes. The tunica albuginea forms a capsule around the testicle and supplies numerous septa, which divide the testicle into approximately 400 lobules. These converge toward the upper pole. Each lobule is associated with two or more seminiferous tubules that produce spermatozoa. These tubules form the rete testis, which connects by straight tubular recti into the epididymis via efferent ductules. The blood supply to the testis is from the internal spermatic arteries, which arise bilaterally from the aorta just below the origin of the renal arteries. These spermatic vessels traverse the inguinal canal, where they anastomose with the cremasteric and vasal arteries, which arise from the hypogastric arteries. The venous return is via a network of small veins called the pampiniform plexus that forms spermatic veins within or proximal to the inguinal canal. The right spermatic vein drains directly to the vena cava, and the left spermatic vein ascends to join the left renal vein. Lymphatic drainage is via retroperitoneal nodes. The testicular nerve plexus travels within the spermatic arteries and veins to the testicles and branches are distributed to the epididymis and vas deferens. Afferent pain fibers from the testicle travel in corresponding plexuses, with their origins in the dorsal roots of the tenth and eleventh thoracic nerves. This afferent innervation plays an essential role in referred pain mechanisms from renal and arterial pain syndromes.

The epididymis has three segments: head, body, and tail. The head is found in the upper pole of the testicle. The body is located posterior to the testicle. The tail is attached to the inferior pole of the testicle. The head of the epididymis consists of convoluted efferent ductules that form lobules. These lobules empty into one duct, forming the body of the epididymis. The vas deferens is a thick, muscular duct 2–3 mm in diameter and approximately 18 inches long that is connected to the epididymis. The vas deferens travels through the spermatic cord and through the inguinal canal, ascending to pass extraperitoneally around the lateral margins of the inferior epigastric artery and then traveling downward to the lateral wall of the pelvis. It crosses the ureter at the level of the ischial spine and then proceeds medially and inferiorly onto the posterior surface of the bladder, where it terminates as the ampulla of the vas deferens. The inferior end of the ampulla narrows and joins the duct; the seminal vesicle, forming the ejaculatory duct, which traverses the prostate to open into the prostatic urethra at the crista urethralis. The vas deferens derives its own blood supply from the hypogastric artery.

SEMINAL VESICLES AND BULBOURETHRAL GLANS

The seminal vesicles are convoluted glandular sacs approximately 4 cm in length and 1 cm in width located lateral to the vas deferens on the posterior bladder wall. They comprise an accessory sexual gland, storing fluid critical for sperm survival, which includes high levels of fructose. The seminal vesicles are supplied by nerves from the vesicle plexus, the prostatic plexus, and the lower portion of the inferior hypogastric plexus. Efferent fibers pass to the ejaculatory ducts in the vas deferens. Contraction of the seminal vesicles and seminal ejaculation are caused by sympathetic innervation, which also constricts the internal urethral spincter and relaxes the detrusor to prevent retrograde ejaculation.

The bulbourethral glands, located on each side of the membranous urethra between the fascia layers of the urogenital diaphragm, have ducts that run distally into the corpus spongiosum before entering into the bulbous urethra. These glands provide a mucoid secretion to seminal fluid.

PERINEUM

The male perineum is divided into the anal and urogenital triangles. The borders include the pubic symphysis anteriorly, ischial tuberosities laterally, and the coccyx posteriorly. The perineal body is located centrally between the bulbous urethra and the anus. A median ridge, the perineal raphe, passes from the anus anteriorly to become the median raphe of the scrotum and the ventral raphe of the penis. The urogenital triangle is marked posteriorly along a border to which Colles' fascia attaches. Below Colles' fascia, the bulbospongiosus muscle is located in the midline surrounding the bulb of the penis. On either side are the ischiocavernosis muscles covering the crura of the penis as they attach to the ischial and pubic arches. The superficial transverse perineal muscles run from the perineal body to the inferior pubic rami. The perineal membrane is located deep to the superficial space. The spincter urethrae surround the membranous urethra and form the external voluntary sphincter. Arterial supply to the region is derived from the internal pudendal artery, which travels from Alcock's canal with the pudendal nerve to supply muscles of the perineum, scrotum, penis, and urethra.

PELVIC AUTONOMIC INNERVATION

Specific mention must be made of the autonomic innervation to the pelvis. The pelvic portion of the sympathetic trunk is continuous with the abdominal portion, descending anteriorly to the sacrum and posteriorly to the rectum. Four to five segments communicate to the sacral and coccygeal spinal nerves as well as branches to the efferent somatic plexus, particularly the pelvic plexus. The pelvic splanchnic nerves constitute the sacral part of the parasympathetic system and are preganglionic fibers from the sacral roots S2–S4. Branches pass to the pelvic plexus and then to the pelvic viscera. There are additional parasympathetic fibers that ascend to the hypogastric plexus and the inferior mesenteric plexus. Somatic nerves from the thoracolumbar cord derive branches to the ilioinguinal and genitofemoral nerves. From the sacral cords arise fibers that lead to the pudendal nerve and the posterior femoral cutaneous nerve.

ANATOMY OF REFERRED PAIN

Referred pain is an especially important component in dealing with disorders of the male genitalia. Sensations in the viscera, which are insensitive to cutting or burning, but do respond to tension or contraction, will be perceived as pain in a region of skin or tissue distal to the organ affected. The afferent fibers from the referred pain site enter the spinal cord at the same segment as those pain fibers from the viscus itself. In the case of renal and ureteral pain, referred discomfort is a common presenting symptom and may be recognized by the patient. The distribution of afferent fibers with autonomic nerves is such that renal pain is felt in either the costovertebral angle, left flank, left lower quadrant of the abdomen, or even the inguinal and scrotal areas. Somatic sensory fibers from the groin, bladder, proximal urethra, and genitalia may enter the cord at the same level as the autonomic fibers from the kidney and portions of the ureter: namely, the tenth thoracic through the second lumbar segments. With ureteral colic, pain is conducted through visceral afferent fibers in a fashion similar to that of the kidney. Colic in the ureter as a results of distention or inflammation is referred to continuous areas innervated by segments T11–L2. This cutaneous referral produces pain that often commences in the back or flank and progresses anteriorly and inferiorly into the area of the groin and genitalia. Ureteral pain may also be perceived in the anterior aspects of the upper thigh, along the femoral branches of the genitofemoral nerve (L1, L2). The testicles may be retracted by activation of the cremasteric reflux via the genital branch of the genitofemoral nerve.

RENAL AND URETERAL PAIN

Pain derived from the kidney and ureter is often perceived as genital pain. It is essential to obtain a good history as to the onset and duration of the pain and an exact description as to the origin, length, duration, and movement of the pain. The history often provides the insight to perform the proper diagnostic studies, which can include intravenous pyelography and/or ultrasound studies of the kidney and ureter to determine if there is obstruction (4). The most common cause of renal and ureteral pain is colic associated with stone passage.

However, it also may be found with severe hematuria or inflammation (5).

Treatment is initiated to relieve pain initially and determine the exact cause of the obstruction. Pain relief is usually required. Narcotics may be administered intravenously or intramuscularly.

Once pain is relieved the patient can usually effectively increase fluid intake. If nausea is present, intravenous fluids are required to allow for hydration. The pain from renal or ureteral pathology will usually be perceived as pain or discomfort in the ipsilateral flank, left lower quadrant, inguinal region, or scrotum. At times pain will also be felt on the anterior thigh of the affected side (6). Antispasmodics are sometimes helpful along with narcotic relief. Anticholinergics may produce relaxation of ureteral spasms or bladder spasms. Heat, including warm tube baths, also at times produces relief. Urinary output should be monitored carefully so that the patient does not become dehydrated or so that the renal unit does not become totally obstructed.

Nerve blocks are not especially effective in the treatment of renal or ureteral pain. The major source of relief of pain is the removal of the offending agent, stone or infection. Establishment of urinary drainage past the obstruction will usually relieve pain. Removal of the stone if present can be accomplished with cystoscopy and basket extraction uretroscopy. The stone may be pushed back to the kidney where it can be removed with extracorporeal shock wave lithotripsy or percutaneous endoscopy and stone removal. Throughout all these procedures it is essential to have adequate urinary drainage, which will prevent further pain.

In many instances renal or ureteral pain will subside with the passage of a stone or the correction of urinary infection. It is important after the pain has subsided that follow-up studies are obtained to make sure that the anatomic integrity of the upper urinary tract has returned to normal.

BLADDER PAIN

Conditions in the male bladder are usually perceived as suprapubic fullness, pain, urinary frequency, hematuria, or urinary incontinence. The pain, however, may be referred to the penis and be felt as perineal or scrotal pain or pain the glan penis. These are aspects of the referred pain induced by the nerve supply from the scrotum passing adjacent to the bladder.

Primary pain caused by the bladder is usually related to urinary drainage. In the male, obstruction may occur with failure to empty completely. Drainage by catheter will usually give instantaneous relief. In those patients not suffering with urinary retention, frequency and spasms are the next most disabling symptom. Anticholinergics and various antispasmodics or analgesics may be used. The primary cause of the pain should be ascertained, whether it be infection, bleeding, or obstruction. In conditions associated with infections, such as cystitis, prompt intervention with appropriate antibiotics will usually cause marked relief in pain within 6–12 hr. Urine cultures should be obtained where possible so definitive antibiotic therapy can be continued so that there is a cure. Once the pain has subsided, diagnostic tests should be undertaken to determine what caused the pain (7). Intravenous pyelography, cystograms, and/or ultrasound of the bladder should be accomplished. Cystoscopy should be performed to ascertain if there are anatomic obstructions or conditions within the bladder that caused the discomfort, such as stones, malignancies, or anatomic obstructions of the ureteral orifices. When there are obstructive elements at the bladder outlet, such as prostate enlargement or urethral obstruction, surgery is required to prevent further pain within the bladder. With inflammatory conditions follow-up urinary cultures are required to establish the fact that infection has been eliminated. In bladders where response is not prompt in inflammatory conditions, biopsies should be obtained since carcinoma in situ may often masquerade as an inflammatory condition.

PROSTATE PAIN

Pain from the prostate is perceived in the external genitalia, including the head of the penis, or may be felt in the scrotum, in the perineum, or even into the anterior thigh (8). Patients sometimes will complain of suprapubic tenderness or aching. Another symptom that will be noticed is pain during ejaculation or shortly after sexual activity. Urinary frequency, urgency, or double voiding may be perceived (9).

A careful history and physical examination will usually reveal that the prostate is the source of the problem. Urinalysis with urine culture is essential since it is often difficult to isolate the offending organism in prostatitis.

On physical examination the abdomen may be slightly distended and there may be tenderness over the bladder. Examination of the external genitalia and scrotum will be essentially normal. Rectal examination, however, will often reveal a swollen or tender prostate and, after prostatic massage, fluid can be derived from the urethra or on postvoiding urine that will produce the offending bacteria (10).

Prostatis may affect men of any age and is not confined to the elderly. The treatment and relief of pain consists of proper introduction of appropriate antibiotics and the use of urinary analgesics and antispasmodics. The patient should be told to soak in warm water and to urinate while sitting in the tub. This often relieves the severe urgency and dysuria associated with prostatitis.

In pain caused by obstruction from the prostate, the symptom complex will usually be that of bladder outlet obstruction. The patient will notice nocturia, frequency, severe urgency, and, at times, double voiding. Double voiding is a symptom complex where the patient voids and within 5–10 min has to void again, with a considerable amount of urine being passed. With an obstructed prostate, use of antispasmodics may cause urinary retention. The primary relief of pain is delivered by urinary diversion with a Foley catheter or a suprapubic cystostomy. Surgery then should be undertaken to relieve the prostatic obstruction. The prostatic obstruction may be caused by benign or malignant causes. Follow-up studies should be done with malignant specimens to properly treat carcinoma of the prostate. The principles of pain management remain, however, to obtain temporary urinary diversion from the bladder and then proceed with elimination of the prostatic obstruction.

Care should be taken, however, to assure that the pain is caused by prostatic obstruction and not prostatic irritation, which is seen in conditions such as prostatitis, prostatosis, and prostatodynia. In these conditions spasms of the prostate will often mimic prostatic obstruction. However, surgery in these patients may remove tissue but the symptom complex will remain. This is especially true of males in the early years where, unfortunately, transurethral resections of the prostate are accomplished but the pain complex continues.

Urodynamics and intravenous pyelography are advised in all patients under 50 years of age who are suffering with symptoms of prostatic pain. If the intravenous pyelogram shows normal upper tracts with no evidence of ureteral obstruction and complete emptying of the bladder, then care should be taken in considering surgery. Urodynamics should also be obtained, which will state whether the bladder is emptying properly. Urine flowmetry can be employed to see if the patient is emptying his bladder in a timely fashion. In prostatic obstruction the flow rates will be very slow, whereas in prostatitis flow will often be faster but possibly interrupted by nerve spasms.

Even after the acute infection has been eliminated from the prostate, many individuals will continue with long-term pain and discomfort in the perineum, genitals, or suprapubic area (11). This symptom complex is often refered to as prostatodynia. Treatment for this condition should be symptomatic, to include analgesics and positive reinforcement. Sometimes the symptom complex becomes very severe and the patients will suffer severe depressive episodes. Referral to a pain center is often required in an effort to teach the individual to live with a chronic pain condition. Far too often physicians believe surgery will correct this symptom complex, which it will not. If there are no signs of obvious bladder obstruction from the prostate or severe active infection, surgery will rarely be curative. Reinforcement to the patient of the benign nature of the condition should be made. Many times patients believe they may have an undiscovered malignancy. Prostatic biopsies to rule out carcinoma of the prostate should be undertaken on those patients who do not respond to conventional therapy.

URETHRAL PAIN

Conditions originating in the urethra are usually perceived by the patient as dysuria, frequency, or pain in the scrotum or perineum. The urethra is usually affected by inflammatory conditions, most often sexually transmitted diseases (12, 13). In this case the patient will also note a urethral discharge on many occasions.

Important in the treatment of the disease is a proper history and good physical examination, including a proper urinalysis and a smear of the urethral secretion (14). When sexually transmitted diseases are present, prompt treatment with appropriate antibiotics will usually produce immediate relief of pain. Urinary analgesics may be used to relieve the dysuria and the frequency. Warm sitz baths are often helpful for the discomfort. In acute conditions severe symptoms such as urinary obstruction may result, which require temporary catheterization or suprapubic cystostomies to relieve bladder outlet obstruction. Urethroscopy will usually diagnose the condition.

The urethra can also be involved in chronic conditions derived from repeated infections or trauma (15). Most notably these conditions can lead to urethral strictures, which are ring-like constrictions of the urethral diameter. The patient will complain of a narrowed stream, increased frequency, and a decreased force of urinary evacuation. In addition to the history, the physician can make the diagnosis by observing the patient void. A thin dribbling or erratic stream will often be indicative of the urethral stricture.

Treatment for urethral strictures consists of proximal urinary diversion by dilating the stricture and inserting a Foley catheter or suprapubic cystostomy. The primary form of therapy for urethral strictures is urethoscopy with internal urethrotomy. This will often open the stricture so that it may be dilated definitively. This is effective for approximately 50% of patients. However, a difficulty with urethral strictures is that they will often recur or reform. In those cases a definitive urethroplasty may be needed in order that the constricted area may be excised and the uretha allowed to heal with a proper caliber (16, 17).

Generally, painful conditions of the urethra can be managed conservatively until definitive diagnostic tests reveal the etiology of the problem.

TESTICULAR AND EPIDIDYMAL PAIN

Pathologic conditions of the testicle and epididymis will usually be perceived as pain within the scrotum or pain in the inguinal area. The patient may also note difficulty voiding as a result of referred pain or dysuria. The patient may also exhibit temperatures and a sense of malaise.

The diagnosis is made by a careful history and physical examination. Urinalysis will often reveal inflammatory conditions associated with early epididymitis or orchitis (18). In young men careful examination has to be made to distinguish between an acute epididymo-orchitis and testicular torsion. Testicular torsion may be intermittent, and when it does occur it is a surgical emergency. Classically, in distinguishing torsion from epididymitis, the patient's testicle is found to be elevated in the scrotum close to the external inguinal ring in torsion. Many times the testicle can be untwisted in a counterclockwise fashion. In epididymitis there is tenderness along the epididymis or the testicle. The testicle will usually hang in a dependent portion of the scrotum.

Certain diagnostic tests can often help distinguish the pain of torsion of the testicle from epididymo-orchitis. In torsion, the urinalysis will usually be normal and there is usually no temperature elevation. Radioactive testicular scans will be diagnostic, showing decreased blood supply to the testicle in the torsion case. An ultrasound of the scrotum can also be helpful. However, it should be emphasized that when the diagnosis is questionable in the young male, scrotal exploration should be done to rule out torsion. If epididymal orchitis is found, there are no serious sequelae. However, if a patient is treated conservatively for an epididymo-orchitis when in fact he has a torsion of the testicle, he will lose the function in that testicle. For medicolegal reasons the physician must be very careful to rule out a torsion.

If surgery is done for torsion, the patient should have an orchiopexy on the contralateral side. Torsion will usually occur on a contralateral side at a later date. To prevent this occurrence both testicles should be fixed properly in the scrotum at the time of the acute problem.

Cancer of the testicle is also a common problem in males 20 to 40 years of age [19]. In most cases the early cancer may be nonpainful. However, it can be associated with acute infection and epididymitis. Therefore, if there is any suspicious mass in the testicle that is associated with epididymitis, the patient should be treated appropriately with antibiotics. It is mandatory to do proper follow-up studies once the acute inflammatory condition has subsided to rule out carcinoma of the testicle. Ultrasonograms of any testicular masses should be obtained in doubtful cases to rule out carcinoma of the testicle. As with torsion, in doubtful cases the testicle should be biopsied. An inguinal exploration is performed with temporary occlusion of the spermatic artery and vein so that the testicle can be delivered into the field. The mass in the testicle then can be viewed and, if it is a tumor, an orchiectomy will be performed. If there is doubt in the surgeon's mind, the testicle can be isolated on sterile towels and a biopsy sent for frozen section. However, it should be emphasized that with any masses that are obviously persistent within the testicle, biopsies should be done after appropriate acute therapy for what is perceived to be epididymitis or orchitis [20].

Trauma to the testicle will also occur as a result of athletic events, accidents, or injuries. In most instances the testicle can be treated by elevation and ice to the scrotum. Immobilization will usually stop bleeding and allow for resolution of the problem. However, testicular scans and ultrasonograms should be done to verify that there is a good blood supply to the testicle. If a portion of the testicle has been fractured, scrotal exploration with excision of the necrotic portion of the testicle and anastomosis of the tunica albuginea will often preserve testicular function. As with the other testicular conditions, a high index of suspicion is required to prevent long-term complications of the testicle [21].

Testicular pain may also be experienced when the testicle appears to be normal with no signs of testicular torsion. This can occur with torsion of the appendices testis. These are small structures that will give temporary pain when twisted, but the testicle will be in a normal position and the testicular scan will be normal.

In dealing with any patient with testicular or epididymal pain, careful physical examination must always be conducted. If the physical examination is normal and there is no tenderness over the testicle or the epididymis, then referred pain must be considered. The prostate gland should be carefully examined since prostatitis will often be perceived as pain in the scrotum or testicle. In certain cases silent renal or ureteral colic will only be perceived as testicular pain. Appropriate radiologic studies will reveal a cause for the ureteral or renal pathology.

SCROTAL PAIN

Pain within the scrotum that is not directly related to the testicle or the epididymis may be caused by referred pain from other structures in the genitourinary tract.

Hydrocele is a benign enlargement of the scrotum that consists of a fluid-filled cavity within the tunica vaginalis that is obliterated from the peritoneum by the processus vaginalis [22]. The fluid can enlarge to cause chronic pain or a heavy dragging sensation within the scrotum. In patients presenting with hydrocele, physical examination of the testicle may not be possible because of the size of the hydrocele. Ultrasound should be done to rule out a testicular neoplasm. If the condition is large and causing marked symptoms, hydrocelectomy should be performed. This operation may be done through the scrotum or through an inguinal approach. The hydrocele sac is excised and sutured so it will not reform.

In an acute situation, relief from pain in the scrotum due to a hydrocele may be obtained by placing ice on the scrotum. Drainage of a hydrocele by needle or syringe aspiration can be done but is not recommended. This will cause an initial decrease in size of the hydrocele but the fluid will usually reform. The hydrocele may become infected, which could then lead to orchitis and epididymo-orchitis.

Varicoceles are another condition that can produce pain and discomfort within the scrotum [23]. Varicocele is a dilated collection of veins usually found on the left side of the scrotum. This is because the left spermatic vein travels upward to drain into the left renal vein. If the valves become incompetent, the patient will notice a sense of fullness and heaviness and a mass in the left side of the scrotum. At times this can be bilateral. The diagnosis can be made by having the patient stand and produce a Valsalva maneuver. This will reduce a large sac-like structure in the scrotum that consists of the dilated veins of the varicocele.

When a patient is having pain from a varicocele, treatment should consist of ice and reduction of exertion. However, long-term relief is best produced by having the varicocele repaired surgically. Not only is this advised for pain relief, but studies have shown that over time the testicle on the affected side will lose substance because of the varicocele (24). The varicocele could also affect fertility by decreasing sperm count and motility. When a varicocele is found, especially in young men, surgery should be recommended to prevent long-term problems and short-term discomfort.

PENILE PAIN

Pain within the penis is commonly associated with inflammatory conditions or obstructive conditions in other areas of the genitourinary tract. Careful histories should be obtained as to the type, etiology, and duration of the pain perceived in the penis. Careful inspection and physical examination should be performed. As discussed in previous sections of this chapter, referred pain may be felt in the penis from the kidney, ureter, bladder, or prostate. If physical examination of the penis is normal then these areas should be considered as primary sources of the pain.

Primary conditions that can cause pain in the penis are varied. In the uncircumcised male, the foreskin can cause irritation or constriction over the glans penis. When the foreskin cannot be retracted the condition is caused phimosis. This can be elicited by pain or tenderness in attempts to retract the foreskin. The treatment in the short term can be ice and mild analgesics. When this condition is present, however, circumcision should be performed.

In many men acute pain will be experienced with paraphimosis, which is a condition in which the foreskin, when retracted, forms a constricting band at the base of the glans penis. The foreskin cannot be replaced over the glans. Treatment of this condition consists of ice and manual retraction to bring the foreskin over the glans. If this is impossible, then xylocaine can be used on the dorsum of the penis to obtain local anesthesia. A dorsal slit is made with a scapel in the constricting band, which will relieve the stenosis, allowing the foreskin to be replaced over the glans. However, the long-term therapy for paraphimosis and phimosis is a properly performed circumcision.

Other conditions that can be experienced in uncircumcised males are chronic irritation of the glans penis. This can produce balanitis or even malignancies of the penis (25). Meatal stenosis may also be produced, leading to a narrow, strictured urinary stream. Condyloma acuminata may form underneath the foreskin also. When these conditions are present, circumcision should be performed to allow for treatment of conditions and to prevent recurrence. Carcinoma of the penis does not occur in males circumcised at birth. Therefore, in any patient who is suffering with conditions of inflammation or pain in the glans penis, circumcision should be considered if the foreskin is present.

Peyronie's disease is a condition of the penis where fibrous plaques form on the tunica albuginea of the corpora cavernosa (26). This condition can be mild and noticed only as a fibrous lump on the penis. However, with progression it may lead to severe pain within the penis and/or penile angulation with erection. If the Peyronie's plaques become large, the penis may angulate 90° with an erection. In progressive cases erectile impotence may occur. The diagnosis of Peyronie's disease is made by good physical examination. In the early stages of this disease conservative treatment with vitamin E or steroid injections may be attempted. Ultrasonic treatment also has been attempted. When the condition becomes severe the only treatment that may be possible is excision or removal of the plaque with grafting of the excised area. This can be done with dermal grafts or various artificial vascular grafts. In many cases with severe penile angulation and deformity the patient only improves with a penile prosthesis (27). The patient should be reassured that Peyronie's disease is not a malignant condition and does not progress to carcinoma of the penis.

Priapism is an emergency condition in which the penis sustains a prolonged painful erection that will not detumesce. This may be seen in patients suffering with chronic diseases such as leukemia or with various congenital diseases such as sickle cell trait or disease (28). The etiology may be unknown, or the condition may be seen in patients who engage in repeated, strenuous sexual activity. When first experienced the management of the pain from priapism should consist of hospitalization with sedation and relief of pain. Insertion of a spinal or caudal anesthetic will often produce detumescence of the penis. Aspiration of the corpora with drainage of the blood from the corpora may also produce detumescence. At other times surgical procedures are required to shunt the blood from the corpus cavernosa to the saphenous vein or to establish drainage from the corpora cavernosa to the corpus spongiosum urethra (29, 30). In either case priapism can be a surgical emergency and the patient should be treated with narcotic pain relief, sedation, and prompt efforts to obtain detumescence of the penis. Prompt efforts at reduction of priapism are important since, if not relieved, the penis will scar. The patient may also suffer with erectile impotence. Prompt surgical treatment with detumescence is essential if erectile ability is to be maintained.

At times the penis will be involved with pain caused from neuralgias involving the ilioinguinal, iliohypogastric, or genitofemoral nerves when they have been traumatized from injuries or previous surgery. The pain may be referred to the penile shaft. Diagnosis should consist of careful inspection to rule out primary etiologies within the penis.

Inflammatory conditions of the penis are becoming very

important. Condyloma acuminata are rapidly becoming one of the more serious sexually transmitted diseases being treated by urologists. The condyloma are caused by human *Papillomavirus* (HPV) strains, which easily disseminated to sexual partners. Most of the condyloma and most HPV strains are benign. However, HPV 16 and 18 are associated with condyloma of the female cervix, which may be a precancerous lesion (31). Therefore, with males exhibiting condyloma of the penis careful treatment of both the patient and the sexual partner should be done to guarantee total treatment. Condyloma have been treated in multiple fashions, including surgical excision and local caustic agents, such as podophyllin and cryosurgery. Recently laser therapy with either the CO_2 or Neodymium YAG laser has proved to be very efficacious in totally removing the condyloma and destroying the virus that surrounds the condyloma in the surrounding normal-appearing skin (32, 33). In any patient who has condyloma a careful inspection should be done of the entire penis, scrotum, and urethra. This is best accomplished by washing the infected areas with a 3–5% acetic acid solution. With magnification the skin is carefully inspected. If suspicious lesions are seen, they should be biopsied to ascertain if condylomas are present. All of these areas should be treated. The discomfort from condylomas is usually associated with itching or bleeding that can occur if the condyloma are within the urethral meatus. When condyloma are within the urethral meatus, urethroscopy should be performed to ascertain that the condyloma have not progressed into the bulbous or prostatic urethra or bladder. The Neodymium YAG laser is very effective in eliminating the condyloma that are within the urethra or that (rarely) occur at the bladder neck and bladder. In patients with dysuria, frequency, or bloody discharge, urethral condyloma should be suspected.

CONCLUSION

The management of pain in the male genitalia is essentially concerned with the proper diagnosis of the etiology of the pain. Local treatments may not be effective because the etiologic agent is in a distal organ. Therefore, the management of pain is primarily concerned with the diagnosis of the etiology. Once this is established, proper treatment can be obtained to relieve the discomfort.

References

1. Bo WJ, Krueger WA: Gross anatomy of the kidney: cross and coronal-sectional anatomy. In M. Resnick M, Parker M (eds): *Surgical Anatomy of the Kidney*. Mount Kisco, NY, Futura Press, 1982, p 1.
2. Tanagho EA: Anatomy of the lower tract. In Walsh P, Gittes R, Perlmutter A, Stamey T (eds): *Campbell's Urology*. Philadelphia, WB Saunders, 1986, p 46.
3. Warwick R, Williams DL: The male urethra. In Warwick R, Williams PL (eds): *Gray's Anatomy*. Philadelphia, WB Saunders, 1973, p 1334.
4. Cameran DD, Azimi F: The value of excretory urography in the diagnosis of acute pyelonephritis. *J Urol* 112:546, 1974.
5. Smith DR, Raney FL: Radiculitis distress as a mimic of renal pain. *J Urol* 116:269, 1976.
6. Dowd JB: Flank pain in non-urologic disease. *Med Clin North Am* 47:437, 1963.
7. Stamey TA: *Pathogenesis and Treatment of Urinary Tract Infections*. Baltimore, Williams & Wilkins, 1980.
8. Meares EM: Prostatitis syndromes: new perspective about old woes. *J Urol* 123:141, 1980.
9. Drach GW, Fair WR, Meares EM, Stamey TA: Classification of benign diseases associated with prostatic pain: prostatitis or prostatodynia. Letter to Editor. *J Urol* 120:266, 1978.
10. Schaeffer AJ, Wendel EF, Dunn JK, Grayhack JT: Prevalence and significance of prostatic inflammation. *J Urol* 125:215, 1981.
11. Meares EM, Stamey TA: Bacteriologic localization patterns in bacterial prostatitis and urethritis. *Invest Urol* 5:492, 1968.
12. Bowie WR: Non-gonococcal urethritis. *Urol Clin North Am* 22:55, 1984.
13. Harrison WG: Gonococcal urethritis. *Urol Clin North Am* 11:45, 1984.
14. Centers for Disease Control: Sexually transmitted disease treatment guidelines. *MMWR* 31:335, 1982.
15. Mitchell TP: Injuries to the urethra. *Br J Urol* 40:649, 1968.
16. Badenoch AW: A pull-through operation for impassable traumatic strictures of the urethra. *Br J Urol* 22:404, 1950.
17. Waterhouse K, Abrahams J, Gruber H, et al: The transpubic approach to the lower urinary tract. *J Urol* 109:486, 1973.
18. Berger RE: Nongonococcal urethritis and related syndromes. *Monogr Urol* 3:99, 1982.
19. Donahue JP (ed): *Testis Tumors*. Baltimore, Williams & Wilkins, 1983.
20. LaNasa JA, Lange EK: Disorders of the scrotum and its contents. In Resnick MI, Older RA (eds): *Diagnosis of Genitourinary Disease*. New York, Thieme-Stratton, 1982, p 433.
21. McDougal WS, Persky L: *Traumatic Injuries of the Genitourinary System*. Baltimore, Williams & Wilkins, 1981.
22. Marshall FF: *The Management of Hydroceles*. AUA Update Series Vol. 1, Lesson 9. Houston, American Urologic Association, 1982.
23. Cockett ATK, Koshiba K: The scrotum and its contents. In Cockett ATK, Koshiba K (eds): *Manual of Urologic Surgery*. New York, Springer-Verlag, 1979, p 221.
24. Takihara H, Sakatoku J, Fujii M, Nasu T, Cosentino MJ, Cockett ATK: Significance of testicular size measurements in andrology. I. A new orchidometer and its clinical application. *Fertil Steril* 39:836, 1983.
25. Baker BH, Spratt JS, Perez-Mesa C, et al: Carcinoma of the penis. *J Urol* 116:548, 1976.
26. Metz P, Ebbehoj J, Uhrenholdt A, Wagner G: Peyronie's and erectile failure. *J Urol* 130:1103, 1983.
27. Malloy TR, Carpiniello VL, Wein AJ: Advanced Peyronie's disease treated with the inflatable penile prosthesis. *J Urol* 125:327, 1981.
28. Baran M, Leiter E: The management of priapism in sickle cell anemia. *J Urol* 119:610, 1978.
29. Ercole CJ, Pontes JE, Pierce JM: Changing surgical concepts in the treatment of priapism. *J Urol* 125:210, 1981.
30. Winter CC: Cure of idiopathic priapism. New procedure for creating fistula in glans and corpora cavernosa. *Urology* 8:389, 1976.

31. Grussendorf-Conen EJ, de Villiers E, Gissman L: Human Papillomavirus genomes in penile smears of healthy men. *Lancet* 76:1092, 1986.
32. Fuselier HA Jr, McBurney EI, Brannan W, Randrup ER: Treatment of condyloma acuminata with carbon dioxide laser. *Urology* 15:265, 1980.
33. Malloy TR, Wein AJ: Laser treatment of bladder carcinoma and genital condylomata. *Urol Clin North Am* 13:121, 1987.

part e
malignant disorders

chapter 32
Physical Management of Malignant Pain

Theresa Ferrer-Brechner, M.D.

The physical management of malignant pain involves the expert orchestration of currently available modalities so that they will provide pain relief commensurate with the natural progression of disease and the now-prolonged life expectancy of patients with cancer. Serious commitment to providing pain relief should last throughout the patient's life expectancy if pain persists or recurs. This review plans to give the clinician who deals with patients suffering from malignant pain the ability to maximize their use of currently available pain-relieving modalities as well as keep them abreast with recently innovated modalities.

Although this chapter is primarily aimed toward the physical management of malignant pain, it by no means ignores the fact that simultaneous psychological evaluation and management is of equal importance. The management of cancer-related pain is best dealt with by an interdisciplinary/multidisciplinary approach between physicians, psychologists, and other health care professionals. This milieu of pain specialists can create a program that has increased chances of maximizing efficacy of physical modalities specific for malignant pain. In dealing with malignant pain, we need to remember that cancer is not a static disease, but progressive at variable rates. Therefore, physical modalities should be planned according to the known natural progression of the disease.

The physical modalities currently available for the treatment of cancer pain are numerous. The choice of modality is influenced largely by the specialty of the physician who happens to be taking care of the patient at the time of pain complaint. The oncologist, who traditionally manages the patient's pain problem initially, needs to master the pharmacologic approach, as well as understand other available options if pharmacologic approaches no longer provide adequate pain relief. To maximize the use of an interdisciplinary approach for malignant pain treatment, the primary physician should fully understand the role of various available modalities, identifying specialists who can lend expertise in performing procedures that are outside his/her scope of practice. Since there are only four or five cancer pain clinics in the entire United States, the responsibility of managing cancer pain primarily falls on internists and oncologists medically managing these patients.

This chapter deals with the physical evaluation and management of patients with malignant pain. Current and recent modes of therapy are presented with the concept of a graduated somatic approach, that is, utilizing less invasive, less risky approaches before more invasive, high-risk modalities are utilized.

PHYSICAL EVALUATION

A competent physical evaluation of the cancer patient with pain includes a thorough neurologic examination; appropriate radiologic workup, including repeat computed tomography (CT) scan and magnetic resonance imaging (MRI); assessment of functional capacity; understanding of pain language; assessment of previous analgesics and adjunctive drugs used; and, if necessary, utilization of prognostic and diagnostic nerve blocks. Although oncologic modalities are no longer utilized, further workup to clearly define the pathophysiology of pain is of paramount importance.

NEUROLOGIC EVALUATION

Neurologic evaluation is necessary to understand the underlying cause of pain. The various causes of pain have been identified by Foley (1), and include the two main causes of pain in the patient with malignancy (Table 32.1): pain secondary to direct tumor invasion, and pain secondary to cancer-directed therapy. It is of paramount importance to determine the predominant cause of the patient's pain, since it will dictate the mode of therapy. For example group I patients primarily suffer from nociceptive pain, and group II from deafferentation pain. The management of these two types of pain are entirely different, the first group responding well to narcotic analgesics, and the second group to drugs such as tricyclic antidepressants and anticonvulsants, but not to narcotic analgesics. Deafferentation pain is characterized by decreased response to pinprick sensation, hyperesthesias, and dysesthesias in the painful area as a result of destruction of large somatic fibers from viral diseases, surgical trauma, chemotherapy, or neural compression. This destruction results in the functional loss of the somatic fibers that normally inhibit small nociceptive C fibers in the periphery of the involved area. Neurologic exam is also necessary to document the extent of neural compression from tumor invasion, and is helpful in planning the extent of neuroablation, as well as documenting the extent of any altered sensory function prior to a neuroablative procedure. In addition, repeated neurologic exam will document any impending neurologic catastrophe, such as spinal cord compression, during the course of treating the pain.

ASSESSMENT OF PAIN EXPERIENCE

Assessment of somatic pain in patients with malignancy is difficult because it is often mixed with "suffering" or the affective/emotional aspect of the pain experience. The patient with malignancy and pain need not be subjected to lengthy methods of assessing pain experience used more commonly in chronic nonmalignant pain. However, semiquantitative methods of assessing pain severity and pain experience must be attempted to appropriately assess the impact on treatment outcome. Some suggestions for easily applicable pain assessment tools for cancer patients are the Pain Visual Analog Scale (2), which measures pain severity, and the McGill Pain Questionnaire (3), which measures the sensory and affective dimension of pain experience. Both of these tests can be easily filled out repeatedly by patients with malignancy and pain.

To successfully physically manage malignant pain, one has to decrease not only the somatic or sensory aspect, but also the affective aspect of pain experience. We have shown that somatic treatments such as pharmacologic treatment and neurolytic blocks only decrease the sensory dimension, and not the affective dimension, of the pain experience (4). Therefore, repeated evaluation of the pain experience during the course of treatment is important in directing changes of therapy.

Another useful method of assessing pain in cancer patients is to use a daily diary, which yields information on medication compliance, sleep patterns, diurnal variation of pain, and types of activities that increase or decrease pain. Assessment of previous analgesics lays important groundwork for planning subsequent pharmacologic tailoring. Types of previous medications used, duration of analgesia, and side effects encountered with each medication should be elicited from the patient.

DIAGNOSTIC NERVE BLOCKS

Prognostic and diagnostic nerve blocks can also be an important aspect of the total evaluation of the patient's pain. The pathophysiology of pain and the extent of dermatomes involved can be determined by the use of carefully administered neural blocking procedures with varying concentrations of local anesthetics. Sympathetic mediated pain secondary to reactive causalgia, lymphatic

Table 32.1
Pain Syndromes Associated with Cancer

I. Due to direct tumor invasion
    A. Bone metastasis
        1. Base of the skull
        2. Sphenoid
        3. Vertebral body
            a. C2
            b. C7–T1
            c. L1
        4. Sacral syndrome
    B. Nerve encroachment
        1. Peripheral nerves: neuropathy
        2. Plexus: branchial, lumbar, sacral
        3. Root: leptomeningeal
        4. Spinal cord: compression

II. Due to therapy
    A. Postsurgical
        1. Radical neck dissection
        2. Thoracotomy
        3. Mastectomy
        4. Phantom limb
    B. Chemotherapy
        1. Neuropathies
        2. Aseptic necrosis of femoral head
        3. Herpes zoster and postherpetic neuralgia
    C. Radiation therapy
        1. Myelopathy
        2. Necrosis
        3. Fibrosis
        4. Secondary tumors

distention, and deafferentation pain can be blocked by sympathetic ganglion blocks. The ganglia can be blocked with low concentrations of local anesthetic (e.g., 0.5% lidocaine or 0.25% bupivicaine), at various locations: for head and neck pain, upper and middle cervical ganglion block; for upper extremities, stellate ganglion block; for lower extremities, paravertebral sympathetic ganglion block. Somatic nerve–mediated pain can be blocked by administration of a higher concentration of local anesthetic (e.g., 1% lidocaine, 0.5% bupivicaine), into somatic nerves or epidural space. This is particularly helpful in determining whether neurolytic somatic nerve blocks can be helpful in patients with pain secondary to multiple rib metastases, chest wall or abdominal wall metastases, or somatic nerve compression due to vertebral metastases.

When determining the prognosis of neurolytic blocks with local anesthetics, appropriate semiquantitative pain scales and careful sensory examination should be documented before and after injection of the local anesthetic. At least 50% reduction in pain and absence of intolerable side effects should be present before chemical neurolysis is entertained. If a patient is a candidate for a neurolytic block, a diagnostic block with local anesthetic should be done 24–48 hr before to determine the volume of neurolytic agent necessary. Prior to any diagnostic block, platelet count, prothrombin time, bleeding time, and thromboplastin time should be determined. This is particularly important in patients receiving epidural blocks, where the danger of epidural hematoma with coagulopathy can lead to severe neurologic deficits if not treated immediately with surgical intervention. In addition, if impending spinal cord compression is suspected, a CT scan or MRI should be done before an epidural or spinal injection is attempted.

PHYSICAL TREATMENTS

Table 32.2 lists the general types of current physical treatments for the alleviation of malignant pain. Description of some of these modalities has been dealt with in previous chapters. Since malignancy is not a stable disease, but is typically progressive, the use of a single modality frequently fails to give a lasting or "permanent" solution to the pain problem. Often, a combination of the various modalities is necessary over the course of the disease. Understanding the life history of the specific cancer inducing the pain will provide better information in orchestrating the various types of physical modalities available for pain control. Recently, a consensus group for cancer pain management suggested a decision tree for managing malignancy pain, taking into consideration various causes of cancer pain, factors that can influence the pain experience, and currently available modalities (5). A synopsis of this algorithm is presented in Figure 32.1.

INDIVIDUALIZED PHARMACOLOGIC TAILORING

In this section, both standard and current novel approaches in drug therapy are discussed as they apply to malignant pain therapy. Although drug therapy has been the mainstay of treatment for malignant pain, it remains the mode most fraught with controversy. Unfortunately, most physicians have been taught primarily to use narcotic analgesics for the relief of acute pain (i.e., postoperative pain, post-trauma pain, pain from procedures). Therefore, physicians expect to use narcotic analgesics only for a limited period of time, becoming increasingly uncomfortable in extending their use for long periods of time in patients with malignant pain. There is difficulty in understanding the individualized development of tolerance with prolonged use. Often patients are labeled "addicted" when the requirements for analgesia naturally increases. Risk of substance abuse with chronic opioid use in patients with chronic noncancer pain or cancer patients has not been substantiated. In reviewing the use of narcotics in a cancer pain clinic, the major factor for increased drug intake is substantiated progression of metastatic disease (6). In addition, monitoring the incidence of narcotic addiction in 39,946 hospitalized medical patients revealed that of 11,882 who received at least one narcotic prep-

Table 32.2
Currently Available Physical Treatments for Malignant Pain

I. Pharmacologic tailoring
   A. Nonnarcotic and narcotic analgesics
   B. Adjuvant drugs
     1. Antidepressants
     2. Anxiolytics
     3. Anticonvulsants
     4. Steroids
     5. Antihistamines
     6. Dextroamphetamine
     7. Phenothiazines
     8. Caffeine
II. Modulation of pain pathway
   A. Central stimulation: periventricular or thalamic capsule stimulation
   B. Dorsal column stimulation
   C. Peripheral stimulation: transcutaneous electrical nerve stimulation, acupuncture
III. Neuroablation
   A. Chemical: injection of neurolytic solutions
     1. Spinal block
     2. Epidural block
     3. Somatic nerve block
     4. Sympathetic ganglion block
     5. Peripheral nerve block
   B. Surgical
     1. Percutaneous or open chordotomy
     2. Surgical rhizotomy
     3. Dorsal root entry zone lesions
     4. Median myelotomy
     5. Hypophysectomy

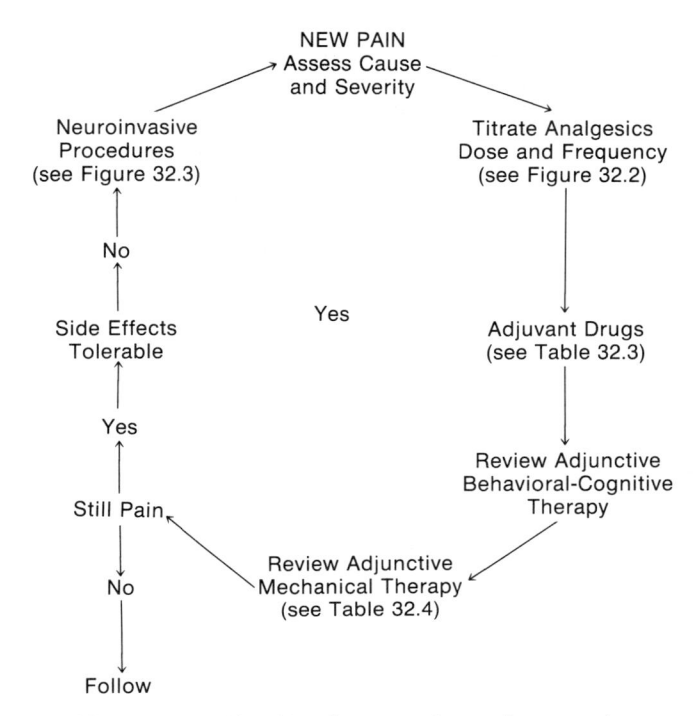

Figure 32.1. Algorithm for managing malignant pain.

aration, there were only 4 cases of reasonably well-documented addiction in patients without prior addiction history (7). For physicians to effectively begin using narcotic analgesia in cancer patients, the fear of inducing addiction in cancer patients should be eradicated.

To effectively use narcotic analgesics for malignant pain, several factors need to be examined: choice of drug; method of administration; route of drug administration; and development of tolerance with prolonged use. In this review, only analgesic studies done in cancer pain are addressed since the review of pharmacology of analgesics for other pain models has been given elsewhere.

Figure 32.2 illustrates the ladder of analgesic drugs for oral use utilized for malignant pain. (a) aspirin-type drugs, including the nonsteroidal anti-inflammatory drugs (NSAIDs); (b) aspirin-type drugs combined with mild narcotics; and (c) narcotic analgesics.

Aspirin-Type Drugs

Nonnarcotic analgesics are used primarily for mild malignancy pain as the first line of analgesic (8, 9). This class includes aspirin, acetaminophen, and NSAIDs. Their use in malignancy pain is limited because aspirin beyond 1300 mg has a "ceiling" effect; therefore further increase in dosage will not increase peak analgesia, but may increase duration (10). In addition, malignancy pain rarely stays at a mild level, but more commonly proceeds to moderate or severe pain. Increasing the dose to more than 4 g/day of aspirin produces gastrointestinal side effects or salicylate intoxication in a majority of patients. Unfortunately, the majority of studies on mild analgesics have been done in postoperative, dental, or other acute pain models, and have rarely been done on patients with malignancy pain.

Acetaminophen has been found to be equieffective and equipotent to aspirin in malignancy pain, and their time-effect curves virtually overlap (11). As with aspirin, a ceiling effect is also obtained past a 1000-mg dose. Acetaminophen has fewer side effects than aspirin, but with overdosage can induce hepatotoxicity. A daily dose over 4-6 g is not recommended because of this dangerous side effect, especially in cancer patients with liver involvement.

Aspirin-Type Drugs with Mild Narcotics

The second step in the analgesic ladder is the use of mild narcotics in combination with aspirin or acetaminophen. A majority of analgesic studies done with this group again have been in postoperative, postpartum, or dental pain models, and not on chronic malignant pain. Moertel et al. probably performed the only study comparing a number of oral analgesics in outpatients with malignant pain (12). Codeine (65 mg) and pentazocine (50 mg) were not significantly different than aspirin (600 mg) and propoxyphene hydrochloride (65 mg) was found to be slightly less effective than aspirin (650 mg).

Combinations of opiate and antipyretics are known to produce analgesia by two mechanisms: opioids bind to opiate receptors in the central nervous system, and the antipyretics act peripherally. Therefore, an additive analgesic effect is produced with this combination, usually substantially greater than when either drug is administered by itself. This combination also results in reduction of side effects. Specifically, in malignant pain, factorial studies indicate that the combination of 600 mg of aspirin and 32 mg codeine clearly produces more significant analgesia than either one alone (13). For those with chronic pain, repetitive dosing of codeine with acetaminophen over a period of 8 days produced a greater analgesic effect than is seen with a single-dose study (14). Although the subjects did not have malignant pain, it demonstrates that differences in efficacy can be secondary to repetitive dosing, common in patients with malignant pain, and that results seen with single-dose acute pain models do not necessarily apply to chronic cancer pain models.

In 100 outpatients with cancer pain who self-administered medications in a drug crossover study, Moertel et al. found that codeine (65 mg), oxycodone (9.76 mg), and pentazocine (25 mg) produced statistically significant increases in the analgesia when added to aspirin, but propoxyphene napsylate added to aspirin failed to increase analgesia (12).

Nonsteroidal anti-inflammatory drugs are known to be more efficacious than aspirin and acetaminophen and are known to enhance narcotic analgesia more than aspirin and acetaminophen. Specifically, in a double-blind study

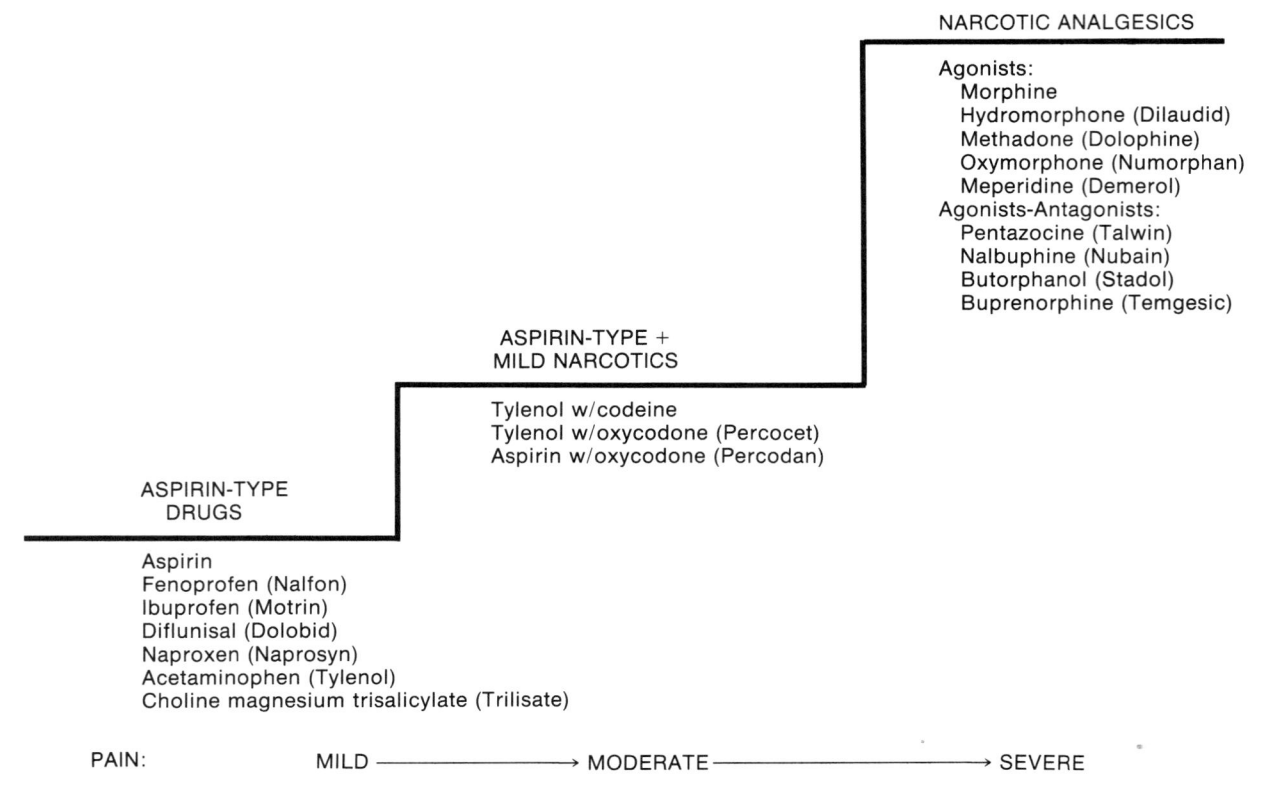

```
                                                    NARCOTIC ANALGESICS
                                                    Agonists:
                                                      Morphine
                                                      Hydromorphone (Dilaudid)
                                                      Methadone (Dolophine)
                                                      Oxymorphone (Numorphan)
                                                      Meperidine (Demerol)
                                                    Agonists-Antagonists:
                                                      Pentazocine (Talwin)
                                                      Nalbuphine (Nubain)
                                                      Butorphanol (Stadol)
                                                      Buprenorphine (Temgesic)

                        ASPIRIN-TYPE +
                        MILD NARCOTICS
                        Tylenol w/codeine
                        Tylenol w/oxycodone (Percocet)
                        Aspirin w/oxycodone (Percodan)

    ASPIRIN-TYPE
       DRUGS
    Aspirin
    Fenoprofen (Nalfon)
    Ibuprofen (Motrin)
    Diflunisal (Dolobid)
    Naproxen (Naprosyn)
    Acetaminophen (Tylenol)
    Choline magnesium trisalicylate (Trilisate)

    PAIN:          MILD ─────────→ MODERATE ─────────────→ SEVERE
```

Figure 32.2. Ladder of commonly used drugs for malignant pain.

in patients with malignant pain, addition of ibuprofen (600 mg) to methadone (2–5 and 5 mg) was clearly superior to methadone given alone in the same doses (15). Although newer NSAIDs have mushroomed, studies on their use for chronic malignancy pain is lacking, despite the fact that research for better analgesics in this area is of priority.

Narcotic Analgesics

Narcotics are the basic mainstay of therapy for managing moderate to severe acute and chronic malignant pain. For a complete review of the principles of various narcotics used in cancer pain, the reader is referred to a recently published guide on the topic (16). This guide promotes nine principles for the individualization of narcotic analgesics:

1. Individualize dose by choosing the route of administration to fit the patient's needs, titrating the dose to analgesia, and respecting the wide variation in optimal analgesic for the cancer patient.
2. Administer the analgesic on a time-contingent, *not* pain-contingent, basis.
3. Become familiar with the dose and time course of potent narcotics.
4. Be aware of the potential hazards of pentazocine (Talwin) and meperidine (Demerol). Pentazocine is an agonist-antagonist drug in oral form and, therefore, will precipitate withdrawal in patients taking pure agonist opioids. Meperidine (Demerol) is short acting and has poor oral to intramuscular potency. Its metabolic by-product, normeperidine, can induce central nervous system stimulation, possibly leading to convulsions (17), especially in patients with compromised kidney function.
5. Recognize and treat side effects appropriately.
6. Use drug combinations that enhance analgesia without increasing side effects.
7. Do not use placebos to assess the nature of the pain.
8. Watch for the development of tolerance and treat appropriately.
9. Be aware of the development of physical dependence and prevent withdrawal.

To remove the myths that hamper most physicians in appropriately prescribing adequate narcotic analgesics in malignant pain, the definitions of tolerance, physical dependence, and psychological dependence ("*addiction*") should be clearly understood. It is inhuman to label cancer patients "addicts," especially if this is the main reason for their undertreatment with analgesics.

Adjuvant Drugs

There are some atypical types of malignant pain that may not respond even to high doses of narcotics. In these situations, the use of adjuvant drugs or procedures becomes of paramount importance (Table 32.3). Merely increasing narcotic dose with this atypical narcotic-resistant pain syndrome will just increase narcotic toxicity without increasing analgesia.

Patients with progressive bone metastasis may require adjuvant use of NSAIDs for their antiprostaglandin E_2 effect, or epidural steroids for painful nerve root or plexus compression resulting in neural edema. Patients with smooth muscle spasm (rectal, pancreatic, parotid, and salivary glands) may also not respond well to narcotics and may require adjuvant anticholinergic drugs such as atropine (0.2–0.4 mg). Deafferentation resulting in neuropathic pain (postherpetic neuralgia, postmastectomy and post-thoracotomy pain), is best treated with the use of tricyclic antidepressants with or without phenothiazine (18, 19). The analgesic effect of amitriptyline is better seen at lower doses (25–150 mg) than their antidepressant effects in patients with chronic pain.

Another group of patients whose pain may not respond well to narcotics are patients with headaches secondary to increased intrathecal pressure. Narcotic administration can cause CO_2 accumulation, which further increases intracranial pressure. This condition is best treated with systemic or oral steroids. Skeletal muscle spasm due to malignant infiltration of the posterior fossa or paraspinal muscles can be best treated with drugs such as Flexeril.

Other adjuvant drugs that can be useful for cancer pain are:

1. Anticonvulsants (phenytoin, carbamazepine, sodium valproate, clonazepam) for brief shooting or lancinating pain secondary to chronic neuralgias such as postherpetic neuralgia, intercostal neuralgia, traumatic neuralgias (20).
2. Dextroamphetamine, which has been shown to increase analgesia when given with narcotics (21) as well as reduce the sedative effects of narcotics in patients with malignant pain.
3. Antihistamines such as hydroxyzine (Vistaril) in a 25–50-mg dose, which has analgesic, antiemetic, and sedative actions and, therefore, is ideal for patients who have pain, anxiety, and nausea.

Drugs that should be avoided in the management of cancer pain are sedative-hypnotic drugs, benzodiazepines, cannabinoids, and cocaine, because of nonexistent or poor analgesic effect in the face of intolerable side effects.

New Techniques in Narcotic Administration

Newer methods of drug delivery have recently been innovated in an attempt to improve the management of cancer pain. These include: (a) sublingual; (b) continuous subcutaneous infusion; (c) transdermal; (d) continuous spinal or epidural opioid infusion; and (e) intraventricular injection. In addition, the use of patient-controlled analgesia (PCA) has innovated the use of intravenous morphine administration, giving the patients better control of their pain. Not all of these methods have undergone adequate clinical trials in patients with malignancy pain.

The sublingual area is rich in blood and lymphatic vessels, making it ideal for rapid absorption (22). The ideal drugs for sublingual administration are methadone, fentanyl, or buprenorphine, because of their high partition coefficient, a measure of lipid solubility. To maximize the proportion of unionized opioids in the sublingual cavity, the pH of the dosing solution can be raised to enhance absorption. The absorption of levorphanol or methadone was significantly increased when the pH of the solution was increased from 6.5 to 8.5 (23).

Continuous subcutaneous infusion (CSCI) can be a relatively simple, safe, and effective method of pain control in children and adults. A portable infusion pump is attached to a 27-gauge butterfly needle and inserted in the subcutaneous tissue, usually in the chest area (24). Most opioids can be used for CSCI except meperidine and pentazocine, which can be irritating to tissues. The ideal volume of infusion seems to be <1 ml/hr to prevent local irritation.

Transdermal delivery, the newest method of opioid delivery, can offer several advantages for patients with chronic malignancy pain. However, absorption of drugs applied to the skin surface is a challenging problem. The opioid must have high lipid solubility to penetrate the skin to the capillaries, adequate water solubility to allow highly concentrated solutions (>1.0 mg/ml) to be incorporated in the reservoir, and a high relative analgesic potency since it reduces the bulk of the reservoir. The ideal drug presently being studied is fentanyl, which is found to appear in the

Table 32.3
Adjuvant Drugs for Malignant Pain

Problem	Adjuvant Drug
Nociceptive pain	
Bone pain	NSAIDs
	L-dopa
Visceral pain	ASA
	Acetaminophen
Deafferentation pain	
Burning pain	Tricyclic antidepressants
Shooting pain	Anticonvulsants
Nausea and vomiting	Hydroxyzine
Sedation	Dextroamphetamine
Painful neural compression	Steroids
Increased intracranial pressure	Steroids

plasma 2–3 hr after application of the patch and reaches steady state plasma level after 12 hr (25).

Continuous spinal or epidural opioid infusion was introduced in the 1970s for the management of acute pain due to postoperative, obstetric, and chronic benign and malignant pain (26). The advantages of centrally administered opioids include a prolonged analgesia with lower doses when compared to systemic opioid administration. In contrast to the use of local anesthetics in the epidural or intrathecal space, opioid analgesia is free of sympathetic motor and proprioceptive adverse effects. Administration of opioids centrally does produce adverse effects of nausea and vomiting, pruritus, and delayed respiratory depression in narcotic-naive patients. The analgesic effects of centrally administered opioids are dose dependent, naloxone reversible, and subject to tolerance development (27). Several factors determine the clinical response to spinal opioids: relative analgesic potency, receptor selectivity pharmacokinetics in cerebrospinal fluid (CSF) and spinal cord, and tolerance to opioids. Although morphine is the most common opioid injected into the epidural or intrathecal space, no controlled studies have compared graded doses of spinal opioid to obtain relative potency estimates. Receptor selectivity for mu, kappa, and delta receptor types in the spinal cord has been studied in animal models. Selection of opioids for specific receptors in the spinal cord can be used to obviate tolerance by switching the patient to another narcotic of different receptor specificity (27). Morphine, the narcotic commonly used for epidural and intrathecal administration, binds primarily to mu receptors. After tolerance to intrathecal morphine developed in rats and primates, administration of DADL, a β-receptor ligand, induced significant analgesia (28). Respiratory depression in a morphine-tolerant cancer patient with an intrathecal bolus of DADL, reversed by naloxone, was recently reported (29).

Pharmacokinetics of intrathecally or epidurally administered opioids is affected by lipid solubility and ionization of the opioid in CSF. In comparing cisternal concentration of morphine and methadone after lumbar subarachnoid injections, morphine reached the cisternal CSF 180 min after injection, whereas methadone did not (30). The lipid solubility of methadone results from its rapid uptake into the spinal cord, leaving little in the CSF to move supraspinally. This results in more rapid, but shorter duration, analgesia with methadone in comparison to morphine.

Opioids can be administered intrathecally or epidurally in single doses, repetitive doses, or continuous infusion. Single-dose injection of morphine and β-endorphin in the intrathecal space at the second and third lumbar space induced peak analgesia in 30 min that lasted for periods averaging 20 hr (31, 32). Cancer patients who were not narcotic naive did not suffer from respiratory depression, hypotension, hypothermia, or catatonia. Chronic intraspinal or epidural opioid infusions can be accomplished by repetitive or continuous infusion into an open or closed system. A catheter can be implanted into the epidural or intrathecal space and connected into an Omaya reservoir or a custom device (33). A high-precision pump with a 50-ml reservoir can be implanted subcutaneously (34). Chronic administration of epidural narcotics leads to tolerance. The average increase of intrathecal morphine dose over a 12-week period was 2–6.6 mg/day (35).

Acute complications include nausea, pruritus, respiratory depression, and urinary retention. Complications with chronic implantation include mechanical problems such as catheter displacement and development of CSF hygromas with fluid collection under the pump and along the catheter tract (34, 36). The use of chronic intrathecal or epidural opioid infusion seems to be ideal if the life expectancy is 2–3 months (37).

Patient-controlled analgesia is a new method for intravenous opioid delivery, where the patient is able to demand an opioid dose directly from a drug-dispensing system that will administer a preset dose of the opioid. By administering small doses by triggering a push-button device at frequent intervals, the patient can theoretically titrate analgesia against pain (38). Thus, PCA is innovative by providing individualized pharmacologic tailoring and patient autonomy. There are several PCA devices commercially available at present. Some ideal characteristics are ease of programmability, availability of a printout, and a sounding device that responds to both active or inactive trigger. Various narcotics have been administered to postoperative patients by this technique (39, 40). The use of PCA has also been compared between intravenous and epidural routes of narcotic administration (41).

MODULATION OF PAIN PATHWAY

Modulation of pain pathway in human beings is performed by stimulation of three sites: the periventricular/periaqueductal gray matter in the brain, the dorsal column in the spinal cord, and the periphery, by percutaneous stimulation (acupuncture) and transcutaneous electrical nerve stimulation (TENS). TENS and acupuncture are considered adjunctive mechanical treatments for malignant pain (see Table 32.4).

Deep brain stimulation has been mainly applied to therapy of chronic noncancer pain (42), and was thought to have minimal application to therapy of pain due to

Table 32.4
Adjunctive Mechanical Treatments

> Physical and occupational therapy
>   Orthotic/prosthetic devices
>   Improve functionality
> Peripheral stimulation–produced analgesia
>   Transcutaneous electrical nerve stimulation
>   Acupuncture

malignancy (43), since a majority of these patients have become tolerant to exogenous opiates. This impression is challenged by a recent study. Seventeen patients with intractable pain secondary to progressive malignancy and tolerant to high doses of systemic or epidural narcotics were treated with electrical stimulation of the brain (44). Thirteen of the 17 patients achieved virtually complete pain relief, and 13 patients withdrew themselves totally from the exogenous narcotics within 2 weeks of deep brain stimulation. This successful analgesia with deep brain stimulation in narcotic-tolerant patients may be secondary to a nonopioid mechanism and not due to the accepted opioid mechanism. Therefore, deep brain stimulation may be an excellent alternative for the relief of intractable pain due to malignancy, even in those unresponsive or tolerant to the analgesic effect of opiates.

Dorsal column stimulation has been used in patients with malignant pain, but is reported to have only 50% efficacy (45). Phantom pain appears to respond better to this treatment than pain due to peripheral nerve lesions and acute pain (46).

Peripheral stimulation–induced analgesia by TENS or acupuncture has not been adequately studied in patients with malignant pain. In a noncontrolled study, TENS was found effective in 96% of patients with malignant pain during the first 10 days, decreasing to 11% by the end of 1 month (47).

NEUROABLATIVE PROCEDURES

Neuroablation can be performed by chemical or neurosurgical techniques (see Fig. 32.3). Neurosurgical techniques for pain control have been covered in Chapter 11 and are not dealt with in this review, with two exceptions.

Neurosurgical Procedures

Two neurosurgical techniques warrant special attention since these procedures have been widely used for the management of malignant pain: percutaneous chordotomy and hypophysectomy.

Percutaneous chordotomy, the interruption of the ascending spinothalamic tract, is usually done with stereotaxic technique at the cervical or thoracic level. After needle position confirmation, a lesion can be made by radiofrequency. In patients with malignant pain, 80% efficacy is reported immediately after the procedure, but this deteriorates to 60% in just a few weeks (48). Chordotomy is ideal in patients with unilateral pain in a dermatomal level below T10–T12, but who still have intact bowel and bladder function, intact motor function, and a life expectancy of 6 months to 1 year. One must use caution in patients with restricted pulmonary function on the ipsilateral side of the pain, since the spinothalamic tract decussates contralaterally, whereas motor fibers do not. If motor fibers to the intercostal nerves on the opposite side are

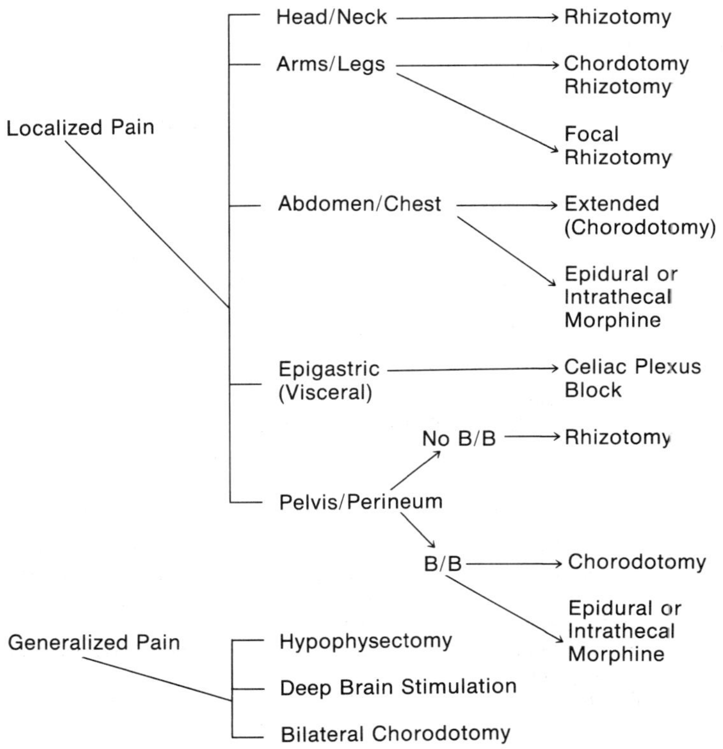

Figure 32.3. Neuroinvasive procedures. Rhizotomy may be surgical or chemical. B/B = bladder and bowel function.

affected by the chordotomy, the remaining normal lung function can deteriorate.

Hypophysectomy has been recommended for the management of pain due to hormone-dependent prostate or breast cancer. This can be accomplished by a transsphenoidal approach with injection of various destructive substances such as alcohol, water, or yttrium (49–51). Success is quoted in between 74 and 94% of patients with malignant pain, but long-term studies to demise have not been carried out.

Chemical Neurolysis

The use of neurolytic blocks by injection of various concentrations of neurolytic agents into the epidural, intrathecal, ganglia, and peripheral nerves has been used for more than 50 years (52). The most common agents used are phenol or alcohol, the concentration and volume being dependent on the site of injection. The type of neurolytic block performed is dependent on the site of injection and the pathophysiology of pain (Table 32.5). Distinguishing between nociceptive and deafferentation pain must be accomplished by neurologic examination and differential nerve blocking procedure prior to chemical neurolysis.

Further deafferentation with neuroablation must be avoided if the cause of pain is due to previous deafferentation, since the pain may get worse 3–6 months later. Neurolysis can be used only if the classic pharmacologic treatment of deafferentation does not produce adequate pain relief, and if life expectancy is less than 3–6 months.

To understand fully the indications and limitations of neurolytic block, discussion of available neurolytic agents and the success and limitations of commonly used neurolytic blocks is necessary.

Alcohol is perhaps the longest used neurolytic agent, initially used by Daglioti in 1936. It is used in concentration of 50–100%, depending on the site of injection (Table 32.6). Phenol, on the other hand, is available in concentrations of 4–10%, dissolved in 10–100% glycerol (Table 32.6). The differences between these two agents are best shown when they are injected intrathecally. One hundred per cent alcohol is hypobaric and 4–5% phenol in absolute glycerin is hyperbaric in relationship to the CSF specific gravity. Therefore, when alcohol is used, the patient is positioned so that the dorsal roots to be blocked are in the most superior position (53). With phenol, the patient is positioned so that the dorsal roots to be blocked are in the most dependent position (54). Alcohol, on injection, produces burning pain, sometimes making it difficult for the patient to maintain their critical position. Phenol, on the other hand, is not painful on injection, and is better tolerated by the patient. Success rates for intrathecal phenol and alcohol do not differ significantly, ranging from 46 to 63% despite decades of use.

Complications of intrathecal neurolysis are primarily those of bladder, bowel, and motor paresis (55). If intact bladder and/or bladder function exists, epidural or intrathecal morphine or percutaneous chordotomy may be a more appropriate alternative.

Epidural neurolysis with phenol or alcohol has been introduced as an alternative to intrathecal block, especially indicated for wide segmental block (56). The ideal application of this technique is in patients with chest or abdominal trunk pain. Concentrations for alcohol used for

Table 32.5
Choices for Neurolytic Block Sites

	Nociceptive pain	Deafferentation pain
Head and neck	Somatic nerve block of peripheral nerves	Upper and middle cervical ganglion block
Upper extremities	Cervical epidural or intrathecal block	Stellate ganglion block
Chest wall and thoracic viscera	Intercostal nerve block	Thoracic epidural or intrathecal block
	Thoracic epidural/ intrathecal block	
Abdomen		
Viscera	Celiac plexus block	Celiac plexus block
Wall	Thoracic epidural/ intrathecal block	
	Intercostal nerve block	
Lower extremities	Intrathecal phenol	Lumbar sympathetic block
	Epidural/intrathecal morphine	
Perineal	Intrathecal block	Caudal block
	Intrathecal/epidural morphine	
	Caudal block	

Table 32.6
Concentrations of Neurolytic Agents

	Alcohol	Phenol
Intrathecal	100%	4–15% in glycerol
Epidural	30%	10% in 10% glycerol
	100%	7% in water
Celiac plexus	50%	—
Sympathetic ganglion	50%	10% in 10% glycerol
Pituitary	100%	7% in water

epidural neurolysis range from 30 to 100%, and for phenol, 6–10%. Meaningful successful outcome of epidural neurolysis has not been adequately studied, but isolated reports indicate wide variations ranging from 33 to 90% success (54, 55, 57).

Another important neurolytic block for malignant pain that warrants special attention is celiac plexus block (58). Celiac plexus block is ideal for relief of malignant pain secondary to pancreatic carcinoma, retroperitoneal metastasis, peritoneal carcinomatoses, colon carcinoma, gastric carcinoma, and liver and spleen capsular distention. The needle is placed anterior to vertebral bodies T12–L1 under fluroroscopic guidance or CT scan and 40–50 ml of 50% alcohol are injected. The reported success rate ranges from 57 to 94% (58, 59).

Unfortunately, a majority of oncologists and surgeons are not aware of this procedure, and continue to manage their patients with narcotics, often aggravating impending colon obstruction with narcotic-induced ileus. Celiac plexus block can also be easily performed under direct vision during an exploratory laparotomy. This is particularly indicated if pancreatic carcinoma is diagnosed during exploration, since no oncologic therapy in the past 30 years has succeeded in prolonging the life expectancy of this group of patients.

ORCHESTRATION OF PHYSICAL TREATMENTS

To orchestrate the physical treatments available for malignant pain, one has to take into consideration several factors: life expectancy, natural history of the patient's malignancy, stage of the disease, rapidity of progression, and acceptability of procedures to the patient and family. Sensitivity to the patient's and family's goals and degree of acceptance of the progressive disease are of paramount importance in planning treatment. Since malignant pain can be stable, progressive, persistent, or recurrent at various stages, the physician placed in charge of controlling the pain should have a commitment to the patient until demise. Modalities should be made available to the patient for the persistent quest for pain relief.

Several principles useful for successful orchestration of modalities are:

1. Be sensitive to the changing needs of the patient as the disease progresses. Increased narcotic intake is associated with sudden progression of the disease, and not due to "addiction" potential in patients with malignant pain.
2. Start with a noninvasive, low-risk approach before proceeding to a more invasive, high-risk approach (see Fig. 32.1).
3. Relief of pain in one area may result in the awareness of pain in other areas.
4. The risk versus benefit ratio in every step should be explained to the patient and family, and the ultimate choice of alternatives be given to the patient.
5. Respect the patient's decision, even if it is not similar to yours. The ultimate goal of treatment is to provide comfort without sacrificing functions important to the patient and his/her family.

The orchestration of physical modalities is best illustrated by an actual case presentation. A 32-year-old female with cervical carcinoma metastatic to the sacral plexus and pelvic area was referred to the pain clinic because of persistent lower pelvic and perineal pain. The patient had undergone a total radical abdominal hysterectomy 4 months prior to admission, received radiation postoperatively, and was presently receiving chemotherapy. The patient still had intact bowel function, but had intermittent urinary incontinence. Computed tomography scan revealed a recurrent tumor anterior to the sacrum, beginning to erode into the sacral bone. The patient was receiving Tylenol with codeine, two tablets every 4 hr, whenever pain became severe. She was averaging 10–15 tablets/day; her pain decreased 30–40% for 2–3 hr after ingestion of the drug. She had become totally inactive, staying in bed most of the day. She took Valium (10 mg) at night for sleep, which only gave her 3–4 hr of sleep until she was awakened by the pain.

The first step in the treatment was analgesic tailoring. The patient was changed to the next step in the analgesic ladder (see Fig. 32.2) and given Percocet, two tablets given on a time-contingent, around-the-clock approach. Valium was discontinued and substituted with amitriptyline, (25 mg before sleep). This maneuver immediately decreased her pain level to 25% as measured by the Visual Analog Scale, a level acceptable to her. She was able to increase her activity during the day, spending more time with her children.

Two months later, she developed acute herpes zoster in her neck and arm after receiving a chemotherapeutic regimen. She was treated with intravenous acyclovir and steroids, but the lesions and pain persisted. On the third week, stellate ganglion block was performed at 3-day intervals, with 0.5% lidocaine and 80 mg Depo-Medrol (60, 61). After three blocks, her lesions resolved and pain subsided dramatically.

The patient did well until 1 month later when her perineal and pelvic pain escalated, with Percocet no longer providing pain relief. Urinary incontinence became complete and an indwelling catheter was inserted. Computed tomography scan showed further erosion of the tumor into the anterior scaral table. The patient still maintained anal spincter control.

Percocet was discontinued and methadone (5 mg, q4h) was started. This provided 50% relief. An epidural catheter was inserted at the L4–L5 level and directed downward. Morphine (5 mg) was injected, producing pain relief for 17 hr. A neurosurgeon was consulted for implantation of an indwelling epidural catheter with a portacath. The patient and family were instructed on how to continue morphine injections into the portacath at home. The patient obtained satisfactory pain relief until 2 months later.

At that time, the dose of epidural morphine was escalated to 20 mg every 6 hr, and failed to produce adequate pain relief. Repeat CT scan revealed further progression of metastasis. Bowel spincter control was lost at this point. Intrathecal phenol injection was presented to the patient as an alternative and was accepted. Phenol (2 ml of 5% in absolute glycerol) was injected intrathecally with the patient in a sitting position, relieving 75% of her pain. She was taught how to use patient-controlled analgesia, and went home with a portable device. She died at home 1 month later, pain free.

References

1. Foley KM: Pain syndromes in patients with cancer. In Bonica JJ, Ventafridda V (eds): *Advances in Pain Research and Therapy*. New York, Raven Press, 1979, vol 2, pp 59–75.
2. Wallenstein SL, Heidrich G, Kaiko R, et al: Clinical evaluation of mild analgesics: the measurement of clinical pain. *Br J Clin Pharmacol* 10(suppl):3195–3275, 1980.
3. Graham C, Bond SS, Gerkovich MM, et al: Use of the McGill Pain Questionnaire in the assessment of cancer pain: replicability and consistency. *Pain* 8:377–387, 1980.
4. Cohen R, Brechner T: The role and timing of neural blockade in the multidisciplinary management of cancer pain. In Gamez Q, Egay L (eds): *Proceedings of the 8th World Congress of Anesthesiology*. New York, Elsevier, 1984, pp 381–386.
5. Cleeland CS, Ratondi A, Brechner T, et al: A model for the treatment of cancer pain. 1:209–215, 1986.
6. Kanner RM, Foley KM: Patterns of narcotic drug use in cancer pain clinics. *Ann NY Acad Sci* 362:162–165, 1981.
7. Porter J, Jeck H: Addiction rate in patients treated with narcotics. *N Engl J Med* 302:123, 1980.
8. Foley KM: The treatment of cancer pain. *N Engl J Med* 313:84–95, 1985.
9. Moertel CC, Ahmann DL, Taylor WF, Schwartaul N: A comparative evaluation of marketed analgesic drugs. *N Engl J Med* 287:815–815, 1972.
10. Wallenstein SL: Analgesic studies of aspirin in cancer patients. In: *Proceedings of the Aspirin Symposium*. London, Aspirin Foundation, 1975, pp 5–10.
11. Houde RW, Wallenstein SL, Beaver WT: Clinical measurement of pain. In deStevens G (ed): *Anglesics*. New York, Academic Press, 1965, pp 75–122.
12. Moertel CG, Ahmann DL, Taylor WF, et al: Relief of pain by oral medications: a controlled evaluation of analgesic combinations. *JAMA* 229:55–59, 1974.
13. Matts SGF: A clinical comparison of panadeine Co, a soluble codeine Co and soluble aspirin in the relief of pain. *Br J Clin Pract* 20:515–517, 1966.
14. Kaiko RF, Foley KM, Gabrinski PY, et al: Central nervous system excitatory effects of meperidine in cancer patients. *Ann Neurol* 13:180–185, 1983.
15. Ferrer-Brechner T, Ganz P: Ibuprofen (Motrin, ®) as an analgesic potentiator of methadone (Dolophene, ®) in cancer patients. *Am J Med* 77(1A):78–83, 1984.
16. Payne R, Max M, Inturrisi C, et al: *Principles of Analgesic Use in the Treatment of Acute Pain and Chronic Cancer Pain: A Concise Guide to Medical Practice*. Washington, DC, The American Pain Society, 1987.
17. Reidenberg MM: Central nervous system excitatory effects of meperidine in cancer patients. *Ann Neurol* 13:180–185, 1983.
18. Watson CT, Evans RV, Reed K, et al: Amitriptyline versus placebo in postherpetic neuralgia. *Neurology* 32:671–673, 1982.
19. Max MB, Culnane M, Schafer SC, et al: Amitriptyline relieves diabetic neuropathy pain in patients with normal or depressed mood. *Neurology* 37:589–596, 1987.
20. Swerdlow M: Anticonvulsant drugs and chronic pain. *Clin Neuropharmacol* 7:51–82, 1984.
21. Forrest WH, Brown BW, Brown CR, et al: Dextroamphetamine with morphine for the treatment of postoperative pain. *N Engl J Med* 296:712–715, 1977.
22. Slattery PJ, Boas RA: Newer methods of delivery of opiates for the relief of pain. *Drugs* 30:539–551, 1985.
23. Inturrisi C: Newer methods of opioid drug delivery. International Association for the Study of Pain, Refresher Courses, August 2, 1987, 27–39.
24. Coyle N, Mauskop A, Maggard J, et al: Continuous subcutaneous infusions of opiates in cancer paitnets with pain. *Oncol Nurs Forum* 13:53–57, 1986.
25. Gourlay GK, Plummer JL, Kowalski DA, et al: An evaluation of the pharmacokinetics and efficacy of transdermal fentanyl in the treatment of postoperative pain. *Pain* Suppl 4:S229, 1987.
26. Cousins MJ, Mather LE: Intrathecal and epidural administration of opioids. *Anesthesiology* 61:276–310, 1984.
27. Yaksh TL, Atchison SR, Durant PAC: Characteristics of action and pharmacology of intrathecally administered D-Ala^2-D-Leu^5-enkephalin. In Foley KM, Inturrisi CE (eds): *Advances in Pain Research and Therapy*. New York, Raven Press, 1986, vol 8, pp 303–314.
28. Lord JAH, Waterford AA, Hughes J, et al: Endogenous opioid peptides: multiple agonists and receptors. *Nature* 267:495–499, 1977.
29. Onofrio BM, Yaksh TL: Intrathecal delta-receptor ligand products analgesia in man. *Lancet* 1:1386–1387, 1983.
30. Payne R, Inturrisi CE: CSF distribution of morphine, methadone and sucrose after intrathecal injection. *Life Sci* 37:1134–1137, 1985.
31. Omaya T, Jen T, Yamaga R: Profound analgesic effects of endorphin in man. *Lancet* 1:122–124, 1980.
32. Wang JK, Nauss LA, Thomas JE: Pain relief by intrathecally applied morphine in man. *Anesthesiology* 50:149–151, 1979.
33. Poletti CE, Cohen AM, Todd DP, et al: Cancer pain relieved by long term epidural morphine with permanent indwelling systems for self administration. *J Neurosurg* 55:581–584, 1981.
34. Coombs, PW, Saunders RL, Pageau MG: Continuous intrapsinal opioid analgesia; technical aspects of an implantable infusion system. *Reg Anaesth* 7:110–113, 1982.
35. Coombs, DW, Saunders RL, Gaylor MS, et al: Relief of continuous chronic pain by intraspinal opioid infusion via an implanted reservoir. *JAMA* 250:2336–2339, 1983.
36. Greenberg HS, Layton PB, Schroeder, et al: Continuous intrathecal morphine for intractable cancer pain. *Neurology* 33(S2):226, 1983.
37. Greenberg H, Enssinger W, Taren J, et al: Benefit from and tolerance to continuous intrathecal infusion of morphine for intractable cancer pain. *J Neurosurg* 57:360–364, 1982.
38. Keeri-Szanto M, Heaman S: Postoperative demand analgesia. *Surg Gynecol Obstet* 134:647–651, 1972.
39. Harmer M, Slattery PS, Rosen M, et al: Intramuscular on

40. Kay B: Postoperative pain relief: use of an on-demand analgesia computer (ODAC) and a comparison of the rate of fentanyl and alfentanyl. *Anesthesia* 36:949–951, 1981.
41. Tamsen A, Sjoestroem S, Hartvig P: The Uppsala experience of patient controlled analgesia. In Foley KM, Inturrissi CE (eds): *Advances in Pain Research and Therapy*. Raven Press, New York, 1986, vol 8, pp 325–331.
42. Young RF, Feldman RA, Kroening R, et al: Electrical stimulation of the brain in the treatment of chronic pain in man. In Kruger L, Liebeskind JC (eds): *Advances in Pain Research and Therapy*. New York, Raven Press, 1984, vol 6, pp 289–303.
43. Mayerson BA, Boethius J, Carlsson AM: Alleviation of malignant pain by electrical stimulation in the periventricular-periaqueductal region: pain relief as related to stimulation sites. In Bonica JS, Liebeskind JC, Albe-Fessard D (eds): *Advances in Pain Research and Therapy*. New York, Raven Press, 1979, vol 3, pp 523–533.
44. Young RF, Brechner T: Electrical stimulation of the brain for relief of intractable pain due to cancer. *Cancer* 57:1266–1272, 1986.
45. Long DM, Erickson DE: Stimulation of the posterior columns of the spinal cord for relief of intractable pain. *Surg Neurol* 4(1):134–141, 1975.
46. Krainick JR, Thoden U: Experience with dorsal column stimulation (DSC) in the operative treatment of chronic intractable pain. *J Neurosurg Sci* 18(3):187–189, 1974.
47. Ventafridda V, Sganzeria EP, Fochi C, et al: Transcutaneous stimulation in cancer pain. In Bonica JJ, Ventafridda V (eds): *Advances in Pain Research and Therapy*. New York, Raven Press, 1979, vol 2, pp 509–515.
48. Rosumoff HF, Carrall F, Brown J, et al: Percutaneous radiofrequency cervical chordotomy technique. *J Neurosurg* 23:639, 1965.
49. Katz J, Levin AB: Treatment of diffuse metastatic cancer pain by instillation of alcohol into the sella turcica. *Anesthesiology* 46(2):115–121, 1977.
50. Lipton S, Miles J, Williams N, et al: Pituitary injection of alcohol for widespread cancer pain. *Pain* 5(1):73–82, 1978.
51. Fitzpatrick JM, Gardiner RA, William JP, et al: Pituitary ablation in the relief of pain in advanced prostatic carcinoma. *Br Med J (Clin Res)* 284:75–76, 1981.
52. Swerdlow J: Subarachnoid and extradural neurolytic block. In Bonica JJ, Ventafridda V (eds): *Advances in Pain Research and Therapy*. New York, Raven Press, 1979, vol 2, pp 325–337.
53. Swerdlow M: Current views on intrathecal neurolysis. *Anesthesia* 33:733, 1978.
54. Ferrer-Brechner T: Epidural and intrathecal phenol neurolyses for cancer pain: review of rationale and techniques. *Reg Anaesth* 8(8):14–20, 1981.
55. Wood K: The use of phenol as a neurolytic agent: a review. *Pain* 5:205, 1978.
56. Colpitts MR, Levy BA, Lawrence M: Treatment of cancer-related pain with phenol epidural block (abstr). In *Proceedings of the World Congress on Pain*, Montreal, 1978. Pain Suppl 4, 1987.
57. Korevaar WC, Kline MT, Donnelly CC: Thoracic epidural neurolyses using alcohol. *Pain* Suppl 4:5133, 1987.
58. Thompson GE, Moore DC, Bridenbaugh LD, et al: Abdominal pain and alcohol celiac plexus nerve block. *Anesth Analg* 56(1):1–5, 1977.
59. Hankemeier U: Neurolytic celiac plexus block for cancer-related upper abdominal pain using the unilateral puncture technique and lateral position. *Pain* Suppl 4:135, 1987.
60. Tenicela R, Lovasek D, Eaglstein W: Treatment of herpes zoster with sympathetic blocks. *Clin J Pain* 1:63–67, 1985.
61. Perkins HM, Hanalon PR: Epidural injection of local anesthetic for the relief of pain secondary to herpes zoster. *Arch Surg* 113:253–254, 1978.

chapter 33
Psychological Management of Malignant Pain

Blake H. Tearnan, Ph.D.
Clay H. Ward, M.S.
Charles S. Cleeland, Ph.D.

THE PROBLEM

Pain due to cancer and its treatment is a major national health problem (1). It has been estimated that hundreds of thousands nationally and millions worldwide are affected. Depending on the type of cancer, as many as one-third of patients with metastatic disease and greater than two-thirds of terminally ill patients report pain severe enough to interfere with their social and physical activity and overall enjoyment of life (2). Cancer pain can also produce disturbances in sleep and appetite, causing adverse effects on health status.

The severity of the problem is reflected in the public's view of cancer as a very painful disease, equal to the pain caused by a myocardial infarction. Survey data suggest a significant minority of patients would delay or avoid treatment because of expected pain (3). Most persons questioned indicated cancer pain would be a sufficient reason to end one's life.

Comprehensive medical management can produce significant reductions in cancer pain. The integration of systemic analgesics, anti-inflammatory drugs, antidepressant medication, palliative radiotherapy and chemotherapy, and destruction of pain fibers by surgery and destructive nerve blocks can result in substantial pain relief. Unfortunately, the range of therapies available at most hospitals and clinics is limited to systemic analgesics alone. Data show only about 50% of cancer patients report good to excellent relief from these medications (4).

The psychological treatment of pain due to cancer might provide relief for patients not responding favorably to traditional or comprehensive medical management. This approach is appealing for several reasons. First, psychological factors often mediate pain perception. Second, behavioral management of pain can be taught by persons representing a wide variety of professional backgrounds. Third, this approach can be applied to other areas of patient distress such as anxiety and depression. Fourth, it may help to increase a patient's sense of mastery over his or her health and environment. Finally, it has no negative side effects. Although empirical support for behavior techniques is lacking (discussed below), their heuristic appeal, bolstered by the success of behavioral treatments of chronic pain and medicine's drawbacks, is promising.

BACKGROUND

The psychological treatment of cancer pain requires a basic understanding of cancer and the physical basis of cancer pain. It is also important for the behavioral clinician to recognize the many differences between assessment and treatment of chronic benign pain and pain of malignant origin. Cancer is a generic term that is used to describe a variety of different diseases that share in common the distortion of cell development leading to invasion of surrounding tissues and metastases. The primary site of cancer (e.g., lung, breast, prostate) determines many of its features, including rate of development, response to medical therapies, spread of disease, and the course, severity, and quality of pain. Foley (5) found that 85% of patients with primary bone tumors and 52% of patients with breast cancer had pain, in contrast to 20% with lymphomas and only 5% with leukemias. Taken as a whole, nearly one-third of all hospitalized cancer patients have pain requiring the use of analgesics and close to two-thirds of terminally ill patients report significant pain (6).

Cancer pain can result from diverse causes because of its multiple and primary metastatic sites. Foley (6) reported 78% of hospitalized cancer patients in pain had pain due to direct tumor involvement, with 50% the result of bone disease, 25% caused by nerve compression, and 3% due to invasion of hollow viscus. She discovered only 19% of patients had iatrogenically produced pain. Similar results were found in patients with advanced cancer (7). Most patients had multiple mechanisms for their pain.

Cancer pain caused by nerve damage or compression is similar in many ways to nerve-related pain of benign origin (7). Treatment-related pain can resemble the neuropathic pain associated with diabetes. Tumor invasion of bone produces pain that is different from most noncancerous pain syndromes. Patients often describe this pain as severe and throbbing. Unfortunately, it appears to be the most difficult type of cancer pain to manage, even with multimodal therapies.

Cancer pain is usually well managed early in the course of the disease or is not present, and immediate postoperative pain is effectively controlled with systemic analgesics. However, as the disease progresses, pain problems increase significantly. Daut and Cleeland (2) found that only 6% of cancer patients with nonmetastatic disease reported pain, whereas 33% of patients with metastases had pain.

The severity of the pain reported by patients with advanced disease is also generally higher than patients at initial diagnosis (2). Pain ratings of severity for the majority of cancer patients are moderate. Patients surveyed rated their pain at its worst close to the midpoint or lower on conventional pain scales. This contrasts with the widely held belief by health care providers and the general public that cancer pain is extremely painful (3). Comparing the severity of pain across different diseases, patients with metastatic cancer rated their worst pain at about the same level as patients with rheumatoid arthritis (2). Both the cancer and arthritic patients rated their worst pain at a significantly lower level than patients with chronic benign pain.

The relationship between pain and life adjustment problems for patients with chronic benign pain is well known. Many of these patients report difficulties in their marriages, work, and recreational activities. They also admit to significant levels of depression and other mood disturbance (8). Surprisingly, cancer pain does not appear to be strongly related to psychosocial problems, negative mood in particular. In one study, patients with advanced disease and moderate to severe pain at initial contact were interviewed and completed ratings of pain severity, mood, and activity (9). Patients completed the same scales for 5 consecutive months. The relationships among pain ratings and mood measures were examined. A significant but small correlation between pain severity and measures of negative mood was found. More compellingly, patients with end-stage disease and poorly controlled pain reported very little mood disturbance at any assessment period. Although these data need to be interpreted in light of several factors (e.g., artifacts of methodology), they appear robust in studies using alternative designs and subjects.

Even though cancer pain has not been strongly linked to adjustment difficulties, on an individual basis there is ample evidence that cancer patients are at risk for developing problems including depression, increased marital stress, fatigue, body image concerns, and anxiety; in many patients these problems are enduring (10). The comprehensive assessment and treatment of the cancer pain patient should be directed at pain reduction and amelioration of significant psychosocial problems.

Most psychologically based therapies for cancer pain are based on a chronic benign pain model where the absence of progressive disease is assumed. The fundamental principles and goals of treatment are helpful to many patients with active disease. However, cancer pain is unique in many ways, which suggests that many therapies currently being used to treat chronic benign pain do not apply or have to be qualified. For example, when pain is persistent but benign, complaints of pain can result in social alienation or may be reinforced by family members. Treatment efforts need to be aimed at discouraging the patient from reporting pain and teaching family members to ignore the patient's pain complaints. Continual reporting of pain that is benign and stable contributes little information that is diagnostically or therapeutically useful. However, patients with cancer pain need to report pain, and medical staff and family members should encourage and listen to their complaints. New pain can signal a change in disease status and reporting of pain is a prerequisite for proper titration of analgesics.

This is not to imply that clinicians should throw the baby out with the bath water by ignoring the role social reinforcement and other positive consequences play in exacerbating and maintaining cancer pain behavior. However, instead of attempting to eliminate the reinforcement of all pain behaviors, extinguishing pain behaviors that are clearly inappropriate or excessive would be an alternative therapeutic goal.

Cancer pain therapies also differ in the use of increased physical activity, which is a mainstay in the rehabilitation of chronic benign pain. Encouraging cancer patients to increase their physical activity can be counterproductive. Some patients experience pain only when active. Patients in pain due to vertebral metastases may endanger themselves if physically active.

The meaning of pain for the cancer patient also differs. More than a reminder of chronic debilitation and discomfort, it represents the presence of a life-threatening disease. The anxiety and uncertainty this may generate can influence the total pain experience and make it more difficult for the patient to cope.

Perhaps the most significant difference is the role analgesic and palliative medications play in the relief of pain. Elimination of analgesic medications has been advocated as an appropriate treatment goal for chronic benign pain patients. This goal is motivated by concern about psychological addiction, physical dependence, and the depressant and mental blurring effects of narcotics. Although it is beyond the scope of this chapter to examine the use of analgesics in chronic pain, it must be emphasized that reduction of the analgesics is rarely a goal for the patient with progressive malignant disease. Quite the contrary, patients need to be taught to recognize the role that analgesics play in pain control and how and when to take them. They also need to be taught how to request needed analgesics so that they are most likely to receive them.

Many cancer patients are undermedicated for pain (11, 12). Physicians are often reluctant to prescribe analgesics in effective doses because of concerns about addiction and the rapid development of narcotic tolerance and respiratory depression. Much of the problem of undermedication, however, has its basis in patients' beliefs and attitudes. For instance, patients may refuse to follow a medication schedule carefully designed to maintain effective blood levels of analgesics, instead taking medications only when pain is unbearable because they do not want to think of themselves as addicts. They may not wish to report that the medications they are taking are not effective because to do so would "bother the doctor." Some patients may want to avoid taking narcotics because of the belief that narcotic dependence is acknowledging that their disease is beyond hope (13).

The psychological management of cancer pain should never be used as a substitute for analgesics. Its use to ease staff's concern about narcotic addiction is rarely in the patient's best interest. If patients volunteer that they want to reduce their analgesics after some success with psychological management, this can be attempted on a trial basis following medical consultation.

Identifying patients appropriate for psychological intervention of cancer pain is a difficult task. There are no empirical guidelines to assist the clinician. Some clinicians have suggested that patients who have pain that is adequately controlled by analgesics with few side effects are poor candidates for behavioral treatment. Few of them are motivated to expend the time and effort to learn behavioral methods. At the other extreme are patients with severe pain that limits their capacity to learn new skills. The best candidates appear to be patients with moderate pain that is not adequately controlled by analgesics.

ASSESSMENT OF THE PAIN PROBLEM

The aim of assessment is twofold. First, the clinician must pinpoint and define the entire domain of pain behaviors across cognitive, overt behavioral, and physiologic response dimensions. Second, stimuli associated with the occurrence and recurrence or exacerbation of the pain behavior need to be identified. This requires a knowledge of frequently occurring controlling variables unique to cancer pain and attention to the multitude of factors that can affect the assessment process and influence a patient's report of pain.

RESPONSE DIMENSIONS
Cognitive Responses

The assessment of cancer pain requires an understanding of the patient's cognitions, including an analysis of cognitive errors and self-statements. Cognitive errors refer to maladaptive patterns of thinking that are unrealistic and distorted. They are assumed to be causally related to the maintenance and exacerbation of the pain complaint and can interfere with treatment. Cancer pain patients can present several different types of cognitive errors. Frequently observed are thoughts that they can do nothing to reduce their pain or that they should have better control over their pain problem than they do, and the belief that pain is inevitable and should be tolerated. Self-statements are thoughts patients may have regarding their pain, such as "the pain is frightening," or "it hurts so bad." Self-statements are internal dialogues patients have that reflect the cognitive appraisal of their pain state. Self-statements differ from cognitive errors in that they have not been analyzed to represent some underlying belief system or faulty logic such as "I will never be able to overcome this problem." Both cognitive errors and self-statements can be assessed during the interview by direct questioning, but often the most reliable method is to have patients self-monitor their pain. The patient is instructed to use pain diaries to record any thoughts or feelings that accompany the pain when it is at its worst (14).

Overt Behavioral Responses

The pain behavior of cancer patients can include the verbal and nonverbal responses patients use to communicate the experience of pain, such as facial grimacing, limping, bracing, and groans. Estimates of physical activity are also useful. Measures of time spent in bed, physical exercise, amount of housework, and the like have all been employed with chronic pain patients (15). Because cancer patients may be physically disabled as a result of their disease or the effects of treatment, the use of activity measures should be limited to the range of behaviors in which patients are physically capable of engaging but that are restricted because of pain.

The amount and type of pain medication usage is another overt behavioral measure of pain that is frequently reported. The milligram dosage per day and the specific type of palliative drug prescribed or taken should be recorded. Because analgesic orders vary with practice setting and patients may not accurately report levels of pain to their physicians prescribing the drugs or take the medications as prescribed, the reliability of medication usage as a measure of the pain experience is questionable.

Overt pain behavior can be collected through direct observation by others, such as nursing personnel, other therapists, and significant others. Simple rating sheets can be constructed for use on a time-sampling basis, or the behaviors can be recorded at the end of a specific time period. Unfortunately, systematic ratings can be costly in terms of observation time, interference with other procedures, and training observers to an acceptable reliability criterion. Although recording sheets used once daily are more convenient and practical, there is some loss of reliability due to memory interference.

The self-report of overt pain behaviors can also be gathered. This includes the self-monitoring of pain behaviors or information obtained from pain behavior inventories or by interview. The problem of reliability with any self-report instrument is well known. However, these measures are easily obtainable, economical, and sometimes the only instruments used, especially with cancer patients. One very useful self-report measure of overt pain behavior is rating of pain interference in activity. It has been shown to be significantly correlated with mood, pain intensity, and physical disability in cancer patients (4).

It deserves mention that any self-report instrument used with cancer patients should be simple and brief. Many patients are quite ill and obtunded because of their disease or high narcotic doses and will not be able to follow complicated instructions, or will be too fatigued to complete lengthy measures. An additional reason for simplicity is patient compliance. Patients do not always share the clinician's enthusiasm for comprehensive data bases.

Sensory-Physiologic Responses

The final response system is physiologic. Measures of heart rate, muscular activity, respiration, and other responses have been used to estimate autonomic arousal and pain severity. Unfortunately, the usefulness of these measures, with the possible exception of muscular activity, is of questionable value, especially in chronic pain. Most reports have not shown a clear relationship between physiologic measures and degree of pain (16).

Instead, clinicians have relied upon patients' descriptions of the sensory-physiologic aspects of their pain, including intensity, temporal aspects, location, and quality (17). Intensity measures are usually simple numeric rating scales of subjective pain intensity. They normally require the patient to rate his or her average, worst, least, and present pain on a 10-point scale or an equivalent visual analogue scale without numeric anchors during a specific time period such as the last week or month. The temporal aspects of the patient's pain are usually assessed for frequency and duration. Most cancer patients will complain of constant, daily pain. However, fluctuations in the pain most likely occur and should be documented. Location parameters of the pain are collected by having patients shade the location of their pain on the front and back of human figures, or simply by describing where the affected area is located. The patient can be asked to indicate if the pain is deep or shallow. Finally, the measure of pain quality is obtained by asking patients to describe their pain using words such as "burning," "stabbing," and "cramping."

Pain quality ratings have been shown to be a useful alternative to assessing pain intensity with cancer patients. Tearnan and Cleeland (18) found that cancer patients who reported high levels of pain intensity tended to use certain sensory words such as "sharp," "gnawing," and "pressing" more frequently than patients who rated their pain intensity lower. In addition, it was found that without the aid of word lists as prompts, patients' word usage overall was limited to a few sensory descriptions. Very few evaluative words and virtually no affective descriptors were used.

Physiologic data can be obtained with the use of sophisticated instrumentation such as electromyographic recordings. Usually, however, patients are simply asked to describe their pain and its location or they are instructed in self-monitoring. Again, the use of some procedures is limited with cancer patients. A great deal depends on the physical status of the patient, as well as what is permissible and appropriate in the setting where the cancer patient is being treated. One method of collecting ongoing pain intensity ratings as well as other measures of pain by nursing and additional health care staff for use with inpatients is to place a recording sheet directly in the patient's chart with clear instructions (19).

PAIN PRECIPITATORS

One of the most important aspects of assessment is examining the relationships among the exacerbation of pain and various cognitive, behavioral, physiologic, emotional, and environmental stimuli. Cognitive stimuli can include any thoughts, beliefs, or images cancer patients have that appear to aggravate or trigger their pain state. Clinicians using numerous examples of verbal and imaginal prompts to systematically explore potential cognitive antecedents will yield more than asking the simple question, "Are there any thoughts or images that seem to make your pain worse?" Examples of cognitive antecedents cancer patients have identified include images of fire, a red-hot poker, or a sharp knife, and thoughts that the pain is all-consuming and out of control and nothing can be done to control it, as well as "I must be weak-minded because I cannot tolerate the pain." Many cognitive antecedents will also be useful in defining the cognitive response of pain. Whether they should be included as antecedent stimuli is based on the presumption that they may also exacerbate or trigger the pain state.

By far the largest category of antecedent stimuli are behaviors cancer patients engage in that contribute to the onset or worsening of pain. These behaviors can include certain bodily movements such as bending, twisting, coughing, and reaching as well as activities such as walking, getting out of bed, eating, standing, and sitting. Cancer patients with vertebral metastases will experience pain with many movements and may have to confine themselves to bed because of the dangers of fracture, whereas patients with prostatic disease may experience pain whenever they engage in weight-bearing activities. Each cancer patient will differ, and only a thorough assessment will uncover the particular behaviors that contribute to the experience of pain.

Physiologic pain precipitants include the disease, but also disease- and treatment-related adverse effects that make patients more vulnerable or intolerant to pain sensation. For example, fatigue, nausea, weakness, and dry mouth are commonly observed. In addition, the ingestion of stimulants or other substances can substantially alter the biochemistry of the patients and modify the pain response.

Emotional upset can also be related to the patient's pain complaint. It is well understood that anxiety and depression can alter the experience of pain. The cancer patient who has just been informed that his or her disease has progressed and metastasized to the lung will undoubtedly be anxious and report higher levels of pain, especially since the pain can serve as a constant reminder of the disease process. Questions that elicit from patients information that the pain is less, the same, or worse when they are relaxed or in a good mood need to be a standard part of the assessment inquiry.

Environmental factors can often precipitate pain, and may are unique to the hospital setting. For example, patients may complain that their pain seems to worsen when they are alone or when the doctors are making their rounds. Frequently, patients state that their pain is hardest to cope with when they are not comfortable because their bed is cold or too hard or there is too much noise in the hallways for them to rest properly (19). Staff or family behaviors can also be correlated with pain.

Antecedent events must be operationally defined and reliability understood between clinician and patient and/or staff. Simplicity and specificity are the rules of a good behavioral description. Too often patients and staff are asked to monitor pain and note the presence or absence of antecedent events without being sure what to look for.

PAIN DIMINISHERS

The next step in the assessment process is exploring factors that help reduce the patients' pain severity. A thorough coverage of pain diminishers needs to include the same general categories used to systematically uncover pain antecedents, that is, cognitive coping strategies that the patient may engage in to help lessen the pain should be examined. These include self-statements, ignoring the pain, reinterpreting the pain, praying, and distraction (15). Cancer patients, like chronic pain patients, will differ in their use of strategies that they find helpful. Common behavioral pain diminishers include bed rest, physical or social activity as distractors, use of heating pads, and warm baths. Medication and alcohol are common physiologic pain reducers. The type of medication, amount, and percentage of pain relief are usually assessed. Finally, environmental events that can diminish pain will vary with the setting and resources the patient is exposed to. For instance, some hospitals provide support groups that many cancer patients find useful in helping to cope with their pain.

CONSEQUENCES

The immediate consequences of the patients' pain behavior need to be assessed to determine if medical staff or significant others are reinforcing behaviors that are clearly inappropriate or excessive. It will be recalled that most pain behaviors emitted by cancer patients should be attended to and strengthened since pain can signal new or recurrent disease and communication of pain is necessary for the titration of analgesics. However, pain behaviors that foster unneeded dependency and helplessness or seem unreasonable may be targets for later intervention.

ONSET, HISTORY, AND DEVELOPMENT

A thorough assessment strategy should examine the onset, history, and development of the pain complaint. This information is important since it helps the clinician put the problem in perspective and may lead to the discovery of antecedent stimuli that were overlooked. The knowledge of previous therapy attempts is also important to know since steps need be taken to correct the inadequacies of past failures and build on previous successes. Analyzing the development of the patient's pain problem will provide clues regarding past coping attempts and over what time frame changes in the pain occurred.

OTHER COMPLICATIONS

Cancer pain can produce adverse changes in mood, work, family, physical activity, and interpersonal relationships (4). These are areas that need to be routinely evaluated to determine the overall impact of the pain problem on the patient's life. These changes, if pronounced, can compromise the patient's response to medical treatment and interfere significantly with the quality of life. They can also amplify the pain experience. Ratings of pain interference in mood, pleasant activities, and overall enjoyment of life can be used in addition to more traditional assessment tools. Interviews with significant others can also provide worthwhile information regarding the impact pain has had on the family and marriage.

FORMULATION

Formulating a treatment plan and making predictions regarding the patient's response to intervention is the final step in the assessment process. This is accomplished by generating several hypotheses about the onset, development, and maintenance of the patient's pain complaint and proposing a treatment intervention based on these conclusions that would most likely result in the desired change. For instance, cancer patients who report that anxiety exacerbates their pain, and report diminished pain after receiving diazepam, might be good candidates for relaxation/biofeedback therapy.

ASSESSMENT INSTRUMENTS

There are numerous instruments that can assist the clinician in the assessment process. Some have been designed specially for pain assessment and others are used primarily for determining the patient's level of mood and personality disturbance. Most are self-report measures. Cancer patients are often unable to complete a comprehensive test battery or lengthy test, such as the Minnesota Multiphasic Personality Inventory (MMPI), because of their medical status. The best assessment tool for this population is one that can be easily understood with minimal instructions and is relatively short. It should require little administrative supervision by psychological staff. Additionally, nurses and other health care staff should find the instrument useful and easily interpretable. Finally, it should include items that sample pain behaviors as well as mood disturbance.

The Pain Research Group at the University of Wisconsin Medical School developed the Wisconsin Brief Pain Inventory (BPI) for the specific purpose of administration to cancer pain patients (20). The BPI is a short questionnaire that usually requires only 10 minutes for the patient to complete. It includes several types of items such as whether or not the patient has had any surgery in the last month; front and back human figures with instructions for the patient in pain to shade the painful area; numeric ratings of worst, average, least, and present pain intensity; requests for the patient to describe any pain diminishers or antecedents that have been associated with pain relief or exacerbation; current pain treatments; and questions regarding response to treatment. In addition, the patient is also instructed to rate several pain adjectives, such as "throbbing" and "burning," on a scale of 0 to 10. Another section of the questionnaire includes several items that ask patients how much they feel their pain has interfered with their mood, general activity, walking ability, normal work, relations with other people, sleep, and enjoyment of life. Finally, the questionnaire contains a shortened version of the Profile of Mood States (POMS) that has been shown to be statistically equivalent to the complete scale (21). The POMS was included to screen for mood disturbance. The BPI has demonstrated respectable validity and reliability and has been shown to be a useful pre- and post-treatment measure (20).

GENERAL ASSESSMENT ISSUES

Several issues need to be addressed when assessing the cancer pain patient. These matters can significantly affect an evaluation, and unless the clinician is cognizant of their presence they can lead to spurious conclusions and/or disrupt the assessment process.

Setting

Most cancer patients in pain are inpatients or outpatients at medical centers. They are receiving ongoing cancer therapy or palliative care, or are being evaluated periodically for recurrence of their disease. In most cases when conventional therapy fails to relieve pain, a member of a liaison service specializing in pain is requested to consult. The role of a consultant in a medical setting is that of an expert who is expected to render an opinion quickly without consuming too much of the patient's time. Under these circumstances, lengthy procedures are unsuitable since the consultant often has to present recommendations after only one session. This necessitates a streamlined version of an ideal assessment. If the consultant is expected to treat the patient, he or she can afford more elaborate procedures but is still limited by the brief residence of inpatients and by the physical and mental incapacitation of many patients.

The clinician should be sensitive to the patient's primary care providers, who may not share their enthusiasm for psychological control of pain and may see the intervention as an interference. Unfortunately, these negative opinions can sometimes be communicated to the patient and compliance reduced. Frequent physician updates on the patient's progress and rationale for particular assessment and treatment protocols can help eliminate many obstacles.

Overcoming a Reluctance to Participate

Cancer pain patients are medical patients. Oftentimes the patient's beliefs about the role of a psychologist or other behavioral clinician run counter to their expectations for being treated for medical problems. As a result, some patients are reluctant to participate in assessment or treatment. DeGood (22) discussed practical ways in which to overcome this barrier and increase compliance with chronic pain patients. His suggestions can be applied to cancer patients in pain. In brief, he first explains to patients that he is a psychologist and reassures them that often pain produces changes in one's life that can affect work, mood, and so forth. According to DeGood, this usually helps to de-escalate the implicit message that "the referral was because the doctor thinks the pain is all in my head." Although the credibility of cancer patients is rarely questioned regarding the organic basis of their pain, they may have a history of diagnostic procedures in which nothing was discovered, and may believe that the severity of the pain and their inability to tolerate it is related to psychological weaknesses. DeGood mentions that this initial explanation also helps challenge the belief that because psychological variables may be correlated with the exacerbation of pain this makes the physical problem less legitimate.

DeGood recommended that the interview initially focus on physical symptoms. This helps reduce the defensiveness of the patient and establish the credibility of the behavioral clinician. He advised that when assessing other aspects of the pain complaint, such as depression, these topics be introduced with a statement to the effect that "pain often makes us feel . . . ." Patients are often reluctant to admit to emotional problems since doing so confirms the belief that something is wrong mentally. Finally, we have found that cancer patients need to be assured that their participation in no way indicates that their medical therapy, including the use of analgesic medications, will be jeopardized.

Factors Affecting the Report of Pain

Numerous factors can influence a patient's report of pain. The clinician should be familiar with the more frequently occurring factors since they can significantly affect how cancer patients communicate their pain. For instance, the patient's history can influence how pain is reported. Patients who have received support in the past from health care professionals for their pain problem and for requesting medication will be more inclined to admit to pain.

Often cancer patients are reluctant to report pain because of beliefs that discourage disclosure (4). One study found that many cancer patients do not complain of pain because they believe there is a social stigma attached to people who do (23). Other patients admit that they do not want to bother their doctor or distract him or her from their medical treatment. Our society also reinforces the notion that a good patient does not complain when in pain and a complainer is one who has lost self-control. Unfortunately, health care professionals sometimes directly reinforce these beliefs (19).

The nature of the pain itself can also influence a patient's report. A patient who has severe pain may be more motivated to admit to pain and request medications than patients experiencing mild or moderate pain. Yet, certain pain locations, such as rectal or genital, can discourage reports of pain because of personal embarrassment (24). Patients will acknowledge pain more readily if it is constant as opposed to episodic. The expectation of pain-free periods can increase the patient's tolerance level (19). Finally, patients experiencing significant interferences in mood and physical activity because of their pain may be more likely to communicate their experience.

The stage of disease may also affect the report of pain. Abrams (25) wrote an intriguing paper in which she observed that cancer patients are less likely to communicate to others as their disease progresses. She found that newly diagnosed patients are optimistic and hopeful concerning treatment and anxiety is lessened by direct answers to questions. As the disease advances, there is a change in what patients desire to know and to whom they direct their questions. Patients develop a fear of abandonment by their physician that is managed by becoming compliant and uncomplaining. In the terminal stages, communication becomes minimal and support from others is more important. Although Abrams did not address the issue of pain communication specifically, the points she raised certainly have many implications for pain assessment.

Other variables influencing the pain report of cancer and chronic pain patients that have been mentioned in the literature include neuroticism (26), level of awareness and education (27), depression and chronicity (28), use of certain medications (29), desire to manipulate treatment (30), and staff support of pain complaints (29). Each of these factors should be considered in the assessment process.

PSYCHOLOGICAL TREATMENT APPROACHES

Psychological interventions have received increasing attention in the management of cancer pain (31–35). These approaches are similar to psychological treatments used in the management of chronic, nonmalignant pain. Although the application of therapies shown to be effective in the management of chronic, nonmalignant pain to the management of cancer pain is a logical extension of theory and clinical practice, it should be reemphasized that cancer pain is distinct in many ways. Consequently, treatments shown to be effective in treating chronic, nonmalignant pain cannot be assumed to be equally efficacious in treating cancer pain. The purpose of this section is to discuss treatment-related issues and briefly outline psychological approaches that appear to have promise in the management of cancer pain. The primary purpose is not to detail or recommend proven techniques, since there is a paucity of empirical literature to support the efficacy of any particular psychological intervention in the management of cancer pain. In many ways, this section is an invitation for research in this area, since empirical research and clinical evaluation of treatment outcome are the first order of business.

Individuals responsible for the delivery of treatment need a certain level of training and sophistication. However, most of these techniques can be implemented by individuals with a wide variety of professional backgrounds who have a core of interpersonal skills typically associated with successful behavioral change (36). Our own experience indicates that oncology nurses can be readily trained to effectively teach and implement the majority of psychological pain control techniques. Hypnosis might be the exception that is reserved for induction by professional psychological or other specially trained staff, but even this restriction is based more on caution than common sense. It seems unlikely that self-hypnosis taught by persons with limited hypnotic training presents major problems when restricted to relaxation and pain control.

Training of staff members in psychological pain management should include an educational component covering psychological assessment, conceptualization, and treatment of cancer pain; a skills acquisition and rehearsal component with behavioral modeling, rehearsal, feedback, and reinforced practice; and training in general factors of behavior change and psychotherapy. Once treatment is implemented, follow-up consultations are important so that treatment effectiveness can be measured and, if necessary, adjustments in the treatment plan recommended. Ongoing assessment and evaluation of treatment effectiveness is especially important given the complex nature and changing clinical presentation of cancer pain.

Ongoing assessment and evaluation is important from another perspective. An assessment that fails to consider ongoing changes in disease, person, or situation variables is often responsible for treatment failure. The spectrum and variety of cancer pain patients necessitates the understanding of the temporal setting and origin of the pain in order to determine the most effective therapeutic approach (5). It is the selection and combination of psychological pain control techniques tailored to the specific characteristics of the individual cancer pain patient that determines successful intervention.

Cancer pain patients experience both acute and chronic pain that may be due to the disease itself and/or its treatment. At least four different types of cancer pain patients can be identified, each with different treatment requirements (5, 33). One group consists of patients with no active disease but chronic, persistent post-treatment pain. These patients are free of active disease, but may have pain due to postsurgical scarring, neuropathy induced by chemotherapy, or postradiation myelopathy or fibrosis. Because the disease has been arrested, these patients are not good candidates for continued narcotic medication. Instead, the treatment approach should be similar to interventions used for patients with chronic, nonmalignant pain.

Patients with acute treatment-related pain or those preparing for cancer therapy that will produce pain represent a second group of pain patients. Pain in these patients is often adequately controlled by properly prescribed analgesics (5). However, some will experience pain that is refractory to traditional medical management. Psychological approaches to pain control might be of benefit to this subgroup of patients. In addition, psychological approaches might also be useful for reducing anticipatory anxiety with patients undergoing painful and frightening treatment procedures.

A third group of cancer patients have chronic pain due to active disease with a prognosis of at least several months. Patients with an indefinite prognosis are often good candidates for psychological pain-control techniques. Most individuals in this group are receiving narcotic and other analgesic drugs. They may want to continue working or managing their households, continue with avocational activities, and/or have an active family life. In order to stay active, they may want to reduce their use of analgesic medications to minimize side effects, primarily mental blurring. Many will elect to learn psychological control techniques to increase their sense of control over some aspect of their disease. Some patients might also want to manage other areas of disease-related discomforts such as nausea, sleep disturbances, and procedurally related anxiety. Unlike the patient with arrested disease, but like the patient preparing for painful treatment procedures, the appropriate use of narcotic medication is important. Issues of addiction, tolerance, dependence, scheduling, and sufficient plasma levels need to be reviewed on an individual basis.

A fourth group of patients are those in the terminal stages of illness. With this group of patients, it is very important to review all available medical management techniques for potential benefit to the individual. Psychological pain-control techniques may still be useful, but it is important to recognize factors that might limit the applicability of some techniques. The patient's ability to concentrate and to remember is often restricted by alliative medications and fatigue. Cognitive functioning may be additionally impaired if brain metastases are present. Sufficient time to implement or teach pain management techniques will also be limited.

At this point, it is not clear which psychological pain control techniques are most effective for each group of cancer pain patients. With the exception of patients in the terminal stages of illness, most psychological approaches to pain management seem applicable. However, research is needed to indicate which techniques are most effective with which patients.

PSYCHOTHERAPY

Psychotherapy as an approach to pain control is based on the assumption that the perception of pain occurs within a personal and interpersonal context. The general premise is that dealing with critical intra- and interpersonal issues will reduce the impact of pain. It has been argued that psychotherapy aimed at relieving the emotional distress, anxiety, or depression associated with either the diagnosis of cancer or cancer pain can often have a favorable influence on the patient's experience of pain (32, 35, 37). Suggested techniques include education and reality orientation, support, reassurance, encouragement, group and family therapy, and activities designed to facilitate enrichment of remaining time such as activities palnning and participation, goal setting, and positive expectations. Unfortunately, there is no direct empirical evidence for the benefits of psychotherapy in reducing cancer pain. Psychotherapy and psychosocial interventions have been shown to be effective in ameliorating emotional distress and improving the quality of life (38–41); however, the direct effect of such interventions on cancer pain has not been demonstrated.

HYPNOSIS

Hypnosis is probably the oldest and most widely used psychological approach to pain management for cancer patients. Numerous clinical reports have appeared in the literature over the last three decades to support its efficacy in treating cancer pain (42–48). Hypnosis has also been reported to be effective in treating emotional distress, anxiety, or treatment-related discomfort in cancer patients (49). Although the literature reports that 20–50% of cancer patients benefit from hypnosis (35), this evidence is largely anecdotal and based on uncontrolled studies.

Hypnotic pain-reduction techniques overlap somewhat with relaxation and cognitive-behavioral techniques. The five major techniques that have been used for analgesia and the treatment of cancer pain are anesthesia, direct diminution, sensory substitution, displacement, and dissociation (50, 51). The technique of anesthesia refers to hypnotic suggestions that render a body area numb and insensitive to pain.

Direct diminution and sensory substitution are techniques that change the meaning of pain so that it is less important and painful. Direct diminution employs suggestions that focus on the lessening of the intensity of the pain. These suggestions often use metaphors, such as turning down the volume or dimming the brightness analogies. Sensory substitution also tries to modify painful stimuli, but the suggestions focus more on creating a sensory substitution or a reinterpretation of the sensation. For example, the painful sensation might be reinterpreted as a sensation such as coldness, tingling, or itching. Barber (51) indicated that both of these techniques are effective and easier to use than anesthesia because they allow the patient to still know the pain is present and the sensations are not necessarily pleasant. Consequently, the suggestion seems more plausible to the patient. Barber also argues that these techniques are most effective when the suggestions incorporate the qualities of the patient's subjective experience of pain.

Displacement suggestions are used to displace the pain from one body area to another. The applicability of this technique is limited primarily to pain that is well localized and painful by virtue of its localization. A change in the quality or intensity is sometimes achieved by changing the location.

Dissociation refers to hypnotic suggestions to create a sense of dissociation from the pain. Often this technique is used with individuals confined to a bed. The suggestions are used to dissociate the body of pain from the patient's awareness. Patients are still able to perceive and describe the pain, but there is less affective involvement and it is less distressing.

Posthypnotic suggestions and self-hypnosis are additional techniques that are used to extend the pain relief. These techniques appear useful in rehabilitation where the goal is to maintain activity levels. Posthypnotic suggestions attempt to establish a cue that initiates the pain-relief experience. For example, one suggestion might instruct the patient that whenever they see a clock they "will discover at the same time how comfortable and relaxed they really feel, as if they are at peace with time." Other posthypnotic suggestions are based on functional cues, such as the perception of pain. Self-hypnosis is thought to be especially effective in creating long-term pain relief (51).

Despite numerous shortcomings, including the absence of comparison groups, a few studies examining the use of hypnosis in the treatment of cancer pain deserve mention. An early uncontrolled study by Butler (52) showed that 5 out of 12 patients benefited from hypnosis and that depth of trance was the critical factor in determining the effectiveness of hypnosis in relieving pain. Depth of trance and a high degree of hypnotic susceptibility have been cited by others as important in hypnotic pain relief (53, 54). Finer (55), however, suggested that depth of trance is not important, but susceptibility is the major determinant of effectiveness. Yet, susceptibility is often uncertain and difficult to predict without actually hypnotizing the patient (55). Clearly, research is needed to resolve the role of depth of trance and individual differences in susceptibility in the use of hypnosis to treat cancer pain.

Kellerman et al. (56) used a hypnotic induction with suggestions of muscle relaxation, rhythmic breathing, and pleasant imagery. When their subjects appeared to be deeply relaxed, they gave posthypnotic suggestions of reduced discomfort, greater mastery during painful medical procedures, and an increased sense of well-being. Based on self-report, the hypnosis was effective in reducing anxiety and discomfort in 16 adolescents undergoing painful medical procedures. Unfortunately, there were no objective behavioral observations of anxiety or discomfort during the procedures and no control groups.

Zeltzer and LeBaron (57) presented data from a controlled study on the use of hypnosis in pediatric cancer patients undergoing bone marrow aspirations and lumbar puncture. Their study included both subjective self-report and objective ratings of anxiety and pain. They compared hypnosis consisting of imagery and fantasy to a nonhypnotic technique of deep breathing, distraction, and practice sessions. Both treatment procedures were effective in reducing pain and anxiety, but hypnosis was significantly more effective.

A study by Spiegal and Bloom (58) evaluated the effectiveness of hypnosis in treating disease-related breast cancer pain. Patients were randomly assigned to a control group, a weekly support group, or a support group with self-hypnosis exercises. The difference between support groups was a 10–15-min weekly training session in self-hypnosis using sensory substitution by having the patients imagine competing sensations in the affected areas. Self-report measures of pain at 4- and 13-month follow-ups revealed that the self-hypnosis group had the lowest pain ratings. However, conclusions regarding the superiority of self-hypnosis are tempered by the facts that both treatment groups showed smaller increases in pain over time compared to the control group and that direct statistical analyses of group means was not reported. Thus, the results suggest that psychological interventions, including self-hypnosis, are effective, but little can be concluded about the comparative benefits of hypnosis.

As stated earlier, controlled studies on the effectiveness of hypnosis in treating cancer pain are lacking. Furthermore, available studies are deficient in ways that limit conclusions regarding the effectiveness of hypnosis in treating cancer-related pain. In addition to the problems common to most research on psychological approaches to cancer pain, such as the absence of control groups and failure to use multimodal and objective pain measures, there are several difficulties specific to hypnosis. A major problem is the lack of standardized and clearly defined hypnotic induction and therapeutic techniques. Hilgard and Hilgard (46) have suggested that research on hypnosis should measure hypnotic susceptibility prior to treatment, clearly define and delineate hypnotic inductions and therapeutic techniques, and use more objective, multimodal measures. A measure of depth of trance would also be useful.

RELAXATION AND BIOFEEDBACK

Relaxation Training

There are several techniques for inducing a state of physiological and mental relaxation, ranging from passive techniques such as yoga and meditation to the more active relaxation technique of progressive muscle relaxation (59). The two most commonly used relaxation procedures are progressive muscle and autogenic relaxation. Progressive muscle relaxation consists of systematically tensing and relaxing 14–16 muscle groups (60–62). The introduction, exact order, and number of muscle groups involved varies, but common to all protocols is approximately 10 sec of tensing followed by 10–15 sec of relaxation. Although therapeutic implementation is relatively easy, a certain degree of training and experience in the techniques is important to ensure effectiveness (60, 62).

Autogenic relaxation is a more passive relaxation technique (63, 64). In autogenic relaxation, the patient is instructed to use self-statements and visual images to achieve relaxation. Typically, autogenic relaxation exercises begin with suggestions of heaviness, warmth, and relaxation of specific muscle groups until the whole body is involved. Often additional phrases are added to quiet emotions and mental states such as "I feel at ease" and "My mind is quiet and calm."

Most relaxation techniques adhere to a format of 6–10 weekly sessions in which the techniques are modeled and rehearsed, coupled with daily home practice for 15–30 min. Patients are often given an audiotape to facilitate home practice; however, it is important to ensure that the individual has mastered the technique. In this respect, audiotapes are best viewed as adjuncts rather than substitutes for supervised instruction where there is a chance to monitor progress, provide feedback, and solve problems that arise. Often relaxation procedures, especially autogenic and meditation techniques, produce a feeling of depersonalization that may be distressing to some individuals. Adequate patient preparation can help prevent any distress associated with feelings of deep relaxation.

Biofeedback

Biofeedback is a technique that uses instrumentation to provide feedback of physiologic responses. The feedback is useful in learning self-regulation of the physiologic response. The most common types of biofeedback are electromyographic (EMG), skin temperature, skin conductance, and electroencephalographic (EEG). Like relaxation techniques, biofeedback is thought to reduce sympathetically mediated responses and/or affective responses, such as anger or anxiety, that induce, facilitate, or maintain the pain.

Relaxation techniques and biofeedback appear to be equally efficacious (65) and are often used in conjunction with each other. Several studies have shown relaxation and biofeedback techniques to be beneficial in the management of side effects from chemotherapy (66, 67) and in treating insomnia secondary to cancer (68). Unfortunately, direct empirical evidence of effectiveness in treating cancer pain is limited to two uncontrolled studies (69, 70). In the first study, the combined use of EMG and EEG biofeedback was evaluated in seven cancer patients (69). Their results showed significant reductions in pain during biofeedback sessions, but generalization of pain reduction to the home environment was only demonstrated in two patients. In a follow-up study using EMG and skin conductance biofeedback on five patients who completed the study, three patients were able to reduce their analgesic medication intake and two patients were able to achieve pain reduction in their daily activities (70). Although these studies were uncontrolled, it is noteworthy that these patients were seriously ill and most were considered to be nonresponders to other pain management approaches.

COGNITIVE APPROACHES

Turk and Rennert (71) have proposed a cognitive–social learning approach to the management of cancer pain. One of the major assumptions of cognitive approaches to pain management is that the experience of pain is based partly on its appraisal and psychological significance to the individual. The individual's evaluation of the pain is influenced by cognitive coping resources, beliefs, attitudes, and other cognitive factors. Negative expectations and anticipatory fears such as unavoidable pain, loss of control, disfigurements, and subjective perceptions of rejection are common among cancer patients. These cognitions will likely have a negative impact on the cancer pain problem and contribute to increased distress. The goal of cognitive approaches to pain management is to modify cognitions, beliefs, and behaviors that may be contributing to the pain problem and to teach specific cognitive coping skills to deal with pain (31). Cognitive techniques have been effective in treating chronic, benign pain problems (14).

Obviously, there is a cognitive component to most forms of psychological pain management. Guided or self-directed imagery, controlled attentional focus, fantasy, and self-statements are commonly used in relaxation training and hypnosis. Howver, cognitive techniques also consist of several additional types of procedures, such as cognitive distraction and attention diversion techniques, and cognitive coping strategies or restructuring. Distraction and attention diversion techniques can be divided into the broad categories of environmental stimulation techniques, such as social activities, and cognitive strategies, such as focusing attention on nonpainful sensations, positive thoughts, pleasant images, or aspects of the environment (14, 31).

Cognitive restructuring and coping strategies generally involve reconceptualization of the pain. The patient's thoughts and feelings associated with the pain experience are evaluated. Thoughts and feelings that have a negative effect on the experience of pain are targeted for change (72). Such cognitive restructuring requires a certain degree of skill in eliciting cognitions contributing to the pain problem, as well as an active collaboration between clinician and patient. Other cognitive techniques include covert self-reinforcement for mastery of acute pain episodes, imagery rehearsal of coping skills, and use of imagery for covert desensitization or exposure to procedures or activities that are painful but necessary for treatment.

BEHAVIORAL APPROACHES

Although operant approaches in treating chronic pain are well established (73) and a mainstay of psychological approaches to treating chronic pain, little attention has been focused on the role of environmental reinforcement on cancer-related pain and pain behavior. Ahles et al. (74) provided some evidence for the operant reinforcement of pain behaviors in cancer patients by significant others. Yet, as noted above, the report of pain is important in the assessment of the disease process and, in most cases, should not be ignored. This is the fundamental difference between cancer pain and chronic, benign pain where pain complaints are of little therapeutic value. This difference will limit the use of operant approaches for cancer pain patients.

Medication scheduling is one area where operant control of cancer pain may be significant. Contingent reinforcement for pain behavior and the experience of pain is often maintained by pain-contingent analgesic administration (73). Often pain-contingent administration of analgesics occurs because of physician and patient concerns about tolerance or dependence. The use of contingent scheduling of medication eliminates reinforcement for the experience or demonstration of pain by subsequent medication-induced pain relief.

Contingent reinforcers for the experience of pain and/or pain behaviors may often be overlooked in cancer pain treatment. Ahles (31) has noted that operant variables are often of little importance for patients in the terminal stages of illness, yet may be an important factor for patients who experience pain for extended periods. Operant factors are likely to be especially important in patients who experience chronic pain but do not have active disease. This area has largely been ignored and needs greater clinical and research attention.

Other behavioral approaches might also be useful in the management of cancer pain either by themselves or in conjunction with other treatment approaches. Incentive programs might be useful to increase compliance with treatment, such as taking medication, home practice of relaxation techniques, and so on. Audiovisual presentations of modeling might be useful in acute treatment-related pain. Contracting to maintain activity level and participation in social events might be beneficial for increasing adaptive functioning despite pain. Exposure, modeling, and other behavioral approaches might be useful in treating pain, as well as anxiety or depression associated with cancer disease and its treatment. Again, these techniques could be effective in reducing pain and suffering in cancer patients but have not been systematically evaluated except in comprehensive treatment packages.

STAFF EDUCATION AND SKILLS TRAINING

In some cases, the focus of treatment is not on the patient but on the staff. As already mentioned, pain-contingent administration of narcotics by staff might be an important factor in maintaining cancer pain. Physician concerns about addiction, respiratory depression, and tolerance can contribute to inadequate control of cancer pain with analgesics. Also, patients might not request pain medication because of aversive reactions by staff to prior requests. The important point is that attitudes and misconceptions by physicians and other health care professionals can interfere with the adminsitration of analgesic medication and how patients cope with their pain (11, 75–77).

Educational and skills training programs focusing on information regarding the administration of narcotics and other analgesic drugs, information on the pathophysiology of cancer pain, and concerns about narcotic addiction, tolerance, and respiratory distress could have a positive impact on the treatment of cancer pain. Hauck (78) found that participation in a 2-hr educational program on cancer pain management resulted in an increase in knowledge about the pharmacology of analgesics and an increase in positive attitudes toward cancer pain patients. Unfortunately, no direct assessment was conducted of pain management, actual behavior toward patients, or the patients' perception of staffs' attitude toward them. Additional research is needed to determine whether such programs actually result in better pain management. In addition to health care professionals, such a program could be extended to patients and their families since they often have similar attitudes, misconceptions, or behaviors that interfere with pain management.

COMPREHENSIVE TREATMENT PACKAGES

Comprehensive treatment programs are likely to be the most effective method for managing cancer pain. One approach has been suggested by Turk and Rennert (71). They outlined a treatment package based on cognitive–social learning principles. They described four components to their treatment package. The first phase is a pretreatment preparation that provides an overview of the program with an introduction to the notion that pain can be influenced by a variety of cognitive, affective, social, and behavioral factors. Patients are also provided with the expectation that specific skills can be learned to minimize the negative impact of these factors on their pain. A secondary purpose of the pretreatment preparation is to reassure patients that such a referral does not indicate that they are crazy or that their pain is "all in their heads." This concern can usually be addressed by emphasizing that all patients with serious disease and pain will experience a variety of stressors that often exacerbate the level of pain (71). In a sense, this initial phase is designed to enhance the patient's motivational level and assess for potential factors that might interfere with their cooperation in the treatment program.

Turk and Rennert (71) described the second phase of treatment as a conceptualization-translation component. The primary goal of this phase is to educate the patient on the multidimensional nature of pain and the rationale behind various treatment procedures. This phase is designed to provide a framework for understanding the interaction between the experience of pain and sensory-physiologic, affective, and cognitive responses. Patients are also taught problem-solving skills and how to break large, overwhelming problems into smaller component parts. This phase of treatment focuses on reconceptualization of nonspecific, vague, and seemingly overwhelming pain-related and non-pain-related problems into specific and concrete problems that can be solved.

The third phase of treatment involves actual training in cognitive and behavioral strategies to reduce pain and minimize stress. Patients are taught relaxation and attention diversion techniques. In addition to focusing on pain reduction, an emphasis of this phase in treatment is to enhance the individual's sense of control and personal mastery. The fourth phase is essentially a continuation of rehearsal and practice to consolidate the pain-control techniques and reinforce a sense of personal control. Turk and Rennert suggested that a stress inoculation procedure is useful at this point in treatment. This involves having the individual imagine himself experiencing pain and then using the previously learned coping techniques. A second technique also used at this time is to have the individual take the role of an instructor and teach the coping techniques to the clinician, who takes the role of a new patient.

A final element of the treatment package is homework tasks of gradually increasing difficulty. For example, the patient might be instructed to practice pain-control techniques only when pain is low at first, then gradually shifting the use of pain-control techniques when pain is more severe. Before-and-after pain ratings are often useful in evaluating the effectiveness of the pain-control techniques. If the techniques are effective in dealing with low levels of pain, then they can be used with increasing levels of pain. The point is to ensure that the patient is experiencing success in order to increase his or her sense of competence and confidence in the techniques. Turk and Rennert (71) reported that this approach to cancer pain management is effective; unfortunately they present no data to support this conclusion. Although the program appears to have face validity for being an effective treatment for cancer pain, conclusions regarding efficacy must await empirical verification.

Jay, Elliot, and colleagues (79, 80) have used cognitive-behavioral interventions to develop a comprehensive treatment approach to treat pain and distress in children undergoing painful medical procedures. Their intervention, labeled the Cognitive Behavior Therapy Package (CBTP), incorporates five behavioral treatment components: filmed modeling, breathing exercises, positive reinforcement, imagery/distraction, and behavior rehearsal (34, 80). In a controlled treatment outcome study, pediatric cancer patients receiving the CBTP showed significantly lower levels of behavioral distress (e.g., crying, screaming), self-reported pain, and physiologic reactivity during bone marrow procedures than either a control or Valium-treatment group (80). This research is praiseworthy, not only because it supports the efficacy of psychological approaches to cancer pain, but also because it represents one of the few controlled treatment outcome studies in this area.

TREATMENT ISSUES

In summary, there are a variety of psychological interventions available for use in the management of cancer pain. The problem is not the lack of approaches but rather the dearth of empirical evidence to confirm efficacy or to establish the applicability and generalizability of psychological approaches to cancer pain. Research on treatment-related acute pain in adult cancer patients has almost been entirely ignored, although some research has focused on treatment-related acute pain in pediatric cancer patients

(34). The studies on disease-related chronic pain are limited by a lack of rigorous scientific methodology, especially appropriate control groups, quantitative and multi-modal pain measures, and evaluation of process variables or mechanisms of change.

Some of the limitations in current research on the psychological management of cancer pain are undoubtedly related to inherent difficulties in conducting research on cancer patients (81) and the incomplete conceptual understanding of important psychological aspects of cancer pain. Although there is ultimately no substitute for controlled treatment outcome studies, one approach to advancing knowledge in this area is through the use of time series methodology (56). Barlow et al. (82) have detailed the application of single-case designs and time series methodology to document change in clinical practice. Since clinicians are currently employing psychological interventions, considerable knowledge could be gained from more systematic evaluation of treatment responses in individuals. Specific interventions could be compared, as well as the efficacy of combined treatments for different types of cancer pain problems and person variables. Such information would be extremely valuable in planning and justifying the commitment of time and resources for controlled treatment outcome studies.

CASE STUDY

A 52-year-old, married male with abdominal cancer and disseminated metastases involving major organs and bony sites was referred to the pain clinic after several months of persistent, poorly controlled pain. During the interview, he rated his current pain level as 8 or 9 on a 0 to 10 scale. He rated his average pain as 8 with a range between 7 and 10. He described his pain as a constant, intense, sharp, stabbing pain. He reported the pain had been getting gradually worse over the last 2 months. He was taking acetaminophen and 30 mg of codeine on a pain-contingent basis.

Assessment of the pain problem focused on cognitive, psychosocial, behavioral, and treatment variables that might be contributing to the pain problem. The patient demonstrated a considerable amount of pain behaviors throughout the interview. He would grimace, brace his arms on the chair, stop his speech to close his eyes, and several times he got out of the chair to pace. Although there was little evidence for operant factors in the pain problem, the patient and his wife had just separated immediately prior to the diagnosis of cancer. He expressed feelings of affection and closeness toward his wife and appeared upset about the uncertainty of his marital status.

The patient presented as a masculine, strong-willed person who was frustrated by his inability to control his pain or prevent it from interfering with his life. He described himself as an active person who had always solved problems by taking charge of things. He demonstrated several cognitive errors and negative self-statements during the interview, such as "I should be able to better control the pain" and "I can't handle it." He also believed that he must "walk off" the pain. He spent a considerable amount of time pacing and little time attempting to relax. Assessment revealed that he had not been taught any relaxation or coping strategies to deal with the pain. Because he believed that he should be able to cope with or tolerate the pain, he was taking only 60 mg of codeine a day.

Several areas needed intervention. First, his medication was switched to a time-contingent schedule rather than an as-needed schedule. He was also started on methadone for better pain control. Pharmacologic issues such as maintenance of plasma levels, tolerance, and dependence were discussed with the patient. His feelings toward the use of medication to control his pain were dealt with so that he was comfortable with the change in treatment plan. Cooperating with the patient's physician was also necessary to get the medication changed since the physician showed some of the same concerns about dependence, tolerance, and scheduling medication on a fixed-time interval.

Given the patient's concern and distress about the status of his marriage, brief psychotherapy was used to help resolve the marital issue. The wife and patient agreed to suspend their plans to separate. The wife became increasingly involved with the patient throughout the treatment program, offering considerable support.

The patient was also instructed in more direct psychological pain-control techniques. One aspect of the intervention focused on education and cognitive restructuring regarding taking a different approach to the pain problem rather than actively trying to overcome it by walking it off. The patient readily acknowledged that his active approach was not effective and seemed to make the pain worse. He was then taught autogenic relaxation and the use of cognitive coping strategies of attention distraction, pleasant imagery, and positive self-statements. Some cognitive restructuring was also necessary to deal with the feelings of frustration and hopelessness from previous attempts to deal with his pain. The patient responded well to this approach to his pain problem. Over a 6-week period his pain ratings dropped to an average of 4 with a minimum rating of 2 and a maximum rating of 8. He also reported improvements in his ability to interact with other people despite some increase in medication side effects.

CONCLUSIONS

The diverse expressions of pain associated with cancer necessitate that behavioral assessment and the resulting psychological treatment plan must be based not only on a thorough understanding of the pain complaint, but also on an adequate knowledge of the disease itself and its stage of progression. In all cases, comprehensive psychological and medical therapies must be evaluated for potential benefit to the patient. The specific needs of cancer patients will require some reorientation by clinicians with experience in treating chronic pain.

Although the lack of controlled studies on the effectiveness of psychological approaches for cancer pain underscores the need for empirical investigation, those who undertake such studies should be aware of the difficulties that they face. Multiple medical therapies for cancer pain are often used simultaneously. Differences in cancer site, stage of the disease, physical basis of pain, and concurrent medical treatments will make equivalent group compositions difficult.

Despite the complexity of the issues, psychological approaches do appear to have a place in the comprehensive management of cancer pain. We suggest that relatively simple behavioral skills training can be surprisingly effective in pain reduction, that a package of different psychological techniques appropriately selected for the individual has distinct advantages over any skill presented in isolation, and that cancer patients, as a group, are well motivated to learn and practice these skills. Psychological approaches do appear to have some advantages over other methods of treating cancer pain, since pain control can be achieved without unpleasant or destructive side effects and, in fact, facilitate life-enhancing and health promoting cognitions and behavior.

References

1. National Institute of Health. *Report of the Panel on Pain to the National Advisory NINDS Council* (NIH 79-1912). Washington, DC, Government Printing Office, 1979.
2. Daut RL, Cleeland CS: The prevalence and severity of pain in cancer. *Cancer* 50:1903–1918, 1982.
3. Levin CN, Cleeland CS, Dar R: Public attitudes towards cancer pain. *Cancer* 56:2337–2339, 1985.
4. Cleeland CS: The impact of pain on the patient with cancer. *Cancer* 54:2635–2641, 1984.
5. Foley KM: Assessment of pain. *Clin Oncol* 3:17–31, 1984.
6. Foley KM: Pain syndromes in patients with cancer. In Bonica JJ, Ventafredda V (eds): *Advances in Pain Research and Therapy* New York, Raven Press, 1979, vol 2, p 59.
7. Schwettmann RS, Shacham S, Cleeland CS: Relating cancer pain to its physical basis. Presented at the annual meeting of the American Pain Society, Chicago, IL, 1983.
8. Turk D, Holzman AD: Chronic pain: interfaces among physical, psychological, and social parameters. In Holzman AD, Turk DC (eds): *Pain Management: A Handbook of Psychological Treatment Approaches*. New York, Pergamon Press, 1986, pp 1–9.
9. Shacham S, Reinhardt LC, Raubertas RF, Cleeland CS: Emotional state and pain: intraindividual and interindividual measures of association. *J Behav Med* 6:405–419, 1983.
10. Telch CF, Telch MJ: Group coping skills instruction and supportive group therapy for cancer patients: a comparison of strategies. *J Consult Clin Psychol* 54:802–808, 1986.
11. Bonica JJ: Cancer pain: a major national health problem. *Cancer Nurs* 1:313–316, 1978.
12. Marks RM, Sacher EJ: Undertreatment of medical inpatients with narcotic analgesics. *Ann Intern Med* 78:173–181, 1973.
13. Twycross RG, Lacks SA: *Symptom Control in Advanced Cancer: Pain Relief*. London, Pitman, 1985.
14. Turk D, Meichenbaum D, Genest M: *Pain and Behavioral Medicine*. New York, Guilford Press, 1983.
15. Keefe FJ, Brown C, Scott DS, Ziesat H: The behavioral assessment of chronic pain. In Keefe FJ, Blumenthal JA (eds): *Assessment Strategies in Behavioral Medicine*. New York, Grune & Stratton, 1982.
16. Hilgard ER: Pain as a puzzle for psychology and physiology. *Am J Psychol* 24:103–113, 1969.
17. Melzack R (ed): *Pain Measurement and Assessment*. New York, Raven Press, 1983.
18. Tearnan BH, Cleeland CS: The use of pain descriptors by patients with cancer pain. Upublished manuscript, The University of Wisconsin, Madison, 1984.
19. McCaffery M: *Nursing Management of the Patient with Pain*, ed 2. Philadelphia, JB Lippincott, 1979.
20. Daut RL, Cleeland CS, Flanery RC: Development of the Wisconsin Brief Pain Questionnaire to assess pain in cancer and other diseases. *Pain* 17:197–210, 1983.
21. Shacham S: A shortened version of the Profile of Mood States. *J Pers Assess* 47:305–306, 1983.
22. DeGood DE: Reducing medical patients' reluctance to participate in psychological therapies: the initial session. *Professional Psychol Res Pract* 14:570–579, 1983.
23. Jacox A, Stewart M: *Psychosocial Contingencies of the Pain Experience*. Iowa City, The University of Iowa Press, 1973.
24. Hardy JD: The nature of pain. *J Chronic Dis* 7:22–51, 1956.
25. Abrams RD: The patient with cancer—his changing pattern of communication. *N Engl J Med* 274:317–322, 1966.
26. Bond MR: Pain and personality in cancer patients. In Bonica JJ, Albe-Fessard D (eds): *Advances in Pain Research and Therapy*. New York, Raven Press, 1976, vol 1, pp 311–316.
27. Moses R, Cividoli N: Differential levels of awareness of illness: their relation to some salient features in cancer patients. *Ann NY Acad Sci* 125:884, 1966.
28. Kremer EF, Block A, Gaylor M: Behavioral approaches to treatment of chronic pain: the inaccuracy of patient self-report measures. *Arch Phys Med Rehabil* 62:188–191, 1981.
29. Kremer EF, Block A, Atkinson JH: Assessment of pain behavior: factors that distort self-report. In Melzack R (ed): *Pain Measurement and Assessment*. New York, Raven Press, 1983.
30. Ignelzi RJ, Kremer EF, Atkinson JH: Patient pain intensity report to different health professionals. Presented at the annual meeting of the Association for Advancement of Behavior Therapy, New York, November 1980.
31. Ahles TA: Psychological approaches to the management of cancer-related pain. *Sem Oncol Nurs* 1:141–146, 1985.
32. Bonica JJ: Cancer pain. In Bonica JJ (ed): *Pain*. New York, Raven Press, 1980, pp 335–362.
33. Cleeland CS, Tearnan BH: Behavioral control of pain. In Holzman AD, Turk DC (eds): *Pain Management: A Handbook of Psychological Treatment Approaches*. New York, Pergamon Press, 1986, pp 193–212.
34. Jay SM, Elliot C, Varni JW: Acute and chronic pain in adults and children with cancer. *J Consult Clin Psychol* 54:601–607, 1986.
35. Noyles R Jr: Treatment of cancer pain. *Psychosom Med* 43:57–70, 1981.
36. Kendall PC, Norton-Ford JD: *Clinical Psychology: Scientific and Professional Dimensions*. New York, John Wiley & Sons, 1982.
37. Bond MR: Psychologic and psychiatric techniques for the relief of advanced cancer pain. In Bonica JJ, Ventatridda V (eds): *Advances in Pain Research and Therapy*. New York, Raven Press, 1979, vol 2, pp 215–222.

38. Feinstein AD: Psychological interventions in the treatment of cancer. *Clin Psychol Rev* 3:1–14, 1983.
39. Ferlic M, Goldman A, Kennedy BJ: Group counseling in adult patients with advanced cancer. *Cancer* 43:760–766, 1979.
40. Gordon WA, Freidenbergs I, Diller L, et al: Efficacy of psychosocial intervention with cancer patients. *J Consult Clin Psychol* 48:743–759, 1980.
41. Shapiro A: Psychotherapy as adjunct treatment for cancer patients. *Am J Clin Hypn* 25:150–155, 1983.
42. Ament P: Concepts in the use of hypnosis for pain relief in cancer. *J Med* 13:233–240, 1982.
43. Barber J, Gitelson J: Cancer pain: psychological management using hypnosis. *Cancer* 30:130–135, 1980.
44. Butler B: The use of hypnosis in the care of cancer patient, part I. *Br J Med Hypn* 6:2–12, 1954.
45. Cangello VM: Hypnosis for the patient with cancer. *Am J Clin Hypn* 4:215–226, 1962.
46. Hilgard ER, Hilgard JR: *Hypnosis in the Relief of Pain.* Los Altos, CA, William Kaufmann, 1975.
47. Koerner ME: Using hypnosis to relieve pain of terminal cancer. *Hypn Q* 20:39–46, 1977.
48. LaBaw W, Holton C, Tewell K, Eccles D: The use of self-hypnosis by children with cancer. *Am J Clin Hypn* 7:308–319, 1975.
49. Hilgard JR, LeBaron S: Relief of anxiety and pain in children and adolescents with cancer: quantitative measures and clinical observations. *Int J Clin Exp Hypn* 30:417–442, 1982.
50. Araoz DL: Use of hypnotic techniques with oncology patients. *J Psychosoc Oncol* 1:47–54, 1983.
51. Barber J: Hypnotic analgesia. In Holzman AD, Turk DC (eds): *Pain Management: A Handbook of Psychological Treatment Approaches.* New York, Pergamon Press, 1986, pp 151–167.
52. Butler B: The use of hypnosis in the care of cancer patient, part II. *Br J Med Hypn* 6:2–12, 1955.
53. Hilgard ER, Morgan AH: Heart rate and blood pressure in the study of laboratory pain in man under normal conditions and as influenced by hypnosis. *Acta Neurol Exp* 35:741–759, 1975.
54. Reeves JL, Redd WH, Storm FK, Minagawa RY: Hypnosis in the control of pain during hyperthermia treatment of cancer. In Bonica JJ (ed): *Advances in Pain Research and Therapy.* New York, Raven Press, 1983, vol 5, pp 857–861.
55. Finer B: Hypnotherapy in pain of advanced cancer. In Bonica JJ, Ventafridda V (eds): *Advances in Pain Research and Therapy.* New York, Raven Press, 1979, vol 2, pp 223–229.
56. Kellerman J, Zeltzer L, Ellenberg L, Dash J: Adolescents with cancer: hypnosis for the reduction of the acute pain and anxiety associated with medical procedures. *J Adoles Health Care* 4:85–90, 1983.
57. Zelter L, LeBaron S: Hypnosis and nonhypnotic techniques for reduction of pain and anxiety during painful procedures in children and adolescents with cancer. *J Pediatr* 101:1032–1035, 1982.
58. Spiegel D, Bloom JR: Group therapy and hypnosis reduce metastatic breast carcinoma pain. *Psychosom Med* 45:333–339, 1983.
59. Woolfolk RL, Lehrer PM (eds): *Principles and Practice of Stress Management.* New York, Guilford Press, 1984.
60. Bernstein DA, Borkovec TD: *Progressive Relocation Training: A Manual For the Helping Professions.* Champaign, IL, Research Press, 1973.
61. Jacobson E: *Progressive Relaxation.* New York, Avon, 1938.
62. Rimm DC, Masters JC: *Behavioral Therapy: Techniques and Empirical Findings,* ed 2. New York, Academic Press, 1979.
63. Norris PA, Fahrion SL: Autogenic biofeedback in psychophysiological therapy and stress management. In Woolfolk RL, Lehrer PM (eds): *Principles and Practice of Stress Management.* New York, Guilford Press, 1984, pp 220–254.
64. Schultz JH, Luthe W: *Autogenic Therapy, Vol 1: Autogenic Methods.* New York, Grune & Stratton, 1969.
65. Silver BV, Blanchard EB: Biofeedback and relaxation training in the treatment of psychophysiological disorders: or, are the machines really necessary? *J Behav Med* 1:217–239, 1978.
66. Lyles JN, Burish TG, Krozely MG, Oldham RK: Efficacy of relaxation training and guided imagery in reducing the aversiveness of cancer chemotherapy. *J Consult Clin Psychol* 50:509–524, 1982.
67. Redd WH, Andrykowski MA: Behavioral intervention in cancer treatment: controlling aversion to chemotherapy. *J Consult Clin Psychol* 50:1018–1029, 1982.
68. Cannici J, Malcolm R, Peck LA: Treatment of insomnia in cancer patients using muscle relaxation training. *J Behav Ther Exp Psychiatry* 14:251–256, 1983.
69. Fotopoulos SS, Graham C, Cook MR: Psychophysiologic control of cancer pain. In Bonica JJ, Ventafridda V (eds): *Advances in Pain Research and Therapy.* New York, Raven Press, 1979, vol 2 pp. 231–243.
70. Fotopoulos SS, Cook MR, Graham C, et al: Cancer pain: evaluation of electromyographic and electrodermal feedback. *Prog Clin Biol Res* 132D:33–53, 1983.
71. Turk DC, Rennert D: Pain and the terminally ill cancer patient: a cognitive social learning perspective. In Sobel HJ (ed): *Behavior Therapy in Terminal Care.* Cambridge, MA, Ballinger, 1981, pp 95–123.
72. Holzman AD, Turk DC, Kerns RD Jr.: The cognitive-behavioral approach to the management of chronic pain. In Holzman AD, Turk DC (eds): *Pain Management: A Handbook of Psychological Treatment Approaches.* New York, Pergamon Press, 1986, pp 31–50.
73. Fordyce W: *Behavioral Methods for Chronic Pain and Illness.* St. Louis, CV Mosby, 1976.
74. Ahles TA, Blanchard EB, Ruckdeschel JC: The multidimensional nature of cancer-related pain. *Pain* 17:277–288, 1983.
75. Bagley C, Falinski E, Garnizo N, Hooker L: Pain management: a pilot project. *Cancer Nurs* 5:191–199, 1982.
76. Jacox AK, Rogers AG: The nursing management of pain. In Marino LB (ed): *Cancer Nursing.* St. Louis, CV Mosby, 1981, pp 381–404.
77. Cleeland CS, Cleeland LM, Dar R, Rienhardt LC: Factors influencing physicians' management of cancer pain. *Cancer* 58:796–800, 1986.
78. Hauck SL: Pain problem for the person with cancer. *Cancer Nurs* 9:66–76, 1986.
79. Jay SM, Elliot CM, Ozolins M, Olson R, Pruitt S: Behavioral management of children's distress during painful medical procedures. *Behav Res Ther* 23:513–520, 1985.
80. Varni JW, Jay SM, Masek BJ, Thompson KL: Cognitive-behavioral assessment and management of pediatric pain. In Holzman AD, Turk DC (eds): *Pain Management: A Handbook of Psychological Treatment Approaches.* New York, Pergamon Press, 1986, pp 168–192.
81. Ahles TA, Cohen RE, Blanchard EB: Difficulties inherent in conducting behavioral research with cancer patients. *Behav Ther* 1:69–70, 1984.
82. Barlow DH, Hayes SC, Nelson RD: *The Scientist Practitioner: Research and Accountability in Clinical and Educational Settings.* New York, Pergamon Press, 1985.

chapter 34
Neurosurgical Treatment of Pain Related to Cancer

Stephen R. Freidberg, M.D.

Pain, a common symptom of disease, is valuable because it may initiate or direct a search for underlying disease. The ideal way to eliminate pain is to treat the underlying disease. However, sometimes the primary underlying disease is not or cannot be treated adequately, and pain persists, becomes chronic, and is the focal point of a wretched existence that requires attention.

Pain caused by benign disease must be differentiated from pain caused by malignant disease. Chronic pain of benign origin presents a specific constellation of symptoms. Frequently, secondary gain occurs either consciously or subconsciously. Does the pain permit a long-desired change in occupation or marital relationship? Is the basic problem severe underlying depression? Surgical attempts at relief of pain of benign origin invariably fail, and the problem is managed best by a behavior modification program in a pain clinic (1).

Chronic pain caused by malignant disease requires a different therapeutic approach. Although the patient is frequently ill and depressed, the evaluation and treatment of pain as an isolated entity are usually fairly straightforward (2). In the last decade, improvements have been made in the treatment of cancer by surgery, chemotherapy, and radiotherapy. These modalities together with a clearer understanding of the mechanism of action and more effective delivery of pain-controlling medication have substantially reduced the need for neurosurgical methods to relieve pain. In some instances, however, a carefully chosen neurosurgical operation provides excellent palliation of pain with low risk and low morbidity (3, 4). Neurosurgical treatment of pain may be *ablative*, with destruction of neural tissue, or *augmentative*, with stimulation of neural tissue or more effective delivery of medication.

To experience pain, a patient must have a peripheral lesion exciting pain receptors. This sensation is transmitted through the central nervous system to the brain, where the stimulus is recorded as pain. Therefore, it is theoretically possible to divide the neural connection between the peripheral nerve and the brain and alleviate the pain. Although ablative surgery is effective in selected patients, unfortunately it is not the solution for all patients. Psychodynamic factors can embellish the sensation of pain, creating a clinical situation that demands treatment (5). Alternatively, some patients may tolerate the pain.

A clinically proved approach to the problem of pain associated with cancer is presented in this chapter. Procedures being investigated, which are currently not appropriate in a general neurosurgical practice, are discussed.

ABLATIVE NEUROSURGERY

Virtually every neural structure has at one time or another been sectioned in an attempt to relieve pain.

PERIPHERAL NEURECTOMY

Peripheral neurectomy (Fig. 34.1*J*) is rarely effective. A lesion is not commonly found in the dermatomic area of a single nerve because of the overlap of innervation from adjacent nerves. Sectioning many nerves, as is possible with intercostal nerves, leaves the denervated area with a

Figure 34.1A–K. Diagrammatic representation of neurosurgical operations for relief of pain. References to each specific section are detailed in the text. (Copyright © 1986, the Lahey Clinic Medical Center, Burlington, MA.)

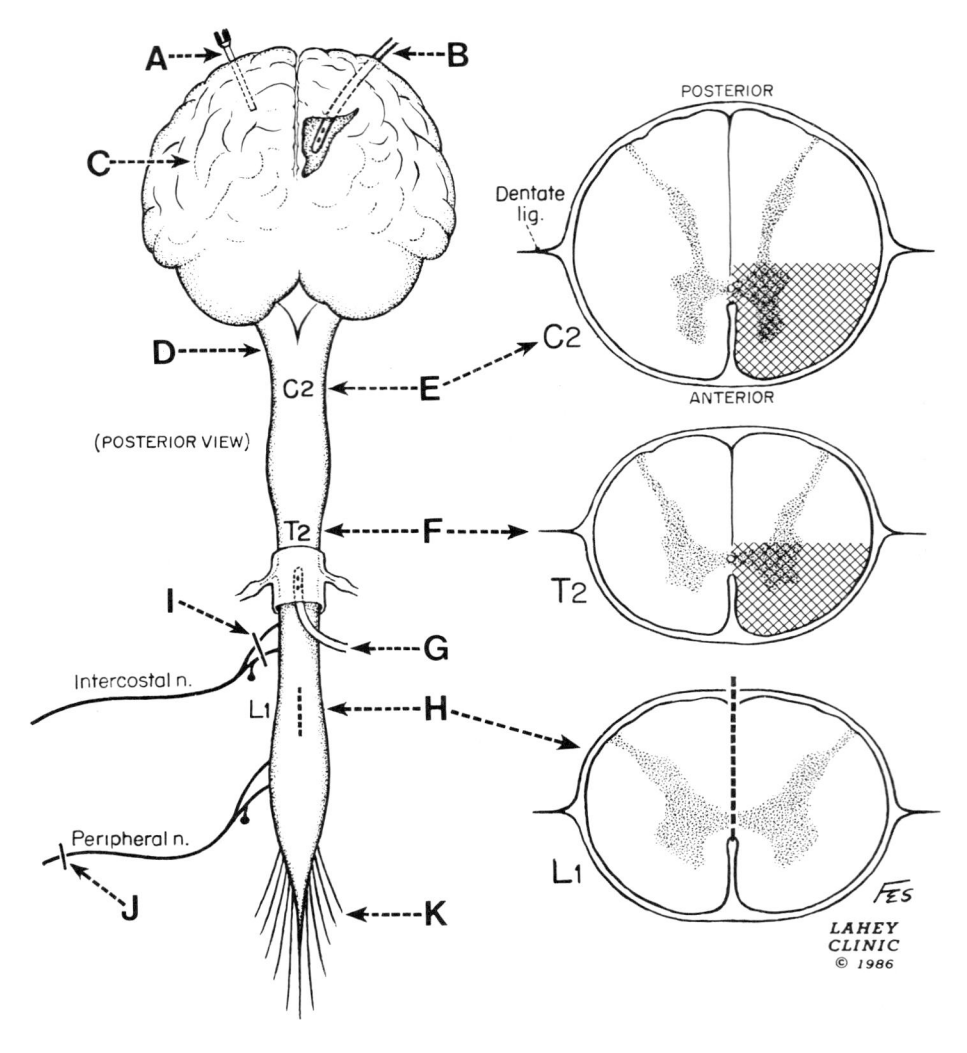

numb sensation and almost certainly with persistent pain. Nerves with important functional innervation in the extremities cannot be sectioned safely.

NERVE ROOT SECTION (RHIZOTOMY)

Nerve root section (Fig. 34.1I) usually does not help relieve pain. No important motor nerves are present at the thoracic level, and the operation is associated with low morbidity. In two series of patients with cancer who underwent thoracic rhizotomy (6, 7), results were disappointing in terms of relief of pain.

Rhizotomy, however, does provide excellent relief of pain in specific limited clinical situations. Infiltration of the brachial plexus in patients with carcinoma of the breast is an extremely painful condition. Section of the dorsal root, if it involves C5, C6, C7, and C8, renders the arm sensory deprived and useless. We have used rhizotomy to treat two patients with invasion of the brachial plexus from carcinoma of the breast, one with an amputation at the shoulder and one who had total loss of function of the brachial plexus as a result of her disease. Dorsal rhizotomy was performed with a long hemilaminectomy on the involved side from C3 to C8, with excellent relief of pain and no change in the clinical status. These results would not have been possible had the patient had a neurologically functioning limb.

Patients with nerve root involvement with epidural cancer may benefit from root section carried out at the time of laminectomy.

A sacral rhizotomy (Fig. 34.1K) performed with alcohol is effective for perianal, perineal, and genital pain associated with carcinoma of the rectum, bladder, or genitalia (4). Sacral rhizotomy is easily carried out in the radiology department with a needle inserted into the L5–S1 interspace under fluoroscopic control. Because alcohol is hypobaric compared with cerebrospinal fluid, the patient is positioned with the head down. Absolute (95%) ethanol is injected in aliquots of 0.25 ml until a maximum of 2 ml is injected or until the sensory level, which begins in the perianal and genital areas (S4 and S5), rises to S2 on the posterior calf. The level will descend to S3 on the posterior thigh several hours after the procedure. The level must not rise to S1 because weakness of plantar flexion of the ankle and sensory loss on the sole of the foot will be produced. A contraindication to this procedure is a short dural sac ending at L5 rather than in the sacrum. In this situation, the S1 roots will be bathed in alcohol. A myelogram using 1 ml of contrast material is always performed before injecting alcohol, and the procedure is stopped if the sac ends at L5. A sacral rhizotomy can be carred out without motor loss, but loss of sphincter control is invariable. Many of these patients already have a colostomy. Bladder function in patients who have had extensive pelvic surgery is frequently compromised, and a permanent Foley catheter may be necessary after rhizotomy. The ideal patient for this procedure is one with both fecal and urinary diversion. Some physicians (8) prefer to perform this operation using hyperbaric phenol mixed with iophendylate (Pantopaque) or glycerin. In selected patients, this procedure provides long-lasting, excellent relief of pain with minimal acceptable morbidity.

COMMISSURAL MYELOTOMY

Commissural myelotomy (Fig. 34.1H) is used in some medical centers for treatment of pain in the pelvic area. An incision is made in the lumbar spinal cord over several segments. The incision sections the commissural fibers in the ventral white matter before they enter the spinothalamic tract. The surgeon must be certain the incision is at the correct level. Although Sourek (9) described the correlation between vertebral and spinal cord levels, a discrepancy may exist, and the cord level selected may not be completely accurate. Even with use of the operating microscope, paraparesis or dorsal column dysfunction is possible. We rarely perform this operation.

Gildenberg and Hirshberg (10) described limited myelotomy at either the level of C1 or the thoracolumbar junction. Schvarcz (11) described an extralemniscal tract in the center of the spinal cord at the cervicomedullary junction. Destroying this tract provided relief of pain. I have no personal experience with the limited myelotomy.

ANTEROLATERAL CORDOTOMY

Anterolateral cordotomy remains the mainstay of treatment to relieve pain associated with cancer (4). The spinothalamic tract is sectioned after the fibers have crossed in the anterior commissure of the spinal cord. The lesion is, therefore, made on the side opposite the pain. Unlike commissural myelotomy, anterolateral cordotomy does not require selecting an exact level, but the level must be sufficiently craniad to the site of the pain to produce a satisfactorily high sensory level to pain and temperature. As always, careful selection of patients is the key to a safe, effective operation, the result of which usually lasts for several years. The sensory loss is well tolerated by the patient.

The appropriate patient for cordotomy is one with pain that is clearly unilateral in the lower part of the body. An open T2 cordotomy (Fig. 34.1F) contralateral to the pain produces a midthoracic sensory level to pinprick and temperature with analgesia. Weakness of the leg on the side of the cordotomy is a possibility. Disturbance in sphincter control is usually transient.

One of the problems related to cordotomy is that pain near the midline, even if dominant on only one side, frequently becomes clinically serious on the opposite side after relief of pain from cordotomy (12). Minor contralateral pain becomes magnified, and the patient requires relief of pain on the other side. Bilateral pain or pain developing on the second side requires bilateral cordotomy, usually carried out at T3 with at least a week between operations. Physiologically, bilateral cordotomy is a more serious operation than unilateral cordotomy. The patient is likely to experience severe autonomic dysfunction with sphincter dysfunction and orthostatic hypotension, which may require elastic stockings and fludrocortisone (Florinef) to maintain blood pressure.

Pain in the upper extremity or in the chest wall produces a more difficult clinical problem than pain in the lower extremity. For pain at the higher level, cordotomy must be performed at C2 (Fig. 34.1E). Because the ventral gray matter of the anterior horn of the spinal cord is sectioned along with the spinothalamic tract, unacceptable motor deficit in the arm is produced if the incision is made at a level where the anterior horn is clinically important. Therefore, the lesion cannot be made between C4 and T1. For pain in the chest wall, a satisfactorily high sensory level can usually be obtained with C2 cordotomy. A problem may arise in the presence of a pneumonectomy on the painful side or damage to the residual lung by tumor or radiation or both. The lung on the nonpainful side may be compromised as a result of chronic lung disease. A C2 cordotomy may interfere with function of the ipsilateral phrenic nerve, which will reduce pulmonary function severely on the nonpainful side (13). Unilateral cordotomy not only interferes with the motor component of respiration but also decreases the central response to inspired CO_2 (14). Krieger and Rosomoff (15) demonstrated the danger of performing bilateral cordotomy at a high cervical level. The dangers of severe pulmonary insufficiency, impairment of automatic control of respiration (Ondine's curse), and autonomic dysfunction make this operation unjustified.

Although cordotomy may be performed at either C2 or T2, a standard open operation by a hemilaminectomy at T2 is preferred (16). The physiologic morbidity associated with cordotomy at T2 is considerably less at this level than at C2. The surgical technique at C2 is the same if the level of pain demands this approach.

Some neurosurgeons (17, 18) prefer to carry out cordotomy with a percutaneous technique using a radiofrequency current to produce a lesion. It can be performed with the patient under local anesthesia, a benefit in an ill patient. The main advantage is the ability to manipulate the lesion while testing the patient, an especially important point if the pain is in the upper extremity or brachial plexus (19). It is extremely difficult to obtain a level this high with open cordotomy. With no operative complications, patients have been satisfied, but when the procedure is unsuccessful, patients become uncomfortable. The incidence of hemiparesis and respiratory difficulty is also higher with percutaneous than with open cordotomy. The high cervical percutaneous procedure is currently reserved for patients with pain high in the upper extremity and in the brachial plexus. Gildenberg and associates (20) described a high thoracic percutaneous technique, and Hardy and coworkers (21) described a microsurgical approach to the anterior cervical area using a variation of Cloward's technique. I have no personal experience with these last two procedures.

MEDULLARY TRACTOTOMY (Fig. 34.1D)

Pain related to cancer of the head and neck is difficult to treat. Fortunately, improved methods of treatment of the underlying disease make this an infrequent clinical problem. Percutaneous trigeminal rhizotomy or posterior fossa trigeminal root section may relieve the pain. However, because of the complex sensory innervation of the face, destruction of the fifth cranial nerve may not be adequate. In this situation, a lesion made in the descending tract of the trigeminal root in the medulla produces satisfactory relief of pain. The open operation was designed by Sjöqvist in 1938 (22). Stereotaxic procedures have been performed since 1972 in interested centers (23).

HYPOPHYSECTOMY

Hypophysectomy (removal of the pituitary gland) effectively relieves bone pain in patients with carcinoma of the breast and prostate. Objective shrinkage of tumor is seen in 50% of patients with breast cancer and in 30% of patients with prostate cancer. Relief of pain, however, is obtained in 70% of patients in each group (24). The mechanism of pain relief is not completely understood but may be related to a hypothalamic mechanism triggered by removal of the pituitary gland. After the pituitary gland has been removed, changes are noted in the pituitary stalk and hypothalamus. Total hypophysectomy is not necessary for pain relief (25). Permanent postoperative diabetes insipidus correlates well with good pain relief (26). Since pain relief is not reversed with injection of naloxone (Narcan), it is probably not mediated through changes in the endorphin system. Moricca (27) carried out hypophysectomy by injection of alcohol into the pituitary gland in patients with a wide variety of malignant processes with uniformly good results. Zervas and Gordy (28) performed the operation with a radiofrequency probe technique. I have carried out hypophysectomy through a transsphenoidal approach.

LESIONS OF THE BRAIN (Fig. 34.1C)
Cingulotomy

A patient's perception of pain may be altered by creating a lesion in the bilateral frontal lobe or cingulum. These lesions do not produce relief of pain but rather apathy, thereby relieving the terror and anxiety brought on by the cancer and the pain. Hurt and Ballantine (29) achieved satisfactory short-term relief of pain after cingulotomy in 18 of 32 patients with cancer, and satisfactory long-term relief of pain was achieved in two of nine. The lesions can be produced by an open or percutaneous technique. Because of the social pressure against leukotomy in the United States, this operation is performed infrequently.

Thalamotomy

Hitchcock and Teixeira (30) reported their experience with lesions produced stereotaxically in the centromedian and basal nuclei of the thalamus and reviewed the literature on thalamotomy for control of chronic pain. They believed the centromedian lesion was associated with the best rate of success for both immediate and long-term results. In all of their eight patients with malignant disease, centromedian thalamotomy yielded complete relief compared with only four of six patients who had basal thalamotomy. If adequate relief of pain was not obtained with unilateral thalamotomy, a contralateral lesion was created with little morbidity. The results of thalamotomy in patients with cancer were better than in those with benign disease.

ALCOHOL BLOCK OF THE CELIAC PLEXUS

Local metastases are common in patients with cancer of the upper abdominal viscera, that is, pancreas, gallbladder, liver, stomach, and colon, and produce pain in the region of the upper abdomen or back or both. This sensation of pain is conducted by the splanchnic nerves, which contain autonomic and pain fibers. The sensation through these fibers can be interrupted by block of the celiac plexus.

Gorbitz and Leavens (31) described the technique of celiac plexus block. It is valuable in patients in whom tumor is confined to the viscera. The injection of alcohol is painful and involves the risk of vascular or visceral perforation. They stressed that the needle should be placed under radiographic control with intravenous neuroleptanesthesia (31). Should a somatic component to the pain be present, further ablative treatment may be necessary after relief of visceral pain by the celiac block.

AUGMENTATIVE NEUROSURGERY (NONABLATIVE PROCEDURES)

The last decade has produced a clearer understanding of the endogenous endorphin system (32). Endorphins are opiates produced in the body that bind to specific receptors in the central nervous system. These are the receptors for opiates administered exogenously and are thought to represent the mechanism by which narcotics relieve pain. Exogenous opiates administered locally to the central nervous system bind with receptors and produce analgesia in doses far lower than with systemic administration and without the severe side effects associated with systemic narcotics. This observation forms the basis of spinal and intraventricular administration of narcotics.

SPINAL MORPHINE

Endorphin receptors are present in the substantia gelatinosa of the dorsal gray matter of the spinal cord (33, 34). Preservative-free morphine sulfate (2–5 mg in 2–5 ml of saline solution) is administered every 8–12 hr in the epidural or subarachnoid space through an indwelling catheter (35) (Fig. 34.1G). When the procedure is effective, the patient experiences relief of pain with little systemic effect. The catheter can be placed percutaneously through a Tuohy needle (Becton-Dickinson, Rutherford, NJ 07070) or by limited laminectomy. The reservoir attached to the proximal portion of the catheter, which is tunneled beneath the skin, varies from a simple externalized Broviac type, to an implanted Ommaya system (American Heyer-Schulte, Division of American Hospital Supply Corporation, Goleta, CA 93117), which requires intermittent and transcutaneous injections, to a totally implantable Infusaid pump (Infusaid, Norwood, MA) (36).

Disagreement exists regarding the optimal method of administering the narcotic. Shetter and colleagues (36) reported less tolerance, and ultimately a lower necessary dose of narcotic, with continuous rather than intermittent infusion. Intermittent instillation using an externalized catheter or an implanted reservoir has the benefits of simplicity and low initial cost. When installed, the device can be serviced by the patient, family member, or visiting nurse. The necessary medication, syringes, and needles are readily available from local pharmacies. The implanted pump is considerably more expensive initially and demands periodic refilling by a physician (37). It does, however, free the patient from having injections several times a day.

Most investigators have used preservative-free morphine. Coombs and associates (38) used hydromorphone (Dilaudid) in a patient sensitive to morphine and changed to clonidine (Catapres) when tolerance to the hydromorphone developed. They hypothesized that different subgroups of drugs may have different profiles of receptor affinity (38). The ability to lower the equivalent dose of medication may prolong the effectiveness of this system and reduce the side effects.

INTRAVENTRICULAR NARCOTICS

In an admittedly preliminary study, Lobato and co-workers (39) produced satisfactory analgesia with intraventricular injection of morphine (Fig. 34.1B). An Ommaya reservoir, which can be inserted with the patient under local anesthesia, is used. The patient's family can be instructed in the method of administering the drug for home use. A dose of 0.5–1.0 mg every 12–24 hr has sufficed in most instances with a low complication rate, few serious side effects, and minimal intolerance. The effect is not reversed by naloxone. The authors therefore postulate that a nonopiate analgesic system is being activated (39). This is currently an experimental approach to relief of pain, but it does hold promise.

ELECTRICAL STIMULATION OF THE SPINAL CORD

In 1965, Melzack and Wall (40) proposed the gate control theory of transmission of pain. They postulated the presence of an inhibitory synapse in the substantia gelatinosa of the dorsal gray matter of the spinal cord, which is activated by stimulation of large myelinated peripheral afferent fibers. The inhibitory synapse acts on the synapse of the small unmyelinated fibers carrying impulses of pain from the periphery to the second-order neuron crossing in the ventral white commissure and forming the ventral spinothalamic tract. This would "close the gate" on the transmission and sensation of pain. With reasoning analogous to that of cordotomy, namely, that the incision need only be cephalad to the level of the pain, a high thoracic or cervical level of implantation was usually chosen. Based on this theory, the medical electronic industry produced an array of sophisticated electronic devices that could stimulate the dorsal spinal cord either epidurally or from the subarachnoid space (41). The totally implanted spinal cord stimulators are powered by the transcutaneous activation of an induction coil. Eventually it was possible to install the electrodes percutaneously with a needle and embed the entire system using local anesthesia (42). Unfortunately, this technique never produced adequate results for the severe pain related to cancer. Some physicians (43, 44) still advocate this as treatment for pain of benign origin.

Transcutaneous nerve stimulation is a simple and harmless widely used modality that stimulates peripheral nerves through the intact skin. The mechanism is probably similar to that of acupuncture. Unfortunately, the technique is not effective for cancer pain (45).

ELECTRICAL STIMULATION OF THE BRAIN (Fig. 34.1A)

Richardson (46) investigated the relief of pain after stereotaxically implanting electrodes into deep brain structures. Stimulation of the periventricular gray and periaqueductal gray matter (PVG-PAG) increases levels of β-endorphins and enkephalins in the ventricular fluid. This effect is reversed by naloxone. He postulated that the β-endorphin is activated by the stimulation, subsequently inhibiting input in the dorsal horn of the spinal cord (46). Activating this system is beneficial for pain produced outside of the central nervous system, that is, pain that enters the central nervous system through the dorsal horn of the spinal cord. Richardson recommended ablative procedures initially for cancer and brain stimulation when ablation is not appropriate, such as pain in the upper extremity, midline area, and head and neck. For pain caused by neural deafferentation, stimulation in the internal capsule produces better results.

Young and Brechner (47) substantiated these findings by stimulating the PVG-PAG in 17 patients with cancer and obtained good results in 13. They noted that relief of pain produced by stimulation of the PVG-PAG lasted several hours longer than the stimulation procedure, implicating a humeral mechanism. Stimulation of thalamic nuclei is helpful for deafferentation pain, does not increase levels of endorphins, and does not result in relief of pain that exceeds the time of stimulation. Stimulation techniques hold promise but at present are being performed in only a few academic centers.

CONCLUSIONS

Pain can be a devastating accompaniment of disseminated cancer. The initial treatment of disease is aimed at the treatment of the tumor either systemically or locally. Analgesics are the first response to the pain. When treatment of the disease and medical treatment of the pain are not effective, neurosurgical procedures judiciously applied can produce gratifying comfort and palliation associated with a low incidence of morbidity and few side effects.

Reference

1. Friedberg SR: The neurosurgeon's approach to pain. In Aronoff GM (ed): *Evaluation and Treatment of Chronic Pain*. Baltimore, Urban & Schwarzenberg, 1985, pp 319–331.
2. Black P: Neurosurgical management of cancer pain. *Semin Oncol* 12:438–444, 1985.
3. Foley KM: The treatment of cancer pain. *N Engl J Med* 313:84–95, 1985.
4. Freidberg SR: Neurosurgical treatment of pain caused by cancer. *Med Clin North Am* 59:481–485, 1975.
5. Cleeland CS: The impact of pain on the patient with cancer. *Cancer* 54(11 suppl):2635–2641, 1984.
6. Loeser JD: Dorsal rhizotomy for the relief of chronic pain. *J Neurosurg* 36:745–750, 1972.
7. Onofrio BM, Campa HK: Evaluation of rhizotomy: review of 12 years' experience. *J Neurosurg* 36:751–755, 1972.
8. Nathan PW, Scott TG: Intrathecal phenol for intractable pain: safety and dangers of the method. *Lancet* 1:76–80, 1958.
9. Sourek K: Commissural myelotomy. *J Neurosurg* 31:524–527, 1969.
10. Gildenberg PL, Hirshberg RM: Limited myelotomy for the treatment of intractable cancer pain. *J Neurol Neurosurg Psychiatry* 47:94–96, 1984.
11. Schvarcz JR: Sterotactic extralemniscal myelotomy. *J Neurol Neurosurg Psychiatry* 39:53–57, 1976.
12. Nathan PW: Results of antero-lateral cordotomy for pain in cancer. *J Neurol Neurosurg Psychiatry* 26:353–362, 1963.
13. Mullan S, Hosobuchi Y: Respiratory hazards of high cervical percutaneous cordotomy. *J Neurosurg* 28:291–297, 1968.
14. Parker JF, Freidberg SR, Andrews JL Jr: Pulmonary dysfunction after unilateral percutaneous cervical cordotomy. *Lahey Clin Found Bull* 26:105–114, 1977.
15. Krieger AJ, Rosomoff HL: Sleep-induced apnea. Part 1: A respiratory and autonomic dysfunction syndrome following bilateral percutaneous cervical cordotomy. *J Neurosurg* 40:168–180, 1974.
16. Spiller WG, Martin E: Treatment of persistent pain of organic origin in the lower part of the body by division of the anterolateral column of the spinal cord. *JAMA* 58:1489–1490, 1912.
17. Mullan S: Percutaneous cordotomy. *J Neurosurg* 35:360–366, 1971.
18. Siegfried J, Kühner A, Sturm V: Neurosurgical treatment of cancer pain. *Recent Results Cancer Res* 89:148–156, 1984.
19. Takaoka Y, Freidberg SR: Electrode carrier for percutaneous cordotomy. *J Neurosurg* 40:786, 1974.
20. Gildenberg PL, Lin PM, Polakoff PP II, Flitter MA: Anterior percutaneous cervical cordotomy: determination of target point and calculation of angle of insertion. Technical note. *J Neurosurg* 28:173–177, 1968.
21. Hardy J, LeClercq TA, Mercky F: Microsurgical cordotomy by the anterior approach: technical note. *J Neurosurg* 41:640–643, 1974.
22. Sjöqvist O: Cited by White JC, Sweet WH: *Pain—Its Mechanisms and Neurosurgical Control*. Springfield, IL, Charles C Thomas, 1955, p 450.
23. Hitchcock ER, Schvarcz JR: Stereotaxic trigeminal tractotomy for post-herpetic facial pain. *J Neurosurg* 37:412–417, 1972.
24. Ramirez LF, Levin AB: Pain relief after hypophysectomy. *Neurosurgery* 14:499–504, 1984.
25. LaRossa JT, Strong MS, Melby JC: Endocrinologically incomplete transethmoidal, trans-sphenoidal hypophysectomy with relief of bone pain in breast cancer. *N Engl J Med* 298:1332–1335, 1978.
26. Levin AB, Katz J, Benson RC, Jones AG: Treatment of pain of diffuse metastatic cancer by stereotactic chemical hypophysectomy: long term results and observations on mechanism of action. *Neurosurgery* 6:258–262, 1980.
27. Moricca G: Chemical hypophysectomy for cancer pain. In Bonica JJ (ed): *Advances in Neurology: International Symposium on Pain*. New York, Raven Press, 1974, vol 4, pp 707–714.
28. Zervas NT, Gordy PD: Radiofrequency hypophysectomy for metastatic breast and prostatic carcinoma. *Surg Clin North Am* 47:1279–1285, 1967.
29. Hurt RW, Ballantine HT Jr: Stereotactic anterior cingulate lesions for persistent pain: a report on 68 cases. *Clin Neurosurg* 21:334–351, 1973.
30. Hitchcock ER, Teixeira MJ: A comparison of results from center-median and basal thalamotomies for pain. *Surg Neurol* 15:341–351, 1981.
31. Gorbitz C, Leavens ME: Alochol block of the celiac plexus for control of upper abdominal pain caused by cancer and pancreatitis: technical note. *J Neurosurg* 34:575–579, 1971.

32. Snyder SH: Opiate receptors in the brain. *N Engl J Med* 296:266–271, 1977.
33. Yaksh TL: Spinal pharmacology of pain and its modulation. *Clin Neurosurg* 31:291–303, 1983.
34. Behar M, Magora F, Olshwang D, Davidson JT: Epidural morphine in treatment of pain. *Lancet* 1:527–529, 1979.
35. Poletti CE, Cohen AM, Todd DP, Ojemann RG, Sweet WH, Zervas NT: Cancer pain relieved by long-term epidural morphine with permanent indwelling systems for self-administration. *J Neurosurg* 55:581–584, 1981.
36. Shetter AG, Hadley MN, Wilkinson E: Administration of intraspinal morphine sulfate for the treatment of intractable cancer pain. *Neurosurgery* 18:740–747, 1986.
37. Krames ES, Gershow J, Glassberg A, Kenefick T, Lyons A, Taylor P, Wilkie D: Continuous infusion of spinally administered narcotics for the relief of pain due to malignant disorders. *Cancer* 56:696–702, 1985.
38. Coombs DW, Saunders RL, Fratkin JD, Jensen LE, Murphy CA: Continuous intrathecal hydromorphone and clonidine for intractable cancer pain. *J Neurosurg* 64:890–894, 1986.
39. Lobato RD, Madrid JL, Fatela LV, Rivas JJ, Reig E, Lamas E: Intraventricular morphine for control of pain in terminal cancer patients. *J Neurosurg* 59:627–633, 1983.
40. Melzack R, Wall PD: Pain mechanisms: a new therapy. *Science* 150:971–979, 1965.
41. Sweet WH, Wepsic JG: Stimulation of the posterior columns of the spinal cord for pain control: indications, technique, and results. *Clin Neurosurg* 21:278–310, 1973.
42. Zumpano BJ, Saunders RL: Percutaneous epidural dorsal column stimulation: technical note. *J Neurosurg* 45:459–460, 1976.
43. Young RF: Evaluation of dorsal column stimulation in the treatment of chronic pain. *Neurosurgery* 3:373–379, 1978.
44. Urban BJ, Nashold BS Jr: Percutaneous epidural stimulation of the spinal cord for relief of pain: long-term results. *J Neurosurg* 48:323–328, 1978.
45. Long DM: Stimulation of the peripheral nervous system for pain control. *Clin Neurosurg* 31:323–343, 1983.
46. Richardson DE: Intracranial stimulation for the control of chronic pain. *Clin Neurosurg* 31:316–322, 1983.
47. Young RF, Brechner T: Electrical stimulation of the brain for relief of intractable pain due to cancer. *Cancer* 57:1266–1272, 1986.

part f
central-peripheral pain

chapter 35
Peripheral Neuropathy

David R. Cornblath, M.D.

This chapter concerns diagnosis and management of those peripheral neuropathies in which pain is frequently a dominant feature. Although the symptom of pain is a sensory phenomenon, the majority of these neuropathies involve both sensory and motor fibers; in some, autonomic nervous system involvement may also be prominent. Pathologically, the majority of these disorders are distal symmetric axonal degenerations (1). A few are systemic vascular disorders with manifestation in the peripheral nervous system. Rarely are demyelinating neuropathies characterized by pain. Entrapment neuropathies and specific mononeuropathies are dealt with in other chapters in this volume.

The chapter discusses three points relevant to the evaluation and treatment of painful peripheral neuropathy. First, because these disorders have in common dysfunction of small myelinated and unmyelinated fibers, patients present with a stereotypical story of the nature of their pain. Examinations of these patients are similar regardless of the underlying etiology of the neuropathy. Second, the differential diagnosis of patients with painful peripheral neuropathy is limited. The section dealing with the individual disorders concentrates on features helpful in diagnosis, because detailed information about the specific disorders can be found in a recent text on the subject of peripheral neuropathy (2). Finally, treatment is directed first at the underlying cause of the neuropathy, but simultaneous treatment of the pain itself can be successful if applied in an appropriate manner.

SYMPTOMS AND SIGNS

The symptoms of pain in patients with peripheral neuropathy are relatively stereotypical. Classically, these may be either positive or negative (3). Individual patients may have both. Positive symptoms may include paresthesias (abnormal spontaneous sensations) such as tingling, the feeling as though novocaine is wearing off, or the feeling that the limb is asleep. More annoying are dysesthesias, in which the presentation of ordinary stimuli results in disagreeable sensation. Dysesthesias constitute the most distressing symptom, because normally the limbs are continually in contact with stimuli. This is particularly troublesome at night when the feet are elevated and the bed sheets touch the feet. The characteristics of dysesthetic pain are distinctive: burning, raw, and searing. It has also been described as an unfamiliar sensation that is located on the skin. Many patients find that activity increases their dysesthesias, and it is these types of symptoms for which patients seek medical attention. Patients may also have negative symptoms, that is, numbness, a "wooden" feeling, or a feeling as though the limb were wrapped in cotton or encased in cement. Some feel as if they are walking on stilts. These symptoms rarely trouble patients because pain is not problematic. When sensory loss is particularly severe, patients find that they are unable to locate their feet unless they look at them. More severe nerve fiber loss is present in patients who injure themselves without their knowledge.

Physical examination of patients with painful peripheral neuropathy almost always reveals distal sensory abnormalities, particularly among those modalities that reflect small myelinated and unmyelinated fiber function (i.e., pain and temperature). Many of these patients have intact large fiber function (i.e., position and vibration sense, strength, and reflexes). Touch is variably affected and may produce dysesthesias. In recording examinations in these patients, several items should be noted. First, does the patient complain of positive or negative symptoms? Second, is the threshold for perception of a stimulus normal or raised at a specific location? Third, are dysesthesias or hyperpathias (abnormally exaggerated responses to a painful stimuli) produced?

Two features are hypothesized to be important in the generation of peripheral nerve pain (4). First, there must be increased impulse generation in nerve fibers. These most likely occur in small myelinated or unmyelinated fibers. Second, unmyelinated fibers must be abnormal for pain to be generated. This may happen either "externally" as in a compressive lesion or "internally" as in a peripheral neuropathy.

What is the evidence for these conclusions? First, microneurographic recordings of human nerves reveal that perception of pain is associated with nerve impulses that are conducted at velocities consistent with C fiber (5). Second, there is morphologic evidence. Dyck and colleagues related pain in the foot to the presence of acute fiber breakdown in myelinated fibers (6). The ratio of remaining large and small fiber was not related to pain. Brown and colleagues found that in patients with painful diabetic neuropathy the number of myelinated fibers was reduced by two-thirds, especially the small myelinated fibers (7). Nevertheless, the total number of unmyelinated fibers was normal, but based on morphologic criteria these were assumed to represent regenerating sprouts, which implied previous fiber breakdown. Said and others found that diabetic patients without spontaneous pain but who indeed do have painless injuries have virtually no unmyelinated fibers and a moderate reduction in the small myelinated fiber population (8). This suggests that the primary problem in pain generation is related to small myelinated and unmyelinated fibers. These data do not allow a clear understanding of the role of large myelinated fibers in the generation of peripheral nerve pain. The gate theory implies that loss of large myelinated fibers alone might leave small myelinated and unmyelinated fibers free to generate painful impulses (9). Fortunately, this does not appear to be the case, as exemplified by Friedreich's ataxia, which is not associated with spontaneous pain (10). Large myelinated fibers play a role in pain modulation, but are not necessary for the generation of pain.

Since pain in peripheral neuropathies depends on abnormalities of unmyelinated and small myelinated fibers, autonomic function, which is subserved by a similar nerve fiber class, may also be affected. In addition to the therapeutic importance of dysautonomia, knowledge that the autonomic nervous system is involved also aids differential diagnosis. Symptoms of orthostatic hypotension, gastrointestinal dysautonomia, impotence, changes in sweat pattern, gustatory sweating, and bladder dysfunction should be sought. This topic is reviewed in a recent monograph (11).

DIFFERENTIAL DIAGNOSIS

As mentioned above, the differential diagnosis in these patients is limited (Table 35.1). In many patients, the correct diagnosis can be obtained from the history and physical examination. Further evaluation, including blood and urine studies, electrodiagnostic testing, and sural nerve biopsies, will be necessary in only a small proportion of patients.

Diabetes is the most common cause of a painful peripheral neuropathy, although not all painful neuropathies are diabetic in origin. In diabetics who develop painful peripheral neuropathy, the history of diabetes is usually well established. In most, the neuropathy begins after many years of suboptimally controlled diabetes. Other "end-organ" disease, retinopathy and nephropathy, is frequently present. A more difficult situation is evident in patients with painful peripheral neuropathy in whom diabetes has not been previously diagnosed but is suspected. Some of these patients have metabolic abnormalities consistent with diabetes and will meet American Diabetic Association criteria. In others, an abnormal glucose tolerance test suggests diabetes. In that situation, it is helpful to include detailed ophthalmologic evaluation, measurement of glycolated hemoglobin, and evaluation of glucose in a 24-hr urine collection. In some patients, the probability that the painful neuropathy is caused by glucose intolerance is further strengthened by the presence of other neurologic complications suggestive of sustained hyperglycemia, such as impotence and carpal tunnel or lateral femoral cutaneous nerve entrapments. In those circumstances, the neuropathy is presumptively related to

Table 35.1
Causes of Painful Peripheral Neuropathy

Diabetes	Ischemia
Malnutrition	Sjögren's syndrome
Alcohol	Dysproteinemias
Amyloidosis	Cancer
AIDS	Porphyria
Toxins	Fabry's disease
Drugs	Insulinoma
Uremia	Mononeuropathies
	Guillain-Barré syndrome

glucose intolerance, and treatment is instituted for that disorder.

The best therapy for painful diabetic peripheral neuropathy is improved glucose control (12). In diabetics previously taking insulin, this may require more frequent administration of insulin therapy or frequent dose adjustments based on glucometer readings. In diabetics previously treated with oral agents or diet, insulin therapy may be necessary. In individuals recently discovered to be diabetic, therapy will be dictated by the degree of abnormal glucose intolerance. These forms of therapy alone may be sufficient to alleviate the pain (13, 14). Moreover, in some patients with diabetic neuropathy, pain may spontaneously resolve (15). Two hypotheses have been proposed to explain this. First, nerve regeneration may occur because of improved glucose control. Second, fibers may continue to degenerate so that spontaneously generated impulses no longer occur. Because these are observed frequently, therapy for the pain should be attempted with short-acting symptomatic drugs. In other patients, pain is continual and aggravating and has to be managed in other ways. The value of aldose reductase inhibitors (16) and myoinositol supplementation (17) in specific treatment of painful diabetic peripheral neuropathy await further study.

Malnutrition from alcoholism, gastrointestinal disease or surgery, improper diet, or other etiologies can cause a painful neuropathy (18). The disorder is characterized by early dysesthesias that then progress to weakness and sensory loss. The soles of the feet are particularly troublesome, and in various disorders associated with malnutrition the term "burning feet" has been used. Deficiency of the B vitamins, especially thiamine, pyridioxine, pantothanic acid, and cyanocobalamin, are most commonly associated with neuropathy. Other dietary constituents such as niacin are also associated with painful neuropathy. In many of these patients, it is difficult to ascribe the neuropathy to a single vitamin deficiency. This occurs because many of these individuals are multiply vitamin-deficient, the symptoms and signs of the individual vitamin deficiencies may overlap, and laboratory measurements of the vitamins may not truly reflect tissue stores or utilization. Treatment involves multivitamin replacement and a high-calorie balanced diet.

Two points deserve further mention. First is the debate concerning the precise role of **alcohol** in the production of peripheral neuropathy. The evidence has been summarized in a recent review (18) and suggests that alcohol alone is not neurotoxic to peripheral nerves. Unfortunately, most alcoholics are also malnourished, which creates difficulty in ascribing cause and effect. Treatment in addition to that mentioned above includes abstinence from alcohol. Second is the "neuropathy" of B_{12} deficiency. Most authorities agree that the peripheral nerve component of B_{12} deficiency is minor and far overshadowed by the spinal cord disease. Thus, the routine treatment of patients with painful peripheral neuropathy with B_{12} injections is unwarranted.

Amyloidosis is another cause of painful peripheral neuropathy. About 30% of patients with amyloidosis have peripheral neuropathy that is usually painful (19). These patients may present with neurologic dysfunction, especially distal dysesthesias, and only when detailed histories are taken is it clear that there is a systemic disorder manifest by weight loss and fatigue. In addition to painful neuropathy, many of these patients have evidence of further neurologic abnormalities such as autonomic insufficiency, impotence, and carpal tunnel syndrome. The presence of a paraprotein in the serum or urine suggests the diagnosis, which is confirmed by biopsy. Of currently available techniques, immunofixation electrophoresis is the most sensitive (20). There is no proven therapy for amyloidosis. The patients have a progressive neurologic decline but usually die from general medical problems.

A neuropathy characterized by painful parasthesis and dysesthesias is reported in patients with **AIDS,** usually in the preterminal stage of the disorder (21). The incidence is unknown. The disorder begins in the toes and proceeds proximally, associated with minor weakness. In autopsy examination of four cases, we have found gracile tract degeneration suggesting a distal axonal degeneration of the primary sensory neurons in the lumbosacral dorsal root ganglia (22). The relationship of this syndrome to human immunodeficiency virus is unknown.

Several **toxins and drugs** can cause a painful neuropathy. Arsenic intoxication presents with an acute gastrointestinal disturbance that is followed by a painful neuropathy (23). There may be remissions, particularly while in hospital, and relapses, suggesting repeated exposure. In general, the neuropathy is a distal axonal degeneration. However, there are reports of patients with a disorder resembling acute inflammatory demyelinating polyneuropathy (Guillain-Barré syndrome) from arsenic intoxication. The diagnosis is confirmed by measurement of arsenic in urine, hair, and nails. Unfortunately, the neuropathy may progress after exposure is discontinued. Thallium intoxication also produces a painful peripheral neuropathy (23). As with arsenic, these patients develop an acute gastrointestinal disturbance followed shortly thereafter by painful neuropathy. Hair loss, which occurs several weeks after the initial intoxication, is a diagnostic finding. Urine collection with measurement of thallium establishes the diagnosis. For both toxic neuropathies, removal of the toxin is the only proven therapy.

Metronidazole (24, 25), misonidazole (26), and nitrofurantoin (27) have been associated with painful peripheral neuropathy particularly when given over a long time. These drug-associated neuropathies reverse when the treatment is stopped provided that the degree of nerve damage is not severe. Nitrofurantoin neuropathy is especially likely to occur in patients with uremia (28) and may mimic uremic neuropathy.

Uremic neuropathy can occasionally be painful, especially at its onset (29). These patients have been uremic for at least several months. Many are improved either by more vigorous dialysis or by transplantation (30).

We and others have seen patients with **Sjögren's syndrome** with painful sensory neuropathy (31). Our patients have been primarily elderly women without a significant prior medical history. On close questioning many have had dry eyes (keroconjunctivitis sicca) and dry mouth (xerostomia) that have been unrecognized for years. The presence of Rh_0 antigen, a weakly positive antinuclear antibody, and an inflammatory lip biopsy are diagnostic. Although nerve biopsies are reported to show chronic inflammation (31), our patients' biopsies have only revealed chronic axonal degeneration. Treatments with corticosteroids have not helped.

Peripheral neuropathies have been associated with **abnormalities of serum proteins** (32). A proportion of these are painful at onset. In many, the neuropathy may precede the signs of a systemic illness so that careful testing of serum and urine for the presence of abnormal proteins is mandatory in patients with painful peripheral neuropathy. The neuropathy associated with multiple myeloma typically presents as a distal symmetric axonal degeneration with pain as a major component. Cryoglobulinemia has also been associated with painful peripheral neuropathy. Clues helpful in diagnosis are distal nerve lesions, Raynaud's phenomenon, bleeding diatheses, and digital ulcers. If suspected, special precautions must be taken in examining serum for the presence of cryoglobulins. Treatment is directed at the underlying cause of the cryoglobulinemia. Macroglobulinemia occurs primarily in elderly patients and presents systemically with fatigue, weight loss, anemia, lymphadenopathy, organomegaly, and an elevated erythrocyte sedimentation rate. The polyneuropathy usually develops after the illness is well established. Immunosupressants and plasmapheresis are the treatments of choice.

A syndrome of progressive sensory loss, areflexia, and ataxia has been described in patients with dorsal root ganglionopathy. Although the majority of these patients do not have pain, occasional patients develop severe painful paresthesias. These may be asymmetric and frequently involve the face. Electrodiagnostic studies are distinctive, with absent sensory action potentials and normal motor conduction studies and electromyography. The differential diagnosis is limited, with an occult **carcinoma**, particularly lung, breast, or ovarian, highest on the list (33, 34).

In **porphyria,** the neurologic phase of the illness may begin with pain (35). Painful paresthesias may occur anywhere on the body and are rapidly followed by weakness frequently involving proximal arms. The patients sometimes mimic those with Guillain-Barré syndrome. A detailed history particularly looking for a positive family history, associated episodes of abdominal pain, or psychiatric disturbance will suggest the diagnosis. The Watson-Schwartz test is diagnostic during an acute episode. Further testing is necessary to define the specific metabolic abnormality. At that point, family studies are mandatory. Treatment of the primary disorder consists of glucose infusion and hematin. Propranolol is useful in controlling the dysautonomia. In treating the pain, it is important to be aware of the list of contraindicated drugs in these patients (36). Chlorpromazine, meperidine, and morphine may be safely used when pain is severe. The former has the advantage of also helping with the psychiatric disturbance that accompanies the illness.

Fabry's disease (ceramide trihexosidase deficiency) is an X-linked genetic disorder in which young men and boys commonly complain of spontaneous pain in the feet and legs (37). The typical patient has spontaneous episodes of distal extremity pain that are brought on by emotional stimuli associated with vasomotor instability of the legs. However, examination may show no evidence of neuropathy. A characteristic rash, renal disease, and evidence of accelerated vascular disease—hypertension, stroke, and myocardial infarction—suggest the diagnosis, which is confirmed by enzyme assay in leukocytes or cultured skin fibroblasts. There is no specific therapy, although enzyme replacement has been attempted.

Patients with **insulinoma** may develop a severe peripheral neuropathy that is frequently painful (38). Although motor signs predominate, painful paresthesias are common. The neuropathy usually develops after an episode of prolonged hypoglycemia in which cerebral symptoms overshadow the neuropathy. Diagnosis is suggested by low random blood sugars and hypoglycemia during a prolonged fast.

Multiple **mononeuropathies** may present with pain in the distribution of the named nerve(s). There are a large number of causes of this syndrome, especially vascular (2). Treatment of the underlying lesion is usually all that is required.

Patients with acute inflammatory demyelinating polyneuropathy **(Guillain-Barré syndrome)** may have pain as one of their presenting complaints (39). Usually this is deep-seated back pain, resistant to nonnarcotic analgesics. No satisfactory explanations exists for this pain, which usually subsides witin a week or two.

TREATMENT

The treatment of pain secondary to a peripheral neuropathy is multifaceted. First and most successful is treatment directed at the peripheral neuropathy per se. In many cases, this is all that is required because this alone relieves the pain. For example, in diabetes, improved glucose control either by more frequent insulin injections or by the use of the subcutaneous insulin pump (14) has been reported to completely alleviate pain. In alcoholic/nutritional neuropathy, abstinence from alcohol and vitamin replacement are usually sufficient to relieve pain.

In several of the disorders listed above, such as drug-induced or toxic neuropathies, pain is a transitory phenomenon. In these and in processes where primary treatment of the neuropathy is expected to eventually alleviate pain, the use of analgesics alone is frequently sufficient. Aspirin, acetaminophen, nonsteroidal anti-inflammatories, and narcotic analgesics are used. Many physicians are reluctant to use narcotics in these cases. However, if it is known that the disorder will be short lived, then hesitancy about the use of these agents is unnecessary.

The third method of treatment is nonmedication therapies that patients try themselves. These include transcutaneous electrical nerve stimulation, immersion of dysesthetic skin in cold water, and the wearing of tight stockings for treatment of dysesthesias that occur in the evening when the feet are elevated. Although none of these modalities has been proven in controlled trials to help patients, individuals may find any or all of them beneficial, so it is worth attempting them in all patients.

Finally, the most difficult problem is the treatment of chronic neuropathic pain. The published literature consists primarily of small controlled studies and anecdotal reports about individual agents. Although many of these are not scientifically rigorous, the reports at least provide a guide to therapy. In using these medications the following principle is applied: a single medication is given until the maximum dose is reached as determined either by evidence of drug toxicity or failure to relieve symptoms. If unsuccessful, that agent is discontinued and a second medicine is given following the same principle. Medications reported effective in treatment of painful peripheral neuropathy include anticonvulsants [carbamazepine (40), phenytoin, and clonazepam], tricyclic antidepressants [amitriptyline (41) and imipramine (42)], and phenothiazines (41). Less well studied agents are calcium channel blockers and intravenous lidocaine (43). These medications can be administered until a satisfactory response to therapy is found. If no single agent is successful, combinations of these medications should be tried. Finally, sympathetic blocks and spinal cord stimulation may be attempted in resistant cases.

As mentioned above in the section on diabetic neuropathy, pain from peripheral neuropathies may spontaneously resolve. This is important information in two ways. First, it can be transmitted to patients and used to reassure them that with time it is likely that they will improve. This is helpful psychologically because patients are frequently depressed at the thought that the pain will last forever. Second, it is worth attempting a trial of medication withdrawal every few months in the hope that the pain will have spontaneously resolved.

References

1. Griffin JW: Peripheral neuropathies. In Rosenberg RA (ed): *Clinical Neurosciences*. New York, Churchill Livingstone, 1983, vol I, p 529.
2. Dyck PJ, Thomas PK, Lambert EH, Bunge R (eds): *Peripheral Neuropathy*, ed 2. Philadelphia, WB Saunders, 1984.
3. Matthews B: *Holmes's Introduction to Clinical Neurology*, ed 3. Baltimore, Williams & Wilkins, 1968.
4. Asbury AK, Fields HL: Pain due to peripheral nerve damage: an hypothesis. *Neurology (Cleveland)* 34:1587–1590, 1984.
5. Torebjork HE, Hallin RG: Identification of afferent C units in intact human skin nerves. *Brain Res* 67:387–403, 1974.
6. Dyck PJ, Lambert EH, O'Brien PC: Pain in peripheral neuropathy related to rate and kind of fiber degeneration. *Neurology (Minneap)* 26:466–477, 1976.
7. Brown MJ, Martin JR, Asbury AK: Painful diabetic neuropathy: a morphometric study. *Arch Neurol* 33:164–171, 1976.
8. Said G, Slama G, Selva J: Progressive centripetal degeneration of axons in small fibre diabetic polyneuropathy. *Brain* 106:791–807, 1983.
9. Melzack RA, Wall PD: Pain mechanisms: a new theory. *Science* 150:971–979, 1965.
10. Dyck PJ, Lambert EH, Nichols PC: Quantitative measurement of sensation related to compound action potential and number and sizes of myelinated and unmyelinated fibers of sural nerve in health, Friedreich's ataxia, hereditary sensory neuropathy, and tabes dorsalis. In Cobb WA (ed): *Handbook of Electroencephalography and Clinical Neurophysiology*. Amsterdam, Elsevier, 1972, vol 9, p 83.
11. Appenzeller O: *Clinical Autonomic Failure*. New York, Elsevier, 1986.
12. Committee on Health Care Issues, American Neurological Association: Does improved control of glycemia prevent or ameliorate diabetic polyneuropathy? *Ann Neurol* 19:288–290, 1986.
13. Archer AG, Watkins PJ, Thomas PK, Sharma AK, Payan J: The natural history of acute painful diabetic neuropathy. *J Neurol Neurosurg Psychiatry* 46:491–499, 1983.
14. Boulton AJM, Drury J, Clark B, Drury J, Ward JD: Continuous subcutaneous insulin infusion in the management of painful diabetic neuropathy. *Diabetes Care* 5:386–390, 1986.
15. Mayne M: The short term prognosis of diabetic neuropathy. *Diabetes* 17:270–273, 1968.
16. Jaspan J, Herold K, Maselli R, Bartkus C: Treatment of severely painful diabetic neuropathy with an aldose reductase inhibitor: relief of pain and improved somatic and autonomic nerve function. *Lancet* 2:758–762, 1983.
17. Green DA, Brown MJ, Brownstein SE, Schwartz S, Asbury AK, Winegrad AL: Comparison of clinical course and sequential electrophysiologic tests in diabetics with symptomatic polyneuropathy and its implications for clinical trends. *Diabetes* 30:139–147, 1981.
18. Victor M: Polyneuropathy due to nutritional deficiency and alcoholism. In Dyck PJ, Thomas PK, Lambert EH, Bunge R (eds): *Peripheral Neuropathy*, ed 2. Philadelphia, WB Saunders, 1984.
19. Kelly JJ, Keyle RA, O'Brien PC, Dyck PJ: The natural history of peripheral neuropathy in primary systemic amyloidosis. *Ann Neurol* 6:1–7, 1979.
20. Datiles T, Humphrey R, Cornblath D, Honcharik M, Johnson R: Monoclonal proteins in peripheral neuropathies. Presented at the Conference on Clinical Immunology, Baltimore, MD, October 10, 1986.
21. Cornblath DR, McArthur JC, Griffin JW: The spectrum of peripheral neuropathies in HTLV-III infection. *Muscle Nerve* 9(suppl):76, 1986.
22. Rance NE, McArthur JC, Landstrom DL, Griffin JW, Cornblath

DR, Price DL: Degeneration of the fasculis gracilis in patients with AIDS. *Ann Neurol* 20:142, 1986.
23. Windebank AJ, McCall JT, Dyck PJ: Metal neuropathy. In Dyck PJ, Thomas PK, Lambert EH, Bunge R (eds): *Peripheral Neuropathy*, ed 2. Philadelphia, WB Saunders, 1984, p 2133.
24. Bradley WG, Karlsson IJ, Rassol CG: Mentronidazole neuropathy. *Br Med J* 2:610–611, 1977.
25. Coxon A, Pallis CA: Metronidazole neuropathy. *J. Neurol Neurosurg Psychiatry* 39:403–405, 1976.
26. Dische S, Saunders MI, Lee ME, Adams GR, Flockhart IR: Clinical testing of the radiosensitizer Ro 07-0582: experience with multiple doses. *Br J Cancer* 35:567–599, 1977.
27. Olivarius B de F: Polyneuropathy due to nitrofurantoin therapy. *Ugeskr Laegerl* 118:753, 1956.
28. Tyler HR: Neurologic disorders in renal failure. *Am J Med* 44:734–748, 1968.
29. Nielsen VK: The peripheral nerve function in chronic renal failure. VII. Longitudinal course during terminal renal failure and regular hemodialysis. *Acta Med Scand* 195:155–162, 1974.
30. Asbury AK: Uremic neuropathy. In Dyck PJ, Thomas PK, Lambert EH, Bunge R (eds): *Peripheral Neuropathy*, ed 2. Philadelphia, WB Saunders, 1984, p 1811.
31. Kaltrieder HB, Talal N: The neuropathy of Sjogren's syndrome: trigeminal nerve involvement. *Ann Intern Med* 70: 751–762, 1969.
32. Mcleod JG, Walsh JC, Pollard JD: Neuropathies associated with paraproteinemias and dysproteinemias: In Dyck PJ, Thomas PK, Lambert EH, Bunge R (eds): *Peripheral Neuropathy*, ed 2. Philadelphia, WB Saunders, 1984, p 1847.
33. Horwich MS, Cho L, Porro RS, Posner JB: Subacute sensory neruopathy: a remote effect of carcinoma. *Ann Neurol* 2:7–19, 1977.
34. Malinow K, Yannakakis GD, Glusman SM, Edlow DW, Griffin J, Pestronk A, Powell DL, Ramsey-Goldman, Eidelman BH, Medsger TA, Alexander EL: Subacute sensory neuropathy secondary to dorsal root ganglionitis in primary Sjogren's syndrome. *Ann Neurol* 20:535–537, 1986.
35. Ridley A: Porphyric neuropathy. In Dyck PJ, Thomas PK, Lambert EH, Bunge R (eds): *Peripheral Neuropathy*, ed 2. Philadelphia, WB Saunders, 1984, p 1704.
36. Eales L, Dowdle EB: Porphyria and dangerous life-threatening drugs. *S Afr Med J* 56:914–917, 1979.
37. Brady RO: Fabry disease. In Dyck PJ, Thomas PK, Lambert EH, Bunge R (eds): *Peripheral Neuropathy*, ed 2. Philadelphia, WB Saunders, 1984, p 1717.
38. Jaspan JB, Wollman RL, Bernstein L, Rubinstein AH: Hypoglycemic peripheral neuropathy in association with insulinonia: implication of glucopenia rather than hyperinsulinism. *Medicine* 61:33–44, 1982.
39. Ropper AH, Shahani BT: Pain in Guillain-Barre syndrome. *Arc Neurol* 41:511–514, 1984.
40. Rull JA, Quibrera R, Gonzalez-Millan H, Castaneda DL: Symptomatic treatment of peripheral diabetic neuropathy with carbamazepine (Tegretol): double blind crossover trial. *Diabetologia* 5:215–218, 1969.
41. Davis JL, Lewis SB, Gerich JE: Peripheral diabetic neuropathy treated with amitriptyline and fluphenazine. *JAMA* 238: 2291–2292, 1977.
42. Kvinsdal B, Molin J, Froland A, Gram LF: Imipramine treatment of painful diabetic neuropathy. *JAMA* 251:1727–1730, 1984.
43. Kastrup J, Angelo HR, Peterson P, Dejgard A, Hilsted J: Treatment of chronic painful diabetic neuropathy with intravenous lidocaine infusion. *Br Med J* 292:173, 1986.

chapter 36
Entrapment and Compression Neuropathies

Stephen R. Conway, M.D.
H. Royden Jones, Jr., M.D.

The terms *entrapment neuropathy* and *compression neuropathy* are often used interchangeably, although they are really separate entities. The term *entrapment* is appropriate to use when mechanical distortion of a nerve occurs within a fibro-osseous tunnel or as a consequence of a constricting fibrous band. With entrapment, nerve damage may result from angulation and stretch as well as compression. The term also implies that the distortion occurs at a particular site that is potentially correctable by surgery (1). In contradistinction, *compression* neuropathies result from pressure applied to a nerve through the skin, as in Saturday night palsy, during operation from retractors, or from soft tissue sources, such as hematomas.

In either entity, nerve damage can result from high-grade pressure exerted over a short period of time or low-grade pressure exerted chronically. For example, ulnar compression neuropathy can occur acutely after coma, administration of anesthesia, or repeated low-grade trauma, such as habitually leaning on the elbows. Similarly, entrapment neuropathies can develop acutely or gradually. Generalized polyneuropathies may predispose to compression (hereditary liability to pressure palsies) or entrapment (as in diabetics). Other systemic conditions, such as rheumatoid arthritis, can result in entrapment syndromes by causing deformities in joints and ligaments.

Two types of pain are characteristic of compression and entrapment syndromes. When sensory fibers from the skin are disrupted, dysesthesias usually occur appropriate to all or part of the cutaneous distribution of the nerve. In addition, poorly localized pain frequently occurs as a result of disruption of sensory afferent nerves from structures, such as joint capsules, that do not have dermatomal representation. For example, deep pain is often a prominent symptom of entrapment of the anterior interosseous nerve (a pure motor nerve) and not infrequently accompanies carpal tunnel syndrome (in addition to the typical sensory dysesthesias).

The diagnosis of entrapment and compression neuropathies is greatly aided by electromyography (EMG), which consists of nerve conduction studies and needle examination of muscle. Nerve conduction studies help to determine the site of nerve compression or entrapment and the presence or absence of conduction block, and the needle examination is useful to estimate the degree of acute and chronic axonal loss if any. With this information an accurate prognosis can be determined. The recovery from pure demyelinative lesions, for example, is likely to be quicker and more complete than the recovery from lesions associated with axonal loss.

MEDIAN NERVE

CARPAL TUNNEL SYNDROME

Carpal tunnel syndrome refers to the constellation of symptoms and signs resulting from compression of the median nerve within the carpal tunnel. It is by far the most common entrapment neuropathy seen in clinical practice and serves as a model for entrapment neuropathies.

Anatomy

The boundaries of the carpal tunnel are formed by the carpal bones and the superficial border of the thick ligamentous flexor retinaculum, which is attached medially to the hamate and pisiform bones and laterally to the trapezium and scaphoid bones. The contents of the canal include the median nerve, blood vessels, and the flexor tendons of the hands and their sheaths. The median nerve gives off its palmar cutaneous branch before entering the tunnel. This branch courses superficial to the flexor retinaculum, and thus its injury during operation can result in persistent pain that can be mistaken for inadequate decompression of the median nerve itself (2). The flexor tendons are surrounded by synovial tissue that permits smooth gliding. The synovial tissue, however, is susceptible to hypertrophy and degeneration, which can narrow the effective space within the canal.

Venous and arterial vessels within the carpal tunnel compose part of a complex interrelated pressure system (3). Any increase in pressure can reduce venous outflow, raise intrafunicular pressure within the nerve, and consequently endanger the flow in the nutrient arteries to the median nerve. When hypoxia reaches a critical level, pain fibers become hyperexcitable and discharge spontaneously. Within the carpal tunnel the median nerve is composed of small funiculi that are well separated by epineural tissue packing (3). These funiculi can be compressed selectively, resulting in symptoms in only a segment of the distribution of the nerve.

Clinical Features

Carpal tunnel syndrome occurs most often in middle-aged women. In Phalen's series (4), the ratio of women to men was 3:1. Of these patients, 58% were between 40 and 60 years of age. The typical history is the gradual development of numbness and paresthesias in the median distribution of the hand (thumb, index finger, middle finger, and radial half of the ring finger). However, Fine and associates (5) reported 25 patient with carpal tunnel syndrome with pain or paresthesia exclusively or predominantly in a single digit. They attributed this to compression of a single fascicle. Phalen (4) observed that many of his patients complained of pain and numbness in the whole hand. He noted, however, that most of them reported the little finger to be spared after careful examination of their hands at night.

The most characteristic symptoms are nocturnal paresthesia and pain. These are most likely caused by the diminished return of blood from the limb during sleep because of hypotonia and lack of movement. Relief is commonly obtained by shaking the hand vigorously "to get the circulation going." Both flexion and extension of the wrists raise the pressure within the carpal tunnel (3). In addition, flexion forces the nerve against the flexor retinaculum. Sleeping with the wrists in the flexed position therefore might be a cause for symptoms at night. Driving, reading a newspaper, and sewing are also common precipitants.

Poorly localized deep aching wrist pain occurs frequently. Occasionally pain may also occur proximally in the forearm, elbow, and shoulder. In one series (6), proximal pain occurred in 57 of 90 limbs in 72 patients with carpal tunnel syndrome. Of the 49 patients in whom surgical correction was performed, 46 experienced relief of proximal symptoms.

Raynaud's phenomenon has been reported (7) to complicate carpal tunnel syndrome and even to antedate the characteristic neurologic symptoms. Phalen (8) believed that the occurrence of Raynaud's phenomenon could be a result of the large sympathetic nerve supply carried by the median nerve. Dawson and associates (9), in their review of one series of 24 patients with carpal tunnel syndrome and Raynaud's phenomenon, noted that four patients had Raynaud's phenomenon in the feet as well and suggested that this group might have a higher incidence of systemic rheumatic disease. The incidence of Raynaud's phenomenon in carpal tunnel syndrome is low, and at least one study (9) suggests that the prognosis for the alleviation of vasospastic symptoms with carpal tunnel release is guarded.

The results of detailed neurologic examination in patients with carpal tunnel syndrome are probably best related to the duration of symptoms. The presence of objective sensory loss is not invariable despite the almost universal complaint of numbness. In Phalen's experience (4) from 1950 to 1970, nearly 70% of patients had decreased sensation in some part of the median distribution of the hand. In many of them this included only the tip of the middle finger. However, with widespread recognition of the syndrome, earlier diagnosis may be associated with a higher percentage of normal examinations even though the patient complains of symptoms in the median nerve distribution. Of Phalen's patients, 60% had Tinel's sign, a tingling sensation radiating out into the hand produced by tapping over the median nerve at the wrist. The wrist flexion or Phalen's test reproduced the symptoms in 80% of Phalen's patients. This maneuver entails unforced flexion of the wrist for 30–60 sec. In this position the median nerve is compressed between the proximal edge of the transverse carpal ligament and the adjacent flexor tendons and radius (4).

Motor signs in the form of thenar weakness or atrophy, particularly involving the abductor pollicis brevis, usually develop after sensory symptoms have been present for a period of time. Weakness is usually an indication of serious nerve compromise and almost always warrants surgical decompression.

Carpal tunnel syndrome must be distinguished most often from radiculopathy of the sixth and seventh cervical roots. Occasionally it must be distinguished from median nerve lesions at the elbow and rarely from spinal cord compression or cerebral lesions that cause sensory symptoms in the hand.

Pathology

The pathology leading to compression of the median nerve is varied but can be divided generally into three types: processes that involve the walls of the tunnel and thus decrease the space for its contents, factors that affect the contents of the tunnel directly, and idiopathic factors (3). The first group includes injuries to the wrist (e.g., dislocation of one of the carpal bones), hypertrophic arthropathy, ganglia of the carpal joints, and thickening of the flexor retinaculum. A small carpal tunnel may predispose the nerve to pressure and ischemia, particularly in occupations requiring repetitive wrist and hand movements. The second group, affecting the contents of the carpal tunnel, includes changes resulting from pregnancy, disorders of the tendon sheaths and bursae, hypertrophic neuropathies, and, rarely, lipomas.

In pregnancy, the increase in total body extracellular fluid probably results in soft tissue swelling within the canal. In most patients, this resolves alter delivery (10). Carpal tunnel syndrome sometimes develops after delivery possibly because of the types of hand movements required in taking care of a baby (11).

Tenosynovitis of the flexor tendons and sheaths may occur in patients with rheumatoid arthritis. The tendons may also swell from a nonspecific tenosynovitis caused by occupational factors. In both instances, the intracanalicular space reserved for the median nerve may be decreased.

In gout, symptoms of carpal tunnel syndrome can result from deposits of urate along the median nerve and flexor tendons. With mild symptoms, medical management alone may be curative (12). Carpal tunnel syndrome may be the presenting symptom of amyloidosis, and staining of the removed tissue for amyloid fibrils at time of surgical decompression has been advocated (13).

Carpal tunnel syndrome had also been reported in association with both hypothyroidism and hyperthyroidism (14). In myxedematous patients, nerve compression is likely caused by thickening of the tendon sheaths by diffuse deposits of hyaluronic acid mucopolysaccharides. A similar process may also occur in patients with Graves' disease because localized myxedema occurs in a small number of these patients (14).

Median neuropathy in the carpal tunnel has been reported in patients with acromegaly and overactivity of the pituitary gland. In one series (15), successful treatment of the pituitary disorder abolished symptoms. In some patients, improvement was evident within weeks, suggesting that nerve entrapment was caused by edematous synovial tissue rather than osseous change. Persistence of symptoms was regarded as evidence for continued hypersomatotropism.

The placement of vascular shunts for hemodialysis has also been reported to cause carpal tunnel syndrome, probably by increasing hyperemia distal to the fistula (16).

Treatment

The treatment of carpal tunnel syndrome is successful in the majority of patients. Conservative measures are usually reserved for patients who have subjective sensory symptoms or reversible systemic conditions such as pregnancy or myxedema. Splinting the wrist is often effective in relieving pain in patients with mild symptoms. Local injection of steroids may provide relief but rarely prolong remission (4).

Most patients in whom conservative management fails are candidates for surgery. The majority of neurologists and surgeons would regard thenar weakness or atrophy as an absolute indication for surgical decompression at any stage. The success rate of surgery has depended on the duration of symptoms. In one series (17), a 97% success rate was obtained in patients with symptoms of less than 6 months' duration, but a failure rate of up to 25% was registered in patients with more prolonged complaints. Incomplete section of the flexor retinaculum is the most common cause for surgical failure.

ENTRAPMENTS OF THE PROXIMAL MEDIAN NERVE

Entrapments of the proximal median nerve are uncommon and usually occur near the elbow. When present, they commonly occur below the elbow in the region of the pronator teres muscle (pronator syndrome) or in the forearm (anterior interosseous nerve syndrome). Less commonly, the entrapment occurs above the elbow as a result of an anomalous band (the ligament of Struthers) running from the supracondylar process to the medial epicondyle (18).

Anterior Interosseous Nerve Syndrome

Anatomy The anterior interosseous nerve is a pure motor branch of the median nerve arising 5–8 cm distal to the lateral epicondyle. It supplies the pronator quadratus, flexor pollicis longus, and flexor digitorum profundus muscles of digits two and three. It carries no fibers for cutaneous sensation but does carry proprioceptive and deep pain fibers from the wrist (19).

Clinical Features Entrapment of the anterior interosseous nerve has been associated with the tendinous origins of the pronator teres, flexor digitorum profundus, and flexor digitorum sublimis muscles (20). Occupational stresses and strenuous exercise requiring repetitive elbow flexion and pronation can lead to compression of the nerve. Trauma to the nerve after intravenous cutdown in the anterior cubital fossa has also been reported (21).

Pain in the proximal forearm may herald the weakness, which has been characterized as a loss of dexterity in pinching. With pinching maneuvers, the index finger may remain hyperextended at the distal interphalangeal joint secondary to weakness of the flexor digitorum profundus muscle, and the thumb may assume a "straight" posture because of weakness of the flexor pollicis longus muscle

(22). The intrinsic muscles of the hand may be affected when a median to ulnar crossover occurs originating from the anterior interosseous nerve (9). However, this is rare. Abduction of the thumb should be normal because the abductor pollicis brevis muscle is innervated by the parent median nerve.

Rupture of the tendons of the flexor pollicis longus or flexor digitorum profundus muscles (not uncommon in rheumatoid arthritis) must be distinguished from entrapment of the anterior interosseous nerve. The patient usually has a history of flexor tenosynovitis or locking of the thumb (9). Occasionally, idiopathic brachial plexitis can result in weakness in an anterior interosseous nerve distribution, sometimes in association with weakness in the shoulder girdle (23).

Treatment The majority of patients with spontaneous anterior interosseous nerve palsy have a satisfactory return of function with conservative therapy (19). Surgical exploration may be indicated after 8–12 weeks if no improvement occurs.

Pronator Syndrome

Pronator syndrome may result from compression of the median nerve proximal to the branching of the anterior interosseous nerve. The three areas in which this occurs are beneath the lacertus fibrosus (bicipital aponeurosis), a thick fascial band extending from the biceps tendon to the forearm fascia; by a tendinous band in the substance of the pronator muscle; and under the fibrous arch of the flexor digitorum profundus.

Clinical Features Typically, patients complain of an aching discomfort in the forearm, numbness in the thumb and index finger, and weakness in the hand. A notable finding at physical examination is tenderness over the proximal part of the pronator teres muscle that is aggravated by pronation of the forearm against resistance (24). Resisted pronation may also result in paresthesias in the distribution of the median nerve. A positive Tinel's sign is often present at the proximal edge of the pronator muscle.

Weakness of the pronator muscle can result if the entrapment is under the bicipital aponeurosis (25). Weakness in other muscles is variable depending on the degree of compression and can be absent. When present, weakness may involve long flexor muscles of the fingers and thumb and the abductor pollicis brevis muscle innervated by the median nerve. Usually, objective sensory loss is poorly defined (9).

Nerve conduction studies rarely show abnormalities localizing the lesion but are useful in excluding carpal tunnel syndrome (24). Needle EMG may be helpful in demonstrating signs of denervation in the forearm above the carpal tunnel but distal to the site of entrapment in the proximal forearm. In many patients, pronator syndrome is associated with activities causing muscular hypertrophy of the forearm. Acute trauma, elbow dislocation, compartmental syndrome, and iatrogenic bleeding into the forearm can also cause compression (9). Surgical decompression may be necessary.

Entrapment at the Ligament of Struthers

Compression of the median nerve by the ligament of Struthers is rare and is usually associated with a supracondylar bone spur. Compression is even more unusual in the absence of a supracondylar bone spur (18).

Clinical Features The symptoms in patients with entrapment at the ligament of Struthers are similar to those in patients with pronator syndrome, including severe pain near the elbow (18). Differentiation between the two syndromes may be aided by the finding of tenderness and pain above the elbow, which is sometimes at the site of bone spurs from which the ligament of Struthers arises. The signs and symptoms can be vague and nonspecific in both syndromes, and testing can be difficult because of pain. Radiography of the elbow demonstrating the bony spur above the lateral epicondyle may be helpful in diagnosis. Surgical excision of the ligament and the bony spur is usually curative.

ULNAR NERVE

ENTRAPMENT AND COMPRESSION OF THE ULNAR NERVE

The anatomic course of the ulnar nerve predisposes it to injury at the elbow and wrist. Compression of the ulnar nerve at the elbow can occur during anesthesia or periods of intoxication or coma. Compression can also occur in bedridden patients or in those who habitually lean on their elbows (26). Most entrapments of the ulnar nerve occur at the elbow as a consequence of degenerative arthritis with tardy ulnar palsy or compression within the cubital tunnel, as is discussed later.

The cubital tunnel is roofed by an aponeurotic band that bridges the two heads of the flexor carpi ulnaris muscle. The ulnar nerve passes under this band medial to the elbow joint, which forms the lateral wall of the tunnel. Cubital tunnel syndrome refers to compression of the ulnar nerve in this fibro-osseous canal.

The term *cubital tunnel syndrome* is currently reserved for ulnar nerve compression in the cubital tunnel not associated with degenerative arthritis of the elbow (27). However, the original report of cubital tunnel compression included two patients with classic tardy ulnar palsy (28), and it was suggested that scarring of the ligamentous joint tissue could cause nerve compression by thickening the floor of the tunnel.

Degenerative arthritis of the elbow resulting in chronic ulnar neuropathy has been termed *tardy ulnar palsy*. Tardy ulnar palsy classically appears years after a traumatic injury to the elbow. In Sunderland's (3) study of 14 patients, 10 experienced fracture from 5 to 30 years or more previously. In four patients, old fractures of the lateral epicondyle were evident. However, the original injury often could not be defined because of bony overgrowth and deformity. The lesion in tardy ulnar palsy results from a combination of friction, progressive interstitial neuritis, and tension across a deformed joint (3). Several of Sunderland's patients experienced a recent additional injury to the elbow or nerve. The symptoms of tardy ulnar palsy are usually progressive; however, several patients in Sunderland's series improved after they avoided excessive use of the arm (3).

Various patterns of motor and sensory loss can occur because the intraneural topography of the nerve is such that selected fiber bundles may be affected. Tingling and numbness of the medial half of the fourth finger and the entire fifth finger are usually the earliest indications of involvement of sensory fibers and were noted in each of Miller's nine patients (27). However, sensory loss is not invariable even in patients with advanced weakness. Pain uncommonly radiates into the field of the ulnar nerve, although it frequently accompanies the elbow disability (3). Of the nine patients, seven complained of pain that was variably characterized as steady, aching, or throbbing. The pain localized to the hand, forearm, shoulder, and elbow. Compression over the cubital tunnel reproduced the pain in six patients. Classically, in patients with advanced disease, atrophy of the ulnar intrinsic muscles occurs, as was noted in each of Miller's nine patients. This was most evident in the first dorsal interosseous muscle with relatively strong ulnar finger and wrist flexion.

No patient with cubital tunnel syndrome in Miller's series (27) had a history of elbow trauma or arthropathy. Several patients had occupations that required repetitive movements of the hands with the elbow in a flexed position. Bilateral symptoms were frequent, and occupational activity tended to worsen the symptoms.

Treatment

The cubital tunnel syndrome must be distinguished from tardy ulnar palsy. Decompression of the cubital tunnel is probably the procedure of choice in the former (29), and transposition of the ulnar nerve (a more complicated operation) is usually recommended for the latter (3). However, neither operation has been evaluated in a controlled fashion. The results of operation for tardy ulnar palsy are variable. An appreciable number of patients experience immediate or lasting improvements in pain and subjective symptoms (tingling and numbness). However, motor function often does not recover or is delayed (3).

In Miller's (27) patients with cubital tunnel syndrome, surgical exploration revealed the ulnar nerve to be compressed by a dense aponeurotic band at the cubital tunnel. At operation, the tunnel was observed with the elbow in 90° flexion and extension. In each instance, the nerve was tightly compressed by the aponeurosis in flexion. Most patients experienced improvement in strength and relief of pain subsequent to decompression of the tunnel.

Several investigators (26, 30) evaluating treatment of ulnar nerve lesions at the elbow have reported patients in whom a macroscopic abnormality was not demonstrated at the time of operation. These patients did not differ clinically in a clear-cut way from patients with the more definable causes of ulnar neuropathy. The cause of some of these patients' lesions may be external compression. Whether or not operation benefits patients in this subgroup is not known, although simple release was reported to be less effective than transposition (26, 30).

Most studies (26, 30, 31) of ulnar neuropathies at the elbow have shown that recovery from pain and weakness is more likely in younger patients without underlying neuropathy and in patients who have had symptoms for less than a year. In our experience and that of others (32), patients in whom compressive ulnar neuropathies develop concomitantly with a surgical procedure tend to fare poorly whether treated surgicaly or conservatively.

ENTRAPMENT AND COMPRESSION OF THE ULNAR NERVE BELOW THE EBLOW

Ulnar nerve lesions below the elbow are uncommon. These occur at several sites. Compression within the forearm is rare and usually occurs in association with fracture, pressure from casts, or a closed compartment syndrome (9). The clinical picture is similar to that of compression at the wrist, although if the lesion is proximal to the dorsal sensory cutaneous branch, numbness over the dorsum of the hand results.

Damage to the dorsal sensory branch may result from blunt trauma or laceration. This branch splits from the parent trunk 6–8 cm proximal to the wrist, curves around the distal ulna, and supplies the dorsum of the hand and fourth and fifth digits. Painful dysesthesias can occur that resemble the quality of pain in lesions of the radial sensory nerve or lateral cutaneous nerve of the thigh.

Entrapment may occur at the wrist. As the dorsal cutaneous nerve exits proximally, sensory loss when present is confined to the palmar surface of the fingers of the fourth and fifth digits and the hypothenar eminence. To enter the hand, the nerve must travel through Guyon's canal, a fibro-osseous tunnel bounded by the transverse and volar carpal ligaments and the bony margins of the pisiform and hamate bones. Unlike the carpal tunnel, Guyon's canal does not contain tendons. Within the canal the nerve bifurcates into a superficial and a deep branch. The superficial branch supplies the palmaris brevis muscle and provides sensation to the hypothenar eminence and palmar surface of the fourth and fifth digits. The deep motor branch loops around the hook of the hamate and supplies the intrinsic muscles of the ulnar innervated hand.

Shea and McClain (33) described three variations in the clinical presentation of ulnar nerve lesions at the wrist. In their series, the symptoms and signs ranged from pure motor to pure sensory depending on where in the canal the nerve was compressed. The pure motor syndrome was most common, and isolated lesions of the superficial volar sensory branch were uncommon.

Lesions of the ulnar nerve at the wrist may be painless or may result in pain radiating to the digits and forearm. Dawson and associates (9) reported on six patients with these lesions occurring with Raynaud's phenomenon; the lesions probably resulted from concurrent thrombosis of the ulnar artery, which also travels through Guyon's canal. Ulnar neuropathy at the wrist has been reported to occur as a result of masses within Guyon's canal, such as ganglia; acute or chronic occupational trauma to the hypothenar eminence (9), such as in electricians (i.e., wire splicer's palsy), cyclists (34), or patients with walking frames (35); or acute laceration or fracture of the carpal bones.

RADIAL NERVE

Radial mononeuropathies can result from compression or entrapment above or below the elbow. Lesions of the proximal radial nerve are considered first.

ENTRAPMENT AND COMPRESSION OF THE HIGH RADIAL NERVE

Anatomy

The radial nerve is a continuation of the posterior cord of the brachial plexus. Branches to the long and medial heads of the triceps muscle arise in the axilla and brachioaxillary angle and run a relatively exposed and superficial course. In comparison, the remaining nerve trunk is more closely applied to the humerus in the spiral groove, explaining why weakness of the triceps muscle frequently results from crutch palsy but not humeral fractures or compressions distal to the axilla. The posterior cutaneous nerve of the forearm, like the branches to the triceps muscle, also lies more superficial and is not directly applied to the humerus. Thus, this nerve can also be spared in humeral fractures.

After winding around the posterior shaft of the humerus, the radial nerve pierces the intermuscular septum, leaving the spiral groove and the protective cover of the triceps muscle. As it continues subcutaneously around the supracondylar region, it is again susceptible to compression before running deep to the brachioradialis and brachialis muscles to the dorsum of the forearm (3).

Clinical Features

Compression of the radial nerve can result if another body lies on top of the arm for prolonged periods ("honeymooner's palsy"). The nerve can also be compressed in the axillary outlet by a crutch or the edge of a chair or bench. The latter types of compression occur most commonly during sleep or as a consequence of intoxication or anesthesia when warning sensations are not perceived. Radial nerve palsy above the elbow rarely results from nontraumatic compression. Compression from musclar effort (36), thickened epineurium (37), fibrous myopathy (38) (caused by drug injection), and tumor has been reported. However, most commonly the cause is traumatic, resulting from external compression or humeral fracture.

Treatment

The treatment of patients with high radial nerve palsy caused by traumatic compression is usually conservative. Patients with wrist-drop should have the wrist splinted in moderate extension to avoid joint stiffness and shortening of inactive muscles. The latent period to recovery depends on the level and type of injury. Patients with first degree nerve injuries that interrupt conduction but not axonal continuity begin to recover in 2–10 weeks. Patients with secondary nerve injuries that cause axonal degeneration may require 8–40 weeks for recovery (3).

Patients with third-degree nerve injuries that cause disruption of the connective tissue wall of the endoneural tube or complete severance of the nerve usually recover imperfectly if at all (3).

The treatment of compression of the radial nerve occurring in association with humeral fracture is controversial because both early exploration and observation have been advocated. The majority of patients recover spontaneously (3, 39). Some injuries occur after closed reduction and result from compression of the intact nerve by fracture fragments. In one study (39), these patients had a good prognosis after surgical exploration. Sunderland (3) recommends immediate nerve exploration for radial nerve injuries associated with complicated and open fractures or injuries resulting after closed reduction or both. This would avoid unnecessary surgery in patients in whom spontaneous recovery is likely to occur (simple nondisplaced fractures). Delayed surgical exploration is probably indicated if no recovery has occurred with conservative measures by 8 weeks.

COMPRESSION OF THE RADIAL NERVE AT OR BELOW THE ELBOW

Posterior Interosseous Nerve Syndrome

Anatomy The posterior interosseous nerve forms at the level of the lateral humeral epicondyle where the radial nerve divides into deep and superficial divisions. It descends as a continuation of the deep branch under cover of the brachioradialis and extensor carpi radialis muscles anterior to the radiohumeral joint but lateral to the biceps tendon. It supplies both the extensor carpi radialis and supinator muscles before passing beneath the tendinous free edge of the supinator muscle, which forms an arch, the arcade of Frohse. Although some disagreement concerning its anatomy exists (21), the arcade is usually agreed to be the region of entrapment. It is dynamic in its proportions, narrowing when the wrist is supinated and extended (3). Distal to the supinator muscle, the nerve supplies the extensor carpi ulnaris muscle and extensor muscles of the fingers and thumb.

Clinical Features Because the sensory branch of the

radial nerve bifurcates just distal to the elbow (before the arcade), entrapment of the posterior interosseous nerve is purely motor and has no associated sensory loss or dysesthetic pain. The radial wrist extensor muscles are also spared because the point of entrapment is distal to their innervation. Thus, wrist-drop is not complete and wrist extension is performed with a radial predilection.

Lesions of the posterior interosseous nerve are rare. Some of these lesions are caused by trauma from fractures of the upper third of the radius or Monteggia's fractures (dislocation of the head of the radius and fracture of the ulna) (3). When not due to trauma, the syndrome usually presents over the course of several days to a week (9). The onset may be associated with pain and tenderness over the lateral epicondyle or in the proximal forearm, although pain is not a feature in many instances. Paralysis may be partial or sequentially involve only certain muscles. The wrist may be spared. For example, Dawson and associates (9) reported on three patients who also had rheumatoid arthritis in whom weakness began in the fourth and fifth fingers before progressing to involve the index finger, long finger, and thumb.

Nontraumatic posterior interosseous nerve compression may result from tumors (usually lipomas) (9, 40). In many instances, the tumor is palpable preoperatively (40). Radiography may also delineate a radiolucent mass. Decompression results in recovery when performed shortly after the onset of symptoms (9). Ganglion cysts and neurofibromas involving the posterior interosseous nerve have also been reported (41, 42). Rarely, rheumatoid synovitis may result in posterior interosseous nerve palsy. The thickened synovia can herniate beneath the supinator muscle, stretching and compressing the nerve.

Idiopathic posterior interosseous nerve syndrome is usually thought to result from compression by the arcade of Frohse, although other structures have been implicated (43). Repeated pronation, supination, and extension of the elbow joint can draw the edges of the arcade taut against the nerve (43). Alternatively, minor trauma can cause edema or synovitis that compresses the nerve against the arcade (9).

Treatment If a mass cannot be demonstrated, operation should be delayed 8–12 weeks to see whether spontaneous recovery occurs. The nerve should be explored if weakness is progressive or nonresponsive to conservative measures (3, 9).

The association of posterior interosseous nerve syndrome with resistant tennis elbow is controversial. Although a subgroup of patients with resistant tennis elbow and forearm pain may have underlying posterior interosseous nerve entrapment, proving who does is difficult. It seems prudent to employ conservative mesures in patients whose results of neurologic and EMG evaluation are normal.

Radial Sensory Neuropathy

Clinical Features Superficial radial sensory neuropathy is usually a result of trauma. The quality of the pain is similar to entrapment of the lateral cutaneous nerve of the thigh (meralgia paresthetica) and is characterized by burning dysesthesia over the dorsoradial aspect of the hand (cheiralgia paresthetica).

The nerve lies freely between the tendons of the brachioradialis and extensor carpi radialis longus muscles and along the dorsoradial aspect of the radius unless the forearm is pronated, causing the tendons to cross (44). Pronation of the wrist, usually with flexion, can thus pinch the nerve and induce or aggravate symptoms. This movement, which also stretches the first dorsal compartment tendons, is the basis for the Finkelstein test used to diagnose De Quervain's extensor tenosynovitis. Thus, entrapment of the radial sensory nerve must be considered in the differential diagnosis of pain in the first dorsal compartment.

Radial sensory neuropathy can result from crush or twisting injuries to the forearm or compression by a tight watchband or handcuffs (45). Tight casts are a frequent cause. Damage to the nerve can also occur after De Quervain's tenosynovectomy, fracture of the radius, and cutdown for intravenous infusion (9, 46). In a series by Dellon and Mackinnon (44), 15% of patients had coexistent injury to the terminal branch of the posterior interosseous nerve, which innervates the dorsal wrist capsule, resulting in additional deep, aching, nonradiating pain.

Treatment Conservative measures are usually effective in treating patients with radial sensory neuropathy. Removal of the offending compression often results in improvement within 6–8 weeks (9). Splinting and injection of hydrocortisone have been advocated as well as neurolysis and proximal nerve resection in patients with intractable pain.

THORACIC OUTLET SYNDROME

Thoracic outlet syndrome has been called "the most controversial entity encountered in the field of peripheral nerve disorders" (47). A number of different clinical entities are commonly grouped together under this heading. The term *thoracic outlet* refers to the area between the base of the neck and the axilla. Thoracic outlet syndrome refers to the symptoms resulting from compression of the subclavian artery or vein or brachial plexus in this region. It can be divided broadly into vascular and neurogenic types. Vascular thoracic outlet syndrome may be arterial or venous. Neurogenic thoracic outlet syndrome has been classified by Wilbourn (47) into four types: classical, true, or motor; atypical; droopy shoulder; and disputed. The need for a disputed category reflects the enormity of the controversy pertaining to this entity. Only the classic and disputed thoracic outlet syndromes are considered here.

VASCULAR THORACIC OUTLET SYNDROMES

Arterial thoracic outlet syndrome can occur when the subclavian artery is repeatedly compressed or traumatized. The resultant symptoms are largely ischemic and are caused by anatomic changes in the artery. Intimal injury resulting in mural thrombosis and atheromatous degeneration can lead to arterial stenosis or the formation of emboli, jeopardizing the affected limb. Ulcerated fingertips or a cool, numb, pale hand with absent pulses can result (48, 49). Rarely, these emboli can travel retrograde to the carotid or vertebral arteries (48).

Venous thoracic outlet syndrome is caused by occlusion of the subclavian or axillary veins. It can also result from repeated compression. It is distinguishable from arterial thoracic outlet syndrome in that it results in a diffusely swollen, bluish arm and dilated veins over the chest and shoulder (47).

Numbness in vascular thoracic outlet syndrome is probably reflective of nerve ischemia and not nerve compression. Usually, the vascular and neurologic syndromes occur independently (50).

NEUROGENIC THORACIC OUTLET SYNDROME

Classic neurogenic thoracic outlet syndrome, although rare, is a well-defined entity. In England, Gilliatt (51) found only 20 patients with this syndrome over 15 years, and in this country, Wilbourn found 15 patients in approximately 9 years (47).

Clinical Features

The clinical, electromyographic, and radiographic features are characteristic (52). Wasting and weakness are usually marked in the thenar eminence, particularly in the median-innervated abductor pollicis brevis muscle. Most patients also experience weakness and wasting of the ulnar-innervated intrinsic muscles of the hand.

Pain and paresthesias commonly radiate to the inner aspect of the forearm. Sensory loss when present is over the inner side of the forearm and can involve the ulnar side of the hand and fingers (52). Sensory symptoms usually precede weakness. In a series by Gilliatt and associates (52) of nine patients, seven experienced pain as an initial symptom, either as an intermittent ache in the arm or forearm or diffuse pain in the limb.

The findings from EMG exclude the carpal tunnel syndrome (53). Median motor and sensory latencies across the wrist are normal, even though the pattern of wasting (thenar eminence) is suggestive of this diagnosis, and ulnar sensory potentials are typically diminished in amplitude. The characteristic radiographic abnormality is an elongated seventh cervical transverse process or rudimentary cervical rib.

Treatment

In the series by Gilliatt and associates (52), the compression was caused by a knife-like fibrous band that lifted and stretched the lower trunk of the plexus so that the nerve fibers from the thoracic outlet were angled sharply backward and downward to enter the axilla. The band extended from the tip of the abnormal cervical process or rib to the scalene tubercle on the first rib. Severing the band resulted in subjective improvement in most patients. However, improvement in strength and muscle wasting was usually minimal.

Although most patients with true thoracic outlet syndrome complain of pain in the arm before weakness develops in the hand, they clearly represent a minute subgroup of all patients with arm pain because classic thoracic outlet syndrome is uncommon. The number of operations performed for thoracic outlet syndrome is thus disconcerting. The majority are performed on patients without the objective neurologic findings or characteristic radiographic abnormalities previously discussed. Gilliatt (51), for example, referred only two patients with pain and paresthesias alone for operation over a 15-year period. Both patients had cervical ribs. Yet, the operation may still be a popular one in some centers, as illustrated by one large surgical series (54) in which operations were performed on patients without objective neurologic findings and with symptoms ranging from hemicranial headache to pseudoangina! Tragically, some experience serious injury to the brachial plexus or subclavian artery as a result of operation (55).

Whether thoracic outlet syndrome is as common as reported depends on whether one is a promoter of the disputed category as truly neurogenic. We agree with Wilbourn (47) that thoracic outlet syndrome

> is a rare or nonexistent entity, usually erroneously diagnosed by physicians venturing out of their field of training and expertise, who are not recognizing carpal tunnel syndrome, cervical radiculopathy, anxiety-tension state, or "compensation disease." The end result is that patients are . . . subjected to needless and potentially harmful surgical procedures while being denied appropriate therapy.

MISCELLANEOUS ENTRAPMENTS OF THE ARM

AXILLARY NERVE

The axillary nerve is a branch of the posterior cord of the brachial plexus. Lesions of the axillary nerve are most often associated with injuries to the shoulder, for example, fractures of the surgical neck of the humerus (3). The nerve can also be stretched after inferior dislocation of the shoulder or when the arm is externally rotated and abducted. Paralysis of the deltoid is the most disabling consequence, limiting abduction of the arm. Cutaneous sensation over the outer aspect of the upper arm can be diminished or normal even with complete denervation of the deltoid (3).

SUPRASCAPULAR NEUROPATHY

Anatomy

The suprascapular nerve originates from the upper trunk of the brachial plexus where the fifth and sixth cervical roots join at Erb's point. It courses laterally deep to the trapezius and omohyoid muscles through the suprascapular notch, a U-shaped structure within the superior border of the scapula.

The suprascapular notch is bridged by the superior transverse scapular ligament, which inserts medially along the edge of the lateral border of the spine and laterally at the scapular neck or scapulohumeral joint capsule (56). The ligament provides an anatomic predisposition to entrapment (57). Shoulder movements that exert traction on the ligament can cause compression of the nerve where it passes through the notch (56).

Clinical Features

The primary symptom of suprascapular nerve entrapment is shoulder pain that is poorly localized but most severe at the posterior and lateral aspects of the shoulder (58). Thus, suprascapular neuropathy must be differentiated from rotator cuff injuries and subacromial bursitis, which can also result from vigorous physical activity involving the shoulder girdle. Physical examination can show weakness of the supraspinatus and infraspinatus muscles, which are abductors and external rotators of the shoulder. The suprascapular nerve has no cutaneous representation.

In addition to musculoskeletal conditions, entrapment of the suprascapular nerve must be distinguished from brachial plexitis and radiculopathy of the fifth or sixth cervical root, which can cause similar symptoms. Dawson and associates (9) cited four features that favor the diagnosis of suprascapular neuropathy: local pain or palpation of the suprascapular notch; relief of pain after anesthetic block of the nerve as it passes through the notch; increased pain from maneuvers that stretch and compress the nerve, such as swinging the arm forward across the chest; and abnormalities seen on EMG that are localized to the infraspinatus and supraspinatus muscles.

Suprascapular neuropathy can result from trauma to the shoulder from either injury to the nerve or damage to the transverse scapular ligament or surrounding tissue. It can also occur spontaneously or as a result of lipomas or ganglion cysts. Backpacking has also been implicated (57).

MUSCULOCUTANEOUS NERVE

Anatomy

The musculocutaneous nerve is a mixed nerve originating from the lateral cord of the brachial plexus at the lower border of the pectoralis minor muscle. It travels obliquely (downward and outward) between the brachialis and biceps muscles before emerging 2–5 cm above the elbow crease as the lateral cutaneous nerve of the forearm.

Clinical Features

The musculocutaneous nerve is rarely injured in isolation because it is deeply situated and well protected for much of its course. Because it is fixed at the coracobrachialis muscle, stretch injuries can result from violent extension of the forearm. Heavy exercise has also been reported as a cause of injury either from contractions of the coracobrachialis muscle or chronic pressure secondary to muscle hypertrophy (59). Lesions of the nerve in the arm can result in weakness of the biceps muscle and dysesthesias over the radial aspect of the forearm.

Injury to the sensory portion of the nerve at the elbow distal to its muscular branches can also occur, probably from compression by the lateral free edge of the biceps aponeurosis. Bassett and Nunley (60) reported on 11 patients in whom symptoms developed after repeated pronation and supination of the forearm (one man inserted 3000 screws in a weekend!) or after hyperextension and pronation of the arm (as might occur after a fall or from an improper tennis swing). Pain over the anterolateral aspect of the elbow was the presenting symptom in every patient. All patients had tenderness over the area where the musculocutaneous nerve exits from beneath the biceps tendon. Ten patients had sensory loss along the radial aspect of the volar part of the forearm, but only those with acute sensory loss had burning dysesthesias in this distribution (60). A majority of these patients required surgical decompression for relief.

Entrapment of the sensory division of the musculocutaneous nerve has been reported to occur spontaneously (9). Injury to the nerve can result from carrying a heavy handbag with the strap across the elbow crease (61). The nerve can also be injured by careless venipuncture where it is located beneath the cephalic and median cephalic veins (between the biceps and brachioradialis muscles) (3).

SYNDROMES OF THE LONG THORACIC AND ACCESSORY NERVES

Scapular winging usually results from lesions of the long thoracic or accessory nerves.

Lesions of the Accessory Nerve

Anatomy The accessory nerve arises from the upper cervical segments and travels cephalad through the foramen magnum before exiting the skull at the jugular foramen. In the neck, it becomes superficial just above the midpoint of the posterior border of the sternocleidomastoid muscle. It courses obliquely across the posterior triangle of the neck to the deep surface of the trapezius muscle to which it is attached (62).

Clinical Features Accessory nerve palsy is associated with weakness of the trapezius muscle and variably with weakness of the sternocleidomastoid muscle. Most lesions develop after surgical procedures involving the posterior triangle of the neck, such as radical neck dissection or biopsy of a lymph node. The nerve can also be injured in sporting accidents. Rarely, accessory nerve palsy develops spontaneously without apparent cause (62). Injury to the accessory nerve results in shoulder pain and instability. The shoulder droops, and abduction of the arm is impaired. The scapula moves so that its superior angle is displaced farther from the midline than its inferior angle. Scapular winging is accentuated by flexion of the arm.

Lesions of the Long Thoracic Nerve

Anatomy The long thoracic nerve is formed from the fifth, sixth, and seventh cervical roots. It courses posterior to the brachial plexus on the scalenus medius muscle over the outer border of the first rib and vertically down the thoracic wall to innervate the serratus anterior muscle. The nerve is attached to both the scalenus medius muscle above and the serratus anterior muscle below, making it susceptible to stretch injuries when the shoulder is depressed or the neck is flexed to the opposite side (3).

Clinical Features In contradistinction to accessory nerve palsy, lesions of the long thoracic nerve cause minimal shoulder deformity at rest and more pronounced scapular winging with use. The inferior angle of the scapula becomes displaced farther from the midline and posterior chest wall than the superior angle. Scapular winging is accentuated by extension of the arm against resistance.

Compression of the nerve can occur during anesthesia if the patient is placed in the Trendelenburg position with poorly positioned shoulder rests that force the shoulder downward (3). Traction injuries can result from carrying heavy objects on the shoulder. Enlarged lymph nodes at the root of the neck and entrance to the axilla or their surgical removal can also result in nerve injury (3).

Lesions of the long thoracic nerve result in shoulder instability and weakness in raising the arm. The serratus muscle normally pulls the scapula forward and assists the trapezius muscle in rotating the scapula outward. Elevating the arm from a position of forward flexion or abduction is thus impaired (3). The weakness can be accompanied by shoulder pain radiating to the arm and neck.

Injuries to the long thoracic nerve can be accompanied by injuries to the brachial plexus or accessory nerve. Thus, winging of the scapula and weakness of the shoulder and arm can have more than one cause. Scapular winging can also result from paralysis of the dorsal scapular nerve to the rhomboid muscles and radiculopathy of the seventh cervical root (63).

LESIONS OF THE PERONEAL NERVE

The hallmark of peroneal nerve entrapment is foot-drop caused by weakness of the tibialis anterior muscle. Weakness of ankle eversion is also usually apparent. The fibers of the peroneal nerve are among the nerves most commonly compressed in the leg. They clinically comprise a distinct group, even in the upper thigh where they form a component of the sciatic nerve. Peroneal fibers split at the apex of the popliteal fossa where the sciatic nerve terminates into its peroneal and tibial divisions. The peroneal division courses laterally around the fibular head to enter a fibro-osseous tunnel bounded by the peroneus longus and fibula (9). The tibial fibers continue as a posterior tibial nerve. For reasons to be discussed, the peroneal division is often affected preferentially in proximal lesions of the sciatic nerve.

The fibers that make up the peroneal nerve are particularly vulnerable to focal lesions at the fibular head. Less often the peroneal components of the sciatic nerve are affected in the proximal thigh and clinically can mimic a primary lesion of the peroneal nerve at the knee. Compression of the peroneal nerve at the fibular head has a tendency to be neuropractic (caused by focal demyelination) (64), whereas lesions of the proximal sciatic nerve often have appreciable axonal loss.

At the fibular head the common peroneal nerve is particularly vulnerable to compression and penetrating injury because the nerve is only covered by skin and superficial fascia adjacent to the periosteum of the fibula (65). Inversion injuries of the ankle can cause damage to the peroneal nerve at the fibula head because the nerve is tethered proximally and has limited longitudinal mobility (66). Other causes of lesions of the peroneal nerve include infarction (64), pretibial myxedema (67), prolonged squatting (68), and tumors.

Prognosis depends on whether there is isolated conduction block due to focal demyelination or concomitant axonal injury present. Prolonged compression, such as that which occurs in someone chronically ill inadvertently crossing the knees or an intoxicated patient laying in one position, is usually associated with a good prognosis because focal demyelination is the major pathophysiologic mechanism. However, if axonal loss occurs, such as from penetrating trauma directly to the nerve, infarction, or sometimes with severe stretch injuries, prognosis for recovery can be one of a long and sometimes guarded course.

LESIONS OF THE SCIATIC NERVE

The sciatic nerve is most prone to injury at its exit in the pelvis at the sciatic notch. Although occasionally these lesions involve both the peroneal and tibial components, frequently a great portion of involvement affects the peroneal fibers. To the inexperienced observer this can mimic a lesion of the peroneal nerve at the fibular head. Predominant involvement of the peroneal fibers in lesions of the proximal sciatic nerve may be due to the presence of fewer and larger funiculi with less connective tissue packing in this portion of the sciatic nerve. It is also believed that the sciatic nerve is less tolerant of displacement because it is tethered at both sciatic notch and fibular head (64). In contrast, lesions of the midthigh usually compromise both peroneal and tibial function equally, probably because they tend to result from violent trauma, and in this position the fibers are equally vulnerable.

Damage to the sciatic nerve at the sciatic notch can result from fracture on dislocation of the hip, penetrating injuries, complications of hip surgery, prolonged pressure on the buttocks during various comatose states, and, rarely, spontaneous or anticoagulant-induced sciatic notch hematoma and primary or metastatic tumors, such as lymphomas.

Injuries caused by hip surgery or fracture are sometimes associated with a poor prognosis. Those arising during prolonged periods of coma can result in persistent disability. Stretch injuries can also occur at the time of operation, requiring utilization of the lithotomy posture. These injuries can also have persistent disabling sequelae. A poor prognosis is associated with axonal damage and inability of the nerve to regenerate over its great length to permit reinnervation. In contrast, if compression lesions mainly affect the myelin without axonal damage, as may be seen in pressure palsy or hip dislocations, the prognosis for full recovery is good, particularly in children (69).

SYNDROMES OF THE FEMORAL NERVE

ANATOMY

The femoral nerve is the largest branch of the lumbar plexus and forms in the abdomen in the substance of the psoas muscle. In the abdomen, it lies behind the ileocecal bowel on the right and sigmoid colon on the left. It innervates the psoas and iliacus muscles, coursing in the groove between them with the iliolumbar vessels before exiting the pelvis beneath the inguinal ligament to enter the thigh. Therefore, when these muscles are unaffected by a lesion to the femoral nerve, the lesion should be distal to the inguinal ligament.

In the thigh, the femoral nerve lies within the femoral triangle lateral to the artery. Several centimeters distal to the inguinal ligament it divides to supply the skin over the anterior thigh, the medial side of the knee, and the proximal part of the leg (via the saphenous nerve) and the innervation to the quadriceps and sartorius muscles (3). Lesions distal to the inguinal ligament can thus be partial because the femoral nerve breaks into numerous motor and sensory branches.

CLINICAL FEATURES

The femoral nerve is susceptible to open and closed injuries. Important causes of nontraumatic injury to the femoral nerve include hematoma and abscess of the iliacus muscle. The location of the nerve in the groove between the iliacus and psoas muscles makes it particularly vulnerable to an expanding mass in this area (43).

Hematomas usually occur as a consequence of anticoagulation or a clotting disorder, such as hemophilia (70). Characteristically, a large, sometimes painful globular swelling develops in the iliac fossa that in some instances extends into the groin. The hip can be flexed, abducted, and externally rotated to reduce tension on the nerve, which is stretched over the hematoma (70). The obturator nerve is classically spared. Treatment is controversial because complete recovery of nerve function has been reported even after large hemorrhage (71). However, with the availability of computed tomography to monitor lesion size a more precise assessment of the results of expectant treatment or surgical decompression may become available to guide management better.

Closed injuries can also occur as a complication of anesthesia. With the patient in the lithotomy position, the femoral nerve can be compressed under the inguinal ligament. Forced extension of the limb or hyperextension of the hip over the edge of a bed during coma can also injure the nerve, probably from undue stretch.

Open injuries to the femoral nerve can result from penetrating trauma, such as stab wound, or procedures involving catheterization of the femoral artery (3). They can also occur during the course of operation. Retraction injury, for example, has been attributed to forced lateral displacement of the psoas muscle (3).

THE SAPHENOUS NERVE

The saphenous nerve can be injured separately, resulting in pain down the medial aspect of the leg to the inner side of the foot or big toe. The point of emergence from the subsartorial fascia about 10 cm above the medial femoral epicondyle is its region of mechanical vulnerability. Entrapment here can mimic orthopedic causes of knee pain (72). Because the pain sometimes can be induced or aggravated by limb movement, it can also simulate intermittent claudication (73).

Isolated involvement of the prepatellar branch of the saphenous nerve can occur spontaneously or from trauma, for example, after medial meniscectomy. Stinging pain or an isolated spot of numbness below the knee can result. Tingling and a feeling like pins and needles can also occur when the knee is bent (74).

ENTRAPMENT OF THE LATERAL CUTANEOUS NERVE OF THE THIGH (MERALGIA PARESTHETICA)

ANATOMY

The nerve is derived from the second and third lumbar roots. In its intrapelvic course it penetrates the psoas muscle and travels obliquely across the iliac fossa to the anterosuperior iliac spine where it exits the pelvis beneath the inguinal ligament. It is particularly vulnerable to compression at the iliac spine where it passes between bone and the ligament and the attachment of the sartorius muscle (3).

CLINICAL FEATURES

The discomfort of meralgia paresthetica is variously described as burning, itching, pricking, or a feeling of coldness or numbness localized over the anterolateral aspect of the thigh. Hyperesthesia can also be present.

The syndrome has been associated with conditions that cause protuberant abdomens, such as pregnancy, obesity, and liver disease. It can also occur as a result of direct trauma, tight jeans, carrying a wallet in the front pocket, or standing at attention (75, 76). Presumably these conditions result in increased pressure on or stretch of the nerve.

Although meralgia paresthetica is usually benign, it rarely results from serious intrapelvic disease, such as retroperitoneal malignant tumor (77). Damage to the nerve can also occur as a result of abdominal surgery.

TREATMENT

Most patients with meralgia paresthetica recover spontaneously within weeks or months (3). Removal of sources of external compression is usually effective. Although local anesthetic block can be successful in providing symptomatic relief, this is rarely necessary because most patients cease to complain about the condition when reassured of its benign nature. Operation on the nerve, such as sectioning the nerve, is not recommended because of the risk of the development of painful neuromas that are worse than the meralgia itself (3). The role of neurectomy, decompression, or transposition has not been defined well for patients in whom conservative therapy fails.

ENTRAPMENT OF THE TIBIAL NERVE (TARSAL TUNNEL SYNDROME)

ANATOMY

The tarsal tunnel is located behind and inferior to the medial malleolus. It is bounded laterally by the bony tibia and medially by the flexor retinaculum (laciniate ligament). In addition to the tibial nerve, its contents include the tendons of the posterior tibial, flexor digitorum longus, and flexor hallucis longus muscles and the tibial artery and vein.

Within the tarsal tunnel or immediately distal to it, the tibial nerve divides into the medial and lateral plantar nerves. The calcaneal branch originates variably above or beneath the flexor retinaculum to supply the skin of the heel and calcaneus. The medial plantar division provides sensation to the plantar surface of the first, second, and third toes and the medial half of the fourth toe. It also supplies the abductor hallucis muscle. The lateral plantar nerve courses obliquely across the foot and supplies sensation to the lateral half of the fourth and fifth toes and innervation to the flexor digitorum brevis and abductor digiti minimi pedis muscles (78).

CLINICAL FEATURES

Foot pain and paresthesias are characteristic of tarsal tunnel syndrome and can be accompanied by sensory loss and Tinel's sign at the ankle (79). The pain is similar to that of carpal tunnel syndrome even to the extent that it occurs at night and can be accentuated or induced by prolonged standing or walking (9, 80). Weakness of the phalanges can also result, impairing the pushing off phase of walking (9). Although the tarsal tunnel syndrome has been likened to the carpal tunnel syndrome, the analogy falls short because tarsal tunnel syndrome is rarely a source of foot discomfort.

Tarsal tunnel syndrome must be distinguished from many other causes of pain in the foot, including painful peripheral neuropathies with which it may be associated. It also must be distinguished from entrapment of the medial plantar nerve in the foot, which has been reported to occur in joggers (81).

The most common cause of tarsal tunnel syndrome is trauma, such as fractures or dislocation of the ankle (9). Other possible precipitants include tenosynovitis; chronic thrombophlebitis; systemic diseases, such as gout, hyperlipidemia (82), hypothyroidism (83), and rheumatoid arthritis; and ganglion cysts.

TREATMENT

The treatment of patients with tarsal tunnel syndrome is initially conservative and may involve arch support, anti-inflammatory medication, or injection of steroids. Precipitating trauma should be removed. Sectioning the laciniate ligament frequently results in relief of symptoms when conservative therapy fails (9, 84).

References

1. Gilliatt RW, Harrison MJG: Nerve compression and entrapment. In Asbury AK, Gilliatt RW (eds): *Peripheral Nerve Disorders: A Practical Approach.* Boston, Butterworth, 1984.
2. Carroll RE, Green DP: The significance of the palmar cutaneous nerve at the wrist. *Clin Orthop* 83:24–28, 1972.
3. Sunderland S: *Nerves and Nerve Injuries,* ed 2. New York, Churchill Livingstone, 1978.
4. Phalen GS: The carpal-tunnel syndrome: clinical evaluation of 598 hands. *Clin Orthop* 83:29–40, 1972.
5. Fin EJ, Wongjirad C, Agrawal S: Single-digit pain and paresthesia: a symptom of early carpal tunnel syndrome. *Ann Neurol* 16:150, 1984 (abstr P144).
6. Cherington M: Proximal pain in carpal tunnel syndrome. *Arch Surg* 108:69, 1974.
7. Serra G, Migliore A, Tugnoli V: Raynaud's phenomenon and entrapment neuropathies (letter). *Ann Neurol* 18:519, 1985.
8. Phalen GS: Reflections on 21 years' experience with the carpal-tunnel syndrome. *JAMA* 212:1365–1367, 1970.
9. Dawson DM, Hallett M, Millender LH: *Entrapment Neuropathies.* Boston, Little, Brown, 1983.
10. Massey EW: Carpal tunnel syndrome in pregnancy. *Obstet Gynecol Surv* 33:145–148, 1978.
11. Tobin SM: Carpal tunnel syndrome in pregnancy. *Am J Obstet Gynecol* 97:493–498, 1967.
12. Murphy F, Beetham WP Jr, Torgerson WR Jr: Carpal tunnel syndrome caused by tophaceous gout: report of two cases with review of the literature. *Lahey Clin Found Bull* 23:18–23, 1974.
13. Mahloudji M: Familial carpal-tunnel syndrome due to amyloidosis (letter). *Lancet* 1:1374, 1968.
14. Beard L, Kumar A, Estep HL: Bilateral carpal tunnel syndrome caused by Graves' disease. *Arch Intern Med* 145:345–346, 1985.
15. O'Duffy JD, Randall RV, MacCarty CS: Median neuropathy (carpal-tunnel syndrome) in acromegaly: a sign of endocrine overactivity. *Ann Intern Med* 78:379–383, 1973.
16. Holtmann B, Anderson CB: Carpal tunnel syndrome following vascular shunts for hemodialysis. *Arch Surg* 112:65–66, 1977.
17. Semple JC, Cargill AO: Carpal-tunnel syndrome: results of surgical decompression. *Lancet* 1:918–919, 1969.
18. Suranyi L: Median nerve compression by Struthers ligament. *J Neurol Neurosurg Psychiatry* 46:1047–1049, 1983.
19. Spinner M: The anterior interosseous-nerve syndrome. *J Bone Joint Surg* 52A:84–94, 1970.

20. Shahani BT: Median nerve entrapments at the elbow. In *1986 AAEE Course E: Entrapment Neuropathies*, Boston September 25, 1986. Rochester, MN, American Association of Electromyography and Electrodiagnosis, 1986, pp 11–12.
21. Finelli PF: Anterior interosseous nerve syndrome following cutdown catheterization. *Ann Neurol* 1:205–206, 1977.
22. Cherington M: Anterior interosseous nerve syndrome straight thumb sign (letter). *Neurology* 27:800–801, 1977.
23. Parsonage MJ, Turner JWA: Neuralgic amyotrophy: shoulder-girdle syndrome. *Lancet* 1:973–978, 1948.
24. Hartz CR, Linscheid RL, Gramse RR, et al: The pronator teres syndrome: compressive neuropathy of the median nerve. *J Bone Joint Surg* 63A:885–890, 1981.
25. Martinelli P, Gabellini AS, Poppi M, et al: Pronator syndrome due to thickened bicipital aponeurosis (letter). *J Neurol Neurosurg Psychiatry* 45:181–182, 1982.
26. Chan RC, Paine KEW, Varughese G: Ulnar neuropathy at the elbow: comparison of simple decompression and anterior transposition. *Neurosurgery* 7:545–550, 1980.
27. Miller RG: The cubital tunnel syndrome: diagnosis and precise localization. *Ann Neurol* 6:56–59, 1979.
28. Feindel W, Stratford J: Cubital tunnel compression in tardy ulnar palsy. *Can Med Assoc J* 78:351–353, 1958.
29. Miller RG, Hummel EE: The cubital tunnel syndrome: treatment with simple decompression. *Ann Neurol* 7:567–569, 1980.
30. Macnicol MF: The results of operation for ulnar neuritis. *J Bone Joint Surg* 61B:159–164, 1979.
31. Harrison MJG, Nurick S: Results of anterior transposition of the ulnar nerve for adult neuritis. *Br Med J* 1:27–29, 1970.
32. Miller RG, Camp PE: Postoperative ulnar neuropathy. *JAMA* 242:1636–1639, 1979.
33. Shea JD, McClain EJ: Ulnar-nerve compression syndromes at and below the wrist. *J Bone Joint Surg* 51A:1095–1103, 1969.
34. Noth J, Dietz V, Mauritz KH: Cyclist's palsy: neurological and EMG study in 4 cases with distal ulnar lesions. *J Neurol Sci* 47:111–116, 1980.
35. Reid RI, Ashby MA: Ulnar nerve palsy and walking frames. *Br Med J* 285:778, 1982.
36. Lotem M, Fried A, Levy M, et al: Radial palsy following muscular effort: a nerve compression syndrome possibly related to a fibrous arch of the lateral head of the triceps. *J Bone Joint Surg* 53B:500–506, 1971.
37. Stöhr M, Reill P: Chronic compression syndrome of the radial nerve above the elbow (letter). *Muscle Nerve* 3:446–447, 1980.
38. Kim LYS: Compression neuropathy of the radial nerve due to pentazocine-induced fibrous myopathy. *Arch Phys Med Rehabil* 68:49–50, 1987.
39. Shaw JL, Sakellarides H: Radial-nerve paralysis associated with fractures of the humerus. *J Bone Joint Surg* 49A:899–902, 1967.
40. Goldman S, Honet JC, Sobel R, et al: Posterior interosseous nerve palsy in the absence of trauma. *Arch Neurol* 21:35–441, 1969.
41. Bowen TL, Stone KH: Posterior interosseous nerve paralysis caused by a ganglion at the elbow. *J Bone Joint Surg* 48B:774–776, 1966.
42. Lallemand RC, Weller RO: Intraneural neurofibromas involving the posterior interosseous nerve. *J Neurol Neurosurg Psychiatry* 36:991–996, 1973.
43. Carfi J, Dong MM: Posterior interosseous syndrome revisited. *Muscle Nerve* 8:499–502, 1985.
44. Dellon AI, Mackinnon SE: Radial sensory nerve entrapment. *Arch Neurol* 43:833–835, 1986.
45. Massey EW, Pleet AB: Handcuffs and cheiralgia paresthetica. *Neurology* 28:1312–1313, 1978.
46. Braidwood AS: Surgical radial neuropathy. *J Bone Joint Surg* 57B:380–383, 1975.
47. Wilbourn AJ: Thoracic outlet syndrome. In *1984 AAEE Course D: Controversy in Entrapment Neuropathies*, Kansas City, MO, September 20, 1984. Rochester, MN, American Association of Electromyography and Electrodiagnosis, 1984, pp 28–38.
48. Fields WS, Lemak NA, Ben-Menachem Y: Thoracic outlet syndrome: review and reference to stroke in a major league pitcher. *AJR* 146:809–814, 1986.
49. Judy KL, Heymann RL: Vascular complications of thoracic outlet syndrome. *Am J Surg* 123:521–531, 1972.
50. Gilliatt RW: Thoracic outlet syndromes. In Dyck PJ, Thomas PK, Lambert EH, Bunge R (eds): *Peripheral Neuropathy*, ed 2. Philadelphia, WB Saunders, 1984, vol 2, pp 1409–1417.
51. Gilliatt RW: Thoracic outlet compression syndrome (letter). *Br Med J* 1:1274–1275, 1976.
52. Gilliatt RW, Le Quesne PM, Logue V, et al: Wasting of the hand associated with a cervical rib or band. *J Neurol Neurosurg Psychiatry* 33:615–624, 1970.
53. Gilliatt RW, Willison RG, Dietz V et al: Peripheral nerve conduction in patients with a cervical rib and band. *Ann Neurol* 4:124–129, 1978.
54. Roos DB: The place for scalenectomy and first-rib resection in thoracic outlet syndrome. *Surgery* 92:1077–1085, 1982.
55. Cherington M, Happer I, Machanic B, et al: Surgery for thoracic outlet syndrome may be hazardous to your health. *Muscle Nerve* 9:632–634, 1986.
56. Aiello I, Serra G, Traina GC, et al: Entrapment of the suprascapular nerve at the spinoglenoid notch. *Ann Neurol* 12:314–316, 1983.
57. Hadley MN, Sonntag VKH, Pittman HW: Suprascapular nerve entrapment: a summary of seven cases. *J Neurosurg* 64:843–848, 1986.
58. Thompson WAL, Kopell HP: Peripheral entrapment neuropathies of the upper extremity. *N Enlg J Med* 260:1261–1265, 1959.
59. Braddom RL, Wolfe C: Musculocutaneous nerve injury after heavy exercise. *Arch Phys Med Rehabil* 59:290–293, 1978.
60. Bassett FH III, Nunley JA: Compression of the musculocutaneous nerve at the elbow. *J Bone Joint Surg* 64A:1050–1052, 1982.
61. Hale BR: Handbag paraesthesia (letter). *Lancet* 2:470, 1976.
62. Eisen A, Bertrand G: Isolated accessory nerve palsy of spontaneous origin. *Arch Neurol* 27:496–502, 1972.
63. Makin GJV, Brown WF, Ebers GC: C7 Radiculopathy: importance of scapular winging in clinical diagnosis. *J Neurol Neurosurg Psychiatry* 49:640–644, 1986.
64. Wilbourn AJ: Peroneal mononeuropathies. In *1986 AAEE Course E: Entrapment Neuropathies*, Boston, September 25, 1986. Rochester, MN, American Association of Electromyography and Electrodiagnosis, 1986, pp 19–28.
65. Berry H, Richardson PM: Common peroneal palsy: a clinical and electrophysiological review. *J Neurol Neurosurg Psychiatry* 39:1162–1171, 1976.
66. Meals RA: Peroneal-nerve palsy complicating ankle sprain. *J Bone Joint Surg* 59A:966–968, 1977.
67. Siegler M, Refetoff S: Pretibial myxedema—a reversible cause

of foot drop due to entrapment of the peroneal nerve. *N Engl J Med* 294:1383–1384, 1976.
68. Koller RL, Blank NK: Strawberry pickers' palsy. *Arch Neurol* 37:320, 1980.
69. Jones HR Jr, Gianturco L: Sciatic neuropathies in children: report of 9 cases. *Ann Neurol* 18:158, 1985 (abstr P157).
70. Nobel W, Marks SC Jr, Kubik S: The anatomical basis for femoral nerve palsy following iliacus hematoma. *J Neurosurg* 52:533–540, 1980.
71. Susens GP, Hendrickson CG, Mulder MJ, et al: Femoral nerve entrapment secondary to a heparin hematoma. *Ann Intern Med* 69:575–579, 1968.
72. Kopell HP, Thompson WAL: Knee pain due to saphenous-nerve entrapment. *N Engl J Med* 263:351–353, 1960.
73. Mozes M, Ouaknine G, Nathan H: Saphenous nerve entrapment simulating vascular disorder. *Surgery* 77:299–303, 1975.
74. Massey EW: Gonyalgia paresthetica (letter). *Muscle Nerve* 4:80–81, 1981.
75. Kaufman J, Canoso JJ: Progressive systemic sclerosis and meralgia paraesthetica (letter). *Ann Intern Med* 105:973, 1986.
76. Massey EW: Meralgia paresthetica: an unusual case. *JAMA* 237:1125–1126, 1977.
77. Flowers RS: Meralgia paresthetica: a clue to retroperitoneal malignant tumor. *Am J Surg* 116:89–92, 1968.
78. Kraft GH: Tarsal tunnel entrapment. In *1986 AAEE Course E: Entrapment Neuropathies*, Boston, September 25, 1986. Rochester, MN, American Association of Electromyography and Electrodiagnosis, 1986, pp 13–18.
79. Oh SJ, Sarala PK, Kuba T, et al: Tarsal tunnel syndrome: electrophysiological study. *Ann Neurol* 5:327–330, 1979.
80. DeLisa JA, Saeed MA; The tarsal tunnel syndrome. *Muscle Nerve* 6:664–670, 1983.
81. Oh SJ, Lee KW: Medial plantar neuropathy: a heretofore unrecognized mononeuropathy. *Ann Neurol* 20:135, 1986 (abstr P46).
82. Ruderman MI, Palmar RH, Olarte MR, et al: Tarsal tunnel syndrome caused by hyperlipidemia: reversal after plasmapheresis. *Arch Neurol* 40:124–125, 1983.
83. Schwartz MS, Macworth-Young CG, McKeran RO: The tarsal tunnel syndrome in hypothyroidism. *J Neurol Neurosurg Psychiatry* 46:440–442, 1983.
84. Kaplan PE, Kernahan WT: Tarsal tunnel syndrome. *J Bone Joint Surg* 63A:96–99, 1981.

chapter 37
Reflex Sympathetic Dystrophy and Causalgia

Nelson Hendler, M.D., M.S.

CLINICAL SIGNS AND SYMPTOMS

Reflex sympathetic dystrophy (RSD) and causalgia are symptom complexes that evoke a great deal of confusion. Very often, physicians do not recognize that these are separate and distinct entities, and commonly assume that they are disorders of the same etiology, as well as responsive to the same treatment. Clinically, this has not proven accurate. Reflex sympathetic dystrophy is a group of symptoms and clinical signs that usually follows a minor injury to a limb. In contradistinction, causalgia is usually associated with peripheral nerve injury, classically from a bullet wound or some other partial nerve damage. In a very fine review article, Payne clearly defined the distinction between causalgia and RSD (1). Clinically, one can make the distinction between the two disorders on the basis of not only signs and symptoms, but also response to treatment.

REFLEX SYMPATHETIC DYSTROPHY

Following the distinction drawn by Payne, one considers RSD as occurring as the result of minor trauma; inflammation following surgery, infection, or lacerations resulting in some degree of swelling in the affected limb; infarctions; degenerative joint disease; frostbite; and burns (1). One should add to this list the possibility of any compression, such as casting or swelling due to injury, that may cause prolonged pressure on peripheral nerves. Additionally, this author has seen at least two or three cases per year of RSD brought about from arthroscopy. Unfortunately, no other reported cases appear in the literature, so this is really a clinical impression garnered from 15 years' experience working with RSD patients.

According to Payne, there seem to be three phases to RSD. Additionally, physicians should recognize that RSD is a symptom complex that is a cluster of symptoms and signs, and that patients do NOT present with all the signs and symptoms during the course of their disease. In fact, very often, they may have only one or two of the signs and symptoms of the disorder.

As described by Payne, the *acute stage* of RSD lasts several weeks, and is characterized by spontaneous pain, usually aching or burning, that follows the distribution of blood vessels or peripheral nerves. The acute stage may manifest as "hyperpathia" (this is described as a painful syndrome of overreaction to a stimulus or after-sensation following a stimulus) and may include hypesthesia or hyperesthesia, (described as a decreased or increased sensation to stimulation, respectively) or dysesthesia (described as an unpleasant abnormal sensation) (1). Associated with these tactile sensations are usually a warm, dry, red skin or cold, blue, sweaty skin, with some swelling, and, surprisingly, increased hair and nail growth. Additionally, the patient has dependent redness and reduced motion in the damaged extremity. This summarizes the acute stage of this disorder, which may last several weeks, and may begin immediately or several days after the onset of the injury.

The second stage of RSD, beginning about 3–6 months after the injury, is called the *dystrophic stage* by Payne (1). During this stage, the patient experiences a burning type of pain, which radiates either above or below the site of the injury, and increased hypersensitivity or hyperalgesia (an exquisite sensitivity to touch or temperature—a most important distinction that is discussed later in the chapter). The patient has changes in the nails on occasion, as well as decreased hair growth. This seems to be a variable finding, and certainly is *NOT* a sine qua non of the diagnosis of RSD. Joints may become stiff, with decreased range of motion and possible thickening, associated with some degree of muscle wasting. Edema may be present, and upon appropriate testing osteoporosis may be noted (1).

The third stage described by Payne is the *atrophic stage*, which usually occurs 6 months or longer after the injury. According to Payne, the patient experiences pain, decreased skin temperature, trophic changes in the skin associated with a smooth glossy skin, stiff fixed joints associated with contractures, increased or decreased sweating in the affected extremity, and demineralization of the bone associated with wasted muscles and reduced strength (1).

CAUSALGIA

Causalgia is usually associated with peripheral nerve injury and severe pain. According to Payne, pain occurring in causalgia follows an injury to a nerve trunk, usually a major proximal nerve branch, and is described as a persistent burning pain, but does not necessarily have to be burning in quality. It is unrelated to associated damage from surrounding tissue, and seems to be worsened by emotional or environmental stimuli. Most importantly, the pain seems to persist more than 5–6 weeks, which seems to be the length of time needed for surrounding tissue to recover from injury. Typically, the injury is due to damage by a bullet, a knife, or other such objects. When the injury is associated with a high-velocity missile, one must consider not only the actual damage to the tissue itself, but hydrostatic effects caused by shockwaves. When one takes into account the fact that the body is made up largely of water, it is easy to see how a high-velocity missile can cause damage not only to the actual tissue that has been penetrated by the missile, but also to surrounding tissue as a result of hydrostatically transmitted shock waves. If the reader desires additional confirmation regarding the hydrostatic effects of high-velocity missiles, he or she is referred to a most amazing book entitled *Split Seconds* (2).

Typically, patients with causalgia report an onset of pain within several hours to a week after the injury, and describe the pain using words such as "stinging," "aching," "burning," or "tingling." Superimposed on the regular pain, patients may experience paroxysms of deep pain (1).

Long clearly made the distinction between causalgia and RSD (3). Causalgia is secondary to partial injury to major mixed nerves, caused by low- or high-velocity missiles, and manifests as trophic changes in the distribution of the nerve associated with extreme hypersensitivity. The pain is diffuse and burning, and true causalgia almost always responds to sympathectomy. Long suggested performing three or more sympathetic blocks, sometimes every day for up to a week or longer, with the expectation that longer relief should follow each subsequent block. With positive responses to sympathetic blocks, he would suggest a sympathectomy (3). On the other hand, RSD usually follows a minor injury and does not involve a major nerve root (3). Frequently, the site of injury is the wrist, and the pain seems to get worse with cold but not with emotional upset, unlike causalgia. Demineralization of the bone occurs, with fibrosis of tendons and sheaths and spasm of the muscle. Dysesthesia suggests that there will be less success with sympathectomy.

THEORY

With the above clinical descriptions in mind, one can then make an effort to define the various anatomic, neuroanatomic, and physiologic bases for these two disorders. Chostine et al. have suggested multiple etiologies for causalgia (4). Various considerations include ephapse, in which there seems to be an erosion of the insulation between nerve fibers, allowing for short-circuiting between somatic afferent fibers and sympathetic efferent fibers, and experimentally produced neuromas, with resultant ephapses occurring both acutely and chronically between myelinated fibers. However, because of the delay in developing the ephapses, which does not correspond to the clinical observations of a relatively rapid onset of RSD and causalgia, the theory of ephapses as the etiology of causalgia has fallen from favor (4). To replace this theory, the concept of nerve sprouts, or free nerve endings that are sparsely myelinated, seems feasible. Axonal sprouting has been noted to occur early after an injury, with a high frequency, and without total axonal disruption (4). The possibility that causalgia is produced by these sparsely myelinated fibers is supported by evidence that the blood-nerve barrier, which is similar to the blood-brain barrier, has been destroyed in the injured nerve (4).

Perhaps the most comprehensive review of the neurophysiologic basis of RSD and causalgia has been advanced by Roberts (5). In his extensive review article, Roberts dealt with the neuroma mechanisms associated with pain of causalgia and RSD. He called these disorders "sympathetically maintained pain (SMP)." His hypothesis regarding SMP is based on two assumptions: "(1) that a high rate of firing in spinal wide dynamic range (WDR) or multireceptive neurons results in painful sensation and (2) that nociceptor response is associated with trauma which can produce long-term sensitization of the WDR neurons." Furthermore, his theory postulates that SMP is mediated by low-threshold, myelinated mechanoreceptors, and that these impulses, which carry messages to the brain, are the result of sympathetic fibers carrying messages from the spinal cord and brain to act upon the receptors, or to act upon the fibers carrying messages to the brain (5). The most important part of this hypothesis is the fact that Roberts does not postulate the need for nerve injury, or for dystrophic tissue. However, before one can more fully appreciate Roberts' theories, one has to explore the basic anatomy of the sympathetic chains.

GROSS ANATOMY

The most startling finding, and one that flies in the face of commonly held beliefs, is a report by Kleiman in which sympathetic chains were found to have communication between them, in up to 80% of cases (6). This is an important finding, since this anatomic consideration is rarely, if ever, discussed in surgical textbooks or clinical papers. This finding also explains why some cases of RSD do not respond to sympathetic denervation, and why, paradoxical as it may seem, some cases do respond to contralateral blocks (i.e., if a patient has pain in the left leg, blocking the right lumbar sympathetic chain may produce relief). Additional anatomy has been described by Allen and Morety (7). When one traces the pathway of the sympathetic nerves, cell bodies are located in the lateral columns of the cervical, thoracic, and lumbar spinal cord. Cell bodies then give off axons, which form the preganglionic fibers of the sympathetic nervous system. From C7 to L2, these fibers are associated with the anterior spinal nerve roots, and leave the spinal cord in this pathway. They then separate from the nerve root and become the white rami communicantes, which then continue on to the paravertebral ganglia, which form a chain running from the skull to the coccyx. From the ganglia themselves postganglionic fibers run back to nerve roots, or become separate nerves supplying various organs. It is important to note that some ganglion cells are found in the anterior roots, as well as the white and gray rami (7). By the same token, some pre- and postganglionic fibers do not pass through sympathetic trunks, which again indicates that there is residual sympathetic innervation due to either normal variants or aberrant fibers that bypass the sympathetic trunk. This anatomic finding explains the failure of some ganglionectomies, and suggests that one might need to do anterior nerve root sections and preganglionic rami sectioning (Smithwick procedure) in patients in whom ganglionectomy has failed (7).

Cervical outflow, coming from the upper portion of the cervical chain, sends fibers to the pupils and the eyelids. These fibers radiate from the upper stellate ganglion, which also supplies various fibers in the head and face. The upper thoracic sympathetic chain receives preganglionic input from upper thoracic roots, and supplies the upper extremity through postganglionic fibers that pass through the brachial plexus (7). The lower extremities receive input from the T11 through L3 nerve roots, forming ganglia, and from the lower two lumbar and upper sacral nerve roots, with gray rami (postganglionic) to the lumbosacral plexus (7).

MICROANATOMY

As described in the gross anatomy portion above, there are various sites along the sympathetic chain where damage can occur to a nerve. Additionally, there are several sites where chemical intervention is possible, notably at the synapses that occur along the sympathetic pathways. Additionally, the various fibers that carry sympathetic messages are important. It has been widely held that C fibers, which are small unmyelinated fibers carrying sensory messages, are responsible for the transmission of pain. However, some theories consider that SMP is mediated by activity in A fibers, since C fiber blockade fails to eliminate pain in patients with SMP (5). Therefore, one must start at the very beginning of the onset of pain, that is the receptor itself, in order to fully understand SMP, RSD, and causalgia.

Originally, it was thought that nociceptor afferents (nerves that carry the message of pain from the periphery to the cord and the brain) were responsible for the continuous pain of SMP, RSD, and causalgia (5, 8, 9). However, in Roberts' paper, he adheres to a theory first advanced by Loh and Nathan (10) that indicates that low-threshold mechanoreceptors are responsible for SMP (5). Roberts takes this position because nociceptor afferents, which are typically considered unmyelinated C fibers, do not have appropriate responses to sympathetic activity and, therefore, both practically and conceptually cannot be included as the receptors that mediate SMP. However, Roberts reported that mechanoreceptors do respond appropriately to both touch and sympathetic activity (5). For causalgia, others have proposed a neuroma formation as the cause of pain. However, Roberts believes that the sympathetic action of a neuroma is not capable of explaining why treatments that occur distal to the injury (in the form of either a nerve block or guanethidine infusion) are able to ameliorate causalgia. However, Roberts used the summation theory, or convergence theory, to say that both the peripheral receptors (in this case, mechanoreceptors) that arise in the neuroma and those that arise in the skin itself are transmitting painful messages to the cord, and that distal blocks eliminate only the mechanoreceptors from the skin, which is not enough to trigger responses in the WDR neurons in the spinal cord. Additionally, the concept of a neuroma causing prolongation of causalgia-type pain does not fit the clinical observation that SMP may occur even in cases in which the nerve is not injured (5).

Ochoa advanced the theory that mechanical A-delta nociceptor endings become sensitized to multiple sensory inputs (11). This gives rise to the thermal hyperalgesia that is seen in RSD. On the other hand, Ochoa believes that there are abnormalities in distal nociceptor fibers that seem to have a low threshold. These low-threshold mechanoreceptors reside within large myelinated fibers, and are non–sympathetic dependent, because they transfer their information to nociceptor pathways proximal to the site of injury. These fibers may account for the mechanical hyperalgesia, manifesting as sensitivity to light touch. The above-mentioned receptors, which are the source of the hyperalgesia seen in RSD, are different than the burning pain receptors seen in causalgia. Ochoa believes that the burning pain of causalgia is mediated by unmyelinated C fibers (11), whereas Payne believes that this pain is due to nerve stretch and axon disruptions (1). Another consideration is the fact that such pain may be mediated by nerve fascicles where all three types of C fibers exist (11). Therefore, in summary, the current thinking seems to suggest that sparsely myelinated C fibers carry the message of burning pain found in causalgia, whereas sparsely myelinated afferent fibers or the A-delta nociceptors may be responsible for pain in RSD.

SYNAPSES

Both synaptic considerations and axonal considerations have been raised as possible factors controlling RSD as well as causalgia. Ephapses, or artificial synapses, have been demonstrated in normal peripheral nerves. The concept of synaptic factors in RSD and causalgia pain was first advanced by Granit et al. when they found that stimulating the motor root of a damaged mixed motor-sensory nerve also produced recordable electrical events in the sensory root (12). According to the review by Payne, the formation of ephapses after nerve injury may allow a short-circuiting or shunting of current from sympathetic fibers coming from the cord to the peripheral nerve into somatic fibers arising at the site of injury, carrying the message of pain back to the cord (1). Unfortunately, these cross-connections between fibers coming from the cord to the periphery, and conversely coming from the periphery to the cord, have been demonstrated in animal models, but not in humans (1). Another consideration is the possibility of an ectopic impulse resulting from alterations in calcium, sodium, and potassium channels (1). In effect, the damaged nerve becomes "epileptic," and the spontaneous discharges from the sensory nerve may give rise to the episodic pain noted in some individuals. This could be due to lowered threshold or heightened mechanical sensitivity.

Neurosynaptic mediation of causalgia and RSD holds great promise for the future. When reviewing the synapses that are present within the sympathetic chain, it is apparent that these provide a potential site of mediation for sensory input. In order to understand synaptic mediation, one must review the anatomy of a synapse per se. Borrowing heavily from Roberts, one can define the functional neuroanatomy, and delineate the location of various synapses (5). First the trauma occurs, with receptors in the skin detecting various components of the trauma. Initially, the C fiber nociceptors carry the message to the dorsal root ganglion, and thence back to the spinal cord neuron, where they synapse. After synapsing with the neuron in the spinal cord, these multiple neurons transmit information to the WDR neurons, which then send messages, via their axons, to the central nervous system or higher levels of the spinal cord. Using Roberts' model, additional light touch activates the mechanoreceptors, which travel in the A fibers rather than in the C fibers. Since the WDR neurons are already sensitized by the C fibers nociceptors, they respond to what is usually subthreshold stimuli to the A fiber mechanoreceptors. These mechanoreceptors travel in the A fiber, reaching a neuron within the spinal cord, which again impinges on the WDR neuron, which in turn again sends messages up the spinal cord to the brain. Sympathetic fibers exist within the lateral portions of the thoracic cord, sending efferent messages to the sensory receptor. These efferent messages (i.e., messages traveling from the cord to the periphery, mainly to the sensory receptors) may occur in the absence of cutaneous stimulation. However, the sympathetic efferent activity, according to Roberts' theory, requires no cutaneous stimulation, and is the etiology of the SMP. In response to this efferent activity, the WDR neurons fire, again sending messages to the spinal cord and brain (5). The key to Roberts' theory is the fact that the WDR neurons in the spinal cord remain sensitized, and they will give a "vigorous response to mechanical stimulation of A fiber mechanoreceptors" even after healing has occurred (5). In this schema, multiple synapses occur within the spinal cord, at the WDR neuron, and in the sympathetic ganglion. Therefore, synaptic regulation can occur at the spinal cord level or at the sympathetic ganglion level.

When reviewing the actual synapse, one must conceptualize a presynaptic area where various chemicals are formulated, becoming neurosynaptic transmitters. The two synaptic transmitters that are of most interest to the study of RSD and causalgia are the indolamines, of which serotonin is an example, and the catecholamines, of which norepinephrine, epinephrine, dopa, and dopamine are examples. In the presynaptic area of the nerve, precursor substances are manufactured into neurosynaptic transmitters, which confer a degree of specificity on nerve transmission. L-Tryptophan becomes 5-hydroxytryptophan, which becomes 5-hydroxytrypamine (serotonin); dopa becomes dopamine, which can be converted to norepinephrine and epinephrine. The specific type of the neurosynaptic transmitter determines whether or not it will occupy a specific postsynaptic receptor site. Biogenic amines, such as the indolamines and catecholamines, are constantly being formulated and broken down by monoamine oxidase. Thus, chemically, the presynaptic area may be described as an area of high flux, with formulation and degradation of the same chemical occurring in a relatively steady state. As electrical impulses travel down the axon, pore diameter changes, altering the permeability of the membrane and causing the release of neurosynaptic transmitters. These synaptic transmitters flow across a minute gap between nerves and occupy postsynaptic receptor sites. The gap, of course, is called the synapse. The postsynaptic receptor sites determine the strength and duration of the electrical impulse that the synapse propagates. This is done by the degree of specificity that the neurosynaptic transmitters have for a particular receptor site. It also depends on the affinity that a specific neurosynaptic transmitter has for a particular receptor site, and whether it is easily displaced or forms a tight bond.

Almost all neurosynaptic transmitters have their activity ended by presynaptic reuptake, that is, the chemical that occupies the postsynaptic receptor site is then taken back into the presynaptic area. Acetylcholine is an exception, being degraded on the postsynaptic receptor site by acetylcholinesterase. Additionally, some small amount of degradation of biogenic amines occurs in the synapse itself by catechol-O-methyltransferase (COMT). It is thought that less than 5% of the chemical degradation of synaptic transmitters occurs in the synapse by COMT, and 95% of the degradation occurs presynaptically, by monoamine oxidase (MAO). Of course, there is constant rebuilding of the neurosynaptic transmitter presynaptically, creating the steady state mentioned earlier.

Obviously, there are multiple ways to modify the synapse. One can inhibit MAO, thereby enhancing the buildup of a monoamine neurosynaptic transmitter, such as the indolamines or the catecholamines. In fact, a class of drugs called MAO inhibitors do exactly that. By the same token, certain drugs can function as MAO exciters, which facilitate the degradation of biogenic amine neurosynaptic transmitters, such as the indolamines (serotonin) and the catecholamines (epinephrine, norepinephrine, dopamine, and dopa). Since the majority of the neurosynaptic transmitters have their activity ended by presynaptic reuptake, one can enhance the synaptic transmission by blocking presynaptic reuptake. This is how tricyclic antidepressants work. Conversely, one can diminish synaptic transmission by facilitation of presynaptic reuptake. Finally, one can work at the receptor end, by utilizing drugs that mimic the action of the presynaptic transmitters and occupy receptor sites, thereby triggering them as if the actual chemical had been released. By the same token, other drugs can be utilized that occupy the receptor sites but have no pharmacologic activity other than to inhibit the presynaptic transmitter from occupying the receptor site. For example, curare effects a total blockade of the acetylcholine receptor. In this sense, these drugs become inhibitors of neurosynaptic transmission. Receptor sites are found not only postsynaptically, but also presynaptically, very often for the same presynaptic neurosynaptic transmitter. As the number and sensitivity of these receptors change, so does the response to the neurosynaptic transmitter itself.

DIAGNOSIS AND TREATMENT OF CAUSALGIA

DIAGNOSIS

With the foregoing theoretical information, the clinical components of RSD and causalgia should be more readily differentiated by appropriate diagnostic studies.

According to both Raja and his coworkers and Payne, causalgia manifests as a burning pain, which is not a consistent finding in RSD (1, 13). Additionally, causalgia patients may experience paroxysms of pain, especially after stress, whether it be emotional or environmental. In an elegant study, Raja and his coworkers found that patients with causalgias rarely have cold hyperalgesia (2 of 9), and they do not have heat hyperalgesia (0 of 9) (13). Additionally, these patients obtain no relief from sympathetic blocks. Raja et al. differentiated various types of hyperalgesia using sensory testing with either Von Frey hairs for touch, a drop of acetone for cold, or laser thermal stimulation for heat (13). Ochoa feels that causalgia is not always sympathetically mediated, and instead is mediated by unmyelinated C fibers (11). Stretch injuries to the nerve or axon disruption of a major nerve branch is one explanation favored by Payne (1). Usually, the causalgia patient has a history of a nerve injury to a peripheral nerve, or surgery, that has damaged the proximal portion of the nerve trunk (1, 13). The causalgia may be related to damage of nerve fascicles where all three types of C fibers exist (11).

TREATMENT

Various authors have reported that sympathetic blocks are or are not effective, with efficacy for sympathectomy being reported as between 12 and 97% (1). No relief with sympathetic blocks was reported by Raja et al. (13). Payne has suggested that a dorsal root entry zone (DREZ) procedure may prove effective (1). Ghostine et al. have suggested the use of phenoxybenzamine (4). They reported 40 consecutive cases of causalgia, all of whom had received nerve injuries from bullet or shrapnel wounds. The Ghostine group noted partial motor paralysis in the distribution of the damaged nerve in 70% of the cases. However, over time these deficits resolved in many of the cases. They also noted vasomotor changes, usually severe vasodilatation and sweating and less often vasoconstriction (4). Rarely were trophic changes noted. The majority of the cases involved the sciatic nerve, median nerve, brachial plexis, cauda equina, and occipital nerve, in descending order. The treatment that Ghostine and his group utilized was phenoxybenzamine, which is a postsynaptic α_1-blocker and a presynaptic α_2-blocker. As mentioned earlier under the etiology of causalgia, nerve sprouts, which are one of the theoretical origins of this disorder, seem to be highly excitable upon the administration of norepinephrine, which can be reversed with α-blocking agents such as phentolamine but are unaffected by β-blocking agents (4). The dosage of the drug used by Ghostine et al. initially was 10 mg three times a day, although this varied from patient to patient. Eventually, maximum dosages of 40–120 mg/day were reached, with treatment lasting 6–8 weeks. Common side effects were orthostatic hypotension in about 45% of the patients and reduced ejaculatory ability in about 8% of the patients. In some instances, treatment lasted as long as 16 weeks. However, it is important to note that the patients were all treated within 2–70 days after the onset of their injury. In order for this treatment to be effective, it is most important that rapid diagnosis and institution of treatment occur. Another possibility for the pharmacologic treatment of causalgia would be the use of clonazepam, which has been reported by Bouckoms and Litman to be effective for "burning" pains (14).

Surgical sympathectomy has been recommended as a treatment for causalgia, after repetitive sympathetic blocks. Additionally, guanethidine, which is a ganglionic blocking agent, has proven effective in treating some forms of causalgia. However, guanethidine must be used with caution because it causes the release of norepinephrine prior to occupying the receptor sites itself, and the time course of the cessation of activity is variable. The fact that one may occlude an affected limb below the site of the causalgia and still achieve effective blocks with guanethidine suggests that its activity is not at the ganglion, but rather on the peripheral sensory nerves, which produces its effect on causalgia (15). Surgical intervention, in the form of surgical sympathectomy, has been used to treat causalgia with variable cure rates, ranging from 12 to 97% (1). However, the variability may be ascribed to lack of precision and diagnosis, with an overlap of RSD with causalgia, or RSD mistakenly diagnosed as causalgia; varying skills in performing blocks; collateral reinnervation of postganglionic sympathetic fibers; and a delay in performing a sympathectomy (1). For causalgia that is not responding to sympathectomy, the possibility of a contralateral sympathectomy has been raised (6).

DIAGNOSIS AND TREATMENT OF REFLEX SYMPATHETIC DYSTROPHY

DIAGNOSIS

The clinical diagnosis of RSD is more complicated than that of causalgia. Some authors believe that there is a very definite set of criteria to establish the diagnosis, whereas other authors think that only several symptoms from a whole list of symptoms complexes need be present to establish the diagnosis of RSD. Kozin and his coworkers have established the criteria for RSD as a patient presenting with pain and tenderness in an extremity associated with vasomotor instability (particular temperature or color changes) *and* generalized swelling in the same extremity (16). The second group of patients they consider are those with pain and tenderness associated with a vasomotor instability *or* swelling in an extremity; they call this group "probable RSD." However, this system lacks precision because it does not take into account the particular type of pain that patients with RSD experience.

Raja and his coworkers define patients as having RSD if they have pain associated with signs of sympathetic hyperactivity (i.e., lower skin temperature, skin discoloration, increased wetting, and some trophic changes) and symptomatic relief after sympathetic blocks, and found that those with RSD also had thermal hyperalgesia either to cold or to heat (13). In contrast, their patients with causalgia did not experience thermal hyperalgesia to heat, and only 2 out of 7 experienced hyperalgesia to cold. Both the causalgia and RSD patients experienced hyperalgesia to mechanical stimulation (13). On the other hand, Ochoa et al. found mechanical hyperalgesia, which they called allodynia, in their patients with RSD (11). Additionally, hypersensitivity to temperature was also found in patients with RSD, whether it be to heat or to cold (11, 13, 17). One proposed mechanism for mechanical hypersensitivity is ectopic α-adrenergic chemosensitivity (18). Another consideration is a secondary abnormality in distal nociceptor fibers that escaped injury, or intact low-threshold mechanoreceptors with large myelinated fibers that are non–sympathetic dependent because of transfer of information to nociceptor pathways proximal to the site of injury (11). Additionally, Ochoa et al. advanced the concept of α-receptor sensitization, whereas others believe that the hypersensitivity of the mechanoreceptors could possibly be a simple nervous system event (11, 17).

TREATMENT

Treatments for the mechanical hypersensitivity or hyperalgesia of RSD have been advanced by several authors, without clear-cut definition. One group of authors believes that sympathectomy may relieve mechanical hyperalgesia, whereas another group of authors reports that sympathectomy does not (11, 19). Another group has advanced the notion that nifedipine, a calcium channel–blocking agent, may prove effective (20). Finally, a group from South Africa suggested that low-dose naloxone, and possibly longer acting naltrexone, may prove effective for reducing mechanical hyperalgesia, because of the existence of a hypergesic kappa system of opiate receptors (21). Again, the area of mechanical hyperalgesia is quite muddy, since all of the patients with either causalgia or RSD had mechanical hypersensitivity (13).

Thermal hypersensitivity to either heat or cold (hyperalgesia) has been reported by several groups (11, 13, 17). The mechanism behind the thermal hypersensitivity is not well elucidated, but one can clinically differentiate mechanical from thermal hypersensitivity by the use of a drop of acetone (13). Patients with RSD in the series studied by Raja et al. had hyperalgesia to cold (3 of 4, as tested by acetone drop) or to heat (4 of 5, as tested using a laser thermal stimulator) (13). Some patients had hypersensitivity and hyperalgesia to both heat and cold, but these patients did not have causalgia, but rather RSD. Of the group of patients with hyperalgesia to temperature change, 6 of 6 got relief with sympathetic blocks or sympathectomy (13). Other authors have reported that nifedipine is effective for treating hyperalgesia (20). Specifically, in 13 patients with pain having a burning character, dysesthesias, and cold intolerance, nifedipine beginning at 10 mg three times a day, and increasing to 30 mg three times a day, proved effective in 7 out of 13 patients

(20). Nifedipine is a calcium channel–blocking agent, and as such may work by dilating blood vessels and antagonizing the effects of norepinephrine on arterial and venous muscle (1). Also, nifedipine may interfere with ectopic impulse formation that occurs in regenerating nerves, by blocking calcium channel protein (1).

The dystrophic component of RSD is more difficult to delineate. Some authors have reported a diffuse or patchy bony demineralization (16), whereas others have reported frank osteoporosis late in the disorder (22). A number of authors have reported molted skin, again late in the disorder (1, 13, 16). Some authors have reported hair loss, again late in the disorder (13, 22). Vague terms such as *vasomotor instability* have also been reported, as well as trophic skin changes (16). The etiology for these components is not well defined, but the consensus seems to be reduced blood flow to the various involved organs. A more precise diagnostic assessment was advanced by Holder and MacKinnon (23). They evaluated patients with RSD, which they defined as diffuse hand pain, diminished hand function, joint stiffness, and skin and soft tissue trophic changes with or without vasomotor instability. They also used three other control groups, including patients with diffuse pain, focal pain, or vascular disease. Holder and MacKinnon found that 22 of the 23 patients who met their criteria for diagnosing RSD had positive delayed image bone scans, 12 of the 23 patients had positive blood pool images, and 10 of the 23 patients had positive radionuclide angiograms (23). Approximately half the patients with RSD had positive early phase bone scans, whereas almost all of the patients with RSD had positive delayed image bone scans (23).

This study compared favorably with work done by Kozin and his group. Kozin and his coworkers found that x-ray is not a useful tool for diagnosing RSD (16). However, they did find that 83% of the patients with RSD had positive static (delayed) bone scans, whereas 69% of the patients had positive flow studies (16). Therefore, it is apparent that between 50 and 69% of patients with RSD will have positive early phase bone scans, but between 83 and 96% of patients will have positive delayed image bone scans (16, 23). Treatment for this component of RSD is difficult to assess. Kozin et al. reported that 90% of patients with a positive bone scan had good to excellent steroid response, beginning with steroids at the level of 60–80 mg/day and tapering them (16). Schott has reported a variety of therapeutic modalities, including steroids, nonsteroidal anti-inflammatory drugs, α- and β-blocking agents, griseofulvin, calcitonin, transcutaneous electrical nerve stimulation, physical therapy, sympathetic blocks, and intravenous guanethidine (22). However, none of these treatments has been studied in a systematized fashion.

Nail brittleness has been reported by Schott (22) and Payne (1) late in the disorder. The etiology of this is not clear, nor is there any clear-cut treatment. Muscle spasm has been reported by a number of authors (3, 6, 22), again without a clear-cut mechanism describing the etiology (1). Interestingly, electromyography (EMG)–nerve conduction velocity studies seem to be relatively negative in RSD (24). The treatments that seemed most effective for muscle spasm were trigger point injections (1) and the use of baclofen (N.H. Hendler, unpublished observations). Baclofen is a GABA-minergic drug that centrally reduces muscle spasm. The inhibition of substance P may be implicated as part of its mechanism for reducing spasm and the pain associated with spasm (21). Soma and quinine have also been tried, with only limited success (N.H. Hendler, unpublished observations). Contractures, usually in the hand, have also been reported (1, 22). The etiology of this is unclear, but is probably related to disuse. Again, there is an absence of positive EMG–nerve conduction velocity studies (24), and the only treatment seems to be preventative, by the use of passive range of motion exercises and physical therapy.

Contralateral involvement has been reported by several authors (6, 22). The etiology for this, in approximately 80% of examined cadavers (6), is cross-communication between the sympathetic fibers and sympathetic chains. Contralateral blocks and denervation have been recommended (6). Edema of the affected limb (1, 22) as well as swelling of a specific joint (16) have been reported. Again, the etiology is unclear. The diagnosis is established by measuring the proximal interphalangeal joint, which averages 12.9 mm larger in the affected hand than in the control hand (16). No treatment has been advanced for this, although nifedipine is suggested to be effective (20). The author has observed some benefit from the use of spironolactone, or carbonic anhydrase inhibitors, but not on a consistent basis.

Lower skin temperature has been reported by a variety of authors (1, 13, 25), but it does not seem to be due to vasospasm (26). Reflex contraction due to altered activity within the afferent and efferent nerves is proposed as the etiology (26). Thermography is an excellent diagnostic tool to document the reduced skin temperature (24, 25). In fact, very often patients with RSD are diagnosed as having psychosomatic disorders, and thermography can be a most convincing diagnostic tool to confirm the otherwise subjective complaint (25). Treatment for lower skin temperature associated with pain is best effected using regional sympathetic blocks employing reserpine (26). It is important to note that these reserpine blocks, or Bier blocks, are not effective for vasospasm, but specifically seem to function best for treating RSD (26). Therefore, vasospasm does not seem to be the etiologic mechanism for the coldness noted in the limb in RSD (26).

Stiffness (1, 23) and tenderness (16) of the joints have been reported; again, the etiology is not clear (1). Very often, the involvement of the joint leads to misdiagnosis and confusion with other diseases that can affect the joint, notably infective arthritis, rheumatoid arthritis, Reiter's syndrome, systemic lupus erythematosus, and arthritides (16). In one series, 71% of the patients with joint tenderness and stiffness had a poor response to stellate ganglion blocks (16). Steroids, notably prednisone (60–80 mg) for 2–4 days, then 40–60 mg for 2–4 days, and then 30–40 mg for 2–4 days, in four equally divided doses), were the initial therapy. Subsequently, the dose was rapidly tapered using a single morning dose of 40 mg, then 30 mg, 20 mg, 10 mg, and 5 mg over 2 or 3 days at each dosage. Using this regimen, 82% of the patients with joint stiffness and tenderness obtained good or excellent relief (16).

An unusual complication of RSD is the appearance of pathologic fractures subsequent to minor trauma (N.H. Hendler, unpublished observations). In patients complaining of persistent pain in the limb that seems to be bony in origin, rather than part of the RSD, it would be imperative to obtain bone scanning to confirm the presence or absence of an undetected break. In the author's experience, one patient with long-standing RSD received a minor trauma (i.e., bumping her ankle while walking in a train) that resulted in a chronic intense worsening of pain in the heel. X-rays of this area were within normal limits, but the pain persisted for several days after the event, and a bone scan was obtained. Only on bone scan did the break in the calcaneus appear, which had been totally missed by routine x-ray. Ninety-five per cent of any breaks present will have a positive bone scan after 72 hr (27). Interestingly, after the fracture is healed, 90% of the bone scans have returned to normal 2 years from the date of the injury (27). Therefore, in patients with RSD who have minor injuries and complain of bony pain, it would be prudent to obtain a bone scan, and not rely on x-rays.

Payne has enumerated many attempted treatments for RSD (1). Unfortunately, there seems to be a lack of systematic investigation for these treatments, and most are based on clinical reports rather than on systematized trials. Reported pharmacologic interventions that may work for causalgia are the use of propranolol, a β-blocking agent; prazosin, an α_1-adrenergic blocking agent; phenoxybenzamine, both an α_1-and an α_2-blocker; and guanethidine, a drug that produces a chemical "sympathectomy." Physical therapy has been advanced for the treatment of RSD, specifically to minimize muscle contractures and joint stiffness. However, it is never a definitive treatment, and should not be considered such. Electrical stimulation of the central nervous system, using either electrodes centrally implanted into the periaquaductal or periventricular gray or epidural stimulators, may prove effective, as might transcutaneous electrical nerve stimulation. Tricyclic antidepressants, nonsteroidal anti-inflammatory drugs, narcotics, and anticonvulsants have all been reported as treating some components of reflex sympathetic dystrophy, with varying degrees of success.

Surgical intervention is a treatment that is reserved until all other modalities of treatment have been attempted. In all cases, the criterion for surgical intervention would be repetitive successes with repeat sympathetic blocks. The most commonly employed surgical interventions are resection of the lower third of the stellate ganglion and resection of the upper two thoracic ganglia; however, some surgeons resect the second through fifth thoracic ganglia in an attempt to treat upper extremity difficulties (7). There are four surgical approaches to upper extremity sympathectomies (7):

1. Above the clavicle (anterior cervical approach).
2. Posterior resection of the transverse processes of ribs 2 and 3, and proximal section of ribs 2 and 3.
3. Anterior transplural entry through the pectoralis muscle to the third intercostal space, pressing the lung, in order to reach the operative area.
4. The axillary approach, which is through a transaxillary incision over the second intercostal space.

Also, a lumbar approach may be made through the external and internal obliques, and then the transversalis muscle, below the 12th rib, behind the kidney; others have suggested a thoracolumbar presacral neurectomy (7). Side effects of surgical approaches are postsympathectomy neuralgia, beginning 7–10 days after surgery, and a postsympathectomy dysesthesia that may last 2–14 weeks, and is described as continuous, severe, and worse at night. Anticonvulsants, such as diphenylhydantoin or carbamazepine, may be used to treat this (7). Dorsal root entry zone procedures, which produce lesions in the dorsal root interrupting the nociceptive pathways in the tract of Lissauer and in laminae I through V of the dorsal horn of the spinal cord, may prove to be an effective modality for treating causalgia for stretch injuries (1).

SUMMARY

In summary, it is quite apparent that a great deal of confusion has arisen regarding the diagnosis of RSD and causalgia. This is evidenced by the lack of uniformity in clinical criteria for establishing the diagnosis. Because of this lack of uniformity, assessment of various articles detailing treatment of RSD and/or causalgia is difficult. What some clinicians take as symptoms of RSD are not always present in their entirety. Unfortunately, if one adheres rigorously to these criteria, proper diagnosis, and more importantly proper treatment, may be withheld. The various clinical symptoms that have been reported as associated with RSD and causalgia are shown in Table 37.1. The author would suggest that a patient be considered as having RSD if he or she has at least one type of hyperalgesia (either mechanical or thermal), lower skin temperature, and the sensation of pins and needles. At a minimum, diagnostic studies that would facilitate the diagnosis of RSD would be thermography and bone scan. Clinical diagnostic studies that would prove important would be testing with a drop of acetone for cold hyperalgesia, and testing using Von Frey hairs for mechanical hyperalgesia. All patients suspected of having RSD should have at least three sympathetic blocks. After that, one should utilize various diagnostic and treatment tech-

Table 37.1
Clinical Symptoms Associated with Causalgia and Reflex Sympathetic Dystrophy

Clinical Symptoms	Mechanism	Diagnostic Studies	Treatment
Causalgia a. Burning pain (1, 13)[a]	a. Unmyelinated C fibers (11)	a. Rarely have cold hyperalgesia (2/7) or heat hyperalgesia (0/9) (13); do have mechanical hypersensitivity (13); use a drop of acetone and Von Frey hairs to test	a. Phenoxybenzamine (4), DREZ (1), sympathectomy 12–97% effective (1), clonazepam (14)
b. Paroxisms of pain (1)	b. Nerve stretch and axon disruption (1)		
c. Partial motor paralysis (70%) (4)	c. Peripheral nerve injury, proximal nerve trunk (1, 13)	c. EMG/nerve conduction velocity studies	c. No relief with sympathetic blocks (13); β-blockers don't work (4)
d. Worse with stress (1)			
e. Vasomotor changes, but rare trophic change (4) (Ghostine, et al.)			
Reflex Sympathetic Dystrophy **Hyperalgesia (allodynia)** a. Mechanical—hypersensitivity to light touch (11)	a. Ectopic α-adrenergic chemosensitivity (18); sensitization of WDR neurons in the spinal cord (5); central nervous system mediated (17); intact low-threshold mechanoreceptor with A-delta afferents (11)	a. All patients have mechanical hypersensitivity; use Von Frey hairs to test (13)	a. Sympathectomy may relieve it (7, 11); sympathectomy did not relieve it (19); low-dose naltrexone may work (21); nifedipine ? (20)
b. Thermal—hypersensitivity to either heat or cold (11, 13, 17)	b. No mechanism delineated	b. Patients have either cold hyperalgesia (3/4), and/or heat hyperalgesia (4/5); use a drop of acetone to test (13)	b. 6/6 got relief with sympathetic blocks or a sympathectomy (13); nifedipine ? (20)
Dystrophy a. Osteoporosis (22)	a. No mechanism delineated	a and b. X-ray did not correlate well with clinical symptoms, but bone scan did (69% abnormal flow images, 83% abnormal static images) (16) (also true for clinical features c, e, and l); if clinically had RSD, 22/23 had positive delay image bone scan (23)	a and b. Maybe calcitonin (22)

Table 37.1
Clinical Symptoms Associated with Causalgia and Reflex Sympathetic Dystrophy

Clinical Symptoms	Mechanism	Diagnostic Studies	Treatment
b. Diffuse or patchy boney demineralization (16)	b. No mechanism delineated		
c. Molted skin (1, 13, 16)	c. No mechanism delineated	c. Thermography (24, 25)	c. Prednisone, 60–80 mg to start (16)
d. Hair loss (13, 22)	d. No mechanism delineated	d. Clinical observation	d. Steroids (16, 22)
e. Vasomotor instability (16)	e. No mechanism delineated	e. History or longitudinal observation (16)	e. Sympathetic blocks (22); steroids (16)
f. Nail brittleness (1, 22)	f. No mechanism delineated	f. Clinical observation	f. Sympathetic blocks (22); steroids (16)
g. Muscle spasm (3, 6, 22)	g. No mechanism delineated	g. EMG biofeedback used as test (25)	g. Trigger point injections (1); baclofen (21)
h. Contractures (1, 22)	h. May be attributed to disuse	h. Longitudinal observation (22)	h. Physical therapy (22)
i. Contralateral involvement (6, 22)	i. Cross-communication between sympathetic chain in 80% of cadavers (6)	i. Effective contralateral block (6)	i. Contralateral sympathectomy (6)
j. Edema (1, 22)	j. No mechanism delineated	j. History and clinical observation	j. Nifedipine (20); spironolactone
k. Lower skin temperature (1, 13, 24, 25)	k. Not vasospasm, but maybe an afferent and efferent reflex arc (26)	k. Thermography (24, 25)	k. Phentolamine (25); Bier block with reserpine (26); guanethidine i.v. (22); sympathetic blocks (13, 22)
l. Joint stiffness (1, 23) and tenderness (16)	l. No mechanism delineated	l. Proximal interphalangeal joint is 12.9 mm greater (average) in affected hand; rheumatoid and connective tissue blood studies (16)	l. Prednisone 60–80 mg to start, 82% not good or excellent relief (16)
m. Pathologic fractures (N. H. Hendler, unpublished data)	m. May be related to osteoporosis or patchy demineralization	m. 72 hours after a break 95% of bone scans are positive; 90% normal 2 years after break (27)	m. Proper casting
n. Pins and needles (25) and dysesthesias (1)	n. No mechanism delineated	n. History	n. Sympathectomy (25)

[a] Numbers in parentheses are references.

niques, depending on the type of complaints that the patient has.

For causalgia, one certainly should establish the diagnosis of burning pain as constantly present, in association with a partial peripheral nerve injury. Electromyographic–nerve conduction velocity studies should be conducted to detect whether or not there is an associated nerve injury. Certainly, patients should receive sympathetic blocks and a trial with phenoxybenzamine.

Regardless of whether a patient has RSD or causalgia, one must be aware of the need to make a distinction between the two diagnoses, because the treatments vary. More importantly, if the patient has even a single symptom of RSD, a diagnostic assessment involving the recommended modalities mentioned above would be warranted, and further diagnostic studies pursued if the diagnosis of RSD is not confirmed. Kozin and his coworkers clearly defined a number of overlapping conditions that may originally be misdiagosed as RSD. Twenty-five per cent of the patients who were found not to have RSD had peripheral neuropathy or trapped peripheral nerves, and half the patients misdiagnosed as having RSD had inflammatory arthritis (16). Therefore, laboratory studies, including erythrocyte sedimentation rate, antinuclear antibody, rheumatoid factor, and the like, should be conducted in patients thought to have RSD but in whom the diagnosis is not complete. In any event, causalgia and RSD require clinical acumen to establish the diagnosis, and persistence in order to effect appropriate treatment. Aggressively pursuing all of the diagnostic studies available, as well as relying on clinical judgment, will provide better care for these patients.

References

1. Payne R: Neuropathic pain syndromes, with special reference to causalgia and reflex sympathetic dystrophy. *Clin J Pain* 2:59–73, 1986.
2. Dalton S: *Split Seconds—The World of High Speed Photography*. Salem, NH, Salem House, 1984, pp 21, 28, 30, 31, 32, 34, 36.
3. Long DM: Pain of peripheral nerve injury. In Youmans J (ed): *Neurological Surgery*, ed 2. Philadelphia, WB Saunders, 1982, vol 6, pp 3634–3643.
4. Ghostine SY, Comair YG, Turner DM, et al: Phenoxybenzamine in the treatment of causalgia (report of 40 cases). *J. Neurosurg* 6:1263–1268, 1984.
5. Roberts WJ: A hypothesis on the physiological basis for causalgia and related pain. *Pain* 24:297–311, 1986.
6. Kleiman A: Causalgia: evidence of the existence of crossed sensory sympathetic fibers. *Am J Surg* 87:839–841, 1954.
7. Allen MB Jr, Morety WH: Sympathectomy. In Youmans J (ed): *Neurological Surgery*, ed 2. Philadelphia, WB Saunders, 1982, vol 6, pp 3717–3726.
8. Bonica JJ: Causalgia and other reflex sympathetic dystrophies. In Bonica JJ (ed): *Advances in Pain Research and Therapy*. New York, Raven Press, 1970, vol 3, pp 141–166.
9. Devor M, Janig W: Activation of myelinated afferents ending in a neuroma by stimulation of the sympathetic supply in a rat. *Neurosci Lett* 24:43–47, 1981.
10. Loh L, Nathan PW: Painful peripheral states and sympathetic blocks. *J Neurol Neurosurg Psychiatry* 41:664–671, 1978.
11. Ochoa J, Torebjorle E, Marchetti P, et al: Mechanisms of neuropathic pain: cumulative observations, new experiments and further speculation. In Fields HL, Dubner R, Cervero F (eds); *Advances in Pain Research and Therapy*. New York, Raven Press, 1985, vol 9, pp 431–450.
12. Granit R, Leksell L, Skoglund CR: Fiber interaction in injured or compressed region of the nerve. *Brain* 67:125–140, 1944.
13. Raja SN, Campbell JN, Meyer RA, et al: Sensory testing in patients with causalgia or reflex sympathetic dystrophy. Abstract presented at 6th Annual Meeting of the American Pain Society, Washington DC, November 6–9, 1986.
14. Bouckoms AJ, Litman RE: Clonazepam in the treatment of neuralgic pain syndrome. *Psychosomatics* 26:933–936, 1985.
15. Hannington-Kiff JG: Relief of causalgia in limbs by regional intravenous guanethidine. *Br Med J* 2:367–368, 1979.
16. Kozin F, Ryan LM, Carerra GF, et al: The reflex sympathetic dystrophy syndrome (RSDS). *Am J Med* 70:23–30, 1981.
17. Meyer RA, Campbell JN, Raja SN: Peripheral neural mechanism of cutaneous hyperalgesia. In Field HL, Dubner R, Cervero F (eds): *Advances in Pain Research and Therapy*. New York, Raven Press, 1985, vol 9 pp 53–71.
18. Devor M: Nerve pathophysiology and mechanisms of pain in causalgia. *J Auton Nerv Sys* 7:371–384, 1983.
19. Hoffert MI, Greenburg PP, Wolskee PJ, et al: Abnormal and collateral innervations of sympathetic and peripheral sensory fields associated with a case of causalgia. *Pain* 20:1–12, 1984.
20. Prough DS, McLeskey CH, Poehling GG, et al: Efficacy of oral nifedipine in the treatment of reflex sympathetic dystrophy. *Anesthesiology* 62:796–799, 1985.
21. Gillman MA, Lichtigfeld RJ: A pharmacological overview of opioid mechanisms mediating analgesia and hyperalgesia. *Neurol Res* 7:106–119, 1985.
22. Schott GD: Neurologic manifestation of bone and joint disease. In Asbury AK, McKhann GM, McDonald WC, et al (eds): *Diseases of the Nervous System*. Philadelphia, WB Saunders, 1986, pp 1523–1537.
23. Holder LE, MacKinnon SE: Reflex sympathetic dystrophy in the hands: clinical and scintigraphic criteria. *Radiology* 152:517–522, 1984.
24. Uematsu S, Hendler N, Hungerford D, et al: Thermography and electromyography in the differential diagnosis of chronic pain syndromes and reflex sympathetic dystrophy. *Electromyog Clin Neurophysiol* 21:165–182, 1981.
25. Hendler N, Uematsu S, Long D: Thermographic validation of physical complaints in "psychogenic pain" patients. *Psychosomatics* 23:283–287, 1982.
26. Janoff KH, Phinney ES, Porter JM: Lumbar sympathectomy for lower extremity vasospasm. *Am J Surg* 150:147–152, 1985.
27. Matin P: The appearance of bone scans following fractures, including immediate and long-term studies. *J Nucl Med* 20:1227–1231, 1979.

chapter 38
Phantom Pain

Peter G. Wilson, M.D.

Phantom pain is an interesting and exasperating phenomenon. In order to properly manage phantom pain it must be put into a proper matrix. In this chapter I give clinical examples of phantom pain that are followed by a description of various types of phantom pain and phantom sensation. At the present time there is no clear etiology for phantom pain, and indeed it may be covered by a multitude of etiologies, but I divide the possible mechanisms into (a) central neurologic, (b) peripheral neurologic, and (c) psychological. I finally go on to look at the myriad of treatments utilizing both our own ongoing study and those of others, which include medical treatment, surgical treatments, pharmacologic treatments, and psychological treatments.

CLINICAL VIGNETTES FOR PHANTOM PAIN

The following three vignettes show three patients at different time frames after amputation. Some deal with the difference in time and some include a differentiation between phantom pain and phantom sensation. Stump pain is not dealt with except in the area of differential diagnosis.

CASE 1

Roy, a 19-year-old boy, had been working unloading newspapers from a truck in the early morning when a drunken driver slammed him into the back of the delivery truck, leaving him on the ground, bleeding. An hour later he was in the hospital. For the next 3 weeks, his leg was in traction with terrible pain, only moderately and intermittently controlled with pain medication, and there was a question as to whether an amputation would be necessary. Finally he was told that surgical debridement of the area would be performed; upon awakening he found that he had a below-the-knee amputation, to which he responded with both rage and relief. A few days later, during house staff rounds, when questioned about pain he said that he did have some pain, but it seemed to be in a "strange place." This was not followed up for a few days until a nurse asked why, if he was in pain, he wasn't asking for pain medication, at which point he timidly mentioned that the pain was in the toes of the foot that he no longer had.

CASE 2

Anne was a 67-year-old widow who had a 10-year history of diabetes that had brought on peripheral vascular problems that caused increasing pain in her lower extremity over the past 2 years. She found herself walking less and less and, over the 6 months before coming into the hospital, less able to sleep at night, gradually ending up in a reclining chair, where she was able to sleep for 3 or 4 hr on a good night. Life was becoming intolerable for both her and her family. When she was finally admitted to the hospital, a large gangrenous area had formed on the sole of her foot, which was both smelly and painful. She was informed by her surgeon that they would be trying a bypass operation, to which she readily agreed. A week later, it was obvious to the surgeons that the bypass was not working and it also was obvious to the patient, because the pain continued unabated even as she was given pain medication. She found herself getting rather droopy on the medication, and rather resentful that the medical staff continued to talk to her about possible amputation. Four weeks after her admission to the hospital she was told that an amputation would be necessary, probably a below-the-knee amputation. After the operation she had numerous complications, including infections and poor healing, complained of a lot of stump pain, and needed large doses of pain medication every 3 hr. Because the surgeon thought that she was requesting too much medication, he arranged for a psychiatric evaluation, and Anne admitted to the psychiatrist that the pain was not so much in the stump, but in that "place where there isn't any leg." She was quite sure that she was crazy, and that if she mentioned this to the staff, she would be "put away." On a follow-up 2 weeks later, the phantom pain was less severe in that it no longer was a constant irritation, and would only arise every 6–7 hr. Anne had also been taught by the staff to take some medication before the pain built up, so that in a 24-hr span she would actually need less of the medication. Three months later on follow-up, she was complaining of occasional phantom pain with numerous phantom sensations during the day, and on 1 year follow-up was commenting that she was having phantom pain about once a week, and phantom sensation every day. Five years after the operation, she was moving well with a prosthesis, was going through her daily activities roughly as she had before the onset of her crippling symptoms, and upon close questioning reported that she now had phantom pain lasting a number of minutes once every 2–3 weeks, and phantom sensations once a week.

CASE 3

Kenneth was a 53-year-old self-employed man, married, with his sister-in-law also living in the apartment. A man who had traveled and lived in various parts of the world, he had suffered from periodic depressions from young adulthood to the present. Over the past 2 years, intermittent claudication of both legs had increased to the point where he could go no more than a half a block before he had to stop. He was no longer able to move about, and did most of his work at his desk and over the phone. His wife, who had always been careful about his diet and the care of both extremities, was horrified when he began developing ulcers on both lower extremities. Sympathectomy on both sides was done, but 4 months later it was obvious that this wasn't doing the job. Thrombotic episodes in both legs were followed by revascularization and creating new channels, but because of recurrent thrombotic episodes, this did not prove fruitful. His surgeons began talking about possible amputation. Kenneth threatened suicide, so they talked less about it. Further bilateral thromboembolic episodes led to a necessity for quick amputations and with his surgeon, wife, and sister-in-law insisting, he had bilateral above-the-knee amputations.

After the operations, he screamed out in pain, and as a result was given massive amounts of Levo-Dromoran and, because of severe depression, large doses of antidepressants. He had bilateral phantom pain and complained loudly about it being helped "only slightly" by the medication. Although he was sad, the depressive symptoms cleared, but the phantom pain remained intense and steady. He was given transcutaneous electrical nerve stimulation (TENS) treatment in the hope that this would decrease the need for medication, but this only helped for short stretches, right after the treatments. Three months later, on follow-up, the pain was nearly as intense as previously, and his wife reported that although he was getting around fairly well in his wheelchair, attempts to give him bilateral prostheses had failed. Because the high dosage of Levo-Dromoran was making him drowsy he tried to take less of the medication, but unfortunately found that the pain was very bad. Hypnosis was attempted but he was a poor subject, so progressive relaxation and desensitization was tried and was also not successful. Another course of antidepressants was initiated, not because the symptoms of depression were so disabling, but in the hope that "it might help with the pain." Doses of up to 300 mg of nortriptyline did not help, either with mood or for pain. At the end of the year, Kenneth was still taking large doses of Levo-Dromoran at times when the pain was "too bad," and he was still complaining of daily ongoing pain and poor sleep at night, because of the pain. On a 4-year follow-up, the pain had decreased so that he was only having pain for about a half hour once or twice a day.

ETIOLOGY OF PHANTOM PAIN

Nearly all postamputation patients develop some kind of sensation in the area where the limb used to be. Jensen and Rasmussen (1) best described these sensations under three primary headings: (a) kinesthetic sensations, (b) kinetic sensations, and (c) exteroseptive sensations. This covers everything from (a) a sense of position, length, and volume of the amputated limb that an amputee has after amputation; to (b) a sense on the part of the amputee that there is movement in the limb ("I moved my foot"); to (c) a pins and needles sensation or numbness in the amputated limb. The pain that is reported can be either in the stump or in the limb that is no longer there. It may be anything from a sharp, knife-like pain that is infrequent to a continuous numbing pain that never leaves day and night.

Although phenomenologically there is agreement about the nature of phantom limb pain, what causes the pain is not at all well understood. There are many theories concerning its etiology, which can be lumped into three groups: (a) the central theories, (b) the peripheral theories, and (c) the psychological theories.

CENTRAL THEORIES

The central theories include Melzack and Wall's gait control theory, which centers around the idea of reverberating circuits and deals mostly with a rostral brainstem. According to Melzack and Loeser (2), it is the reticular activating system that exerts an inhibitory influence on the somatosensory projection system. With an amputation, many peripheral fibers are destroyed, the input is reduced, inhibition is decreased, and synchronous self-sustaining activity develops at all neuronal levels. Pain occurs when output from these self-sustaining neurons reaches the cortical level.

Riddoch (3) hypothesized that a cortical representational body image develops over time as a result of peripheral input from all the senses. After amputation, this perception remains unaltered and cortical cells independent of peripheral impulses are then responsible for the phantom phenomena. Others see the pain owing its existence to a thalamic or subthalamic lesion, and indeed phantom pain shows some characteristics identical with thalamic pain. Unfortunately none of the medullary or cerebral causes describe all or even most of the phantom pains, and it has never been possible to provoke pains by stimulating either the cortex or certain parts of the midbrain.

PERIPHERAL THEORIES

The peripheral theories (4) hypothesize that the pain is caused by persistent sensation of the nerve endings in the stump. The amputee then feels that these sensations are assigned to the parts of the body that were originally innervated by the severed nerves. Not infrequently, abscesses or scar tissues have been found to trigger the pain, but unfortunately the pain persists long after the injury has healed or after the scar tissue has been removed. Again, many questions are not answered by this peripheral theory, including the fact that amputees under 6 years old do not seem to have phantom pain (5), but, more important, the fact that the pain does not follow the distribution of the severed nerves.

PSYCHOLOGICAL THEORIES

Most people do not believe that psychological factors are the sole cause of phantom limb pain, but there are studies that seem to indicate that emotional factors are among the risk factors causing phantom pain. Many studies have been done looking at the personality structures of patients with phantom pain (6), and many risk factors have been found by various people to have an impact on the presence of pain. Unfortunately, none of these studies has been duplicated, although some, such as that by Parkes (7), hold promise. In Parkes' study, the following were highly predictive of persistent phantom pain:

1. The appearance of stump or phantom pain within 3 weeks.
2. Illness that had lasted longer than 1 year prior to the amputation and persisted after surgery.
3. Unemployment not due to pain.
4. Rigid and compulsively self-reliant personality types.

The first three are measurable, the fourth difficult to measure. Others have looked closely at the concept of denial (8) or the denial of the loss of a body part (9). Here again there is a question of whether high denial or low denial is really very good.

TIME COURSE OF PHANTOM PAIN

Before going on to treatment, it is important to look at the time course of phantom limbs and phantom pain. Ambroise Paré (10) first described phantom limb pain in 1551, and Weir Mitchell (11) in 1872 used the phrase "phantom limb." Most people will have phantom sensations and as a rule if there are going to be changes they will usually occur in the first 1–2 years after the amputation. It is a common phenomenon that "telescoping" occurs; there seems to be a shrinkage of the phantom, meaning that the extremities seem to fade more and more into the stump. Frequently at the end of a year, telescoping is complete. The level of the amputation does not seem to have any influence on telescoping; as one patient put it, "as my toes got closer and closer to the top stump, they kept their size and I finally ended up feeling like the toes were right on top of the stump, same size." There are tremendous variations in the rate of diminishing of the phantom sensation, and studies by Parkes (7) and Lunn (12) see a precipitous decrease of these sensations over a year's time. Everyone agrees, though, that the longer the phantom sensations and phantom pain last (13), the longer they are bound to stay and the greater the chances that they are going to be there permanently. In our own study (14) of 40 patients followed over 7 years, all 40 patients on being questioned closely at the end of 7 years reported phantom sensation, and 15% reported intermittent low-level pains. It was of interest that even after years the phantom limb experiences did not conform to any peripheral nerve supply.

There are many factors that make a difference in the phantom sensation and especially in phantom pain. Rest, stump movement, heat or cold, and elevation of the stump will frequently relieve the pain, whereas psychopathology, hitting the stump, weather changes, and pain in other parts of the body will make the pain worse (1).

TREATMENT OF PHANTOM PAIN

Since the etiology of phantom pain is not known, treatment becomes a "pick and choose" situation. Sherman et al. reported 68 treatment methods of which they alleged 43 are successful (15). However, there are a number of areas of agreement as to what will make for a better prognosis.

PREOPERATIVE PREPARATION

At the top of the list is preoperative preparation, which should certainly include the warning to patients that phantom sensations are probable and phantom pain occasional. This preparation should also include evaluation of the patient's personality type and previous surgical experiences and a thorough discussion of the meaning of the loss (16). Since the amputated member will have to be buried, there should be a discussion of the care and disposal of the part. The details of the surgical procedure should be left to what the patient wants to hear and not how little or how much the physicians wish to mention. Some patients are most interested in knowing all the details, whereas others will stop you after a number of sentences and say they have had enough. In either case the patient's wishes should be followed, unless there seems to be maladaptive denial. At this preoperative meeting the rehabilitation program should be stressed; in a number of programs the prostheticist or the rehabilitation team come and talk to the patient. Postoperatively the patient should be allowed to mourn the loss, and counterproductive coping mechanisms using counterphobic and denial mechanisms should be looked for and addressed early. Some studies seem to indicate that early return to work and maximal use of prosthesis reduce the risk of developing phantom limb pain (14), and other studies seem to indicate that counseling of the family is helpful to the situation and perhaps may have an impact on phantom limb pain risk.

MEDICAL AND ELECTROSTIMULATION TREATMENT

A second area of general agreement is that medical treatment and electrical stimulation should be tried before the surgical treatments are attempted.

Transcutaneous electrical nerve stimulation was used with good results in about half the patients studied by Thodon et al. in 1979 (17). Spinal cord stimulation and deep brain stimulation have been tried in a number of patients, sometimes with spectacular results (18). Mundinger and Neumuller (19) in 1981 used a combination of deep brain stimulation and TENS that worked in about half their patients. The reasons for using these electrostimulations are that they are nontraumatic and can be repeated. In a number of studies local anesthetics and nerve blocks have been useful, seeming to work for about one-third to one-half of the patients (20). Analgesics, especially salicylates, are frequently used, but seem to be more useful in keeping the pain under some kind of control than eliminating it. Recently, propranalol (21) has been used with some success, and a number of studies have shown that carbamazepine (22) is of great help. Various neuroleptics have been tried without much success, and the use of tricyclic antidepressants (23) as a help in chronic pain is well known.

PAIN MEDICATION

This brings us to a discussion of pain and the philosophy of pain treatments. Perry (24) has shown that doctors tend to undermedicate patients with pain, partly out of ignorance of pharmacokinetics, partly out of fear of addicting the patient, and sometimes as a way of differentiating themselves from the person in pain. No matter how we look at pain, though, it is real, and although it certainly has both objective and subjective components, it is something that deserves treatment. This becomes especially important in phantom pain because the patient tends to see the pain as "crazy" ("How can you have pain in an area that isn't there?")—a viewpoint that not infrequently is shared by the surgical staff for their own reasons. Well-known studies by Twycross (25) have shown that pain medication taken regularly and in adequate doses means that frequently patients will be taking less of the medication over a 24-hr period and the effect will be greater. Fears of addicting patients have proven to be unfounded. This brings us directly to the issue of narcotics, and Jensen and Rasmussen's (1) excellent statement that "resistant pains are not to be accepted until narcotics have been tried." They have found that the vast majority of patients can manage on a fixed morphine dose for many years without becoming addicted.

SURGICAL TREATMENT

In surgical therapy both local and central procedures have been done. The peripheral surgical procedure includes the excision of neuromata (26), which seems to be most effective for stump pain. Even here the percentage of cure is small and this procedure is only useful when there are very positive indications for the presence of neuromata. Unfortunately, this procedure is frequently used when the signs and symptoms of neuromata are not that clear. Occasionally, more extensive amputation has been tried to see if this will help with the phantom pain, but this is usually ineffective.

Rizodomy (27) used to be fairly popular but is now nearly entirely abandoned. Cordotomy (28) was fairly popular in the 1940s but because a rather low number of patients improved the treatment is not done frequently nowadays. Sympathectomy (29) was done frequently in the 1950s but in at least three-quarters of the patients there was recurrence of the pain within 6 months. Midbrain lesions, thalamotomy, prefrontal lobotomies and cortical oblations have been done in the past, probably out of frustration, and did not prove to be of much use.

PSYCHOLOGICAL TREATMENT

The psychological treatments have proven to be of only limited use. Relaxation techniques in our own group proved to help in the general well-being of the patient but did not seem to help much with the pain. Biofeedback techniques (30) have been reported as occasionally effective in individual patients but have not been useful in large groups. Hypnosis (31) was one of the treatments of choice in the 1950s and seemed to hold promise. It unfortunately does not seem to work over long periods of time and has been reported infrequently. Psychotherapy (32) by itself was reported to be of limited help in the 1950s, and again there were indications that the treatment improved the general well-being of the patient but had little effect on the pain. Educational counseling used in conjunction with tricyclics frequently is of more use in chronic pain than intensive psychotherapy. It is nevertheless important for patients to realize that they are understood and that the doctors feel that the pain is real. Work with the family should follow the same lines.

PHYSICAL THERAPY AND OTHER MODALITIES

Physical therapy started early after the amputation seems to be of great use in keeping the phantom pain within limits (15), and there are studies that seem to indicate that early physical therapy may actually decrease the risk of the phantom pain. Ultrasound, heat, and peripheral stimulation have been reported as useful in certain individuals and certainly are safe enough to use. In many reports the pain seems to decrease over short stretches of time, and this is not to be denigrated.

CONCLUSION

We are really at the beginning of studying patients with phantom limb pains, and it is hoped that more prospective studies like those of Parkes will be done in which researchers look at the patient thoroughly both physiologically and psychologically and begin preoperatively to follow these patients for many years. In our own study patients interviewed after 7 years report occasionally having phantom sensations; some report phantom pain. It is crucial that we do not denigrate the pain, that we treat it with all the forces that we can marshall, going from one treatment to the other until we hit something that works. With proper studies perhaps we will be able to predict those people who are most at risk for phantom pain; after that studies of various treatments can be made so that eventually we will be able to match the patient and the appropriate treatment.

References

1. Jensen TS, Rasmussen P: Amputation. In Wall P, Melzack R (eds): *Textbook of Pain*. New York, Churchill Livingstone, 1984, pp 402–412.
2. Melzack R, Loeser JD: Phantom body pain in paraplegics: evidence for a central pattern generating mechanism for pain. *Pain* 4:195–210, 1978.
3. Riddoch G: Phantom limbs and body shape. *Brain* 44:197–222, 1941.
4. Livingston WK: *Pain Mechanism: A Physiologic Interpretation of Causalgia and Its Related States*. New York, Macmillan, 1944.
5. Simmel ML: The absence of phantoms for congenitally missing limbs. *Am J Psychol* 74:467–470, 1961.
6. Scott LE, et al: Preoperative predictors of postoperative pain. *Pain* 15:283–293, 1983.
7. Parkes CM: Factors determining the persistence of phantom pain in the amputee. *J Psychosom Res* 17:97–108, 1973.
8. Schilder P: *The Image and Appearance of the Human Body. Studies in the Constructive Energies of the Psyche*. London, Kegan Paul, 1935.
9. Zuk GH: The phantom limb: a proposed theory of unconscious origins. *J Nerv Ment Dis* 124:510–513, 1956.
10. Parè A: *The Works of That Famous Chirurgion, Ambrose Paré*. London, R. Cotes, 1649.
11. Mitchell SW: Phantom limbs. *Lippincott's Magazine Popular Lit Sci* 8:563–569, 1871.
12. Lunn V: *Om Legemsbevidstheden*. Copenhagen, Munksgaard, 1948.
13. Sherman R, Sherman C: Prevalence and characteristics of chronic phantom limb pain among American veterans: results of a trial survey. *Am J Phys Med* 62:227–238, 1983.
14. Wilson PG, Krebs MJS, Cohen DEI: Risk factors in amputation. *Vasc Surg* (in press).
15. Sherman RA, Sherman CJ, Gall N: A survey of current phantom limb pain treatment in the United States. *Pain* 8:85–89, 1980.
16. Langer E, Jania IL, Wolfer JA: Reduction of psychological stress in surgical patients. *J Exp Soc Psychol* 11:155–165, 1975.
17. Thoden U, Gruber RP, Krainick J-U, Huber-Muck L: Langzeitergebnisse transkutaner nervenstimulation bei chronish neurogenen schmerzzustanden. *Nervenarzt* 50:179–184, 1979.
18. Krainick J-U, Thoden U, Riechert T: Pain reduction in amputees by long-term spinal cord stimulation. *J Neurosurg* 52:346–350, 1980.
19. Mundinger F, Neumuller H: Programmed transcutaneous (TNS) and central (DBS) stimulation for control of phantom limb pain and causalgia: a new method for treatment. In Siegfried J, Zimmermann M (eds): *Phantom and Stump Pain*. Berlin, Springer-Verlag, 1981, pp 167–178.
20. Sherman RA: Published treatments of phantom limb pain. *Am J Phys Med* 59:232–244, 1980.
21. Marsland AR, Weekes JWN, Atkinson RL, Leong MG: Phantom limb pain: a case for beta blockers? *Pain* 12:295–297, 1982.
22. Doupe J, Cullen CH, Chance GQ: Post-traumatic pain and the causalgic syndrome. *J Neurol Neurosurg Psychiatry* 7:33–48, 1944.
23. Elliott F, Little A, Milbrandt W: Carbamazepine for phantom-limb phenomena. *N Engl J Med* 295:678, 1976.
24. Perry S: Undermedication for pain. *Psychiatr Ann* 14:960, 1984.
25. Twycross RG: Diseases of the central nervous system: relief of terminal pain. *Br Med J* 4:212, 1975.
26. Baumgartner R, Riniker C: Surgical stump revision as a treatment of stump and phantom pains. Results of 100 cases. In Siegfried S. Zimmermann M (eds): *Phantom and Stump Pain*. Berlin, Springer-Verlag, 1981, pp 148–155.
27. White J, Sweet W: *Pain and the Neurosurgeon: A Forty-Year Experience*. Springfield, IL, Charles C Thomas, 1969.
28. Siegfried J, Cetinalp E: Neurosurgical treatment of phantom limb pain: a survey of methods. In Siegfried J, Zimmermann M (eds): *Phantom and Stump Pain*. Berlin, Springer-Verlag, 1981, pp 148–155.
29. Kallio KE: Permanency of results obtained by sympathetic surgery in the treatment of phantom pain. *Acta Orthopaed Scand* 19:391–397, 1950.
30. Sherman R: Case reports of treatment of phantom limb pain with a combination of electromyographic biofeedback and verbal relaxation techniques. *Biofeedback Self Regul* 1:353, 1976.
31. Siegel EF: Control of phantom limb pain by hypnosis. *Am J Clin Hypn* 21:285–286, 1979.
32. Postone N: Phantom limb pain. *Psychiatry Med* 17:57–70, 1987.

chapter 39
Postherpetic Neuralgia

John R. Satterthwaite, M.D.

Herpes zoster, or "shingles," is an infectious viral disease commonly encountered in primary medical practice. It is estimated that over 300,000 new cases occur each year in the United States (1). Most of these spontaneously resolve and require only symptomatic treatment during the acute illness. The acute infectious stage can usually be limited with treatment by antiviral agents, which limit viral replication (2). Neuritic symptoms, resulting from incomplete but usually permanent sensory neural damage, can often be controlled or reduced by corticosteroids, analgesics, and nerve blocks. The lesions dry up and crust and the pain usually resolves. Unfortunately, there does exist a percentage of the population in whom the lesions resolve but the pain persists and, in fact, often becomes more severe. This is especially true in the elderly, who have a higher incidence of experiencing excruciating, unrelenting pain long after the acute illness has resolved. This protracted painful syndrome is known as postherpetic neuralgia, one of the most excruciatingly painful of the chronic pain syndromes.

Postherpetic neuralgia has been called the most common cause of intractable, debilitating pain in the elderly (3). Its intensity and duration create such suffering that many consider suicide as a means of escaping its ravages. In fact, it has been said that postherpetic neuralgia is the leading cause of suicide in chronic pain patients over the age of 70 (3). In order to appropriately manage these patients, a knowledge of the pathophysiology and epidemiology is essential in understanding the clinical course and treatment options in this disease.

ACUTE HERPES ZOSTER (SHINGLES)

Herpesvirus varicellae, commonly called varicella-zoster virus, is a DNA virus in the same group as herpes simplex, Epstein-Barr virus, and cytomegalovirus. The primary infection in nonimmune individuals is chickenpox. It is estimated that 95% of all children have been exposed to chickenpox by age 15 (4). As the chickenpox infection resolves, the virus enters the peripheral sensory nerve receptors and is transmitted via the sensory nerves to the dorsal root ganglia of the spinal nerves and extramedullary ganglia of the cranial nerves. Upon entry into the ganglia, the virus becomes dormant but retains its infectious capability (5). As a percentage of the viruses revert to an infectious state, they are quickly destroyed by the cellular immune system before clinical infection becomes evident. As long as the immune system remains intact, the reactivation of these viruses is blocked (6, 7).

Herpes zoster is a viral infection resulting from reactivation of the dormant varicella-zoster virus. Although the mechanism of reactivation is not entirely clear, it appears that a decrease in cellular-mediated immunity allows reactivation of the dormant virus in the dorsal root ganglia or extramedullary ganglia (8). As this reactivation progresses, immunity is stimulated by an active segment or segments sufficient to suppress other areas from activity but not enough to stop the initial reactivation. This likely explains the characteristic unilateral, segmental vesicular eruption that is seen most frequently (9). Reactivation of the virus is due to a fall in host cell-mediated immunity, which may be due to trauma, infection, chronic illness, malignancy, radiation therapy, chemotherapy, or immunosuppression therapy (10). Frequently there is no identifiable cause for the reactivation.

Upon multiplication of the virus, it spreads within the ganglia, causing neuronal necrosis and inflammation characterized by intense lymphocytic infiltration, endothelial proliferation, focal hemorrhage, and ganglion sheath inflammation (6). As the infection continues, the virus subsequently enters the sensory nerve and is transported along the neuron to the nerve endings, where it is released. The virus then enters the corium and epidermal cells, where it multiplies, causing the characteristic cutaneous lesions to be formed (11).

On microscopic examination there is noted to be an intense necrotizing inflammation of the dorsal root, dorsal horn, and peripheral nerve axons with peripheral nerve demyelination and destruction of large-fiber neurons (11, 12). Examination of the skin lesions shows the characteristic intranuclear inclusion bodies, giant cell formation, epidermal cell edema, and inflammation of the corium (11).

Patients with malignant neoplasms are most susceptable to herpes zoster. This is especially true of the lymphomas, and it is estimated that up to 25% of patients with Hodgkin's disease will develop herpes zoster (13).

Many times there is no identifiable explanation for the decrease in immunity. Herpes zoster is extremely uncommon in the young, healthy patient and much more common in the elderly, in whom the incidence is said to be in the range of 0.5–1.0% (5, 14). There is a gradual decrease in cellular-mediated immunity as a person ages such that levels may decrease enough to allow reactivation (15). This may help to explain the increasing incidence with age. No seasonal variations or differences with regard to race, sex, or ethnic background have been reported (16). Persons who have never had chickenpox may develop the disease if exposed to an individual with acute herpes zoster vesicles; however, it is extremely rare to develop herpes zoster solely from exposure to a patient with chickenpox.

CLINICAL MANIFESTATIONS

The preeruptive stage is usually characterized by fever, headache, lymphadenopathy, malaise, and progressively increasing pain with hyperesthesia and paresthesias over the involved dermatome for up to 14 days during the initial ganglionitis (17, 18). This is followed by erythematous dermatitis and subsequently by the characteristic maculopapular rash. This rash then evolves into clear fluid–filled vesicles over the next 72 hr. These vesicles can range from small isolated clumps to a confluent rash involving the entire dermatomal area in the form of a band; thus the name zoster or "girdle" (17). The location of the eruptions of herpes zoster seem to correlate well with those of chickenpox (6) (Table 39.1). Eruptions are occasionally encountered outside the affected dermatome, but in less than 1% do they occur bilaterally (17). Contrary to the old belief, bilateral herpes zoster eruptions are obviously not a sign of impending death.

The entity "zoster non herpete," herpes zoster infection without the eruption, has been a topic of debate for many years, particullarly with regard to the actual existence of this disorder. Pain without the cutaneous rash may represent an isolated viral ganglionitis with no peripheral spread, or possibly the eruption has been isolated and in small clusters and no residual scarring can be grossly detected.

Table 39.1
Average Distribution of Herpes Zoster Skin Lesions[a]

Distribution	Percentage
Cranial	15
(Ophthalmic division of the trigeminal nerve)	(10)
Cervical	12
Thoracic	55
Lumbar	14
Sacral	3
Generalized	1

[a] From Loeser JD: Postherpetic neuralgia: a review of pathophysiology and treatment. Presented at the Annual Meeting of the American Pain Society, Washington, DC, November 8, 1986.

Secondary infection is possible in acute herpes zoster; however, this is not that common and routine antibiotic therapy is not necessary, except in herpes zoster ophthalmicus, unless definite evidence of infection exists (19). Without treatment, and in the absence of superimposed bacterial infection, the vesicles progress to cloudy fluid-filled pustules, with eventual crusting and scab formation within 2–3 weeks and gradual resolution into irregular pink scars. These ultimately become the characteristic hypopigmented, anesthetic scars, which persist for many years.

Pain is slight or absent in children and young adults. Elderly patients seem to have more pain with the vesicular stage than the younger ones. It is frequently described as aching, burning, shooting, stabbing, or soreness. Regardless of the extent of the eruptions, pain will most likely involve the entire sensory dermatome affected.

There is usually no visceral involvement with spinal nerve infection; however, there may be a much greater incidence of motor involvement than has been previously realized (20, 21). If motor neurons in the anterior horn cells become involved, muscular weakness or palsies can develop. Motor loss is not uncommon in cranial and cervical herpes zoster, but is less frequent in truncal zoster. The facial nerve is the most common site of clinically detectable motor involvement (16). Inflammation of the geniculate ganglion may lead to involvement of the external ear and ear canal or of the soft palate and to the loss of taste (Hunt's syndrome). This is often accompanied by seventh nerve paralysis.

The most serious complications exist with involvement of the trigeminal nerve. Ten to 15% of reported cases of herpes zoster involve the ophthalmic division of the trigeminal nerve (22). It is the most commonly involved single nerve in herpes zoster, especially in older patients

(10). In herpes zoster ophthalmicus, the sensory nucleus of the fifth cranial nerve, the meninges, trigeminal ganglion, and cerebral blood vessels may be affected. Most frequently the infection involves the supraorbital and supratrochlear branches of the frontal nerve, with vesicles occurring on the forehead and upper lid. This is accompanied by pain in the distribution of the nerves as well as headache and weakness of the periorbital and lid muscles. Vesicles are deep, and residual scarring of the lids is a common complication leading to impaired vision due to contractures. No ocular involvement is noted unless the nasociliary branch of the semilunar ganglion is affected (10). This occurs in 50% of patients with herpes zoster ophthalmicus and can lead to conjunctivitis, scleritis, iridocyclitis, extraocular muscle palsies, ptosis, and mydriasis, which can cause permanent damage to the cornea, sclera, or ciliary body (10). Involvement of the nasociliary branch can be determined by the presence of Hutchinson's sign, the presence of vesicles on the lateral edge and tip of the nose.

Cutaneous and visceral dissemination are more common with herpes zoster ophthalmicus than with other forms of herpes zoster (10). Central nervous system complications include Bell's palsy, encephalitis, myelitis, peripheral sensory neuropathy, or motor neuropathy (10). This results from direct viral extension to the spinal cord, brainstem, or cavernous sinus and may occur prior to the appearance of the vesicular eruption. Aggressive treatment of ophthalmic herpes zoster is required in order to prevent these complications as well as later problems such as lid contractures, glaucoma, blindness, and postherpetic neuralgia (10).

If the virus spreads along the posterior spinal nerve root, patients may also develop myelitis or meningitis.

Involvement of the sympathetic ganglia may result in a secondary reflex sympathetic dystrophy.

The overall course of herpes zoster usually ranges from 10 days to 6 weeks. This also is age related, with the younger patients healing faster.

COMPLICATIONS

Ocular complications of herpes zoster have been previously mentioned. Most complications of the disease occur during the eruptive stage and are related to the viral infection. Secondary bacterial infection may cause sepsis, fever, chills, and pyoderma. Neurologic sequelae include meningitis, myelitis, encephalomyelitis, paresis, and sensory and motor neuropathies with palsies or paralysis.

In immunocompromised patients, there is an increased incidence of dissemination as the viral infection spreads to adjacent dermatomal areas. As this progresses, fever and increasing debilitation may occur. With dissemination comes the associated threat of visceral involvement. The highest morbidity and mortality occur with visceral spread, and the gastrointestinal tract is a common site. Pericarditis, endocarditis, hepatitis, and encephalitis may also be seen. Less frequently, varicella pneumonia may occur in compromised patients, and this diagnosis carries a high rate of morbidity and mortality (23). In general, if the disease remains localized for 4–7 days, dissemination is much less likely (23).

The most commonly seen complication of herpes zoster is the chronic pain problem of postherpetic neuralgia.

DIAGNOSIS

In the initial stages prior to the eruptions, acute herpes zoster may frequently be misdiagnosed. More common diagnoses such as herpes simplex, pleurisy, herniated intervertebral disks, cardiac disease, cholecystitis, and other acute visceral illnesses are often suspected. Peripheral nerve blocks may frequently be helpful in differentiating herpes zoster pain from visceral pain. It is usually only when the eruption appears that the diagnosis is made with increased certainty.

Occasionally, rickettsial infections, impetigo, mycoplasmas, coxsackievirus, or a localized herpes simplex eruption may be confused with herpes zoster (17). Laboratory correlation is then necessary to differentiate the two diseases. Isolation of the virus from vesicles prior to crusting or demonstration of the antigen in vesicular fluid will greatly assist in the diagnosis. Other confirmatory tests include rising serum antibody titers and demonstration of typical eosinophilic intranuclear inclusions in tissue biopsies or vesicle fluid (24).

Routine laboratory findings are usually normal with the exception of a slightly raised leukocyte count. In central nervous system infections, the cerebrospinal fluid pressure and protein are slightly elevated and CSF (cerebrospinal fluid) sugar is normal. A mild pleocytosis may also be noted.

TREATMENT

Treatment of herpes zoster in the acute stage should be directed toward patient comfort, local skin care with prevention of secondary infection of the lesions, and prevention of postherpetic neuralgia. Calamine lotion or Burow's solution applied topically offer local relief. Local care of the lesions with steroid creams and bandages also helps to decrease inflammation and discomfort.

Frequently, nonnarcotic analgesics such as aspirin and acetaminophen are sufficient to control mild pain. Codeine-containing analgesics, propoxyphene, and oxycodone may be used for more severe pain and usually suffice to control pain in most cases. Stool softeners should be used in the elderly to prevent narcotic-induced constipation.

Use of strongly addicting major narcotics should be avoided except in cases of severe pain uncontrolled by the above-mentioned drugs. Severe pain should also serve as a warning to the clinician that there is a strong potential for the development of postherpetic neuralgia (19). Aggressive treatment with modalities thought to decrease the incidence of postherpetic neuralgia should be considered in addition to analgesics.

Antibiotics

Although the cutaneous lesions may become secondarily infected, prophylactic antibiotics are generally not recommended (19). Systemic and topical antibiotics should be reserved for documented pyoderma or infection. When ocular involvement is present and corneal scarring is feared, prophylactic topical ophthalmic antibiotics should be considered (10).

Corticosteroids

Systemic corticosteroid therapy is the current most common treatment for herpes zoster, but the use of corticosteroids is not without controversy (19). For some time, corticosteroids have been the primary weapon utilized by physicians in treating acute herpes zoster. Numerous references may be found in the literature regarding the effectiveness of steroids in the treatment of acute herpes zoster and the possible preventative effect against postherpetic neuralgia.

Elliot, in 1964, studied 20 patients over the age of 50 using a regimen of prednisone (60 mg/day for 1 week, 30 mg/day the next week, and 15 mg/day the third week). These patients were compared to a group of 10 untreated patients. All patients were experiencing severe pain. Average duration of pain in the treated patients was 3.5 days after treatment started as compared to 3.5 weeks in the untreated group (25, 26).

Perhaps the most significant evidence of steroid effectiveness was in a study by Eaglstein et al. at the University of Miami in 1970 (27). This was the first age-controlled, double-blind study that showed the effectiveness of triamcinolone in reduction of pain duration. Thirty-four patients over age 60 with severe pain were randomly assigned into two groups, one receiving triamcinolone, the other lactose tablets. Study patients were dosed with triamcinolone (48 mg/day for 1 week, 24 mg/day the next week, then 16 mg/day the third week). Median duration of pain in the treated group was 6 weeks, compared with 10 weeks in the untreated group. Each group had one patient with pain lasting over 1 year. Skin healing and pain intensity were not affected.

In 1980, Keczkes and Basheer used 40 mg of prednisolone daily for 10 days, tapering the dose over the following 3 weeks in 40 patients over age 50 (28). They also noted faster relief of pain in the treated group by about one-half over a similar group treated with carbamazepine (400 mg/day). Although the results were statistically significant, the study was not blind and patients were hospitalized during the study. It does, however, help support the results of other studies with similar results.

Another use for steroids is topical application of steroid creams on the cutaneous lesions. This often helps decrease the local tissue reaction (10, 19). Topical steroids are used in herpes zoster ophthalmicus to reduce local cellulitis and inflammation in the eyelids to avoid scarring and resultant frozen upper lid (10). Systemic steroids may also be used for ophthalmic zoster as outlined above.

Subcutaneous infiltration of steroids has also been used to decrease pain and aid in healing of the lesions. This will be discussed later.

Concern has been expressed regarding the use of steroids and the risk of disseminated herpes zoster (29–33). Most studies have found no basis for this fear. Disseminated herpes zoster occurs commonly in patients with hematologic and other malignancies and has been seen to occur in up to 2% of otherwise normal patients (14). There is no evidence that this overall incidence is increased with short-term systemic steroids (33) as opposed to long-term corticosteroid therapy (34).

Antiviral Agents

Acyclovir Perhaps the most promising treatment for acute herpes zoster is the antiviral drug acyclovir, which selectively inhibits viral DNA nucleotidyltransferase (10, 35, 36). Results from early studies have demonstrated a marked reduction in the time of viral shedding, skin healing, and partial pain reduction. In a 1979 study of 23 patients with malignancy and herpes zoster, Selby et al. showed a reduction in new lesion formation and systemic spread, with pain relief within 24 hr, using intravenous acyclovir at a dose of 5 mg/kg administered every 8 hr for 5 days (37). These findings were confirmed by the Collaborative Acyclovir Study Group, which showed faster symptomatic relief and prevention of lesion progression in a double-blind study of immunocompromised patients (38). Although the incidence of postherpetic neuralgia was lower in the study group, this was not statistically significant. Other evidence exists supporting the ineffectiveness of acyclovir in the prevention of postherpetic neuralgia (39). The drug was well tolerated and without any adverse clinical side effects.

Oral acyclovir is currently being evaluated in the treatment of herpes zoster. In a small study, oral acyclovir in a dose of 200 mg five times daily for 5 days showed rapid resolution of the rash if treatment was started within 24 hr of the initial eruption (40). Although neither control nor study patients developed postherpetic neuralgia, oral treatment may also be promising as an agent to arrest the disease if administration is initiated early (40). More investigation is needed on this subject.

Cytosine Arabinoside (ARA-C) Cytosine arabinoside was one of the first antiviral agents studied in the management of acute herpes zoster (17). Conflicting results and frequent untoward side effects, especially persistent neurologic deficits, have caused this treatment to essentially be abandoned.

Adenine Arabinoside (ARA-A) Adenine arabinoside (Vidarabine) is incorporated into viral and host DNA and has been effective in treatment of immunocompromised patients. It was first reported in 1976 in a well-controlled study in immunocompromised patients (41). Rapid resolution of the disease, rapid cutaneous healing, and a decrease in pain duration and intensity were noted. Although the incidence of postherpetic neuralgia was equal to that of the control group, its duration was shortened.

Perhaps the best benefit of ARA-A is the lowered incidence of disseminated herpes zoster with early therapy (42). It is very effective in preventing visceral complications in hematologically compromised patients but relatively ineffective in treating them (42). Its use appears to be most beneficial in patients with disseminated herpes zoster, hematologic malignancies, or those who are otherwise immunocompromised (42). Treatment is most efficacious if begun within the first week following the eruption (10). Treatment is by 12-hr infusion over 5 days. There is some central nervous system, hepatic, and renal toxicity.

Idoxuridine Topical idoxuridine 40% in dimethyl sulfoxide (DMSO) has been reported to shorten pain duration and the acute vesicular stage in acute herpes zoster (30, 43). In order to be effective this is applied as a paste four times a day for the first 4 days following appearance of the vesicles. A double-blind study by Juel-Jensen et al. supports the acute pain reduction and faster healing (32). DMSO is not easily available in the United States.

Topical idoxuridine has also been used in the treatment of ophthalmic herpes zoster (10). Again, this requires linen soaked in DMSO with 40% idoxuridine applied as above.

Systemic idoxuridine is associated with significant systemic toxicity.

Interferon Interferon is a vital component of the body's normally functioning immune system. Early studies have shown high-dose therapy with interferon to be effective in decreasing local disease progression and systemic spread and diminishing the severity of postherpetic neuralgia (44). Although its limited availability limits its usefulness, early consideration should be given to this therapy in severely immunocompromised patients and children with malignancies.

Zoster Immune Globulin Zoster immune globulin has been shown to prevent varicella in susceptable individuals (45, 46). Its primary use has been in the prevention of varicella in children and immunocompromised patients exposed to chickenpox. There is no evidence that it is effective in altering the course of established herpes zoster (46) or in prevention of postherapeutic neuralgia (45).

Adenosine Monophosphate (AMP) Patients with herpes zoster have abnormally low levels of cyclic AMP in their serum (47). Several studies have been performed to evaluate the effectiveness of AMP on DNA virus infections (47–49). In a double-blind, age-controlled, crossover study using 100 mg of AMP injected intramuscularly every other day for 3 weeks, reduction of viral shedding and pain duration were demonstrated when compared to placebo treatment (2). Average pain duration was 3 weeks with no recurrence in 18–24 months of follow-up. Minimal side effects were noted.

Amantadine In a double-blind, controlled study, amantadine was shown to shorten the duration of vesicle formation and severe pain, implying effectiveness on the incidence of postherpetic neuralgia, but this was not defined (50, 51). Amantadine (200 mg/day for 28 days) has been considered effective in patients who are unable to take corticosteroids (52).

Other Antiviral Agents In a brief clinical trial, cimetadine (300 mg by mouth four times daily) provided rapid relief of itching, pain, and crusting of the skin lesions in four patients with cancer (53). This was thought possibly to be due to the antipruritic effect of H2 receptor antagonism, which may also inhibit suppressor T cells, restoring the natural immune response (54–57). Pain relief and crusting of lesions were noted within 48 hr. Further evaluation may be warranted.

Thymidine analogs have some inhibitory effect on the varicella virus, and the antivaricella effects of other antiviral agents, such as isoprinine, ribavirin, and BUDA, are under investigation.

Antidepressants and Tranquilizers

Tricyclic antidepressants and phenothiazine tranquilizers are widely used substances in the therapy of severe pain due to acute herpes zoster as well as postherpetic neuralgia. Although their serotonin effect may contribute to a central pain relief mechanism in acute herpes zoster, their antidepressant effect is also beneficial in this stage. The advent of newer antiviral agents with early pain relief may decrease the use of these drugs in the acute phase. Their use may also be effective in patients who do not respond to other types of pain relief.

Anticonvulsants

Anticonvulsants, primarily phenytoin and carbamazepine, are used to lessen the sharp, paroxysmal pains seen in both acute herpes zoster and postherpetic neuralgia (58, 59). Their primary use is in postherpetic pain, but they can be used in the acute infection if the paroxysmal pain does not respond to analgesics. They should be used cautiously because of the potential for blood dyscrasias.

Nerve Blocks

Nerve blocks have been utilized extensively in the treatment of pain in herpes zoster. Numerous attempts have been made to treat herpes zoster and prevent postherpetic neuralgia using all forms of somatic and sympathetic nerve blocks (60).

Perhaps the most frequently used blocks involve local infiltration of the acute eruptions. This was described by Epstein, who injected procaine with 0.2% triamcinolone subcutaneously in the areas of the eruptions and areas of pain and itching (61). He reported relief in almost 100% of the cases with a reduction in the incidence of postherpetic neuralgia. Response was predictable and complications minimal.

Peripheral somatic nerve blocks have been successful in temporary treatment of the acute pain; however, no evidence exists that they assist in avoiding postherpetic neuralgia.

Since the acute inflammation is primarily located in the nerve roots, much work has been directed toward blocks in the nerve root area. The epidural route has been studied with much success in relieving the acute pain and shortening the duration of the infection (62). Perkins and Hanlon achieved excellent relief in patients with herpes zoster of less than 7 weeks' duration using epidural blocks (63). Pain was relieved, lesions dried up rapidly, and no development of postherpetic neuralgia was noted. Fothergill et al. reported 113 patients age 14-93 who underwent epidural injections, with immediate, permanent pain relief in 110 (64). Postherpetic neuralgia developed in two of the three failures. In 192 patients over age 60, 12 (6.25%) developed postherpetic neuralgia, which is less that the usual 50-60% (64). Immediate relief of pain and prevention of postherpetic neuralgia was also noted in 100% of 113 patients with herpes zoster of less than 10 weeks' duration by Schreuder, who injected 8-12 ml of bupivacaine 0.25% with methylprednisolone (80 mg) epidurally (65). Although patients have been injected with epidural local anesthetics combined with steroids, the additional effect of steroids has not been documented.

Much attention is now being directed toward sympathetic blocks as an extremely effective method of treating acute herpes zoster (9, 66). Although the exact pathophysiology of pain in herpes zoster and postherpetic neuralgia remains unknown, the role of the sympathetic nervous system is receiving more attention. Inflammation of the posterior root ganglia may increase sympathetic efferent activity, causing increased segmental vasoconstriction and increased pain (67, 68). Vasospasm and sympathetic sensitization of peripheral and central pain mechanisms may be relieved temporarily and possibly reversed by early sympathetic blockade. The earliest evidence of sympathetic blockade efficacy was noted in the 1930s when patients suffering from herpes zoster and reflex sympathetic dystrophy were administered sympathetic blocks for their reflex sympathetic dystrophy (9). It was noted that the herpes zoster eruptions in these patients dried and crusted within 2-3 days and their pain was immediately relieved. If these blocks were performed within the first 3 weeks following the eruption, there was rapid resolution of the acute illness and a decreased incidence of postherpetic neuralgia (62, 66). In 1938, Rosenak pioneered the use of sympathetic blocks in acute herpes zoster, noting rapid resolution of the eruptions and a decreased incidence of postherpetic neuralgia (69). In 1969, Colding studied 300 patients who underwent sympathetic blocks during the acute stage, again noting pain relief and a reduction in the incidence of postherpetic neuralgia (70). This was later reproduced in 483 patients (68).

Mani et al. studied sympathetic blocks and noted a decrease in the duration of the acute infection if blocks were performed within the first 4 weeks following the onset (71). Riopelle et al., in 1984, noted brief and lasting relief with sympathetic blocks but no overall change in the incidence of postherpetic neuralgia (72). They believed that this was related to the intensity of the acute pain. All patients studied who developed postherpetic neuralgia had severe pain in the acute phase (72).

Trigeminal and ophthalmic herpes zoster appear to be especially amenable to treatment with sympathetic blocks (73, 74). Ipsilateral bupivacaine 0.25% stellate ganglion blocks within the first 3 weeks have been extremely successful in immediately stopping the pain, and the vesicular lesions crust within 48 hr (74, 75). Early use of stellate ganglion blocks should be considered in all patients with nasociliary ganglion involvement in an attempt to prevent ocular involvement and subsequent complications leading to vision loss (3). This has been duplicated in our own personal experience. When treatment is initiated after 3 weeks, the success rate drops rapidly (66, 75).

Stellate ganglion blocks can be used for facial, cervical, and thoracic lesions to T4. Below T4, the epidural route is preferred for sympathetic block because thoracic paravertebral sympathetic blocks are difficult to perform and have more complications (66).

POSTHERPETIC NEURALGIA

Severe pain during the acute eruptions and especially continuation of pain following resolution of the crusting stage of acute herpes zoster should raise the suspicion of postherpetic neuralgia. There is evidence that the greater the severity of acute pain, the greater the likelihood of developing postherpetic neuralgia (72). It is extremely rare for pain to subside and then recur following a period of complete pain remission (J.D. Loeser, personal communication).

The definition of postherpetic neuralgia varies. Numerous references exist regarding the time frame required before the pain can be classified as postherpetic neuralgia. These range from pain continuing after the crusting of the lesions (76) to pain lasting longer than 1-2 years following resolution of the acute disease (77). In general, the most common classification of postherpetic neuralgia requires pain persistence for 4-8 weeks following resolution of the acute stage of herpes zoster (28).

The overall incidence of postherpetic neuralgia is 18-35% of all herpes zoster patients (78, 79). Age is a major factor in the development of postherpetic neuralgia and its duration. Herpes zoster is more common in the elderly, their pain is usually more intense with longer duration, and they are more likely to develop postherpetic neuralgia (79-82). Postherpetic neuralgia is rarely seen in patients under age 30 and even then usually spontaneously resolves within 1-2 weeks (8). The frequency of occurrence of postherpetic neuralgia gradually increases to about 10% of all patients under age 50 and usually resolves spontaneously in less than a year. In patients over age 50 the likelihood of developing postherpetic neuralgia increases dramatically and, by age 60, 50% may develop the syndrome with little or no spontaneous remission (83). Over age 70, the percentage is increased 1% per year (57).

There is no difference in the incidence with regard to sex (84).

Postherpetic neuralgia is more common following herpes zoster ophthalmicus than truncal herpes zoster (16). Postherpetic neuralgia is extremely common following herpes zoster in patients with diabetes mellitus (79, 85).

PATHOPHYSIOLOGY

Postherpetic neuralgia is a form of deafferentation pain; however, its exact pathogenesis remains obscure (83). There appears to be a dysfunction of both central and peripheral neural mechanisms. Microscopic examinations in acute herpes zoster patients have demonstrated destruction of peripheral nerve endings, peripheral neural demyelination and axonal destruction, neuronal death in the sensory ganglion with secondary wallerian degeneration in the posterior columns, neural necrosis in areas of the anterior and posterior horn of the spinal cord, and damage of the spinothalamic tract, thalamus, and sensory cortex. These areas are eventually replaced with areas of neural fibrosis. Although the damage may be extensive, the extent of neurologic damage does not correlate well with predicting the development of postherpetic neuralgia (12). Pain in this acute phase is thought to be due to an inflammation of the dorsal root ganglion with abnormal dorsal horn discharges (28). In the chronic phase, fibrosis of the dorsal horn and ganglion may cause pain, and this is perpetuated by central mechanisms (28).

Several theories have been proposed over the years that attempt to explain the pain mechanisms of postherpetic neuralgia. In 1959, Noordenbos demonstrated large-fiber demyelination and neural destruction in the peripheral nerve with resulting preponderance of small unmyelinated fibers (86). Intraneural edema and vasoconstriction resulting from the acute inflammation have been implicated in the destruction of these large peripheral fibers (3). Haas described a gate control theory of pain based on the destruction of large-fiber modulation in the peripheral nerve (87). He also noted that large fiber regeneration was much slower than small fiber regeneration and that regenerated large fibers were much smaller than their original size, thus leaving a proportionately larger number of small fibers. Pain carried to the central nervous system via small unmyelinated fibers is modulated at the cord level by input from large myelinated fibers. It is thought that this large fiber loss results in a loss of inhibitory input to the spinal cord (88). This leads to a relative increase in the sensitivity of small fibers to even light touch. This may help explain the prevalence of this syndrome in the elderly, because their neurophysiologic responses to injury are decreased (89) and they have proportionately fewer large fibers in peripheral nerves than their younger counterparts (67). Many elderly patients also have small vessel disease that may increase the tendency toward peripheral neural ischemia, which may aggravate this destruction as well as slow recovery from peripheral neural ischemia and edema following the acute phase. Vasoconstriction and ischemia could also explain the efficacy of early sympathetic blocks in disease resolution.

Head demonstrated pathologic changes and destruction in the dorsal horn of the spinal cord extending for several segments (90). Wall and Gutnick demonstrated spontaneous activity, increased sensitivity to mechanical stimulation, and increased sensitivity to α-adrenergic agonists and sympathetic efferents in experimental nerve transections (91). Chronically deafferentated second-order neurons respond indiscriminately to inputs from adjacent dermatomes. This reafferentation presumably involves activity in the wide-dynamic-range neurons. Recent investigations by Roberts and Foglesong support this and may help explain why the pain of herpes zoster can be lessened by sympathetic blocks (92). They have described peripheral sympathetic stimulation of mechanoreceptors, increasing their sensitivity to light touch. They have also detected this stimulation in wide-dynamic-range neurons in the dorsal horn area. Wide-dynamic-range neuron signals are coded as pain signals arising in the damaged dermatome (93). Spontaneous discharges following loss of peripheral input from this area have been detected (94, 95). These may be responsible for the hyperpathia and paroxysms of pain seen in postherpetic neuralgia. It is conceivable that this hypersensitivity of peripheral and central pain transmitters combined with loss of normal large fiber modulation acts in the production of the pain of postherpetic neuralgia and the production of a central pain pathway.

As time progresses, the central processes proceed rostrally. Electrical changes have been detected in the midbrain, thalamus, and sensory cortex following peripheral deafferentation (96, 97). As this centralization progresses, pain becomes more resistant to conventional treatment and pain tolerance lessens.

Prolonged pain commonly causes anxiety and profound depression in postherpetic patients, thereby further reducing endogenous pain control and increasing pain levels (98). Endogenous pain control mechanisms become more ineffective because they are cortically stimulated and negatively influenced by increasing emotional stress.

All of these factors must be considered when developing a treatment regimen.

SYMPTOMS AND PAIN CHARACTERISTICS

The pain of postherpetic neuralgia is usually described as a continuous aching and burning with frequent paroxysms of sharp, shooting pains in a radicular pattern corresponding to the affected dermatome (16). Characteristically there are two discrete elements to postherpetic pain. The first is a continual aching, burning superficial pain associated with hyperpathia and dysesthesias. This is dramatically increased by light touch. The second is a feeling of constricting tightness along the affected area associated with itching and a feeling of formication. These are accompanied by episodic lancinating pains shooting out in a radicular pattern corresponding to the affected dermatome (16). There is no definite urnal pattern to the occurrence of the hyperpathia and sharp pains, but frequently they are more severe at night, causing interruption of sleep. They can be spontaneous, but are most frequently associated with light touch, especially from clothing (99). Intensity varies but the pain is always present. There are no pain-free intervals. Some movements, light touch, and temperature extremes will aggravate the pain. Often, there is an area in the affected dermatome that, when stimulated, will act as a trigger to the pain. This is usually in one of the hypopigmented areas of scarring. Examination will frequently show decreased sensation to pinprick but hypersensitivity to light touch. Pressure in this area does not increase the pain and, in fact, pressure applied in certain areas may reduce pain by counterirritation (100). Many patients have accidentally discovered this technique and will rub these areas constantly.

Classic physical findings include a unilateral, dermatomal, hypopigmented area of skin that is without sensation to pinprick but extremely painful to light touch (16). Virtually all patients have residual scarring with characteristic skin pigmentary changes. Areas of skin between these scars may be extremely hypersensitive. Patients complain of an inability to wear clothing and altered sleep patterns due to paroxysms of severe, sharp, shooting pain superimposed on a baseline continuous, dull, burning, ache of varying intensity. They also complain of an associated tightness as if a constricting band was around the area.

Alterations in mood, personality, activity levels, and social interactions are common. Patients are frequently visibly depressed, teary-eyed, and, at times, desperate for even brief relief.

TREATMENT

There is no known, consistently reliable, preventative therapy or definitive treatment for permanent relief of established postherpetic neuralgia (10, 84). Much debate exists over the optimal therapy of postherpetic neuralgia in the literature. Every field of medicine has its own ideas of treatment protocols. Unfortunately, much of the literature evolved over the past 50 years lacks age control, double-blind design, and follow-up. Another problem with selected studies is determining whether relief is from treatment or the natural course of the disease in the specific patient. Spontaneous resolution of pain is possible during treatment, thereby causing false assumptions as to the efficacy of the involved treatment regimen. There are, however, studies that strongly suggest that the best treatment of postherpetic neuralgia is early, aggressive treatment of acute herpes zoster infections (19). Shortening the duration of the acute viral phase combined with adequate pain relief may act to minimize the potential for postherpetic sequelae (19). The primary goal in treating established postherpetic neuralgia should be to afford the patient as much relief as possible until the disease runs its course. This can be as short as 6 months to 1 year and as long as 15–20 years (73).

Antiviral and Anti-inflammatory Agents

Although these agents perform well in the treatment of acute herpes zoster and have been shown to aid in its prevention, antiviral and anti-inflammatory agents are of minimal benefit in established postherpetic neuralgia (9).

Analgesics

Postherpetic neuralgia often does not respond adequately to traditional narcotic analgesic agents (22, 100). The most frequently prescribed analgesics used in primary care treatment of postherpetic neuralgia are usually simple oral analgesics such as codeine-containing combinations, propoxyphene, and nonnarcotic synthetic compounds. These are subsequently replaced with stronger narcotic medications. These analgesics may relieve a portion of the pain but are rarely effective in relieving the hyperpathia and dysesthesias (67). Long-term use of narcotic analgesics for pain in postherpetic neuralgia is to be discouraged because pain relief is incomplete, tachyphylaxis is common, and the risk of addiction is very real.

Propoxyphene appears to be very effective in the treatment of hyperpathic pain syndromes. A trial of propoxyphene may be beneficial. This should be given at regular 4-hr intervals, rather than as needed, since for best effect, constant blood levels must be obtained.

Antidepressants, Tranquilizers, and Anticonvulsants

Tricyclic antidepressants have been successfully used to treat postherpetic neuralgia as well as other chronic painful syndromes, and pain relief is considered independent of the antidepressant effect (101). It is believed that tricyclics exert their pain-relieving effect by blocking reuptake of serotonin at serotonergic synapses, and norepinephrine in the descending pain-inhibitory pathways existing between the midpons and dorsal horn of the spinal cord (99, 102).

In 1965, Woodforde and associates reported 11 of 14 patients receiving amitriptyline experienced good to complete pain relief within 2–4 weeks of oral therapy (103). In 1982, Watson and associates performed a double-blind, placebo-controlled crossover study using amitriptyline in postherpetic neuralgia patients (101). Sixteen of 24 patients had good to excellent pain relief with a median dose of 75 mg/day. Serum concentrations were far below therapeutic levels for depression and pain relief was not considered to be due to the antidepressant effect (101, 104). This is frequently observed in clinical practice, where high-dose tricyclics are relatively ineffective in relieving pain. Institution of therapy should be at low doses of 10–25 mg/day and gradually increased, realizing that it may take 2–4 weeks to detect any improvement (9). Drowsiness and dry mouth are frequent side effects and make bedtime administration more practical.

Perhaps the most effective analgesia can be obtained using combination therapy with tricyclic antidepressants and phenothiazine tranquilizers (105–107). In 1973, Taub reported an improved effectiveness of amitriptyline when combined with phenothiazines (perphenazine, fluphenazine, chlorprothixene, or thioridazine (108). The exact analgesic mechanism of action of phenothiazines is not known. Perhaps it may be due to the dopamine antagonist effects, anxiolytic properties, potentiation of tricyclic effects, or some other mechanism (22).

Perhaps the most widely used and clinically most effective phenothiazine is fluphenazine (Prolixin). Initial doses in the range of 2–4 mg/day in combination with amitriptyline appear to be extremely effective in pain reduction. Care should be taken in the elderly population to avoid extrapyramidal side effects.

Tricyclic drugs have also been used in combination with anticonvulsants with good results (22). Anticonvulsants such as carbamazepine and phenytoin have been used in the treatment of other neuralgic disorders, such as tic douloureux. Anticonvulsants are thought to produce analgesia by raising the threshold for repetitive firing of first- and second-order neurons involved in nociception (99). Other studies suggest activation of pain-suppression pathways in the central nervous system (109).

Results using anticonvulsants alone have been limited, and combination therapy with tricyclics is recommended (22). Davis found that carbamazepine relieved only the lancinating pain and not the persistent burning ache (58). In a combination study, Hatangdi et al. administered carbamazepine (600–800 mg) or phenytoin (300–400 mg) with nortriptyline (50–100 mg) in divided doses to 34 patients (105). Of the original 34 patients, 30 had 90% good to excellent pain relief. Pain relief with intravenous injection of 1–1.5 mg/kg lidocaine was used as a predictor of response to oral anticonvulsant therapy.

Raftery reported substantial relief with sodium valproate in combination with amitriptyline (59). Amitriptyline seemed to be most effective in reducing the burning and hyperpathia, whereas the sharp, shooting pain responded to sodium valproate.

Side effects of anticonvulsants are more serious and include bone marrow depression, hepatic dysfunction, ataxia, diplopia, confusion, vertigo, nausea, lymphadenopathy, and nystagmus. Combination therapy may also cause urinary retention.

Other Medical Therapies

Baclofen (Lioresal) is another medication that has been utilized in postherpetic neuralgia (110). It is a muscle relaxant, antispastic drug that acts by inhibiting both monosynaptic and polysynaptic reflexes at the cord level. Gradual titration of dose to effect is recommended.

Chlorprothixene (Taractan) (111) and carbidopa-levodopa (Sinemet) (112) have also been used but are frequently ineffective if other medication regimens have failed (9).

Numerous other medical therapies have been tried over the years in an effort to effectively treat postherpetic neuralgia. Oral and topical vitamin E, vitamin B_{12}, B complex, pimozide, ergot derivatives, vincristine iontophoresis, mephenesin, l-tryptophan, protamide, intravenous local anesthetics, autologous blood transfusion, and even hypnosis all have proponents; however, there is minimal evidence at present to support any degree of improved effectiveness over the previously discussed therapies (16).

In the author's experience, amitriptyline and fluphenazine in combination with phenytoin or carbamazepine offer the best relief in patients who will respond to oral medication management (see Table 39.2). An idealized protocol for management begins with amitriptyline (25–75 mg/day) usually administered at bedtime to take advantage of the sedative effect. Most patients complain of insomnia and tricyclics may help combat this problem. Two to 3 weeks of treatment are required to evaluate effectiveness of tricyclics in pain relief. If ineffective alone, fluphenazine (2–4 mg/day in two to three divided doses) is added. Continued burning pain and hyperpathia may respond to gradual increases in amitriptyline over several weeks in 25–50 mg/day increments either at bedtime or two divided doses (in the morning and at bedtime).

Consideration should be given to anticonvulsants if sharp, intermittant, lancinating pains continue. Effectiveness of anticonvulsants can be evaluated by short-term response to intravenous lidocaine (1.0–1.5 mg/kg administered in a bolus). If this is effective, phenytoin or carbamazepine should be started in the doses listed above.

This is an idealized protocol since most practitioners treating postherpetic neuralgia begin these three medications simultaneously when the diagnosis is made in order to expedite treatment. Early aggressive treatment is

Table 39.2
Some Recommended Doses

Propoxyphene Compound 65	One 3–4 times/day
Amitriptyline	25–75 mg/day
Nortriptyline	50–100 mg/day
Fluphenazine (Prolixin)	2–4 mg/day in divided doses
Phenytoin	200–400 mg/day in divided doses
Carbamazepine	500–1000 mg/day in divided doses
Sodium valproate	200 mg 2–3 times/day
Chlorprothixene (Taractan)	50 mg q 6 h for 5 days
Carbidopa-levodopa (Sinemet 25/100)	1 tablet 3 times a day increasing to a maximum of 6 tablets/day
Baclofen (Lioresal)	5–15 mg 3 times/day
Nifedipine	20–60 mg/day in divided doses

considered to be most beneficial in providing effective relief (19).

Nerve Blocks

Nerve blocks are widely used in the management of postherpetic neuralgia as diagnostic, prognostic, and therapeutic tools (72). The effectiveness of therapeutic nerve blocks in postherpetic neuralgia appears related to the stage of the disease in which they are utilized. Early use of nerve blocks may give protracted relief by limiting input into damaged areas of the spinal cord, thus decreasing the potential for development of self-perpetuating central pain mechanisms. This may be especially true in the case of sympathetic blocks. However, as the syndrome becomes more established, nerve blocks become less effective because of centralization of pain-initiating mechanisms (113). Because of the complex pathologic changes in the nerve, spinal cord, and central nervous system, most relief is transient and the long-term therapeutic effectiveness of nerve blocks alone is minimal because of tachyphylaxis. Unlike acute herpes zoster, in which pain can be effectively managed by local or regional anesthetic blocks, the most beneficial effect in advanced postherpetic neuralgia is usually temporary relief of severe pain, which allows the patient and physician time to begin other therapeutic measures.

Local Infiltration Local subcutaneous infiltration of "hot spots" and trigger areas on the skin (areas of intense burning and itching that trigger intense pain when stimulated) appears to be an extremely popular technique. This technique is supported by Moya and associates in Miami (23). The affected areas are outlined and injected with 0.25% bupivacaine with 0.2% triamcinolone or 16 mg dexamethasone in 50 ml 0.25% bupivacaine. This is injected subcutaneously once or twice a week for 3–4 weeks until relief is obtained. Good relief and low complication rate are cited advantages (23). Early utilization of this technique may afford prolonged relief and avoid further, more aggressive therapy (23).

Peripheral Nerve Blocks Because pain patterns are dermatomal, the most frequently used nerve blocks have been peripheral somatic blocks. These may help to decrease noxious input from damaged nerve fibers and provide transient relief; however, long-term relief is less likely. Repetitive intercostal or paravertebral blocks have been advocated to relieve pain and possibly offer a cure in selected cases. If performed early in the course of the disease process, a series of nerve blocks may provide relief while the syndrome runs its course, but whether the relief obtained is due to the block or to natural resolution of the disease is unknown.

Dorsal root selective nerve blocks are performed to evaluate the effectiveness of dorsal rhizotomy, surgical neurectomy, or chemical neurolysis in the treatment of the disease. Technical difficulty and complications prevent their general use as routine analgesic blocks. In most cases, the epidural route is preferred.

Epidural Blocks Because of the pathologic changes in the dorsal columns as well as peripheral nerves, much attention has been given to the role of epidural blocks in pain management (64, 84). Epidural steroid injections have been used for many years as a treatment modality for radicular pain. In a well-controlled study, Forrest obtained progressive relief of pain using a series of weekly epidural injections over 3 weeks using bupivacaine 0.5% with methylprednisolone 80–120 mg (114). Eighty-six per cent of patients were pain free after 6 months. This was verified with a 1-year follow-up. Perkins and Hanlon studied five patients with postherpetic neuralgia using bupivacaine 0.25% and methylprednisolone administered epidurally (63). Only one injection was given per patient, and pain relief was reported as less than 50% in all patients. Epidural bupivacaine 0.25% with epinephrine can also provide temporary relief in severe pain (16).

Epidural and Spinal Opiates Epidural and subarachnoid morphine have been used in the treatment of postherpetic neuralgia with mixed results. Favorable results have occasionally surfaced, but experience is limited (9).

Sympathetic Blocks With recent evidence further implicating the sympathetic nervous system in the propagation of postherpetic neuralgia, sympathetic nerve blocks are becoming more popular in evaluation and treatment (9). Many claims have been made regarding the effectiveness of early sympathetic blocks in relieving postherpetic pain. For example, Colding found that 50% of 67 patients treated with sympathetic blocks obtained pain relief or marked improvement in pain levels (68). Bonica obtained good relief in a series of paravertebral sympathetic blocks if pain duration was less than 2 months (115).

As mentioned earlier, sympathetic blocks in early herpes zoster have an impressive therapeutic effect, with rapid resolution of the acute illness and prevention of postherpetic neuralgia. Utilization of sympathetic blocks early in the postherpetic phase may also have an improved pain-relief potential. It has been our clinical experience and the experience of others that sympathetic blocks performed within the first 3–6 months of the syndrome greatly improve chances for pain relief or at least diminution of pain to controllable levels. Milligan and Nash reported 77 cases of postherpetic neuralgia with pain duration of 1 year or less (73). Seventy-five per cent were improved and 40% pain free following stellate ganglion block. In patients with pain over 1 year, only 44% were improved with 22% pain free. All but 6 patients were over age 60.

Perhaps sympathetic blocks prevent further changes in central pain perpetuation or decrease ongoing pain reflexes, or the response is just coincidence. No matter what the reason, the chances of decreasing future suffering in just one patient justifies the use of sympathetic blocks in all who may be at risk.

We have also clinically noted that recurrent pain following dorsal rhizotomy and peripheral neurectomy frequently responds favorably to sympathetic blocks. The mechanism of this pain relief is unclear at this time and further study is necessary.

Neuroablative Procedures

Sympathectomy (Chemical and Surgical) Patients in whom sympathetic blocks have been temporarily effective may respond to oral sympatholytic medications. Regitine, phenoxybenzamine, and guanethadine are the most popular oral agents in the treatment of sympathetic dystrophy and may be tried in postherpetic patients. Gradual titration of dosage is recommended to avoid hypotensive complications.

Recent information regarding the effectiveness of nifedipine in the management of sympathetic hyperactivity has led to increased utilization of this drug in reflex sympathetic dystrophy (116). The author has used this medication in sympathetic dystrophy with good results. Although we have used it in a few postherpetic patients, no definite information is yet available as to its overall efficacy in the management of postherpetic pain.

Patients who respond consistently to sympathetic blocks but fail to maintain relief on medications and continue to have recurrence of pain may be candidates for surgical sympathectomy. Evidence of an effective and consistent response to several previous sympathetic blocks should be mandatory prior to this procedure.

Neurolytic Blocks Neurolytic blocks have been performed in patients in whom prognostic peripheral or epidural blocks have provided significant pain relief (117). Ethyl alcohol 50%, absolute alcohol, or phenol 6% have been used for neurolysis. Duration of effect ranges from 2 months to 2 years.

Cryoanalgesia Temporary neurolysis can be obtained using cold-induced lesions of the nerve under direct vision. The nerve is exposed under local anesthesia and frozen. In a small series of patients with trigeminal postherpetic neuralgia, cryoanalgesia provided about 6 weeks' relief of pain (118). No long-term pain relief was noted.

Dorsal Rhizotomy Peripheral neurolysis can also be accomplished by radiofrequency rhizotomy of the dorsal root ganglion (9). A prognostic local anesthetic block should be performed prior to rhizotomy. The results of rhizotomies and neurolysis in general have been gratifying with regard to short-term benefits but long-term effectiveness varies (119). Most relief lasts less than 24 months, and in our experience, many of these patients usually return with increasing hyperpathia, burning, and dysesthesias within 6–12 months of treatment. Further deafferentation and centralization of pain origination appear to be responsible for this recurrence of pain (120). Sympathetic stimulation of central pain pathways may also play a role in this recurrence; however, this most likely represents further cord destruction at the second-order neuron level in the dorsal horn (113).

Dorsal Root Entry Zone (DREZ) Lesions Dorsal root entry zone lesions have been performed in postherpetic patients in order to relieve long-standing pain (83). This surgical procedure involves radiofrequency destruction of the DREZ of the spinal cord, thereby destroying the damaged dorsal horn and also preventing pain transmission from the peripheral nerve (83). The ablation of second-order neurons in this area of the spinal cord stops the origination of pain from this area. Although initial results were quite promising, subsequent results and long-term follow-up have been less encouraging as to long-term pain relief, especially in patients with advanced postherpetic neuralgia (D.E. Kennemore, personal communication). This is most likely due, again, to further centralization of the pain process.

Cordotomy Percutaneous or open cordotomies interrupt ascending pain fibers in the spinothalamic tract. This procedure has occasionally been shown to result in significant pain relief when other modalities have failed (119).

Medullary Tractotomy Medullary tractotomy divides pain fibers traveling from the orofacial region and replaces cordotomy in craniofacial postherpetic neuralgia (9). As with cordotomy, tractotomy has the best success rate among surgical procedures for craniofacial pain. There is some risk involved with both procedures. Patients may also have return of their pain within 1–2 years following surgery (9).

Cingulumotomy and Frontal Lobotomy These surgical procedures alter the central perception of pain but have not been proven particularly effective to date in relieving the pain of postherpetic neuralgia (121, 122).

Counterirritation Techniques

Transcutaneous Electrical Nerve Stimulation (TENS) Transcutaneous electrical nerve stimulation has been found to be somewhat effective in providing relief in some patients refractory to other types of treatment (88, 123). In our experience TENS has been effective in pain reduction when the unit is used after adequate skin desensitization. Use of TENS can increase pain if the skin is initially hyperpathic. We have found TENS to be most effective when applied following a series of epidural somatic/sympathetic blocks in conjunction with oral medications. Multiple electrode placements may be necessary for optimal relief.

Because of its ease of use, relative lack of side effects, and low cost, a TENS trial is certainly justified.

Dorsal Column and Thalamic Stimulation A newer form of invasive counterirritation involves implantation of dorsal column or thalamic neural stimulators. These devices are implanted to block pain-conducting pathways and stimulate endorphin production (124). Evidence to date of the effectiveness of these procedures in the treatment or postherpetic neuralgia is limited.

Ice Therapy Local ice therapy and ethyl chloride spray have been used in an attempt to temporarily relieve pain. This is thought to potentiate activation of remaining large fibers, causing inhibition of pain transmission (9). Mechanical vibration and application of tight binders over the area have also been tried to increase large fiber activity (9).

Acupuncture Acupuncture has been tried in postherpetic neuralgia and has been generally found to be of minimal therapeutic value. One well-controlled study concluded that acupuncture was of little or no benefit in this disease (125).

Ultrasound Ultrasound has been used over the affected dermatome in the treatment of postherpetic neuralgia with minimal success (126). In theory, application of peripheral neural stimulation will replace the large fiber input into the spinal cord and "close the gate" to pain perception (88). In practice this has not been successful in long-term relief of pain (126).

Psychological Treatment

An especially important aspect in the treatment of postherpetic neuralgia is psychological and emotional support. Chronic unrelenting pain is a major factor in the destruction of emotional stability. Severe depression is present in over 50% of patients suffering from postherpetic neuralgia (23). Suicidal ideations are common. Psychological support is extremely helpful in these patients. Drastic alterations in life-style, comfort level, and interpersonal relationships, with limitations to social activities, personal habits, and mobility, aggravate already elevated stress levels. Stress management, relaxation, and counseling can reduce anxiety and help the patient cope with the pain and life-style alteration. Behavior modification can prevent the establishment of chronic pain behavior states and allow the patient to adapt and lead a more productive life in spite of discomfort. Unless the chronic pain state is managed, organic treatment will be less successful when psychological stresses potentiate the suffering of the pain experience. Generalized physical deconditioning also accompanies periods of severe pain or illness, and a physical rehabilitation program should be incorporated into the psychological therapy in order to allow the patient to realize that many of his/her limitations are self-imposed.

SUMMARY

In summary, postherpetic neuralgia is a severe, poorly understood syndrome that affects primarily elderly and debilitated individuals. Treatment of the established syndrome is extremely difficult and minimally successful. The best treatment for this problem appears to be early aggressive treatment of the acute herpes zoster infection, with special attention being paid to those individuals in the high-risk groups for developing postherpetic neuralgia. Until we understand more about the pathophysiology of postherpetic neuralgia, aggressive therapy of all herpes zoster patients is the only potential method of treating postherpetic neuralgia. Accurate predictions as to who will develop postherpetic neuralgia are impossible. Prevention is the key to eradicating this most severe of chronic pain syndromes. It is much better to overtreat a herpes zoster patient than to condemn him/her to a life of misery and suffering.

Reference

1. Ragozzino MW, Melton LJ, Kurland LT, etal: Risk of cancer after herpes zoster. *N Engl J Med* 307:393, 1982.
2. Sklar SH, Blue WT, Alexander EJ, et al: Herpes zoster: the treatment and prevention of neuralgia with adenosine monophosphate. *JAMA* 253:1427–1430, 1985.
3. Winnie AP: Panel on herpes zoster. American Society of Regional Anesthesia 8th Annual Meeting Orlando, FL, March, 1983.
4. Dolin R, Reichman RC, Mazur MH, et al: Herpes zoster-varicella infection in immunosuppressed patients. *Ann Intern Med* 89:35, 1978.
5. Hope-Simpson RE: The nature of herpes zoster: a long term study and a new hypothesis. *Proc R Soc Med* 58:9–20, 1965.
6. Oxman MN: Herpes zoster. In Braude AI, Davis CE, Fierer J (eds): *Medical Microbiology and Infectious Diseases*. Philadelphia, WB Saunders, 1981, pp 1663–1671.
7. Ray CG: Chickenpox (varicella) and herpes zoster. In Petersderf RG, Adams RD, Braunwald E, et al (eds): *Harrison' Principles of Internal Medicine*, ed. 10 New York, McGraw-Hill, 1983, pp 1121–1124.
8. Harnisch JP: Zoster in the elderly. Clinical, immunological, and therapeutic considerations. *J Am Geriatr Soc* 22:789–793, 1984.
9. Borowsky S, Shetter AG: Treatment of pain due to herpes zoster infection. *Arizona Med* 42(C1):16–19, 1985.
10. Liesegang TJ: Herpes zoster ophthalmicus. *Int Ophthalmol Clin* 25:77–96, 1985.
11. Ghatak NR, Zimmerman HM: Spinal ganglion in herpes zoster. *Arch Pathol* 95:411–415, 1973.
12. Zacks SI, Langfitt TW, Elliot FA: Herpetic neuritis. A light and EM study. *Neurology* 14:744–750, 1964.
13. Schimpff S, Serpick A, Stoller B, et al: Varicella-zoster infection in patients with cancer. *Ann Intern Med* 76:241, 1972.
14. Ragozzino MW, Melton LJ, Kurland LT, et al: Population-based study of herpes zoster and its sequelae. *Medicine (Baltimore)* 61:310–316, 1982.
15. Gershon AA, Steinberg SP: Antibody responses to varicella-zoster virus and the role of antibody in host defense. *Am J Med Sci* 282:12–17, 1981.
16. Loeser JD: Herpes zoster and postherpetic neuralgia. *Pain* 25:149–164, 1986.
17. Reuler JB, Chang MK: Herpes zoster: epidemiology, clinical features, and management. *South Med J* 77:1149–1156, 1984.
18. Frengley JD: Herpes zoster—a challenge in management. *Primary Care* 8:715–731, 1981.
19. Dickinson JA: Should we treat herpes zoster with corticosteroid agents? *Med J Aust* 144:375–380, 1986.
20. Thomas JE, Howard FM: Segmental zoster paresis—a disease profile. *Neurology* 22:459–466, 1972.
21. Malloy MG, Goodwill CJ: Herpes zoster and lower motor neurone paresis. *Rheumatol Rehabil* 18:170–173, 1979.
22. Thompson, M, Bones M: Nontraditional analgesics for the management of postherpetic neuralgia. *Clin Pharm* 4:170–176, 1985.
23. Mayne GE, Brown M, Arnold P, Moya F: Pain of herpes zoster and postherpetic neuralgia. In Raj PP (ed): *Practi-*

cal Management of Pain. Chicago, Year Book, 1986, pp 345–361.
24. Veien N: Cytologic examination and viral and bacterial culture in herpes simplex, herpes zoster, and varicella. Cutis 22:61, 1978.
25. Elliot FA: Treatment of herpes zoster with high doses of prednisone. Lancet 2:610–611, 1964.
26. Elliot FA: Shingles. Lancet 2:170–171, 1968.
27. Eaglstein WH, Katz R, Brown JA: The effects of early corticosteroid therapy on the skin eruptions and pain of herpes zoster. JAMA 211:1681–1683, 1970.
28. Keczkes K, Basheer AM: Do corticosteroids prevent postherpetic neuralgia? Br J Dermatol 102:551–555, 1980.
29. (Anonymous): Shingles: a belt of roses from hell (editorial). Br Med J 1:5, 1979.
30. Juel-Jensen BE: Herpes simplex and zoster. Br Med J 1:406–410, 1973.
31. (Anonymous): Disseminated herpes zoster (editorial). JAMA 188:749, 1964.
32. Juel-Jensen BE, MacCallum FO, McKenzie AMR, Pike MC: Treatment of zoster with idoxuridine in DMSO. Results of double-blind controlled trials. Br Med J 4:774–780, 1970.
33. Merselis JG, Kaye D, Hook EW: Disseminated herpes zoster: a report of 17 cases. Arch Intern Med 113:679–686, 1964.
34. Mazur MH, Dolin R: Herpes zoster at the N.I.H.: a 20 year experience. Am J Med 65:738–744, 1978.
35. Hirsch MS, Schooley RT: Treatment of herpes virus infections Part 1. N Engl J Med 309:963–970, 1984.
36. ADIS Editors and Consultants: Acyclovir. A review of its pharmacodynamic properties and therapeutic efficacy. Curr Ther 25:13–20, 1984.
37. Selby PJ, Powles RL, Jameson B, et al: Parenteral acyclovir therapy for herpes virus infections in man. Lancet 2:1267–1270, 1979.
38. Balfour HH Jr, Bean B, Laskin OL, Ambinder RF, Meyers JD, Wade JL, Zaia JA, Aepplie D, Kirk LE, Segretti AC, Keeney RE, and the Burroughs Wellcome Collaborative Acyclovir Study Group: Acyclovir halts progression of herpes zoster in immunosuppressed patients. N Engl J Med 308:1448–1453, 1983.
39. Peterslund NA, Ipsen J, Schonheyder H, et al: Acyclovir in herpes zoster. Lancet 2:827–830, 1981.
40. Finn R, Smith MA: Oral acyclovir for herpes zoster [letter]. Lancet 2:575, 1984.
41. Whitley RJ, Ch'ien LT, Dolin R, et al: Adenine arabinoside therapy for herpes zoster in the immunosuppressed. N Engl J Med 294:1193–1199, 1976.
42. Whitley RJ, Soong SJ, Donlin R, et al (NIAID Collaborative Antiviral Study Group): Early vidarabine therapy to control the complications of herpes zoster in immunosuppressed patients. N Engl J Med 307:971–975, 1982.
43. Dawber R: Idoxuridine in herpes zoster; further evaluation of intermittant topical therapy. Br Med J 2:526–527, 1974.
44. Merigan TC, Rand KH, Pollard RB, et al: Human leukocyte interferon for the treatment of herpes zoster in patients with cancer. N Engl J Med 298:981–987, 1978.
45. Stevens DA, Merigan TC: Zoster immune globulin prophylaxis of disseminated zoster in compromised hosts. Arch Intern Med 140:52–54, 1980.
46. Groth KE, McCullough J, Markes SC, et al: Evaluation of zoster immune plasma—treatment of cutaneous disseminated zoster in immunocompromised patients. JAMA 239:1877–1879, 1978.
47. Sklar SH, Wigand JS: Herpes zoster. Br J Dermatol 104:351–352, 1981.
48. Blue WT, Winland RG, Stobbs DG, et al: Effects of adenosine monophosphate on the reactivation of latent herpes simplex virus type-1 infections of mice. Antimicrob Agents Chemother 20:547–548, 1981.
49. Sklar SH, Buimovici-Klein E: Adenosine in the treatment of recurrent herpes labialis. Oral Surg 48:416–417, 1979.
50. Galbraith AW: Treatment of acute herpes zoster with amantadine hydrochloride. Br Med J 4:693–695, 1973.
51. Galbraith AW: Prevention of postherpetic neuralgia by amantadine hydrochloride. Br J Clin Pract 37:304–306, 1983.
52. Balfour RI, Bridenbaugh LD: Postherpetic neuralgia. Bull Mason Clin 33:17, 1979.
53. Mavlight GM, Talpaz M: Cimetidine for herpes zoster. N Engl J Med 310:318–319, 1984.
54. Talpaz M, Medina JE, Patt YZ, et al: The immune restorative effect of cimetadine adminstration in vivo on the local graft versus host reaction of cancer patients. Clin Immunol Immunopathol 24:155–160, 1982.
55. Rocklin RE, Breard J, Gupta S, Good RA, Melmon KL: Characterization of the human blood lymphocytes that produce a histamine-induced suppressor factor (HSF). Cell Immunol 51:226–237, 1980.
56. Jorizzo JL, Sams WM Jr, Jegasothy BV, Olansky AJ: Cimetidine as an immunomodulator: chronic mucocutaneous candidiasis as a model. Ann Intern Med 92:192–195, 1980.
57. Weick JK, Donovan PB, Najean Y, et al: The use of cimetidine for the treatment of pruritis in polycythemia vera. Arch Intern Med 142:241–242, 1982.
58. Davis EH: Clinical trials of tegretol in trigeminal neuralgia. Headache 9:77–82, 1969.
59. Raftery H: The management of postherpetic pain using sodium valproate and amitriptyline. J Irish Med Assoc 72:399–401, 1979.
60. Lilley J-P, Su WP, Wang JK: Sensory and sympathetic nerve blocks for postherpetic neuralgia. Reg Anesth 11:165–167, 1986.
61. Epstein E: Triamcinolone-procaine in the treatment of zoster and post-zoster neuralgia. California Med 115:6–10, 1971.
62. Bauman J: Treatment of acute herpes zoster neuralgia by epidural injection or stellate ganglion block. Anesthesiology 51:223, 1979.
63. Perkins HM, Hanlon PR: Epidural injection of local anesthetic and steroids for the relief of pain secondary to herpes zoster. Arch Surg 113:253–254, 1978.
64. Fothergill WT, Ninaber V, Thick GC: A treatment of herpes zoster. Practitioner 229:747–749, 1985.
65. Schreuder M: Pain relief in herpes zoster. S Afr Med J 61:820–821, 1983.
66. Cousins MJ, Bridenbaugh PO: Neural Blockade in Clinical Anesthesia and Management of Pain. Philadelphia, JB Lippincott, 1980, pp 363, 632.
67. Lipton S: Postherpetic neuralgia. In Lipton S (ed): Relief of Pain in Clinical Practice. London, Blackwell Scientific Publications, 1979, pp 231–248.
68. Colding A: Treatment of pain: organization of a pain clinic. Treatment of acute herpes zoster. Proc R Soc Med 66:541–543, 1973.
69. Rosenak S: Procaine injection treatment of herpes zoster. Lancet 2:1056–1058, 1938.
70. Colding A: The effect of regional sympathetic blocks in the

treatment of herpes zoster. *Acta Anaesthesiol Scand* 13:113–141, 1969.
71. Mani M, Keh L, Lee KN, Winnie AP, Salem R, Collins VS: Sympathetic blockade for herpes zoster. *Am Soc Anesthesiol San Francisco* 4:469, 1976.
72. Riopelle JM, Naraghi M, Grush KP: Chronic neuralgia incidence following local anesthetic therapy for herpes zoster. *Arch Dermatol* 120:747–750, 1984.
73. Milligan NS, Nash TP: Treatment of postherpetic neuralgia. A review of 77 consecutive cases. *Pain* 23:381–386, 1985.
74. Rosenak SS: Paravertebral block for the treatment of herpes zoster. *NY State J Med* 56:2684–2687, 1956.
75. Winnie AP: The patient with herpetic neuralgia. In Moya F, Gion H (eds): *Postgraduate Seminar in Anesthesiology, Program Syllabus.* Miami Beach, 1983, pp 165–170.
76. Oxman MN: Herpes zoster. In Braude AI, Davis CE, Fierer J (eds): *Medical Microbiology and Infectious Diseases.* Philadelphia, WB Saunders, 1981, pp 1663–1671.
77. Yardley DE, Schwartz RA, Adams HG: Herpes zoster. *Am Fam Physician* 28:138–144, 1983.
78. Kass Eh, Aycock RR, Finland M: Clinical evaluation of aureomycin and chloramphenicol in herpes zoster. *N Engl J Med* 246:167–172, 1952.
79. Brown GR: Herpes zoster: correlation of age, sex, distribution, neuralgia and associated disorders. *South Med J* 69:576–578, 1976.
80. Burgoon CF Jr, Burgoon JS, Baldridge GD: The natural history of herpes zoster. *JAMA* 164:265–269, 1957.
81. DeMoragas JM, Kierland RR: The outcome of patients with herpes zoster. *Arch Dermatol* 75:193–196, 1957.
82. Rogers RS III, Tindall FP: Geriatric herpes zoster. *J Am Geriatr Soc* 19:495–504, 1971.
83. Friedman AH, Nashold BS, Ovelman-Levitt J: Dorsal root entry zone lesions for the treatment of postherpetic neuralgia. *J Neurosurg* 60:1258–1262, 1984.
84. Robinson PN, Fletcher N: Postherpetic neuralgia. *J R Coll Gen Pract* 36:24–28, 1986.
85. McCullouch DK, Fraser DM, Duncan LPJ: Shingles in diabetes mellitus. *Practitioner* 226:531–532, 1982.
86. Noordenbos W: *Pain. Problems Pertaining to the Transmission of Nerve Impulses Which Give Rise to Pain. Preliminary Statement.* Amsterdam, Elsevier, 1959, pp 6–10.
87. Haas LF: Postherpetic neuralgia, treatment and prevention. *Trans Ophthalmol Soc NZ* 29:133–136, 1977.
88. Nathan PW, Wall PD: Treatment of postherpetic neuralgia by prolonged electrical stimulation. *Br Med J* 3:645–647, 1974.
89. Price RW: Herpes zoster. An approach to systemic therapy. *Med Clin North Am* 66:1105–1118, 1982.
90. Head H: The pathology of herpes zoster and its bearing on sensory localisation. *Brain* 3:353–523, 1900.
91. Wall PD, Gutnick M: Ongoing activity in peripheral nerves: the physiology and pharmacology of impulses originating from a neuroma. *Exp Neurol* 43:580–593, 1981.
92. Roberts WJ, Foglesong ME: Nociceptive spinal neurons responsive to sympathetically induced afferent activity. Presented at the Annual Meeting of the American Pain Society, Washington, DC, 1986.
93. Melzack R, Loeser JD: Phantom body pain in paraplegics: evidence for a central "pattern generating mechanism" for pain. *Pain* 4:195–210, 1973.
94. Loeser JD, Ward AA: Some effects of deafferentation on neurons of the cat spinal cord. *Arch Neurol* 17:629–636, 1976.
95. Loeser JD, Ward AA, White LE: Chronic deafferentation of the human cord neurons. *J Neurosurg* 29:48–50, 1968.
96. Devor M, Wall PD: Reorganization of spinal cord sensory map after peripheral nerve injury. *Nature* 276:75, 1978.
97. Wall PD, Eggerr MD: Formation of new connections in adult rat brain after partial deafferentation. *Nature* 232:542, 1971.
98. Casey KL: The neurophysiologic basis of pain. *Postgrad Med* 53:58–63, 1973.
99. Stein JM, Warfield CA: Herpes zoster and postherpetic neuralgia. *Hosp Pract* 17:96A–96O, 1982.
100. Friedman AH, Nashold BS: Dorsal root entry zone lesions for the treatment of postherpetic neuralgia. *Neurosurgery* 15:969–970, 1984.
101. Watson PC, Evans RJ, Reed K, et al: Amitriptyline vs placebo in postherpetic neuralgia. *Neurology* 32:671–673, 1982.
102. Lee R, Spencer PJJ: Antidepressants and pain: a review of the pharmacological data supporting the use of certain tricyclics in chronic pain. *J Int Med Res* 5(suppl 1):146–156, 1977.
103. Woodforde JM, Duyer B, McEwen BW, et al: Treatment of postherpetic neuralgia. *Med J Aust* 2:869–872, 1965.
104. Watson CPN: Therapeutic window for amitriptyline analgesia. *Can Med Assoc J* 130:105–106, 1984.
105. Hatangdi VS, Boas RA, Richards EG: Postherpetic neuralgia: management with antiepileptics and tricyclic drugs. In Bonica JJ, Albe-Fessard D (eds): *Advances in Pain Research and Therapy.* New York, Raven Press, 1976, vol 1, pp 583–587.
106. Kocher R: Use of psychotropic drugs for the treatment of severe pain. In Bonica JJ, Albe-Fessard D (eds): *Advances in Pain Research and Therapy.* New York, Raven Press, 1976, vol 1, pp 579–582.
107. Taub A, Collins WR Jr: Observations on the treatment of denervation dysesthesia with psychotropic drugs: postherpetic neuralgia, anesthesia dolorosa, peripheral neuropathy. In Bonica JJ (ed): *Advances in Neurology.* New York, Raven Press, 1974, vol 4, pp 309–315.
108. Taub AT: Relief of postherpetic neuralgia with psychotropic drugs. *J Neurosurg* 39:235–239, 1973.
109. Hitchcock E, Teixeira M: Anticonvulsant activation of pain suppressive systems. *Appl Neurophysiol* 45:582–593, 1982.
110. Steardo L, Leo A, Marano E: Efficacy of baclofen in trigeminal neuralgia and some other painful conditions. A clinical trial. *Eur Neurol* 23:51–55, 1984.
111. Nathan PW: Chlorprothixene (Taractan) in postherpetic neuralgia and other severe chronic pains. *Pain* 5:367–371, 1978.
112. Kernbaum S, Hauchecorne J: Administration of levodopa for relief of herpes pain. *JAMA* 246:132–134, 1981.
113. Sweet WH: Deafferentation pain after posterior rhizotomy, trauma to a limb, and herpes zoster. *Neurosurgery* 15:928–932, 1984.
114. Forrest JB: Management of chronic dorsal root pain with epidural steroid. *Can Anaesth Soc J* 25:218–225, 1978.
115. Bonica JJ: Thoracic segmental and intercostal neuralgia. In Bonica JJ (ed): *The Management of Pain.* Philadelphia, Lea & Febiger, 1953, pp 861–867.
116. Prough DS, McLeskey CH, Poehling GP, Koman LA, Weeks DB, Whitworth T, Semble EL: Efficacy of oral nifedipine in the treatment of reflex sympathetic dystrophy. *Anesthesiology* 62:796–799, 1985.
117. Neuendorf TL: Epidural phenol in the treatment of postherpetic neuralgia. *J Am Osteopath Assoc* 86:75–77, 1986.
118. Barnard D, Lloyd J, Evans J: Cryoanalgesia in the manage-

ment of chronic facial pain. *J Maxillofac Surg* 9:101–102, 1981.
119. White JC, Sweet WH: *Pain and the Neurosurgeon: A Forty-Year Experience.* Springfield, IL, Charles C Thomas, 1969, pp 380–386, 472, 477.
120. Denny-Brown D, Adams RD, Fitzgerald PJ: Pathologic features of herpes zoster; note on "geniculate herpes." *Arch Neurol Psychiatry* 51:216–231, 1944.
121. Hitchcock ER, Schvarez JR: Stereotaxic trigeminal tractotomy for postherpetic facial pain. *J Neurosurg* 37:412–417, 1972.
122. Sugar O, Bucy PC: Postherpetic trigeminal neuralgia. *Arch Neurol Psychiatry* 65:131–145, 1951.
123. Lond D: Pain of peripheral nerve injury. In Youman JR (ed): *Neurological Surgery.* Philadelphia, WB Saunders, 1982, pp 3634–3643.
124. Mundinger F, Salamao JF: Deep brain stimulation in mesoencephalic lemniscus medialis for chronic pain. *Acta Neurochir Suppl* 30:245–258, 1980.
125. Lewith GT, Field J, Machin D: Acupuncture compared with placebo in postherpetic neuraliga. *Pain* 17:361–368, 1983.
126. Payne C: Ultrasound for postherpetic neuraliga. A study to investigate the results of treatment. *Physiotherapy* 70:96–97, 1974.

part g musculoskeletal and joint pain

chapter 40
Chronic Joint and Connective Tissue Pain

Roger B. Traycoff, M.D.

Successful management of pain in patients with rheumatic diseases requires an understanding that pain is as much an experience as a sensation and that arthritis is a symptom, not a diagnosis. A patient's response to a nociceptive stimulus is, in part, a consequence of past experience, learned behavior, and environmental reinforcers. Failure to recognize the importance of emotional factors may lead to inappropriate therapy. Treatment should be disease rather than symptom oriented. Empiric therapy is seldom appropriate, often leading to suboptimal results.

The two major determinants of pain behavior are the intensity of the stimulus and the patient's interpretation of the meaning of the pain. In rheumatic diseases, the source of nociception is frequently obvious and questions of somatization are not often raised. The emotional components of pain behavior may not be appreciated. Physicians focus on physical findings, having a tendency to treat the disease rather than the patient. To optimally manage these patients, one must understand the natural history of the disease untreated, and be aware of the psychological and socioeconomic consequences of chronic debilitating illnesses. The importance of having a good relationship with patients cannot be overemphasized; patient satisfaction and compliance are affected by perceptions of disease and expectations regarding treatment.

Most failures in managing the pain of rheumatic diseases arise from: (*a*) inability to make a correct diagnosis, (*b*) failure to educate the patient, (*c*) poor compliance with therapeutic regimens, and (*d*) inappropriate use of drugs. Successful management of patients with rheumatic diseases requires an understanding of disease mechanisms, a knowledge of drug pharmacokinetics and pharmacodynamics, and a sense for the patient's expectations and beliefs. It would be incorrect to use potentially toxic drugs to treat a patient whose disease has a high probability of spontaneous remission. Similarly, it would be inappropriate to treat a chronic progressive illness symptomatically when agents that can alter the disease process are available for use.

In the most basic construct, pain associated with rheumatic disease can be divided into (*a*) inflammatory and noninflammatory and (*b*) systemic and nonsystemic based on pathophysiology. Pain due to an inflammatory process is best treated with anti-inflammatory drugs rather than simple analgesics or opiates. There is little evidence that simple analgesics such as acetaminophen or propoxyphene are of value in treating the pain of synovitis. Conversely, data are lacking to support the use of corticosteroids in the treatment of noninflammatory joint disease.

Nonsteroidal anti-inflammatory drugs (NSAID) are the mainstay of therapy, having both analgesic and anti-inflammatory properties. However, it should be recognized that they are not true analgesics (1). NSAID are more correctly classified as antialgesics than analgesics because they act by raising the threshold for firing of free nerve endings rather than by altering the transmission of pain or the response to stimuli.

Using opiates to treat pain of rheumatic origin is inappropriate because of potential problems with the development of tolerance and physical dependence. The short-term benefit of their use is outweighed by problems with escalating dose requirements and loss of efficacy. Potent opiates are rarely used for treating rheumatic diseases except in the presence of major trauma. Even then, most musculoskeletal pain will respond to immobilization and therapy with anti-inflammatory drugs.

Acute and chronic pain differ. In most instances acute pain is self-limited, in contrast to chronic pain, where resolution is uncertain and outcome may be in doubt. When treating chronic disease, it is important to establish a relationship with the patient that promotes wellness and discourages dependency. This can be accomplished by patient education. One should not be overly optimistic to avoid creating unrealistic expectations. However, a pessimistic approach may cause patients to seek alternate care, becoming prey to the use of unproven remedies.

The major variables in treating pain are: (a) the underlying disease process. (b) the patient's expectations, and (c) the drugs available for use. Having a correct diagnosis is a prerequisite for effective therapy. Pain not associated with inflammation can be treated with simple analgesics, low doses of salicylates, or anti-inflammatory doses of NSAIDs. Pain arising from an inflammatory process should be treated with high doses of salicylates or NSAIDs. Psychotropic drugs such as benzodiazepines and tricyclic antidepressants are used as adjuctive therapy, recognizing that their effects are primarily symptom directed. Tricyclic antidepressants are used to treat depression and "fibrositis-like" symptoms (2). They are particularly useful in treating patients with nonarticular rheumatism. Benzodiazepines such as diazepam should only be used for treating patients with "trait anxiety" (3). They are not appropriate for chronic use because of their potential for causing physical dependence, which may increase rather than decrease pain behavior.

The goals of therapy are to relieve pain, preserve function, and prevent joint destruction. Pain relief is best achieved by controlling inflammation. Educating patients and encouraging them to participate in the treatment process are important to ensure compliance and continuity of care. Emphasis on wellness and promoting self-help are important. Referrals for physical and occupational therapy and the use of arthritis support groups should be considered part of the treatment plan. Reliance on drug therapy alone should be discouraged because outcome may relate to variables other than pain control.

APPROACH TO DIAGNOSIS

Having a correct diagnosis is a prerequisite for optimal therapy. An empiric approach to management is seldom appropriate because it may lead to either over- or under-treatment. Therapy should be disease specific as well as symptom directed.

The first question is whether the pain has an anatomically definable basis, that is, is it articular, periarticular, muscular, or neurogenic in origin. The absence of confirmatory physical findings does not preclude a physical basis for pain complaints. The diagnosis of psychogenic pain is suggested by finding inconsistencies in the history and physical examination. Psychogenic pain is rare, but somatization with exaggerated pain behavior is not. Many patients will have a somatic source of nociception complicated by a somatoform disorder. Pain is as much an experience as a sensation, being affected by learned behavior, environmental reinforcers, and secondary gain.

Localization of the pain is invaluable. In rheumatic diseases pain is most often articular in origin. It is characteristically associated with decreased and painful range of motion. Erythema and swelling are apparent particularly when examining appendicular joints. Axial joints such as hips and shoulders seldom have clinical evidence of synovitis presenting with pain and decreased range of motion.

Not infrequently, it is difficult to distinguish articular from periarticular pain syndromes. In these cases, intra-articular injections of local anesthetic and corticosteroid can be diagnostic. Failure to relieve pain following intra-articular injection of local anesthetic is good evidence against the diagnosis of arthritis, assuming that there is no coexistent extra-articular source of pain. When the diagnosis is unclear, infiltration block of extra-articular structures with local anesthetics can be of great diagnostic value, confirming or refuting the presence of tendinitis, bursitis, or enthesopathy.

Pain descriptors are also diagnostically important. Articular and bursal pain is usually described as aching, cramping, or throbbing. Neuritic pain is characterized by numbness, tingling, or burning. The presence of hyperesthesia, dysesthesia, and allodynia suggests either deafferentation pain or reflex sympathetic dystrophy.

The relationship of pain to activity is important. Pain that is present only with activity suggests a mechanical or vascular etiology. Pain present both with activity and at rest is often inflammatory in nature. Pain that is worse at night or during periods of rest should suggest the possibility of tumor, infection, or neuropathy. Pain that is unrelated to position or activity and not responsive to therapy should suggest the possibility of central pain or psychogenic pain.

The second question is whether the underlying disease process is localized or is a manifestation of an underlying systemic disease. The possibility of multisystem disease is raised when one takes the history and performs the physical examination. The laboratory can provide additional evidence for systemic involvement, and help distinguish among the various rheumatic diseases. Serologic markers are particularly helpful in defining the subsets of "lupus-like" syndromes.

The third question is whether the patient's response to the nociceptive stimulus is appropriate. It should be understood that we see pain behavior, not pain. The patient's complaints should be taken at face value; pain is whatever the patient says it is. Therapy should be disease rather than symptom directed. The goals are to decrease suffering and to treat the underlying disease process.

HISTORY AND PHYSICAL EXAMINATION

The history of the present illness and the physical examination are the foundation of the diagnostic process. The history will suggest whether the disease is: (a) systemic or regional, (b) acute or chronic, (c) inflammatory or noninflammatory, or (d) psychogenic in etiology. A history of weight loss, photosensitivity, Raynaud's phenomenon, dermatitis, or polyserositis should suggest the diagnosis of systemic lupus erythematosus, or one of its variants. A history of ocular or genitourinary symptoms should suggest the diagnosis of Reiter's syndrome. A history of diarrhea or abdominal pain should raise the possibility of enteropathic or reactive arthritis. Complaints of back pain or stiffness not relieved by rest should suggest the diagnosis of spondyloarthropathy.

The physical examination will confirm and characterize abnormalities suggested by the history. It should be performed in a systematic and thorough manner, with particular emphasis on the musculoskeletal system. The examiner should note any swelling, tenderness, decreased range of motion, deformities, or signs of inflammation on joint examination.

Extra-articular manifestations of rheumatic diseases should be recognized because of their diagnostic significance. Cutaneous involvement is a feature of psoriatic arthritis, Reiter's syndrome, systemic lupus erythematosus, and systemic vasculitis. Finding subcutaneous nodules should suggest the diagnoses of rheumatoid arthritis, rheumatic fever, or amyloidosis. Conjunctivitis or iritis are features of spondyloarthropathies such as Reiter's syndrome, ankylosing spondylitis, and enteropathic arthritis. The presence of tophi are diagnostic of gout. Pitting of the nails is a sign of psoriatic arthritis, and clubbing a clue to hypertrophic osteoarthropathy. The presence of enthesopathy, tenosynovitis, or axial skeleton involvement should suggest the diagnosis of spondyloarthropathy. Decreased range of motion of the lumbar spine and decreased chest expansion are clues to ankylosing spondylitis.

LABORATORY ANALYSES

Laboratory studies should be used to confirm rather than make diagnoses. None of the available serologic tests have perfect sensitivity or specificity. The basic laboratory evaluation should include an erythrocyte sedimentation rate, hemogram, urinalysis, and a SMAC profile or its equivalent. An elevated erythrocyte sedimentation rate confirms the presence of an inflammatory process. Anemia is a clue to systemic disease and a marker for chronicity. The finding of autoimmune hemolytic anemia should suggest the diagnosis of systemic lupus erythematosus. Leucopenia and thrombocytopenia are features of systemic lupus erythematosus; their presence would be evidence against the diagnosis of rheumatoid arthritis. The finding of hypercalcemia in a patient with rheumatic complaints should suggest the diagnosis of hyperparathyroidism, and the possibility of pseudogout. Hyperuricemia, although not diagnostic of gout, is a helpful clue to urate arthropathy. The finding of proteinuria or hematuria on urinalysis should suggest the possibility of glomerulonephritis due to systemic lupus erythermatosus or vasculitis.

Special studies such as rheumatoid factors, antinuclear antibodies, tissue typing, and serum complement levels may be helpful in the differential diagnosis of rheumatic diseases. Rheumatoid factors are markers for chronic antigenic stimulation. They are not a specific marker for rheumatoid arthritis, being found in other autoimmune diseases, including systemic lupus erythematosus, scleroderma, Sjögren's syndrome, polyarteritis nodosa, mixed connective tissue disease, and amyloidosis. Rheumatoid factors have also been identified in patients with chronic infections or chronic liver disease, and in the elderly with no identifiable disease. The value of finding a rheumatoid factor is that it makes the diagnosis of spondyloarthropathy unlikely. Testing for antinuclear antibodies by indirect immunofluorescence is a useful screen for systemic lupus erythematosus; however, the test lacks specificity. Antinuclear antibodies have been reported to be present in patients with scleroderma, mixed connective tissue disease, rheumatoid arthritis, or autoimmune liver disease. Antinuclear antibodies are often drug induced, occuring in the absence of disease. A positive test for antinuclear antibodies is not diagnostic of systemic lupus, but a negative result in a symptomatic patient is good evidence against the diagnosis. Patients whose test for antinuclear antibodies is positive should have additional studies performed. Testing for antibodies against ribonucleoprotein (RNP), Smith antigen, and soluble cytoplasmic antigens (SSA and SSB) can be helpful.

Synovial fluid analysis has an important role in the diagnosis of arthropathies. Fluid should be routinely sent for white cell and differential counts, and screening for crystals by compensated polarized microscopy. Gram stains, cultures, and lactic acid levels should be done when infection is a consideration. Measurements of synovial fluid protein, glucose, and complement levels are not usually diagnostically helpful. Tissue typing for the presence of human leukocyte (HLA) B27 is of little value in screening for the spondyloarthropathies. The high prevalence of HLA B27 in the normal population limits its specificity as a diagnostic test. A negative study also has limited value because a significant percentage of patients with spondyloarthropathies are HLA B27 negative.

Measurement of serum complement levels has limited diagnostic value. In most rheumatic diseases, the serum complement levels are normal or elevated. The presence of hypocomplementemia may be a clue to the presence of immune complex disease. Usually one measures the total hemolytic complement level (CH50), and the C3 and C4 component levels. A very low total hemolytic complement level is a marker for a hereditary complement deficiency. A low C3 level with a normal C4 level should suggest alternative pathway activation. A low C4 level with either a normal or low C3 level should suggest classic pathway activation as seen with immune complex disease.

DRUG THERAPY

SIMPLE ANALGESICS

Acetaminophen, dextropropoxyphene, and codeine are useful in the treatment of noninflammatory rheumatic pain. There is little evidence to support their use in treating inflammatory joint disease. Nevertheless they are often used empirically either in combination with other drugs or as sole agents. Acetaminophen combined with codeine or propoxyphene is favored because using a centrally acting drug with a peripherally acting analgesic results in synergism (4). Codeine and propoxyphene should not be administered as single agents because they are no better analgesics than aspirin or acetaminophen. Similarly, combining aspirin with acetaminophen or aspirin with a NSAID usually provides little additional analgesia. Pain relief from combining peripheral-acting analgesics is usually not additive, but the side effects appear to be increased in frequency and severity.

Acetaminophen has a dose-response curve similar to that of aspirin. It is frequently administered to patients with degenerative joint disease, to patients with nonarticular rheumatism, and to patients who are intolerant of salicylates or NSAIDs. The major limitation of acetaminophen is its having a flat dose-response curve; in single-dose studies, increasing doses above 1000 mg provides no additional analgesia. Daily doses greater than 4000 mg have been associated with hepatotoxicity (5). Patients who chronically abuse alcohol appear to be at greatest risk for the development of hepatic necrosis.

Acetaminophen can be used in combination with codeine or propoxyphene to provide short-term analgesia. The major problems with the use of analgesic combinations containing opiate derivatives are the development of tolerance and physical dependence. Addiction is a real but most likely overstated risk.

SALICYLATES

For many years, salicylates have been the favored drug for treating inflammatory joint disease. Although none of the newer NSAIDs has been shown to be superior to aspirin in the treatment of rheumatoid arthritis, the efficacy of aspirin for treating pain of other inflammatory arthropathies is less clear. Aspirin may be less effective for treating Reiter's syndrome and ankylosing spondylitis. Gout and pseudogout appear to respond better to NSAIDs than to salicylates.

Many formulations of salicylates are available (Table 40-1), yet aspirin remains the salicylate of choice in most instances. The major advantages of using nonaspirin salicylates are ease of administration, better patient tolerance, and fewer side effects. The major disadvantages are greater cost, less flexible dosing schedules, and unpredictable absorption when administered orally.

Table 40.1
Salicylates Used in Treatment of Inflammatory Joint Disease

Drug	Dose (mg)	Daily Dose (mg)	Frequency
Aspirin	325	2500–5000	q.i.d.
Encaprin	325		b.i.d.
	500		
Easprin	975		q.i.d.
Cama	500		q.i.d.
Ascriptin	325		q.i.d.
Ecotrin	325		q.i.d.
Salts of salicylic acid			
Choline salicylate (Arthropan)	325	300–5000	q.i.d.
Choline magnesium trisalicylate (Trilisate)	500	3000	b.i.d.
Salicylsalicylic acid (Disalcid)	500, 750	3000	b.i.d.
Diflunisal (Dolobid)	500	1000	b.i.d.

Both the analgesic and the anti-inflammatory effects of salicylates have flat dose-response curves. Analgesic doses of aspirin range from 650 to 1000 mg; anti-inflammatory doses range from 3.5 to 5.0 g daily. A therapeutic blood level for anti-inflammatory effects is between 15 and 20 mg/dl. Data are lacking on the relationship between analgesia and salicylate blood levels in the absence of inflammation. Pain relief in inflammatory joint disease is probably due to the anti-inflammatory rather than analgesic effects of salicylate. When treating pain with low doses of aspirin, one must administer it every 4 hr. As the dose is increased, the elimination half-life increases as a result of saturation of hepatic enzymes; therefore, at higher doses the frequency of administration can decrease to every 8–12 hr (6). The exponential increase in salicylate blood levels seen with increasing dose means that small changes in dose can cause large changes in salicylate blood levels. Increasing the daily dose of aspirin by one or two tablets may result in toxicity. Tinnitus, although a useful marker for salicylate toxicity, may not be present in all cases. Salicylate levels should be measured in children and the elderly to document therapeutic blood levels.

NONSTEROIDAL ANTI-INFLAMMATORY DRUGS

Nonsteroidal anti-inflammatory drugs are the cornerstone for treating inflammatory joint disease. When treating rheumatoid arthritis, the choice between salicylates and NSAIDs is a matter of preference; none of the NSAIDs has been shown to be superior to aspirin. This may not be true for other rheumatic diseases. For example, aspirin has little value in treating crystal-induced synovitis.

A major limitation of NSAIDs is their having flat dose-response curves; increasing the dose beyond the recommended level will not increase efficacy. In addition, they act on only one component of the inflammatory response, inhibition of prostaglandin synthesis, which limits their ability to suppress inflammation (7).

Nonsteroidal anti-inflammatory drugs can be divided into five groups based on chemical classes (Table 40.2). They differ more in pharmacokinetics than pharmacodynamics (Table 40.3). Drugs such as ibuprofen, fenoprofen, tolmetin, and meclofenamate have short elimination half-lives, and must be administered every 6–8 hr. Sulindac and naproxen have longer elimination half-lives and can be given twice a day. Piroxicam, which has the longest elimination half-life (30 hr), is administered once daily.

Most of the side effects of treatment relate to inhibition of prostaglandin synthesis (8). The side effect profiles of NSAIDs appear to be similar, and dose related. The exception is meclofenamate, which has a greater tendency to cause diarrhea. Phenylbutazone and indomethacin may be more ulcerogenic than other NSAIDs, which may relate to their potency in inhibiting cyclo-oxygenase. All of the

Table 40.2
Chemical Classes of Nonsteroidal Anti-inflammatory Drugs

Chemical Group	Elimination Half-time (hr)
Indole derivatives	
Indomethacin	1.5–2
Sulindac	18
Tolectin	1
Phenylpropionic acids	
Ibuprofen	1–3
Naproxen	12–15
Fenoprofen	2–3
Ketoprofen	2–3
Pyrazolones	
Phenylbutazone	29–176
Oxyphenbutazone	29–176
Fenamates	
Mefenamic acid	4
Meclofenamate	2–4
Oxicams	
Piroxicam	21–70

Table 40.3
Pharmacokinetics of Nonsteroidal Anti-inflammatory Drugs

Duration of Action	Recommended Daily Dose (mg)
Short acting	
Fenoprofen (Nalfon)	1200–2400
Ibuprofen (Motrin, Rufin)	1200–3200
Indomethacin (Indocin)	75–200
Tolmetin (Tolectin)	800–1600
Meclofenamate (Meclomen)	200–400
Intermediate acting	
Naproxen (Naprosyn)	750–1000
Sulindac (Clinoril)	300–600
Long acting	
Piroxicam (Feldene)	10–20
Phenylbutazone (Butazolidin)	300–400
Oxyphenbutazone (Tandearil)	300–400

NSAIDs have the potential for causing bronchospasm in salicylate-sensitive asthmatics.

As a group, the NSAIDs can adversely affect renal function by decreasing prostaglandin-dependent renal blood flow. Indomethacin appears to have a greater potential for this than other NSAIDs, and sulindac appears to have the least (9). Patients at greatest risk are those with compromised renal function from either volume contraction or intrinsic renal disease. Diabetics may be at greater risk for the development of hyperkalemia from hyporeninemic hypoaldosteronism caused by inhibition of prostaglandin E synthesis. Immune-mediated nephropathy may be more common with fenoprofen, but has been described with other agents. Patients who develop edema while taking aspirin will also be intolerant of NSAIDs. Phenylbutazone is unique in that it promotes fluid retention by two mechanisms: inhibition of prostaglandin synthesis and its aldosterone-like effects on the renal tubules.

CORTICOSTEROIDS

Corticosteroids are potent anti-inflammatory agents, but have no intrinsic analgesic properties. They are only useful for treating pain associated with inflammation. Corticosteroids do not prevent joint destruction, or alter disease progression. The major risks associated with chronic use are osteoporosis, avascular necrosis of bone, hypertension, glucose intolerance, and cataract formation. There is no evidence that one class of corticosteroid is more efficacious than another. Differences relate more to tissue half-life and potency (Table 40.4). Dexamethasone is the most potent corticosteroid, having the longest duration of action. Shorter acting corticosteroids are favored because the risk of suppressing the hypothalamic-pituitary-adrenal (HPA) axis is low when they are used in doses of

Table 40.4
Corticosteroids Used in Treatment of Inflammatory Joint Disease

Duration of Action	Potency	Equivalent Doses (mg)
Short Acting		
Hydrocortisone	1	20
Prednisone	4	5
Methylprednisolone	4	4
Intermediate acting		
Triamcinolone	5	4
Long Acting		
Betamethasone	25	0.6
Dexamethasone	30	0.75

7.5–10 mg/day (prednisone equivalents). There may be a relationship between side effects and duration of axis suppression. Alternate day corticosteroid therapy may decrease the risk of axis suppression, but is usually less effective in treating inflammatory joint disease. The major factor determining axis suppression is the duration of exposure to corticosteroid. For this reason, single daily dose regimens are preferred. Multiple daily doses are more effective in decreasing inflammation, but are also more likely to cause HPA axis suppression. The advantage of less HPA axis suppression with daily single-dose therapy is lost when doses of prednisone or its equivalent exceed 15 mg/day.

The role of corticosteroids in the treatment of inflammatory joint disease is controversial. The major question is whether the benefits outweigh the potential risks. Low-dose corticosteroids have a role in the treatment of rheumatoid arthritis (10), which is in contrast to the crystal-induced arthropathies and the spondyloarthropathies, where corticosteroids are infrequently used. Corticosteroids are rarely administered systemically in acute gout because their use may prolong an attack. Many physicians believe that corticosteroids have little place in treating the spondyloarthropathies. This may relate to the need to justify their use in diseases where the probability of remission is high and the risks of joint destruction are low. The use of corticosteroids in this setting would potentially expose the patient to undue risks.

Systemic lupus erythematosus is one of the few rheumatic diseases where there is little controversy over the appropriateness of corticosteroid therapy. Questions relate more to dose regimens than to appropriateness of use. Corticosteroids may be effective in treating pain due to pleuritis, pericarditis, and abdominal serositis. However, most patients with arthritis can be successfully treated with salicylates when used in high doses.

Intra-articular corticosteroids are useful in treating acute flares of synovitis involving one to several joints. Their use often leads to rapid relief of pain and swelling, but the duration of relief is highly variable. When used infrequently, the risks appear to be low. Chronic use may be associated with progressive joint deterioration.

Although there is little controversy regarding the effectiveness of intra-articular corticosteroids in the treatment of inflammatory joint disease, their efficacy in treating osteoarthritis is controversial (11). They may relieve pain in osteoarthritis when there is a significant inflammatory component to the arthritis. Most of the patients who respond will have effusions or a history of joint stiffness similar to that of patients with rheumatoid arthritis but of shorter duration. Patients with osteoarthritis who have no evidence of synovitis generally have little relief of pain following intra-articular injections.

Perhaps the most successful use of depot corticosteroids is in treating bursitis and tenosynovitis. Many patients will have rapid relief of symptoms following injection. The risks of single injections are small. The major complications are infection and fat atrophy, both of which can be minimized by using meticulous technique. As with other therapies, excessive use increases the risk of side effects. When used too frequently, patients may become cushingoid from systemic absorption of corticosteroids.

OSTEOARTHRITIS

Osteoarthritis is a chronic articular disease characterized by degeneration of cartilage, sclerosis of subchondral bone, and osteophyte formation. It is not a single disease, but rather an expression of a final common pathway leading to joint destruction. Most oligoarticular disease probably arises from trauma or developmental abnormalities.

Osteoarthritis can be divided into primary and secondary based on etiologic factors, and into oligoarticular and generalized on the basis of numbers of joints involved. Oligoarticular osteoarthritis primarily involves weight-bearing joints such as the hips and knees. It rarely affects the shoulders or elbows in the absence of antecedent trauma. Generalized osteoarthritis involves the distal interphalangeal joints, the proximal interphalangeal joints, the large weight-bearing joints, and the spine.

Primary osteoarthritis can be subdivided into primary generalized osteoarthritis and erosive osteoarthritis. Secondary osteoarthritis is classified by disease associations. It may be secondary to trauma, developmental abnormalities, or metabolic diseases. Among the metabolic diseases associated with osteoarthritis are diabetes mellitus, ochronosis, acromegaly, hypothyroidism, and Wilson's disease.

Most patients with osteoarthritis present with complaints of pain and stiffness. The pain is characteristically aggravated by activity and relieved by rest. Patients may complain of stiffness and aching following immobilization. Typically, this discomfort is relieved by movement. Most of the pain occurs late in the day as a consequence of excessive use. Physical examination of the joints shows bony overgrowth, decreased range of motion with crepitus, and the absence of synovitis. Signs of systemic disease are typically lacking.

Pain in osteoarthritis arises from involvement of both articular and periarticular structures. Pain-sensitive areas in the joint include the capsule, articular fat pads, and subchondral bone (12). Extra-articular pain can arise from ligaments, tendons, and bursae. Pain from muscle fatigue due to chronic mechanical stress may also contribute to discomfort.

Early osteoarthritis is generally painless since articular cartilage is aneural. The role of microfractures in subchondral bone as a source of pain is unclear since x-ray changes of osteoarthritis may be present in patients having no articular complaints. The fact that subclinical inflammation is commonly seen in specimens of synovial membrane suggests that synovitis may be a source of pain. The possibility that rest pain in osteoarthritis is due to intraosseous venous engorgement has also been raised (13).

TREATMENT

Treatment of osteoarthritis is symptomatic since there is no known cure for the disease. Therapy must be individualized to meet the needs of the patient. It can be divided into three areas: (a) physical and occupational therapy, (b) drugs, and (c) surgery. Optimal management requires an accurate diagnosis of the sources of pain and identification of the factors contributing to the pain behavior.

The goals of therapy are to relieve pain, to preserve function, and to prevent joint destruction. Relief of pain can be achieved by a combination of drugs, physical therapy, and surgical intervention. Patients must understand the nature and prognosis of their disease as well as the treatment options. Education will help dispel unrealistic expectations and do much to improve patient compliance. An educated patient is less likely to abuse medications or seek alternate care.

Drug Therapy

Salicylates and NSAIDs are the mainstay of therapy because of their analgesic and anti-inflammatory properties. Treatment is palliative; there is little evidence these drugs have any effect on the underlying disease process. The end point is relief of pain.

Mild osteoarthritis is usually treated with simple analgesics such as acetaminophen or low-dose salicylates. Acetaminophen is administered orally in doses of 650 mg every 4-6 hr as needed. Aspirin is prescribed in analgesic doses of 2-3 g/day in divided doses. Patients with more severe pain can be treated with aspirin or acetaminophen combined with either codeine or propoxyphene administered on an as-needed basis.

Nonsteroidal anti-inflammatory drugs and high-dose salicylates are used for treating patients unresponsive to simple analgesics. They appear to be most effective where there is clinical evidence of synovitis. Although there are no convincing data to suggest that one NSAID is superior to another, indomethacin may be the exception. It may be more effective in treating the subset of patients with osteoarthritis who have coexistent crystal-induced synovitis. Patients having hydroxyapatite deposition disease or subclinical pyrophosphate arthropathy may respond better to indomethacin than to salicylates.

Intra-articular Corticosteroid Injections

Intra-articular corticosteroids are widely used for treating articular pain unresponsive to treatment with NSAIDs. However, there is controversy over the appropriateness of their use. Data from controlled studies are contradictory, with some studies showing efficacy (14) and others showing no benefit compared to placebo (15).

Questions regarding potential adverse effects on articular cartilage have also been raised (16). There are anecdotal reports of patients developing "Charcot-like" joints following repeated intra-articular injections of corticosteroids. Studies of the effects of corticosteroids on articular cartilage from animals are also contradictory. Intra-articular corticosteroids inhibit articular proteoglycan synthesis in rabbit, but not in primate, cartilage. Taken together, these data indicate that intra-articular corticosteroids are useful in treating a subset of patients with osteoarthritis and that they have a significant potential for causing side effects if used inappropriately. In practice, their use should be limited to patients who have not responded to either NSAIDs or high doses of salicylates. Intra-articular corticosteroids should not be administered more frequently than every 4 months and then only if the duration of benefit from the previous injection lasted more than 4 weeks. Short-term relief of pain does not justify the use of repeated injections.

Physical Therapy

The major use of physical therapy is to correct postural abnormalities and to strengthen deconditioned muscles that are contributing to pain. Assistive devices such as canes, walkers, and crutches help relieve pain by decreasing weight bearing on symptomatic joints. Correction of biomechanical abnormalities to decrease load is important. Weight reduction for the obese patient may be helpful. Application of heat and cold to symptomatic areas may give short-term relief by relieving muscle spasm. Physical measures combined with exercise can decrease joint contractures and increase range of motion. Major limitations of physical therapy are high cost, availability, and poor patient compliance with exercise programs in outpatient programs.

RHEUMATOID ARTHRITIS

Rheumatoid arthritis is a chronic multisystem disease characterized by polyarthritis and a variety of extra-articular manifestations such as subcutaneous nodules, serositis, pulmonary fibrosis, and vasculitis. The disease may be either seropositive or seronegative. Only 70% of patients have serum rheumatoid factor titers greater than 1:60. The prognosis of the disease is highly variable and the course, in most patients, is not predictable. The presence of subcutaneous nodules, high titers of rheumatoid factor, and the early appearance of joint erosion indicate a poor prognosis and the need for aggressive therapy.

The treatment of pain in rheumatoid arthritis is synonymous with suppression of inflammation; control of synovitis will result in control of pain. The exception is where coexisting degenerative arthritis is causing pain from irritation of nociceptors in subchondral bone; pain will persist despite intensive anti-inflammatory drug therapy. Also, many patients with rheumatoid arthritis may have a fibrositis-like syndrome in addition to synovitis. Corticosteroids and NSAIDs are not effective in treating these noninflammatory pain syndromes. Successful management of myofascial pain requires conditioning and muscle stretch exercises, trigger point injections, and at times the use of tricyclic antidepressants.

Successful management of pain requires an accurate diagnosis with localization of the pain generators. Extraarticular pain syndromes such as bursitis, tenosynovitis, enthesopathy, and entrapment neuropathies may be present in addition to arthritis. Failure to identify these entities will lead to suboptimal results. Many of these syndromes are poorly responsive to NSAIDs and salicylates, requiring treatment with corticosteroids. One must also recognize when articular pain is arising from noninflammatory causes. Using remittent drugs to treat "burned-out" rheumatoid disease would be inappropriate.

DRUG TREATMENT

When treating rheumatoid arthritis, one must have a sense for the disease untreated. The natural history of nodular erosive disease is persistence of symptoms. In contrast, patients with "probable" rheumatoid arthritis may have spontaneous remissions, or persistence of symptoms without progression to joint destruction. When the prognosis is in doubt, therapy should begin with salicylates or NSAIDs. These drugs should be used in maximally recommended doses to obtain their anti-inflammatory effects. A NSAID should be given for at least 10–14 days before changing to another drug because of lack of efficacy. The end point is not only relief of pain but a decrease in inflammation. If three consecutive NSAIDs do not provide adequate suppression of inflammation, it is unlikely that a fourth one will be effective. Changing from one class of NSAIDs to another, although conceptually appealing, usually does not result in increased efficacy. Before discontinuing a drug because of lack of benefit, one must confirm that the patient is taking the medication as prescribed. Patient compliance is important in assessing response to therapy. This can be easily done by comparing the number of times a patient obtains refills of medication to the expected number of requests.

If the patient does not have significant relief of pain from NSAIDs, or has had symptoms for more than 6–9 months, one should consider adding a remittent drug to the therapeutic regimen. The choice of drug will vary depending on one's training and experience. Usually, either antimalarial drugs or chrysotherapy are considered. Auranofen, an oral gold compound, is often administered before treatment with parenteral gold or penicillamine because it is potentially less toxic (17). Remittent drugs are slow to act, requiring from 3 to 6 months before significant benefit is seen. The end point is a decrease in inflammation, not a decrease in pain. Remittent drugs may have a significant placebo effect. Patients may claim to be improved yet have no change in physical findings. Therefore, one needs to document improvement before committing a patient to a prolonged course of therapy. If no progress has been made after 3 months of therapy, one should change to another remittent drug.

Auranofin is a trialkylphosphine gold complex that can be administered orally. It has a lower frequency of mucocutaneous and renal toxicity than parenteral gold compounds. The major side effect is diarrhea. There is little correlation between auranofin blood levels and therapeutic efficacy (18). The usual dose is 3 mg given orally twice a day.

Parenteral gold compounds include aurothioglucose and aurothiomalate (19). Both drugs have similar efficacy and potential toxicities. Aurothiomalate differs in causing a nitratoid reaction characterized by acute vasodilation and cutaneous flushing following intramuscular injection. Parenteral gold is usually administered in doses of 25–50 mg weekly to a cumulative dose of 1000 mg. Patients are then placed on long-term maintenance therapy since most patients will have an exacerbation of arthritis following discontinuation of treatment. The relationship between the dose of gold and efficacy is unclear. There is no difference in response when comparing the 10-mg weekly doses to the traditional 50-mg weekly dose. Doses higher than 50 mg/week appear to increase toxicity without confering additional benefit.

The major toxicities of parenteral gold are mucocutaneous and renal. Patients frequently develop stomatitis or dermatitis, requiring cessation of therapy. Renal toxicity presents as proteinuria; the major risk is the development of nephrotic syndrome. Renal biopsy findings have been variable, ranging from a focal proliferative glomerulonephritis to membraneous nephropathy.

Penicillamine is also used for treating rheumatoid arthritis unresponsive to NSAIDs (20). It is administered orally in doses of 375–1000 mg/day. Therapy is begun at doses of 125–250 mg daily, and increased by 125 mg every 2–4 weeks. By gradually increasing the dose, the frequency of intolerance is significantly decreased. Major side effects are rash and loss of taste. Proteinuria is a common complication with a potential for progressing to nephrotic syndrome. Thrombocytopenia is also seen. Anemia and leucopenia are less frequently noted. Blood studies should be done at least every 2–4 weeks during the first 6 months of therapy, and then at least every 4–6 weeks thereafter. Side effects such as myasthenia gravis, Goodpasture's syndrome, breast gigantism, and lupus-like syndrome should be anticipated.

Azathioprine can also be used, but may not be the drug of next choice because of its oncogenic potential (21). It has been approved for use in the treatment of rheumatoid arthritis. Nevertheless, patients who are cigarette smokers or who have a strong family history of cancer may not be good candidates for treatment because of their having a greater risk of developing a neoplasm while taking an immunosuppressant drug. The possibility of azathioprine playing a permissive role by impairing immune surveillance cannot be discounted.

The use of methotrexate (22) and alkylating agents such as cyclophosphamide (23) should be reserved for cases in which the indications are clear and incontrovertable. Recent studies using methotrexate have shown it to be effective and well tolerated in many patients. It is usually administered in doses ranging from 5 to 25 mg/week. The major side effects are stomatitis and gastrointestinal upset. Problems with abnormal liver function tests are common; however, the risk of hepatic fibrosis in this setting appears to be low. Patients with diabetes mellitus and alcoholics appear to have greater risks of liver toxicity following treatment with methotrexate. If there is a question about underlying liver disease, a percutaneous liver biopsy should be performed prior to beginning treatment. Patients having no risk factors may not need a liver biopsy at outset. However, all patients should be biopsied after taking a cumulative dose of 2000–3000 mg. The absence of abnormal liver function tests cannot be taken as evidence against the presence of hepatic damage.

There is no consensus on the use of corticosteroids in rheumatoid arthritis. They are usually given in low doses to treat patients who are candidates for remittent drugs, but not as first-line therapy. All patients taking corticosteroids should be placed on calcium supplements to prevent the development of osteoporosis; the exception is patients with absorptive hypercalcemia, who are at risk of nephrolithiasis.

Corticosteroids can be administered orally, parenterally, or intra-articularly. Prednisone, the most commonly used drug, is usually administered in doses of 5–7.5 mg daily. Split doses are more effective than single daily doses, but have a higher frequency of side effects. Depot corticosteroids are occasionally useful when one does not want to commit a patient to oral steroid therapy. Long-acting drugs such as triamcinolone acetonide can be used in doses of 30–60 mg intramuscularly. Long-term use is associated with the development of a cushingoid habitus with all the complications of chronic corticosteroid use.

Corticosteroids can be administered intra-articularly to treat oligoarticular flares of synovitis. The risk of damage to articular cartilage is most likely overstated and does not appear to be a major problem when injections are repeated less frequently than every 4–6 months. Complications such as infection and fat atrophy at the injection site are uncommon. The incidence of infection, when using a sterile no-touch technique, is approximately 1:20,000 injections. It is important to avoid overdistending the joint during injection since excessive pressure will result in extravasation of drug into the subcutaneous tissue, increasing the risk of developing fat atrophy. The joint should be aspirated prior to injection. If the joint fluid is not removed, the corticosteroid crystals will be suspended in synovial fluid and not reach the site of inflammation.

Antimalarials are useful in treating refractory synovitis (24). Controlled studies have confirmed their efficacy. Eye exams should be performed prior to beginning therapy and repeated every 4–6 months to identify subclinical retinopathy. Doses of chloroquine should not exceed 6 mg/kg/day; doses of hydroxychloroquine should not exceed 4 mg/kg/day. Doses should be decreased in patients with impaired renal function.

PHYSICAL THERAPY

Physical therapy has a role in treating patients with rheumatoid arthritis (25). It provides short-term relief of symptoms, promoting a sense of wellness and helping to maintain function. However, there are a few data to show that physical therapy has any effect on the progression of disease. Major problems with expense and poor patient compliance limit its use. Patients instructed by physical therapists seldom continue their exercises in an unsupervised setting. Nevertheless, the patient should be encouraged to see a therapist on a regular basis to prevent the development of contractures and damage to joints because of improper usage.

THE "STEP-CARE" APPROACH

Rheumatoid arthritis is treated by a "step-care" approach whereby patients are given a series of potentially remittent drugs on a trial-and-error basis. Typically, patients will have taken a number of drugs to which there was an initial response, but subsequent loss of efficacy. Drug-induced remissions may be lost following discontinuation of treatment; therefore, maintenance therapy is almost always indicated. The exceptions are methotrexate and the cytotoxic drugs, because of their potential for cumulative toxicity. Methotrexate has a risk of causing hepatic fibrosis and possibly interstitial pulmonary disease. Cyclophosphamide has the potential for causing hemorrhagic cystitis and carcinoma of the bladder.

CRYSTAL-INDUCED ARTHRITIS

Crystal-induced arthritis, in contrast to other forms of arthritis, has well-defined etiologies. The major effector cells are neutrophils rather than mononuclear cells. These arthritides are articular diseases that lack systemic manifestations. There is no evidence that they respond to remittent drugs or benefit from immunosuppressive therapy. Treatment is limited to anti-inflammatory drugs and uric acid–lowering agents when appropriate.

GOUT

Gout is perhaps the best understood of the crystal-induced diseases. It arises as a consequence of hyperuricemia and crystal deposition. Monosodium urate crystals are the phlogistic agent. Treatment of acute attacks requires suppression of inflammation. Effective treatment requires normalization of serum uric acid levels and depletion of the total body urate pools.

PSEUDOGOUT

Pseudogout, or calcium pyrophosphate dihydrate deposition disease, is caused by deposition of calcium pyrophosphate dihydrate crystals in articular cartilage. Acute attacks of arthritis arise from shedding of preformed crystals into joints, where they induce an inflammatory reaction similar to that seen with gout. The disease typically presents as an acute arthritis resembling gout, but can also present as pseudorheumatoid arthritis, pseudo-osteoarthritis, pseudoneuropathic arthritis, and asymptomatic chondrocalcinosis. It can be idiopathic, familial, or associated with metabolic diseases such as hyperparathyroidism, hemochromatosis, hypothyroidism, ochronosis, or Wilson's disease. Treatment of calcium pyrophospate dihydrate deposition disease is palliative since there is no known cure.

HYDROXYAPATITE DEPOSITION DISEASE

Hydroxyapatite deposition disease is also pleomorphic. It can present as an acute inflammatory arthritis, a chronic painful degenerative arthropathy, or periarthritis. Periarticular disease includes bursitis, tendinitis, and tenosynovitis. Hydroxyapatite crystals have been implicated in the "Milwaukee shoulder" syndrome, a chronic degenerative arthritis of the shoulders characterized by degeneration of the rotator cuff, joint space narrowing, and the presence of microspheres containing hydroxyapatite crystals. These crystals have also been implicated in both the periarthritis and destructive arthropathy seen in patients on chronic hemodialysis.

TREATMENT

All forms of crystal-induced arthritis respond in part to NSAIDs (26). Phenylbutazone and indomethacin are perhaps the most effective agents. However, other NSAIDs have also been reported to be effective. Doses of NSAIDs used for treating acute attacks of gout are generally 25% higher than the doses used for treating rheumatoid arthritis. Pain associated with crystal-induced synovitis responds poorly to simple analgesics, salicylates, and opiates. Relief can only be obtained by suppression of inflammation.

Colchicine is effective in the treatment of both acute gout and pseudogout when administered intravenously (27). The usual dose is 2 mg in 20 ml of saline administered over 20 min. Additional 1-mg doses can be given every 3–6 hr if needed, to a maximum of 4 mg/24 hr. When treating gout, colchicine can also be administered orally in doses of 0.6 mg every 1–2 hr until a maximum of 12 tablets is given or side effects occur (28). Most patients obtain relief after 2–3 doses. Oral colchicine is not considered to be effective in the treatment of either acute or chronic pseudogout.

The choice between a NSAID and colchicine is arbitrary since both regimens are effective. Intravenous colchicine is preferred by many physicians for the treatment of acute gout, whereas a NSAID is preferred for the treatment of pseudogout. Colchicine is useful in patients with a history of peptic ulcer disease because it has no ulcerogenic potential. It should be avoided in patients with intercurrent diarrheal disease, chronic renal insufficiency, or bone marrow dysfunction. Colchicine is primarily excreted by the kidneys and therefore tends to be retained in patients with impaired renal function. Accumulation may lead to suppression of marrow function with resultant anemia or leucopenia.

Nonsteroidal anti-inflammatory drugs are effective and usually well tolerated. Indomethacin and phenylbutazone are most commonly used because of their efficacy and a long history of use. Phenylbutazone can never be considered a drug of first choice since other agents with less significant risks are available. Indomethacin may be the NSAID of choice in treating acute attacks of gout or pseudogout.

Oral corticosteroids have little place in the treatment of crystal-induced arthritis. Systemic corticosteroid therapy will suppress an acute attack, but often there is an exacerbation of the arthritis upon discontinuation of therapy. This is in contrast to intra-articular corticosteroid injections, which are useful in treating monoarticular arthritis unresponsive to either colchicine or NSAIDs.

Acute attacks of gout should not be treated with agents that lower the serum uric acid because of their risk of exacerbating an attack. In general, one should not begin therapy to lower the serum uric acid until the attack has completely subsided; then either allopurinol or a uricosuric drug can be given along with colchicine or a NSAID. Colchicine is usually given in a dose of 0.6 mg three times a day for 3–6 months as prophylaxis to prevent an exacerbation of arthritis while lowering the serum uric acid level (29).

The treatment of chronic gout requires continuous therapy to lower the uric acid. The goal is to reduce the total urate pool to normal. This can be done by using either allopurinol (30) or a uricosuric agent. Allopurinol is usually administered at doses of 200–300 mg daily. Divided doses of allopurinol are not required because of the long elimination half-life of oxypurinol, its active metabolite. On occasion, doses of 600–800 mg/day may have to be given to maintain a uric acid level below 7 mg/dl. Patients who are taking high doses of allopurinol or taking thiazide diuretics concurrently may be at risk for developing the Stevens-Johnson syndrome or hepatotoxicity. Similarly, patients with impaired renal function may tend to accumulate the drug because of decreasd renal clearance.

In most cases the choice between allopurinol and a uricosuric agent is a matter of preference. The exceptions are patients with a history of nephrolithiasis and patients who are overexcreters, that is who excrete more than 1000 mg of uric acid per day on a regular diet. These patients should be treated with allopurinol rather than a uricosuric agent because drugs enhancing renal excretion of uric acid have a risk of causing nephrolithiasis.

Probenecid and sulfinpyrazone are the commonly used uricosuric agents. Like allopurinol, they should not be given during an acute attack of gout. Probenecid is usually given in an initial dose of 250 mg/day, with the dose being gradually increased to 1.0–1.5 g/day, over 7–10 days (31). It must be administered in divided doses because of its short elimination half-life. Therapy with sulfinpyrazone is initiated at 50 mg twice daily and gradually increased to 200–800 mg in divided doses (32). The uricosuric effects of both probenecid and sulfinpyrazone are blocked by salicylates. Therefore, one should administer NSAIDs rather than salicylates when using these drugs. Sulfinpyrazone also has an effect on platelet function and on the metabolism of both wafarin and tolbutamide. Appropriate dose adjustments for these drugs should be made.

SPONDYLOARTHROPATHIES

The spondyloarthropathies include ankylosing spondylitis, Reiter's syndrome, psoriatic arthritis, and enteropathic arthritis. The diseases classified as spondyloarthropathies share features of enthesopathy, sacroiliitis, iritis, seronegativity (i.e., lacking rheumatoid factors), and an association with the histocompatibility antigen HLA-B27.

ANKYLOSING SPONDYLITIS

Ankylosing spondylitis is a chronic inflammatory disease that primarily involves the axial skeleton. It typically presents as back pain. The pain characteristically involves the low back or buttocks. The onset is often insidious without a history of antecedent trauma or precipitating event. It is inflammatory in character, being associated with morning stiffness and improvement with activity. There may be an associated arthritis involving predominantly large joints such as the hips, shoulders, knees, and ankles. Involvement of the small joints of the hands and feet is less common. Small joint involvement is typically asymmetrical. Enthesopathy is a characteristic feature of the disease. Patients may complain of chest pain due to involvement of costosternal and costochondral joints. Extra-articular complications such as iritis, conjunctivitis, and prostatitis may be seen as an early manifestation of the disease, providing a clue to the diagnosis. Late complications such as apical pulmonary fibrosis, aortic insufficiency, and cardiac conduction defects are uncommon.

REITER'S SYNDROME

Reiter's syndrome is defined by the triad of arthritis, conjunctivitis, and urethritis. There may be an associated stomatitis, balanitis, keratodermia, prostatitis, or diarrhea. The arthritis typically involves the large weight-bearing joints of the lower extremities. Tenosynovitis and enthesopathy are common features of the disease. Achilles tendinitis, plantar fasciitis, and costochondritis are commonly seen, helping to distinguish incomplete Reiter's syndrome from rheumatoid arthritis. Extra-articular manifestations such as aortic insufficiency, pericarditis, and cardiac conduction defects are uncommon. Rarely one sees pleuritis or neurologic involvement with peripheral and cranial neuropathies.

PSORIATIC ARTHRITIS

Psoriatic arthritis is defined as a seronegative arthritis occuring in patients with psoriasis. Arthritis involving the distal interphalangeal joints and classic arthritis mutilans, although characteristic, are not the most common manifestation of the disease. It typically presents as an asymmetric oligoarthritis. A small percentage of patients will have a rheumatoid arthritis–like pattern or will present with apparent ankylosing spondylitis. Extra-articular manifestations are uncommon. Conjunctivitis, iritis, and scleritis are seen in a minority of patients. Ocular involvement is strongly associated with sacroiliitis and the presence of the HLA B27 histocompatibility antigen.

ENTEROPATHIC ARTHRITIS

Arthritis is a major manifestation of inflammatory bowel disease. It is typically seen with Crohn's disease and ulcerative colitis, but is also a feature of Whipple's disease, intestinal bypass arthropathy, and reactive arthritis following enteric infections. These diseases are typically nonerosive and nondeforming. There is an association between the presence of arthritis and activity of the inflammatory bowel disease. Enteropathic arthritis usually presents as an acute oligoarthritis predominantly involving the joints of the lower extremities. Upper extremity involvement does occur, but is less frequent. An association between spondylitis, iritis, and HLA B27 is reported.

TREATMENT

As a group, the spondyloarthropathies are difficult to treat. With the exception of a subset of patients with psoriatic arthritis, there is no evidence that therapy with remittent drugs such as gold compounds is of any value. Therapy is limited to NSAIDs, physical therapy, and intra-articular corticosteroid injections. Remittent drugs such as antimalarials, gold compounds, and penicillamine have little value in treating patients with ankylosing spondylitis, Reiter's syndrome, or enteropathic arthritis. Physicians are less likely to treat these patients as aggressively because the prognosis of the spondyloarthropathies is better than that of rheumatoid arthritis.

The choice of anti-inflammatory drug is empiric. Patients with spondyloarthropathies may respond more favorably to treatment with NSAIDs than to salicylates. In general, one should begin therapy with the drug with the least side effects and change to less well tolerated drugs only after less toxic regimens have been tried. Phenylbutazone may be the most effective drug in many of these patients, but it is not favored as an initial choice because of its potential for causing agranulocytosis or aplastic anemia.

Corticosteroids are seldom appropriate for treating the spondyloarthropathies, with the exception of psoriatic arthritis, where they are often used for treating skin manifestations. Patients with Reiter's syndrome and those with ankylosing spondilitis appear to respond less well to corticosteroids than patients with rheumatoid arthritis. In addition, the prognosis of these diseases appears to be more favorable and therefore physicians are reluctant to treat with corticosteroids. There is no evidence that corticosteroids will prevent ankylosis or alter the progression of disease.

In summary, therapy of the spondyloarthropathies is empiric. One usually begins therapy with either aspirin or a NSAID. When aspirin is used, it should be administered in maximally tolerated doses. Therapeutic blood levels should be documented to confirm compliance. Aspirin should be given with meals and antacids to decrease the development of gastric erosions. Patients with a history of peptic ulcer disease may be given H2 blockers at bed time to decrease HCl-induced gastric damage due to salicylates. If a NSAID is administered, it should be given in maximally recommended doses for at least 2-3 weeks before changing to another drug. The end point of therapy is suppression of inflammation as well as relief of pain.

Some patients with Reiter's syndrome and others with ankylosing spondylitis have chronic disease that is refractory to treatment with NSAIDs and salicylates. These patients may be treated with cytotoxic drugs. Methotrexate and azathioprine are the most frequently used agents; however, data on their efficacy are lacking. There is no evidence that antibiotics have any role in the treatment of reactive arthritis due to venereal or enteropathic infection.

Some patients with psoriatic arthritis may respond to therapy with gold compounds. Others may be unresponsive, requiring treatment with cytotoxic agents. Methotrexate is the favored drug because it is effective in treating not only the arthritis, but the cutaneous manifestations as well. Only patients with chronic potentially disabling disease should be considered for therapy.

Methotrexate is usually administered on a weekly rather than daily schedule. Doses range from 5 to 25 mg/week, with usual doses being from 5 to 7.5 mg/day. Methotrexate is absorbed well both orally and parenterally. The major factor determining toxicity is duration of exposure rather than dose. Therefore, a single daily dose is to be preferred. Alternatively, the drug can be administered every 12 hr for 3 consecutive doses. Daily administration is associated with significant risk of toxicity. Patients with impaired renal function should not be given methotrexate because of the risk of accumulation. Patients taking aspirin are also at greater risk for toxicity. Potential drug interactions with probenecid and sulfonamides are also important.

CONNECTIVE TISSUE DISEASES

The connective tissue diseases are a heterogeneous group that includes systemic lupus erythematosus, mixed connective tissue disease, progressive systemic sclerosis, and the systemic vasculidities. Pain most commonly arises from serositis and arthritis. Serositis manifests itself as pleuritis, pericarditis, and peritonitis. Patients present with complaints of chest and abdominal pain.

Systemic lupus erythematosus is a chronic immunologically mediated multisystem disease characterized by the presence of multiple autoantibodies. It occurs most frequently in young women of childbearing age. Females are affected 7-10 times as often as males. The clinical manifestations of systemic lupus erythematosus are varied. Typically, patients will present with musculoskeletal complaints, and be diagnosed as having arthritis. It is usually polyarticular, involving small joints of the hands, the wrists, and the knees. The arthritis is nonerosive but can be deforming, having an appearance similar to rheumatoid arthritis.

Patients may also have articular complaints due to avascular necrosis of bone. This is usually seen in patients treated with corticosteroids. Patients complain of pain in the hips, knees, or shoulders. The pain of avascular necrosis generally does not respond to treatment with anti-inflammatory drugs.

Cardiopulmonary complaints are very common. Pleuritic pain can occur with or without effusions. Pericarditis, a common cardiac manifestation, occurs in approximately one-third of patients; patients complain of substernal chest pain that is typically aggravated by lying supine. Friction rubs are commonly heard, providing a clue to the diagnosis.

Abdominal pain is also seen in systemic lupus erythematosus. It may be due to aseptic peritonitis or mesenteric vasculitis. Ascites has been noted in up to 60% of patients who come to aytopsy, suggesting that peritoneal involvement is more common than clinically recognized. Mesenteric vasculitis with abdominal pain is uncommon, but may present as acute pancreatitis or ischemic bowel syndrome with perforation.

Mixed connective tissue disease and Sjögren's syndrome have many features in common with systemic lupus erythematosus. Clinical features are protean, involving almost every organ system. These patients may present with complaints of joint, chest, or abdominal pain.

The natural history of these diseases is variable and unpredictable. The initial choice of therapy will depend on the severity of the illness and the type of organ involvement. Pain arising from arthritis and serositis frequently responds to treatment with high-dose salicylates. The doses required to suppress articular inflammation range from 3.5 to 5.0 g daily. A few of these patients may develop a salicylate-induced hepatitis, which usually subsides following discontinuation of the drug. In these cases, antimalarial drugs may be used to suppress the arthritis. Hydroxychloroquine is usually used in doses of 200–400 mg/day. The major risk is retinal damage with the potential for blindness. The risk of retinal damage is dose related, and serious toxicity is rare if the patient is monitored appropriately. Baseline eye exams should be done before beginning treatment and repeated every 4–6 months thereafter. Nonsteroidal anti-inflammatory drugs can also be used but are more likely than aspirin to cause side effects requiring discontinuation of therapy. Ibuprofen has been associated with central nervous system dysfunction and aseptic meningitis. Nonsteroidal anti-inflammatory drugs have also been reported to cause significant impairment of renal function. This may range from a decrease in renal blood flow to acute renal failure due to interstitial nephritis.

Corticosteroid therapy is indicated for severe systemic manifestations of the disease. It is not usually needed for the treatment of either arthritis or serositis. If pain is unresponsive to treatment with either salicylates or nonsteroidal anti-inflammatory drugs, prednisone can be administered in doses of 5–10 mg/day as a single morning dose. Divided doses of corticosteroids, although potentially more effective, are more likely to cause suppression of the HPA axis, causing obesity, hypertension, and glucose intolerance.

EXTRA-ARTICULAR PAIN SYNDROMES

Extra-articular pain syndromes can mimic arthritis. These include tendinitis bursitis, and periarthritis. Recognition is imperative for optimal management. The character of the pain is variable, but it is generally described as aching, stabbing, or throbbing. Diagnosis is made by physical examination. The history, although suggestive, is often inconclusive. The diagnosis is confirmed by infiltration block using a local anesthetic. The local anesthetic should be infiltrated in the area of maximal tenderness. Assuming accurate placement, immediate relief of pain will confirm the diagnosis. Failure to relieve pain indicates either an incorrect diagnosis or improper injection technique. A depot corticosteroid can be mixed with the local anesthetic at the time of injection.

ROTATOR CUFF TENDINITIS AND SUBACROMIAL BURSITIS

Rotator cuff tendinitis, a common cause of shoulder pain, can be acute, subacute, or chronic. Characteristically patients complain of pain in the deltoid area rather than the shoulder. A painful arc is typically noted between 60° and 100° of abduction, but other motions may be painful as well. The diagnosis is easily confirmed by injection of local anesthetic into the subdeltoid area using a lateral approach (33).

BICIPITAL TENDINITIS

Patients with bicipital tendinitis frequently complain of pain in the area of the bicipital groove. The discomfort is reproduced by resisted supination of the hand with the elbow flexed. There is generally significant tenderness over the biceps tendon. There will be immediate relief of pain following infiltration of the synovial sheath surrounding the biceps tendon (33).

LATERAL EPICONDYLITIS

Pain in lateral epicondylitis is localized to the dorsal aspect of the proximal forearm, with maximal tenderness over the insertion of the extensor muscles on the lateral epicondyle. Flexion and extension of the elbow is usually free and painless. Resisted wrist extension and supination will reproduce the pain. Patients can be treated by splinting of the wrist, by local injections of corticosteroid, and rarely by surgery. A small number of patients have entrapment of the deep radial nerve at the arcade of Frohse mimicking lateral epicondylitis. The differential diagnosis is facilitated by injection of local anesthetic, that is, conduction block of the deep radial nerve at the arcade of Frohse (34).

DE QUERVAIN'S TENDINITIS

In de Quervain's tendinitis there is localized tenderness over the radial styloid associated with inflammation of the abductor pollicis longus and extensor pollicis brevis tendons. The diagnosis is suggested by a positive Finkelstein's test (i.e., pain on lateral deviation of the wrist with the thumb adducted). Treatment includes NSAIDs, immobilization, and local injection of corticosteroid. Patients who do not respond to conservative therapy should be considered for surgical treatment (35).

ANSERINE BURSITIS

Anserine bursitis is characterized by pain and tenderness in the region of the insertions of the medial collateral ligament and the sartorius muscle on the medial aspect of the proximal tibia. The pain, arising in the distribution of the infrapatellar branch of the saphenous nerve, can be felt along the medial aspect of the knee and proximal leg. Anserine bursitis is best treated with local injections of corticosteroid and local anesthetics; it is poorly responsive to treatment with NSAIDs (36).

ACHILLES TENDINITIS

Pain in the heel associated with erythema and tenderness is diagnostic of Achilles tendinitis or retrocalcaneal bursitis. In most cases, it is due to chronic trauma from ill-fitting shoes, but can be a manifestation of an underlying spondyloarthropathy. Pain associated with trauma will respond to rest. However, pain due to enthesopathy will usually require treatment with NSAIDs or local injection of corticosteroid (37).

POLYMYALGIA RHEUMATICA

Polymyalgia rheumatica is a syndrome of diffuse proximal myalgias occurring in elderly patients (38). The onset can be acute or subacute. A subset of these patients has giant cell arteritis. Another subset has rheumatoid arthritis presenting with proximal joint involvement. The diagnosis is one of exclusion. Patients typically have a Westergren sedimentation rate of at least 50 mm/hr. Laboratory findings are nonspecific. The anemia of chronic disease, an elevated serum alkaline phosphatase level, and polyclonal hypergammaglobulinemia are frequently seen. Patients may have age-related antinuclear antibodies and rheumatoid factors, but lack other serologic markers for autoimmune disease.

The diagnosis of giant cell arteritis is suggested by a history of headache, scalp tenderness, jaw claudication, or visual disturbance. In most cases the physical examination is normal, but in a small percentage of patients there will have to be palpable abnormalities of the temporal arteries. The diagnosis is confirmed by temporal artery biopsy.

The response to treatment with corticosteroids is also helpful diagnostically. Most patients will have a dramatic decrease in pain and stiffness within hours of beginning treatment with 7.5–10 mg of prednisone or its equivalent. Pseudopolymyalgia as seen with rheumatoid arthritis will have a less impressive response to corticosteroids. A failure to obtain significant pain relief with low-dose prednisone should cause one to question the diagnosis of polymyalgia.

The term *polymyalgia rheumatica* is most likely a misnomer. There is little evidence that pain is of muscular origin. Muscle enzymes, electromyograms, and muscle biopsies are reported to be normal. Pain may arise from involvement of proximal joints such as shoulders and hips. The presence of synovitis is suggested by reports of increased uptake of radioisotopes in the shoulder region, and by reports of an oligoarticular arteritis being present in many patients.

There is controversy over the need for high dose corticosteroid therapy in patients with polymyalgia rheumatica having no evidence of giant cell arteritis. Proponents of "high-dose" therapy argue that a negative biopsy does not rule out arteritis, and therefore all patients should be treated as though they had the disease. Others argue that many patients with polymyalgia rheumatica do not have arteritis and that the use of high-dose corticosteroid therapy is unnecessary. Inappropriate use of corticosteroids in high doses will lead to increased morbidity and mortality from adverse effects of corticosteroids. In these cases, a negative temporal artery biopsy is reassuring.

The end point in patients with both polymyalgia rheumatica and giant cell arteritis is suppression of inflammation as evidenced by normalization of the erythrocyte sedimentation rate. These patients are usually given from 45 to 60 mg of prednisone daily for 1 month, followed by gradual tapering of the dose over 3–6 months while maintaining a normal erythrocyte sedimentation rate. Patients who have no evidence for arteritis can be treated symptomatically. The end point is relief of pain. These patients are usually given from 7.5 to 10 mg of prednisone daily for control of symptoms, with tapering of the dose as tolerated. A small percentage of these patients will have subclinical arteritis; therefore, one should be prepared to increase the dose of corticosteroid when symptoms of vascular disease first appear. The major risk of inadequately treated giant cell arteritis is blindness. All patients should be given supplemental calcium to decrease the risk of corticosteroid-induced osteopenia. A minimum of 1000 mg of elemental calcium should be administered daily.

References

1. Capetola RJ, Rosenthale ME, Dubinsky B, McGuire JL: Peripheral antialgesics—A review. *J Clin Pharmacol* 23:545–556, 1983.
2. Rosenbaum JF: The drug treatment of anxiety. *New Engl J Med* 306:401–404, 1982.
3. Ward NG, Bloom VL, Friedel RD: The effectiveness of tricyclic antidepressants in the treatment of coexisting pain and depression. *Pain* 7:331–341, 1979.
4. Beaver WT: Combination analgesics. *Am J Med* 77(3A):38–53, 1985.
5. Bonkowsky HL, Mudge GH, McMurtry RJ: Chronic hepatic inflammation and fibrosis due to low dose paracetamol. *Lancet* 1:1016–1018, 1978.
6. Levy G, Tsuchiva T: Salicylate accumulation kinetics in man. *N Engl J Med* 287:430–432, 1972.
7. Ferreira SH: Peripheral analgesia: mechanisms of the analgesic action of aspirin-like drugs and opiate antagonists. *Br J Clin Pharmacol* 10:2379–2455, 1980.
8. Blackshear JL, Napier JS, Davidman M, Stillman MI: Renal complications of nonsteroidal antiinflammatory drugs: identification and monitoring of those at risk. *Semin Arthritis Rheum* 14:163–175, 1985.
9. Swainson CP, Griffiths P: Acute and chronic effects of sulindac on renal function in chronic renal disease. *Clin Pharmacol Therap* 37:298–300, 1985.
10. Byron MA, Mowat AG: Corticosteroid prescribing in rheumatoid arthritis—the fiction and the fact. *Br J Rheum* 24:164–166, 1985.
11. Friedman DM, Moore MA: The efficacy of intraarticular corticosteroids for osteoarthritis of the knee. *Arthritis Rheum* 21:556–559, 1978.

12. Wyke B: The neurology of joints in osteoarthritis. *Ann Rheum Dis* 19:257–261, 1981.
13. Arnold CC, Lemper RK, Linderholm H: Intraosseous hypertension and pain in the knee. *J Bone Joint Surg* 57B:360–363, 1975.
14. Hollander JL: Treatment of osteoarthritis of knee. *Arthritis Rheum* 3:564–569, 1960.
15. Wright V, et al: Intraarticular therapy in osteoarthritis: comparison of hydrocortisone acetate and hydrocortisone tertiary butylacetate. *Ann Rheum Dis* 19:257, 1960.
16. Butler M, et al: A new model of osteoarthritis in rabbits III. Evaluation of antiarthrosic effects of selected drugs administered intraarticularly. *Arthritis Rheum* 26:1380, 1983.
17. Davis P, Harth M (eds): Proceedings—therapeutic innovation in rheumatoid arthritis: worldwide auranofin symposium. *J Rheum* 9(suppl 8):1–209, 1982.
18. Champion GD, et al: Auranofin in rheumatoid arthritis. *J Rheum* 9(suppl 8): 137, 1982.
19. Cooperating Clinics Committee of the American Rheumatism Association: A controlled trial of gold salt therapy in rheumatoid arthritis. *Arthritis Rheum* 16:353–358, 1973.
20. Dixon A St J, et al: Synthetic D(−) penicillamine if rheumatoid arthritis. Double blind controlled study of a high and low dose regimen. *Ann Rheum Dis* 34:416–421, 1975.
21. Hunter T, et al: Azathioprine in rheumatoid arthritis: a long term follow up study. *Arthritis Rheum* 18:15–20, 1975.
22. Kremer JM, Lee JK: The safety and efficacy of the use of methotrexate in long term therapy of rheumatoid arthritis. *Arthritis Rheum* 29:822–831, 1986.
23. Cooperating Clinics Committee of the American Rheumatism Association: Controlled trial of cyclophosphamide in rheumatoid arthritis. *N Engl J Med* 283:883–889, 1970.
24. Adams EM, et al: Hydroxychloroquine in the treatment of rheumatoid arthritis. *Am J Med* 75:321–326, 1983.
25. Robinson HS, et al: Evaluation of a province-wide physical therapy monitoring service in an arthritis control program. *J Rheum* 7:387, 1980.
26. Kelly WN, Fox IH: Gout and related disorders of purine metabolism. In *textbook of Rheumatology*, ed 2. Philadelphia, WB Saunders, 1985, pp 1382–1388.
27. Wallace SL: The treatment of the acute attack of gout. *Clin Rheum Dis* 3:133–143, 1977.
28. Wallace SL: Colchicine. *Semin Arthrtis Rheum* 3:369, 1974.
29. Yu TF, Gutman AB: Efficacy of colchicine prophylaxis in gout. *Ann Intern Med* 35:179–192, 1961.
30. Brewis I: Single daily dose allopurinol. *Ann Rheum Dis* 34:256–259, 1975.
31. Yu TF: Milestones in the treatment of gout. *am J Med* 56:676–685, 1974.
32. Emmerson BT: A comparison of uricosuric agents in gout with special reference to sulfinpyrazone. *Med J Aust* 1:839–844, 1963.
33. Cogen L, et al: Medical management of the painful shoulder. *Bull Rheum Dis* 32:88–92, 1982.
34. Goldie I: Epicondylitis lateralis humeroepicondyalgie or tennis elbow. *Acta Chir Scand (Suppl)* 339:1+, 1964.
35. Muckart RD: Stenosing tendovaginitis of abductor policis longus and extensor pollicis brevis at the radial styloid (de Quervain's disease). *Clin Orthop* 33:201–207, 1964.
36. Larsson LG, Baum J: The syndrome of anserine bursitis. *Arthritis Rheum* 28:1062–1065, 1985.
37. Sheon RP, Moscowitz RW, Goldberg VM: *Soft tissue rheumatic pain: recognition, management, prevention.* Philadelphia, Lea & Febiger, 1982, pp 219–222.
38. Healy LA, et al: Polymyalgia rheumatica and giant cell arthritis. *Arthritis Rheum* 14:138–141, 1971.

chapter 41
Single-Muscle Myofascial Pain Syndromes

David G. Simons, M.D.

This and the next chapter together provide a solid basis for managing chronic myofascial pain syndromes (MPSs). Myofascial trigger points (TrPs) may occur in any skeletal muscle in response to strain by acute or chronic overload. Each of the body's approximately 500 skeletal muscles can develop TrPs that produce a referred pain pattern characteristic of that muscle. Each pattern becomes part of a single-muscle myofascial pain syndrome. Each single-muscle syndrome is responsive to appropriate treatment. To successfully deal with the multiple complex interwoven factors encountered in a chronic MPS, one should identify each single-muscle syndrome and every perpetuating factor, approaching them as discrete and soluble but interacting problems. The goal is to identify and treat the *cause* of the pain, not just the symptom of pain.

The process begins with the recognition of the composite single-muscle syndromes that together comprise the total myofascial pain picture as reported by the patient. This chapter first describes how to recognize an *acute* single-muscle syndrome due to TrPs. Next, it presents the distinctive characteristic pain patterns, stretch positions, and vapocoolant spray patterns of many of the common single-muscle syndromes throughout the body. The following chapter shows how this essential information is applied to manage a complex *chronic* MPS due to TrPs.

RECOGNITION OF A SINGLE-MUSCLE SYNDROME

Janet G. Travell is the pioneer responsible for first organizing these syndromes in a clinically useful way (1).

Myofascial TrPs are equally common in men and women (2), and are a frequent source of musculoskeletal pain in children (3). One study reports a sample of 200 Air Force recruits without pain complaint who, by age 19, had developed points of tenderness that fit the current definition of latent TrPs in the shoulder-girdle musculature (2). Many of these TrPs referred pain on stimulation. These latent TrPs tend to become active with the stresses of adult life and with the gradual deterioration of muscular function in time. Latent TrPs, although less irritable than active TrPs, at times may have any or all of the characteristics of active TrPs *except* the clinical complaint of pain. With chronicity, satellite TrPs tend to develop in muscles located in pain reference zones that exhibit true muscle spasm. Also with chronicity, secondary TrPs may develop in muscles in the same functional unit (4).

The diagnosis of MPS due to myofascial TrPs depends on eight clinical characteristics (4). All eight clinical features emphasize the fact that this is primarily an affliction of muscle:

1. History of the onset and its cause
2. Distribution of the pain
3. Restriction of motion
4. Mild, muscle-specific weakness
5. The focal tenderness of a TrP
6. The palpable taut band of muscle in which a TrP is located
7. A local twitch response to snapping palpation
8. Reproduction of the referred pain pattern on more sustained mechanical stimulation of the TrP.

These first four characteristics are frequently very helpful, and the last four can be essential, for making the diagnosis.

HISTORY OF ONSET

By history, the onset of pain is often sudden and associated with a clearly remembered muscular strain, but the onset may be gradual, resulting from repetitive physical stress. The *distribution* of referred pain (or altered sensation) is more significant than the kind of pain. Pain referred from TrPs is usually described as dull, constant, and aching but may be described as shooting or stabbing, rarely as burning. Altered sensation is occasionally described as numbness and is substantiated by examination (5). Intensity is variable from hour to hour and from day to day. A newly activated TrP may spontaneously revert to a latent TrP. However, in the presence of serious perpetuating factors newly activated TrPs persist as chronically active or intermittently active, pain-producing TrPs. In addition, they are likely to multiply as satellite and secondary TrPs (4). Characteristically, pain symptoms are closely related to changes in the activity of or in the demands on the involved muscle.

DISTRIBUTION OF PAIN

Referred pain patterns are the key to identifying which muscle, or muscles, are most likely to be causing the myofascial pain. Examples in the next section show that each muscle has its own characteristic pain pattern (4). The sketchy pain drawings usually requested of patients are generally useless for identifying mysofacial TrPs.

Accurately drawn referred pain patterns are the initial key to locating the TrPs. A *precise drawing* that includes the patient's complete pain distribution is essential. Each area of pain should be delineated by the patient with *one finger* on the body, and should be drawn by the examiner on an anatomically accurate body form, such as those designed for this purpose (4); the drawing is then corrected or confirmed by the patient. Leading questions are scrupulously avoided. The local tenderness *elicited* in response to pressure applied by the patient on a TrP must be carefully distinguished from the pain and tenderness *referred* to that area by a distant TrP. Patients often need help from the examiner to make these important distinctions.

When pain involves several parts of the body, it is important to number the pain areas in the sequence of their appearance, to distinguish between pains that occur at different times and to group together those that are experienced together in association with an activity or position. The known pain pattern of each muscle is then applied in reverse to identify the muscle or muscles that are most likely to be causing that piece of the patient's total pain picture. The importance of obtaining a complete and accurate pain drawing at the initial visit, as well as obtaining drawings that identify any changes at subsequent visits, cannot be overemphasized.

A myofascial TrP usually refers *tenderness* as well as pain to the zone of referred pain, which often confuses both the unwary examiner and the patient.

RESTRICTION OF MOTION

On examination, patients consistently have some painful limitation of the stretch range of motion. Passive lengthening of a muscle harboring TrPs causes pain when the muscle is forcibly stretched beyond its restricted range of motion. Also, strong voluntary contraction of an involved muscle, especially in the shortened position, is likely to be painful.

MUSCLE-SPECIFIC WEAKNESS

The involved muscle shows some degree of rachety weakness without atrophy. When carefully examined, it acts as if it is reflexly inhibited from maximal contraction.

FOCAL TENDERNESS

Exquisite focal tenderness of the TrP is identified by the jump sign—a vocalization by and withdrawal *of the patient*. This spot tenderness is an essential feature of both a TrP and a tender point (TeP).

Algometers are becoming widely used to quantify TrP and TeP sensitivity in clinical studies (6–10). Fischer designed a family of convenient spring-type pressure algometers (11–13) that are commercially available. Reeves and associates (14) have established the reliability of Fischer's pressure threshold meter (11). Jensen and associates developed and validated an electronic strain-gauge unit that is also being produced commercially (10). Schiffman and associates (15) have developed and tested an electronic strain-gauge unit with a blunt probe. When the probe is pressed across the TrP in a taut band, this unit simulates snapping palpation and returns considerable tactile feedback to the examiner. This algometer is especially well suited to the study of local twitch responses and should soon be commercially available.

PALPABLE TAUT MUSCLE BAND

The palpable band associated with a TrP is a dependable and totally objective finding. The TrP is the point of maximum tenderness along the course of a taut band in an involved muscle. The rope-like taut band (sometimes described more like a nodule) can be palpated if the muscle is sufficiently close to the skin. The tense fibers that comprise the palpable band are most easily distinguished from the normally relaxed fibers surrounding them by stretching the muscle gently just short of, or to the onset of, resistance. This degree of stretch maximizes the palpable differences in tension between taut and normal fibers.

LOCAL TWITCH RESPONSE

Firm snapping palpation across, or needle penetration into, an active TrP usually evokes a local twitch response of the fibers in the taut band. This response is an objective sign and has been observed only in response to abrupt mechanical stimulation of TrPs. It was recently studied electromyographically by Fricton and associates (16). This objective local twitch response is seen as a transient dimpling of the skin near the more distant tendinous attachment of the muscle or is felt as a transient contraction of only the fibers in the taut band, without contraction of the muscle fibers surrounding the taut band.

REPRODUCTION OF REFERRED PAIN

Mildly painful sustained pressure on an active TrP usually reproduces or increases the referred pain from that TrP, if the TrP is not already activated to maximum intensity. This confirms to both the patient and the examiner that this TrP is responsible for at least part of the patient's pain. In this way one can piece together the total pain distribution of patients with multiple TrPs that project multiple, often overlapping, single-muscle referred pain patterns. Each pattern contributes its own portion of the total pain distribution. It is noteworthy that sometimes a TrP may refer analgesia instead of pain (5).

SUMMARY

In summary, the first four of the above features are helpful in making a *clinical* diagnosis: the dependence of symptoms on muscular strain and muscular activity; the specificity of the referred pain and tenderness patterns initiated by each skeletal muscle; painful restriction of the stretch range of motion; and some weakness of involved muscles without atrophy.

The remaining four features are essential for making the diagnosis of myofascial TrPs for *research* purposes. Clinically, focal exquisite TrP tenderness is always present and a taut band is palpable whenever the muscle is accessible. The last two features, the local twitch response and the referred pain response, have been considered pathognomonic of TrPs (4). A possible exception would be if the pain can be referred from some TePs of fibromyalgia. These last two responses are most vigorous in the most active TrPs, but sometimes can be elicited from latent TrPs. An exquisitely tender TrP may be too sensitive for the patient to permit the application of sufficient pressure to elicit a local twitch response.

Only active TrPs are responsible for *clinical* pain complaints. Latent TrPs, although less irritable, may have any or all of the other characteristics of active TrPs, including local twitch responses and the reproduction of that TrP's referred pain pattern when the TrP is firmly compressed.

PATHOGENESIS OF TRIGGER POINTS

Although the pathogenesis of myofascial TrPs has not been fully documented, pathophysiologic mechanisms are well established that can account for the distinctive clinical characteristics of TrPs, and these mechanisms have been extensively discussed (17). The local tenderness of the TrP can be explained by sensitization of group III and/or group IV muscle afferents (18). Initiation of referred pain by the TrP is explicable by the same process of nerve sensitization. The central nervous system pathways of referred pain may depend on one or more of the four known mechanisms by which pain may be referred (17, 19).

The electrically silent palpable hardness of the taut band and its associated local twitch response are more difficult to explain. The same mechanism that causes the contraction without action potentials in McArdle's disease, if applicable locally at the TrP, could account for shortened muscle fibers. One possibility is that such a mechanism is sustained by an energy crisis locally in the muscle. This mechanism is substantiated by recent studies of "fibromyalgia" patients, many of whom had TrPs that referred pain (20). Studies have demonstrated reduced and disturbed oxygen tension (21), a deficit of high-energy phosphates with an excess of low-energy phosphates (22), and ragged red and moth-eaten fibers under light microscopy (23). The latter are found in muscles experiencing impaired metabolism.

ACUTE SINGLE-MUSCLE SYNDROMES

This section presents many of the common single-muscle syndromes found throughout the body. Every skeletal muscle has the potential to develop myofascial TrPs. The key to each syndrome is recognition of the referred pain pattern characteristic of that muscle. The syndromes are grouped according to the region of the body to which pain is referred. This referred pain is the pain for which the patient seeks relief. Detailed instructions in the principles of stretch and spray that apply to individual muscles are found in the next section.

HEAD AND NECK PAIN

A number of neck muscles, including the upper trapezius, sternocleidomastoid, splenii, and suboccipital muscles, refer pain strongly to the head. These muscles are often largely responsible for headache diagnosed as "tension" headache or "muscle tension" headache (24). Masticatory muscles frequently cause temporal, maxillary, and jaw pain, also earache and toothache; cutaneous facial muscles sometimes contribute to facial pain (4).

The masticatory muscles that are active during closure of the lower jaw include the masseter, temporalis, medial pterygoid, and upper division of the lateral pterygoid. The digastric and lower division of the lateral pterygoid muscles primarily open the jaw. The masseter and temporalis muscles are most likely to be responsible for ear pain, temporal headache, and hypersensitivity of the teeth to pressure, heat, and cold. Pain and tenderness referred to a normal tooth has resulted in the extraction of an innocent tooth when the myofascial origin of the pain was not identified. The lateral pterygoid muscle often is involved when pain and/or dysfunction include the temporomandibular joint.

The normal range of jaw opening is easily tested by the patient's ability to insert a tier of their first three knuckles of the nondominant hand between the incisor teeth (4). Masticatory muscles are most responsive to stretch-and-spray therapy when the patient is supine. When the patient is seated, the head should be tilted fully backward rather than upright to eliminate antigravity reflexes.

Upper and Lower Trapezius

The **upper trapezius** is probably the muscle that most commonly develops myofascial TrPs. Trigger points in the clavicular section project pain to the back of the neck and to the temporal region (Fig. 41.1A) (1, 25). Upper trapezius TrPs (black arrows) are likely to be activated and perpetuated by lack of support for the elbows when sitting; this happens much of the time when the person's upper arms are short in relation to torso height so that the elbows fail to reach the chair's armrests (4). Persistent avoidable elevation of the shoulders as a result of emotional tension commonly abuses this muscle.

For relief of upper trapezius TrPs, the patient should be seated and *relaxed*; the shoulder on the side to be stretched is anchored by the patient's grasping the chair seat or placing the hand under the thigh. The spray is applied (dashed arrows, Fig. 41.1A) upward from the acromion over the upper section of the trapezius muscle, including pain reference zones in the posterolateral aspect of the neck, behind the ear, and around to the temple and mandible. The muscle is placed in the maximum lengthened position by passively tilting the head and neck toward the side opposite the involved muscle with the face turned toward the side of the involved muscle. An effective home program of self-stretch has the supine patient place the head in the stretch position and gently but firmly add stretch tension exerted by the opposite hand.

The **lower trapezius** TrP (Fig. 41.1B) is usually found in the inferior margin of the lower trapezius muscle about where it crosses the vertebral border of the scapula. This TrP refers pain and tenderness to the upper trapezius muscle, generating satellite TrPs there. Such satellite TrPs rarely respond until the primary TrP, in the lower trapezius, is first inactivated.

The stream of vapocoolant spray is applied for TrPs in the lower trapezius muscle as shown by the dashed arrows in Figure 41.1B. Stretch is applied as indicated by the curved white arrow. The operator may pull the patient's elbow across the chest, lifting slightly to fully protract and elevate the scapula. Stretch is smoothly coordinated with unidirectional parallel sweeps of the spray. The patient should perform this same stretch as a self-stretch home exercise, preferably seated under a hot shower (4).

Sternocleidomastoid

The clavicular and sternal divisions of the sternocleidomastoid muscle present distinctively different pain patterns. The two divisions also refer different kinds of autonomic phenomena and differ in stretch positions.

Myofascial TrPs of the **clavicular division** refer pain *bilaterally* across the forehead. Referral across the midline is unusual for myofascial TrPs. Pain may also be referred deep in the ear, and close behind the ear (Fig. 41.1C) (4, 25). Postural instability, spatial disorientation, and dizziness may occur when the patient suddenly increases the tension in this muscle by flexing the neck, looking up, or turning over in bed.

A stream of vapocoolant is directed upward above the clavicle to cover the muscle, the occiput, and forehead (Fig. 41.1C). To stretch this division of the muscle, the patient anchors the hand under the chair seat or fixes the hand under the thigh. The operator cradles the patient's head against the operator's torso to provide head support. In this way, the patient relaxes and lets the operator gradually extend the head backward and sidebend it (Fig. 41.1C).

The **sternal division** refers pain to the occiput, to the vertex, to the cheek, around the eye, and to the throat (Fig. 41.1D). Its lowermost TrPs can refer pain downward over the sternum. Motor and autonomic concomitants are narrowing of the palpebral fissure, scleral injection, lacrimation, and coryza.

Following initial sweeps of spray, the sternal division is stretched by gently rotating the face to the same side and tipping the chin downward to the acromion. As this movement proceeds slowly, the spray is directed along the length of the muscle from the sternum to the mastoid process, including the back of the head (dashed arrows in Fig. 41.1D). Before the operator directs the sweeps immediately above the eye, the patient's eye is covered with an absorbent pad and the patient closes the eye tightly. Spray in the eye is fiercely painful for about 2 min but causes no permanent damage. Accidentally spraying the ear drum is also startling but painful only because of impact and cold.

Masseter and Temporalis

The superficial division of the masseter muscle refers pain to the face and upper or lower molar teeth (Fig. 41.1E), whereas TrPs in the temporalis muscle refer pain to any of the upper teeth and over the temporal bone and eyebrow in finger-like projections (Fig. 41.1F). Trigger points in the deep masseter may cause earache and ipsilateral tinnitus.

The masseter, temporalis, and medial pterygoid muscles may be stretched and sprayed together by combining the spray patterns (dashed arrows) of Figures 41.1E and F. The operator applies the spray over the lower jaw and continues in parallel sweeps upward behind the ear, then covering the cheek, temporal region, and eyebrow. For self-stretch, the supine patient places the fingers on the posterior molars and gently pulls downward, applying long axis distraction, and then pulls slightly forward. To fully stretch the posterior temporalis fibers, the mandible also should be pulled to the opposite side.

Figure 41.1. Location of TrPs (*solid black arrows*) and pain patterns (*solid black and black stipples*), stretch positions, and spray patterns (*dashed arrows*) for muscles that cause head and neck pain. The *curved white arrows* show the direction of pressure applied to passively stretch each muscle and the *dashed arrows* trace the path of parallel sweeps of vapocoolant spray to release the tension and permit stretch of each muscle. In *H*, the broken arrow in the pain pattern deep to the ear indicates pain deep in the head radiating to the back of the eye. (From Simons DG: Myofascial pain syndromes. In Basmajian JV, Kirby RL (eds): *Medical Rehabilitation*. Baltimore, Williams & Wilkins, 1984, pp 314, 315.)

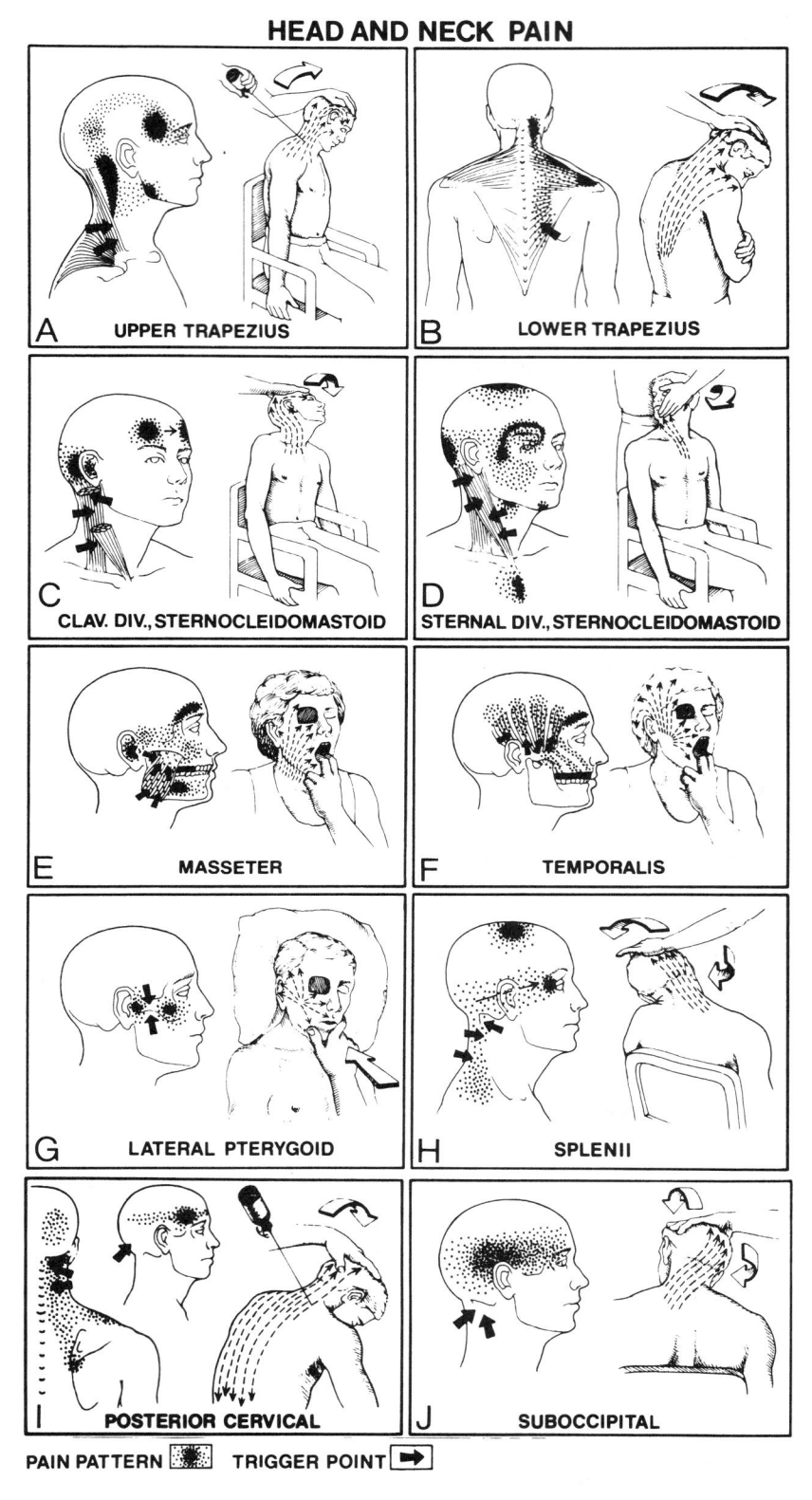

Lateral Pterygoid

The lateral pterygoid (Fig. 41.1G) is difficult to stretch (4). It is inaccessible to ischemic compression. Alternate treatment techniques such as injection or ultrasound usually must be used.

Splenii

Myofascial TrPs in the splenius capitis and cervicis muscles refer deep-seated head pain, as in Figure 41.1H. Stretching these muscles requires combined head and neck flexion, sidebending of the head, and rotation of the face toward the opposite side, as illustrated. The patient's hand must anchor the torso, as for the upper trapezius. Relaxation during stretch and spray is facilitated for most muscles by having the patient slowly exhale with the eyes directed downward (26).

Posterior Cervical Muscles

Semispinalis cervicis and capitis TrPs refer pain to the occiput and to the temporal region (Fig. 41.1I). Multifidus TrPs are found deep in the paraspinal mass, often at the C5 and C6 levels; they refer pain to the suboccipital area and toward the scapula. These posterior cervical pain patterns are likely to appear together. Multifidus TrPs often initiate satellite TrPs in the suboccipital muscles.

For treatment of the posterior cervical muscles, the head and neck are flexed against the chest while bilateral parallel sweeps of spray are directed as in Figure 41.1I, starting at the base of the neck.

Suboccipital Muscles

The suboccipital muscles project pain inside the head and to the upper part of the face (Fig. 41.1J). They, the scalene, and the sternocleidomastoid muscles are commonly the cause of persistent whiplash symptoms following a rear-end collision. These muscles are responsive to stretch and spray, and to massage or pressure therapy (27). Injection of the lateral suboccipital muscles is not recommended because of TrP proximity to the external loop of the vertebral artery (4).

The stream of spray is applied as in Figure 41.1J. Stretch of the medial suboccipital muscles combines slight flexion of the head on the neck with rotation of the face to the opposite side (curved arrows, Figure 41.1J). To stretch the lateral suboccipital muscles, the head is flexed slightly and tilted on the neck toward the opposite side; only head movement on the cervical spine stretches these muscles.

SHOULDER AND UPPER EXTREMITY PAIN

Myofascial TrPs in some muscles of the neck, shoulder girdle, and upper extremity refer pain to the ipsilateral upper torso and upper extremity (Fig. 41.2). Persistent shoulder pain due to myofascial TrPs commonly follows trauma (28), such as a dislocated shoulder, fracture, or soft tissue injury in a fall (4).

Painful restriction of sidebending of the neck is likely to be caused by scalene and/or upper trapezius TrPs. The levator scapulae is more likely to restrict rotation than is the sternocleidomastoid muscle. Subscapularis TrPs often severely restrict abduction and external rotation of the arm at the shoulder. Moderate restriction of abduction may be caused by TrPs in the more vertical, lower sternal and abdominal fibers of the pectoralis major muscle or in the triceps brachii muscle. Myofascial TrPs in the long slack latissimus dorsi muscle minimally restrict forward flexion of the arm. Those in the infraspinatus, teres minor, and posterior deltoid muscles restrict internal rotation at the shoulder.

Scaleni

Any of the three scalene muscles can refer pain to the anterior, lateral, and posterior shoulder girdle regions and also down the length of the upper extremity to the index finger, skipping the elbow (Fig. 41.2A) (1, 29). Tension due to TrPs in the anterior and middle scalene muscles can also entrap the lower trunk of the brachial plexus, which often causes symptomatic neurapraxia of the ulnar nerve (4).

For relief, the jet stream of vapocoolant spray is directed downward over the scalene muscles and over their complete referred pain pattern, including the hand and upper back, while all of these muscles are passively lengthened by sidebending the head to the opposite side. The face position of Figure 41.2A places maximum stretch on the posterior scalene. Rotating the face toward the involved side emphasizes stretch of the anterior scalene muscle. Simple sidebending of the neck stretches chiefly the middle scalene. A self-stretch program and correction of mechanical perpetuating factors, such as paradoxical respiration (4), are usually necessary for sustained relief.

Levator Scapulae

A "stiff neck" syndrome with restricted rotation of the neck is commonly caused by active TrPs in the levator scapulae muscle (30). This muscle refers pain as in Figure 41.2B (4, 31).

The sweeps of spray extend downward, over the muscle and its referred pain pattern. The operator must simultaneously press the shoulder down and back to stabilize it and press the head forward and to the opposite side with one arm while applying sweeps of spray with the other hand (Fig. 41.2B). Instead, he or she may apply shoulder pressure and spray with one arm and assist stretch with the other. Full stretch combines flexion, sidebending, and rotation of the neck to the opposite side.

The neck must always be protected, particularly where there is hypermobility, loss of cervical lordosis, or cervical joint degeneration. When a levator stretch is needed, it is best done by stabilizing the head and neck and then moving the scapula downward and into lateral rotation.

Deltoid

The free borders of the anterior and posterior deltoid muscle are more common sites of TrPs than is the middle deltoid. Pain from deltoid TrPs, like pain from the gluteous maximus muscle, is referred locally (Fig. 41.2C and D).

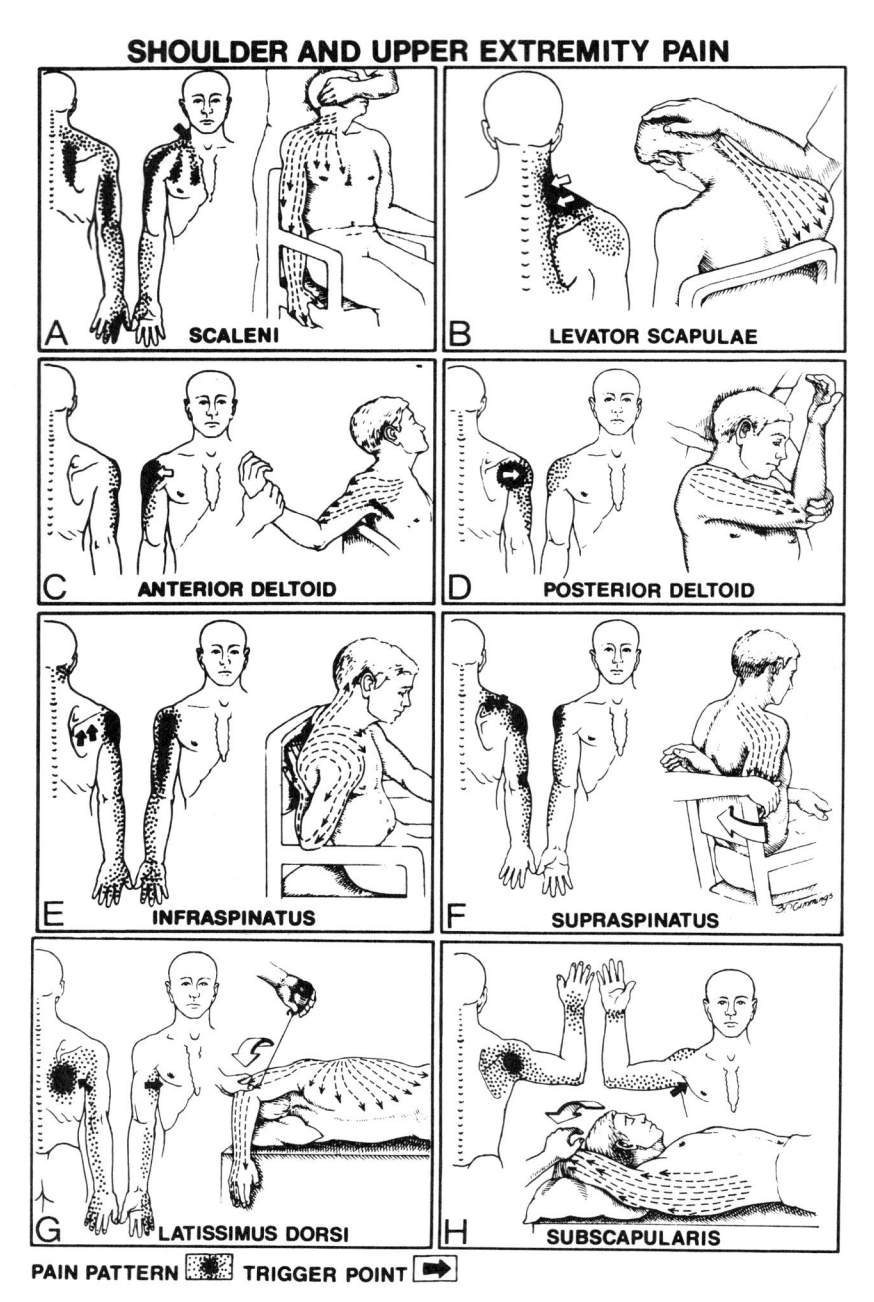

496 Pain Management in Selected Disorders/Section 3

Figure 41.2. Location of TrPs (*short straight black, or white arrows*) and pain patterns (*solid black and stipples*), stretch positions, and spray patterns (*dashed arrows*) for eight muscles producing shoulder and upper extremity pain. The *curved white arrows* identify the direction(s) of pressure applied to stretch the muscle. The *dashed arrows* trace the impact of the stream of vapocoolant spray applied to release the muscular tension during stretch. (From Simons DG: Myofascial pain syndromes. In Basmajian JV, Kirby RL (eds): *Medical Rehabilitation*. Baltimore, Williams & Wilkins, 1984, pp 315, 316.)

Spray is directed distalward over the muscle and over its pain pattern (Fig. 41.2C and D). Maximum stretch of the anterior deltoid (Fig. 41.2C) requires both horizontal extension and external rotation of the arm. Stretch of the posterior deltoid (Fig. 41.2D) brings the elbow as far across the chest as possible. Additional stretch may be achieved by using internal rotation rather than the external rotation shown in Figure 41.2D.

Infraspinatus

The pain commonly referred from TrPs in the infraspinatus muscle is distinctive for its penetration deep into the shoulder joint (Fig. 41.2E) (31, 32).

The sweeps of spray follow the dashed arrows in Figure 41.2E. The seated patient reaches behind the back as high as possible toward the scapula and then leans back against the chair to relax. The arm is progressively repositioned passively until full range of motion is achieved.

Supraspinatus

The supraspinatus muscle usually projects pain and tenderness (Fig. 41.2F) to the middeltoid region and to the elbow, which the infraspinatus and scaleni patterns skip. Supraspinatus TrPs sometimes activate satellite TrPs in the deltoid muscle.

The spray path is shown as dashed arrows in Figure 41.2F and continues to the wrist. Full stretch is difficult to attain because the body obstructs pure adduction. The difficulty is circumvented by alternately adducting the arm behind and in front of the torso, as for the deltoid stretch.

Latissimus Dorsi

Myofascial TrPs in the long slack latissimus dorsi (Fig. 41.2G) are particularly troublesome to the patient because no positioning of the arm seems to relieve that pain. The TrPs causing the pain are easily overlooked. Referred pain from both the latissimus dorsi (Fig. 41.2G) and serratus posterior superior (see Fig. 41.4D) projects to the scapular area. The serratus posterior superior muscle refers pain more cephalad in relation to the scapula and deep into the chest. Pain into the chest is not characteristic of latissimus dorsi TrPs.

For the latissimus dorsi muscle, vapocoolant is applied from the TrP in the direction of referred pain to cover the *entire* muscle and its pain pattern, as in Figure 41.2G.

Full stretch can be attained seated, but patient relaxation is improved in the side-lying position and downward tilting of the pelvis is more easily achieved. Effective stretch of the latissimus dorsi (Fig. 41.2G) requires essentially the same arm position as for the subscapularis (Fig. 41.2H). Therefore, subscapularis TrPs may have to be released first to attain full stretch of the latissimus dorsi.

Subscapularis

Myofascial TrPs (black arrow in Fig. 41.2H) in the subscapularis muscle are often the key to a frozen shoulder syndrome. Active TrPs in this muscle severely restrict both abduction and external rotation of the arm (4, 33). This severe limitation of motion encourages TrPs in the other shoulder girdle muscles and leads to the frozen shoulder. Pain referred from the subscapularis concentrates on the back of the shoulder and frequently includes a "band" of pain and tenderness around the wrist.

Treatment begins with upsweeps of the spray that cover the side of the chest and axilla, as in Figure 41.2H. The sweeps include *all of the scapula*, especially its vertebral border, which is not shown in the figure. Sweeps of spray are continued to include the wrist. Stretch employs gentle, progressive abduction and external rotation of the arm at the shoulder.

Biceps Brachii

Referred pain from biceps brachii TrPs radiates upward to the shoulder anteriorly and sometimes downward to the elbow (Fig. 41.3A). Bicipital tendinitis may sometimes be relieved by inactivation of TrPs in the long head of the biceps brachii.

The stream of vapocoolant is directed as in Figure 41.3A. The long head of the biceps brachii crosses two joints and for full stretch requires elbow extension, horizontal extension of the arm at the shoulder, and pronation of the forearm, as illustrated. The in-doorway stretch is strongly recommended for the patient's home program (4).

Brachialis

The brachialis muscle, remarkably, projects pain strongly to the base of the thumb (Fig. 41.3B). It is noteworthy that the supinator (Fig. 41.3D), brachioradialis (33), and adductor pollicis (33) muscles also refer pain and tenderness to the thumb area. The stream of spray is applied distally over the brachialis muscle and to cover the thumb and then cephalad over the biceps, which is its upper pain reference zone (4). The brachialis is stretched only by extension of the forearm at the elbow. Myofascial TrPs in the muscle are readily palpated by pushing the distal biceps aside, and they respond well to injection (Fig. 41.3B).

Triceps Brachii

Five TrP locations in the three heads of the triceps muscle refer individual pain patterns (4) that are combined in Figure 41.3C. Because the long head is a two-joint muscle, its TrPs restrict simultaneous flexion at the elbow and at the shoulder. The long head of the triceps is a commonly overlooked cause of shoulder dysfunction. The taut bands of the long head TrPs are readily identified by pincer palpation of its belly just above midarm adjacent to the humerus. The muscle is examined for taut bands by encircling the long head, inserting the tips of the finger and thumb between the muscle and the humerus. The taut bands are detected by rolling the muscle fibers between the fingertips (4).

The spray is applied in parallel sweeps (Fig. 41.3C). Full stretch requires simultaneous two-joint flexion as illustrated, a position seldom assumed in daily activity.

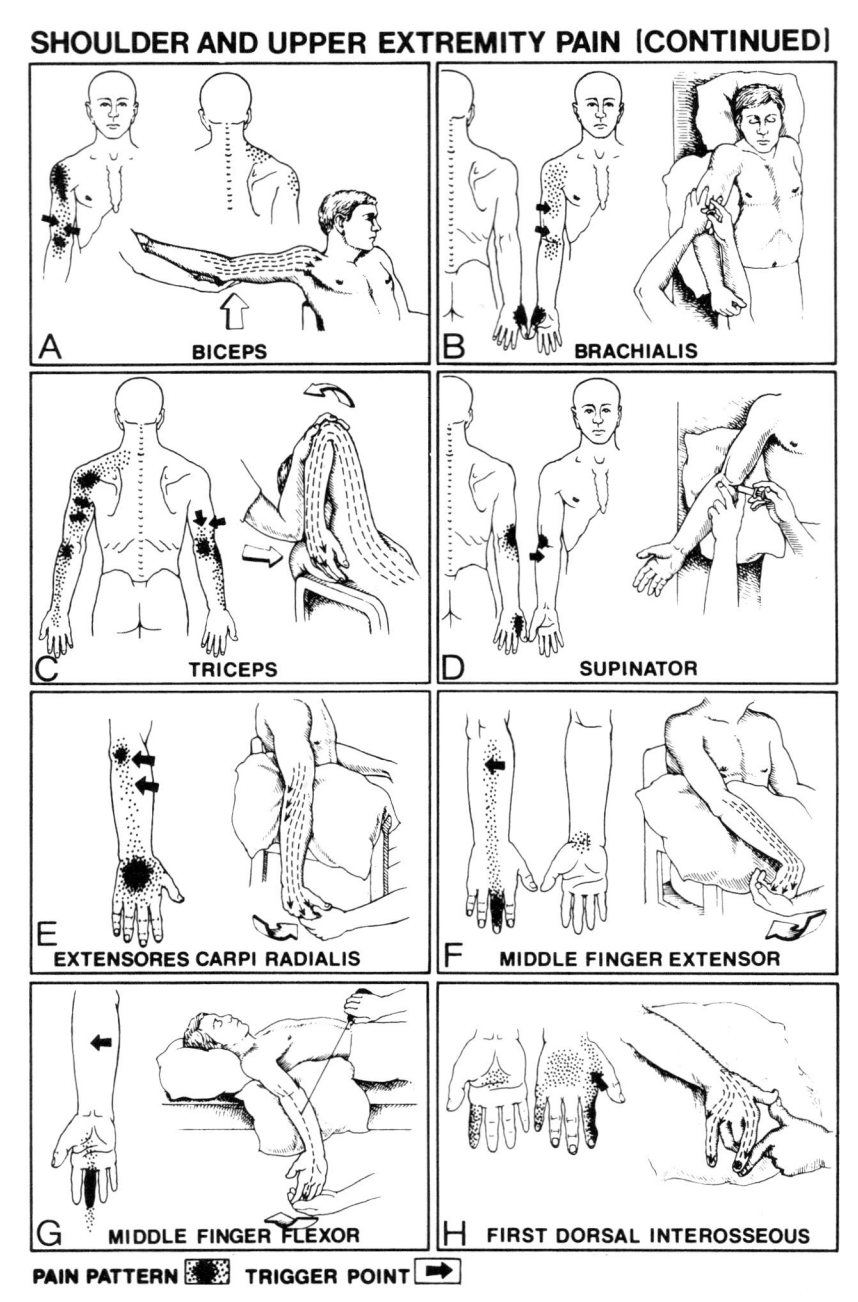

498 Pain Management in Selected Disorders/Section 3

Figure 41.3. Location of TrPs (*short straight black arrows*) and pain patterns (*solid black and stipples*), stretch positions, and spray patterns (*dashed arrows*) for eight muscles responsible for shoulder and upper extremity pain. The *curved white arrows* identify the direction(s) of pressure applied to passively stretch the muscle. The *dashed arrows* trace the impact of parallel sweeps of vapocoolant spray applied to release the muscular tension during stretch. (From Simons DG: Myofascial pain syndromes. In Basmajian JV, Kirby RL (eds): *Medical Rehabilitation.* Baltimore, Williams & Wilkins, 1984, pp 316, 317.

Supinator

Active TrPs in the supinator muscle are often responsible for "tennis elbow" or "epicondylitis." The supinator refers pain and tenderness to the lateral epicondyle and also to the dorsal web space of the thumb (Fig. 41.3D).

The stream of vapocoolant is directed distalward over the muscle, then back and around to cover the lateral epicondyle and finally is continued distally over the dorsum of the forearm and thumb. Stretch requires combined extension at the elbow and pronation of the hand (4). Injection of the most common TrPs in the medial border of the muscle is illustrated in Figure 41.3D. The radial nerve should be avoided when injecting these TrPs (4). The extensor muscle mass on the dorsum of the forearm distal to the lateral epicondyle frequently also develops TrPs as part of the "tennis elbow" syndrome. These TrPs are readily identified by taut bands and local twitch responses.

Extensores Digitorum and Carpi Radialis

The hand and finger extensors that comprise the extensor muscle mass are strongly activated by a vigorous grip. Active TrPs in these muscles frequently cause the hand grip to be painful and measurably weakened; a cup or a glass may unexpectedly drop from the grasp. The extensor carpi radialis refers pain and tenderness to the lateral epicondyle and dorsum of the hand (Fig. 41.3E). Active TrPs in the finger extensors refer pain to the dorsal surface of the corresponding finger, as illustrated in Figure 41.3F.

The stream of spray is applied over the muscles and includes the wrist and fingers. Effective stretch of all of these muscles requires full flexion of the wrist *and fingers*, as illustrated.

Flexores Digitorum

The patterns of pain referred from the flexores digitorum sublimis and profundus are similar. Each section of these muscles refers pain to the corresponding finger; Figure 41.3G presents an example. Patients with TrPs in this muscle may describe the pain as extending to the tip of the finger, occasionally shooting beyond the tip.

Vapocoolant spray is applied distalward, as in Figure 41.3G. The wrist and fingers must be extended simultaneously for a full stretch.

Interossei of Hand

Myofascial TrPs of the interossei are relatively common. The dorsal interossei are readily palpable against the metacarpal bones. Interosseous TrPs refer pain along the side of the digit that corresponds to the distal attachment of that muscle. In addition, the first dorsal interosseus usually projects pain across the hand and into the little finger (Fig. 41.3H). In some patients interosseus TrPs are an important contributing cause of Heberden's nodes, which may be aborted early in their development by inactivation of the responsible interosseous TrPs.

The stream of vapocoolant spray is applied distalward with stretch by adduction of the index finger, as in Figure 41.3H. Frequently injection is required.

TRUNK AND BACK PAIN

Muscles of the chest and abdomen frequently exhibit misleading viscerosomatic and somatovisceral interactions. A viscerosomatic example is the development of satellite TrPs in the pectoralis major muscle in response to an acute myocardial infarction or to myocardial ischemia (4). Another example is the appearance of TrPs in the external oblique muscle of the abdomen secondary to pain referred into that region by gastrointestinal ulcer disease (34).

A somatovisceral example is the cardiac arrhythmia associated with the "arrhythmia TrP" in the right pectoralis major muscle (4).

Pectoralis Major and Minor

The pectoralis minor muscle and the more horizontal fibers of the sternal division of the pectoralis major muscle commonly refer pain that closely mimics cardiac ischemia (Fig. 41.4A) (4, 25). The lateral, nearly vertical lower fibers of the pectoralis major refer pain and *tenderness* to the breast (Fig. 41.4B), causing severe breast hypersensitivity that, in either sex, may render clothing contact intolerable.

For either of the pectoral muscles, vapocoolant is first directed upward and laterally over the muscle and its referred pain pattern as in Figure 41.4A and B.

Stretch is applied to the sternal division of the pectoralis major, as illustrated by the curved white arrow in Figure 41.4A, whereas stretch is applied to the pectoralis minor by retraction of the scapula with backward traction on the arm. The nearly vertical thoracic fibers along the lateral border of the pectoralis major are partially stretched by the intermediate position shown in Figure 41.4B. They are fully stretched by *full* flexion of the arm at the shoulder. This fully flexed position also stretches the anterior costal fibers of the latissimus dorsi. Therefore, when it, too, is tense, the latissimus dorsi also must be released, as in Figure 41.2G, to achieve full pectoralis range of motion.

For lasting inactivation of pectoralis TrPs, a head-forward, round-shouldered posture, which maintains the pectoral muscles in the shortened position, must be corrected. In the seated position this poor posture is spontaneously improved without muscle strain by use of a comfortable lumbar support, a towel roll or small pillow placed against the small of the back at waistline level (4). This ensures the maintenance of a full normal lumbar curve.

Serratus Anterior

Although the serratus anterior is not considered a respiratory muscle, its active TrPs restrict chest expansion and cause shortness of breath (4). Figure 41.4C portrays its referred pain pattern.

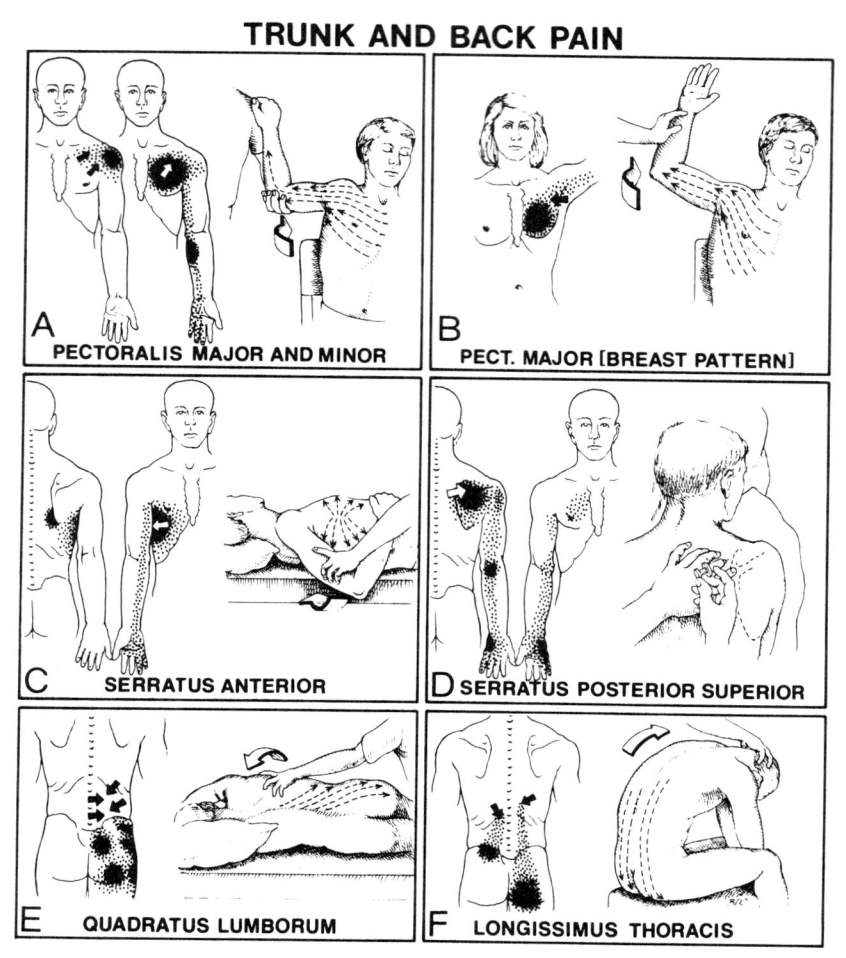

500 Pain Management in Selected Disorders/Section 3

Figure 41.4A–F. Location of TrPs (*short straight white* or *black arrows*) and pain patterns (*solid black and stipples*), stretch positions, and spray patterns (*dashed arrows*) for 10 muscles that cause trunk and back pain. The *curved white arrows* identify the direction(s) of pressure applied to stretch the muscle. The *dashed arrows* trace the impact of the stream of vapocoolant spray applied to release the muscular tension during stretch. (From Simons DG: Myofascial pain syndromes. In Basmajian JV, Kirby RL (eds): *Medical Rehabilitation*. Baltimore, Williams and Wilkins, 1984, pp 317, 318.)

Chapter 41/Single-Muscle Myofascial Pain Syndromes 501

G LOWER THORACIC ILIOCOSTALIS **H** **I** UPPER LUMBAR ILIOCOSTALIS

J MULTIFIDUS **K** EXTERNAL OBLIQUE

L **M** UPPER AND LOWER RECTUS ABDOMINUS **N** McBURNEY'S POINT

PAIN PATTERN TRIGGER POINT ➡

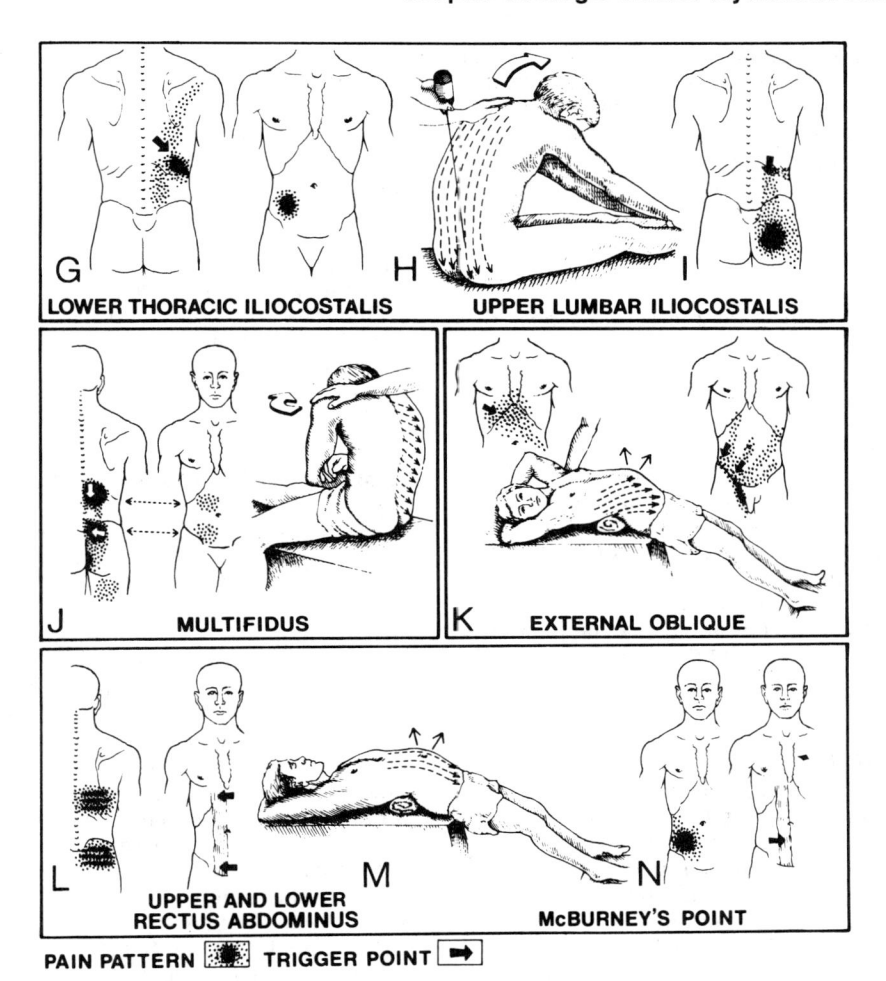

Figure 41.4G–N.

Vapocoolant is applied in radial sweeps (Fig. 41.4C) that should cover the lower half of the scapula. The serratus anterior may be stretched with the patient supine, as illustrated in Figure 41.4C, or comfortably seated in an armchair. Self-stretch is performed when seated by using the uninvolved arm to reach behind the torso and pull on the distal humerus of the involved side to strongly retract the scapula.

Serratus Posterior Superior

The enigmatic referred pain of the serratus posterior superior (Fig. 41.4D) is threateningly deep and frequently projects into and through the upper chest, suggesting visceral disease. Positioning of the arm often provides no relief. To palpate serratus posterior superior TrPs, the scapula must be fully protracted in order to uncover the lateral ends of the muscle (4). The tenderness of these TrPs is palpated through the trapezius and rhomboid muscles against the ribs. Some release of the muscle can be obtained by manual stretch, but stretch is frequently unsatisfactory. Trigger points in this muscle usually require ischemic compression or local injection, as illustrated in Figure 41.4D. When injecting, one should direct the needle nearly parallel to the skin surface and always toward a rib, not toward an intercostal space, to be sure of avoiding a pneumothorax.

Quadratus Lumborum

The quadratus lumborum muscle is one of the most common sources of musculoskeletal low back pain (25, 35, 36) and is commonly overlooked (37), partly because effective palpation requires unusual positioning of the patient. Active TrPs in the quadratus lumborum project pain to the sacroiliac joint, lower buttock, and lateral hip regions (Fig. 41.4E) (31, 35, 38). Satellite TrPs often generated in the posterior section of the gluteus minimus muscle cause a secondary sciatica-like pain pattern (see Fig. 41.5D) that further misleads the diagnostician. Bilateral quadratus lumborum TrPs are common and produce pain that extends bilaterally across the sacroiliac regions.

For precise examination of the quadratus lumborum muscle, the side-lying patient is positioned to open a space between the twelfth rib and the crest of the ilium. Space is provided by elevating the rib cage and tilting the pelvis downward on that side. The examination position is nearly the stretch position of Figure 41.4E, except that the upper leg lies behind the lower leg and the uppermost knee rests on the examining table (29, 35, 38).

The vapocoolant spray is directed distally to cover all of the lumbar area and buttock, emphasizing the sacral and sacroiliac joint region, especially when that region is reported as painful. Two stretch positions may be required (35). One is the leg-forward position shown in Figure 41.4E, which tilts the pelvis away from the ribs and rotates it forward. The other is the leg-back position (29, 35), which places the upper leg behind the lower leg, reverses the rotation on the thoracolumbar region, and simultaneously lengthens the adjacent iliopsoas muscle. To release restricting tension in the latter muscle, spray is directed downward over the abdomen, close to the midline, and over the inguinal region and the inner thigh to completely cover the skin representation of the muscle and its pain reference zones (35, 38). The iliopsoas muscle can, itself, be an important source of referred pain (33, 36).

Injection of TrPs in the quadratus lumborum is effective, but requires careful technique and appreciation of the regional anatomy involved (29, 35).

Quadratus lumborum TrPs are usually perpetuated by a short leg and/or a small hemipelvis. Both are correctable by appropriate heel and butt lifts, which are often *essential* for lasting relief of this myofascial pain syndrome (4, 35, 38).

Thoracic and Lumbar Paraspinal Muscles (4, 38)

In the midthoracic region, the most medial paraspinal muscle, the spinalis, lies against the spinous processes. Next laterally is the superficial longissimus, one of the longest muscles in the body. It extends from the occiput to the sacrum. The superficial and most lateral paraspinal fibers, the iliocostalis, attach to the ribs. Bilaterally, the direction of the deeper paraspinal muscles, the multifidi and rotatores, presents an inverted "V" configuration; the deeper they lie the shorter they are, and the more diagonal is their course. The deepest, the rotatores, course between adjacent vertebrae at nearly a 45° angle. To adequately stretch these fibers one must often mobilize adjacent vertebrae by using a manual medicine technique, such as strongly rotating and flexing the spine simultaneously.

Taut bands and local twitch responses are easily identified in the longissimus fibers. These TrPs refer pain distally many segments removed, sometimes reaching the distal buttock (Fig. 41.4F).

Lower thoracic iliocostalis TrPs refer pain as in Figure 41.4G, whereas Figure 41.4I shows the pain pattern of upper lumbar iliocostalis TrPs. The multifidi refer pain locally (Fig. 41.4J). The rotatores frequently refer pain to the midline at the same segmental level. Generally, thoracolumbar paraspinal muscles refer pain caudalward (Fig. 41.4G), so that the spray is applied bilaterally downward, including the buttocks (Fig. 41.4H). Multifidus TrPs respond to a shorter, more angulated unilateral spray pattern (Fig. 41.4J).

Stretch position for the longissimus is shown in Figure 41.4F, with the patient's feet on the floor and the legs spread apart far enough that the arms can dangle freely between them. The patient must allow the wrists and elbows to flex in a relaxed manner as the fingers encounter the floor. The parallel sweeps of spray should also cover the gluteus maximus muscle (Fig. 41.4F and I), because it is stretched by the full hip flexion. Relaxation and stretch of the iliocostalis may be augmented by rotating the patient's chest to the opposite side.

For stretch of the multifidi, full rotation is applied toward the involved side (Fig. 41.4J), preferably without flexion. Injection is often necessary for the deepest diagonal muscles. In the thoracic region the needle must be angled medially toward the spinous processes to avoid a pneumothorax.

Caution must be used in stretch of the lumbar paraspinals. Normal lumbar lordosis must not be compromised. If hypermobility is present, rhythmic stabilization exercise in the neutral position is preferable.

Abdominal Muscles

Myofascial TrPs in the abdominal external oblique muscle may refer pain locally, into adjacent areas, and sometimes across the midline (Fig. 41.4K), (4, 25, 39). Those TrPs close to the thoracic or pelvic attachment of the rectus abdominis muscle commonly refer pain *horizontally* across the back at nearly the same level as the TrP (Fig. 41.4L). A McBurney's point TrP in the rectus abdominis may convincingly simulate the pain and tenderness of appendicitis (Fig. 41.4N). Tensing the abdominal muscles by elevating both feet in the supine position easily permits differentiation of visceral from abdominal wall tenderness. This tensing of the abdominal muscles augments TrP tenderness and protects the viscera from the pressure of palpation (40). If the patient has a suspected back problem that prevents this maneuver, he or she can, instead, strongly contract the abdominal muscles while supine by exerting downward extension of the upper limbs against resistance.

The spray pattern for TrPs in the rectus abdominis muscles is illustrated in Figure 41.4M. Stretch of the abdominal wall muscles is achieved by positioning the patient as in the same figure and having the patient protrude the abdomen by taking a deep breath and contracting the diaphragm while relaxing the abdominal wall muscles. The patient must not hold the breath (close the glottis). The rotation movement that should be added to stretch the external oblique muscle (Fig. 41.4K) is not required to stretch the rectus abdominis.

LOWER EXTREMITY PAIN

Generally, TrPs in lower extremity muscles refer pain locally and/or distally. However, the adductor muscles also refer pain proximally. Since patients commonly identify gluteal pain as low back pain, gluteal muscle TrPs are likely to contribute to a "low back pain" complaint (39).

Gluteus Maximus

Like the deltoid muscle, gluteus maximus TrPs are easily palpated for taut bands and show vigorous local twitch responses. The gluteus maximus generates local referred pain that concentrates mainly over the sacrum and inferior surface of the buttock (Fig. 41.5A).

The patient is placed in the side-lying position for stretch and spray (Fig. 41.5A). The vapocoolant spray is directed distally, as illustrated, while the thigh is progressively flexed by bringing the knee toward the chest. Active gluteal TrPs are commonly associated with tight hamstring muscles; these would also need to be released by stretch and spray (see Fig. 41.6C) to achieve full range of hip motion and lasting relief.

Gluteus Medius

TrPs in the gluteus medius refer pain (Fig. 41.5B) along the crest of the ilium posteriorly and over the sacrum; pain may also extend across the buttock and over the upper thigh posteriorly.

The line of impact of the stream of vapocoolant spray extends from the crest of the ilium distalward over the upper *half of the thigh* as indicated in Figure 41.5B. For passive stretch, the thigh is flexed nearly 90° and progressively adducted as the spray is applied. Pulling backward on the anterior superior iliac spine augments the stretch. The Dudley J. Morton foot configuration, when present, is a perpetuating factor and should be corrected (4, 35, 39).

Gluteus Minimus

The anterior and posterior portions of the gluteus minimus project separate referred pain patterns. The anterior TrPs refer pain to the thigh laterally and also to the buttock, as in Figure 41.5C, whereas TrPs in the posterior part of the muscle refer pain to the lower extremity posteriorly, as in Figure 41.5D. This pattern suggests an S1 radiculopathy or "sciatica." Adding to the confusion, gluteus minimus TrPs may be perpetuated by an S1 radiculopathy.

Location of the sweeps of spray for release of TrPs in the anterior portion of the muscle and its stretch position are portrayed in Figure 41.5C. For TrPs in the posterior portion, they are shown in Figure 41.5D. In neither case is it necessary to fully bend the knee, but if the knee is straight, hamstring tension may block full hip flexion. The gluteous maximus muscle is included in the posterior spray pattern to release restricting TrPs that it may harbor.

Piriformis

Active piriformis TrPs restrict both adduction and internal rotation of the thigh at the hip. Tenderness is elicited by external or rectal palpation (39). Figure 41.5E shows the piriformis referred pain pattern and the vapocoolant is directed as illustrated. For stretch, the thigh of the side-lying patient is flexed at the hip to nearly 90° and internally rotated as the knee is lowered gently to increase adduction at the hip, as depicted in Figure 41.5E. Gravity can be used to facilitate adduction by allowing the leg to hang over the edge of the treatment table. The gluteus maximus muscle also should be sprayed if it is blocking full range of movement.

Tension caused by taut bands due to TrPs in the piriformis muscle may entrap the peroneal part or all of the sciatic nerve, depending upon anatomic variations, as the nerve passes through instead of around the muscle (39).

Adductores Longus and Brevis

In addition to the pattern in Figure 41.5F, pain from either the long or short hip adductors may be referred

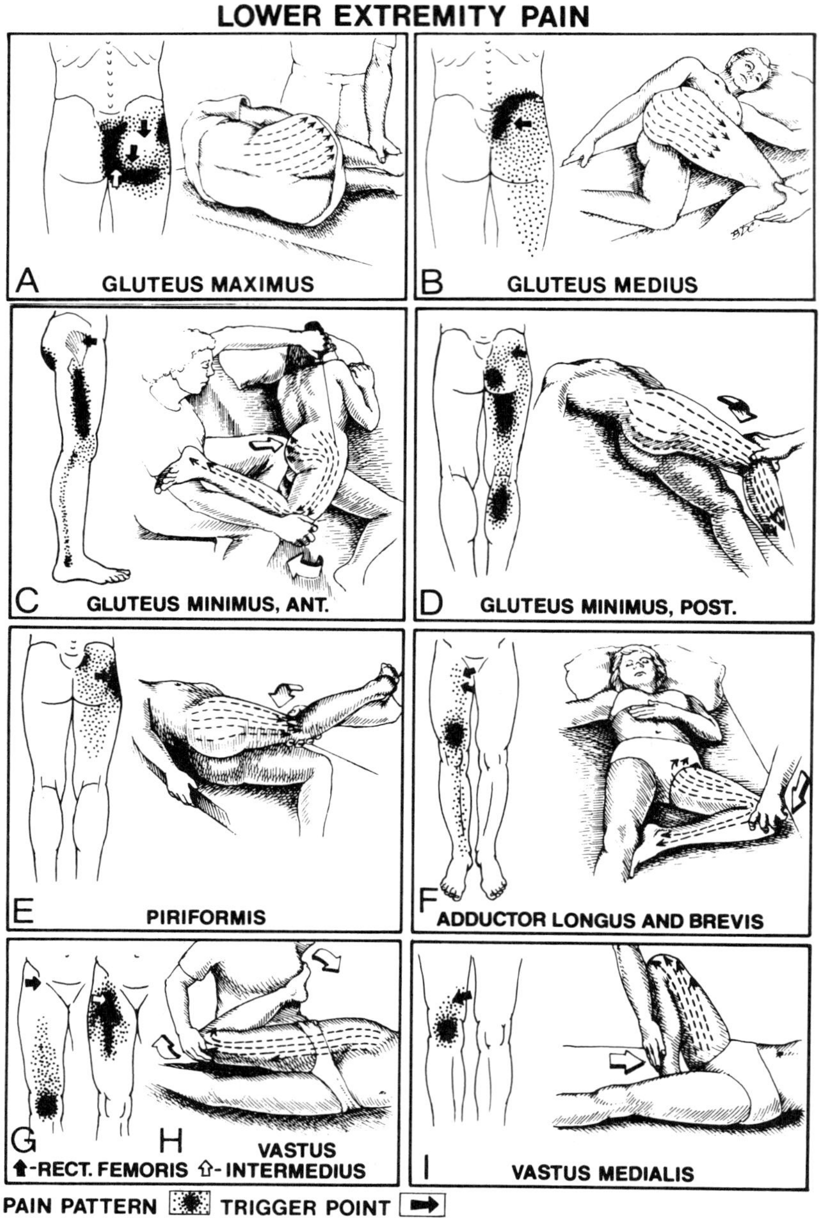

LOWER EXTREMITY PAIN

Figure 41.5. Location of TrPs (*short straight black* or *white arrows*) and pain patterns (*solid black and stipples*), stretch positions, and spray patterns (*dashed arrows*) for nine muscles responsible for lower extremity pain. The *curved white arrows* identify the direction(s) of pressure applied to stretch a muscle. The *dashed arrows* trace the impact of the stream of vapocoolant spray applied to release the muscular tension during stretch. (From Simons DG: Myofascial pain syndromes. In Basmajian JV, Kirby RL (eds): *Medical Rehabilitation*. Baltimore, Williams & Wilkins, 1984, pp 318, 319.

upward throughout the groin (1, 33). Active TrPs in these muscles markedly restrict abduction of the thigh.

To inactivate TrPs in these muscles, sweeps of the vapocoolant that overlap in the midthigh are directed proximally as well as distally (Fig. 41.5F). As the spray is applied, the muscle is gradually lengthened by placing the patient in the position shown in Figure 41.5F and gently helping the knee downward toward the examining table (white arrow).

Quadriceps Femoris

Active TrPs in the **rectus femoris** muscle are usually located at the proximal end of the muscle near the solid black arrow in Figure 41.5G. They project pain to the front of the knee, as shown in the same figure.

Vastus intermedius TrPs are found in the area near the small white arrow in Figure 41.5G; they lie deeper and more distal than the rectus femoris TrP and refer pain intensely over the upper thigh anteriorly.

Vastus medialis TrPs refer pain (Figure 41.5I) to the anteromedial aspect of the knee and to the patellar area. When this muscle is suddenly overloaded, its TrPs may reflexly inhibit contraction without pain, giving rise to the buckling knee syndrome.

The TrPs found distally in the anterior portion of the **vastus lateralis** muscle (solid black arrow, Fig. 41.6A) are frequently multiple and difficult to eliminate; they refer pain intensely and extensively as shown in Figure 41.6A. The TrPs found more proximally in the posterior portion of the vastus lateralis are located near the small white arrow on the right lower extremity shown at the left side of Figure 41.6B, and usually refer pain vertically in a local pattern.

To inactivate TrPs in the rectus femoris, the patient lies on the unaffected side, as in Figure 41.5H. The parallel sweeps of vapocoolant are directed distally, as illustrated, and the knee is flexed *while extending the hip*. For release of TrPs in the other three quadriceps muscles, the spray is applied distalward over each muscle as shown in Figure 41.5H and I. Knee flexion alone, regardless of hip position, stretches all three vasti, but not the rectus femoris.

Biceps Femoris

Pain is referred to the biceps femoris from TrPs that are located near the tip of the black arrow in Figure 41.6B. Release of hamstring tightness is most easily attained by initially directing the spray upward over the adductor magnus and inguinal region of the supine patient while horizontally abducting the thigh at the hip without raising the leg (not illustrated). The lower extremity is then elevated to bring the thigh directly from the abducted position to the 90° flexed position while the spray is applied over the true "hamstring" muscles in the pattern of Figure 41.6C.

Soleus

The TrPs in the soleus, a second-layer, single-joint muscle (Fig. 41.6D), cause referred heel pain and *tenderness* that frequently are mistaken for symptoms caused by a heel spur. Occasionally, TrPs in this muscle also project pain to the sacroiliac joint region on the same side, as illustrated elsewhere (35, 39).

The prone patient is positioned and vapocoolant is directed as in Figure 41.6D, over the entire muscle. Progressive downward dorsiflexion pressure is then applied firmly (curved white arrow) to the ball of the foot. Self-stretch of this muscle is accomplished by standing with the heel flat on the floor and progressively *bending the knee*. Self-stretch of the gastrocnemius is similar, but requires that the knee remain straight.

Gastrocnemius

Myofascial TrPs are usually found in the gastrocnemius, a superficial, two-joint muscle, in either the medial (Fig. 41.6E) or lateral (not shown) border of the muscle. The TrPs in either head refer pain essentially as seen in the same figure (31, 35). These TrPs render walking uphill especially painful and commonly cause nocturnal calf cramps.

For treatment, the patient lies prone with the knee straight and the foot dorsiflexed at the ankle, as in Figure 41.6E. The stream of spray is directed distally over all of the muscle and includes the foot, which is firmly dorsiflexed by the operator's knee in order to apply the necessary force in the direction of the curved white arrow in Figure 41.6E. As with all other muscles, the pressure applied should NEVER be painful, but applied only to the point of beginning discomfort.

The patient is taught how to self-stretch the gastrocnemius muscle by standing with the knee straight on the affected side and with the involved leg behind the other leg while shifting the pelvis and body forward. As the forward knee bends the ankle of the affected leg dorsiflexes with the rear knee fully extended. The *heel remains solidly on the floor*.

Tibialis Anterior

The tibialis anterior dorsiflexes and inverts the foot. Its TrPs (black arrow in Figure 41.6F) refer pain as illustrated, concentrating on the great toe (1, 31).

To release anterior tibial TrPs, the patient lies supine and spray is directed distalward over the muscle, as shown in Figure 41.6F. This muscle is passively lengthened by simultaneously plantar flexing and slowly everting the foot (white curved arrow, Fig. 41.6F).

Peroneus Longus and Brevis

The adjacent peroneus longus and brevis muscles have similar functions and essentially the same referred pain pattern. The TrPs in the peroneus longus (black arrow in Fig. 41.6G) are usually a few centimeters distal to the common peroneal nerve where it passes over the fibula beneath the peroneus longus muscle, just distal to the fibular head (1). Peroneus brevis TrPs are more distal, approximately midleg (35).

For both muscles, treatment begins with application of vapocoolant spray in the pattern shown in Figure 41.6G.

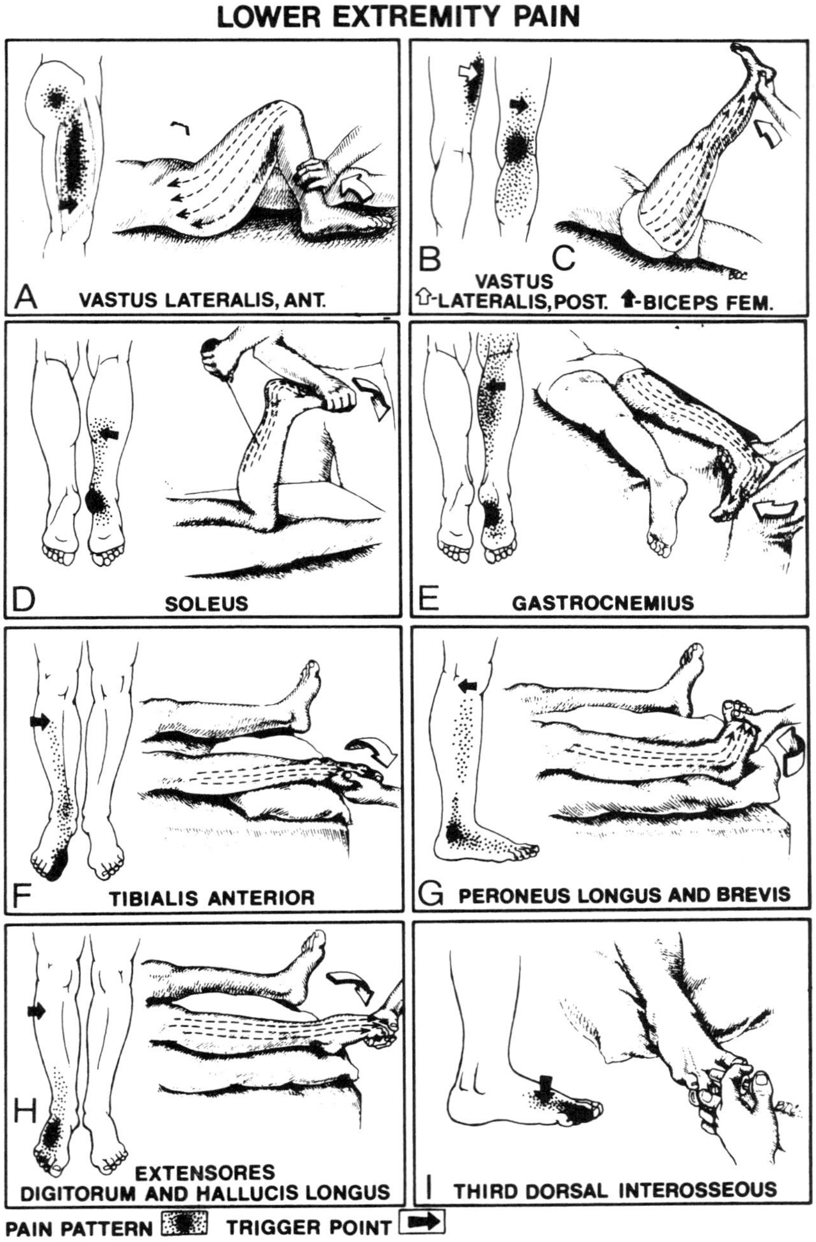

506 Pain Management in Selected Disorders/Section 3

LOWER EXTREMITY PAIN

A VASTUS LATERALIS, ANT.
B VASTUS LATERALIS, POST. C BICEPS FEM.
D SOLEUS
E GASTROCNEMIUS
F TIBIALIS ANTERIOR
G PERONEUS LONGUS AND BREVIS
H EXTENSORES DIGITORUM AND HALLUCIS LONGUS
I THIRD DORSAL INTEROSSEOUS

PAIN PATTERN   TRIGGER POINT

Figure 41.6. Location of TrPs (*short straight black* or *white arrows*) and pain patterns (*solid black and stipples*), stretch positions, and spray patterns (*dashed arrows*) for 10 muscles causing lower extremity pain. The *curved white arrows* identify the direction(s) of pressure applied to stretch the muscle. The *dashed arrows* trace the impact of the stream of vapocoolant spray applied to release the muscular tension during stretch. In *B*, both are right lower extremities. (From Simons DG: Myofascial pain syndromes. In Basmajian JV, Kirby RL (eds): *Medical Rehabilitation.* Baltimore, Williams & Wilkins, 1984, pp 319, 320.)

The foot of the supine patient is plantar flexed and inverted (curved white arrow in Fig. 41.6G).

Tension caused by the taut bands of TrPs in the peroneus longus muscle can compress the deep peroneal nerve against the underlying fibula. This sometimes results in loss of sensation in the common peroneal nerve distribution with partial foot-drop weakness. When the TrPs are released, these symptoms, which are due to neurapraxia, resolve in minutes to days. This myofascial syndrome is perpetuated by the instability and stress of walking on the "knife-edge" of a long second metatarsal bone (D.J. Morton foot configuration) (4, 35).

Extensores Digitorum and Hallucis Longus

Active TrPs in the extensores digitorum and hallucis longus muscles, like those of the peroneal muscles, refer pain that includes the dorsum of the foot laterally (Fig. 41.6H). In addition, pain may extend further distally to the toes.

Vapocoolant is applied distalward in the pattern shown in Figure 41.6H; both muscles are stretched by simultaneously plantar flexing the foot and all toes.

Interossei of the Foot

As in the hand, foot interosseous TrPs are not rare. These TrPs, like those in the hand (4), refer pain distally to the side of the digit corresponding to the attachment of the involved muscle, as illustrated for the third dorsal interosseus in Figure 41.6I. These TrPs are commonly associated with the hammer toe that, if not too long-standing, can be alleviated by inactivating the corresponding interosseous TrPs. The taut bands and TrPs are exquisitely tender. They are readily palpable against the metatarsal bones and, therefore, easily injected (Fig. 41.6I). Stretch and spray alone may not be adequate therapy for these muscles.

Acknowledgment The author gratefully acknowledges the thoughtful and meticulous review of the manuscript by Janet G. Travell, M.D. and Lois Statham Simons, R.P.T., M.S.

References

1. Travell J, Rinzler SH: The myofascial genesis of pain. *Postrad Med* 11:425–434, 1952.
2. Sola AE, Rodenberger ML, Gettys BB: Incidence of hypersensitive areas in posterior shoulder muscles. *Am J Phys Med* 34:585–590, 1955.
3. Bates T, Grunwaldt E: Myofascial pain in childhood. *J Pediatr* 53:198–209, 1958.
4. Travell JG, Simons DG: *Myofascial Pain and Dysfunction: The Trigger Point Manual.* Baltimore, Williams & Wilkins, 1983.
5. Langs HM: Myofascial pain and analgesia. *Pain Suppl* 4:S297, 1987 (abstr 570).
6. Jaeger B, Reeves JL: Quantification of changes in myofascial trigger point sensitivity with the pressure algometer following passive stretch. *Pain* 27:203–210, 1986.
7. Crook J, Tunks E. Norman G, et al: A comparative study of tenderness thresholds in trigger points and non-trigger points in normal and fibromyalgia patients. *Pain Suppl* 4:S307, 1987 (abstr 509).
8. Scudds RA, McCain GA, Rollman GB, et al: Changes in pain responsiveness in fibrositis patients after successful treatment. *Pain Suppl* 4:S353, 1987 (abstr 677).
9. Tunks E, Norman G, Kalaher S, et al: Validity and reliability of the clinical use of a pressure algometer in the study of trigger points. *Pain Suppl* 4:S307, 1987 (abstr 590).
10. Jensen K, Andersen HO, Olesen J, et al: Pressure-pain threshold in human temporal region. Evaluation of a new pressure algometer. *Pain* 25:313–323, 1986.
11. Fischer AA: Pressure threshold meter: its use for quantification of tender spots. *Arch Phys Med Rehabil* 67:836–838, 1986.
12. Fischer AA: Pressure tolerance over muscles and bones in normal subjects. *Arch Phys Med Rehabil* 67:406–409, 1986.
13. Fischer AA: Tissue compliance meter for objective, quantitative documentation of soft tissue consistency and pathology. *Arch Phys Med Rehabil* 68:122–125, 1987.
14. Reeves JL, Jaeger B, Graff-Radford SB: Reliability of the pressure algometer as a measure of myofascial trigger point sensitivity. *Pain* 24:313–321, 1986.
15. Schiffman E, Fricton J, Haley D, et al: A pressure algometer for myofascial pain syndrome: reliability and validity. *Pain Suppl* 4:S291, 1987 (abstr 558).
16. Fricton JR, et al: Myofascial pain syndrome: electromyographic changes associated with local twitch response. *Arch Phys Med Rehabil* 66:314–317, 1985.
17. Simons DG: Myofascial pain syndrome due to trigger points. In Goodgold J (ed): *Rehabilitation Medicine.* St. Louis, CV Mosby, 1988 (in press).
18. Mense S, Schmidt RF: Muscle pain: which receptors are responsible for the transmission of noxious stimuli? In Rose FC (ed): *Physiological Aspects of Clinical Neurology.* Oxford, Blackwell Scientific Publications, 1977.
19. Institute of Medicine: *Pain and Disability: Clinical Behavioral and Public Policy Perspectives.* Washington DC, National Academy Press, 1987.
20. Bengtsson A, Henriksson K-G, Jorfeldt L, et al: Primary fibromyalgia—a clinical and laboratory study of 55 patients. *Scand J Rheumatol* 15:340–347, 1986.
21. Lund N, Bengtsson A, Thorborg P: Muscle tissue oxygen pressure in primary fibromyalgia. *Scand J Rheumatol* 15:165–173, 1986.
22. Bengtsson A, Henriksson K-G, Larsson J: Reduced high-energy phosphate levels in painful muscle in patients with primary fibromyalgia. *Arthritis Rheum* 29:817–821, 1986.
23. Bengtsson A, Henriksson K-G, Larsson J: Muscle biopsy in primary fibromyalgia. *Scand J Rheumatol* 15:1–6, 1986.
24. Graff-Radford SB, Reeves JL, Jaeger B: Management of chronic headache and neck pain: effectiveness of altering factors perpetuating myofascial pain. *Headache* 27:186–190, 1987.
25. Sola AE: Treatment of myofascial pain syndromes. In Benedetti C et al (eds): *Advances in Pain Research and Therapy.* New York, Raven Press, 1984, vol 7, pp 467–485.
26. Lewit K: Postisometric relaxation in combination with other methods of muscular facilitation and inhibition. *Manual Med* 1:101–104, 1986.
27. Rubin D: An approach to the management of myofascial trigger point syndromes. *Arch Phys Med Rehabil* 62:107–110, 1981.
28. Reynolds MD: Myofascial trigger points in persistent posttraumatic shoulder pain. *South Med J* 77:1277–1280, 1984.

29. Simons DG: Myofascial pain syndromes due to trigger points: 2. Treatment and single-muscle syndromes. *Manual Med* 1:72–77, 1985.
30. Travell J: Rapid relief of acute "stiff neck" by ethyl chloride spray. *J Am Med Wom Assoc* 4:89–95, 1949.
31. Sola AE: Trigger point therapy. In Roberts JR, Hedges JR (eds): *Clinical Procedures in Emergency Medicine*. Philadelphia, WB Saunders, 1985.
32. Reynolds MD: Myofascial trigger point syndromes in the practice of rheumatology. *Arch Phys Med Rehabil* 62:111–114, 1981.
33. Simons DG, Travell JG: Myofascial pain syndromes. Wall PD, Melzack R (eds): In *Textbook of Pain*. London, Churchill Livingstone, 1984, pp 263–276.
34. Melnick J: Trigger areas and refractory pain in duodenal ulcer. *NY State J Med* 57:1073–1076, 1957.
35. Travell JG, Simons DG: *Myofascial Pain and Dysfunction: The Trigger Point Manual, Vol. II*. Baltimore, Williams & Wilkins, in process, est. 1989.
36. Zohn DA: The quadratus lumborum: an unrecognized source of back pain, clinical and thermographic aspects. *Orthop Rev* 15:87–92, 1985.
37. Sola AE, Williams RL: Myofascial pain syndromes. *Neurology* 6:91–95, 1956.
38. Simons DG, Travell JG: Myofascial origins of low back pain. 2. Torso muscles. *Postgrad Med* 73:81–92, 1983.
39. Simons DG, Travell JG: Myofascial origins of low back pain. 3. Pelvic and lower extremity muscles. *Postgrad Med* 73:99–108, 1983.
40. Slocumb JC: Neurological factors in chronic pelvic pain: trigger points and the abdominal pelvic pain syndrome. *Am J Obstet Gynecol* 149:536–543, 1984.

chapter 42
Chronic Myofascial Pain Syndrome

David G. Simons, M.D.
Lois Statham Simons, M.S., R.P.T.

This and the preceding chapter provide a basis for managing the *chronic* myofascial pain syndrome (MPS). The goal is to eliminate the multiple *causes* of the pain rather than deal with it only as a symptom. The previous chapter summarized the identification and treatment of a single-muscle MPS due to trigger points (TrPs). Such a single syndrome can multiply by the addition of satellite and secondary TrPs that arise and persist because of perpetuating factors. A chronic MPS develops from these additional, but treatable, TrP syndromes. Management of this complex problem is simplified by resolving the total myofascial pain picture into its single-muscle components and by correcting the perpetuating factors. By identifying the myofascial syndromes muscle by muscle, one can recognize the pieces of the puzzle that comprise the total pain picture and proceed to manage each one individually.

This chapter first examines two kinds of perpetuating factors, systemic and mechanical. Then it reviews treatment techniques used to inactivate myofascial TrPs: stretch and spray, other physical methods, and injection with stretch. Next, it compares myofascial TrPs with two other closely interrelated but separate conditions, fibrositis/fibromyalgia and articular dysfunction. Finally, it summarizes how all of these issues are addressed in the care of a patient who has a chronic MPS due to TrPs.

Chronic pain that has not been attributable to an organic disease process is a major unsolved problem of the health care system in this country (1). This unsolved problem accounts for the popularity of pain management clinics that help the patient to *live with* his or her pain. Too often, the clinics do frustratingly little to teach the patient how to *relieve* the pain (1). Fields pointed out, "The most common persistent and disabling pains are those of musculoskeletal origin (2), with which this chapter is concerned.

Many directors of chronic pain programs have come to recognize two basic facts concerning their patients. First, few if any of these patients have only one condition that is responsible for their suffering. There are multiple *interacting* factors. Second, no two patients are alike. Thus, the success of a chronic pain program hinges on:

1. Identification of which of a multitude of sources are significant contributors to the suffering of the individual patient.
2. Estimation of the relative importance of the sources of suffering with an understanding of the interactions in the patient.
3. Effective therapy of the major causes applied in an order and combination that respects their interactions.

We have much to learn.

If the health care provider is to relieve the patient's chronic pain, that provider must address issues and apply therapeutic measures that were previously overlooked. A well-known disease like rheumatoid arthritis may be well managed, but the chronic myofascial TrPs may have been overlooked (3). Key answers must not have been part of conventional medical training; otherwise conventional medicine would have solved the problem.

Apparently, myofascial pain syndromes are a much more common cause of chronic pain than is generally appreciated. In a comprehensive pain center, myofascial TrPs were considered the primary cause of pain in 85% of the patients admitted to the program (4). In a dental clinic for patients with chronic head and neck pain, over half of the patients were found to have a primary diagnosis of myofascial pain syndrome (5). In a general practice of internal medicine, 10% of all patients, and 31% of those presenting with a pain complaint, had myofascial TrPs that were primarily responsible for their symptoms (6).

We owe Janet G. Travell, M.D., a great debt of gratitude for her clinical genius, research, and dedication that have established the diagnosis and management of myofascial pain. She published in 1952 the first compendium of individual pain patterns characteristic of the muscles most commonly responsible for myofascial pain throughout the body (7). This early work has been the key to understanding and managing acute single-muscle myofascial pain syndromes. Dr. Travell was the first to decipher the causal relationship between persistent myofascial TrPs that cause a chronic MPS and the multiple factors that perpetuate those TrPs. She clearly identified this relationship in 1976 (8) and described many perpetuating factors in detail in 1983 (9).

PERPETUATING FACTORS

Perpetuating factors act clinically like the missing link that converts an acute single-muscle syndrome into a chronic pain syndrome. These factors may be systemic or mechanical. Systemic factors are a frequent problem and they increase the irritability of the skeletal muscles throughout the body. Mechanical factors are equally ubiquitous and they overload and aggravate TrPs in specific muscles, depending on which muscle or muscles are overstressed (9).

In our experience, a patient with chronic pain due to myofascial TrPs nearly always has one, and often several, perpetuating factors that must be resolved before the myofascial components of the pain can be managed as single-muscle syndromes. Patients whose myofascial pain picture has remained essentially *static* for months or longer may not have serious perpetuating factors; specific myofascial local treatment can give these patients lasting relief. Patients in whom myofascial TrP symptoms have been *progressive* in time and who respond to treatment only temporarily, at best, consistently have perpetuating factors that must be resolved. Their primary TrPs generate satellite and secondary TrPs as previously described (9).

Generally, one stress activates a TrP and other factors perpetuate it. Prior to activation of a TrP, existing perpetuating factors usually cause negligible symptoms. For example, a leg length discrepancy of 6 mm (1/4″) may have caused no symptoms throughout most of a lifetime; however, when quadratus lumborum TrPs are activated by an accident or repetitive strain, the leg length difference becomes the perpetuator of the newly established TrPs. For lasting relief of the pain referred from the quadratus lumborum TrPs, the previously innocuous leg length discrepancy must be corrected.

The presence of significant perpetuating factors is confirmed by a poor response, or no response, to a trial of specific myofascial therapy applied to the muscle causing the myofascial pain. Although the initial response may be good, the symptoms soon return, sometimes in hours, more often in days. Lack of any response to the therapeutic trial may mean that treatment was applied to a latent TrP and not to the active TrP that was responsible for the pain. Occasionally, severe perpetuating factors render myofascial TrPs so extremely irritable that even gentle stretch and spray does not relieve the TrPs, and in fact may aggravate them.

SYSTEMIC FACTORS

Systemic perpetuating factors can aggravate TrPs in any muscle and increase the irritability of all skeletal muscles. These systemic factors render the muscles more vulnerable to the development of initial, secondary, and satellite TrPs (9). Major systemic factors include enzyme dysfunction because of nutritional inadequacy, metabolic and endocrine dysfunction, chronic infection or infestation, and psychological stress.

Correction of a significant perpetuating factor reduces irritability of the muscles. The patient has less pain. The responsiveness of the muscles to specific myofascial therapy improves.

Skeletal muscles are energy engines. They convert the energy stored in adenosine triphosphate (ATP) to mechanical movement. Understandably, *anything* that interferes with energy metabolism of the muscle tends to compromise this energy function and increase muscle irritability.

Enzyme Dysfunction and Nutritional Inadequacy

The nutritional inadequacies that most commonly are found to perpetuate myofascial TrPs are insufficient B-complex vitamins, particularly B_1, B_6, B_{12}, and folic acid. Other nutritional inadequacies that perpetuate TrPs are low serum levels of the electrolytes potassium or calcium and insufficiency of major minerals such as zinc, copper, iron, and essential trace minerals. The effect of prolonged inadequacies (low normal or marginal stores) of many of these nutrients is a relatively unexplored field of medicine.

A vitamin is an essential nutrient not synthesized by the body. It serves as a coenzyme to many apoenzymes that are supplied by the body. In the absence of the vitamin coenzyme, the metabolic step performed by that apoenzyme is blocked. The effect of this blockage depends on how critical to body chemistry are the functions served by that enzyme. A summary of the enzymatic functions of each of these vitamins has been reviewed in detail (9).

Vitamin *deficiency* is signaled by abnormally low laboratory values, often by the excretion of abnormal metabolites, and by characteristic symptoms ascribable to a lack of that vitamin. Vitamin *inadequacy* is identified by laboratory values in the lower quartile of the normal range. Abnormal metabolites may be demonstrable in the blood and urine. Laboratory values for vitamins in the lower range of normal are *not optimal* values. The usual basis for selecting laboratory control subjects does not screen out individuals with marginal insufficiency, including many who show chemical evidence of abnormal vitamin-dependent enzyme function (10). Laboratory values in the lower quartile of "normal" may be seriously suboptimal and are clinically responsible for increased irritability of the muscles. Clinically, correction of the inadequacy reduces muscle irritability and improves its responsiveness to therapy. Table 42.1 summarizes the clinical distinctions between a vitamin deficiency and a vitamin inadequacy.

Experience with patients shows that the lower these serum values are within the lower quartile of the "normal" range, the more likely it is that the inadequacy will perpetuate TrPs. Other than pain, vitamin inadequacies cause clinical complaints that are often subtle and nonspecific; mental and physical functions are suboptimal.

The prevalence of unrecognized vitamin *deficiency* is remarkably high, especially in hospital patients. Among 120 hospital patients, 88% had abnormally low levels in one or more of 11 vitamins (11). Despite this high prevalence, the history of dietary intake was inadequate in only 39%. More than half of the patients were low in two or more vitamins. Serum folate, which was the most common vitamin deficiency, was low in 45% of these patients. Symptoms of vitamin deficiency were clinically apparent in only 38% of them (11).

If vitamin *deficiency* can be this common, how much more common must be vitamin *inadequacy*? Well-controlled studies have yet to be conducted that answer this question definitively. If inadequacy is indeed common, and if such inadequacies perpetuate myofascial TrPs, then one would expect a large proportion of chronic myofascial pain patients to have vitamin inadequacy. In fact, over half of the patients referred to a myofascial pain clinic had vitamin B_{12} inadequacy, folate inadequacy, or both (D.G. Simons, unpublished data, 1987). Shealy (12) measured blood vitamin levels in 150 patients with chronic pain; he found that 80% of smokers and 35% of nonsmokers were deficient in vitamin B_6. A *deficiency* of any of the four B vitamins is nearly always a serious perpetuator of myofascial TrPs; an *inadequacy* usually is a perpetuator. A recent study of inpatients with chronic pain (13) found insufficient blood levels of vitamins B_1, B_2, and folate. After pharmacologic supplementation with 12 vitamins for 12 days, the greatest pain relief was reported in those patients who registered the highest blood levels of vitamins B_1, B_6, B_{12}, and folic acid.

The common assumption that a well-balanced diet fully satisfies the metabolic need for a vitamin ignores loss of the vitamin during food preparation, impaired absorption, inadequate utilization, increased metabolic requirement, and increased excretion or destruction within the body (14). The wide variation in the requirements of individuals for essential nutrients, including vitamins, is well established (15). The official recommended dietary allowance (RDA) (16) is often considered the maximum amount anyone should need. That does not hold true for many chronic myofascial pain patients. As an extreme example, a few babies with a specific enzyme deficiency require megadose supplements of a vitamin coenzyme (e.g., B_{12}) for survival (17). These individuals have a severe congenital deficiency of an apoenzyme that requires that vitamin as its coenzyme. These congenital enzyme defects have been reviewed from the myofascial point of view (9). A minor degree of the same defect (poor genetic penetrance) could explain why some middle-aged patients gradually develop increased susceptibility to TrPs.

The Water-Soluble Vitamins The B-complex vitamins and vitamin C are water soluble. They have remarkably low toxicity because an excess is quickly excreted in the urine; the safety of all of these water-soluble vitamins is not questioned at 10 times the recommended dietary allowance (18).

Thiamine Inadequacy of thiamine (vitamin B_1) reveals its essential roles in nerve function and energy metabolism. Insufficiency causes increasingly severe loss of vibration sense at progressively more distal sites on the upper and lower extremities. The need for thiamine depends on the rate of energy expenditure. The daily RDA is 0.5 mg/1000 kcal of energy expenditure (16). Intact energy metabolism is essential to normal muscle function. The two life-threatening symptoms of severe thiamine deficiency are the disabling nervous system dysfunction of dry beriberi and the heart muscle failure with *severe* skeletal muscle weakness (19) of wet beriberi. Vitamin B_1 deficiency is well known in the alcoholic and heavy social drinker.

Pyridoxine Remarkably so, pyridoxine (vitamin B_6) is a jack of all trades; it is an essential coenzyme for more than 60 apoenzymes in human metabolism. It is a metabolic necessity for the synthesis and degradation of numerous amino acids, including the methionine-to-cysteine pathway. It activates phosphorylase, which release glucose from glycogen. It is essential for the synthesis of many neurotransmitters, is required for normal cell

Table 42.1
Distinctions Between Vitamin Deficiency and Vitamin Inadequacy

Vitamin Deficiency	Vitamin Inadequacy
Subnormal laboratory values	Lower quartile and marginal laboratory values
Excretion of abnormal metabolites	Abnormal metabolites possible
Characteristic deficiency symptoms	Nonspecific or mild symptoms
Loss of function	Impaired function

reproduction, and is needed in the synthesis of at least 10 hormones (20).

Exactly which B_6-related enzyme dysfunctions increase the irritability of muscles is not yet clear. However, clinically, that irritability is relieved by correction of vitamin B_6 deficiency and inadequacy. Several drug classes increase the demand for vitamin B_6 and can easily cause inadequacy. These classes include antitubercular drugs, oral contraceptives, the chelating agent penicillamine, anticonvulsants, corticosteroids, and excessive alcohol consumption (20-23). Since laboratory testing for serum levels of vitamins B_1 and B_6 is so expensive and vitamin supplements are relatively inexpensive, when necessary, a pragmatic compromise is to prescribe a balanced B-complex supplement instead of measuring their values.

Both vitamins B_1 and B_6 are widely distributed in nature, but in relatively small amounts. Both are easily destroyed in food preparation. Vitamin B_1 (thiamine) is quickly leached out of food during washing and is destroyed in boiling. Likewise, pyridoxine suffers substantial losses during cooking and is quickly destroyed by ultraviolet light (sunlight) and oxidation (as when food is held on a steam table in a cafeteria).

Cobalamin and Folate The strongly interacting pair cobalamin (vitamin B_{12}) and folate play an essential role in the synthesis of deoxyribonucleic acid (DNA) that is required for the maturation of erythrocytes and, therefore, for oxygen transport. Vitamin B_{12} is also essential to normal fat and carbohydrate metabolism, which maintains the integrity of the spinal cord and peripheral nervous system (17).

Deficiency of both vitamin B_{12} and folate characteristically causes megaloblastic anemia, but only vitamin B_{12} deficits produce catastrophic peripheral nervous system disease. When anemia that is caused by vitamin B_{12} deficiency is treated with folic acid (because blood values were not measured), the hematologic picture reverts to normal but neurologic deficits progress. Therefore, the Federal Drug Administration limits nonprescription folic acid preparations to the RDA value of 400 μg/dose. Unfortunately, this approach compromises adequate supplementation of folate and does not adequately solve the problem addressed.

Both vitamins are critical for normal muscle function. Laboratory tests for serum vitamin B_{12} and folate are readily available. Therefore, chronic myofascial pain patients who respond poorly to treatment should be tested for both.

The serum level of both vitamin B_{12} and folate should be known before initiating treatment with either. Metabolic interdependence of folate and vitamin B_{12} results can precipitously lower the serum folate level, depleting what initially appeared to be an adequate reserve, and supplementation with only folic acid can deplete vitamin B_{12} reserves.

The amount of vitamin B_{12} in the diet is rarely deficient except in *strict* vegetarians. This vitamin is ordinarily synthesized only by bacteria (17). Daily ingestion of 3-5 μg of cobalamin is sufficient when absorption and metabolic utilization are normal. Dietary cobalamins and cyanocobalamin must be converted by the body to the only metabolically useful form, hydroxocobalamin. Some patients are seriously deficient in enzymes required to convert the other forms of cobalamin to the hydroxo- form; these patients respond only to supplements of hydroxocobalamin and not to cyanocobalamin.

On the other hand, folates are found in many foods, particularly leafy green vegetables (foliage), but at most in limited amounts. Compounding this scarcity, folates are largely destroyed by processing and cooking. Lack of folate is the most common vitamin deficiency and is especially frequent in elderly persons who eat institutional cafeteria-style meals.

Serum values in the lower quartile of normal for either vitamin should be supplemented to reach at least midnormal levels. An initial oral supplement of 2 mg of folic acid three times daily should elevate the folate level to midnormal range within 2-3 weeks. One milligram daily usually maintains this blood level. A daily 1-mg (1000-μg) oral supplement of vitamin B_{12} usually restores the serum level to midnormal within 4-6 weeks and maintains it there. Oral administration, if the vitamin is absorbed, avoids the necessity for injection. This dose is several hundred times the RDA, but totally innocuous, even if injected.

Ascorbic Acid The importance of adequate stores of water-soluble ascorbic acid (vitamin C) to prevent ecchymoses in those patients receiving injection therapy has been reviewed (9). This vitamin is essential to normal muscle function and, when inadequacy is corrected, relieves postexercise soreness and stiffness. Large supplements of several grams a day ause no problems. Five hundred milligrams of timed-released vitamin C ingested daily usually provides an ample supply to prevent capillary fragility and to reduce postexercise soreness.

The Fat-Soluble Vitamins The fat-soluble vitamins A, D, and E are well stored and can readily reach toxic levels. Above-normal serum vitamin A levels appear to be another source of increased muscular irritability. Therefore, chronic MPS patients taking a daily *total* (including dietary) of more than 10,000 IU of vitamin A should have their serum level tested. The National Academy of Science recommends physician supervision for ingestion of more than 10,000 I.U. daily (16).

Metabolic and Endocrine Dysfunction

Like the vitamin inadequacies discussed above, metabolic factors of gout, anemia, low electrolyte levels, and hypoglycemia increase muscle irritability and aggravate symptoms caused by TrPs; so do the endocrine disorders of hypometabolism and estrogen deficiency.

Since the monosodium urate crystals of **gout** are less soluble in the acidic media of injured tissues than in blood, they tend to deposit in areas of local injury or of metabolic distress such as TrPs. Chronic myofascial pain patients with a gouty diathesis often respond to treatment only when the hyperuricemia is under control. Generally, these patients respond better to injection than to stretch and spray. Vitamin C in relatively large amounts (1–4 g/day) is an effective uricosuric agent (24). The hyperirritability of myofascial TrPs subsides remarkably with uricosuric therapy in most patients with serum uric acid levels that are in the excessive, or even the high "normal," range.

Regardless of the cause for **anemia**, from the muscle's point of view the resultant hypoxia is a serious metabolic problem because the muscle depends on oxygen to sustain the oxidative metabolism that is essential for meeting its energy needs.

The presence of abnormally **low electrolyte levels** of ionized calcium and potassium can seriously disturb muscle function by increasing muscle irritability; these electrolytes play critical roles in the contractile mechanism. Serum ionized calcium, not merely total calcium, is the essential measure. Unfortunately, the total calcium found on the usual automated blood chemistry battery or profile correlates poorly with the level of serum ionized calcium (25).

The presence of **hypoglycemia** intensifies metabolic distress in muscles (26) and clearly aggravates myofascial TrPs. Therapy by stretch or injection is best deferred whenever patients are hypoglycemic. Treatment then is likely to aggravate rather than relieve the pain. A packet of powdered drinking gelatin in fruit juice provides a handy source of carbohydrate and enough protein to avoid subsequent hypoglycemia.

Evidence for **hypometabolism** (subclinical hypothyroidism) was reported in 13% of healthy elderly individuals (27) and is found in some treatment-refractory patients with pain due to myofascial TrPs. When inadequate metabolism is suspected, first, adequate serum folate and vitamin B_1 levels must be assured because these vitamin inadequacies can cause symptoms mimicking those of low thyroid function. Hypometabolism is a controversial diagnosis because the usual laboratory test results for thyroid function are low-normal, but still within "normal" limits in these patients. The patient often has marginally low L-triiodothyronine (T_3) uptake and low to midrange L-thyroxine (T_4) by radioimmunoassay (RIA). In these patients, low thyroid function is clearly revealed by a low basal metabolic rate (28) if the test is properly performed, or by a low basal body temperature (29), and by clinical symptoms of inadequate thyroid function. Thyroid insufficiency is confirmed therapeutically by the response to thyroid supplementation (28). When insufficiency is present, thyroid supplementation results in serum cholesterol decrease, basal metabolism or basal temperature normalization, decrease in irritability of the muscles, and return of normal energy and stamina (9, 30).

Basal temperature readings are obtained by having the patient place an ovulation thermometer in the axilla daily for 10 min in the morning before arising after sleep. The mean basal temperature over 3–4 days normally averages at least 36.1°C (97.0°F). The lower the basal temperature is under this value, the more vulnerable the patient is to hyperirritable TrPs in the muscles and often to depression. Usually, women who ovulate are at the basal (low point) of their cycle for only 3–5 days immediately following menses.

Thyroid supplementation should be avoided in patients with cardiac arrhythmias or myocardial disease that compromises cardiac reserve. Thyroid medication increases the load on the heart and also the requirements for vitamin B_1 and estrogen. It tends to increase blood pressure. Overmedication causes symptoms of hyperthyroidism. Adjustment of dosage in these patients depends primarily on the clinical responses to therapy. The site of metabolic dysfunction is apparently at the level of cellular utilization and is poorly reflected in serum levels of thyroid hormone.

Thyroid supplementation for those patients who meet the criteria described by Sonkin (28) remains controversial among endocrinologists, but it is of critical importance to those patients in whom this factor is a major perpetuator of disabling myofascial pain.

Chronic Infection and Infestations

Viral disease, bacterial infection, and parasitic infestation can also perpetuate TrPs.

During any systemic **viral illness,** including the common cold or attack of "flu," the irritability of myofascial TrPs is likely to increase markedly. One of the most common viral perpetuators is an outbreak of herpes simplex virus type 1; however, neither herpes simplex virus type 2 (genital herpes) nor herpes zoster is known to aggravate TrPs. Herpesvirus type 1 causes the common fever blister, aphthous mouth ulcer, canker sore, or cold sore. Isolated vesicles filled with clear fluid may also appear on the skin of the body or extremities. Lesions similar to those in the mouth have been reported in the esophagus. The symptoms of vomiting and diarrhea strongly implicate similar gastrointestinal involvement.

No drug is known to completely cure these infections of herpes simplex virus type 1, but a multipronged treatment approach can greatly reduce the frequency and severity of recurrences. A daily dose of 300–500 mg of niacinamide reinforces mucous membrane resistance. Three tablets (or 1 packet) of viable lactobacillus two or three times daily for at least a month helps to reestablish normal intestinal flora, which reduces the danger of an intestinal viral outbreak. Rubbing an antiviral ointment, such as Vira-A, into the skin or on mouth lesions three times daily accelerates their resolution.

Chronic **bacterial infection** tends to exacerbate muscle irritability. Persistent infection, such as an abscessed tooth, infected sinus, or chronic urinary tract infection, can perpetuate TrPs. Acute sinusitis may become chronic due to blockage caused by allergy. Normal erythrocyte sedimentation rate and C-reactive protein tests help to eliminate the possibility of chronic infection.

The danger of a **parasitic infestation** is of concern in travelers exposed to substandard sanitation and in active male homosexuals. The most common infestation was fish tapeworm, until pollution of fresh water greatly reduced fishing; next is giardiasis; and less common, but likely to be more serious, is amebiasis. The first two can seriously impair absorption of and consume vitamin B_{12}; amebae may produce myotoxins that are absorbed systemically. The diagnosis of infestation is investigated by stool examinations for occult blood, ova, and parasites on at least three samples. Serologic testing is available for amebiasis.

Post-traumatic Hyperirritability Syndrome

The chronic myofascial pain perpetuated by the post-traumatic hyperirritability syndrome causes great suffering, is poorly understood, and is difficult to manage. This group of patients responds to strong sensory stimuli much differently than most patients. Patients with this syndrome have incurred a major impact to the body and/or head. The trauma characteristically has been an automobile accident or fall that was sufficiently severe to have disrupted consciousness and inflicted damage to the sensory pathways of the central nervous system. These patients experience constant pain that is augmented by normally inconsequential sensory stimuli, including a loud noise, vibration, prolonged physical activity, and emotional stress. The constant pain is also augmented by severe pain from other sources. An augmented state then persists and may take days or weeks to return slowly to the previous level of activation. During augmentation, the muscles exhibit an increased hyperirritability of TrPs.

After onset, coping with pain has suddenly become the focus of life for these patients, who previously had paid no special attention to pain. If they exceed their restricted limit of activity, they experience a marked increase in pain and fatigue that depletes their vital energy and severely limits their activity. Suppressing pain is exhausting to the patient.

Also, in patients with post-traumatic hyperirritability, augmentation of symptoms is associated with a marked increase in sensitivity to subsequent stimuli. Not only are they then in more pain, but they are more vulnerable to further activation by strong stimuli. This increased vulnerability of the sensory system also subsides slowly. Recovery to the previous degree of vulnerability may also take hours, days, or weeks depending on the intensity of the stimulus and the severity of the reaction to it. The inciting sensory input appears to modulate the excitability of the arousal system. These patients are vulnerable to major extension of their injury and intensification of their symptoms by additional trauma that to most people would be minor.

The most effective management approach found so far has been to inactivate all identifiable TrPs and to correct perpetuating factors. The patients must learn to pace themselves and stay within their stress tolerance. Elimination of stimuli that exacerbate symptoms is a prime goal. Occasionally, when necessary, the sensory system can be reset to baseline by pharmacologically suppressing central nervous system excitability through one night. To date, barbiturates have been most effective.

Psychological Stress

Recently a committee of the National Academy of Sciences agreed that among chronic pain patients malingering is rare, at most accounting for only a small percentage (1). Much difference of opinion is generated by the question: "Is the chronic pain an expression of the patient's psychological dysfunctions or is the pain driving the patient crazy?" If an organic cause of the pain is not obvious, it is tempting to conclude that the symptoms are psychogenic. This relieves the health care professional, but not the patient.

Patients who suffer a serious chronic MPS that is undiagnosed and untreated are strongly impacted psychologically. They are confronted with a severe inescapable pain of unknown origin and of uncertain prognosis that is devastating to their vocational, social, and private lives. Worst of all, family and physicians are questioning their psychological integrity until they begin to question their own sanity. The future is an ominous, impenetrable dark cloud. The ensuing depression aggravates the pain and reinforces uncertainty and a sense of hopelessness (1). The most important service one can render these patients is to recognize their treatable myofascial pain and to make an unambiguous diagnosis with a convincing demonstration and explanation of active TrPs. As patients learn self-treatment and self-management techniques they gain control of the pain; the pain no longer controls them and victimizes their lives.

Employment status is the most significant factor for predicting which patients in chronic pain rehabilitation programs will improve. Loss of employment is clearly a stronger perpetuating factor than ongoing litigation (1). When patients reorient their primary focus of attention from being productive members of society to becoming full-time pain patients, they develop a new self-image that shifts from function orientation to sickness orientation. Psychologically it is of utmost importance to preserve the patient's self-respect and function orientation through vocational activity.

MECHANICAL FACTORS

Systemic perpetuating factors may relate to any or all of the skeletal muscles. However, each *mechanical* perpetuating factor relates to specific muscles. The columns in Table 42.2 identify specific perpetuating stresses and the muscle or muscle group that is most likely to be affected by that stress. Major mechanical factors include anatomic variations, seated and standing postural overload, and vocational stress.

Anatomic Variations

Two common and closely related anatomic variations are a **short leg** and/or a **small hemipelvis** (9). These variations often must be corrected by a heel lift, a butt lift,

Table 42.2
Muscles Often Affected by Specific Mechanical Perpetuating Factors

Stress	Muscles	References
Anatomic variations		
Short leg and/or small hemipelvis	Quadratus lumborum	9 (Chap. 4), 31, 32, 33 (Chap. 4)
	Iliopsoas	32, 33 (Chap. 5)
	Thoracolumbar paraspinals	9 (Chap. 48), 31
	Shoulder girdle and neck-righting	9 (Chaps. 7, 19, 20)
	Masticatory	9 (Chaps. 8–12)
Short upper arms or armrests too low	Levator scapulae	9 (Chaps. 4, 19)
	Upper trapezius	9 (Chap. 6)
	Scaleni	9 (Chap. 20)
	Rhomboids	9 (Chap. 27)
	Triceps brachii	9 (Chap. 32)
Long second metatarsal (D.J. Morton foot configuration)	Peroneus longus	9 (Chap. 4), 33 (Chap. 20)
	Vastus medialis	33 (Chap. 14)
	Gluteus medius	33 (Chap. 8)
Seated postural stress		
Hard smooth mat	Foot intrinsics	33 (Chap. 27)
Seat too high from floor	Hamstrings	33 (Chap. 16)
	Soleus	33 (Chap. 22)
Back unsupported	Quadratus lumborum	32, 33 (Chap. 4)
(no backrest contact, poor lumbar support, no scapular contact)	T-L paraspinals	9 (Chap. 48)
	Pectoralis major	9 (Chap. 42)
	Rhomboids	9 (Chap. 27)
Standing postural stress		
Head-forward posture	Pectoralis major	9 (Chap. 42)
	Rhomboids	9 (Chap. 27)
	Posterior cervicals	9 (Chap. 16)
Slanted running surface	Quadratus lumborum	32, 33 (Chap. 4)
	Scaleni	9 (Chap. 20)
	Sternocleidomastoid	9 (Chap. 7)
Vocational stress		
Shoulder elevation	Upper trapezius	9 (Chap. 6)
	Levator scapulae	9 (Chap. 19)
Arm elevation	Supraspinatus	9 (Chap. 21)
	Deltoid	9 (Chap. 28)
Hand supination	Supinator	9 (Chap. 36)
Grasp	Finger extensors	9 (Chap. 35)
	Finger flexors	9 (Chap. 38)
	Wrist extensors	9 (Chap. 34)
	Wrist flexors	9 (Chap. 38)

or both for lasting relief of low back (32) and sometimes head, neck, and shoulder pain due to myofascial TrPs. To ensure appropriate correction, evaluation of these variations must be conducted with the patient in a functional standing or seated position. An effective technique for determining and making the required correction is described in detail (9).

The relatively common phenomenon of **short upper arms** is frequently an unrecognized perpetuator of TrPs in the shoulder elevator muscles. This anatomic variation is corrected by providing elbow rests or pads that modify the furniture to fit the individual (9).

The **long second metatarsal,** or D.J. Morton foot configuration, throws the foot off balance as a result of a knife-edge support during toe-off. This instability disturbs gait and overloads lower extremity muscles. The muscles most affected are primarily the peroneus longus and secondarily the vastus medialis and gluteus medius. This anatomic variation is compensated by inserting a toe pad under the head of the short first metatarsal bone to place the foot on a tripod base (9, 33).

Seated Postural Stress

This ubiquitous muscular stress may be induced by a small hemipelvis as noted above, by a hard smooth mat under an office chair, by a chair seat too high for heels to reach the floor, by lack of a firm back support, by lack of lumbar support, by low armrests, and by a persistent head-forward posture.

Use of a **hard smooth mat,** such as plexiglass, allows the office chair with free-rolling casters to glide whenever its occupant changes position or exerts the slightest pressure against the desk. Frequently, the intrinsic foot muscles and long toe flexors must try to grasp the slick surface; this repeated and prolonged but unconscious effort overloads and perpetuates TrPs in these muscles.

A **chair seat too high** for that individual's leg length leaves the heels dangling off the floor. This causes under-thigh compression of the hamstrings and chronic shortening of the soleus muscle as the toes drop toward the floor. Both postural effects perpetuate TrPs in the corresponding muscles and can be avoided by providing a suitable footrest (book, pillow, or small footstool). A desk surface that is too high can be corrected by shortening the legs of the desk, or by elevating the seat height with appropriate adjustment of footrests.

A chair with **inadequate back support** may be the result of a poor seat design that renders the seat too long from front to back, that has a flat back that provides no lumbar support, that supplies no scapular contact, or that has a backrest with inadequate backward angulation. When the seat is too long from front to back, the backs of the knees are solidly engaged against the front of the seat, but the buttocks do not reach the backrest. The backrest should always be contoured to support a normal lumbar lordosis; otherwise, the patient must place a pillow or roll in the small of the back to provide this support. This lumbar support also helps to correct the head-forward posture (9). This repositioning facilitates balancing the head over the shoulders with minimal muscular effort.

The **armrests** must provide solid elbow support. If their height is not adequate, the armrests should be elevated or padded to provide the needed support.

The troublesome **head-forward posture** is further relieved by placing the work or reading material on a slant board and, for those who require reading glasses, by tilting the *lenses* of the eyeglasses (9). Papers that are placed to one side require a crooked neck position that aggravates TrPs. Placing the work on a secretary's desk stand in front and nearly at eye level relieves this aggravation. Scapular contact with the backrest and backward angulation of the backrest help to carry the weight of the head and shoulders and to stabilize the spine, relieving the quadratus lumborum and paraspinal muscles.

The forward head position is a powerful mechanical perpetuator of TrPs, especially in some neck and shoulder-girdle muscles. This posture, with loss of the normal cervical lordosis, is also associated with a variety of painful cervical articular dysfunctions.

Standing Postural Stress

The **head-forward posture** that produces chronic muscular strains when standing is aggravated by shifting body weight backward onto the heels. Conversely, this posture is spontaneously improved and effortlessly held by shifting the center of gravity forward over the balls of the feet while emphasizing lumbar lordosis. This positioning allows the head to remain erect, balanced over the shoulders without muscle and joint strain. It elevates the chest and swings the scapulae backward to their normal resting position. This repositioning unloads the rhomboid muscles by relieving the persistent shortening of the pectoral muscles (9). This improved posture lessens the load on the posterior cervical muscles, which in the head-forward posture must support the weight of the head against the pull of gravity.

A **slanted walking or running surface** is common on the seashore or on a banked circular track. It produces the same effect as a short leg (9) and tilts the pelvis to one side. Contraction of the quadratus lumborum and/or paraspinal muscles must hold the spinal curvature that is required to compensate for the lateral tilt of the pelvis. This sustained contraction while on the feet causes a persistent overload that perpetuates TrPs in these mucles.

Vocational Stress

A work situation that encourages or requires sustained **shoulder elevation** commonly overloads the upper trapezius and levator scapulae muscles, which perpetuates their TrPs. Typists and other workers who must hold their hands in a sustained elevated position tend to persistently shrug their shoulders. For correction, the body should be raised or the work lowered.

Similarly, prolonged **arm abduction** overloads the supraspinatus and deltoid muscles. Suitable elbow support relieves the strain. The supraspinatus and upper trapezius muscles develop chronic myofascial syndromes when subjected to frequent repetitive movements that overload those muscles. When tested electromyographically, these painfully involved muscles had less endurance and more rapid onset of fatigue than nonpainful muscles. The authors (33) accounted for these findings by alteration in muscle metabolism due to ischemia.

Forceful or repetitive **forearm supination** will full extension at the elbow readily overloads the supinator muscle, as when playing tennis or turning a screwdriver (9). Full extension at the elbow eliminates the more forceful supinator function of the biceps brachii muscle. This repetitive motion with the forearm extended may activate TrPs in the supinator muscle, producing symptoms that frequently are labeled epicondylitis or tennis elbow. To decrease load on the supinator muscle, the forearm should be less than fully extended at the elbow when forcefully supinating the forearm.

Repeated or sustained **strong grasp** often activates TrPs of the finger extensors because these extensors function vigorously during grasp. The patient with TrPs of the finger extensors complains of a weak and painful grip. Items like a cup or glass are likely to slip unexpectedly out of the grasp, apparently due to unpredictable TrP-induced reflex inhibition of muscle contraction. The supinator muscle is frequently involved along with the wrist and finger extensors.

INACTIVATION OF TRIGGER POINTS

When the composite myofascial pain pattern of the patient with chronic MPS is analyzed into its component single-muscle syndromes, the TrPs responsible can then be managed, one muscle at a time, as single-muscle syndromes. This section presents the basic treatment principles applicable to most muscles. Details for individual muscles are summarized in the preceding chapter and described elsewhere (9, 32, 33).

In this section, first the principles of stretch and spray are summarized. Then, other physical methods such as postisometric relaxation, ischemic compression, and massage are noted. Finally, the technique of injection and stretch is reviewed.

STRETCH AND SPRAY

Treatment of an acute or chronic MPS by stretch and spray is one of the simplest, quickest, and least painful ways to inactivate the TrPs. Stretch and spray can be used alone or frequently is applied immediately after TrP injection. This postinjection application ensures inactivation of any remaining TrPs in that muscle. Stretch and spray also is valuable for complex cases that involve many muscles in one or more regions of the body (35). Since muscles within one functional group interact strongly, stretch and spray permits release of several closely related muscles at one time.

The procedure of passive stretch and intermittent spray should cause little or no discomfort and should not excite reflex spasm. Complete voluntary relaxation while the muscle is lengthening is essential. The alarming cold stimulation produced by the vapocoolant spray on skin receptors over the muscle and its pain reference zone is needed to block reflex spasm and pain (8). The restoration of normal full stretch length of the muscle *inactivates* the TrP mechanism.

Vapocoolant spray is applied in one-directional parallel sweeps in a jet stream to the skin. When the skin is cold to the touch, rewarming should precede a repeat application of vapocoolant. Excessive cooling (frosting) of the skin and cooling of the underlying muscle should be *avoided*. Fluori-Methane (Gebauer Chemical Co., 9410 St. Catherine Ave., Cleveland, OH 44104) is more effective and much safer than ethyl chloride. Ethyl chloride is undesirably colder, is a potentially lethal general anesthetic, and is flammable and explosive. Fluori-Methane is none of these. Parallel sweeps of Fluori-Methane spray should be applied slowly at 10 cm (4 in)/sec. The spray pattern should cover the entire length of the muscle, progressing in the direction of and *including* the referred pain zone. The bottle is held about 45 cm (18 in) from the skin to allow the vapocoolant that starts at room temperature in the bottle to cool by evaporation before impacting the skin. The optimal angle of impact of the spray is about 30° (9).

To obtain the complete relaxation that is essential for effective passive stretch, the seated patient should be positioned comfortably with *all* limbs and the back and head well supported. The recumbent position is preferable, if it permits full stretch of the affected muscles. One or two sweeps of spray should precede the passive stretch to inhibit the pain and stretch reflexes. To take up any slack that develops while applying spray, the operator maintains gentle, smooth, *steady* tension on the muscle. He or she should carefully *avoid* force strong enough to produce pain and avoid any jerky or rapid rocking motions that could activate TrPs.

Treatment by stretch and spray is not complete until the skin has been rewarmed for several minutes by a moist hot pack or a wetproof heating pad. Then the patient should slowly execute several cycles of active range of motion through both the *fully shortened* and *fully lengthened* positions of the muscle group under treatment. Emphasis is placed on gently but surely reaching maximum range of motion in each direction. A more detailed description of the stretch and spray procedure is available (9).

One particularly effective way of facilitating relaxation is to ask the patient to slowly take a deep breath, and then gradually and completely to exhale through pursed lips. During this long, slow, and maximal exhalation, the muscles tend to relax and are more easily lengthened. Inhalation usually is facilitated by having the patient look up, and exhalation by having the patient look down toward the feet (36). The effects of simultaneously looking down and exhaling are additive in facilitating relaxation. The Lewit stretch technique (postisometric relaxation) (37), described below, may be combined with stretch and spray or used as an alternate method of lengthening the muscle.

OTHER PHYSICAL METHODS

Muscle lengthening can be achieved in several ways: by stretch and spray, as described above; by postisometric relaxation; by the use of reciprocal inhibition; by ischemic compression; and by deep friction massage. Additional modalities are sometimes used. Low-intensity ultrasound is valuable when applied directly to the TrP. This approach may be effective when the TrP is otherwise inaccessible. Some find electrical stimulation over the TrP helpful; high-voltage galvanic stimulation is reported to be effective in the hands of those accustomed to its use.

Postisometric Relaxation

The technique of alternating voluntary contraction with passive stretch for releasing tight muscles has been identified by many names. Physical therapists are likely to refer to this as contract-relax or rhythmic stabilization (38). Osteopathic physicians speak of muscle energy techniques (39).

Postisometric muscular relaxation as described by Lewit and Simons (37) is simple and effective. The effects are additive when it is combined with the stretch-and-spray technique. This stretch technique is routinely taught to patients as a home program of self-treatment for specific muscle syndromes. The muscle is gently lengthened to the onset of resistance (end of slack) and held there isometrically. For the next 3–7 sec, either the operator or the patient provides fixed resistance against which the patient contracts the muscle *gently* and *isometrically* at approximately 10% of maximal effort. While the *same position* is passively maintained, the patient "let's go" (relaxes the contracting muscle). Only after the patient has thoroughly relaxed is the muscle again *slowly, gently,* and passively lengthened, taking up all the slack that has developed. Gravity is used to provide the stretch force whenever possible. Elongation of the muscle should be painless. This contract-relax cycle may be repeated three to five times. Full release of tension usually occurs after the second or third cycle. Relaxation is facilitated by coordinating respiration (37) and eye movements (36) as described above, under "Stretch and Spray."

Ischemic Compression

Ischemic compression, sometimes called "thumb therapy," is painful but noninvasive and effective (40). Pressure that directly compresses a peripheral nerve must be avoided. This technique may be applied either by the operator or as self-treatment by the patient. Constant pressure is applied directly to the taut band on the spot of greatest tenderness (the TrP) with a steady, moderately painful (tolerable) pressure. As the pain eases, the pressure is increased to maintain approximately the same level of discomfort. When the TrP is no longer painful (after 15 sec to 1 min of pressure) the pressure is released and full active range of motion performed. For the greatest effect, stretch and spray and then moist heat may be applied following ischemic compression.

Immediately after release, the blanching of the skin due to pressure is quickly replaced by a persistent reactive hyperemia. If the pressure produces a similar hyperemia at the TrP, the increased perfusion should contribute to recovery. The procedure is less painful, but takes longer, if the therapist applies less pressure repeatedly on successive days. Treatment is repeated until TrP tenderness is obliterated and the referred pain disappears.

Massage

Deep muscle massage (deep friction or stripping massage) is another way to inactivate TrPs in superficial muscles. This massage requires lubrication of the skin and the application of *firm* bilateral thumb pressure against the taut band while sliding the thumbs *slowly* progressively along its length. Fluid content of the band is "milked out" by the pressure between the thumbs. A sense of increased resistance and accumulation of fluid is experienced at the TrP. This procedure may be repeated several times until the tenderness and tautness of the palpable band are relieved and the TrP no longer refers pain. The slowly progressive "milking" action eliminates the sense of induration. This technique is effective but painful and is usually followed by local muscle soreness for a few days. In experimental studies, each massage treatment session caused a transient myoglobinemia until the abnormal tension and tenderness were relieved (41, 42).

INJECTION AND STRETCH

Injection of muscle TrPs is selected initially when the joint movement is mechanically blocked, as in the case of the coccygeus muscle, or when the muscles cannot be stretched fully, as in the case of the lateral pterygoid muscle (9). Injection is useful for releasing TrPs unresponsive to the foregoing noninvasive methods. Dry needling (9, 43) and isotonic saline injection (9, 44) also are effective; however, without a local anesthetic, dry needling is more painful. Isotonic saline for injection usually contains 0.9% of the preservative and *local anesthetic* benzyl alcohol. The flushing effect of the injected fluid on sensitizing agents may also be important. Reduction of local TrP tenderness depends more on penetration of the TrP by the needle than on which substance, if any, is injected (44).

Needle penetration of the skin is less painful when the needle is inserted rapidly with a flick of the wrist after the antiseptic alcohol has dried. To make insertion painless, the site may be chilled for 6–8 sec with a stream of Fluori-Methane spray applied in a figure-of-eight pattern. The needle is inserted in the crossover region of the spray pattern (9, 45). The skin is chilled just short of frosting; frosting causes an unnecessarily painful sting.

The essence of effective needle therapy is the *mechanical disruption* of the self-sustaining TrP mechanism. The critical role of penetrating the TrP with the needle was demonstrated experimentally (44). To do this requires precise localization of the TrP before injection. The injection of 0.5% procaine in isotonic saline *without epinephrine* reduces the consistently severe and sometimes intolerable pain of TrP penetration. Importantly, the 0.5% concentration ameliorates the pain but preserves the tenderness to palpation of any remaining TrPs. Continuous injection of small amounts of procaine during needle insertion further reduces the sensory impact of needle contact with the TrP. The preservation of local TrP tenderness permits palpation for and detection of any TrPs that were missed, so that they, too, can be injected without withdrawing the needle, thereby avoiding additional skin penetrations.

The local analgesic effect of the 0.9% concentration of benzyl alcohol preservative permits the substitution of this saline for procaine injection in those few patients who are allergic to procaine. Lidocaine in 0.5% solution is less desirable than procaine but, if necessary, can be used. Long-acting local anesthetics such as bupivacaine should be avoided because they obliterate the tenderness of remaining TrPs and produce muscle necrosis, which is unnecessary. Necrosis is not caused by 0.5% procaine or lidocaine (46).

For injection, the patient should be recumbent, to prevent psychological syncope. When injecting muscles over the ribs, needle penetration between the ribs must be scrupulously avoided because it can easily cause a pneumothorax.

The first step in the injection of a tender TrP is to palpate its taut band between the fingers with the TrP localized accurately between the finger tips. The needle is then inserted precisely into the TrP (9). Needle contact with the TrP is confirmed by a jump response *of the patient* and/or a local twitch response *of the taut band* in the muscle. Probing with the needle should continue until such a response has been obtained or the region has been fully explored with the needle. Tenderness to palpation and the local twitch response can no longer be elicited following successful inactivation of a TrP. The tautness of the band may or may not disappear. Digital pressure is applied during and after injection to ensure hemostasis.

The injection is supplemented by a stretch-and-spray procedure and by a moist hot pack or pad to inactivate any remaining TrPs. The moist heat helps to minimize postinjection soreness that otherwise may last for 2–3 days. The patient should be alerted that aspirin or acetaminophen (Tylenol) relieves this soreness.

It is most important to conclude with several cycles of active range of motion that reach both the fully shortened and the fully stretched positions of the treated muscles, as described for stretch and spray. Repetition of this slow, but complete, range of movement helps greatly to reestablish normal function. The same stretching and range of motion exercises are routinely instituted as a home program. This home stretching program often makes a critical difference for maintaining the increased range of motion obtained by treatment.

CONFUSINGLY SIMILAR CONDITIONS

The pathophysiology of three of the most common, yet least recognized, causes of musculoskeletal pain has yet to be established. The three appear to be closely intertwined. They are myofascial TrPs (9); fibromyalgia (47–49); which was first called fibrositis (50–52); and articular dysfunction (53). To date, not one of the three has a reliable diagnostic laboratory or imaging test. Each diagnosis must be made by history and a directed physical examination. In each, the critical information would be missed on the usual history and routine physical examination. The examiner must know what questions to ask, what specific evidence to look for, and how to examine for each, and must take the time to look. The symptoms and findings that distinguish these three are based only on clinical experience. To be sure of any one of them, at this time, the examiner should be conversant with all three.

Investigators of one of these three conditions are very likely to include in their study a significant number of patients who are suffering from at least one of the other two conditions. In this event, their conclusions are as likely to be confusing as helpful. It now looks as if these three conditions have distinctively different causes, which can, and often do, produce confusingly similar clinical pictures. However, each of the three responds best to significantly different therapeutic approaches. Many patients doubtless have a combination of two or all of these conditions and, when treated for only one of them, respond poorly. Included in this circle of confusion are many additional diagnoses that also are likely to include patients with myofascial TrPs. A few of the most common of these additional diagnoses include nonarticular rheumatism (54), muscular rheumatism (55), osteochondrosis (56, 57), bursitis (9), tendinitis (9), and occipital neuralgia (58). For many others, see Simons [59, 60 (Table I)] and Reynolds (61).

MYOFASCIAL TRIGGER POINTS

A single-muscle syndrome due to myofascial TrPs starts with a focal disorder in *one muscle* as a result of acute or repeated overload stress. This condition is clearly myogenic, not psychogenic. However, this pain and tenderness are felt not at the TrP but at a distance. This referred pain, which appears in a characteristic pattern for each skeletal muscle (7, 9, 33, 60), seems inexplicable to practitioners unacquainted with these patterns. These TrPs may cause pain early in life (62) and occur with nearly equal frequency in men and women (63). A chronic MPS that proliferates over time due to systemic perpetuating factors is not so obviously myogenic; this chronic myofascial condition may look confusingly like fibrositis/fibromyalgia (64). Myofascial TrPs are distinguished clinically by eliciting referred pain and tenderness, by locating the palpable taut bands containing the TrP, and by demonstrating local twitch responses of the taut bands. When myofascial TrPs are recognized as an acute syndrome, and if there are no serious perpetuating factors, the pain is quickly and easily relieved.

FIBROSITIS/FIBROMYALGIA

It is increasingly clear that the second condition, fibrositis/fibromyalgia, is primarily a *systemic* disease that targets the muscles and the collagen of the dermal-epidermal junction (60). Fibrositis is characteristically a disease of women between 40 and 60 years of age. Less than 15% of fibrositis patients are men (52). In 1972, leading the recent resurgence of interest in fibrositis, Smythe (65) characterized fibrositis in terms of psychogenic rheumatism. Some still consider fibrositis or fibromyalgia as partly, if not predominantly, psychogenic (66–68). However, others recently have found no psychological difference compared with other chronic painful conditions (69). In 1977, Smythe and Moldofsky (51) redefined fibrositis as a nonrestorative sleep syndrome that was previously described by Moldofsky et al. (70). The redefined fibrositis was characterized by multiple diffuse tender points (TePs) at prescribed locations. In 1981, Smythe (71) updated this redefinition of fibrositis that, in essence, has been adopted by rheumatologists. This acceptance was confirmed at a recent symposium (72). Yunus and associates (49) in the following year renamed and modified Smythe's redefinition of fibrositis as primary fibromyalgia and increased the number of patients incorporated in the new term by reducing the number of TePs required to make the diagnosis. *Primary fibromyalgia*, is rapidly gaining recognition (48, 67, 72–75). It is less of a misnomer than the term *fibrositis*.

Smythe (76) now identifies essentially two different syndromes characterized by TePs in muscles: fibrositis, which he characterized as essentially a painful nonrestorative sleep syndrome with TePs; and another syndrome that causes referred pain. If Smythe's concept is correct—and there is rapidly accumulating evidence that these are two distinct conditions—one would expect to see a spectrum of patients. Those at one end would be pure fibrositis/fibromyalgia, those at the other end, pure MPS due to TrPs; a large group in the middle should have various proportions of both. Evidence for such a spectrum was observed by Bengtsson and associates (77).

The TePs of fibromyalgia patients have been distinguished from TrPs by identifying as TrPs those tender spots that caused referred pain when compressed (77). Other authors do not mention how they distinguish TrPs from TePs, if at all (49, 52, 74, 78). Both TrPs and TePs are always tender; TePs do not always (if ever) refer pain. Using only the referred pain criterion for TrPs, Bengtsson and associates (77), found that 35 of 55 primary fibromyalgia patients (64%) had both TePs and TrPs. Nine of the patients (16%) exhibited only TePs; 11 (20%) exhibited only TrPs. If only myofascial TrPs project referred pain and the fibromyalgic TePs do not, very likely this and possibly all fibromyalgia studies have included a mixed population of patients with both fibromyalgia and chronic MPS. On the other hand, if fibromyalgic TePs do refer pain, for experimental purposes it is essential that TrPs be unambiguously identified using other criteria. Myofascial TrPs can be unambiguously distinguished from TePs by their location in a palpable taut band and by the local twitch response of that band to snapping palpation.

Numerous investigators present evidence that fibromyalgia is a systemic disease involving both skin and muscle. Both Caro (79) and Bengtsson (73) have reported collagen changes at the dermal-epidermal junction characterized by abnormal deposition of immunoglobulin G (IgG). Bartels and Danneskiold-Samsøe (80) reported abnormal collagenous constrictions like rubber bands around muscle fibers in *nontender* muscles of fibrositis patients. Crook and associates (74) concluded that the abnormal muscle tenderness of fibromyalgia patients is much more widespread than only the prescribed spots of muscular tenderness. They confusingly called these tender spots TrPs (74). Others have reported clear indications of an energy crisis in nontender muscles of fibromyalgia patients (67, 73, 75, 81). These studies do not clarify which of these findings would or would not be found in patients with only myofascial TrPs. Only hypothesized mechanisms provide guidelines.

Current literature indicates that infrared thermography is useful for substantiating the common finding of circulatory disturbance in the skin associated with already diagnosed myofascial TrPs (82, 83). It is clear that thermography cannot at this time be used as a primary diagnostic tool (84). No studies are known to date that effectively distinguish the thermographic patterns of myofascial TrPs from those of TePs in fibrositis/fibromyalgia.

ARTICULAR DYSFUNCTION

The third condition, articular dysfunction, is marked by a loss of joint "play" and/or normal mobility (85). Karel Lewit (36, 86) emphasized that articular dysfunction, particularly in joints involving transitional vertebrae, causes musculoskeletal pain that is characteristically associated with tenderness and increased tension of specific muscles. These articular symptoms and dysfunctions are relieved by mobilization of the restricted joint and by restoration of normal range of motion in the associated muscles that can restrict motion of the joint.

James W. Fisk (87) also noted the importance of strong interactions between some joint dysfunctions and the muscles. Clinically, it is becoming increasingly clear that joint dysfunction can be a potent perpetuator of myofascial TrPs, if not the initial cause of some myofascial pain syndromes. The reverse is also true: the shortening and tension of muscles caused by myofascial TrPs can block mobilization or quickly undo its beneficial effects. Often, both conditions must be treated together for lasting relief.

An overlooked painful articular dysfunction of another kind is the recently reported *instability* of spondylolisthetic or retro-olisthetic lumbar vertebra (88). The painfulness is relieved by strengthening the deep spinal rotator muscles (O. Friberg, personal communication, 1987).

Radiculopathy is often associated with myofascial TrPs (9, 89) and osteochondrosis (56). However, the myofascial component may not abate simply with resolution of the neuropathy; additional specific myofascial therapy may be required to inactivate persistent TrPs.

MANAGEMENT APPROACH

This section explores how one can identify the multiple pieces that comprise the complex puzzle of a chronic MPS and emphasizes the importance of treating the whole patient, not just the TrPs.

First, this section provides guidelines for distinguishing

acute and recurrent pain as compared with the suffering of chronic pain. A clear distinction is drawn between pain and suffering. Finally, the approach to management emphasizes resolution of the sources of the pain while eliminating factors that intensify the suffering.

ACUTE PAIN, RECURRENT PAIN, AND CHRONIC PAIN

The distinctions among acute versus recurrent pain versus chronic enigmatic pain are not always simple and clear-cut, as pointed out by Addison (90). The patient with acute pain usually recognizes a cause for the pain and expects it to be temporary. Recurrent acute pain is similar; the patient again expects relief within a reasonably short period of time.

Addison (90) characterized chronic enigmatic pain (his "chronic pain syndrome") as pain that:

1. Rarely serves a biologic function.
2. Is associated with the development of chronic pain behaviors.
3. Presents with a lack of pathophysiologic mechanisms to account for the pain and with a lack of physical findings that are diagnostic of a well-recognized organic disease.

Obviously, disabling pain that persists, but that serves no discernible biologic function, will cause serious psychological difficulties and modify the patient's behavior. The failure to find an organic cause for the pain is, in many cases, a matter of overlooked diagnoses, which the preceding sections have detailed. In addition, there is no reason to assume that we already know all of the diseases that exist. We may not yet know how to recognize the organic cause of the patient's pain. That approach is far different from concluding decisively that the pain is due primarily to an aberration of the patient's psyche. The latter is true occasionally, but this conclusion should be reached *only* in the face of unambiguous, overwhelming evidence. To hastily reach this conclusion often does the patient a disastrous injustice (1).

A committee of the National Academy of Sciences concerned with chronic pain of enigmatic origin (1) concluded that identifying decrements in the patient's function at all levels was the most reliable means to verify serious chronic pain and suffering. The committee concluded that categorizing a patient as having "chronic pain syndrome" served no useful purpose. It obscured the need to better understand the diverse and multifactorial nature of enigmatic chronic pain.

Increasingly, a distinction is being drawn between the chronic pain per se and its affective dimension, suffering. Price and associates (91) underscored evidence that the relationship between measures of the sensory and affective dimensions in different types of clinical pain is powerfully influenced by the psychological context in which the pain is experienced. Since there is no objective measure of pain per se (1), one *must* accept the patient's description of his or her suffering at face value. The only appropriate question is why the patient experiences that degree of suffering. The suffering is caused by much more than pain sensation alone (91, 92). The clinical distinction between pain and suffering is blurred because patients tend to describe their suffering in terms of pain sensations. Unexplained persistence of the pain adds on psychological, social, behavioral, and vocational losses, all of which intensify suffering.

Causes of Chronic Enigmatic Pain

To identify organic causes of pain in a patient with chronic enigmatic pain one must discover overlooked diagnoses. When conducting the history and physical examination, one should be looking for clues that will identify each pain problem as primarily musculoskeletal, neurologic, cardiovascular, other viscerogenic, or, rarely, psychogenic. Musculoskeletal sources that are frequently overlooked are covered in this and the preceding chapter. The remaining known causes are covered in other chapters of this volume. Usually, much of the patient's pain is of myofascial origin, but some of it is not. The myofascial component is resolved into its single-muscle syndromes and each is dealt with as described previously. The remaining causes are corrected or managed by appropriate specialists.

The following analysis of which muscles developed myofascial TrPs as the result of motor vehicle accidents presents one example of the effect of major trauma on the muscles. Failure to inactivate the TrPs and to correct their perpetuating factors in the immediate postaccident period makes accidents a fertile source of chronic MPS. Baker (93) reported on 100 successive patients who had sought medical help for symptoms related to a single motor vehicle accident. He tallied the frequency of myofascial TrPs in 36 minutes for each of four directions of impact. Table 42.3 summarizes Baker's results; they identify which muscles are most likely to be involved in a patient who experienced an auto accident.

The following interpretation of Baker's data (93) is based on the fact that lengthening contractions are more likely to overload muscles than are shortening contractions (94, 95). His results show that in head-on collisions the head extensors were most likely to be overloaded. The impact of the head-on collision is often anticipated. These extensors could have been overloaded by resisting the anticipated forward movement of the head in response to initial deceleration. On the other hand, rear-end collisions are more likely to have taken the patient by surprise. The fact that the extensor muscles also most commonly developed TrPs in this reverse situation suggests that the muscles were overloaded chiefly when they attempted to resist forward head motion later during the subsequent deceleration phase as the car stopped.

Broadside impact would not always be anticipated. The impact usually produces an initial acceleration phase, followed very shortly by a rapid deceleration phase as the sideward motion stops. Although muscles on both sides of the body developed TrPs after broadside impacts, the muscles on the left were more likely to develop TrPs following impact from the left and muscles on the right were more likely to be involved following impact from the right (Table 42.3). The muscles most commonly involved were those that would be subjected to lengthening contraction during the subsequent deceleration, not during initial acceleration.

In the same paper, Baker (93) noted that extensor digitorum muscles of drivers, who have the steering wheel available for support, were more likely to develop TrPs than were the same muscles of passengers, with one exception. In head-on collisions where passengers would be likely to grasp the dashboard, they were as likely to develop extensor digitorum TrPs as were the drivers. Baker observed that in all of these patients, a number of muscles were free of TrPs: the biceps and triceps brachii, tibialis anterior, lateral gastrocnemius, lateral hamstrings, wrist and finger flexors, abdominals, and mid- and posterior deltoid.

Intensification of Suffering

A number of factors influence the suffering of patients with chronic pain. One of the most important is the patient's orientation. Suffering is ameliorated when the patient is function oriented and attention is focused on activities. Conversely, pain orientation intensifies the suffering. Because pain orientation affects the patient's responses so adversely, the reasons for pain orientation should be identified and addressed. The reasons are frequently multiple and have evolved from fear of the unknown cause of the pain and deep frustration with health care professionals for failing to explain and relieve the pain. This fear and frustration then lead to hopelessness and depression, loss of vocational activity, denigration of status in the family, and an escalating need for income. A patient with poor coping skills is quickly overwhelmed by this situation. Impoverishment of social life, waning of sexual activity, financial distress, development of pain and sickness behaviors, and iatrogenic drug addiction frequently follow. Each of these factors should be identified as such and appropriate corrective actions taken to begin the long hard climb back to function.

In many patients with chronic pain of enigmatic origin, a crucial factor is their fear of the future. They can find no satisfactory explanation for the cause of their pain and no one has been able to relieve it; therefore, they have no idea how rapidly or severely it will progress or how much more disabling it will become. Most important, it denies them any reason to plan for the future, which destroys hope. This situation understandably leads to frustration and anger, and the hopelessness often feeds a growing depression. Identification of the *cause* of the pain is the critical first step on the road to recovery.

Function Versus Pain Orientation

When patients have an outstanding lawsuit or pending application for disability, the question arises as to how great an impediment this is to their improvement. Frequently, finding an answer is as simple as asking these

Table 42.3
Muscles Most Likely to Develop Trigger Points in 100 Consecutive Patients with Symptoms Related to a Single Motor Vehicle Accident (Driver and Passenger Data Combined)[a]

Muscle	Frequency of Involvement %	Most Likely Side[b]	Muscle	Frequency of Involvement %	Most Likely Side[b]
Deceleration (head on) (N=16)			Acceleration-deceleration (rear end) (N=52)		
Splenius capitis	94	B	Quadratus lumborum	79	R
Quadratus lumborum	81	R	Splenius capitis	77	L
Semispinalis capitis	75	L	Semispinalis capitis	62	L
Vastus medialis	69	B	Sternocleidomastoid	52	R
Infraspinatus	63	R	Infraspinatus	46	B
Sternocleidomastoid	56	B			
Levator scapulae	50	R			
Broadside from driver's side (N=16)			Broadside from passenger's side (N = 16)		
Quadratus lumborum	81	B	Splenius capitis	75	R
Splenius capitis	69	L	Semispinalis capitis	69	B
Semispinalis capitis	63	L	Quadratus lumborum	63	R
Levator scapulae	56	L	Levator scapulae	44	R
Infraspinatus	50	L	Extensor digitorum	44	R

[a] Summarized from Baker BA: The muscle trigger: evidence of overload injury. *J Neurol Orthop Med Surg* 7:35–43, 1986.
[b] Side on which the listed muscle was most likely to have developed active trigger points. All muscles showed some bilateral involvement. L = predominantly left side; R = predominantly right side; B = nearly equal bilateral involvement.

patients. One should find out what the remuneration expectations are and how critical the potential income is to their future. Frequently, expectations of remuneration are grossly inflated. Helping them to recognize reality can be tremendously beneficial in achieving functional orientation.

One should discuss candidly with the patient the fact that any improvement in his or her symptoms and function as a result of treatment will compromise the financial rewards of the suit. Some patients welcome a face-saving opportunity to forego treatment until the suit has been settled. After this conversation, it is much easier to discuss motivations openly and sympathetically.

Coping

Patients with inadequate or sick coping repertoires are frequently dependent on their pain symptoms to fill in the gaps. Poor coping skills may lead to unhealthy family relations, poor financial management, poor nutrition, and the like. By encouraging patients to verbalize and look for the stresses that aggravate their pain, it is possible to focus on improving those coping skills that will be of most immediate benefit.

FINDING PIECES OF THE PUZZLE

To resolve the enigma of chronic myofascial pain, one must identify the pieces of the puzzle that comprise the patient's *total* pain picture. All too frequently, patients receive fragmented health care in which each specialist focuses on one point of view or organ system, yet no one integrates the whole picture, including all aspects of the patient's functioning. When there are multiple interacting factors, someone needs to be concerned with all of them and their interactions to coordinate their management. Every patient should know clearly the name of the doctor whom the patient considers to be primarily responsible for his or her health care.

One effective approach to unraveling the complexities of a chronic MPS is to separately identify and number all of the patient's pain problems. A separate problem is distinguished by its own time and circumstances of onset, its own distribution of pain, and the tendency for that distribution of pain to become more severe or regress in response to a stress or remedy. When successive pain problems evolve one from another, one looks for perpetuating factors. When the pain problems have distinct independent origins, the problems more likely have unrelated causes that may or may not be influenced by perpetuating factors.

HISTORY

While conducting the history and physical examination, one needs to distinguish the organ system responsible for *each* pain problem. If the pain relates strongly to locomotor activity and body positioning, it is probably musculoskeletal in origin. In that case, the examiner should query and examine for the presence of myofascial TrPs, fibrositis/fibromyalgia, and articular dysfunction, separately or in combination.

To resolve difficult cases, the history should be comprehensive and detailed. All available past medical records, including a recent complete physical examination, should be reviewed. Of concern are past illnesses, hospitalizations, serious diseases, surgeries, accidents, injuries, and the organ system review. Gastrointestinal symptoms may be somatovisceral manifestations of abdominal wall TrPs (9, 96). A complete current history that explores all relevant issues is facilitated by a questionnaire (Table 42.4) that serves as a reminder and guide for more detailed questioning.

Concerning the major items in Table 42.4, the **vocational** status is one of the most critical. Every effort should be made to maintain the individual in active employment. The **pain** section helps to put the patient's pain in perspective. One must be sure to which pain the patient's answers apply. The patient's perception of what causes the pain influences strongly the response to treatment, especially compliance with self-stretch exercises. Some are seriously worried about cancer but are hesitant to mention it, unless asked. A convincing demonstration to the patient that the pain is of muscular origin, and reassurance that it is not caused by cancer, provides tremendous relief and helps greatly to refocus attention from pain to function. The **dietary** history helps to assess the likelihood of vitamin and other nutrient inadequacies, which are common perpetuating factors. **Sleep** disturbance, when secondary to myofascial TrPs, returns to normal with relief of the disrupting myofascial pain. Unrefreshing sleep is an important feature of fibrositis. A COMPLETE listing of all **medications,** vitamins, and remedies that the individual takes can give valuable insight into the medical care the individual is receiving. It clearly reveals medical conditions that are currently under treatment and often reveals unnecessary drug clutter that may contribute to iatrogenic disease. The history of **previous treatment** provides valuable clues as to the cause of the pain by noting which therapies alleviated symptoms and which did not. **Exercise** is considered essential to optimal health in general and to unimpaired function of the musculoskeletal system in particular. Well-conditioned muscles are less vulnerable to myofascial TrPs. The **personal** section helps one to understand how much disruption in life-style and function the pain is causing and elucidates the emotional effects of the pain. The last question identifies the activities that are important to the patient and are disrupted by the pain. Useful goals for the treatment program come from this list.

The examiner next completes the pain drawing on a body form as described in the preceding chapter under the heading, "Recognition of a Single-Muscle Syndrome." The *sequence* of numbered pain problems is carefully correlated, problem by problem, with the past and current medical history. It is impressive how clearly many pa-

Table 42.4 Patient Information Questionnaire

IDENTIFICATION:
Name _____ Date _____
SSN _____ Age ____ Sex ____
Home telephone_____

VOCATIONAL:
Occupation_____
    Right ____ or left ____ handed
I am still working ____ or I last worked:
    ____ weeks ago
    ____ months ago
    ____ years ago
I stopped work because _____
_____
_____

PAIN:
  Check pain in the following areas:
Right Left
____ ____   Headache
____ ____   Neck pain
____ ____   Shoulder pain
____ ____   Arms, forearms, & hands
____ ____   Chest
____ ____   Abdomen
____ ____   Upper back
____ ____   Mid and low back
____ ____   Hips, buttocks, & groin
____ ____   Legs and feet
* Please **PUT A STAR** in front of worst pain
  When did your pain first start?
____ weeks ____ months ____ years ago
  How did pain start?
____ suddenly ____ gradually
  Describe event that started the pain:
_____
_____

  How long have you had pain at the present level of severity?
    ____ weeks ____ months ____ years
  Pain is present: (mark one)
    ____ only during activity, or
    ____ sometimes at rest, or
    ____ all the time
  What do you think causes your pain?
_____
_____

  My typical pain level is _____
(0 to 10, if 10 worst pain possible)
  Pain is increased by: _____
_____
_____
_____

I get relief by: _____
_____
_____
_____

I have pain ____ % of my waking hours.

DIET:
Typical breakfast: _____
_____
_____

Typical lunch: _____
_____
_____

Typical dinner: _____
_____
_____

I often eat: _____
___ red meat ___ chicken ___ fish
___ bread ___ cereals ___ cheese
___ yogurt
What vegetables: _____
_____
_____

What fruits: _____
_____
_____

How much milk per day? _____
How many cups of coffee and/or tea daily? _____
How many glasses/cans of other caffeine drinks? _____
  I snack on: _____
_____

I avoid: _____
_____

SLEEP:
____ I sleep well, no trouble
____ I have occasional difficulty
____ I have frequent difficulty
____ I always have insomnia
I usually wake up feeling:
___ refreshed ___ better ___ as tired as when I went to bed
  When I get up in the morning my muscles:
___ are no stiffer than usual
___ are stiff and take ___ hours to loosen up

Table 42.4 (*continued*)

Sleep position: _____

MEDICATIONS:
List *ALL* of the medications you take
or use either regularly or occasionally:
(include vitamins and home remedies)

_____

PREVIOUS TREATMENT FOR PAIN:
I have seen the following kind of
specialists and health care providers
concerning this pain problem (include
approximately when and results):

_____

Exercise:
I get exercise by: (how often)

_____

Personal:
I smoke ___ packs per day. I don't smoke ___
I do ___ do not ___ drink alcoholic beverages
I am ___ married ___ single ___ separated ___ divorced ___ other
Sexually active? (problems ?) _____

I live:
___ with my spouse and ___ family members
___ with a friend   ___ alone
I am ___ satisfied ___ dissatisfied with this arrangement

Most of the time lately I feel:
(CHECK ONE WORD IN EACH COLUMN)
___ happy   ___ anxious ___ worried   ___ depressed
___ neutral ___ neutral ___ neutral   ___ neutral
___ sad   ___ relaxed ___ satisfied ___ enthusiastic

Disability benefits:
___ Receive compensation for _____
___ Have applied for (increased) benefits
___ No application pending
___ Have lawsuit pending

What are you unable to do because of pain that you want to do? _____

---

tients can distinguish among several pain problems with regard to the circumstances at onset, the distress each causes, and the relative degrees of threat they impose. When the patient indicates a pain level, the examiner must be sure to which pain problem it applies.

Throughout this history, the examiner attempts to sort out the contribution of organic disease and the contribution of learned and interactive pain behaviors. Patients with chronic pain characteristically suffer from a mixture of both. What is causing the patient's *pain*? What contributes to the patient's *suffering*?

PHYSICAL EXAMINATION

A minimal physical examination of the patient with pain problems that are primarily musculoskeletal should include hands-on examination of the muscles. Surprisingly, this critical step is too frequently overlooked. After a careful history, the physical examination substantiates suspected findings and resolves ambiguities. Techniques have been fully described to examine the patient for myofascial TrPs (9), for fibrositis/fibromyalgia (49, 71), and for articular dysfunction (53).

LABORATORY TESTS AND IMAGING

The following laboratory studies are routinely performed to help identify perpetuating factors in patients with a progressive MPS. The complete blood count screens for marginal anemia and for a macrocytosis that may reflect a vitamin B_{12} and/or folate inadequacy. An elevated erythrocyte sedimentation rate or C-reactive protein serves as a nonspecific warning of possible chronic infection. Normal values help to eliminate this possibility.

Chemistry Battery

The chemistry battery is most useful for detecting marginal hyperuricemia, low serum potassium or calcium (ionized calcium must be ordered separately and is more meaningful than total calcium), and elevated cholesterol that would relate to low thyroid function. A thyroid battery that includes T_4 and T_3 by RIA, T_3 uptake, T_4–resin T_3 uptake index, and thyroid-stimulating hormone helps to identify the commonly recognized thyroid deficiencies. The battery is indicated if clinical symptoms and signs of inadequate thyroid function are present.

Vitamin Studies

Serum vitamin B_{12} and/or folate values in the lower quartile of the normal laboratory values have been found to be perpetuators of myofascial TrPs in many patients. Vitamins B_1 and B_6 levels should also be obtained, if financially feasible. Plasma ascorbic acid should be determined if the clinical findings suggest low tissue reserves. Vitamin A should be tested if a total of more than 10,000 IU of vitamin A has been ingested daily for a period of time.

Imaging

Radiographs, computed tomography scans, and magnetic resonance imaging are rarely helpful for the identification of the three commonly overlooked musculoskeletal conditions. Imaging can be important for detecting perpetuating factors. Thermography is useful for documenting clinically diagnosed myofascial pain due to TrPs (84).

MANAGING THE PIECES

In patients with chronic MPS, one must balance therapy addressed to the origin of the pain with management of its psychological and behavioral complications. With both approaches, the focus of attention is directed toward function rather than pain.

Recovery from the complex interacting factors that comprise chronic pain is an incremental process. One can think of the patient as climbing up a ladder. Steps taken with one foot correspond to *resolution of causes of the pain*. Steps with the other foot represent *correction of factors that intensify the suffering*. For improvement of the patient as a whole, both feet must make stepwise progress.

APPROACH

The most effective first step usually is to select the most severe pain problem, or the major one that appears most likely to respond to treatment, and use it to test the therapeutic response in order to demonstrate to the patient the muscular origin of the pain. This is done: (*a*) by reproducing a myofascial referred pain pattern by pressing on the TrP, and (*b*) by immediate treatment that provides at least partial relief of the pain using specific myofascial therapy applied to the muscle. The operator makes sure that the patient understands the myofascial origin of the pain and understands that relief was provided by therapy that affected only the muscles and not the nerves or bones. To emphasize the muscular origin of the pain, the patient may be reminded of Dr. Janet Travell's quote, "Broken bones heal; injured muscles learn." By having patients note the exact positioning before and after stretch, they can see for themselves the increase in range of motion. Later, they can relate that increase in function to a corresponding reduction in pain.

Frequently, among patients suffering chronic pain, the origin of the pain is of more concern than the pain itself. Recognizing the muscular cause of the pain and learning how to relieve it themselves gives them control and is profoundly reassuring. Concurrently, the patient is screened for perpetuating factors; any mechanical factors that are apparent are corrected promptly, especially those that would perpetuate the specific pain syndrome selected for initial treatment.

With regard to the behavior issues, one starts correcting or neutralizing major reinforcers of pain or sick behavior. The spouse or significant other is often the key and should become involved in the treatment program. In the case of patients with a high proportion of sick or pain behavior, it may be wise to deal with the causes of the pain only on a prescheduled time-contingent basis.

This holistic approach is likely to require the coordinated efforts of a team of health care professionals. Many physical therapists have developed expertise in the specific manual myofascial treatment techniques and in the treatment of articular dysfunctions. Social workers and psychologists are experts at dealing with coping skills and remedial behavior. A physician must deal with the systemic perpetuating factors and administer TrP injections, if needed.

Continuing specific myofascial therapy (stretch-and-spray, injection, and other stretch techniques) is based on the response to previous therapy sessions. In patients with chronic myofascial pain, one must also locate and resolve perpetuating factors. For instance, correction of the commonly found foward head posture is essential. The patient comes to appreciate the fruitlessness of continued treatment until perpetuating factors are under control.

When a myofascial pain diagnosis has been established, complete failure of response to local treatment may be due to attention having been focused erroneously on a latent TrP instead of the active TrP responsible for the pain. It also is possible that the patient had several active TrPs that referred pain to the same area from different muscles and that not all of the active TrPs were inactivated.

It is essential that a detailed drawing of the pain under treatment be recorded at each visit so that changes in the referred pain pattern are clearly documented. Marked reduction in the pressure sensitivity of previously treated myofascial TrPs and disappearance of the corresponding pain pattern represents progress. The patient who is aware only of continuing residual pain may not appreciate the improvement. The recorded changes in the pain pattern assure both the patient and the clinician of the progress.

Many times, a previous pain reemerges because a less irritable TrP is now uncovered, like peeling off an outer layer of onion. Apparently, the central nervous system can attend to only a limited number of outstanding sources of pain at one time and a previously subliminal pain replaces that which was eliminated.

When the patient shows evidence of both myofascial TrPs and fibrositis/fibromyalgia, the myofascial TrPs are treated as such and the fibromyalgia is treated as outlined by Goldenberg (48). If the patient has a combination of myofascial TrPs and articular dysfunction, generally progress is made by releasing the tight muscles. The joint is then mobilized, followed by inactivation of any remaining TrPs. Neither treatment by itself succeeds in many of the patients who suffer from both conditions.

DRUGS

Pain cocktails are used successfully to detoxify patients on excessive analgesic or narcotic medication. Tricyclic compounds, such as amitriptyline or doxepin hydrochloride, are most effective in relatively small doses, 50–75 mg at bedtime for improving sleep and reducing pain sensitivity. Primary antidepressant action requires larger doses. Sleep may also be improved by 50 mg of the soporific antihistiminic dimenhydrinate (Dramamine) taken at bedtime. A nonsteroidal anti-inflammatory drug (NSAID) may be tried for temporary pain relief, but generally, when taken orally, they are of little or no help in relieving myofascial pain due to TrPs. The NSAID diclofenac, which is a prostaglandin antagonist, when injected in the TrP was more effective than lidocaine (97).

PATIENT EDUCATION

Characteristically, one muscular stress activates a TrP and a totally different factor, or factors, perpetuate it. The patient must understand this difference. Gradually, patients learn which of their muscles cause(s) a particular pain pattern and what movements overload those muscles, perpetuating the TrPs. These patients appreciate learning how to relieve the pain by self-stretch and how to avoid overloading the muscles. Patients must restructure their activities to avoid repetitive movement or sustained contraction that overloads and perpetuates TrPs in their muscles.

The patients are encouraged, whenever possible, to continue *what* they are doing by learning *how* to do it without overloading muscles. They learn to use, not abuse, their muscles. Correction of an anatomic or postural perpetuating factor frequently requires change of patient behavior; unless the patient fully understands the relationship between the pain and the perpetuating factor, he or she will soon revert to previous activity patterns and then wonder why the pain has returned.

INDUSTRIAL CASES

Although specific myofascial therapy appears to restore the muscle to its preinjury tolerance for stress in some patients, there is mounting evidence that in other patients inactivation of an active TrP leaves a latent TrP that is more vulnerable to reactivation than before injury. This poses a serious problem for many industrial cases where vocational rehabilitation is the critical issue. After inactivation of the TrPs, the patient is unable to do the same job in the same way that he or she did before. Often the gap between functional capacity and muscular demands of the job can be bridged by a combination of: (a) modifying the job to reduce muscle strain, (b) conditioning of the muscles with exercises to increase activity tolerance, and (c) regular performance of stretching exercises to minimize irritability of the TrPs.

Unemployed patients often can be transitioned back to employability through volunteer activities that place comparable demands on their muscles. This transition is now facilitated by work hardening and is practiced chiefly by occupational and sometimes by physical therapists.

The great tragedy is that often a complex chronic MPS could have been quickly and readily resolved initially, while still acute. If only it had been recognized and properly treated as myofascial, including correction of any perpetuating factors, much suffering and disability could have been averted.

Acknowledgments The senior author expresses an enormous debt of gratitude to Janet G. Travell, M.D., and to the fellow members on the Institute of Medicine Committee on Chronic Pain and Disability (1) for helping him to better understand chronic pain from the patient's point of view. The authors are deeply grateful to Dr. Travell for thoughtful review and constructive criticism of the manuscript and to Bernadette Jaeger, D.D.S., for her helpful suggestions.

References

1. Institute of Medicine: *Pain and Disability: Clinical, Behavioral and Public Policy Perspectives.* Washington, DC, National Academy Press, 1987.
2. Fields HL: *Pain.* New York, McGraw-Hill, 1987, pp 209–214.
3. Reynolds MD: Myofascial trigger point syndromes in the practice of rheumatology. *Arch Phys Med Rehabil* 62:111–114, 1981.
4. Fishbain DA, Goldberg M, Meagher BR, et al: Male and female chronic pain patients categorized by DSM-III psychiatric diagnostic criteria. *Pain* 26:181–197, 1986.
5. Friction JR, Kroening R, Haley D, et al: Myofascial pain syndrome of the head and neck: a review of clinical characteristics of 164 patients. *Oral Surg* 60:615–623, 1985.
6. Skootsky S: Incidence of myofascial pain in an internal medical group practice. Presented at the Annual Meeting of the American Pain Society, Washington, DC, November 6–9, 1986.

7. Travell J, Rinzler SH: The myofascial genesis of pain. *Postgrad Med* 11:425–434, 1952.
8. Travell J: Myofascial trigger points: clinical view. In Bonica JJ, Albe-Fessard D (eds): *Advances in Pain Research and Therapy.* New York, Raven Press, 1976, vol 1, pp 919–926.
9. Travell JG, Simons DG: *Myofascial Pain and Dysfunction: The Trigger Point Manual, Vol I.* Baltimore, Williams & Wilkins, 1983.
10. Azuma J, Kishi T, Williams RH, et al: Apparent deficiency of vitamin B_6 in typical individuals who commonly serve as normal controls. *Res Commun Chem Pathol Pharmacol* 14:343–348, 1976.
11. Baker H, Frank O: Vitamin status in metabolic upsets. *World Rev Nutr Diet* 9:124–160, 1968.
12. Shealy CN: Vitamin B_6 and other vitamin levels in chronic pain patients. *Clin J Pain* 2:203–204, 1987.
13. Siebert GK, Gerbershagen HU, Mäder, et al: Vitamin-status of inpatients with chronic cephalgia and effects of a 12 day-vitamin supplementation. *Pain Suppl* 4:S298, 1987 (abstr 572).
14. Wood B, Breen KJ: Clinical thiamine deficiency in Australia; the size of the problem and approaches to prevention. *Med J Aust* 1:461–462, 464, 1980.
15. Williams RJ: *Physicians Handbook of Nutritional Science.* Springfield, IL, Charles C Thomas, 1975, pp 48, 70–82.
16. National Research Council, Committee on Dietary Allowances: *Recommended Dietary Allowances,* ed. 9. Washington, DC, National Academy of Sciences, 1980.
17. Hillman RS: Vitamin B_{12}, folic acid, and the treatment of megaloblastic anemias. In Gilman AG, Goodman LS, Gilman A (eds): *The Pharmacological Basis of Therapeutics,* ed 6. New York, MacMillian, 1980, pp 1331–1346.
18. Danford DE, Munro HN: Water-soluble vitamins: the vitamin B complex and ascorbic acid. In Gilman AF, Goodman LS, Gilman A (eds): *The Pharmacological Basis of Therapeutics,* ed 6. New York, MacMillan, 1980, pp 1560–1582.
19. Neal RA, Sauberlich HE: Thiamin. In Goodhart ME, Shils ME (eds): *Modern Nutrition in Health and Disease,* ed 6. Philadelphia, Lea & Febiger, 1980, pp 191, 193–196.
20. Sauberlich HE, Canham JE: Vitamin B_6. In Goodhard RS, Shils ME (eds): *Modern Nutrition in Health and Disease,* ed 6. Philadelphia, Lea & Febiger, 1980, pp 219–225.
21. Rose DP: Oral contraceptives and vitamin B_6. In *Human Vitamin B_6 Requirements.* Washington, DC, National Academy of Sciences, 1978, pp 193–201.
22. Stead WW: Tuberculosis. In Wintrobe MM, Thorn GW, Adams RD, et al: *Harrison's Principles of Internal Medicine,* ed 7. New York, McGraw-Hill, 1974, p 867.
23. Theuer RC, Vitale JJ: Drug and nutrient interactions. In Schneider HA, Anderson CE, Coursin DB (eds): *Nutritional Support of Medical Practice.* New York, Harper & Row, 1977, pp 209, 300, 302.
24. Kelley WN: Gout and other disorders of purine metabolism. In Isselbacher KJ, Adams RD, Braunwald E (eds): *Harrison's Principles of Internal Medicine,* ed 9. New York, McGraw-Hill, 1980, pp 479–486.
25. Avioli LV: Calcium and phosphorus. In Goodhard RS, Shils ME (eds): *Modern Nutrition in Health and Disease,* ed 6. Philadelphia, Lea & Febiger, 1980, pp 298–305.
26. Lehninger AL: *Biochemistry.* New York, Worth, 1970, pp 383–550.
27. Cooper DS: Subclinical hypothyroidism. *JAMA* 258:246–247, 1987.
28. Sonkin LS: Endocrine disorders, locomotor and temporomandibular joint dysfunction. In Gelb HG (eds). *Clinical Management of Head, Neck and TMJ Pain and Dysfunction.* Philadelphia, WB Saunders, 1977, pp 140–180.
29. Barnes E: Basal temperature versus basal metabolism. *JAMA* 119:1072–1074, 1942.
30. Travell J: Identification of myofascial trigger point syndromes: a case of atypical facial neuralgia. *Arch Phys Med Rehabil* 62:100–106, 1981.
31. Simons DG: Myofascial pain syndromes due to trigger points: 2. Treatment and single-muscle syndromes. *Manual Med* 1:72–77, 1985.
32. Simons DG, Travell JG: Myofascial origins of low back pain. 2. Torso muscles. *Postgrad Med* 73:81–92, 1983.
33. Travell JG, Simons DG: *Myofascial Pain and Dysfunction: The Trigger Point Manual, Vol II.* Baltimore, Williams & Wilkins, in process, est. 1989.
34. Hagberg M, Kvarnström S: Muscular endurance and electromyographic fatigue in myofascial shoulder pain. *Arch Phys Med Rehabil* 65:522–525, 1984.
35. Simons DG: Myofascial pain syndromes due to trigger points: 1. Principles, diagnosis, and perpetuating factors. *Manual Med* 1:67–71, 1985.
36. Lewit K: Postisometric relaxation in combination with other methods of muscular facilitation and inhibition. *Manual Med* 2:101–104, 1986.
37. Lewit K, Simons DG: Myofascial pain: relief by post-isometric relaxation. *Arch Phys Med Rehabil* 65:452–456, 1984.
38. Knott M, Voss DE: *Proprioceptive Neuromuscular Facilitation.* New York, Hoeber, 1968, pp 97–99.
39. Mitchell FL Jr, Moran PS, Pruzzo NA: *Evaluation and Treatment Manual of Osteopathic Muscle Energy Procedures.* Valley Park, MO, Mitchell, Moran and Pruzzo, Associates, 1979,
40. Simons DG: Myofascial pain syndromes. In Basmajian JV, Kirby RL (eds): *Medical Rehabilitation.* Baltimore, Williams & Wilkins, 1984, pp 209–215, 313–320.
41. Danneskiold-Samsøe B, Christiansen E, Anderson RB: Myofascial pain and the role of myoglobin. *Scand J Rheumatol* 15:154–178, 1986.
42. Danneskiold-Samsøe B, Christiansen E, Lund B, et al: Regional muscle tension and pain ("fibrositis"): effect of massage on myoglobin in plasma. *Scand J Rehabil Med* 15:17–20, 1983.
43. Lewit K: The needle effect in the relief of myofascial pain. *Pain* 6:83–90, 1979.
44. Jaeger B, Skootsky SA: Double blind, controlled study of different myofascial trigger point injection techniques. *Pain Suppl* 4:S292, 1987 (abstr 560).
45. Weeks VD, Travell J: How to give painless injections. In *AMA Scientific Exhibits.* New York, Grune & Stratton, 1957, pp 318–322.
46. Benoit PW, Belt WD: Some effects of local anesthetic agents on skeletal muscle. *Exp Neurol* 34:264–278, 1972.
47. Bennett RM: Fibromyalgia. *JAMA* 257:2802–2803, 1987.
48. Goldenberg DL: Fibromyalgia syndrome: an emerging but controversial condition. *JAMA* 257:2782–2787, 1987.
49. Yunus M, Masi AT, Calabro JJ, et al: Primary fibromyalgia. *Am Fam Physician* 25:115–121, 1982.
50. Campbell SM, Bennett RM: Fibrositis. *DM* 32(11):653–722, 1986.
51. Smythe HA, Moldofsky H: Two contributions to understanding of the "fibrositis" syndrome. *Bull Rheum Dis* 28:928–931, 1977.
52. Wolfe F: The clinical syndrome of fibrositis. *Am J Med* 81:(Suppl 3A):7–14, 1986.

53. Lewit K: *Manipulative Therapy in Rehabilitation of the Motor System.* Stoneham, MA, Butterworth, 1985.
54. Fassbender HG: Non-articular rheumatism. In *Pathology of Rheumatic Diseases.* New York, Springer-Verlag, 1975, pp 303–314.
55. Miehlke K, Schulze G: Der sogenannte Muskelrheumatismus. *Internist* 2:447–453, 1961.
56. Popelianskii IaIu, Bogdanov EI, Khabirov FA: [Algesic trigger zones of the gastrocnemius muscle in lumbar osteochondrosis (clinicopathomorphological and electromyographic analysis)] (Russian). *Zh Nevropatol Psikhiatr* 84:1055–1061, 1984.
57. Popelianskii IaIu, Zaslavskii ES, Veselovskii VP: [Medicosocial significance, etiology, pathogenesis, and diagnosis of nonarticular disease of soft tissues of the limbs and back] (Russian). *Vopr Revm* 3:38–43, 1976.
58. Graff-Radford SB, Reeve JL, Jaeger B: Myofascial pain may present clinically as occipital neuralgia. *Neurosurgery* 19:610–613, 1986.
59. Simons DG: Muscle pain syndromes—Parts I and II. *Am J Phys Med* 54:289–311, 1975; 55:15–42, 1976.
60. Simons DG: Myofascial pain syndrome due to trigger points. In Goodgold J (ed): *Rehabilitation Medicine.* St. Louis, CV Mosby, 1987 (in press).
61. Reynolds MD: The development of the concept of fibrositis. *J Hist Med Allied Sci* 38:5–35, 1983.
62. Bates T, Grunwaldt E: Myofascial pain in childhood. *J Pediatr* 53:198–209, 1958.
63. Sola AE, Rodenberger ML, Gettys BB: Incidence of hypersensitive areas in posterior shoulder muscles. *Am J Phys Med* 34:58–590, 1955.
64. Simons DG: Fibrositis/fibromyalgia: a form of myofascial trigger points? *Am J Med* 81(suppl 3A):93–98, 1986.
65. Smythe HA: Non-articular rheumatism and the fibrositis syndrome. In Hollander JL, McCarty DJ (eds): *Arthritis and Allied Conditions,* ed 8. Philadelphia, Lea & Febiger, 1972, pp 874–884.
66. Egle UT, Schwab R, Rudolf ML, et al: Illness behaviour and defense mechanisms of patients with psychogenic pain: rheumatoid arthritis and fibrositis syndrome. *Pain Supl* 4:S324, 1987 (abstr 624).
67. Henriksson KG, Bengtsson A, Larsson J, et al: Muscle pain with special reference to primary fibromyalgia (PF). *Pain Suppl* 4:S294, 1987 (abstr 564).
68. Landrø NI, Winnem M: Psychodiagnostic evaluation of patients with myofascial pain syndrome (fibrositis). *Pain Suppl* 4:S419, 1987 (abstr 808).
69. Clark S, Campbell SM, Forehand ME, et al: Clinical characteristics of fibrositis: II. A "blinded," controlled study using standard psychological tests. *Arthritis Rheum* 28:132–137, 1985.
70. Moldofsky H, Scarisbrick P, England R, et al: Musculoskeletal symptoms and Non-REM sleep disturbance in patients with "fibrositis syndrome" and health subjects. *Psychosom Med* 37:341–351, 1975.
71. Smythe HA: Fibrositis and other diffuse musculoskeletal syndromes. In Kelley WN, Harris ED Jr, Ruddy S (eds): *Textbook of Rheumatology.* Philadelphia, WB Saunders, 1981, vol 1, pp 485–493.
72. Bennett RM (ed): The fibrositis/fibromyalgia syndrome: current issues and prospectives. *Am J Med* 81(Suppl 3A):1–115, 1986.
73. Bengtsson A: Primary fibromyalgia: a clinical and laboratory study. Linköping: Linköping University Dissertations, No. 224, 1986.
74. Crook J, Tunks E, Norman G, et al: A comparative study of tenderness thresholds in trigger points and non-trigger points in normal and fibromyalgia patients. *Pain* suppl 4:S307, 1987, (abstr 509).
75. Lund N, Bengtsson A, Thorborg P: Muscle tissue oxygen pressure in primary fibromyalgia. *Scand J Rheumatol* 15:165–173, 1986.
76. Smythe H: Tender points: evolution of concepts of the fibrositis/fibromyalgia syndrome. *Am J Med* 81(suppl 3A):2–6, 1986.
77. Bengtsson A, Henriksson K-G, Jorfeldt L: Primary fibromyalgia, a clinical and laboratory study of 55 patients. *Scan J Rheumatol* 15:340–347, 1986.
78. Tunks E, Norman G, Kalaher S, et al: Validity and reliability of the clinical use of a pressure algometer in the study of trigger points. *Pain* suppl 4:S307, 1987 (abstr 590).
79. Caro XJ: Immunofluorescent detection of IgG at the dermalepidermal junction in patients with apparent primary fibrositis syndrome. *Arthritis Rheum* 27:1174–1179, 1984.
80. Bartels EM, Danneskiold-Samsøe B: Histological abnormalities in muscle from patients with certain types of fibrositis. *Lancet* 1:755–757, 1986.
81. Bengtsson A, Henriksson K-G, Larsson J: Reduced high-energy phosphate levels in painful muscle in patients with primary fibromyalgia. *Arthritis Rheum* 29:817–821, 1986.
82. Fischer AA: Diagnosis and management of chronic pain in physical medicine and rehabilitation. In Ruskin AP (ed): *Current Therapy in Physiatry.* Philadelphia, WB Saunders, 1984, pp 131–134.
83. Fischer AA: Correlation between site of pain and "hot spots" on thermogram in lower body. *Postgrad Med Custom Communications,* March:99, 1986.
84. Simons DG: Myofascial pain syndromes: Where are we? Where are we going? *Arch Phys Med Rehabil* 69:207–212, 1988.
85. Mennel JM: *Joint Pain.* Boston, Little, Brown & Company, 1964.
86. Lewit K: Chain reactions in disturbed function of the motor system. *Manual Med* 3, 1987 (in press).
87. Fisk JW: *Medical Treatment of Neck and Back Pain.* Springfield, IL, Charles C Thomas, 1987, pp 65, 69.
88. Friberg O: Lumbar instability: a dynamic approach by traction-compression radiography. *Spine* 12:119–129, 1987.
89. Rubin D: An approach to the management of myofascial trigger point syndromes. *Arch Phys Med Rehabil* 62:107–110, 1981.
90. Addison RG: Chronic pain syndrome. *Am J Med* 77:54–58, 1984.
91. Price DD, Harkins SW, Baker C: Sensory-affective relationships among different types of clinical and experimental pain. *Pain* 28:297–307, 1987.
92. Melzack R: *The Puzzle of Pain.* New York, Basic Books, 1973, pp 22–24, 153–179.
93. Baker BA: The muscle trigger: evidence of overload injury. *J Neurol Orthop Med Surg* 7:35–43, 1986.
94. Evans WJ, Meredith CN, Cannon JG, et al: Metabolic changes following eccentric exercise in trained and untrained men. *J Appl Physiol* 61:1864–1868, 1986.
95. McCully KK, Faulkner JA: Injury to skeletal muscle fibers of mice following lengthening contractions. *J Appl Physiol* 59:119–126, 1985.
96. Melnick J: Trigger areas and refractory pain in duodenal ulcer. *NY State J Med* 57:1073–1076, 1957.
97. Frost A: Diclofenac versus lidocaine as injection therapy in myofascial pain. *Scan J Rheumatol* 15:153–156, 1986.

selected topics
section 4

chapter 43
Pain Problems in Primary Care Medical Practice

Troy L. Thompson II, M.D.
Richard L. Byyny, M.D.

Most patients with acute or chronic pain initially seek out a primary care physician (e.g., a general practitioner or family physician, general internist, or obstetrician-gynecologist) to evaluate and treat their condition. Pain complaints make up a large percentage of primary care practices; in fact, persistent pain is the most common chief complaint bringing patients to see primary care physicians. Headaches, abdominal pains, and low back pain are among the most common types of pain complaints in primary care practices (1, 2). Low back pain is especially common in those involved in work-related disability claims, and chronic low back pain is the most common reason given for work absenteeism in the United States. Chronic low back pain alone accounts for almost 20 million physician visits annually in the United States alone, and compensation to "chronic low back cripples" accounted for about 40% of disability payments in California in one year. Headaches are estimated to account for about 12 million physician visits annually (3–5). The differential diagnosis of lower back and spinal pain is discussed in Chapter 27, and headache pain is discussed thoroughly in Chapters 19, 20, and 21.

APPROACH TO THE PAIN PATIENT

Patients with chronic pain are probably the most challenging group for primary care, as well as other types of physicians. The evaluation of chronic pain is complex since virtually any biomedical or psychiatric disorder may present as or be associated with complaints of somatic discomfort and pain (6). Also, since many serious illnesses, such as cancer, may initially present with vague pains, a pain complaint whose source cannot be readily identified, but which persists, especially if it worsens, may be very frightening to the physician as well as to the patient. The primary care physician is presented with a dilemma in such clinical situations. Does he do a basic history and physical examination and routine laboratory studies, then "wait it out" to see if the pain complaints persist and become more specific? To do so may lead to progression of a potentially treatable disorder. However, to do the opposite would often have adverse consequences of a different type. That is, it would be very expensive and time consuming to thoroughly work up each pain complaint that a primary care physician saw. In fact, if the average primary care physician sees about 50 patients per day, it would not be possible to completely evaluate each patient because of time constraints. After a basic evaluation, the primary care physician could refer patients with pain complaints to a specialist in the organ system or bodily region that seems most likely to be etiologic. However, this would also become expensive and time consuming, and that specialist might then refer the patient to yet another specialist, and so on, resulting in an escalating spiral of cost, time, and diagnostic procedures and their associated morbidity.

Most primary care physicians usually take a "middle of the road" approach to patients with chronic pain complaints. If the type of pain may be associated with severe pathology, diagnostic efforts are undertaken to rule that out. However, if the pain complaints appear to be benign in nature, most take a "wait and see" approach. Reevaluation appointments every 1–2 months and supportive and symptomatic therapies are the most common management approaches. In part, this approach is due to the repeated observations made by primary case physicians that many pains that bring patients to see them will improve spontaneously if they follow the patient. "Tincture of time" is indeed very effective for many benign and self-limited conditions (biomedical and psychiatric) and is much less costly financially for most patients.

Another reason that primary care physicians often initially adopt a conservative approach for pain symptoms is that they have witnessed morbidity and sometimes mortality due to vigorous diagnostic and possibly to therapeutic procedures. A vivid example of this is the patient with persistent "belly pain" who doctor shops until he eventually finds a physician who will perform an exploratory laparotomy. The typical scenario is that the pain may improve temporarily after the surgery, even if the surgery did not reveal any specific pathology. More often during the past, occasionally an appendectomy or cholecystectomy might be performed "since we were in there anyway" or possibly in hopes that some not grossly evident pathology in those tissues might be related to the pain complaints. However, after several weeks or months the abdominal pain would often return, sometimes in a slightly modified form, as if to convey to the physician "the last surgery did modify the original pain, so another surgery would probably help this pain as well." The well-meaning surgeon, who of course spent many long years learning his skills to relieve patients' suffering, may decide to "go back in again to see if I missed something or if something has become more evident since the previous surgery." The naive surgeon may not realize that if nothing specific was found on the initial exploratory surgery, it is not very likely that another surgery will be more revealing, if only vague, persistent pains are present or if the pains are atypical of any known pathology. Surgeons trained in recent decades are usually fairly sophisticated regarding psychological factors involved with patients who repeatedly seek surgery. However, the occasional anecdotal report of an unexpected "pick up" and treatment coup or cure on a repeat surgery may be used to rationalize "taking another look." Therefore, some primary care physicians make a valiant attempt to keep their chronic pain patients away from surgeons at all costs. In recent years, most primary care physicians have realized that neurosurgical procedures may be effective for some chronic pain patients. In such cases, the primary physician may consult with a neurosurgeon, especially in a referral center, that deals with a number of chronic pain patients.

ADAPTIVE ASPECTS OF PAIN

The physician may develop almost a knee-jerk aversive response to chronic pain patients. These patients are often very difficult to diagnose, because of the tremendous differential diagnosis of almost any chronic pain complaint, and to treat, because of the wide variation in individuals' responses to pain and to pain treatments. However, the primary physician should remind himself that the pain pathway is usually very adaptive and essential to the health and well-being of organisms. Pain is often the earliest signal that an incipient disease process is present. The type and distribution of pain may allow the physician to diagnose a treatable condition promptly, before further tissue damage occurs or before some illnesses, such as cancer, spread and become more difficult or impossible to effectively treat.

The importance of pain sensation to the individual may be further appreciated by considering people who have a congenital absence of pain (7). These individuals are prone to multiple physical injuries and cannot recognize pain as an early warning sign of illness or disability. In fact, out of frustration that they will be injured anyway, some patients with a congenital absence of pain may resort to self-injury, possibly because that gives them some degree of control over the trauma that they sustain. Pain sensation is one of the means by which individuals learn to differentiate themselves from the outside world and to establish their boundaries. Without such feedback, the individual may not develop in a psychologically normal manner and will have a distorted body image.

SOCIOCULTURAL VARIABLES OF PAIN BEHAVIOR

Illness and pain are sometimes thought to be inflicted on someone for wrongdoing. The powerful psychological and sociocultural associations between pain, guilt, and punishment may be further appreciated when it is realized that the word "pain" is derived from the Latin word "*poene*" and the Greek word "*poine*," both of which mean penalty or punishment. Some religious subcultures believe illness and pain are inflicted because the person has sinned. Therefore, these people may believe that they deserve to be ill and to have pain, as though a cure or analgesia might cut short the punishment they deserve because of some real or imagined transgression or sin. Pain is still inflicted as a means of punishment in some cultures and families. Floggings or other forms of physical injury are still used some places as punishment for crimes. Some families still inflict pain, such as through spankings, to punish their children (5, 8, 9).

The primary care physician usually recognizes that many individuals who present to his office with a variety of pain complaints are the "worried well." In fact, no organic explanation of pain could be found in 75% of medical patients who presented with pain as their chief complaint (10). Some individuals are so frightened of physical damage, illness, disability, or deformity that they seek out a physician at the earliest development of even a minor pain. Often these patients suffer from hypochondriasis, anxiety, depression, or some other psychiatric disorder, of which their preoccupation with and extreme sensitivity to pain is one symptom (11). In some of the milder cases, reassurance and education of the patient may suffice. If the patient can be assured that the pain should remain mild and be transient and that they should make a follow-up appointment if it persists even slightly, many patients will require nothing further. More severe psychiatrically associated forms of pain are discussed later.

An individual's response to pain is determined by a complex interaction of psychological, personality, familial, social, and cultural factors (12–14). The degree of perception and amount of complaints about a pain may be affected widely by a number of subjective, emotional, and largely unmeasurable factors. This is important for the primary care physician to realize, since this is different than many other disorders that he typically treats. For most other medical disorders there is some type of laboratory quantification available that may somewhat parallel the degree of illness, control of the illness, or effectiveness of treatment. That is clearly not the case with pain. Some individuals pay great attention to a small amount of physical trauma, while others may amaze the physician with their degree of denial or stoicism about massive trauma or illness. In part, the individual's reactions to pain and adaptation to chronic pain may relate to sociocultural factors.

Some cultures, religions, and families place greater or lesser emphasis on pain complaints (15). For example, patients of lower socioeconomic status are more likely to ascribe pain to physical rather than psychosocial causes than are patients of higher socioeconomic classes (16). Zborowski (17) discussed several stereotypes of cultures as they relate to the pain-associated behaviors in those cultures. These should not be taken too literally. Clearly, many individuals and families with roots in the cultures discussed do not demonstrate the stereotyped responses to a significant degree. However, the stereotypes may be used to remind the physician to evaluate the sociocultural, including familial, factors that may be amplifying chronic pain in patients. Also, the physician will be able to provide better care if he realizes that the meanings of pain and illness and expected illness and pain-related behaviors vary widely between cultures, and even among families who are part of the same subculture (18).

In his research in a large metropolitan veterans' hospital, Zborowski identified four stereotyped groups that he related to their responses to pain: Irish, Italian, Jewish, and "old American" ethnic groups. He believed the Italian and Jewish subcultures tended to be more expressive of pain that they were experiencing. It is important for the primary physician to realize that seemingly exaggerated responses to pain may be due to the patient doing what is expected within his culture, and that his behaviors do not represent psychiatric illness. These individuals might be more likely to be "a mental case" and in need of psychiatric evaluation and treatment if they did not respond in a vivid, expressive manner. The Irish and "old American" subgroups may be much more stoic about their expressions of pain. Their family and friends may value "a stiff upper lip" and view crying or any other emotional expression as a sign of weakness.

The potential risks and benefits of fitting into either extreme of reactivity are obvious. The overly expressive subgroups may come running to the doctor repeatedly with what turn out to be minor complaints. It is not likely that a pain-related illness will go unevaluated in these subgroups, but the physician may become weary of having them appear in his office, especially if he does not understand these sociocultural factors. There is a risk with the overly expressive subgroups that a "boy who cried wolf" situation may develop. That is, if the patient has a thick chart of negative findings, the physician may be less attentive and less vigorous in his evaluation when the patient presents with a bona fide medical disorder. The patient who has been labelled a crock or hypochondriac will obviously die of some biomedical disorder (11, 19).

Some primary care physicians have had experiences where the chronically somatizing patient actually complained less when he developed a biomedical disorder (sometimes including severe conditions such as myocardial infarction or ruptured appendix) than he did with his multiple psychologically based physcan complaints. Some of these patients report exactly the same experiences. For example, a patient reported his ruptured appendix and subsequent peritonitis were less painful and disabling than his usual abdominal distress, which was due to functional bowel syndrome.

On the other hand, the stoic subtypes also run some risks. They may be admired and liked by physicians, who often are also hard-working individuals who deal with stress in their lives by redoubling their efforts and forging ahead. It is hard for a physician to recognize a behavior pattern as potentially pathologic or maladaptive if he shares it with the patient. The stoic may be viewed as the ideal patient by the physician, whereas the emotionally expressive patient may be labeled as whining, whimpering, and generally to be avoided. Paradoxically, the more the emotionally expressive patient and his family are avoided or not engaged emotionally, the more they tend to demonstrate the characteristics that many physicians hate. Thereby, a vicious cycle may be established.

However, the stoic may not seek medical help until an illness has progressed to a severe degree. The stoic may keep going with a chronic condition until he is literally unable to get himself to the doctor's office. The stoic may rationalize this avoidant behavior by feeling that he cannot really be sick if he has not yet seen a doctor; so avoiding the doctor magically protects him from illness and means his condition must be temporary and minor. The stoic may be brought to the emergency room by family, friends, or in an ambulance when he is no longer able to get up or loses consciousness. Even then, it is striking that the stoic and his family or friends—who also, of course, tend to be stoics—may apologize for causing the physician and emergency room staff any trouble. These individuals appear to be self-reliant and hyperindependent on the surface. Underneath, they may be terrified of illness and of needing to be dependent on anyone. Their fear of pain may be second only to their fear of death, so they may try to completely deny the possibility of both. They fear passivity, and once diagnosed as having an illness often resolve to fight it to the end. Athletic or war metaphors, such as "I am going to show this thing who is boss," or ". . . defeat it," are common during the treatment of stoics. Family and friends may describe the patient with pride as always being a fighter. Another risk for stoics and their families is that they may not know when or be unable to let go when "they are beaten," to borrow one of their metaphors. As a result, they may spend a great deal of time and money and experience a lot of frustration seeking exotic cures and repeated evaluations by multiple medical experts or nonmedical "healers," sometimes including quacks and charlatans.

If pain becomes unbearable, the stoic may prefer to withdraw from family and friends rather than "letting them see me like this." It may be equally unbearable for the family and friends to see the previously "strong and proud" individual break down and cry. Crying may be viewed as effeminate in a man and also a sign of weakness in a woman.

Stoics may also be more likely to request an operation for their condition than more emotionally expressive groups. They tend to view illness more in mechanical terms and, therefore, will seek a "mechanical" cure. They will often use mechanical metaphors, such as "the old ticker isn't firing right, so I need a new set of spark plugs put in," to describe their need for a cardiac pacemaker, and so forth.

The stoic may also be more reluctant to accept the primary physician's recommendation of a consultation from another specialist. The stoic may wish to view his physician as he views himself, self-reliant and in need of no outside help. The more emotionally expressive groups may have the opposite response. They may seek the opinions of several specialists and read medical literature to see if their physician "knows what he's doing." If the physician is not aware of the emotional needs that are being met by the latter behaviors of these patients, he may feel insulted, become angry, and want to have even less to do with these patients and their families. Additional sociologic and cultural aspects of pain are discussed in more detail in Chapter 4.

PERSONALITY AND SECONDARY GAIN FACTORS

For some patients, chronic pain may relate to or amplify a number of their psychological characteristics. Those who develop a specific psychiatric disorder in response to the stress of chronic pain are discussed later. However, chronic pain is often associated with secondary gain, which may take a variety of forms. Some chronic pain patients may reap interpersonal gains from their pain, such as by receiving more love or attention from family and friends because they are sick. Occasionally, a patient may wish, either consciously or subconsciously, to remain ill to prevent some event, such as the breakup of a marriage or a child leaving home. This is sometimes confirmed by a spouse who may say "I would leave him in a minute if he got well" or "I was getting ready to leave just before he became ill, but I couldn't live with myself if I left an ill man," or by similar types of comments made by others. For some, chronic illness may serve a social purpose. They may receive more attention and a degree of specialness or group identification as a result of their illness or disability. Automobile license plates or other insignia are sometimes used by members of such groups, presumably at least in part to convey to the world that they wish to be regarded as distinguished and deserving of honor or some form of special treatment.

Financial secondary gain may also result from some forms of chronic pain and disability. This may escalate to create an awesome Catch-22, especially for the lower class or lower middle income individual. They may be able to receive as much or occasionally more compensation for maintaining their disability as they could by working full-time at their usual occupation. Many individuals understandably would choose to have their time to themselves, with the "price" being an occasional visit to the physician and disability review board, rather than working full-time, if their compensation will be at least equal from these two alternatives. Another Catch-22 aspect of some disability compensation programs is that they view patients as either fully disabled or fully able to work. If the patients become somewhat rehabilitated and would be able to work part-time and possibly gradually increase their workload, they may be threatened with totally losing their disability payments the first day they work part-time. Many disability review agencies have become more enlightened in this respect in recent years. They have realized that if they gradually encourage the patient to increase part-time work and slowly decrease disability payments proportionately, many patients will prefer at least some part-time work to having nothing structured to do. This titrated approach may even allow some financial incentive for the patient to do part-time work. Some disability agencies have learned such a flexible and gradual behavior modification approach can save them a great deal of money in the long run and facilitate more patient recovery than a rigid, either-or policy (5). Legal aspects of pain and Social Security disability and workers' compensation law are discussed in Chapters 48 and 49, respectively.

Chronic pain or illness may paradoxically be welcomed by individuals with some types of personalities, and this may be a form of personal secondary gain. If a person feels like a failure, the chronic pain may provide a "way out" when he does fail or feels like a failure. He may be able to say to himself and others that he could have succeeded if it had not been for the chronic disability or discomfort. Some of these patients have referred to their pain as "an old friend" (20), because it is something that has become personified as a useful part of their personality that they can count on during a time of need. The "old friend" may serve as a psychological crutch that may be utilized in many ways depending upon the situation. The psychological evaluation of chronic pain patients is further discussed in greater detail in Chapter 6, and psychological testing of chronic pain patients is discussed in Chapter 45.

The physician who is alert for patients who have a combination of several of the psychosocial, familial, and cultural risk factors for developing chronic pain discussed above may be able to intervene promptly. Early recognition and intervention with such patients may prevent a vicious cycle from being established, which produces a chronic pain syndrome patient and family. Clearly, an "ounce of prevention is worth a pound of cure" regarding chronic pain patients. Early recognition of such patients is further discussed in Chapter 46.

PAIN PATHWAYS AND MODIFICATION OF PAIN PERCEPTION

The primary care physician must continually remind himself that chronic pain is not a simple stimulus-response type of reaction, although this fact has been know for many years (21). When he learned the pain pathway in medical school, it may have appeared fairly straightforward. However, much about it remains to be understood. Specifically, many psychosocial and physiologic factors are able to alter the perception of pain through mechanisms that largely remain mysterious. Probably the most important factor for the physician to remember in evaluating chronic pain patients is that their degree of disability usually relates to a combination of biopsychosocial factors (6, 22). There may certainly be exceptions to this statement, such as the patient who has severe persistent pain due to a proven serious illness, such as metastatic cancer to bone, pancreatic carcinoma, or so forth. However, these patients usually are not as difficult for the physician to manage as are patients with chronic pain for which no definitive diagnosis has been made or for whom their degree of pain complaints appear to greatly exceed the biomedical trauma that is evident.

What initiates the transmission of pain impulses and the exact pain pathway is not fully known. Substance P may be the primary neurotransmitter of afferent nociceptors, which initiate the pain pathway (23). There are two types of peripheral nerve fibers associated with pain transmissions: large, myelinated A fibers, which conduct impulses rapidly and are associated with sharp pain sensations; and small, unmyelinated C fibers, which transmit impulses more slowly and are associated with dull pain (9). The A fibers may be more involved with acute traumatic pain and lead to the spinal reflex withdrawal, if possible, of the traumatized part from the source of injury. The C fibers may become more involved in chronic pain states. Therefore, there appear to be neuroanatomic as well as psychological differences between acute and chronic pain (24, 25).

The fundamental neuroanatomic pain pathway consists of pain stimuli traveling through pain fibers into the dorsal root zone of the spinal cord. At that point, pain fibers divide into ascending and descending branches that run in Lissauer's tract (the posterolateral fasciculus) in the spinal cord. Within two vertebral segments, they appear to leave this tract to synapse with posterior horn neurons. The exact connections and types of interneurons or other structures on which they may impinge or by which they may be affected at this level are not fully known. However, it is believed that alternations in the perception of pain may begin to occur (possibly through gateway or T-cells or other systems that are discussed later) at this level. The pain stimuli then cross anterior to the spinal cord's central canal in the anterior white commissure. They then course rostrally in the lateral spinothalamic tract. The pain fibers then supply input to parts of the limbic system (reticular formation) and to several thalamic nuclei, including the ventral posterolateral (VPL) nucleus of the thalamus, and to the hypothalamus. It is not clear, although it is possible, that the limbic system (which is closely related to the individual's level of alertness and has been described as a type of "rheostat" for cortical activity level) and possibly thalamic nuclei may be able to influence the transmission of pain stimuli at this level. Fibers then relay pain impulses from the thalamus to the secondary somatic sensory area of the cerebrum, and some fibers go directly from the VPL nucleus to the primary somatic sensory area.

For severe and intractable chronic pain, nerve blocks and neurosurgical and neuroablative procedures have been used at virtually every level of the pain pathways described above. Neurosurgical transection of the spinothalamic and spinoreticular formation pathways may initially cause pain relief in up to 85% of patients (26). However, many of these patients redevelop painful sensations within a few months. This suggests that pain pathways may exist or develop in other than the anterolateral quadrant of the spinal cord (6, 27, 28). Nerve blocks, neuroablative techniques, and spinal surgery are discussed further in Chapters 10, 11, and 12, respectively.

Two basic types of pain sensation exist, and chronic pain usually has more characteristics of the second type. The first is *fast pain*, which is reported as sharp or pricking and has little emotional counterpart. The second is termed *slow pain*, which may be reported as a burning sensation. The fast pain pathways appear to be more somatotopically arranged and allow such pain to be sharply localized. Slow pain appears to be closely integrated with emotional factors, possibly in the thalamic and hypothalamic regions, and is not organized in a manner that allows precise spatial or temporal information processing.

Descending pathways from the cerebral cortex and other higher structures may partly modify pain perception by having effects at the posterior horn or in the reticular formation. However, in humans, pain is not consciously perceived until the impulses reach the thalamus, but pain will be perceived if the cortical projection areas have been destroyed but the thalamus has remained intact. The parietal cortex is primarily where the source of pain is localized and its intensity is perceived. Memory regions and cortical association areas may also play a role in amplifying or diminishing the reaction to pain perception. If the person has memories or past experiences with a similar type of pain, the reaction may be diminished if those experiences were benign or greatly increased if significant psychological or physiologic trauma resulted.

Most individuals have approximately the same threshold for the perception of pain. However, that threshold may be decreased by almost half in most individuals, and even more in some, by several techniques or interventions. These include acupuncture, biofeedback, relaxation techniques, hypnosis, and imagery training (6, 29, 30). A pleasant or euphoric mental state may also decrease pain perception. Analgesics and placebos may diminish the pain threshold (1, 13). Approximately one-third of individuals with clear-cut pain secondary to physiologic trauma have significant pain relief secondary to a placebo (31). A critical point for the physician to realize is that response to placebo in no way rules out or diminishes the probability that a biomedical disorder underlies the pain. It is not clear how placebo effects may be taking place; some persons' beliefs that relief will be forthcoming may lead them to be able to produce neurophysiologic changes that diminish pain perception. This may occur through effects the cortex has on lower central nervous system functions, or a positive, optimistic mood might increase endorphin levels.

The endorphins are compounds that were named for "endogenous morphine." The central nervous system, through as yet incompletely understood mechanisms, does appear to have the capacity to produce its own analgesia (32). The capacity to do this and the effectiveness of such a system undoubtedly would vary somewhat between individuals. Possibly those individuals who have a more pronounced placebo response or who are responsive to biofeedback or some other techniques may in fact have a better or more responsive endorphin system (6). For example, 30–40% of postsurgical patients report little or no pain and require few or no analgesics. Might these be the individuals who are able to mobilize their endorphin systems? Since about the same percentage of people are placebo responders, are these the same people in both groups? Might some people be able to mobilize their endorphins in response to one situation but not another?

The endorphin system seems to be concentrated in regions of the brain, especially the periaqueductal and perinventricular gray matter, that parallel the distribution of opiate receptors in the brain (33). It has also been found that naloxone (an opioid antagonist) may reverse the effects of placebo analgesia, which further suggests that placebos may operate by activating the endogenous opioid system in placebo-responsive individuals (28).

The state of other neurotransmitter systems may also affect pain perception and tolerance. Depressed individuals are often much more responsive to pain stimuli. Since the noradrenergic and serotoninergic systems have been associated with some types of depression, disruption or stress upon those systems may make the patient less resilient in managing painful stimuli. In fact, serotonergic neurons have also been found to interact with the endorphin system. Since most tricyclic antidepressants act in part by increasing the synaptic levels of serotonin, this effect may relate to the benefit of tricyclics for some pain patients (34). Tricyclics may also help some pain patients by increasing the cortical inhibition of pain perception or responsiveness, in addition to their activities on the catecholamines (9). Malfunction in the dopamine system may be associated with schizophrenia, and some schizophrenics seem to be able to suffer significant injuries yet experience relatively little or no pain. Anxious and panic disorder patients may be exquisitely sensitive to pain, and disruption in their γ-aminobutyric acid neurotransmitter systems may be related to those disorders. Many of these neurotransmitter systems are inhibitory or facilitatory of other systems in various regions of the brain; therefore, an effect on one might eventually have multiple effects that could alter the person's perception or tolerance of pain.

Melzack and Wall proposed a gate control theory, which has received a lot of attention and debate, in which they postulate a "gateway" type of cell in the spinal cord that might be opened or closed to allow or prevent pain stimuli from passing through and reaching higher levels in the nervous system. If these "gating" or transmitting neurons (or T-cells) are in the spinal cord, they could alter the number of pain stimuli reaching the level of the thalamus, and thereby alter pain perception. These T-cells (to be differentiated from immunologic T-cells) are hypothesized to exist in the substantia gelatinosa of the spinal cord and to be affected by large peripheral afferent nerve fibers as well as by higher nervous system activity. The degree of modulation of the inflow of pain impulses may be affected by the relative activity of inhibitory A fibers and facilitatory C fibers, as well as by descending influences from the brain (35, 36).

Transcutaneous or dorsal column electrical stimulators may operate to diminish pain perception by stimulating peripheral fibers that partially close or overload these gating cells (37). Some dentists use "white noise" generators to diminish the pain perceived during dental procedures, and these presumably operate in a similar manner but at the level of cranial nerves. It is hypothesized that the sensory nerves have a limited capacity to carry stimuli, including pain impulses. If some nonpainful form of stimulation bombards a region from which painful stimuli are arising, presumably the pain impulses will have to compete for the sensory nerves' capacity to transmit them, and the number of painful stimuli "getting through" might be thereby diminished. It is not clear that a specific gating type of neuron, which incidentally has not been identified anatomically, would even need to exist. If the sensory nerves are continually bombarded with electrical stimuli, it might make sense that they would be less responsive to any single type of stimulus, including pain, that also was feeding into their pathway. However, the opposite type of response to continual sensory bombardment and overload might hypothetically occur; that is, the neurons might develop a hypersensitivity response, especially if the stimulation is stopped, in which even a small stimulus would lead to an exaggerated response. This might be similar to kindling phenomena leading to a seizure, in which, because of a gradual buildup of seizure predisposing factors, an otherwise minor event may trigger a full-blown seizure—a "straw that broke the camel's back" type of situation.

Transcutaneous stimulators may also be effective, at least in part, by stimulating the patient's endorphin system. This possibility is supported by the observation that naloxone (an opioid antagonist) may reduce the effectiveness of treatment by transcutaneous electrical nerve stimulation, especially of a high-frequency type (38). Neural stimulation techniques are discussed in more detail in Chapter 12.

It is clear that the perception of and reaction to painful stimuli may be significantly affected by the psychological meaning that the pain has for the individual. In fact, the degree of pain experienced and need for analgesia may be much more strongly related to the psychological meanings of the injury and pain than to the actual amount of physiologic trauma present. Beecher (39) performed elegant research in demonstrating this point. He found that many soldiers who experienced significant wounds in battle complained of little or no pain and refused morphine when it was offered. Civilians who experienced similar wounds, often even due to the same type of injury, such as a gunshot wound, tended to complain of much more pain and to request more analgesia. In fact, only one-third of the soldiers accepted analgesic when offered as compared to 80% of civilians. Beecher explained these differences as due to the very different meanings that the injuries had to these two groups. If the soldiers were alert and able to refuse analgesia, there was a good chance that they would survive the wound, and it would be their "ticket home," whereas, if they had not been wounded, they knew they might have gone on to be more severely wounded or killed in battle. Therefore, there might understandably be a certain degree of relief associated with the wound. Some soldiers have stuck a leg or arm out of their foxhole when they have heard a shell coming in with the hope that they will sustain a minor shrapnel wound by doing so. Again, the injury in such a case might be life-saving and would be partially welcomed. On the other hand, there are usually little or no positive personal or social consequences of being wounded as a civilian; therefore, their injury is seldom desired and tends to have few positive associated features. Furthermore, Pavlov was able to train dogs to look forward to a minor wound or other traumatic stimuli if it was linked to being fed. Some individuals also learn to control others by threatening or carrying out self-injurious acts. The wrist cutter or other person who threatens suicide may learn that this is a dramatic and sometimes effective way of getting the attention of others, and getting them to do what he wants when all other avenues have failed.

PAIN DISORDERS SEEN AND MANAGEMENT BY PRIMARY CARE PHYSICIANS

A number of the more common and persistent disorders that bring patients to see a primary care physician with pain complaints are listed in Table 43.1. However, this is far from inclusive, and the patient with any medical condition that produces pain is most likely to be seen initially by a primary care physician. As is apparent from reviewing Table 43.1, a comprehensive history and physical examination and thorough laboratory screening are essential parts of the evaluation of chronic pain patients. The physician should assure that he knows seven key aspects of the pain symptoms (40):

1. The exact location and if any migration occurs
2. Its quality and severity at onset
3. The typical duration and course the pain follows
4. If the quality fluctuates during its course
5. What is the severity and how the severity varies during its course
6. Any factors that alleviate or aggravate the pain or precipitate its onset
7. Any other signs or symptoms that may be associated with the pain

Chronic pain patients tend to be very complex and difficult to diagnose; therefore, the primary care physician may understandably become frustrated when no specific diagnosis can be made and no treatment seems to help. At such times, the primary physician may be tempted to "turf" the patient to other physicians, especially to multiple subspecialists, or to other professionals interested in treating pain. In such situations, the physician's frustration may be revealed through calling the patient a "referred pain," a "crock," or other such terms (3, 19). The primary physician may wish to send the patient for a consultation, but it is generally better for the patient if a primary physician continues to "quarterback" and coordinate the total health care efforts (41). Otherwise, a "committee" of often poorly communicating subspecialists may each be trying to take care of one part of the problem. The image of four blind men describing an elephant comes to mind in this regard; each describes what he feels (the

Table 43.1
Common Pain Disorders Seen by Primary Care Physicians[a]

Headache disorders
    Tension (muscle contraction) headaches
    Vascular (migraine or cluster) headaches
    Psychogenic
Abdominal disorders
    Irritable (functional) bowel syndrome
    Peptic ulcer disease
Musculoskeletal disorders
    Low back pain
    Rheumatoid or other forms of arthritis
    Myofascial pain
Psychiatric disorders
    Depression, atypical depression
    Hypochondriasis
    Anxiety, panic disorders
    Conversion symptoms
    Compensation neurosis
    Malingering
    Delusions due to psychosis (e.g., dementia, schizophrenia)
Ischemic disorders
    Angina pectoris
    Peripheral vascular disease (e.g., claudication)
Neoplastic disorders
    Direct invasion or compression of nerves
    Metastases causing invasion or compression of other structures
Neurologic disorders—nerve lesions
    Post-traumatic neuritis
    Causalgia
    Postoperative neuromas
    Amputation stump (phantom) pain
    Coccydynia
    Scar pain
    Nerve entrapments
    Postherpetic neuralgia—shingles
    Trigeminal neuralgia—tic douloureux
    Sympathetic dystrophy (e.g., shoulder-hand syndrome)
    Spastic states
    Thalamic pain
Other categories
    Temporomandibular joint (TMJ) syndrome (bruxism)
    Dental, nasal, sinusoidal, ophthalmologic, or otologic pain
    Gout
    Chronic pancreatitis

[a] Adapted from Boyd DB, Merskey H, Nielsen JS: The pain clinic: An approach to the problem of chronic pain. In Smith WL, Merskey H, Gross SC (eds): *Pain: Meaning and Management.* Jamaica, NY, SP Medical & Scientific Books, 1980, p 161; and from Thompson TL II: Headache. In Kaplan HI, Sadock BJ (eds): *Comprehensive Textbook of Psychiatry,* ed 4. Baltimore, Williams & Wilkins, 1985, p 1203.

trunk, an ear, a leg, and the tail), but no one puts together the entire picture. Balint referred to such leaderless group efforts at health care as a "collusion of anonymity"; if asked, the patient may not know who is his doctor. In fact, the patient does not have an identified, single doctor (42).

Sometimes out of frustration, the primary physician may conclude that the patient's pain must all be psychogenic (6). The physician may be tempted to tell the patient "it's all in your head, and you should see a psychiatrist." The physician can never be sure that the pain is purely psychogenic, so for medicolegal as well as humanistic reasons, it is recommended that such statements not be made. The patient may be told that nothing specific has yet appeared and that it is doubtful, although this cannot be said with 100% certainty, that anything serious or life-threatening is causing the pain. The physician may then suggest that the patient consult with a psychiatrist to see if some psychiatric medications might relieve the secondary anxiety and depression and that psychotherapy might be considered to learn how to better cope with the ongoing pain and how to adapt the other aspects of his life to the pain as well as possible.

If the primary physician assures the patient that he will continue to evaluate and follow his pain medically at regular intervals, most patients will be willing to accept psychiatric consultation or referral. Problems tend to arise if the primary physician says or implies that he does not need to see the patient further and that psychiatric care is all that is needed. The patient may rightly feel abandoned by that approach and, as mentioned earlier, if a biomedical disorder eventually appears that explains or relates to the pain, the physician will at least look bad professionally and, in today's litiginous society, may end up with a malpractice suit. It is useful to remember that at least 10% of pain patients who are referred to specialized pain clinics for evaluation and treatment are eventually found to have what was a covert biomedical disorder underlying their pain (3, 9).

The physician should also remember that there does not have to be either a biomedical or a psychosocial etiology to the pain. Even if the pain began as purely psychogenic, the patient may develop a biomedical condition that produces pain. This is especially likely if the chronic pain condition persists for a number of years. Therefore, even if a patient has a good response to psychiatric treatment and the psychiatrist concurs that the pain was psychogenic, if some degree of pain persists, at least a periodic physical reexamination is recommended.

The primary physician should also realize that many patients, possibly especially chronic pain patients, because of the length of time involved and failure of usual therapies, attempt to treat themselves before seeking medical help. Over-the-counter drugs, alcohol, and many illicit drugs with actual or reputed analgesic properties are multibillion-dollar-per-year businesses. The patient may be reluctant or embarrassed to spontaneously mention such self-treatment behaviors to the physician; therefore, the physician should routinely ask during the initial evaluation and then at least periodically reassess such substance use or abuse. If a patient is addicted to some form of analgesia, the addiction should be treated before any other form of psychiatric treatment is offered. If an addicting level of an analgesic has not been successful in relieving the pain, it is not very likely that adding another analgesic would do so.

Because of the frequency of substance abuse in chronic pain patients, the physician should also be alert for signs of withdrawal. Withdrawal may need to be more protracted than with other patients, because sensitivity to pain may increase during withdrawal. Anxiety, agitation, and insomnia also often appear during withdrawal, which may make the pain less tolerable.

PSYCHIATRIC DISORDERS IN PRIMARY CARE CHRONIC PAIN PATIENTS

Chronic pain may either result from or develop in response to a wide range of psychiatric conditions. Some of the most common of those are listed in Table 43.1. Pare is thought to have said that "There is nothing that abateth so much the strength as paine." In fact, ongoing pain may be so emotionally stressful that the term pain shock has been developed to describe the constellations of psychiatric distress symptoms that may develop. The depressed, anxious, agitated patient, or the patient who is chronically tired because of insomnia may also have decreased activity levels in general, which may lead to muscle atrophy and deconditioning and thereby to worsening of some types of pain (3). Therefore, careful psychiatric evaluation is recommended as early as is possible during the care of any chronic pain patient who is not responding to standard treatment approaches. A psychiatric consultant also may collaborate with the primary physician in the ongoing management of the pain patient and his family (43, 44).

Thorough psychiatric evaluation of a group of chronic pain patients revealed that 98% had an associated psychiatric disorder, including somatoform disorder (30%), substance abuse (19%), affective disorder (15%), psychological factors affecting physical condition (10%), adjustment disorders (8%), and several other disorders (2–4% each). Thirty-seven per cent of these patients also had a personality disorder, including histrionic (30%), dependent (25%), borderline (15%), and narcissistic (10%), and one patient had each of several other types. Therefore, a wide range of psychiatric and personality disorders may be associated with chronic pain symptoms (1, 45). However, this point is debatable, and some believe that most chronic pain patients do not fit into standard psychiatric diagnostic categories (46).

Some Minnesota Multiphasic Personality Inventory (MMPI) studies have found chronic pain patients to have an increased rate of scoring in the "neurotic triad," which includes high scores on hysteria, hypochondriasis, and depression. Other pain patients have been found to have the "conversion V" pattern on the MMPI, which is created by high scores on the hysteria and hypochondriasis scales and a low score on depression (3). A critical factor to consider is whether these chronic pain patients would have had these patterns premorbidly and to what degree the patterns may have been created or amplified by the chronic pain.

DEPRESSION

Chronic pain frequently leads to depression, and depression may predispose a person to develop chronic pain (47). Some patients with atypical depressive illness develop pain as their major or only symptom, as a so-called depressive equivalent. This begins to occur more frequently in young adult and middle-age years but may continue to increase in frequency with aging. These patients have an increased incidence of a personal or family history of depression (48). In the elderly, "pseudodementia" may actually be due to depression, and depression frequently is not accompanied by standard vegetative symptoms (changes in appetite, weight, sleep, energy level, and so forth). In a younger person, depression that is not associated with depressed mood and vegetative signs may be termed "atypical." However, for the elderly an "atypical" depression may be much more typical and somatic complaints, including pain, are commonly associated with depression. The reported increase in hypochondriasis in the elderly may be in part due to an increase in depression that is not diagnosed and effectively treated.

In any patient known or suspected of having depression associated with chronic pain, the depression should be treated vigorously. Although the use of psychotropic medications in pain management is the focus of Chapter 8, this topic is discussed to some degree in this chapter, in part because primary care physicians frequently use psychotropic drugs to treat pain patients and because primary physicians treat many more patients with psychiatric conditions than do all mental health care professionals combined (49). This would include treatment with imipramine (150 mg/day) or its equivalent of another cyclic antidepressant for at least 4–6 weeks. Shorter trials, even though serum levels are within the therapeutic range, may be ineffective. If the patient has had no side effects at that level, a serum level determination may be useful in titrating the dosage into the therapeutic range. If adverse side effects persist at a usual dosage level, a serum level may also be useful to assure the lowest dosage is being given that will lead to a serum level within the therapeutic range. Physicians may be reluctant to increase the antidepressant dosage to an effective level in elderly or medically debilitated patients. Many potentially treatable depressions have persisted because the physician did not give an effective dosage. Tricyclics are safe for cardiac patients, except for a couple of months after myocardial infarction, unless a conduction defect or persistent dangerous arrhythmia is present (50). An untreatable depression, especially with chronic pain, has much more morbidity than judicious use of tricyclics in these patients (51).

If the depression is not responsive to tricyclics, a monoamine oxidase inhibitor (MAOI) or electroconvulsive therapy (ECT) should be considered (52, 53). Stimulants also have been successfully used in some depressed pain patients. Dextroamphetamine may facilitate the response to morphine in some patients with acute pain, such as postoperatively (54). Postoperative pain management is specifically discussed in Chapter 44. Methylphenidate may provide prompt antidepressant effects in some patients; the dosage is titrated upward from 5 mg, generally not to exceed 30 mg/day. Some patients with chronic pain may seek narcotics, hoping for an antidepressant effect, and this may lead to excess narcotic use and addiction and also to poor results in treatment of the depression (55). Therefore, any narcotic-seeking patient should be specifically evaluated for an underlying depression, as well as other psychiatric disorders. Chronic pain as a variant of depression is discussed further in Chapter 16.

Psychotically depressed patients may develop nihilistic delusions relating to disease and decay. They may be sure that they have cancer or some other potentially deforming, painful, and/or terminal illness. Patients with other types of psychotic illnesses, such as schizophrenia, may also develop pain as part of their symptom picture. It is often useful to ask the patient what he believes is causing the pain. A psychotic individual will sometimes relate a clearly bizarre and unrealistic explanation. However, the fact that a person has a known psychotic illness does not mean his pain complaints, especially if new or different, should not be taken seriously. Obviously, chronically psychotic individuals at some time in their lives are likely to develop pain due to a biomedical illness. Stories abound of psychotic individuals "ignoring" the pain of an acute myocardial infarction or other usually very painful conditions.

MUNCHAUSEN SYNDROME

It is not possible to classify all patients with Munchausen syndrome as psychotic, although some probably are. However, this is a subgroup that the physician should consider among chronic pain patients, especially if the patient has had multiple diagnostic or exploratory procedures or traveled to medical centers far and wide to be treated. One sometimes useful diagnostic aspect of Munchausen patients is that they tend to be "psychiatry-ophobic." Most patients with chronic pain will not react violently to the suggestion of psychiatric consultation by the physician if it is not done in a context of implying that "it's all in their head," or that "they are crazy," or unless it appears that the primary physician wants to "bow out" of continuing to treat the patient. However, even the mention of a psychiatrist may lead the Munchausen patient to leave against medical advice. Although Munchausen syndrome is often classified as a factitious disorder, it should not be regarded as consciously controlled malingering, as might occur with a drug addict or person desiring undeserved disability compensation. Munchausen syndrome is a serious and potentially lethal disorder if repeated procedures and surgeries are performed (56, 57).

GRIEF

Grieving individuals may sometimes develop pain symptoms as part of their mourning process. Sometimes the pain will appear to originate from the bodily region in which the illness occurred that caused the death of their loved one. At other times the pain may occur in symbolically important areas, such as the chest, representing a "broken heart" or "heartache." Of course, such individuals should be medically evaluated, since there is an increased risk of morbidity and mortality during the acute grief process (58).

POST-TRAUMATIC STRESS DISORDER

Post-traumatic stress disorder (PTSD) may account for about 10% of patents seeking treatment at some pain clinics, especially veterans' hospitals. However, these patients often have other psychiatric disorders as well, including depression, anxiety, and substance abuse (59). Patients with a number of neuroses or personality disorders may have pain as one of their symptoms. Hysterical paralysis or pain is probably the most classic example, in which the patient may develop symptoms that do not correspond to neurologic pathways (such as stocking or glove paralysis, anesthesia, or pain). Hysterical patients are somewhat more likely to develop conversion disorders, but others with no overt hysterical (e.g., flamboyant, seductive, theatrical, center-of-attention) traits may also develop conversion symptoms.

BORDERLINE OR NARCISSISTIC PERSONALITY DISORDER

Patients with borderline or narcissistic personality disorder also are at increased risk for developing chronic pain syndromes (60, 61). The borderline may feel empty, hollow, and chronically bored; they may describe "preferring to feel pain than to feel nothing." These patients sometimes inflict pain upon themselves as a way of determining that they are alive, have boundaries, are not empty, or for other distressing psychiatric reasons. Borderlines commonly slash their wrists but may also injure themselves in other ways to "feel real" or "to snap back into reality." Many Munchausen patients have some borderline features.

Narcissistic patients may become intensely involved with their appearance, wish for perfect bodily functioning, and be very frightened of physical vulnerability, disability, or illness. Because illness poses such a threat, they may present to the physician with what otherwise would appear to be small and inconsequential complaints, including pain. Their grandiosity is a psychological defense against feeling incredibly vulnerable.

ALEXITHYMIA

Chronic pain patients have been found to have a significant incidence (about 33%) of alexithymia, the inability to verbalize and discuss their emotional states and a relatively concrete style of thinking. Older patients have also been found to be more alexithymic, which may be one factor in geriatric patients' expressing emotional distress more often through somatic complaints (62). Patients with a wide variety of psychosomatic-type disorders may have an increased tendency to have alexithymic features. In a sense, that appears to be logical; that is, if they cannot express their emotions verbally and through their actions, those emotional states may be more likely to go through somatic channels. They are not psychologically minded and are not good counseling or psychotherapy candidates, at least not without a lot of groundwork. Therefore, ongoing supportive management is often the best care that can be provided. However, that may be very successful and should not be minimized.

Patients with hypochondriasis often have alexithymic features. It may be infuriating to physicians when they see glaring examples of sources of psychosocial stress in the patient's life, but, upon trying to make connections between those and the patient's somatic symptoms to the patient, is rewarded with a blank stare or denial of any connection. In fact, part of the patient's problem may be just that; he cannot perceive and correctly evaluate emotional factors in his life. If the physician begins to become angry at such patients and begins to think of them as "crocks" or label them with other perjorative terms, this should be used as a diagnostic clue that hypochondriasis or some other alexithymic disorder may be present (4, 19).

SOMATOFORM DISORDERS

Hypochondriasis is one of the most common of the somatoform disorders, which simply means that emotional distress is expressed through the form of somatic complaints. Somatization disorder is another term that is frequently used to describe this general group of patients. A differential diagnostic point is that although both patients with somatization disorder and hypochondriasis may have multiple physical complaints that cannot be related to any biomedical disorders, patients with hypochondriasis often have a more pronounced fear of having a serious illness. The somatization disorder patient will not have la belle indifference, as might the classic hysterical patient with conversion symptoms, but they are not usually as continually anxious and frightened as the patient with hypochondriasis. The chief complaint of hypochondriacal patients is their fear of multiple serious illnesses, whereas the somatization disorder patient tends to have many physical complaints without the same degree of desperation.

The best approach for the primary care physician to take with patients with a somatoform disorder, after a careful history, physical exam, and screening laboratory studies, is calm reassurance and offering to continue to follow them regularly. Many of these patients will not initially respond to reassurance, but the form that the reassurance takes may make a difference. It is not reassuring to these patients to be told "There is nothing wrong with you." That is also not accurate. There is something wrong with them; they have a somatoform disorder, such as hypochondriasis. However, they should not be told that they have hypochondriasis either, becase the layman's knowledge and reaction to the diagnosis of hypochondriasis is usually that it means "There's nothing wrong with you."

Therefore, the primary physician may need to give these patients some license to be at least a little sick and to somewhat adopt the "sick role" in their relationships. Actually, the physician does not have to "let" them do this; they have already done it. However, the physician should try not to get into a struggle with them right away to get them out of the sick role. For one, it will not work. They are in the sick role and complaining of multiple somatic complaints because they need to do so; that is the best avenue that they have available in their personality repertoire to express their psychosocial distress. If the primary physician can back off from confrontation and instead form a supportive relationship with these difficult patients, that will usually be the best treatment for them. Their repeated "doctor shopping," multiple referrals, and getting placed in "revolving doors" of many health care agencies may gradually diminish.

Somatizing and hypochondriacal patients who develop pain as their primary symptom have sometimes been classified as "pain prone." Pain-prone individuals also have been described by a number of names, not all complimentary (63). George Engel coined the term when he referred to individuals with certain past life experiences and personality traits that make them susceptible to use or in need of pain for underlying psychodynamic reasons as "pain-prone" patients (64). Sternbach has classified a subgroup of these patients as "lower back losers" (65). Szasa has termed similar groups "les hommes douloureux" (66). A common characteristic of patients fitting into these classifications is that their pain usually has some component of unconscious secondary gain. However, over 50% of chronic pain patients may not fit into criteria for a pain-prone disorder (46). Keep in mind that the secondary gain paradoxically may be punishment that they feel they deserve. Also, paradoxically, some individuals feel very guilty, subconsciously if not consciously, for being successful. If they become too successful, they feel they must balance it out by some pain or suffering (8).

A variant of the above groups are sadomasochistic individuals. These patients receive some pleasure from suffering. They may feel that they deserve to suffer and, therefore, feel pleasure that they are on course (although it is an unhealthy and destructive path) for their lives. Others come to associate pain with certain types of pleasure, such as sexual activities, so they can only feel the full extent of pleasure possible if pain is associated with the experience.

NONPHARMACOLOGIC MANAGEMENT CONSIDERATIONS

If the patient is in the middle of a lawsuit, disability determination, divorce, or other situation that may be closely related to the pain symptoms, the physician should be conservative in his treatment approaches. Once the secondary gain associated with such situations is resolved, regardless of outcome, the physician will be able to evaluate the situation more clearly.

It has been demonstrated that encouragement and instruction of patients may reduce postoperative pain (67). If a procedure is going to be performed, taking a few minutes to explain what will be done and answering any questions they may have about it may greatly reduce patients' anxieties. A person who is anxious is much more likely to be sensitive to any painful stimulus and to overreact to it. If the patient knows what to anticipate, he may be able to be much more cooperative, which also may save time during the procedure. Chapter 18 contains a much broader discussion of cognitive and behavioral aspects of pain management.

Chapter 17 contains a detailed discussion of contingency management. However, this is such an important and often overlooked area in the treatment of chronic pain patients that a few comments of special relevance to primary care physicians are made here (6, 68). Just as Skinner discovered with rats and pigeons, almost any behavior may be increased or decreased in frequency if the rewards or punishments associated with it are great enough and persistent. If a chronic pain patient receives more attention, money, or anything else that he values because he has chronic pain, it follows that all of the attitudes and behaviors associated with chronic pain will increase. Likewise, if the person receives more benefits from displaying active, healthy, pain-free behaviors, those will be reinforced. The more a person talks about and becomes preoccupied with his chronic pain, the more his world becomes centered around the pain. Healthy people avoid him, so he becomes surrounded with those who are also preoccupied with his (or their) pain, for a multitude of their own psychological reasons.

Therefore, a contingency plan must be set up so the chronic pain patient receives more "goodies" for being active and trying to carry on a health life-style than for acting ill and debilitated. Such a plan may initially seem illogical and even cruel to spouses, other family members, and employers. However, each of these groups of significant others should be counseled to reward the patient more for healthy behaviors and ignore or give as little positive feedback as possible to pain-related behaviors or comments. Gradually, the patient may thereby become less focused on the pain and more involved in healthier aspects of his life.

PAIN CLINICS

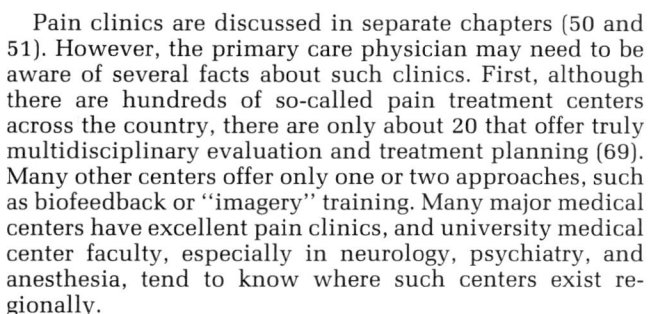

Pain clinics are discussed in separate chapters (50 and 51). However, the primary care physician may need to be aware of several facts about such clinics. First, although there are hundreds of so-called pain treatment centers across the country, there are only about 20 that offer truly multidisciplinary evaluation and treatment planning (69). Many other centers offer only one or two approaches, such as biofeedback or "imagery" training. Many major medical centers have excellent pain clinics, and university medical center faculty, especially in neurology, psychiatry, and anesthesia, tend to know where such centers exist regionally.

A comprehensive pain center should involve evaluation by at least an internist or other primary care physician, neurologist, and psychiatrist. Many other health care professionals may be involved in some centers, including psychologists, social workers, an anesthesiologist if nerve blocks are being considered, a neurosurgeon if neuroablative procedures might be indicated, or multiple other specialists depending upon the site and type of pain. Physical medicine and rehabilitation (PM and R) services may be overlooked, but may be of great help for some chronic pain patients. Conditioning and exercise programs may help patients compensate for and lessen a number of musculoskeletal etiologies of pain (70). The benefits of PM and R services for chronic pain patients are discussed in more detail in Chapter 13.

THE "DRUG" DOCTOR AS AN ANALGESIC

Balint has given physicians a very useful conceptualization, which may be especially helpful to chronic pain patients (9, 42). He recommended that the physician view himself as a "drug" that he prescribes for the patient's well-being. The doctor-patient relationship may be a major asset for physicians in treating pain. Comforting by "laying on of hands" and an appropriate "bedside" manner are usually essential to a good outcome. The physician may overlook the fact that for all of our technologic advances, the doctor-patient relationship is still one of the most powerful parts of our therapeutic armamentarium. The doctor is still the most commonly used "drug" in medical practice. The physician must understand the "pharmacology" of this powerful "drug," its side-effects and potential benefits, and how to determine its correct dosage and schedule of administration for various types of patients. Too much or too little "doctoring" may increase symptomatology. In managing pain, perhaps more than in other aspects of medical care, the doctor-patient relationship must be regularly utilized to its full therapeutic efficacy to be maximally effective.

Models of the doctor-patient relationship include: the active-passive model, where the physician assumes total responsibility; the guidance-cooperation model, such as when the doctor recommends an approach and the patient chooses to comply; and the mutual participation model, in which the physician and the patient together select the diagnostic and therapeutic approach for an illness (71). Whatever model is chosen, its utility hinges upon its appropriateness to the given clinical situation. Success usually depends upon the doctor's ability to gain the trust of the patient he hopes to help. The doctor must listen not only to what the patient says, but to what is being transmitted nonverbally. The ideal relationship is one in which both the doctor and the patient can communicate freely about the patient's fears and wishes, as well as about medical facts. The physician should work to diagnose problems in the doctor-patient relationship and then manage those, as well as managing the patient's medical problems.

ANALGESIC USE FOR CHRONIC PAIN

It is not the primary purpose of this chapter to discuss analgesics. Analgesic and anti-inflammatory medications are the focus of Chapter 7, and a number of special considerations in pharmacologic pain management are discussed in Chapter 9. A number of other sources also discuss these issues in detail (72–75). However, Table 43.2 contains a basic classification of prescribed analgesic agents. In deciding about which pharmacologic agents to use, an essential question is whether you are dealing with "malignant" or "benign" pain (6, 9). Patients with "malignant" pain, due to cancer or other chronic biomedical conditions, may require narcotic or other powerful analgesics, nerve blocks, and neuroablative procedures to control their pain. Malignant forms of pain are thoroughly dis-

Table 43.2
Classification of Analgesics[a]

Centrally active
  Narcotic agonists, naturally occurring
    Morphine
    Codeine
  Narcotic agonists, synthetic agents
    Diamorphine
    Diamophine
    Dihydrocodeine
    Meperidine
    Methadone
    Propoxyphene
  Narcotic partial agonists
    Nalorphine
    Pentazocine
    Buprenorphine
    Butorphanol
    Cyclazocine
  Narcotic antagonists
    Naloxone
    Naltrexone
Peripherally active
  Nonsteroidal anti-inflammatory agents
    Salicylic acid derivatives
    Phenylalkanoic acid derivatives
    Pyrazolone derivatives
    Aniline derivatives
    Anthranlilic acid derivatives

[a] From Chapman CR, Bonica JJ: *Chronic Pain.* Kalamazoo, MI, The Upjohn Company, 1985, p 56, with permission from the publisher and authors.

Table 43.3
Guidelines for the Use of Narcotic Analgesics in Pain Management[a]

1. Start with a specific drug for a specific type of pain.
2. Know the pharmacology of the drug prescribed.
   a. Duration of the analgesic effect.
   b. Pharmacokinetic properties of the drug.
   c. Equianalgesic doses for the drug and its route of administration (see Tables 43.4 and 43.5).
3. Adjust the route of administration to the patient's needs.
4. Administer the analgesic on a regular basis after initial titration of the dose.
5. Use drug combinations to provide additive analgesia and reduce side effects [e.g., nonsteroidal antiinflammatory drugs, antihistamine (hydroxyzine), amphetamine (Dexedrine)].
6. Avoid drug combinations that increase sedation without enhancing analgesia [e.g. benzodiazepine (diazepam) and phenothiazine (chlorpromazine)].
7. Anticipate and treat side effects.
   a. Sedation.
   b. Respiratory depression.
   c. Nausea and vomiting.
   d. Constipation.
8. Watch for the development of tolerance.
   a. Switch to an alternative narcotic analgesic.
   b. Start with one half the equianalgesic dose and titrate the dose for pain relief.
9. Prevent acute withdrawal.
   a. Taper drugs slowly.
   b. Use diluted doses of naloxone (0.4 mg in 10 ml of saline) to reverse respiratory depression in the physically dependent patient, and administer cautiously.
10. Do not use placebos to assess the nature of pain.
11. Anticipate and manage complications.
    a. Overdose.
    b. Multifocal myoclonus.
    c. Seizures.

[a] From Foley KM: The treatment of cancer pain. *N Engl J Med* 313:84–95, 1985; reprinted by permission.

cussed in Chapters 32 through 34. The physician should not hesitate to use large doses of narcotics if that is what is required to manage these patients' pain. Patients with chronic "benign" pain should generally be prescribed appropriate psychotropic agents, such as antidepressants, stimulants, or neuroleptics, and psychotherapy (76).

The patient with severe "malignant" pain may need quite large dosages of narcotics to achieve pain control. The physician should not shrink from prescribing what is required for pain relief in these patients. These patients may need large dosages and therefore usually tolerate much larger dosages than other patients. For example, if morphine is steadily titrated upward, a maintenance dosage may be determined for a terminal cancer patient who is in severe pain that will allow the patient to be basically pain free while still being alert mentally. This may be preferable in most situations to extensive nerve blocks or neurodestructive surgeries.

However, for a number of reasons, physicians are often reluctant to prescribe adequate dosages of narcotics, which is probably not accidentally also the case for other central nervous system drugs, such as antidepressants and anxiolytics (6, 9). An important study by Marks and Sachar demonstrated that many medical inpatients with bona fide biomedical etiologies, such as acute myocardial infarction, for their pain were consistently undertreated with narcotic analgesics (77). Faulty pharmacologic knowledge regarding analgesics was one factor in this underprescribing. One-third of the physicians overestimated the duration of action of meperidine, 27% exaggerated its addiction potential in medical settings, and over three-fourths underestimated the likelihood of meperidine withdrawal symptoms if a patient has received it for an extended period of time. About one-fifth of the physicians had exaggerated and inappropriate fears of causing addiction, including in terminal cancer patients, and would not increase meperidine to effective levels in such patients. Fourteen per cent preferred to decrease analgesic dosage or give placebos to such patients.

A major factor in the underutilization of these, and probably other central nervous system and emotional responsivity-altering, drugs is a strong emotional stigma associated with their use. It is as though some physicians believe that only bad physicians prescribe large dosages of these drugs, regardless of the clinical situation (78). There may also be an underlying belief that if they were better physicians their patient would not need these drugs. Of course, a paranoia factor may also operate in which they fear one of their patients will become addicted, and word will spread through their colleagues and community that they are a "dope pusher who gets patients hooked on narcotics." If the physician initiates a slow withdrawal before discharge and receives prompt psychiatric or substance abuse consultation if this is a problem for the patient, such ongoing prescribed analgesic addiction can almost always be avoided or short-circuited with a prompt treatment program. Additional guidelines for the use of narcotic analgesics in pain management are listed in Table 43.3.

The nonnarcotic analgesics are very effective in treating most acute and mild to moderate pain (Tables 43.2 and 43.4). They are first-line drugs in most cases unless the pain is very severe and needs nearly complete efficacy (e.g., pain from renal colic or cholecystitis). In these cases, one would usually choose a narcotic analgesic (Table 43.5). Aspirin (650 mg/day) is the most efficacious oral

Table 43.4
Oral Non-narcotic and Narcotic Analgesics for Mild to Moderate Pain[a]

	Equianalgesic Dose (mg)[b]	Duration (hr)	Plasma Half-Life (hr)	Comments
Aspirin	650	4–6	3–5	Standard for non-narcotic comparisons; gastro-intestinal and hematologic effects limit use in patients with cancer
Acetaminophen	650	4–6	1–4	Weak antiinflammatory effects; safer than aspirin
Propoxyphene	65[c]	4–6	12	Biotransformed to potentially toxic metabolite norpropoxyphene; used in combination with non-narcotic analgesics
Codeine	32	4–6	3	Biotransformed to morphine; available in combination with non-narcotic analgesics
Meperidine	50	4–6	3–4	Biotransformed to active toxic metabolite normeperidine; associated with myoclonus and seizures
Pentazocine	30	4–6	2–3	Psychotomimetic effects with escalation of dose; available only in combination with naloxone, aspirin, or acetaminophen (US)

[a] From Foley KM: The treatment of cancer pain. N Engl J Med 313:84–95, 1985; reprinted by permission.
[b] Relative potency of drugs, as compared with that of aspirin, for mild to moderate pain.
[c] Some investigators have reported that a much larger dose (propoxyphene, 130 mg; codeine, 60 mg) is effective in patients with mild to moderate pain.

Table 43.5
Oral and Parenteral Narcotic Analgesics for Severe Pain[a]

	Route[b]	Equianalgesic Dose (mg)[c]	Duration (hr)	Plasma Half-Life (hr)	Comments
Narcotic agonists					
Morphine	IM	10	4–6	2–3.5	Standard for comparison; also available in slow-release tablets
	PO	60	4–7		
Codeine	IM	130	4–6	3	Biotransformed to morphine; useful as initial narcotic analgesic
	PO	200[d]	4–6		
Oxycodone	IM	15			Short acting; available alone or as five mg dose in combination with aspirin and acetaminophen
	PO	30	3–5	—	
Heroin	IM	5	4–5	0.5	Illegal in US; high solubility for parenteral administration
	PO	60	4–5		
Levorphanol (Levo-Dromoran)	IM	2	4–6	12–16	Good oral potency, requires careful titration in initial dosing because of drug accumulation
	PO	4	4–7		
Hydromorphone (Dilaudid)	IM	1.5	4–5	2–3	Available in high-potency injectable form (10mg/ml) for cachectic patients and as rectal suppositories; more soluble than morphine
	PO	7.5	4–6		
Oxymorphone (Numorphan)	IM	1	4–6	2–3	Available in parenteral and rectal-suppository forms only
	PR	10	4–6		
Meperidine (Demerol)	IM	75	4–5	3–4 Normeperidine 12–16	Contraindicated in patients with renal disease; accumulation of active toxic metabolite normeperidine produces central nervous system excitation
	PO	300[d]	4–6		
Methadone (Dolophine)	IM	10		15–30	Good oral potency; requires careful titration of the initial dose to avoid drug accumulation
	PO	20			
Mixed agonist-antagonist drugs					
Pentazocine (Talwin)	IM	60	4–6	2–3	Limited use for cancer pain; psychotomimetic effects with dose escalation; available only in combination with naloxone, aspirin, or acetaminophen; may precipitate withdrawal in physically dependent patients
	PO	180[d]	4–7		
Nalbuphine (Nubain)	IM	10	4–6	5	Not available orally; less severe psychotomimetic effects than pentazocine; may precipitate withdrawal in physically dependent patients
	PO	—			
Butorphanol (Stadol)	IM	2	4–6	2.5–3.5	Not available orally; produces psychotomimetic effects; may precipitate withdrawal in physically dependent patients
	PO	—			
Partial agonists					
Buprenorphine (Temgesic)	IM	0.4	4–6	?	Not available in US; no psychotomimetic effects; may precipitate withdrawal in tolerant patients
	SL	0.8	5–6		

[a] From Foley KM: The treatment of cancer pain. *N Engl J Med* 313:84–95, 1985; reprinted by permission.
[b] IM denotes intramuscular, PO=oral, PR=rectal, and SL=sublingual.
[c] Based on single-dose studies in which an intramuscular dose of each drug listed was compared with morphine to establish the relative potency. Oral doses are those recommended when changing from a parenteral to an oral route. For patients without prior narcotic exposure, the recommended oral starting dose is 30 mg for morphine, 5 mg for methadone, 2 mg for levorphanol, and 4 mg for hydromorphone.
[d] The recommended starting doses for these drugs are listed in Table 43.4.

analgesic. It is as effective as standard dosages of codeine in relieving cancer pain. Acetaminophen may be substituted for aspirin; however, this drug has a lower therapeutic-toxic ratio than aspirin. The nonsteroidal anti-inflammatory agents are commonly used peripherally acting analgesics. It is often wise to use peripherally acting compounds, since the earlier the intervention in the pain pathway, the more effective the treatment may be (79). The nonsteroidals are thought to act by blocking the metabolism of arachidonic acid to prostaglandins, as well as by possibly having central nervous system effects (80).

Several of the nonsteroidal anti-inflammatory drugs have been used for their analgesic effects. However, this class of drugs does not seem to be more efficacious than aspirin or acetaminophen. There is little evidence that nonsteroidal anti-inflammatory drugs have fewer side effects than does aspirin when it is administered correctly. Aspirin should be prescribed at two or three 325-mg tablets with each meal and should be taken while patients are eating their meals. American men and women frequently do not eat three meals a day, but they should be counseled to do so when taking aspirin. They should also have a snack or a glass of milk with any additional dosages. Given in this way, one usually achieves excellent analgesic effects with few side effects. The major side effect is upper gastrointestinal irritation. Effects of aspirin on platelets usually have little importance in most of our pain patients (9).

In prescribing narcotic analgesia, it is critical to give the patient a sufficient amount of narcotic to provide adequate pain relief. The optimal analgesic dose of morphine is 10 mg/70 kg of body weight. This dose will relieve pain in 65% of patients. Increasing the dose to 15 mg will relieve pain in another 10%, but the increased dosage markedly increases side effects (81).

One of the most common errors in opiate use is failure to evaluate the efficacy of the "first dose." Physicians tend to assume that the "usual therapeutic dose" should be adequate for all patients, and it is common for them to label the nonresponder as a complainer or a potential addict. An effective dose of opiate given at appropriate intervals should be determined and then continued. Usually 2–3 mg of morphine sulfate or 15–25 mg of demerol hydrochloride, given intravenously every 20 min until analgesia is accomplished, will be effective. The total dosage of narcotic is usually less when opiates are given every 3–4 hours during the early postoperative period (82). Side effects may preclude therapeutic doses, but often decreasing the dose will alleviate side effects and will provide adequate analgesia. Hypoventilation is usually not a problem with analgesic doses, because the pain results in respiratory stimulation, which counterbalances the depressant effect of these drugs (83).

It is usually best not to use opiates "as needed" if there will be persistent pain, but to administer an effective dose regularly. In fact, analgesics should almost always be prescribed on a regular schedule based upon the particular analgesic's duration of action, rather than the patient's request. If the analgesics are given as needed, some patients will try to suffer through the pain or allow the pain to escalate to a severe degree before asking for analgesia. Some stoics, discussed earlier, may never ask for analgesia, regardless of the pain severity, or view it as a "moral or personal defeat" if they have "to give in and admit they need a pill." Regular analgesia will decrease anxiety and the fear and sensitivity to pain and may cause the patient to ultimately use less analgesia to control his pain. Regular analgesia orders also dissociate experiencing increasing pain from receiving pain relief. The latter point is important in contingency management and behavior modification approaches. That is, the patient should not learn that he needs to increase his suffering or disability to receive the attention and treatments that are needed (3, 9).

Opiates may be combined with other analgesics to enhance analgesic activity, to reduce opiate dosage, or to counteract side effects of the opiates and improve tolerance. Combination of opiates and nonnarcotic analgesics have additive analgesic activity but different side effects and usually less central depression. Combination of opiates with minor tranquilizers may potentiate the analgesic effect of the opiate. This may result in a lower dose of opiate for analgesia and less respiratory depression and opiate-induced nausea and vomiting (84–87). The tricyclic antidepressant compounds may be effective for carotidynia, atypical facial pain, and migraine prophylaxis, possibly as a result of vasoconstrictive properties (88–90). Corticosteroids and tetrahydrocannabinol are used in some patients as analgesics (91).

References

1. Hackett TP: The pain patient: evaluation and treatment. In Hackett TP, Cassem NH (eds): *Massachusetts General Hospital Handbook of General Hospital Psychiatry.* St Louis, CV Mosby, 1978, p 41.
2. Thompson TL II: Headache. In Kaplan HI, Sadock BJ (eds): *Comprehensive Textbook of Psychiatry,* ed 4. Baltimore, Williams & Wilkins, 1985, p 1203.
3. Thompson TL II: Chronic pain. In Kaplan HI, Sadock BJ (eds): *Comprehensive Textbook of Psychiatry,* ed 4. Baltimore, Williams & Wilkins, 1985, p 1212.
4. Thompson TL II, Steele BF: The psychological aspects of pain. In Simons RC (ed): *Understanding Human Behavior in Health and Illness,* ed 3. Baltimore, Williams & Wilkins, 1985, p 60.
5. Long DM: The evaluation and treatment of low back pain. In Hendler NH, Long DM, Wise TN (eds): *Diagnosis and Treatment of Chronic Pain.* Littleton, MA, John Wright–PSG, 1982, p 31.
6. Reuler JB, Girard DE, Nardone DA: The chronic pain syndrome: misconceptions and management. *Ann Intern Med* 93:588–596, 1980.
7. Dubovsky SL, Groban SE: Congenital absence of sensation. *Psychoanal Study Child* 30:49–73, 1975.
8. Engel GL: Guilt, pain, and success. *Psychosom Med* 24:37–48, 1962.
9. Luce JM, Thompson TL II, Getto CJ, et al: New concepts of

chronic pain and their implications. *Hosp Pract* 14:113–123, 1979.
10. Devine R, Merskey H: The description of the pain in psychiatric and general medical patients. *J Psychosom Res* 9:311–316, 1965.
11. Rhine MW, Thompson TL II: Hypochondriasis. In Simons RC (ed): *Understanding Human Behavior in Health and Illness*, ed 3. Baltimore, Williams & Wilkins, 1985, p 73.
12. Wise TN: Pain—the most common psychosomatic problem. *Med Clin North Am* 61:771–780, 1977.
13. Strain JJ: The problem of pain. In Strain JJ (ed): *Psychological Care of the Medically Ill*. New York, Appleton-Century-Crofts, 1975, p 93.
14. Webb WL Jr: Chronic pain. *Psychosomatics* 24:1053–1063, 1983.
15. Weisenberg M, Kreindler ML, Schachat R, et al: Pain: anxiety and attitudes in black, white and Puerto Rican patients. *Psychosom Med* 37:123–135, 1975.
16. Hollingshead AB, Redlich FC: *Social Class and Mental Illness*. New York, John Wiley & Sons, 1958.
17. Zborowski M: *People in Pain*. Philadelphia, Jossey-Bass, 1969.
18. Smith WL, Merskey H, Gross SC (eds): *Pain: Meaning and Management*. Jamaica, NY, SP Medical & Scientific Books, 1980.
19. Lipsitt DR: Medical and psychological characteristics of "crocks". *Int J Psychiatry Med* 1:15–25, 1970.
20. Perman J: Pain as an old friend. *Lancet* 1:633–636, 1954.
21. Livingstone WK: What is pain? *Sci Am* 196:59–72, 1943.
22. Engel GL: The need for a new medical model: a challenge for biomedicine. *Science* 196:129–136, 1977.
23. Von Euler US, Pernow B (eds): *Substance P*. New York, Raven Press, 1977.
24. Hendler NH: The four stages of pain. In Hendler NH, Long DM, Wise TN (eds): *Diagnosis and Treatment of Chronic Pain*. Littleton, MA, John Wright–PSG, 1982, p 1.
25. Foley KM, Posner JB: *Pain*. American Academy of Neurology Review Book. Minneapolis, American Academy of Neurology, 1978, p 199.
26. Nathan PW: Results of antero-lateral cordotomy for pain in cancer. *J Neurol Neurosurg Psychiatry* 26:353–362, 1963.
27. White JC, Sweet WH: *Pain, Its Mechanisms and Neurosurgical Control*. Springfield, IL, Charles C Thomas, 1955.
28. Levine JD, Gordon NC, Fields HL: The mechanism of placebo analgesia. *Lancet* 2:654–657, 1978.
29. Melzack R: How acupuncture can block pain. In Weisenberg M (ed): *Pain: Clinical and Experimental Perspectives*. St. Louis, CV Mosby, 1975, p 251.
30. Hilgard ER, Hilgard VR: *Hypnosis in the relief of pain*. Los Altos, CA, William Kaufmann, 1975.
31. Beecher HK: *Measurement of Subjective Responses: Quantitative Effects of Drugs*. New York, Oxford University Press, 1959.
32. Snyder SH: Opiate receptors and internal opiates. *Sci Am* 236:44–56, 1977.
33. Pert A, Yaksh T: Sites of morphine induced analgesia in the primate brain: relation to pain pathways. *Brain Res* 80:135–140, 1974.
34. Lindsay PG, Wyckoff M: The depression-pain syndrome and its response to antidepressants. *Psychosomatics* 22:571–577, 1981.
35. Melzack R, Wall PD: Pain mechanisms: a new theory. *Science* 150:971–979, 1965.
36. Melzack R: *The Puzzle of Pain*. New York, Basic Books, 1973.
37. Campbell JN, Long DM: Transcutaneous electrical stimulation for pain: efficacy and mechanism of action. In Hendler NH, Long DM, Wise TN (eds): *Diagnosis and Treatment of Chronic Pain*. Littleton, MA, John Wright–PSG, 1982, p 77.
38. Proudfit HK, Anderson EG: Morphine analgesia: blockade by raphe magnus lesions. *Brain Res* 98:612–618, 1975.
39. Beecher HK: Relationship of significance of wound to pain experience. *JAMA* 161:1609–1613, 1956.
40. Morgan WL Jr, Engel GL: *The Clinical Approach to the Patient*. Philadelphia, WB Saunders, 1969.
41. Byyny RL, Thompson TL II: The roles of the primary care general internist. In Thompson TL II, Byyny RL (eds): *Primary and Team Health Care Education*. New York, Praeger, 1983, p 13.
42. Balint M: *The Doctor, His Patient, and the Illness*, ed 2. New York, International Universities Press, 1964, p 1.
43. DeVaul RA, Zisook S: Chronic pain: The psychiatrist's role. *Psychosomatics* 19:417–421, 1978.
44. Merskey H: The role of the psychiatrist in the investigation and treatment of pain. In Bonica J (ed): *Advances in Pain Research and Therapy*. New York, Raven Press, 1983, vol 5, p 249.
45. Reich J, Tupin JP, Abramovitz SI: Psychiatric diagnosis of chronic pain patients. *Am J Psychiatry* 140:1495–1498, 1983.
46. Bouckoms AJ: Recent developments in the classification of pain. *Psychosomatics* 26:637–645, 1985.
47. Mersky H, Boyd D: Emotional adjustment and chronic pain. *Pain* 5:173–178, 1978.
48. Magni G, Bertolini C: Chronic pain as a depressive equivalent. *Postgrad Med* 73:79–85, 1983.
49. Regier DA, Goldberg ID, Taube CA: The de facto US mental health services system: a public health perspective. *Arch Gen Psychiatry* 35:685–693, 1978.
50. Vieth RC, Raskin MA, Caldwell JH, et al: Cardiovascular effects of tricyclic antidepressants in depressed patients with heart disease. *N Engl J Med* 306:954–959, 1982.
51. Cahn J, Herold M: Pain and psychotropic drugs. In Soulairac A, Cahn J, Charpentier J (eds): *Pain*. New York, Academic Press, 1968, p 335.
52. Anthony M, Lance JW: Monoamine oxidase inhibition in the treatment of migraine. *Arch Neurol* 21:263, 1969.
53. Mandel MR: Electroconvulsive therapy for chronic pain associated with depression. *Am J Psychiatry* 132:632–636, 1975.
54. Forrest WH Jr, Brown BW Jr, Brown CR, et al: Dextroamphetamine with morphine for the treatment of postoperative pain. *N Engl J Med* 296:712–715, 1977.
55. Halpern LM: Psychotropic drugs in the management of chronic pain. *Adv Neurol* 4:539–545, 1974.
56. Ford CV: The Munchausen syndrome: a report of 4 new cases and a review of psychodynamic considerations. *Int J Psychiatry Med* 4:31–45, 1973.
57. Spiro HR: Chronic factitious illness: Munchausen's syndrome. *Arch Gen Psychiatry* 18:569–579, 1968.
58. Parkes CM, Benjamin B, Fitzgerald RG: Broken heart: a statistical study of increased mortality among widowers. *Br Med J* 1:740–743, 1969.
59. Benedikt RA, Kolb LC: Preliminary findings on chronic pain and posttraumatic stress disorder. *Am J Psychiatry* 143:908–910, 1986.
60. Gross RJ, Doerr H, Caldiorla D, et al: Borderline syndrome and incest in chronic pelvic pain patients. *Int J Psychiatry Med* 10:79–96, 1981.

61. Blazer DG: Narcissism and the development of chronic pain. *Int J Psychiatry Med* 10:69–71, 1981.
62. Postone N: Alexithymia in chronic pain patients. *Gen Hosp Psychiatry* 8:163–167, 1986.
63. Blumer D, Heilbronn M: Chronic pain as a variant of depressive disease: the pain-prone disorder. *J Nerv Ment Dis* 170:381–416, 1982.
64. Engel GL: "Psychogenic pain" and the pain-prone patient. *Am J Med* 26:899–918, 1959.
65. Sternbach RA: *Pain Patients*. New York, Academic Press, 1974.
66. Szasz T: *Pain and Pleasure*. New York, Basic Books, 1957.
67. Egbert LD, Battit GE, Welch CE, et al: Reduction of postoperative pain by encouragement and instruction of patients. *N Engl J Med* 270:825–827, 1964.
68. Fordyce WE: An operant conditioning method for managing chronic pain. *Postgrad Med* 53:123–128, 1973.
69. Black RG: The clinical management of chronic pain. In Hendler NH, Long DM, Wise TN (eds): *Diagnosis and Treatment of Chronic Pain*. Littleton, MA, John Wright–PSG, 1982, p 211.
70. Reischer MA, Spindler HA: The use of physical medicine and rehabilitation in the management of pain. In Hendler NH, Long DM, Wise TN (eds): *Diagnosis and Treatment of Chronic Pain*. Littleton, MA, John Wright–PSG, 1982, p 235.
71. Szasz TS, Hollender MH: A contribution to the philosophy of medicine: the basic models of the doctor-patient relationship. *Arch Intern Med* 97:585–592, 1956.
72. Halpern LM: Analgesic drugs in the management of pain. *Arch Surg* 112:861–869, 1977.
73. Stimmel B: *Pain, Analgesia, and Addiction: The Pharmacological Treatment of Pain*. New York, Raven Press, 1983.
74. Brena SF, Chapman SL (eds): *Management of Patients with Chronic Pain*. Jamaica, NY, SP Medical & Scientific Books, 1983.
75. Fordyce WE, Brockway JO: Chronic pain and its management. In Usdin G, Lewis JM (eds): *Psychiatry in General Medical Practice*. New York, McGraw-Hill, 1979, p 352.
76. Merskey H, Hester RA: Treatment of chronic pain with psychotropic drugs. *Postgrad Med* 48:594–598, 1972.
77. Marks RM, Sachar EJ: Undertreatment of medical inpatients with narcotic analgesics. *Ann Intern Med* 78:173–181, 1973.
78. Perry S: The undermedication for pain: a psychoanalytic perspective. *Bull Assoc Psychoanal Med* 22:77–94, 1983.
79. Levine J: Pain and analgesia: the outlook for more rational treatment. *Ann Intern Med* 100:269–276, 1984.
80. Ferreira SH: Site of analgesic action of aspirin-like drugs and opioids. In Beers RF Jr, Basset EG (eds): *Mechanisms of Pain and Analgesic Compounds*. New York, Raven Press, 1979, p 309.
81. Lasagna L, Beecher HK: The optimal dose of morphine. *JAMA* 156:230–234, 1954.
82. Roe BB: Are postoperative narcotics necessary? *Arch Surg* 87:912–915, 1963.
83. Pflug AE, Murphy TM, Butler SH, et al: The effects of postoperative peridural analgesia on pulmonary therapy and pulmonary complications. *Anesthesiology* 41:8–17, 1974.
84. Keats AS, Telford J, Kurosu Y: "Potentiation" of meperidine by promethazine. *Anesthesiology* 22:34–41, 1961.
85. Moertel CG, Ahmann DL, Taylor WF, et al: A comparative evaluation of marketed analgesic drugs. *N Engl J Med* 286:813–815, 1972.
86. Moertel CG, Ahmann DL, Taylor WF, et al: Relief of pain by oral medications: a controlled evaluation of analgesic combinations. *JAMA* 299:55–59, 1974.
87. Bonica JJ: Fundamental considerations of chronic pain therapy. *Postgrad Med* 53:81–85, 1973.
88. Raskin NW, Prusiner S: Carotidynia. *Neurology* 27:43–46, 1977.
89. Moore DS, Nally FF: Atypical facial pain. *J Can Dent Assoc* 41:396–401, 1975.
90. Gomersall JD, Stuart H: Amitriptyline in migraine prophylaxis. *J Neurol Neurosurg Psychiatry* 36:684–690, 1973.
91. Regelson W, Butler JR, Schulz J, et al: Delta-nine tetrahydrocannabinol as an effective antidepressant and appetite stimulating agents in advanced cancer patients. In Braude MCT, Szara S (eds): *The Pharmacology of Marijuana*. New York, Raven Press, 1976, p 763.

chapter 44
Postoperative Pain Management

Thomas K. Henthorn, M.D.
Tom C. Krejcie, M.D.

It should be noted that in attempts to manage patients experiencing acute pain, the emphasis is on prevention, because if pain can be effectively managed in the acute phase, the muscle guarding and dysfunction that may result tend to be avoided or at least reduced. Preventing progressive amplification of the pain cycle thereby permits the body's normal healing processes to occur without the encumbrances created by secondary pain factors.

Although there is always an overlap between the pathophysiology and treatment for chronic and acute pain, the aim of this chapter is entirely concerned with the management of acute postoperative and post-traumatic pain.

The management of postoperative pain is generally overlooked once the "important" business of surgical diagnosis, operative procedure, and anesthetic management are settled. If the physician in charge does not assume an active role in the analgesic management of the patient, the role is relegated to the junior house staff (or routine orders) who in all likelihood are uninformed and unmotivated to devote much time and effort to what for them is just one aspect of postoperative management.

Finally, the emphasis of this chapter is on the description of the possible alternatives for therapy of adults; however, some of these same modes of therapy may be applied, in theory, to the pediatric population.

ANATOMY AND NEUROPHYSIOLOGY OF ACUTE PAIN

Noxious stimuli affect their high-threshold receptors in the skin, subcutaneous tissue, fascia, periosteum, blood vessels, and viscera. The resulting impulses from these nociceptors are known as noxious or nociceptive impulses at all points in their transmission prior to reaching the cortex of the conscious human. Nociceptive impulses will, when processed by the cerebral cortex, give rise to the perceptual-emotional experience called pain.

Transmission, or nociception, of these impulses originating in the nociceptors occurs via small A-delta and C fibers to the spinal cord, where they synapse in the dorsal horn. The signal is then projected over multiple pathways of the neuroaxis (Fig. 44.1). Those to the anterolateral horn stimulate preganglionic neurons of the sympathetic or parasympathetic systems, whereas transmissions to the anterior horn stimulate somatic motor neurons. These are in addition to the traditional pain-transmitting spinothalamic tracts made up of axons of neurons located in various laminae of the dorsal horn.

The spinothalamic system is actually divided into the neospinothalamic tract and the paleospinothalamic tract. The rapidly conducting neospinothalamic tract has the capacity, via its discretely organized primary projection to the somatosensory cortex, to process discriminative information regarding the site, intensity, and duration of a stimulus resulting in the perception of a sharp, well-localized pain. On the other hand, nociceptive impulses transmitted by the paleospinothalamic tract, composed of diffusely projecting fibers, provoke suprasegmental reflex responses affecting ventilation, circulation, and endocrine function. This multisynaptic system, unlike the neospinothalamic tract, lacks somatotropic organization, resulting in the slowly transmitted impulses being perceived as poorly localized, dull, aching, and burning pain. The paleospinothalamic system may also provoke the powerful "fight or flight" mechanism.

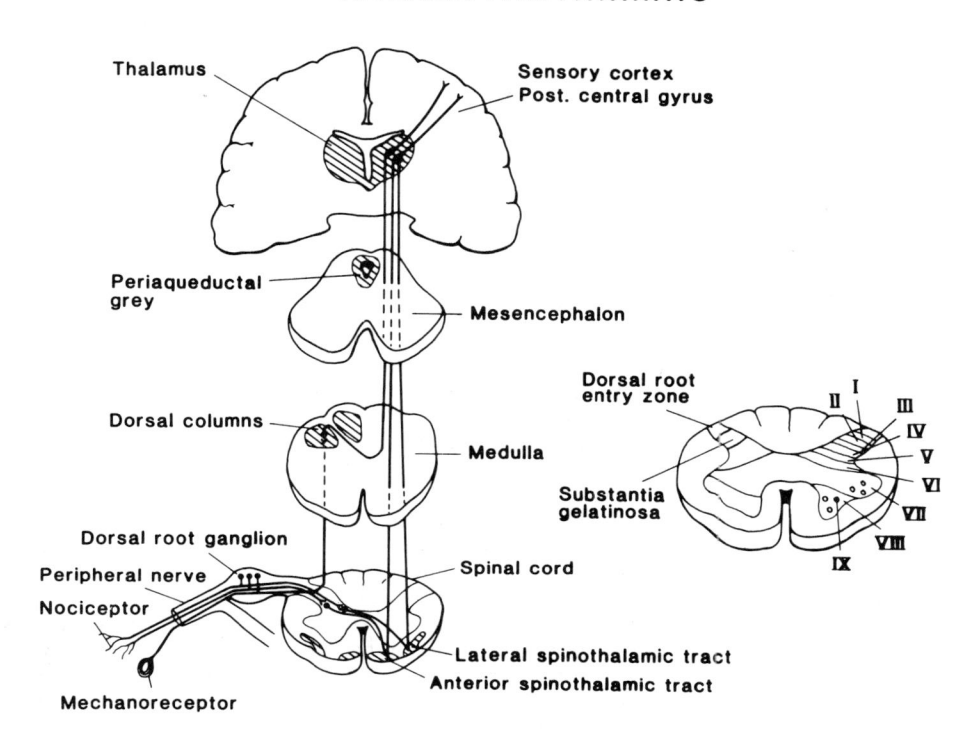

Figure 44.1. Afferent pain pathways and organization of dorsal horn laminae. (From Raj PP: Basic function and organization of the nervous system. In Raj PP (ed): *Practical Management of Pain.* Chicago, Year Book, 1986, p 56.)

MODULATION OF NOCICEPTION

This system of nociceptive transmission can be modulated at multiple points along its course, resulting in either amplification or inhibition of the signal. The release of intracellular substances into the extracellular space lowers the threshold of the local nociceptors. Furthermore, peripheral input into the dorsal horn is modulated by temperature, sympathetic function, blood flow, and the chemical environment, whereas modulation within the dorsal horn is also affected by local, segmental, and suprasegmental influences.

Inhibition of nociception can result from the influence of supraspinal descending neural systems. One of the most powerful of these systems contains axons that comprise the dorsolateral funiculus and receives signals that originate from neurons in the periaqueductal and periventricular gray matter. Stimulating this region of the midbrain produces a profound analgesia that can be blocked by naloxone.

PATHOPHYSIOLOGY OF POSTOPERATIVE PAIN

Segmental responses are the result of nociceptive impulses being transmitted from the dorsal horn to the anterior horn or anterolateral horn and include skeletal muscle spasm, vasospasm, and a decrease in gastrointestinal and genitourinary tract activity. Skeletal muscle spasm initiates a vicious cycle of spasm leading to pain and more spasm. Pain resulting from a lowered nociceptor threshold is a direct consequence of vasospastic ischemia causing local tissue hypoxia, acidosis, and the production and retention of endogenous pain-producing metabolites. Incisional skin trauma initiates a cutaneovisceral reflex that worsens the surgically induced dysfunction. An organized approach to the pathophysiologic responses to nociceptive impulses is presented in Table 44.1.

Hypoventilation and stimulation of the hypothalamic autonomic centers are categorized as suprasegmental responses to nociceptive impulses. Autonomic hyperactivity produces an increase in centrally mediated sympathetic tone and a resultant increase in cardiac output, peripheral vascular resistance, and circulating catecholamines, which in turn further increase sympathetic tone.

The actual perception of pain, overt skeletal muscle activity, and emotional responses all result from cortical stimulation. Although skeletal muscle activity is actually manifested by voluntary or involuntary immobilization, the psychodynamic mechanisms that produce fear and anxiety probably facilitate transmission of the nociceptive impulses throughout the central nervous system. Consequently, these highly complex interactions produce the complex physiologic, behavioral, and affective responses that characterize the pathophysiology of acute pain. Appropriate and efficacious acute pain therapy involves

Table 44.1
Stratification of Response to Nociceptive Impulses Following Intraabdominal Surgery[a]

I. Cortical responses
   A. Pain perception
   B. Psychodynamic mechanism—fear and anxiety
   C. Motivational
   D. Discriminative
   E. Overt voluntary motor activity/inactivity
II. Suprasegmental autonomic responses
   A. Endocrine (stress) response
   B. Alteration of ventilation
   C. Increased sympathetic tone with liberation of catecholamines and further increases in sympathetic tone
   D. Tachycardia → increased cardiac output
   E. Hypertension (as a result of C and D)
III. Segmental reflex responses
   A. Cutaneosomatic/somatosomatic responses
     1. Increased muscle spasm
     2. Ischemia
     3. Hyperhydrosis
   B. Cutaneovisceral/somatovisceral responses
     1. Bronchospasm
     2. Bronchiolar spasm
     3. Decreased gastrointestinal motility
       a. Distention
       b. Nausea
       c. Vomiting
     4. Decreased urinary function → oliguria
   C. Cutaneovascular responses → vasospasm
   D. Viscerocutaneous responses → results similar to A
   E. Visceroviscerall responses → results similar to B
IV. Local (microscopic) tissue responses
   A. Decreased circulation due to vasospasm and muscle spasm
     1. Decreased oxygen supply
     2. Decreased nutrient supply
     3. Retention of metabolites → lowered nociceptor threshold
     4. Cellular damage → liberation of pain substances
   B. Decreased lymphatic drainage → edema
   C. Muscle fatigue
   D. Inflammation

[a] Modified from Bonica JJ: Introduction, Pathophysiology of Pain. In *Current Concepts in Postoperative Pain*. New York, HP Publishing Co, 1978, p 10.

intervening early in an effort to block the pain cycle and thereby decrease its sequelae.

PHARMACOLOGY OF SYSTEMIC ANALGESICS

The systemic administration of analgesic drugs is by far the most common means of treating postoperative pain (1). It is also the most likely mode of therapy to be inadequate for relief of this pain (1–3). The failure of these drugs almost always lies not with the properties of the drug itself, but with some aspect of the way it is prescribed or administered (2, 4). The effective use of these drugs can be realized only if their clinical pharmacology is understood by those practitioners making therapeutic decisions about pain therapy. Reliance on standard recipes or nursing procedure is no substitute for rational application of the pharmacokinetic and pharmacodynamic information that is increasingly being made available.

NARCOTICS

Opioid or narcotic analgesic agents are drugs that specifically bind with opiate receptors to produce any of a variety of effects. These effects include analgesia, respiratory depression, mood alteration, gastrointestinal immotility, miosis, and cardiovascular changes, especially increased venous capacitance. Opioids have been used for centuries to reduce surgically induced pain and anxiety. This remains the most frequent use for these drugs. Morphine was produced from opium early in the last century and has proven to be a highly efficacious analgesic for a variety of pain states. Although potency may vary, the opiates that have been introduced over the years, and continue to be introduced, have not exceeded the efficacy of morphine. Drugs with equal efficacy to morphine are referred to as "pure" narcotic agonists, some of which are listed in Table 44.2. Narcotics with less efficacy are called partial agonists or partial agonist-antagonists; these are discussed later in this section.

Despite the availability of several narcotic agonists of proven efficacy in controlling pain, inadequate relief of postoperative pain remains a problem (1–4). The traditional approach to postoperative pain relief has been to administer narcotics to patients by intermittent intramuscular injection. This approach is often inadequate for several reasons. The primary reason is that patients differ in their requirement for narcotics. In addition, there is a common tendency to overestimate the potency, duration of action, and addiction potential of these drugs. As a result, physician orders may be inadequate because either too small a dose or too long an interval between doses is prescribed (4).

In an attempt to allow for some variability in patient requirement, it is common to prescribe opiates for the relief of acute pain as "p.r.n." This comes from the Latin *pro re nata* (according as circumstances may require), but is sometimes seen as "per RN"—that is, when the nurse is convinced that there is a real need for a narcotic that outweighs the concerns for addiction potential or side effects (e.g., respiratory depression, sedation, constipation) and that this nonemergent request does not seriously interfere with completion of other important duties (4, 5). These concerns have been addressed. It has been repeatedly shown that dependence is a rare event, occurring in fewer than 0.1% of hospitalized patients (6–8). Regarding the concern for the side effects of opiates used

Table 44.2
Approximate Pharmacokinetic and Pharmacodynamic Values for Common Narcotic Agonists

Opiate Agonist	Approx. Dose Equiv. to 10 mg Morphine	Effective Plasma Conc. (ng/ml)	Volume of Distribution (liters/kg)	Clearance (liters/min)	Elimination Half-Life (hr)
Morphine	10 mg	21	4.0	0.8–1.5	2.5–4
Meperidine	100 mg	550	3.5	0.9	3–4
Fentanyl	100 µg	1–2	3.5	1.0	3–5
Alfentanil	500 µg	10–20	0.7	0.45	1.5–2.5
Methadone	10 mg	58	7.0	0.15	24–48

for pain therapy, the observation has been made that this concern is "extravagant" and has "drastically" limited treatment on a scale that is unparalleled in medicine (9). Keats has addressed the logistic issue in a study in which it was shown that the amount of narcotic a patient received was directly proportional to the amount of nursing staff available to the patient (10).

Patients require differing dosages of opiates for a variety of reasons. The factors governing variability can be divided into two general categories: pharmacokinetic (differences in rate of absorption, tissue distribution, and elimination) and pharmacodynamic (differences in response to identical concentrations presented to the active tissue site, or biophase).

Biophase concentrations, although rarely sampled, are generally considered to reflect blood or plasma concentrations, particularly during steady state conditions. Most plasma concentration versus effect data for narcotic agonists have dealt with meperidine. Studies with other opiate agonists [morphine (11), fentanyl (12), alfentanil (13, 14), methadone (15), and ketobemidone (16)] have been consistent with the general pharmacologic principles that have been delineated with the meperidine model. Austin et al. examined plasma meperidine concentrations and pain scores at regular intervals during every-4-hr dosing with intramuscular meperidine (17). The data from three patients in Figure 44.2 illustrate some important findings. First, the concentration-response curves are quite steep, with dramatic changes in pain score occurring over a narrow concentration range. Second, there is a fourfold difference in the plasma concentration required for complete pain relief between patients A and C. Patient B had an intermediate sensitivity to the drug. Studies by Tamsen et al. in which patients self-administered small intravenous doses of meperidine on demand gave a similar picture, as shown in Figure 44.3 (18). Each patient tended to maintain plasma meperidine concentrations within a narrow range, suggesting that the concentration-response relationship is as steep as that demonstrated by Austin et al. (17). Additionally, the concentrations "selected" by patients could vary considerably. Thus, whereas intrasubject concentration variation should be small, intersubject variation should be expected to be large. Although traditional thought has ascribed large intersubject variability to a host of physical and psychosocial factors, recent evidence from Tamsen and coworkers has shown an inverse relationship between narcotic requirement and endorphin levels sampled from the cerebrospinal fluid of postoperative patients (19).

Pharmacokinetic variability can also account for differences in dosage requirement. Unfortunately, there are few studies that offer much guidance in making dosing adjustments for this type of variability. However, if the clinician is alert and expects these sources of variation, proper dose titration for a desired clinical effect is more likely.

The pharmacokinetics of absorption can be highly variable. The principle determinant of absorption from intramuscular injections is muscle blood flow. Several factors may cause the postsurgical patient to have diminished muscle blood flow. Such a decrease is particularly likely in patients who have suffered significant physiologic perturbations during their surgical procedure. Not only may

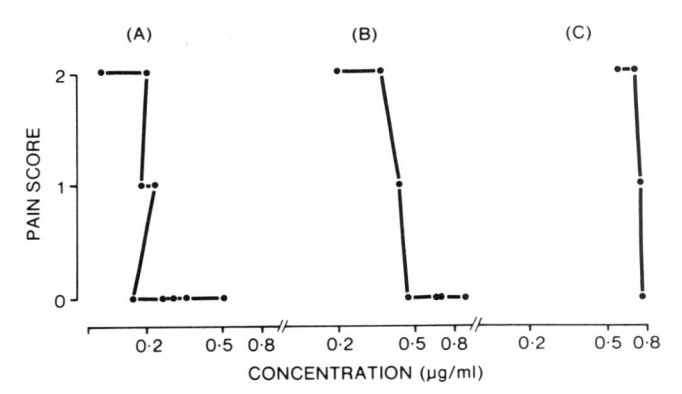

Figure 44.2. Plasma meperidine concentration versus response data for three postoperative patients. *Solid circles* represent measured plasma meperidine concentrations and the corresponding pain score when the sample was obtained. Note the differences in concentration corresponding to vertical portion of the curves for each patient. These differences represent interindividual pharmacodynamic variation. (From Austin KL, Stapleton JV, Mather LE: Relationship between blood meperidine concentrations and analgesic response: a preliminary report. *Anesthesiology* 53:460–466, 1980.)

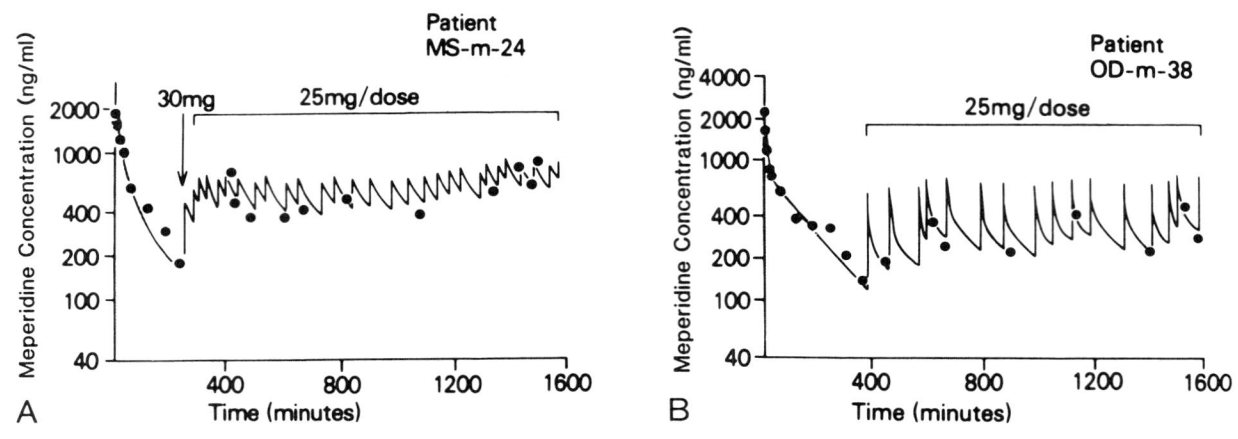

Figure 44.3A and B. Plasma concentrations of meperidine for two patients following a single dose (approximately 150 mg) for surgery and with 25-mg bolus-demand doses for PCA postoperatively. *Solid circles* represent measured plasma meperidine concentrations and *solid lines* are computer-generated estimates of the changes in plasma concentration with time. Note the increased demand frequency and higher "trough" levels of patient A. (Modified from Tamsen A, Hartvig P, Fogerland C, et al: Patient-controlled analgesic therapy: Part II. Invidual analgesic demand and analgesic plasma concentrations of pethidine in postoperative pain. *Clin Pharmacokinet* 7:164–175, 1982).

these patients obtain subtherapeutic plasma concentrations because of poor absorption, but there is the danger that significant depression of sensorium and respiration may occur when muscle perfusion is restored and the narcotic depot is rapidly absorbed. Mather et al. have shown that absorption rates of meperidine have great interindividual variation following intramuscular injection, resulting in large differences in plasma concentrations and levels of pain relief (20). Similarly, oral absorption is dependent on splanchnic blood flow and gastric emptying, both of which may be adversely affected by the effects of surgery and anesthesia, especially when the insults are major. Significant liver dysfunction may lessen the first-pass metabolism, markedly increasing bioavailability. Such findings have led to the recommendation that oral meperidine doses be reduced in patients with cirrhosis (21).

Reductions in function of the major drug-clearing organs, the liver and kidney, may result in reducing drug clearance. Because of the relationship

$$Css = DR/Cle \qquad (44.1)$$

where steady state plasma concentration (Css) is equal to the ratio of dosing rate (DR) to elimination clearance (Cle), one can see that higher drug concentrations will result if standard doses are given to patients with impaired clearing capacity.

All of the major narcotic agonists undergo extensive hepatic metabolism with minimal renal excretion of the parent drug. The two general categories of metabolism, the phase I oxidation and reduction reactions and the phase II conjugations, respond differently to hepatic insults. As a general rule, oxidative metabolic pathways are susceptible to functional impairment when hepatic disease is present. One should be alert to the possibility of reduced elimination clearance as well as reduced first-pass metabolism following oral administration when phase I–metabolized drugs, such as an fentanyl and meperidine, are given (21–23). On the other hand, glucuronidation pathways are more robust and seem to resist the influence of hepatic disease. Morphine, which undergoes glucuronidation, has normal clearance in cirrhotics (24).

Impaired renal function does not directly reduce the elimination clearance of the narcotic analgesics. The uremic state can, however, indirectly impair liver function and diminish hepatic metabolism. There is some evidence that morphine clearance is reduced in renal failure, perhaps by some indirect mechanism (25).

In the 72 hr during which acute postoperative pain management is a concern, it is unlikely that significant levels of metabolites of the narcotic analgesics could accumulate. Chronic administration of meperidine, however, can lead to the accumulation of its metabolite, normeperidine, which causes cerebral excitation leading to irritability and even seizures (26). The conjugated metabolites of morphine (morphine 3- and morphine 6-glucuronide) exceed the levels of the parent drug with chronic oral therapy (because of the lower clearance of these conjugates) and may be particularly high if the patient has renal failure and cannot excrete these water-soluble compounds (27). Morphine 3-glucuronide appears to be pharmacologically inert and although morphine 6-glucuronide has analgesic effects in rats, it is uncertain whether or not this metabolite has any significant effect in humans (27).

OPIATE PARTIAL AGONISTS AND PARTIAL AGONIST-ANTAGONISTS

A variety of opiate drugs with limited agonist activity have been introduced in the past few decades. They have been touted as offering the advantage of analgesic efficacy similar to that of the opiate agonists but having a reduced potential for serious side effects such as addiction and respiratory depression. Because narcotic addiction is not an issue in the postoperative patient, one need not be influenced by claims of lower or absent addiction potential. The partial agonist-antagonists butorphanol, pentazocine, and nalbuphine and the partial agonist buprenorphine are the common analgesics available in parenteral form for postoperative pain therapy. In contrast to the pure agonists, these drugs have been shown to have a ceiling for respiratory-depressive effects (28, 29). However, they also demonstrate a ceiling in their analgesic potency (4, 30, 31). They are capable of antagonizing the analgesic (32), respiratory-depressive (33), and electroencephalographic effects (34) of pure narcotic agonists. A particularly cloudy clinical picture may result when a pure opiate agonist is given to a patient who has already received one of the mixed agonist-antagonists or vice versa. Although these drugs may have a place in the treatment of relatively minor pain that may follow some superficial or extremity operations, the authors do not recommend their routine use for most surgical patients.

NONSTEROIDAL ANTI-INFLAMMATORY ANALGESICS

Since the introduction of aspirin in 1899, nonsteroidal anti-inflammatory agents have been used to treat minor surgical pain. Although aspirin remains the standard to which others are compared, it is no longer the most common minor analgesic in surgical practice. Rather, the powerful opiate agonists are the drugs of choice for severe or even moderate postoperative pain and the nonsteroidal anti-inflammatory analgesics are generally relegated to oral administration following relatively minor procedures such as dental surgery or episiotomy. This is because these agents have a plateau of analgesic efficacy and are effective only if the pain stimulus is not too strong (35). The number of operations performed on an outpatient basis has increased dramatically over the past few years and so, not surprisingly, has interest in these analgesics because many of the newer anti-inflammatory analgesics have been demonstrated to have greater efficacy than aspirin and acetaminophen (35). Because it may be unacceptable in many situations to administer parenteral narcotics to postsurgical outpatients, it is expected that these anti-inflammatory analgesics will be utilized to an increasing degree for treating postoperative pain.

The nonsteroidal anti-inflammatory drugs are thought to act peripherally rather than centrally as the opiates do. By inhibiting the cyclo-oxygenase enzyme system they prevent the metabolism of arachidonic acid to its endoperoxide intermediates, which would then be converted to thromboxanes, prostacyclines, and prostaglandins. These interact with other local mediators to produce erythema, edema, and pain (Table 44.1). Much remains unknown about other antinociceptive mechanisms, but a central action and the possibility of other peripheral mechanisms have been suggested (35).

Ibuprofen (400 mg), indoprofen (200 mg), naproxen (400 mg), diflunisal (500 mg), and ketorolac (10 mg) (36) given orally all appear to have efficacy superior to that of aspirin (650 mg) or, in some cases, aspirin plus codeine in postsurgical patients (35). Some recent studies indicate that with larger parenteral doses of nonsteroidal anti-inflammatory drugs, efficacy similar to that of morphine can be achieved in postoperative patients. Ketorolac (30 mg) given intramuscularly has been shown to be as effective as morphine (12 mg) (37). Lysine acetylsalicylate by continuous intravenous infusion (1.8 g over 5 min followed by 1.8 g over 6 hr) was as effective as a continuous infusion of morphine (10 mg over 5 min followed by 10 mg over 6 hr) (38). These parenteral anti-inflammatory agents are currently investigational but may prove to be viable alternatives to the traditional opiates in the treatment of postoperative pain.

SEDATIVE DRUGS USED AS ADJUNCTS TO ANALGESICS

A component of the discomfort of the postoperative period is often the attendant anxiety. This can often heighten the interpreted intensity of pain or the emotional reaction to it; thus an aggravating cycle, difficult to interrupt with analgesics alone, may ensue (39). Sedative drugs, although of no use for treating acute pain alone, may, in combination with an opiate, accomplish the desired goal of abating both the patient's pain and his focus on or anxiety concerning that pain. Drugs that have been used in this way are promethazine (25–50 mg) (40), hydroxyzine (25–100 mg) (41), dextroamphetamine (5–10 mg) (42), and benzodiazepines [diazepam (5–10 mg), oxazepam (15 mg), or midazolam (1–5 mg)] (43). Promethazine, hydroxyzine (painful when given intramuscularly), and droperidol (1.25–2.5 mg) are also antiemetics and may help counter the nausea that frequently accompanies opiate use (44). Although it is common practice to order some of these drugs in fixed combination with a narcotic analgesic, prudence would dictate their addition only when indicated. Most patients simply will not require these mood-altering drugs, whereas others may experience significant exaggeration of some of the side effects of concomitantly administered narcotics (sedation, respiratory depression).

METHODS OF SYSTEMIC ANALGESIC ADMINISTRATION

Selection of the appropriate systemic drug for a postoperative patient is important, but represents only the first step in the pharmacologic treatment of postoperative pain. The clinician must next decide how the drug will be given and how the effectiveness of the therapy will be assessed so that changes and adjustments can be made to suit a given patient. In deciding how the drug will be given one must consider both the route of administration and the dosing schedule.

ROUTES OF DRUG ADMINISTRATION

The route of drug delivery is often dictated by the drug formulations that are available or by patient considerations such as the availability of intravenous access or the ability of the patient to take medication orally. Most often the clinician chooses a particular approach in order to take advantage of the special properties that a route may offer. Understanding the pharmacokinetic properties associated with various routes of drug administration is essential to planning drug therapy and the interpretation of subsequent events.

Intravenous Drug Administration

To exert a systemic effect the drug must first reach the systemic circulation so that it may then be carried to the tissue sites of action. Understanding the fate of drugs given directly into the circulation is helpful in understanding the time course of events following other methods of systemic drug administration.

The fate or *disposition* of a drug injected intravenously involves the processes of *distribution* to body tissues and *clearance* by the organs of elimination. Drug distribution is governed by the laws of mass action, which drive blood and tissue concentrations towards an equilibrium. The physicochemical properties of drugs and the physiologic (i.e., tissue perfusion) state of the patient are both important factors in drug distribution. Highly lipid-soluble opiate analgesics, such as fentanyl, methadone, or meperidine, move across capillaries into and out of tissues rapidly, with the amount of blood flow to any particular tissue determining the extent and rate. The highly perfused tissue of the central nervous system (CNS) equilibrates rapidly with the blood concentrations of these lipophilic drugs, so changes in the intensity of narcotic effects will quickly follow changes in plasma drug concentrations (14, 15). Following a rapid intravenous injection, concentrations in the blood and CNS will fall as distribution of drug continues to the large reservoir of less well perfused, pharmacologically inert tissues (e.g., skeletal muscle). The apparent size of the total tissue reservoir is termed the volume of distribution. This is usually only a theoretic volume and varies from drug to drug, depending on a variety of factors. Under most circumstances the process of distribution to this volume approaches completion in 0.5–1.5 hr. If drug concentrations fall below effective levels during this phase of disposition the pharmacologic effect dissipates. The termination of drug effect, therefore, is often a result of drug distribution, not drug elimination alone. Thus it is common to observe a 0.5–1.0-hr duration of action following intravenous injection of a therapeutic dose of many drugs.

After distribution is complete, plasma drug concentrations continue to decrease, albeit more slowly, due solely to drug elimination. There are two terms used to describe the kinetics of elimination: elimination half-life and elimination clearance. Elimination clearance is expressed as volume per unit time and is a direct measure of the elimination processes. Its importance during drug therapy is expressed in Equation 44.1, which shows that the eventual or steady state plasma concentration is determined by the ratio of dosing rate and elimination clearance.

Elimination half-life is the time required for the plasma drug concentration to decrease by one-half. This can be measured only after the drug distribution processes are complete. Half-life, which is dependent on the ratio of the distribution volume to elimination clearance, is often erroneously equated with duration of action, but it is only one of several factors that are predictive of how long a drug may act.

Elimination half-life is, however, directly related to the time required to reach 90% of the eventual steady state plasma concentration for a drug given on a fixed schedule or by infusion. The time required to reach 90% of the eventual steady state concentration can be calculated by multiplying the half-life by 3.3. Knowing this, one can predict that meperidine (half-life = 4 hr) given at 50 mg every 3 hr would approach a maximum steady state concentration in about 13 hr (i.e., after four doses), whereas with methadone (half-life = 36 hr) given at 10 mg every 12 hr a maximum steady state would be approached in about 5 days (i.e., after 10 doses). This has important implications when evaluating patients for analgesic efficacy and side effects after making dosage adjustments; maximum effect is approached in 3.3 half-lives.

The time to peak effect following a rapid intravenous injection or bolus infusion is dependent on the rate of rise of the CNS tissue concentration and the rate of decline of the plasma concentration, both of which are affected by the physicochemical properties of a drug (45). Fentanyl will reach a peak in 2–4 min following an intravenous bolus compared with a peak effect for morphine that occurs in 5–10 min. This time requirement is important clinically when one is titrating to an effect. With either patient-controlled or clinician-controlled administration, time must be allowed to observe the eventual effect of a dose before additional increments are given. This time can be shorter for lipophilic drugs such as fentanyl or meperidine, and may be as short as 1–2 min following an intravenous bolus of the new fentanyl congener, alfentanil (14, 45).

Gourlay and colleagues have elegantly made use of these pharmacokinetic principles in the treatment of postoperative pain with methadone (15). As shown in Table 44.2, methadone has a long elimination half-life (approximately 36 hr) because of its low clearance and large volume of distribution. Methadone is also lipid soluble, allowing rapid plasma-to-brain equilibration. Effective doses given parenterally have generally resulted in short durations of action (46) despite the prolonged elimination half-life as plasma concentrations fall below effective levels during the distributive phase (i.e., before the terminal elimination phase). It is not feasible to give a dose that would result in an effective level after the distributive processes yield a pseudoequilibration of tissue concentrations so that the slow, elimination phase could be exploited to produce a long-lasting effect. Such a dose would necessarily be large and initially result in high plasma concentrations that are associated with respiratory depression and excessive sedation. In the report by Gourlay et al. (15) a relatively large methadone dose (20 mg intravenously) was given at the start of anesthesia. The patient's ventilation was then supported during the operation. The plasma methadone concentrations fell as a result of distribution during surgery so that by the time of arrival in the recovery room they were near effective levels. Smaller 5-mg doses were given incrementally in the recovery room so that the dose could be titrated to allow for individual variability (range: 1–3 doses). Because subsequent decreases in plasma methadone concentration were during the slow, elimination phase, these investigators observed a mean duration of action of 21 hr.

Another means of providing prolonged action is by continuous infusion of a drug. Hug, in an editorial (47), called for increased efforts in defining the pharmacokinetics and pharmacodynamics of analgesics so that infusions could be rationally designed to maintain plasma concentrations at an effective analgesic level while avoiding toxicity. As suggested in Equation 44.1, the critical pieces of information needed to devise an infusion are the target concentration (Css) and the elimination clearance (Cle). These variables, given for some narcotics in Table 44.2, when multiplied will yield the proper infusion rate (DR) for the average patient. Unfortunately, many postoperative patients are not average and, as discussed above in some detail, considerable variability in effective plasma concentration and elimination clearance should be expected. Nevertheless, in a very straightforward manner Duthie and colleagues (12) gave a continuous fentanyl infusion of 100 μg/hr for 24 hr for postoperative analgesia and found it effective. Given an elimination clearance for fentanyl of 1.0 liter/min (Table 44.2), one could predict a mean steady state plasma concentration of 1.7 ng/ml; Duthie et al. found their 45 patients ranged between 1 and 3 ng/ml (12). Because steady state levels are not approached before 3.3 drug half-lives have elapsed, some provision for reaching these levels sooner (i.e., with a loading dose) must be made. In the study of Duthie et al. (12) the anesthesia for surgery was narcotic (fentanyl) based, thus obviating the need for a loading scheme. When a narcotic has not been used during the course of anesthesia, loading should be accomplished with incremental intravenous bolus doses of the narcotic in the recovery room. Additionally, some feedback mechanism to adjust the infusion rate needs to be incorporated in the overall treatment plan.

Intramuscular Drug Administration

The process of intramuscular drug absorption is generally first order. That is, a constant fraction of the remaining dose is absorbed at any given time. This results in a continuously diminishing amount of drug entering the circulation. Because absorption and tissue distribution take place concurrently, the result is a delayed and reduced peak plasma concentration despite absolute bioavailability that is usually equal to the intravenous route.

The resultant buffering of peak concentrations and effect has allowed larger, longer acting doses to be given and has generally made the intramuscular route appear safer than the intravenous route. However, the rate of the absorption process is dependent on skeletal muscle blood flow. As previously mentioned, hypoperfusion of skeletal muscle is not a rare event in postsurgical patients. A reduced rate of absorption will delay the peak plasma concentration. It may be difficult to ascertain whether the reduced efficacy seen shortly after injection, in an affected patient, is due to poor absorption (pharmacokinetic factor) or a decreased sensitivity (pharmacodynamic factor). The treatment for the former is allowing more time to elapse, whereas for the latter it is the administration of more drug. By giving more drug into a hypoperfused muscle, one runs the risk of observing a relative overdose if blood flow is suddenly restored, the absorption rate constant increases, and a much larger fraction of the drug remaining in the muscle reaches the circulation in a short time.

The merits of traditional intramuscular narcotic administration are mainly its low cost and simplicity. Almost by design, the plasma concentrations are not maintained constant, but swing widely between subtherapeutic (a requirement of most intermittent "as needed" regimens) and therapeutic and sometimes higher. Figure 44.4 graphically shows the time course of the plasma concentrations resulting from this mode of administration and the resultant toll in the time the patient must endure pain at one extreme and risk sedation and respiratory depression at the other.

In an attempt to mimic continuous infusions, regular timed intramuscular injections have been advocated in an attempt to avoid the unnecessary intervals of subtherapeutic plasma concentrations and the expense of infusion pumps. Welchew has shown that 4-hourly intramuscular morphine (10 mg) gave pain scores and side effects (sedation and nausea scores) similar to on-demand fentanyl (48).

Subcutaneous Drug Administration

Because of the difficulties in maintaining intravenous catheters, particularly in outpatients, subcutaneously placed needles offer a reasonable alternate route for delivering drug either by continuous infusion (49) or by

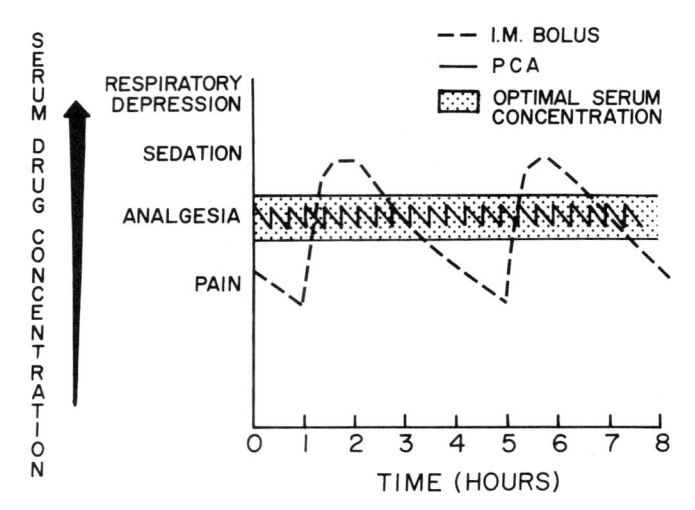

Figure 44.4. Idealized serum drug concentration versus time curves for intramuscular administration (*dashed line*) and intravenous PCA (*solid line*). The vertical axis includes measures for both narcotic concentration and effect. Note the relationship of the idealized concentration lines with optimal serum concentrations that avoid pain and sedation. (From Bennett RL, Griffen WO: Patient controlled analgesia. *Contemp Surg* 23:75–84, 1983.)

frequent intermittent bolus doses. As with intramuscular injections, absorption will delay the peak concentration and effect. A small 23- or 25-gauge needle can be placed subcutaneously, taped in place, and attached to the administration set of the delivery device. It is usually recommended that the needle be reinserted at a new site on a daily basis.

Oral Drug Administration

Oral administration is most often preferred because it is convenient, painless, and superficially appears to be nontechnical. Whenever feasible, patients and physicians will select this route. However, it is fraught with technical difficulties that may jeopardize success. Therefore, alternate routes of administration when treating postoperative or other acute pain states are encouraged. Nevertheless, oral administration of analgesic drugs may be an acceptable choice following many types of operations.

Absorption from the gastrointestinal tract is far more complex than intramuscular or subcutaneous absorption, where tissue blood flow is the chief regulating influence. Since mucosal surface area is so important in determining the rate of absorption from the gastrointestinal tract, passage of the drug from the stomach to the duodenum, where there is a severalfold increase in mucosal surface area, drastically improves drug absorption. Delayed gastric emptying, as sometimes accompanies surgery or trauma, may limit the effectiveness of a dose of analgesic.

After gastric or intestinal absorption, the drug is carried via the portal system to the liver, where metabolism may occur before the drug can gain access to the systemic circulation. This is called first-pass metabolism. It is significant for those drugs with moderate or high hepatic elimination clearance or extraction (i.e., hepatic clearance greater than about 300 ml/min). If normal adult liver blood flow is about 1500 ml/min, then a drug with a hepatic elimination clearance of 300 ml/min would have 20% of the dose lost on first pass; one with a clearance of 900 ml/min would lose 60%. Morphine, with a hepatic clearance of about 850 ml/min, loses a little over one-half of an oral dose to first-pass metabolism. Therefore, most patients will require about two to three times their usual intramuscular morphine dose when it is given orally (27). With some drugs, significant oral dose reductions are required in the presence of hepatic disease because the first-pass effect may be reduced (vide supra) (21).

As mentioned earlier in the chapter, because of the larger dose requirement due to first-pass metabolism, oral administration will result in the production of a larger quantity of metabolites that may [e.g., meperidine (26)] or may not [e.g., morphine (27)] require clinical consideration.

Transdermal Drug Administration

Transdermal drug administration has proven to be a viable means of delivering several drugs such as nitroglycerine and scopolamine. As with other routes requiring absorption, this method requires a predictable blood flow at the dermal application site. However, transdermal administration differs from other routes requiring absorption in that the absorption process is not first order (oral, subcutaneous, or intramuscular absorption are), where a constant fraction of the dose is absorbed at any given time, but is zero order (like an intravenous infusion), where a constant amount is delivered over any given time regardless of the amount remaining in the drug depot. Thus, following application of a "drug patch," concentrations will begin an exponential rise toward a steady state concentration. It will reach 90% of this steady state in 3.3 half-lives. Therefore, unless the anesthetic for the operation was narcotic based and the patient already had significant narcotic plasma concentrations, it may be necessary to give a narcotic "loading" dose when starting transdermal treatment. Such transdermal dosage forms have been successfully used in postoperative pain management with fentanyl (50), but this therapy is still in the investigational stages.

Patient-Controlled Analgesia

Systemically administered narcotic analgesics, although frequently used in the treatment of acute postoperative pain, are not commonly used in a manner that can provide optimal analgesia. One factor responsible for inadequate analgesia is the interindividual variation in narcotic requirements. The minimum effective analgesic concentration (MEAC) in plasma is only one variable affecting the ability to obtain satisfactory postoperative analgesia in any given patient. The MEAC can vary by 21% within a given patient over time and as much as eightfold between patients (11, 16–20). For this reason alone, it is not surprising that "standard" orders for narcotic administration in the postoperative period will seldom provide optimum analgesia.

As mentioned above, the multiple factors affecting drug absorption rates or bioavailability can be circumvented by direct intravenous administration. However, because of the rapid peak levels (and effect) obtained following intravenous bolus administration and the subsequent redistribution to terminate effect, it is usually not a practical utilization of available manpower to administer narcotic analgesics in this manner except in the setting of an intensive care unit or recovery room. Therefore, the use of a machine controlling the intravenous administration of a narcotic either as an intermittent bolus or continuous infusion, or some combination of the two, while having the patient directly or indirectly altering the rate of administration, results in a highly successful modality for providing an optimum level of postoperative analgesia.

A method for providing intermittent demand bolus administration is available and in current use. A method for providing a patient demand–based alteration in the administration rate of a continuous infusion is currently under investigation. It is hoped that this latter mode of administration would further minimize both the peaks and troughs in plasma drug concentrations as well as the repeated and frequent patient intervention, particularly during intervals of sleep. However, with this technique, there is continued concern that the patient must be allowed to "surface" regularly so that the system continues to be patient controlled rather than machine controlled. If a high continuous administration rate were to be established, respiratory depression might occur during sleep or during periods of lesser stimulation. In fact, in the interest of safety, it may be best if some degree of pain is maintained. It has clearly been shown, in most patient-controlled analgesia (PCA) studies, that patients do not try to abolish all pain, but rather settle for a tolerable level of analgesia. Perhaps they are balancing all sensory inputs and selecting an acceptable level of comfort, while minimizing distressful side effects.

The rational approach to PCA is based not only on the choice of the analgesic, but also on the route of administration, incremental dose, and concomitant therapy.

Route of Administration The intravenous, intramuscular, sublingual, oral, rectal, and epidural routes have all been used in conjunction with investigating the efficacy of PCA. For intramuscular injection, a recommended approach is to sterilely place a Teflon catheter in the nondominant deltoid muscle and connect this to an On-Demand Analgesia Computer (ODAC) (51). Using this technique, a lock-out period of 20 min was used to allow patient appreciation of one dose prior to permitting a repeat dose. The authors have no experience with this technique because intravenous access is commonly available in the postoperative setting and is the route of administration to be considered in the remainder of this section. PCA via the oral route is actually the proper terminology for analgesic therapy of the nonhospitalized patient and is most commonly used with aspirin or acetaminophen.

Choice of Agents Multiple drugs have been individually applied using a PCA technique. Most commonly employed have been the narcotic analgesics, but antipyretic analgesics (nonsteroidal anti-inflammatory agents) have also been used. Most experience has been with morphine, but fentanyl (48), nalbuphine (52), buprenorphine (53), and meperidine (18) have been successfully used. Whereas a rapidly eliminated drug such as alfentanil might be useful in an ODAC designed to alter an infusion rate based on patient demand, a bolus-demand technique using alfentanil would be unacceptable to the patient because of the resulting frequent demand rate. Essentially any drug that is efficacious and can relieve pain in the clinical circumstances in which it is currently used can probably be satisfactorily used in an ODAC for PCA.

Another unrecognized advantage of PCA is the ability to concomitantly administer a sedative/tranquilizer, anxiolytic, or antiemetic without the usual concern for adjusting the dose of the narcotic analgesic in an effort to prevent undue sedation or respiratory depression. As noted previously, a significant component of postoperative pain is either anxiety or a dose-limiting side effect of the analgesic that precludes its optimum use by the patient. As seen in the example for postoperative orders (Table 44.3), the authors routinely make available droperidol as an effective

Table 44.3
Suggested Patient-Controlled Analgesia (PCA) Orders

1. No i.m. or i.v. narcotics, hypnotics, or sedatives shall be ordered or administered except by order of the Pain Control Service.
2. Syringe preparation for _____ ODAC device:
   Syringe size: _____ ml
   Analgesic: _____
   Drug volume: _____ ml
   Drug concentration: _____ _____ g/ml
3. Replace syringe as needed for up to 72 hr
4. PCA parameters:
   Demand dose: _____ ml
   Lockout interval: _____ min
   Dose limit (if relevant): _____ ml/ _____ hr
5. Droperidol (2.5 mg i.m. q 6 hr as needed) for nausea/vomiting
6. For inadequate analgesia, questions, problems, or desire to discontinue PCA prior to:
   Date _____
   Contact: _____
   Page # _____ Phone # _____

antiemetic. This butyrophenone produces (in higher doses) a state of quiescence with reduced motor activity, reduced anxiety, and indifference to the surroundings. In addition to its antiemetic property, it exhibits mild α-blocking properties that may be beneficial, because not infrequently patients have some degree of elevated blood pressure in the early postoperative period. The usual concern with the use of such adjuncts is their unpredictable synergistic effect when combined with a narcotic analgesic, particularly with a drug such as droperidol, which may exert its effect for up to 6 hr. However, PCA gives patients the ability to adapt to these changes and alter their demand for the narcotic on an individual basis.

Loading As discussed in the section on pharmacokinetics, the effect of a small intravenous bolus dose of drug will diminish rapidly. It is only with repeated doses over several hours that the tissues, to which the agent redistributes, reach equilibrium so that with a diminishing concentration gradient the duration of effect of each bolus may be expected to increase. This fact, coupled with the notion that pain is "easier to prevent than to treat," dictates that an initial dose, larger than the programmed demand dose, should be administered to "load" the patient when PCA therapy is first initiated. Although using intermittent bolus doses (1 mg every 10 min for morphine) may accomplish this goal, the patient might easily get frustrated during the first hour of self-administration. Although not as common, this same scenario may become apparent, to a lesser degree, after a period of sleep.

Lock-Out Interval For any given drug, its chemical characteristics, pharmacokinetics, and pharmacodynamics will define the time of onset for a particular route of administration. An appropriate interval (10 min for morphine), during which a subsequent bolus dose will not be administered regardless of patient demand, must be selected to allow for patient appreciation of the effect of the previous dose prior to a repeat dose, thereby preventing an "overshoot" of both concentration and effect.

Bolus Demand Dose The bolus dose should be selected to give the patient a noticeable effect within the lock-out time and a reasonable duration of action, and yet avoid increasing the resultant concentration to a level that consistently produces unwanted side effects. The efficacy of PCA can be improved considerably by simply doubling the demand bolus dose of the narcotic. While dramatically decreasing the patient self-assessed pain score, this should increase the total drug requirement only slightly. A recommended bolus dose for morphine would be 1–2 mg, whereas that for fentanyl would be approximately 10–30 μg.

Summary A very complete summary of the PCA experience in the United States and Europe has been compiled by Harmer et al. (54). The authors recommend referring to this text prior to initiating this form of postoperative pain management.

INTRATHECAL AND EPIDURAL OPIATES

Quite soon after the demonstration of the "selective block" caused by opiate agonist effects at the spinal cord level, intrathecal and epidural administration of narcotic agonists for the treatment of chronic and acute pain states became almost commonplace. Narcotic agonists, such as morphine, were shown to have stereoselective binding at both pre- and postsynaptic receptors mainly in the substantia gelatinosa of the dorsal horn of the spinal cord, where nociception is modulated. Inhibition of neuronal cell excitation here produces the so-called selective block of pain conduction (55). Because spinal (intrathecal and epidural) administration of narcotics promised substantial theoretical advantages over similar administration of local anesthetic drugs (avoidance of motor, sensory, and autonomic block) or systemic administration of narcotic analgesics (longer duration, better analgesia, and avoidance, in most cases, of the central side effects of sedation and respiratory depression), this form of pain therapy gained almost overnight popularity.

Numerous early reports substantiated the efficacy of this approach for treating postoperative pain (56–58). However, although the number of patients studied in these reports was sufficient to demonstrate efficacy, it was insufficient to accurately identify and assess risk. Case reports began to appear indicating that in a few rare cases slow cephalad transport of drug causes sedation and respiratory depression 8–15 hr after spinal administration (59, 60). Gustafsson et al. (61) reported a nationwide survey in Sweden involving over 6000 cases in which spinal opiates had been used for treating postoperative pain. They estimated the incidence of ventilatory depression to be 0.25–0.40% and 4–7% when epidural and intrathecal morphine were used, respectively. They identified several risk factors, including advanced age (>70 years), large intrathecal doses (2–5 mg morphine), preoperative pulmonary compromise, concomitant administration of systemic narcotics, and use of morphine rather than meperidine, as increasing the likelihood of encountering this serious side effect.

In order to better understand the risks and avoid side effects, more needs to be known about the fate of drugs injected intrathecally and epidurally. Despite recent research efforts, no pharmacokinetic model exists that can predict brain cerebrospinal fluid (CSF) concentrations and responses following spinal administration of drug. However, a framework for understanding the pharmacokinetic and pharmacodynamic events is realized when a basic physiologic model is referred to.

As shown in Figure 44.5, drug injected intrathecally will mix within the spinal subarachnoid CSF (the volume of which is approximately 30 ml). It will also diffuse into the spinal cord and meninges, be absorbed into the sys-

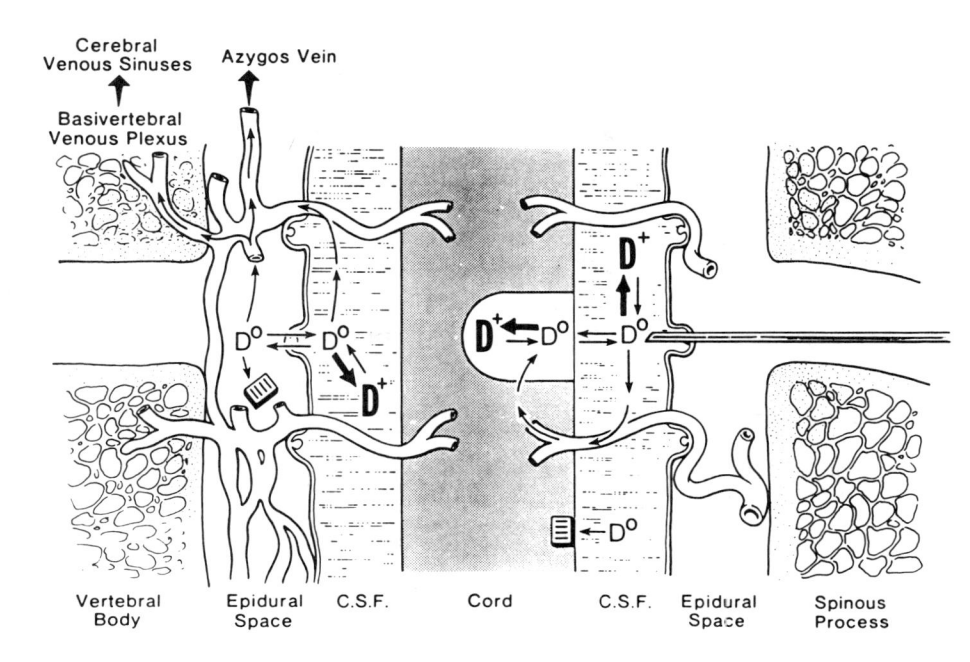

Figure 44.5. Schematic of physiologic/pharmacokinetic model used to describe the fate of drug D°=un-ionized/lipophilic and D⁺=ionized/hydrophilic forms) when deposited into the spinal cerebrospinal fluid (C.S.F.). Un-ionized form of drug is depicted interacting with receptors and nonspecific binding sites (*lined rectangles*) and being cleared from the C.S.F. through arachnoid granulations and by entering blood vessels to reach the systemic circulation. Ionized drug remains in the spinal C.S.F. and is cleared by passive bulk flow to the intercranial C.S.F. (From Cousins MJ, Mather LE: Intrathecal and epidural administration opioids. *Anesthesiology* 61:276–310, 1984.)

temic circulation, and slowly travel rostrally with passive CSF flow (which is approximately 2.0 ml/min) (62). These processes comprise the mechanisms of spinal CSF clearance and may be considered to be in competition; the degree to which any one occurs is largely dependent on the physicochemical properties of the drug. Highly ionized, hydrophilic drugs such as morphine slowly diffuse into cord and meningeal tissue and will tend to be transported cephalad to the brain in the CSF because uptake into the systemic circulation is also slow. Un-ioinized, lipid-soluble drugs such as fentanyl, methadone, hydromorphone, and meperidine will rapidly diffuse into spinal cord and meningeal tissue and readily cross capillary membranes to reach the systemic circulation, leaving less drug in the CSF for passive, rostral transport and making respiratory depression unlikely as well as limiting the spread of analgesia. Morphine will thus have a longer duration of action, because its spinal CSF clearance is lower, being largely dependent on passive CSF transport; it tends to provide a larger area of analgesia; and it has a higher likelihood of exerting centrally mediated side effects than the more lipid-soluble drugs (62).

Drugs injected into the epidural space will have a fate similar to those injected intrathecally once the drug reaches the spinal subarachnoid space (presumably via arachnoid granulations in the dural cuff region and dural membrane penetration). Ability to enter the CSF also increases with an increase in lipid solubility, so that the more lipophilic drugs will have a more rapid onset of action. Conversely, clinical evidence indicates that for the more hydrophilic morphine, onset of analgesia is slow, its duration is prolonged, and the "band" of analgesia is widely distributed. This model and evidence imply that for hydrophilic narcotic agonists, it is the dose of the agent rather than the spinal level of epidural injection that determines the anatomic extent of the analgesia.

Although some drug enters the CSF, most drug injected into the highly vascular epidural space is vigorously absorbed into the systemic circulation. The resulting opiate plasma concentrations are sufficient to produce opiate effects (63). The effects seen soon after epidural injection of opiates are probably wholly or partly a result of systemic, not spinal, action. Another theory put forth to explain early central effects of epidural narcotics purports that following absorption into the epidural venous plexus, under conditions of raised intrathoracic pressure, blood flow and drug could also be transported up the vertebral venous system directly to the brain, in addition to the drug's normal entry into the inferior vena cava via the azygous vein (55).

Following epidural administration, redistribution, rather than systemic clearance, is probably more important in reducing plasma levels of these agents, which gain access to the systemic circulation and thus reduce the risk of respiratory depression. With the exception of a drug such as methadone (elimination clearance of only approximately 150 ml/min and plasma elimination half-life of 24–48 hr), the ratio of the epidural dosing rate to plasma clearance (Eq. 44.1) will yield a low steady state plasma concentration. For methadone the epidural dosing rate will result in relatively higher plasma concentrations at steady state, and because of the long half-life, accumulation to this level will not occur for several days.

Contraindications to subarachnoid or epidural narcotic administration include increased intracranial pressure, drug allergy, infection at the site of injection, and coagulopathy (a relative contraindication).

INTRATHECAL ADMINISTRATION OF NARCOTICS

Intrathecal morphine has been shown to reliably relieve postoperative pain for up to 24 hr following a single injection (62). Although doses have ranged as high as 20 mg, more recent reports indicate that excellent analgesia for similar durations are obtained with doses in the 0.25–0.5-mg range (58, 59). Because higher brain CSF concentrations should result and respiratory depression be more likely with larger doses, it is recommended that the lower effective doses be used.

Despite the fact that subarachnoid administration is pharmacokinetically "cleaner" (i.e., the time and percentage of drug reaching the spinal CSF is precisely known and there is no significant systemic absorption), only in a minority of instances is this route of spinal opiate administration chosen [about 1.5% in the Swedish survey (61)]; the remainder have used epidural injections. As is discussed below, placement of an epidural catheter affords the advantage of dose titration to allow for interindividual variability as well as repeat doses without the increased risk that may accompany repeated needle placements or insertion of an indwelling intrathecal catheter. However, for operations in which a subarachnoid block is used the addition of 0.25–0.5 mg of morphine to the local anesthetic has proven to be effective in providing about 24 hr of pain relief and did not appear to affect the local anesthetic block in any way (64, 65).

EPIDURAL ADMINISTRATION OF NARCOTICS

Choice of Agent

Various drugs have been used for postoperative epidural analgesia, including local anesthetics, pure agonist narcotics, and the partial agonist and partial agonist-antagonist narcotics. Because many of these are experimental and not approved for epidural use, contain preservatives, or both, sufficient data are not yet available to properly evaluate their relative safety and efficacy. Preliminary evidence and experience to date suggests that the highly lipid-soluble agents may be preferable from a safety standpoint, because rostral spread is limited (vida supra), but may not provide adequate thoracic analgesia when administered into the lumbar epidural space for this same reason. At this time either preservative-free morphine or hydromorphone seems to provide adequate postoperative analgesia for upper abdominal and thoracic surgery, and fentanyl or sufentanil provides safer (less respiratory depression) analgesia for lower abdominal and lower extremity pain.

Catheter Placement

Because of the increased technical difficulty and magnitude of complications related to placing and maintaining thoracic epidural catheters, placement of catheters into the epidural space higher than the lumbar level cannot be recommended for routine postoperative analgesia.

Routine Use

As opposed to transcutaneous electrical nerve stimulation (TENS) for somatic pain management, epidural narcotics are effective in relieving both somatic pain (orthopedic surgery) as well as visceral pain (thoracoabdominal surgery). Furthermore, there may exist a synergism between local anesthetic agents and narcotics that would make coadministration most efficacious. The relative merits of any of a number of methods of postoperative pain relief have yet to be elucidated. However, the use of an intravenous narcotic infusion or PCA, or regular intramuscular narcotic injections can provide analgesia less invasively, require less technical skill, and possibly have an equivalent or lower incidence of side effects or complications as compared to spinal opioid administration. Thus, the potential advantages of superior analgesia with spinal narcotics has to be justified in individual cases against the risks involved.

Taking all of this discussion into consideration and using the following guidelines, narcotic epidural analgesia has been found to be a very satisfactory method of postoperative pain management. A standardized form for orders prevents confusion and increases acceptance. An example of routine postoperative orders is reproduced in Table 44.4. A lumbar epidural catheter is placed either prior to or following the surgical procedure. The choice is dependent on logistical considerations, manpower, and obviously whether or not the epidural catheter can or will be used to provide a component of the surgical anesthesia. One-half hour prior to the end of the surgical procedure, fentanyl (100 μg in 10 ml of saline) injected into the catheter as a bolus and a continuous infusion of fentanyl (1000 μg in 100 ml of saline) at the rate of 0.5 μg/kg/hr is initiated. In the event of inadequate analgesia, noting the time to peak effect (up to 30 min), a repeat 100-μg bolus is given with an increase in the infusion rate up to a maximum of 1.0 μg/kg/hr. If there is any question that the catheter may be malpositioned, one can inject a bolus dose of an analgesic concentration of a local anesthetic agent (1–2% lidocaine). This maneuver will not only clarify the level of blockade, and likewise verify catheter position, but will also enable one to "catch up" with the patient's pain, which may be difficult to do with the narcotic alone (66). Among the advantages of this technique are that a continuous infusion decreases the incidence of tolerance and a lipophilic, rapid-onset drug decreases rostral CSF migration of drug. However, because rostal spread is lessened, use of a lipophilic narcotic may not be as efficacious as the administration of a continuous epidural infusion of morphine following a thoracotomy. Finally, because of the

Table 44.4
Suggested Epidural Narcotic Orders

1. Patient has epidural catheter for postoperative analgesia. Bolus of (e.g., fentanyl 100 μg qs to 10 ml NS) given at _____ (time).
2. Pharmacy to prepare _____ ml of _____ (drug) at a concentration of _____ mg/ml to run at an infusion rate of _____ ml/hr. Dose = _____ mg/hr.
3. No p.o./i.m./i.v. narcotics, sedatives, or antiemetic medications without order from Pain Control Service.
4. Naloxone, 1 ampule of 0.4 mg at bedside at all times.
5. Maintain i.v. access while epidural infusion is in use.
6. Orders for nausea. (e.g., naloxone 0.1 mg i.v.—may be repeated q 10 min × 4 if needed; call Pain Control Service if ineffective)
7. Orders for pruritus. (e.g., same as above for nausea)
8. Orders to monitor respiratory rate. (e.g., apply vital sign monitor to patient and set respiratory rate alarm to 8/min; record respiratory rate q 1 hr)
9. Orders for respiratory depression. (e.g., for respiratory rate of 8/min or less, given naloxone 0.4 mg i.v. stat, then contact _____ ; For respiratory rate less than 12/min contact/ _____)
10. For inadequate analgesia, or questions/problems with the epidural catheter, contact _____ .

continued concern regarding respiratory depression, appropriate patient surveillance must be provided. A very comprehensive review of spinal opioids has been assembled by Cousins and Mather (62) and is recommended reading for those interested in pursuing this form of postoperative analgesia.

Tolerance

Tolerance is a problem often observed when spinal narcotics are used. There are three separate methods that can be used to combat the problem of tolerance. The first is alternating antinociceptive agents that are known to act on different systems (e.g., opioids versus baclofen activation of a γ-aminobutyric acid system versus ST-91, an α_2-adrenergic agonist). The second method entails the continuous administration of the narcotic rather than intermittent exposure of the receptors to high concentrations from repeat bolus doses of the drug. The third reflects recent evidence that there are at least two populations of spinal opioid receptors, and that it might be possible to maintain spinal opioid analgesia for prolonged periods by alternating opioid agonists of different receptor characteristic as tolerance develops.

SIDE EFFECTS OF SPINAL OPIATES

There are three groups of side effects or complications associated with the administration of epidural opioids aside from those related to the placement and extended use of an epidural catheter. These include, in order of increasing concern: (a) nausea/vomiting and pruritus, (b) urinary retention, and (c) sedation and respiratory depression.

Similar side effects are observed whether the opiates are injected into the intrathecal or epidural spaces. In general the effects are seen more frequently and may be more severe when the intrathecal route is chosen (61). Most of what follows applies to both routes, but when significant differences occur, they will be mentioned.

Respiratory Depression

The complication of greatest concern is respiratory depression. Following epidural administration of narcotics, one may encounter acute and/or delayed respiratory depression, thus giving rise to the term *biphasic respiratory depression*. Because it is customary to carefully observe patients for the first 30–60 min following epidural injections, acute ventilatory depression occurring in a monitored patient, although of concern, does not command the attention and respect garnered by reports of respiratory depression or arrest occurring up to 15 hr later. As mentioned above, early respiratory depression can be explained on the basis of significant plasma narcotic levels occurring as a result of absorption into the systemic circulation from the epidural space. Because absorption from the CSF is slower and intrathecal doses are much smaller, early respiratory depression by this mechanism should not occur.

Delayed respiratory depression was reported following the use of intrathecal morphine (59, 60) in the same year, 1979, as the first report of its therapeutic use (67). These reports have been followed by many others. It appears that the opioid-naive surgical patient is at much greater risk than the more tolerant cancer patient (68). With morphine, the onset of respiratory depression occurs 6–11 hr following injection and can last for up to 24 hr (62). It is generally responsive to naloxone (intravenous doses of 0.1–0.2 mg repeated every 2 min until attaining the desired effect), without sacrificing the spinal analgesic effect. Because the respiratory depression will last longer than the antagonism of the intravenous doses of naloxone, a continuous naloxone infusion should be started at a rate of 5 μg/kg/hr titrated to maintain eupnea, and continued for at least 24 hr.

When used for postoperative analgesia any of the following factors may contribute to the onset of delayed respiratory depression:

1. The concomitant administration of parenteral opioids other than those injected into the epidural space. This includes premedication or intraoperative administration as well as parenteral administration of narcotics after the analgesia provided by the epidural opioid has "worn off."

2. The residual effect of other centrally acting depressants administered during anesthesia.
3. An alteration or increase in drug transfer to the CNS via venous or CSF distribution. Increased intrathoracic pressure from airway obstruction, grunting, or positive pressure ventilation as well as increased intra-abdominal pressure are all mechanisms by which rostral CSF flow may be augmented. These same pressure changes may cause epidural venous blood flow to be redirected through basivertebral veins to the brain.
4. Accidental dural puncture or delayed catheter migration through the dura would result in direct injection of a relative overdose (approximately 5–10 times) of the narcotic into the CSF.
5. Patient factors, such as advanced age and pulmonary insufficiency, have been found to increase risk.

Although the expected incidence of delayed respiratory depression can be made very low by attention to the predisposing factors, some provision for detecting its onset must be made. Measures to be taken will vary from institution to institution and may even vary within an institution. Some have found devices that detect and measure respiratory rate to be useful, whereas others have relied on frequent observation. Nurses in units that care for these postoperative patients must be properly trained concerning the clinical course following spinal narcotic injections and instructed that naloxone and apparatus to artificially support ventilation should be readily available and used whenever decreased ventilatory rates or sedation are detected.

Nausea and Vomiting

Nausea may be observed in 15–50% of cases of epidural morphine administration and perhaps more frequently when the same narcotics are given intrathecally. Vomiting will occur in only about one-quarter of those reporting nausea. Onset of nausea and vomiting is noted to coincide with the onset of trigeminal analgesia approximately 6 hr after epidural or intrathecal injection, and so, like respiratory depression, this side effect probably results from rostral migration of drug, in this case to the vomiting center and the chemoreceptor trigger zone.

The incidence appears to decrease with repeated doses and in chronic treatment of cancer patients. Systemic opioids and pain itself may cause nausea and vomiting in postoperative patients. Although nausea has also been reported after epidural fentanyl administration, the incidence, like that for respiratory depression, is much lower because of its lipophilicity and minimal central spread. Treatment of this side effect may be accomplished with naloxone or nalbuphine (69).

Urinary Retention

The incidence of urinary retention has been reported to be similar to that of nausea and vomiting, with 39% of postoperative patients requiring catheterization of the bladder in one study (70). Urinary retention, although not life-threatening, is a problem for patients not requiring urethral catheterization for other reasons. One hypothesis regarding the inability to void involves inhibition of acetylcholine release from efferent postganglionic neurons innervating the detrusor muscle, due to binding at opioid receptors. Hence, both naloxone and/or bethanechol can relieve urinary retention in some subjects. Likewise, urinary retention subsides with subsequent exposures to the narcotics, is seen more often in volunteers than in postoperative surgical patients, and is rare in those with chronically treated cancer pain.

Pruritis

Pruritis may occur in 50–75% of postoperative patients given spinal opiates, although fewer than one-quarter of these may require treatment. The pruritis, although not apparently related to histamine release (because it can even occur following fentanyl administration), is thought to be due to a widespread alteration in sensory modulation, particularly in regions of the upper cervical cord. Pruritis has been treated with promethazine and nalbuphine (69).

Summary

Pruritis, nausea, vomiting, and bladder dysfunction can all often subside with subsequent doses of the narcotic as an adaptation to the changes in sensation or the brain's tolerance to these side effects (much like that seen with respiratory depression). Although specific therapy, such as the administration of droperidol for nausea, may be effective, all side effects are antagonized by intravenous naloxone or nalbuphine without diminishing the analgesia provided by the spinal narcotic. However, nalbuphine may cause increased sedation, especially in the aged. Furthermore, the incidence of all side effects, with the possible exception of urinary retention, can be diminished by the administration of highly lipid-soluble drugs such as fentanyl, thereby reducing the concentration of the agent presented via the CSF to the upper cord and brain.

PERIPHERAL NERVE BLOCKS

INTERCOSTAL NERVE BLOCKS

Intercostal nerve blocks have been useful for the treatment of postoperative pain in patients undergoing thoracotomies as well as for those having upper abdominal operations such as cholecystectomies. The major advantage is the relief of pain without the CNS side effects that may accompany systemically administered opiates. As discussed above, analgesia is important following these operations in order to permit satisfactory chest physiotherapy, for clearing pulmonary secretions, and maintaining functional residual capacity. Kaplan et al. (71) have shown that intercostal nerve blocks both significantly alleviate postoperative pain following thoracotomy and improve pulmonary function, and advocated its use whenever possible. Galway and coworkers (72) also found good pain relief but did not show any improvement in pulmonary function in the postoperative period.

The 11 intercostal and one subcostal (beneath the 12th rib) nerves are mixed motor and sensory, and are formed from their respective spinal nerve roots and travel in the subcostal grooves with the intercostal arteries and veins. A collateral intercostal motor nerve splits from the main nerve and travels between the inner and innermost intercostal muscles along the lower margin of the intercostal space. Branches of the main intercostal nerve are given off that supply the skin over the lateral aspects of the thorax and abdomen. The upper six intercostal nerves pass anteriorly and end up as the interior cutaneous branch that supplies the skin over the anterior chest and the parietal pleura; the lower six do the same for the anterior abdomen and the parietal peritoneum as well as the abdominal muscles.

For treatment after abdominal procedures the patient is placed in either the prone or the lateral position. The injection must be made proximal to the origin of the lateral perforating branches, which arise near the midaxillary line. This should be repeated at four or five interspaces if the wound is clearly unilateral and at matching contralateral interspaces if the wound extends to the midline.

With thoracotomies the surgeon can inject the local anesthetic solution under direct vision from within the chest. For adequate analgesia it is usually necessary to block four or five nerves at the level of the thoracotomy wound and two at the level of the drainage tube site.

Loder showed that the addition of dextran to a 1% lidocaine solution significantly extended the duration of anesthesic block (73). Kaplan et al. (71) demonstrated that this principle was applicable to intercostal blocks with 0.75% bupivacaine by addition of an equal volume of low molecular weight dextran 40. This mixture produced 36 hr of analgesia, whereas bupivacaine with saline produced a block of 12 hr duration. In the study of Galway and coworkers (72) in which poor results were obtained, both 0.5% bupivacaine and 1% lidocaine provided only about 3 hr of pain relief.

An anatomic study by Nunn and Slavin (74) demonstrated that fluid injected into the intercostal space could easily spread superiorly and inferiorly behind the parietal pleura. In a case report O'Kelly and Garry (75) used this information to give continuous analgesia to a patient with fractured ribs via an epidural catheter left in the intercostal space. They were able to provide analgesia from the fourth to the tenth segment with injections of 20 ml 0.5% bupivacaine. Similar spread of 20 ml of radiopaque fluid corroborates that the analgesia is a result of direct spread of the local anesthetic. Murphy went on to use the technique for postoperative pain relief following cholecystectomy and renal surgery (76). Restelli et al. (77) have described a variation of this technique in which a catheter is inserted during thoracotomy.

Kvalheim and Reiestad (78) have described a novel intrapleural approach for blocking intercostal nerves for postoperative pain following cholecystectomy and renal and mammary operations. Their technique calls for insertion of a Touhy needle in an anesthetized patient laying in the lateral position. The insertion site is between the eighth and ninth rib and the angle is about 45° (not perpendicular as with Murphy's technique). After "walking" off the lower border of the upper rib and advancing the 3 mm into the intercostal space, the trocar is removed and a freely sliding, glass syringe is attached to the needle. These are then advanced together until the parietal pleura is punctured and confirmation is achieved when the negative pleural pressure draws in the syringe's plunger. An epidural catheter can then be inserted 4–6 cm and 20 ml 0.5% bupivacaine injected to provide effective analgesia for 6–24 hr, at which time similar "top-up" doses can be given.

BRACHIAL PLEXUS BLOCK

Selander (79) has advocated that postoperative analgesia following upper extremity surgery be maintained with a brachial plexus sheath catheter for a continuous technique analogous to the continuous intercostal technique above. This form of analgesia is particularly advantageous in that the accompanying sympathetic block, which can be maintained for several days, enhances graft survival.

A catheter can be threaded into the brachial plexus sheath from either the axillary, interscalene, or infraclavicular approaches. Improved success in gaining access to this space is associated with the use of the short-bevel needle, which produces a "click" when this tissue plane is entered. Confidence is increased if one obtains a concomitant loss of resistance. A catheter can be inserted through the needle using a specially designed kit or over the needle if standard intravenous catheters (at least 6.4 cm in length) are used.

SURGICAL WOUND PERFUSION

A recent report has shown that injection of 10 ml of 0.5% bupivacaine or saline directly into a drainage catheter (placed between the peritoneum and muscle layer along the entire length of a Kocher subcostal incision for cholecystectomy) every 4 hr provided excellent pain relief (80). Although some patients experienced complete freedom from pain, they still suffered the usual fall in vital capacity. The fact that saline was as effective as bupivacaine in relieving pain and reducing narcotic requirement was explained in terms of the wound irrigation displacing humoral agents such as histamine and vasoactive peptides, which are thought to contribute to postoperative pain.

FIELD BLOCKS

Field blocks are often used to provide analgesia following relatively minor procedures such as inguinal herniorrhaphy or augmentation mammoplasty. The pain following such operations is generally the most intense during the first 8–12 hr. Injecting 0.25–0.5% bupivacaine with 1:200,000 or 1:400,000 epinephrine in a wide area and down to the fascial plains to block the nerve branches supplying the area can often produce significant analgesia for the first postoperative day and may obviate or reduce the need for other postoperative analgesic medications.

Field block for inguinal herniorrhaphy is made effective by injecting 20–30 ml of 0.5% bupivacaine with 1:200,000 epinephrine in a series of fan-like injections deep to the external oblique muscle in order to block the ilioinguinal and iliohypogastric nerves.

Another form of field block is the instillation of 40 ml of 0.25% bupivacaine into the intra-articular space following knee arthroscopy. This technique is also useful for outpatients.

TRANSCUTANEOUS ELECTRICAL NERVE STIMULATION

Transcutaneous electrical nerve stimulation (TENS) is the practice of applying controlled low-voltage electrical pulses to the nervous system by passing electrical current through the skin. Initially, TENS was implemented as a screening procedure to assess the potential efficacy of dorsal column stimulators, placed surgically, in an effort to obtain relief of chronic pain. Although TENS was not successful as a screening tool, it was noted to provide a degree of local analgesia. Since that time TENS has become another treatment modality within the available armamentarium of a comprehensive program for chronic pain management (Chapter 12) while gaining increasing acceptance in the treatment of postoperative pain.

APPLIED PHYSIOLOGY

The physiology and pathophysiology of nociceptive impulse transmission, modulation, and perception has been described above. An explanation of TENS is but an extension of this neurophysiology.

The rationale for the use of electrical stimulation to produce analgesia is based on two seperate mechanisms responsible for inhibition of nociception. The particular mechanism that applies might best be explained on the basis of the type of electrical signal delivered to the affected region. In general, these two mechanisms are best explained as a neuromodulation technique based on the gate control theory of pain first described by Melzack and Wall (81). This theory postulates that large myelinated A-beta fiber activity inhibits nociceptive transmission (closes the gate), whereas activity in the smaller A-delta and C fibers facilitates nociception (opens the gate). It has been demonstrated that large myelinated fibers have a low threshold to electrical stimulation. One form of TENS, by delivering a series of impulses to and conducted by these large fibers, closes the spinal gate and thus the transmission of nociceptive impulses to the spinothalamic tract.

Cortical, and particularly midbrain, structures are the origins of descending fibers that are part of an inhibitory neural system blocking transmission at several different levels in the CNS. The cortical origins of descending fibers further modulate the spinal gating mechanisms and account for cognitive processes influencing pain perception. The second mechanism thought to explain stimulation-produced analgesia (SPA) involves those inhibitory neurons that are part of a larger neural system that is selectively stimulated by morphine-like substances and blocked by the narcotic antagonist naloxone. Opiate receptors have been identified in the substantia gelatinosa (laminae II and III of the dorsal horn) and the periaqueductal gray matter of the brain (Fig. 44.1). The former is the proposed site of the spinal gating mechanism and the latter is thought to be the origin and central control trigger for the descending antinociceptive fibers of the dorsolateral funiculus. It is therefore theorized that a second form of TENS results in SPA by effecting a release of endogenous morphine-like ligands in the brain.

In fact, these two separate mechanisms of action may play a part in the analgesic effects of TENS, which, as stated, depend on the type of stimulation delivered. For low-intensity, high-frequency stimuli (conventional TENS), the stimulation of the large myelinated A-beta fibers closes the gate to transmission of noxious impulses. This more peripheral mechanism is not blocked by naloxone (82). As an alternative, high-intensity, low-frequency stimulation (acupuncture-like TENS) may cause release of endorphins that subsequently attach to receptors and thereby inhibit nociception. In fact, this second theory is consistent with the observations that TENS is ineffective in patients with a history of prolonged narcotic use (83) and that other patients will respond to this high-intensity stimulus, administered for brief periods, with prolonged periods of pain relief.

PRACTICAL CONSIDERATIONS

Although TENS devices are manufactured and marketed by various companies, there have only recently been standards developed for the manufacture and marketing of TENS units. The Neurosurgery Committee of the Association for the Advancement of Medical Instrumentation (AAMI) has established standards governing labeling of the devices, electrical safety, and performance requirements as well as terminology.

Most stimulators produce either a symmetric or an asymmetric biphasic output in an effort to prevent iontophoresis or electrolysis (i.e., transfer of ions from the skin to the electrode and back). This biphasic current must be delivered equally in each phase of the wave, with the asymmetric wave being more comfortable for the patient. The frequency (given in pulses per second) the pulse width (in microseconds), and the pulse amplitude are the variables that, along with electrode placement, determine the mechanism of action and efficacy of this mode of therapy. The goal of selecting the optimum parameters for conventional (high-frequency) TENS is to specifically elicit recruitment of the large, densely myelinated afferent nerve fibers (as consistent with the aforementioned peripheral gate control theory of pain) to effect control of pain. Briefly, conventional TENS for postoperative analgesia is delivered through sterile pre-gelled electrodes applied to the skin approximately 1 cm away from the suture line. Initial parameters include a pulse width varying between 60 and 150 µsec with a stimulus frequency of 80–150 pulses/sec and an amplitude of 12–20 mA (that current that provides analgesia without muscle contractions). Initial settings at the low end of these ranges usually provides excellent clinical benefit. Conventional (high-frequency, low-amplitude) stimulation can provide rapid onset, continuous analgesia for 48–72 hr.

Alternately, acupuncture-like TENS, because of the alleged stimulation of endogenous opiate release, does not require selective recruitment of afferent nerve fiber classes. Rather, results are only obtained with recruitment of motor fibers and the resultant visible muscle twitches. Therefore, stimulation parameters include a pulse width of 200–300 µsec at a rate of 1–4 pulses/sec. In this instance, as opposed to those recommended for conventional TENS, amplitude is adjusted to produce visible muscle twitches within the tolerance levels of the patient. Whereas conventional TENS has an immediate onset of analgesia, low-rate TENS does not produce immediate relief but may be delayed by as much as 30 min. Furthermore, the application of stimulation should be limited to no longer than about 45 min, to avoid residual muscle fatigue and concomitant soreness. The duration of analgesia usually persists for a prolonged period of time as is consistent with the release and binding of a hormone rather than electrical events of the nervous system, which take place in seconds or milliseconds.

A hybrid of these two techniques is best described as pulse-train or burst TENS with, likewise, an effect and mechanistic explanation consistent with a combination of the two more widely used techniques just described. Parameters for pulse-train TENS include five pulses each of 200–300 µsec in duration delivered over 100 msec at a frequency of 1–4 pulse-trains/sec and at an amplitude sufficient to produce visible muscle twitches. Because with this mode of delivery of the stimuli the muscle twitches will occur at a lower current setting, pulse-train TENS will provide a more comfortable sensation for the patient.

These types of therapy can easily be delivered by any one of many different TENS devices currently available. However, several different options should be available on the particular device being employed. First, in order to deliver acunpuncture-like TENS, the device must be capable of delivering rates as low as a single pulse per second. Likewise, the device must be capable of delivering one of various waveforms of adjustable width. Those generating spike waveform energy usually have external variables limited to pulse rate and amplitude. These types offer less flexibility and fewer applications. Although several different waveforms are available from various manufacturers, no one waveform has proven to be better than any other in TENS therapy. However, constant-current rather than constant-voltage generators have several advantages. For any given waveform, one that is biphasic with a zero net DC current will reduce skin reaction and increase patient comfort. Finally, the more advanced devices offer automatic variation in set parameters to minimize nerve adaptation or accommodation (more frequently seen with conventional TENS). By incorporating modulating features that automatically alter the frequency, pulse width, or delivered current amplitude within a present range, these units restore effectiveness, increase tolerance to stronger stimuli, and delay accommodation. A book by Mannheimer and Lampe (84) is an invaluable teaching resource and reference for the novice or expert wishing to pursue the use of this modality in the treatment of acute, primarily musculoskeletal pain. The use of TENS appears to offer a number of advantages in the treatment of acute pain because the problems of respiratory depression, sedation, orthostatic hypotension, drug reaction, drug delivery, and urinary retention can be avoided. Likewise, not only are the cognitive aspects of pain diminished, but there is ample evidence to show that the segmental and suprasegmental responses are also blocked, thereby lessening postoperative trauma-related complications and morbidity.

CRYOANALGESIA

Cryotherapy is gaining increasing popularity in the management of chronic pain. This is primarily because of the recent introduction of cryotherapy needle probes and their attendant apparatus that allow this modality to be implemented using a percutaneous approach similar to that used for other major nerve blocks with local anesthetics or neurolytics. Earlier probes required direct visualization of the nerve and application of a relatively large probe. Although this method for producing analgesia was found to be efficacious for post-thoracotomy pain (85, 86), extension of this technique for other types of acute pain seems impractical. First, the nerve block has a duration (one to several months) greatly exceeding the usual duration of acute pain (48–72 hr). Second, the resulting nerve block is myocutaneous, or nondifferential, and will block motor function as well as sensory perception. Finally, the resolution of the block by nerve regeneration within an intact sheath may be accompanied by a prolonged period of hypesthesia. Clearly, further investigation of these techniques must be completed before cryoanalgesia will gain widespread application.

References

1. Anonymous: Postoperative pain (editorial). Br Med J 2:517–518, 1978.
2. Utting JE, Smith JM: Postoperative analgesia. Anaesthesia 34:320–332, 1979.

3. Anonymous: Postoperative pain (editorial). *Br Med J* 2:664, 1976.
4. Mather LE: Pharmacokinetic and pharmacodynamic factors influencing the choice, dose and route of administration of opiates for acute pain. In Bullingham RES (ed): *Clinics in Anaesthesiology*. London, WB Saunders, 1983, vol 1, no 1, pp 17–40.
5. Weis OF, Sriwatanakul K, Alloza JL, et al: Attitudes of patients, housestaff, and nurses toward postoperative analgesic care. *Anesth Analg* 62:70–74, 1983.
6. Porter J, Jick H: Addiction in rare patients with narcotics (letter). *N Engl J Med* 302:123, 1980.
7. Miller RR: Clinical effects of parenteral narcotics in hospitalized patients. *J Clin Pharmacol* 20:165–171, 1980.
8. Marks RM, Sacher EJ: Undertreatment of medical inpatients with narcotic analgesics. *Ann Intern Med* 78:173–181, 1973.
9. Angell M: The quality of mercy (editorial). *N Engl J Med* 306:98–99, 1982.
10. Keats AS: Postoperative pain: research and treatment. *J Chronic Dis* 4:72–83, 1956.
11. Dahlstrom B, Tamsen A, Paalzow L, et al: Patient-controlled analgesic therapy. Part IV: pharmacokinetics and analgesic plasma concentrations of morphine. *Clin Pharmacokinet* 7:266–279, 1982.
12. Duthie DJR, McLaren AD, Nimmo WS: Pharmacokinetics of fentanyl during constant rate I.V. infusion for the relief of pain after surgery. *Br J Anaesth* 58:950–956, 1986.
13. Ausems ME, Hug CC Jr, Stanski DR, et al: Plasma concentrations of alfentanil required to supplement nitrous oxide anesthesia for general surgery. *Anesthesiology* 65:362–373, 1986.
14. Scott JC, Ponganis KV, Stanski DR: EEG quantitation of narcotic effect: the comparative pharmacodynamics of fentanyl and alfentanil. *Anesthesiology* 62:234–241, 1985.
15. Gourlay GK, Willis RJ, Wilson PR: Postoperative pain control with morphine: influence of supplementary methadone doses and blood concentration-response relationships. *Anesthesiology* 61:19–26, 1984.
16. Tamsen A, Bondesson V, Dahlstrom B et al: Patient-controlled analgesic therapy: Part III. Pharmacokinetics and analgesic plasma concentrations of ketobemidone. *Clin Pharmacokinet* 7:252–265, 1982.
17. Austin KL, Stapleton JV, Mather LE: Relationship between blood meperidine concentrations and analgesic response: a preliminary report. *Anesthesiology* 53:460–466, 1980.
18. Tamsen A, Hartvig P, Fagerlund C etal: Patient-controlled analgesic therapy: Part II. Individual analgesic demand and analgesic plasma concentrations of pethidine in postoperative pain. *Clin Pharmacokinet* 7:164–175, 1982.
19. Tamsen A, Sakurada T, Wahlstrom A, et al: Postoperative demand for analgesics in relation to individual levels of endorphins and substance P in cerebrospinal fluid. *Pain* 13:171–183, 1982.
20. Mather LE, Lindop MJ, Tucker GT: Pethidine revisited: plasma concentrations and effects after intramuscular injection. *Br J Anaesth* 47:1269–1275, 1975.
21. Neal EA, Meffin PJ, Gregory PG, et al: Enhanced bioavailability and decreased clearance of analgesics in patients with cirrhosis. *Gastroenterology* 77:96–102, 1979.
22. Klotz U, McHorse TS, Wilkinson GR, et al: The effect of cirrhosis on the disposition and elimination of meperidine in man. *Clin Pharmacol Ther* 16:667–675, 1974.
23. McHorse TS, Wilkinson GR, Schenker S: The effect of acute viral hepatitis in man on the disposition and elimination of meperidine. *Gastroenterology* 68:775–780, 1975.
24. Patawardhan RV, Johnson RF, Hoyumpa A, et al.: Normal metabolism of morphine in cirrhosis. *Gastroenterology* 81:1006–1011, 1981.
25. Moore RA, Sear JW, Bullingham RES, et al: Morphine kinetics in renal failure. In Foley KM, Inturrisi CE (eds): *Advances in Pain Research and Therapy*. New York, Raven Press, 1986, vol 8, pp 65–72.
26. Inturrisi CE, Umans JG: Meperidine biotransformation and central nervous system toxicity in animals and humans. In Foley KM, Inturrisi CE (eds): *Advances in Pain Research and Therapy*. New York, Raven Press, 1986, vol 8, pp 143–153.
27. Sawe J: Morphine and its 3- and 6-glucuronides in plasma and urine during chronic oral administration in cancer patients. In Foley KM, Inturrisi CE (eds): *Advances in Pain Research and Therapy*. New York, Raven Press, 1986, vol 8, pp 45–55.
28. Nagashima H, Karamanian A, Malovany P, et al: Respiratory and circulatory effects of intravenous butorphanol and morphine. *Clin Pharmacol Ther* 19:738–745, 1976.
29. Romagnoli A, Keats AS: Ceiling effect for respiratory depression by nalbuphine. *Clin Pharmacol Ther* 28:478–485, 1980.
30. Murphy MR, Hug CC Jr: The enflurane sparing effect of morphine, butorphanol, and nalbuphine. *Anesthesiology* 57:489–492, 1982.
31. Kay B: On-demand nalbuphine for post-operative pain. *Anaesthetist* 32(suppl):366–367, 1983.
32. Fragen RJ, Caldwell N: Acute intravenous premedication with nalbuphine. *Anesth Analg* 56:808–812, 1977.
33. Latasch L, Probst S, Dudziak R: Reversal by nalbuphine of respiratory depression caused by fentanyl. *Anesth Analg* 63:814–816, 1984.
34. Freye E, Hartung E, Segeth M: Nalbuphine reverses fentanyl-related EEG-changes in man. *Acta Anaesthesiol Belg* 35:25–36, 1984.
35. Cooper SA: New peripherally-acting oral analgesic agents. *Annu Rev Pharmacol Toxicol* 23:617–647, 1983.
36. McQuay HJ, Poppleton P, Carroll D, et al: Ketorolac and acetaminophen for orthopedic postoperative pain. *Clin Pharmacol Ther* 39:89–93, 1986.
37. O'Hara DA, Fragen RJ, Kinzer M, et al: Intramuscular ketorolac tromethamine as compared to morphine sulfate in postoperative pain. *Anesthesiology* 65:A187, 1986.
38. Jones RM, Cashman JN, Foster JMG, et al: Comparison of infusions of morphine and lysine acetyl salicylate for the relief of pain following thoracic surgery. *Br J Anaesth* 57:259–263, 1985.
39. Beecher HK: Anxiety and pain (editorial). *JAMA* 209:1080, 1969.
40. Keeri-Szanto M: The mode of action of promethazine in potentiating narcotic drugs. *Br J Anaesth* 46:918–924, 1974.
41. Hupert C, Yacoub M, Turgeon LR: Effect of hydroxyzine on morphine analgesia for the treatment of postoperative pain. *Anesth Analg* 59:690–696, 1980.
42. Forrest WH, Brown BW, Brown CR, et al: Dextroamphetamine with morphine for the treatment of postoperative pain. *N Engl J Med* 296:712–715, 1977.
43. Yang JC, Clark WC, Ngai SH, et al: Analgesic action and pharmacokinetics of morphine and diazepam in man: an evaluation by sensory decision theory. *Anesthesiology* 51:495–502, 1979.
44. McKenzie R, Wadhwa RK, Lim Uy NT, et al: Antiemetic

effectiveness of intramuscular hydroxyzine compared with intramuscular droperidol. *Anesth Analg* 60:783–788, 1981.
45. Hug CC Jr: Lipid solubility, pharmacokinetics, and the EEG: are you better off today than you were four years ago? (editorial). *Anesthesiology* 62:221–225, 1985.
46. Beaver WT, Wallenstein SL, Houde RW, et al: A clinical comparison of the analgesic effects of methadone and morphine administered intramuscularly, and of orally and parenterally administered methadone. *Clin Pharmacol Ther* 8:415–426, 1967.
47. Hug CC Jr: Improving analgesic therapy (editorial). *Anesthesiology* 53:441–443, 1980.
48. Welchew EA: On-demand analgesia. *Anaesthesia* 38:19–25, 1983.
49. Goudie TA, Allen MWB, Lonsdale M, et al: Continuous subcutaneous infusion of morphine for postoperative pain relief. *Anaesthesia* 40:1086–1092, 1985.
50. Holley FO, van Steenis C: Transdermal administration of fentanyl for postoperative analgesia. *Anesthesiology* 65:A548, 1986.
51. Harmer M, Slattery PJ, Rosen M, et al: Intramuscular on-demand analgesia: double-blind controlled trial of pethidine, buprenorphine, morphine and meptazinol. *Br Med J* 286:680–682, 1983.
52. Lehmann KA, Tenbuhs B: Patient-controlled analgesia with nalbuphine, a new narcotic agonist-antagonist, for the treatment of postoperative pain. *Eur J Clin Pharmacol* 31:267–276, 1986.
53. Chakravarty K, Tucker W, Rosen M, et al: Comparison of buprenorphine and pethidine given intravenously on demand to relieve postoperative pain. *Br Med J* 2:895–897, 1979.
54. Harmer M, Rosen M, Vickers MD: *Patient-Controlled Analgesia*. Oxford, Blackwell Scientific Publication, 1985.
55. Yaksh TL: Spinal opiate analgesia: characteristics and principles of action. *Pain* 11:293–346, 1981.
56. Graham JL, King R, McCaughey W: Postoperative pain relief using epidural morphine. *Anaesthesia* 35:158–160, 1980.
57. Mathews ET, Abrams LD: Intrathecal morphine in open heart surgery. *Lancet* 1:543, 1980.
58. Bromage PR, Camporesi EM, Chestnut D: Epidural narcotics for postoperative analgesia. *Anesth Analg* 59:473–480, 1980.
59. Glynn CJ, Mather LE, Cousins MJ, et al: Spinal narcotics and respiratory depression. *Lancet* 2:356–357, 1979.
60. Liolios A, Andersen FH: Selective spinal analgesia. *Lancet* 2:357, 1979.
61. Gustafsson LL, Shildt B, Jacobsen K: Adverse effects of extradural and intrathecal opiates: report of a nationwide survey in Sweden. *Br J Anaesth* 54:479–486, 1982.
62. Cousins MJ, Mather LE: Intrathecal and epidural administration opioids. *Anesthesiology* 61:276–310, 1984.
63. Chauvin M, Samii K, Schermann JM, et al: Plasma pharmacokinetics of morphine after I.M., extradural and intrathecal administration. *Br J Anaesth* 54:843–847, 1981.
64. Katz J, Nelson W: Intrathecal morphine for postoperative pain relief. *Reg Anesth* 6:1–3, 1981.
65. Nordberg G, Hedner T, Mellstrand T, et al: Pharmacokinetic aspects of intrathecal morphine analgesia. *Anesthesiology* 60:448–454, 1984.
66. Chambers WA, Sinclair CJ, Scott DB: Extradural morphine for pain after surgery. *Br J Anaesth* 53:921–925, 1981.
67. Wang JK, Nauss LA, Thomas JE: Pain relief by intrathecally applied morphine in man. *Anesthesiology* 50:149–151, 1979.
68. Zenz M, Schappler-Scheele B, Neuhans R, et al: Longterm peridural morphine analgesia in cancer pain. *Lancet* 1:91, 1981.
69. Henderson SK, Cohen H: Nalbuphine augmentation of analgesia and reversal of side effects following epidural hydromorphone. *Anesthesiology* 65:216–218, 1986.
70. Lanz E, Theiss D, Riess W, et al: Epidural morphine for postoperative analgesia: a double-blind study. *Anesth Analg* 61:236–240, 1982.
71. Kaplan JA, Miller ED, Gallagher EG: Postoperative analgesia for thoracotomy patients. *Anesth Analg* 54:773–777, 1975.
72. Galway JE, Caves PK, Dundee JW: Effect of intercostal nerve blockade during operation on lung function and the relief of pain following thoracotomy. *Br J Anaesth* 47:730–735, 1975.
73. Loder RE: Local anesthetic solution with longer action. *Lancet* 2:346–347, 1960.
74. Nunn JF, Slavin G: Posterior intercostal nerve block for pain relief after cholecystectomy. *Br J Anaesth* 52:253–259, 1980.
75. O'Kelly E, Garry B: Continuous pain relief for multiple fractured ribs. *Br J Anaesth* 53:989–991, 1981.
76. Murphy DF: Intercostal nerve blockade for fractured ribs and postoperative analgesia: description of a new technique. *Reg Anesth* 8:151–153, 1983.
77. Restelli L, Movilia P, Bossi L, et al: Management of pain after thoracotomy: a technique of multiple intercostal nerve blocks. *Anesthesiology* 61:353–354, 1984.
78. Kvalheim L, Reiestad F: Interpleural catheter in the management of postoperative pain. *Anesthesiology* 61:A231, 1984.
79. Selander D: Catheter technique in axillary plexus block. *Acta Anaesthesiol Scand* 21:324–329, 1977.
80. Thomas DFM, Lambert WG, Williams KL: The direct perfusion of surgical wounds with local anaesthetic solution: an approach to postoperative pain? *Ann R Coll Surg* 65:226–229, 1983.
81. Melzack R, Wall PD: Pain mechanisms, a new theory. *Science* 50:971–979, 1965.
82. Abram S, Reynolds A, Cusick J: Failure of naloxone to reverse analgesia from transcutaneous electrical stimulation in patients with chronic pain. *Anesth Analg* 60:81–84, 1981.
83. Solomon R, Viernstein M, Long D: Reduction of postoperative pain and narcotic use by transcutaneous electrical nerve stimulation. *Surgery* 87:142–146, 1981.
84. Mannheimer JS, Lampe GN: *Clinical Transcutaneous Nerve Stimulation*. Philadelphia, FA Davis, 1984.
85. Katz J, Nelson W, Forest R, et al: Cryoanalgesia for postthoracotomy pain. *Lancet* 1:512–513, 1980.
86. Nelson KM, Vincent RG, Bourke RS, et al: Intraoperative intercostal nerve freezing to prevent post-thoracotomy pain. *Ann Thorac Surg* 18:280–285, 1974.

chapter 45
Psychological Testing

Laurence A. Bradley, Ph.D.
Karen O. Anderson, Ph.D.
Larry D. Young, Ph.D.
Tracy Williams, A.B.

There were few available guidelines when the principal author first became interested in evaluating chronic pain patients in 1975. Sternbach (1) had developed a typology of Minnesota Multiphasic Personality Inventory (MMPI) profiles and a list of "pain games" associated with these patients. Fordyce and his colleagues had begun to demonstrate how operant conditioning could increase or reduce pain behavior (2, 3). However, many health care professionals still were unaware of the work of these investigators.

Fortunately, hundreds of studies regarding the psychological assessment of chronic pain patients have appeared since 1975. These studies have been summarized in a series of reviews (e.g., 4–8). The present chapter provides a representative and critical review of the empirical literature published during the past several years regarding the psychological evaluation of chronic pain. In addition, the chapter offers suggestions concerning the assessment procedures that should be available to all persons who study or provide health care to chronic pain patients.

Given the multidimensional nature of pain (9), it has been suggested that psychological assessment of chronic pain patients should include the evaluation of overt motor behaviors, cognitive-verbal responses, and physiologic responses (5, 10). The following discussion is organized according to this evaluation schema.

MEASUREMENT OF OVERT MOTOR BEHAVIORS

Fordyce and his colleagues (2, 3, 11–15) have produced an important series of papers that have demonstrated the benefits of using overt motor behaviors as measures of pain. The primary benefit associated with the evaluation of overt motor or pain behaviors is that they provide the clinician with quantifiable data regarding the disability shown by patients in physical mobility and other activities that are directly related to functioning in vocational, social, and leisure endeavors (8). Romano et al. (Chapter 6) already have described Fordyce's approach to the measurement of overt motor behaviors. Therefore, this section examines several relatively recent approaches to the measurement of these behaviors using (*a*) direct behavioral observations, (*b*) automated measurement devices, (*c*) self-monitored observations, and (*d*) self-reports of functional disability.

DIRECT BEHAVIORAL OBSERVATIONS

Fordyce (12) originally proposed that health care providers could record patient's overt motor behaviors on an intermittent basis during specific time periods. Two groups of investigators, however, recently have developed standardized protocols for measuring behaviors such as grimacing, bracing, guarded movement, and rubbing of painful body parts. Keefe and Block (16) produced the first of these protocols, which required chronic low back pain patients to perform for video recording a 10-min standardized series of activities (i.e., walking, sitting, reclining, and standing). Two trained observers independently viewed the video recordings and noted the frequencies of guarding, bracing, rubbing, grimacing, and sighing behavior during 20-sec observation periods. In a series of studies employing this measurement protocol, Keefe and Block reported impressive evidence of the protocol's interrater reliability, construct validity, and discriminant validity.

Our research team has successfully modified the protocol for use with rheumatoid arthritis (RA) patients (17–19). We have shown that RA patients' motor behaviors are correlated with self-reports of functional disability (17) as well as with subjective and objective measures of disease activity (18); unlike self-reports of pain intensity, the motor behaviors are independent of self-reports of depression (17, 19).

Keefe and his colleagues recently modified their original protocol for use with osteoarthritis patients (20) and patients with head and neck cancer (21). They also have demonstrated that trained observers may generate reliable and valid frequency counts of chronic low back pain patients' motor behaviors during their physical examinations without using obtrusive video recording equipment (22). Similar to the findings with RA patients, low back pain patients' motor behaviors are correlated with physical examination evidence of disk disease. However, in contrast to RA patients, low back pain patients' behaviors also are associated with self-reports of depression after controlling for physical examination results (23).

Other groups of investigators have developed standardized protocols for measuring both verbal and motor behaviors indicative of pain (24–26) and motor behaviors associated with functional capacity (27–29). Each of the protocols cited above provide quantifiable and relatively objective measures of pain-related behaviors. These protocols also may be used to identify specific behaviors as targets for behavioral treatments and to assess treatment outcome (24).

It should be noted that the recent Report of the Commission on the Evaluation of Pain (30) has recommended to the U.S. Congress that effort should be devoted to developing measures of *behavioral* manifestations of pain and disability. These measures then may be used in future determinations of persons' eligibility for Social Security disability benefits for impairment due primarily to pain. Thus, it is anticipated that health care providers, particularly those involved in disability determinations, will have to become skilled in assessing patients' overt motor behaviors indicative of pain and functional disability. It will be necessary, however, for health care providers to (*a*) maintain for future use the videotape or other objective records of patient behavior if the assessment results are challenged by patients or officials, and (*b*) provide evidence of the reliability and accuracy of the behavioral measurements using conservative indices such as the Kappa coefficient (31) or the phi coefficient (32) and reliability checks of observers (4, 8).

AUTOMATED MEASUREMENT DEVICES

Concerns regarding the reliability of observers' recordings of patient behavior and the generalizability of patient behavior during limited observation periods have led some investigators to produce devices for the automated measurement of overt motor behavior. Cairns and his colleagues (33) developed the first automated device for the measurement of patient "uptime." The device, which resembled a large clock, was mounted on a patient's bed. It automatically recorded and graphically displayed to the patient the amount of time spent out of bed each day. The disadvantage associated with this method, of course, was that the patient could sit or recline in areas other than the bedroom while the device recorded uptime.

Sanders (34) attempted to overcome the deficiencies of the recorder described above by developing an inexpensive, portable automatic device for measuring patient uptime. The recorder consisted of a miniature electronic calculator that was modified to interface with a mercury tilt switch mounted on a patient's thigh with an elastic bandage. Recently, Follick and his colleagues (35) produced an improved version of this device. The improvements included resistance to recording error associated with rapid or vigorous movements, accurate recording of time spent lying down regardless of body position, and the capability of recording time spent sitting as either "downtime" or "uptime."

Both Sanders (34) and Follick and colleagues (35) have provided positive evidence of the reliability and concurrent validity of their automated recording devices. However, the clinical utility of these devices is limited by the need for close supervision of patients, especially those with limited mechanical skills, high levels of emotional distress, or cognitive impairments (35).

Keefe and Hill (36) have described the use of an electromechanical device for the recording of patients' gait patterns that may have somewhat greater clinical utility than the uptime recorders described above. This device consisted of two pressure-sensitive insoles fitted into a patient's left and right shoes that were connected to a coupler worn at the waist. A record of the patient's gait was recorded on a polygraph as the patient walked a 5-m course three times. As expected, it was found that chronic low back pain patients displayed poorer gait symmetry and greater levels of guarded movement and total pain behavior [evaluated by Keefe and Block's (16) method] relative to normal controls. In addition, patients receiving disability payments or using narcotic medication showed more abnormal patterns on gait parameters such as stride length and single limb support time compared to patients without financial compensation or narcotic medication.

The use of the electromechanical device described by Keefe and Hill (36) requires greater time and technological sophistication on the part of health care professionals than do the other automated recorders noted above. However, it may prove to be particularly useful for physical therapists and other rehabilitation staff because it offers very precise information regarding normal and abnormal parameters of patient gait. Thus, as with overt motor behaviors evaluated by direct observation, these gait parameters may be used both for identifying treatment targets and evaluating treatment outcomes.

In summary, little attention has been devoted to the development of automated measurement devices relative to direct observation methods. Moreover, because of the great skill demands placed upon both patients and staff by the use of automated devices, our research group concurs with Follick and his colleagues (35) that these devices be used primarily for research purposes at the present time. Health care providers who employ these devices should do so only in conjunction with other behavioral assessment methods described in this section.

SELF-MONITORED OBSERVATIONS

Patient self-monitoring of behavior is a commonly used method in chronic pain assessment (8, 37). Self-monitoring has two major advantages over most of the direct observation and automated measurement techniques described earlier. First, self-monitoring requires little additional training of health care staff members and patients. Furthermore, self-monitoring allows for the continuous recording of a wide variety of behaviors in addition to uptime, downtime, and abnormal body movements in environments other than the hospital (8).

The majority of the self-monitoring techniques described in the chronic pain assessment literature are very similar to the daily activity diaries advocated by Fordyce (12). This diary consisted of a standard form on which outpatients recorded on an hourly basis the amount of time spent reclining, sleeping, sitting, and walking or standing as well as medication intake. The amount of time recorded in each behavioral category and the amount of medication intake could be calculated at the end of an initial assessment period in order to help determine appropriate treatment plans (5). The patients also could be asked to continue self-monitoring during treatment and follow-up periods to suggest modifications in treatment and to evaluate outcome.

Although early investigators tended to assume that self-monitoring would produce reliable and accurate recordings of behavior (e.g., ref. 1), several studies have shown low levels of association between inpatients' self-monitored recordings and relatively objective measures of medication intake (38, 39) and activity levels or social behavior (40, 41). These low correlations may have been due to impression management efforts by the patients as well as impaired cognitive functioning secondary to depression (42), narcotic medication dependence (43), or traumatic head/neck injury (44). However, Follick and his colleagues (45) have demonstrated high levels of association (r's ranging between .83 and .94) between outpatients' self-monitored recordings of medication use, uptime, and downtime and the relatively objective measures of these variables produced by spouse observations and an automated measurement device (35). It should be noted that two factors might account for the different results produced by Follick and colleagues (45) and those of previous investigators. First, Follick et al. examined the self-monitored recordings of outpatients in their home environments, whereas the other investigators used inpatients' recordings. Moreover, the former investigators primarily used as criterion measures relatively intrusive spouse recordings, whereas the latter employed unobtrusive treatment staff recordings and urine levels of medication. Thus, it is not clear to what extent the high concordance levels reported by Follick and colleagues were due to patients' knowledge that their behavior was being recorded by their spouses.

In summary, despite the early optimism regarding the accuracy and reliability of chronic pain patients' self-monitored observations, the results of most recent studies make it clear that these observations must be compared with some external criterion (e.g., unobtrusive recordings of patient behavior or medication screens) before they can be accepted as reliable or valid. Furthermore, health care providers and investigators may wish to defer using self-monitoring procedures with patients suffering from even subtle cognitive impairment due to depression, head injury, or narcotic medication dependence.

SELF-REPORTS OF FUNCTIONAL DISABILITY

Despite the emphasis upon the assessment of overt motor behaviors described earlier in this section and the emphasis upon changing these behaviors in many pain treatment programs (see Chapters 18 and 19), only recently have investigators devoted attention to measurement of functional disability in activities of daily living. The Sickness Impact Profile (SIP; 46) has shown particular promise as a disability measure with chronic back pain patients. For example, the SIP provides a profile of patient functioning in several areas (e.g., ambulation, mobility, body care, movement) that can provide targets for behavioral intervention (47). In addition, research with arthritis patients has shown the measurement efficiency of the SIP to be equal or superior to that of several other instruments with respect to change in patient mobility, global functioning ability, and social functions (48). Follick and his colleagues also have produced positive evidence regarding the concurrent validity and sensitivity to change of the SIP scores produced by chronic back pain patients (49). Similar findings have been reported for a 24-item scale derived from the original 136-item SIP (50, 51).

Other investigators have attempted to develop their own measures of functional disability. These measures include the Activity Pattern Indicators (52), Pain Behavior Scale

(53), Chronic Illness Problem Inventory (54), Dartmouth Pain Questionnaire (55), and the West Haven-Yale Multidimensional Pain Inventory (56). Most of these instruments evaluate variables such as stressful life events; subjective estimates of pain, mood, and self-esteem; and functional disability. Although the multidimensional character of the instruments probably makes them appealing to health care providers, it should be noted that none of the disability scale components has been validated using the SIP or other accepted devices as criterion measures. Thus, it is recommended that both health care providers and investigators use the SIP or other well-validated disability measures (e.g., Functional Status Index, Health Assessment Questionnaire, Index of Functional Impairment) to measure the functional impairments of chronic pain patients. The multidimensional measures noted above (52–56) also may be used to generate outcome data; however, additional validation research is required before the disability scale components of these measures may be accepted as adequate outcome measures.

DISCUSSION

The measurement of overt motor behaviors is a very practical approach to patient evaluation because it provides information regarding disability in physical mobility and other activities directly related to functioning in vocational, social, and leisure activities as well as other activities of daily living (4). This information may be used both to identify targets for treatment interventions and to evaluate treatment efficacy. There are, however, several problems associated with behavioral measurements. First, the reliability of direct observations and self-monitored recordings of patient behavior must be reexamined at various intervals in order to ensure that observers or patients produce accurate and consistent measurements. Our research group, for example, finds it necessary to evaluate approximately every 2 months the reliability of the trained raters who observe our video recordings of arthritis patient behavior. Frequent reliability checks may make it difficult for some health care providers to use the direct observation and self-monitoring methods described in this section.

The second problem associated with behavioral measurements is that it is not known to what extent direct observations, automated measurement recordings, and self-monitored observations are affected by reactivity. *Reactivity* refers to patient initiation of behavior change due to the assessment procedure alone.

The third problem is that behavioral measurements cannot provide information regarding the sensory or affective dimensions of the patient's pain experience, which might indicate the presence of some underlying pathology (4, 57). Neither can behavioral measurements evaluate some of the qualitative aspects of the patient's activities, such as the degree to which daily activities are appropriately paced or are inappropriate given the status of the patient's physical injuries or disease.

Despite the problems inherent in the measurement of overt motor behaviors, it is recommended that health care providers and investigators use at least one of the assessment techniques described in this section. Functional disability measures such as the SIP, for example, are readily available and require little patient and staff time for administration. It also is very easy to devise self-monitoring diaries; instructing patients to complete these diaries usually is neither difficult nor time consuming. However, self-monitored recordings should be validated against more objective behavioral measures. Finally, most investigators may acquire the resources necessary to perform direct observations of patient behavior or use automated measurement devices. It is anticipated, then, that the majority of treatment outcome studies in the future will include at least one relatively objective measure of patient behavior.

MEASUREMENT OF COGNITIVE-VERBAL RESPONSES

The major portion of the chronic pain assessment literature has been devoted to studies of patients' affective responses and perceptions of pain. However, some attention also has been devoted to assessment of patients' coping strategies and cognitive distortions as well as to their interactions with family members. The following discussion examines the current literature concerning each of these topics.

AFFECTIVE RESPONSES

Sternbach (1) has noted that relatively acute pain tends to be associated with autonomic nervous system responses that are indicative of anxiety (e.g., increased heart rate and blood pressure). However, as pain progresses to a chronic state, anxiety responses tend to habituate and the vegetative signs of depression and hypochondriasis (e.g., disturbances of sleep, appetite, and sexual drive; irritability; withdrawal of interests; somatic preoccupation) tend to be displayed. A large number of studies, therefore, have been performed regarding the utility of various psychometric instruments in evaluating the personality attributes and behavior of chronic pain patients. The MMPI is the instrument that has been used most frequently in these studies (4, 12). Indeed, the use of the MMPI with chronic low back pain patients has been the subject of two recent reviews (58, 59). The following discussion examines the MMPI assessment literature that has appeared since the publication of these reviews and includes literature concerning chronic pain syndromes and psychometric instruments not discussed in the original reviews.

Minneosta Multiphasic Personality Inventory

A large number of investigators have attempted to use the MMPI to differentiate between pain of organic and pain of psychogenic origin (e.g., ref. 60–63). Both positive and negative evidence has been generated regarding the

MMPI's ability to discriminate between organic and psychogenic pain. However, all of these studies have been compromised by two serious methodologic problems (4). First, there is little evidence that physicians may reliably or accurately classify chronic pain patients according to organic or psychogenic etiology. In addition, all of the studies have used repeated univariate data analyses that were likely to have (a) produced significant differences between patient groups due to chance alone, or (b) failed to identify significant interactions between patient groups and the MMPI scales. It is not surprising, then, that recent studies with relatively sophisticated methodologies have not shown MMPI differences between patients classified by pain etiology (e.g., refs. 64–66). It now is generally agreed that it is inappropriate to use the MMPI to differentiate between organic and psychogenic pain (4, 5, 58, 59, 67).

Several investigators have argued that clinical interpretation of chronic pain patients' MMPI profiles is made difficult by the content of the MMPI items. Naliboff and his colleagues (68, 69), for example, have demonstrated that chronic pain patients produce MMPI profiles that are quite similar to those produced by patients with chronic illnesses such as hypertension and diabetes. These investigators also have shown that between 20 and 31% of the variance in patients' Hypochondriasis, Depression, and Hysteria scale scores was determined by self-reports of functional disability. Similar findings have been reported by Watson (70) and Pincus and his colleagues (71) in studies of patients with diverse pain syndromes and rheumatoid arthritis, respectively.

There recently has been an effort to develop novel approaches to the interpretation of chronic pain patients' MMPI profiles. Ahles and his colleagues (72), for example, have demonstrated that the prevalence of "psychologically disturbed" profiles among primary fibrositis patients was markedly reduced by using norms recently developed with contemporary adults (73, 74). Prokop (75) and Moore and colleagues (76) have shown that interpretation of chronic pain patients' scores on the Hysteria and Schizophrenia scales is aided by examining the Harris and Lingoes subscales (described in 77). Examining the patients' subscale responses revealed that their scores on the Hysteria and Schizophrenia scales were determined largely by complaints of physical dysfunction or depression.

Bradley, Prokop, and their colleagues have used hierarchical clustering methods to delineate replicable and relatively homogeneous MMPI profile subgroups among patients with chronic low back pain (78) and multiple pain complaints (79). They have suggested that MMPI profile interpretations would be improved by attempting to identify the behavioral correlates associated with each of the subgroups and the treatments that might be optimal for each subgroup (4, 78). It was anticipated that substantial variation would be found in the subgroup types and their respective behavioral correlates identified by various investigators given the patient differences that exist across treatment settings (80, 81). Generally, however, attempts to replicate the profile subgroups originally derived by Bradley and Prokop have been quite successful using diverse samples of chronic pain patients (e.g., refs. 82–87) and headache patients (88). Several of these studies have demonstrated that the profile subgroups differ significantly from one another on variables such as duration of pain and number of hospitalizations (84), pain intensity ratings (86), degree of physical activity restriction and deterioration in marital communication and social relationships (83, 86, 87), headache frequency (88), and Research Diagnostic Criteria (89) evidence of major depression (90). The studies noted above generally have found that profile subgroups featuring elevated clinical scales show greater disruptions of daily activities than subgroups with relatively unelevated scales. Bradley and Van der Heide (86), however, found that profile subgroups with elevations primarily on the Hypochondriasis, Depression, and Hysteria scales reported greater affective disturbance and disruption of daily activities than did subgroups with elevations both on these three scales and Psychopathic Deviancy, Psychasthenia, and Schizophrenia.

Three investigations have examined the degree to which MMPI profile subgroup membership might predict treatment outcome (84, 87, 91). Each of the investigations delineated profile subgroups within samples composed primarily of chronic back pain patients that closely resembled those derived by Bradley et al. (78). Two studies showed that profile subgroup membership did not predict outcome in multimodal pain management programs (84, 91). However, McCreary (87) reported that chronic back pain patients' responses to conservative orthopedic management could be predicted accurately by subgroup membership. Hit rates ranged from 61 to 99% among the male patients and from 65 to 89% among the females.

The mixed evidence regarding the predictive validity of MMPI profile subgroups is consistent with the positive (92–97) and negative (98–101) results produced by studies of the predictive validity of single or multiple MMPI scale scores. The inconsistent evidence regarding the predictive validity of both profile subgroup membership and single or multiple scale scores may be attributed in large part to methodologic problems such as (a) heterogeneous patient samples, (b) heterogeneous outcome criteria, (c) heterogeneous surgical and nonsurgical treatments, and (d) outcome judgments of unknown reliability.

Another factor that might account for some of the predictive error associated with profile subgroup membership is excessive variability within subgroups (102). Henrichs (102) recently replicated the MMPI profile subgroups derived both by Bradley et al. (78) and Armentrout et al. (83). However, a large number of patients within each subgroup were classified as outliers when Sines' (103) criterion for determining subgroup membership was applied. Nevertheless, application of this criterion produced subgroups that were very homogeneous with regard to behavioral correlates and responses to surgical or nonsurgical treatment. It may be possible, then, to improve the predictive power of MMPI profile subgroup membership by further refinement of the subgroups after their initial derivation by clustering methods.

Finally, it should be noted that there is some evidence that work status outcome of patients with diverse chronic pain syndromes may be accurately predicted by a combination of patients' pretreatment pain intensity levels, ratings of concern about the effects of work, and Hysteria scale scores (104). Thus, it may be possible to use multiple regression analysis to identify those variables in addition to subgroup membership that best predict treatment outcome.

Other Assessment Instruments

Given the problems associated with the clinical interpretation and the predictive validity of the MMPI, several alternative instruments have been developed or tested for use with chronic pain patients. These include the Illness Behavior Questionnaire (IBQ; 105, 106), pain drawing (107), Back Pain Classification Scale (BPCS; 108), Symptom Checklist-90 (SCL-90; 109), and Millon Behavioral Health Inventory (MBHI; 110). This section examines critically the utility of these instruments. Major attention is devoted to the IBQ since, relative to the other measures, it has been studied most frequently.

Pilowsky (111, 112) adopted Mechanic's (113) term *illness behavior* and developed the concept of abnormal illness behavior as a unifying label for all cognitive, affective, and behavioral disturbances associated with chronic pain. In order to develop a measure of this construct, Pilowsky and Spence (105) administered a 55-item questionnaire to 100 patients with chronic pain of diverse etiologies. A factor analysis of the patient's responses produced seven independent dimensions: (a) General Hypochondriasis, (b) Conviction of Disease, (c) Psychological versus Somatic Focus of Disease, (d) Affective Inhibition, (e) Affective Disturbance, (f) Denial of Life Problems Unrelated to Pain, and (g) Irritability. The patients' scores on the derived factor scales then were entered in a clustering procedure that produced three relatively normal patterns of scores and three patterns indicative of abnormal illness behavior (106).

There were many psychometric weaknesses associated with the development of the IBQ, including the lack of reliability data and the use of inappropriate factor-analytic procedures (4). Although a series of studies has demonstrated that patients with various chronic pain syndromes or symptoms without organic pathology produce higher IBQ scores than controls (114–121), several recent factor-analytic investigations have raised questions concerning the factor structure and scoring of the IBQ (122–125). Another factor-analytic study (126) of the 62-item IBQ (127) produced six independent factors that closely resembled the factors originally derived by Pilowsky and Spence (105). These were (a) Health Worry, (b) Illness Disruption, (c) Affective Inhibition, (d) Affective Disturbance, (e) Avowed Absence of Life Problems, and (f) Irritability. It also was found, however, that each of the factor scales was correlated significantly with the Eysenck Personality Inventory Neuroticism Scale (128). Thus, although the IBQ might be able to discriminate chronic pain patients from normal controls (e.g., refs. 119, 120), the instrument might measure primarily anxiety or other neurotic features rather than patterns of abnormal illness behavior.

Keefe and his colleagues (129) recently addressed the question of whether IBQ scores predict pain behavior patterns independently of demographic and medical status variables such as pain duration, number of prior surgeries, and disability status. Using the method of observing overt motor behaviors (16) described earlier, it was found that Affective Inhibition, Affective Disturbance, and Irritability were particularly significant predictors of chronic low back pain patients' pain behavior and pain intensity ratings. The design of this study, however, prevented the investigators from determining if IBQ scores predict pain behavior independently of both demographic and medical status variables *as well as* neuroticism.

Another approach to measuring abnormal illness behavior is to ask patients to mark on an outline of a human figure the areas in which they experience pain. The "pain drawing" is included in many chronic pain assessment batteries (e.g., refs. 55, 130). Ransford and colleagues (107) have developed a system for scoring the pain drawing based on criteria such as the degree to which the anatomic distribution of painful sites is reasonable. Various investigators have produced both positive (131–133) and negative evidence (134) regarding the validity of the scoring system. It has been reported consistently, however, that the number of body areas identified as painful is positively correlated with psychological disturbance (132, 135).

Leavitt and his colleagues have performed a series of studies concerning the degree to which patients' choices of verbal pain descriptors may accurately discriminate between (a) low back pain patients with little or no pathophysiology and marked psychological disturbance and (b) patients with definite pathophysiology and no psychological disturbance (108, 136, 137). It has been reported that 13 verbal descriptors, termed the Back Pain Classification Scale (BPCS), correctly predicted patient membership in these two categories at levels significantly above the base rate (108, 138). It also has been shown that BPCS scores were associated significantly with low back pain patients' improvement ratings and work status following conservative orthopedic management or surgery (133). Similar to work with the IBQ, however, efforts to cross-validate the original findings reported by Leavitt and colleagues have produced both positive (139) and negative results (140). In addition, Biedermann and his colleagues (140) have shown that patients' BPCS scores are not reliable over 5-day test-retest intervals. The classification of 35% of the patients changed over the assessment period.

Several investigators have begun to evaluate the utility of two measures with chronic pain patients that originally were designed for use with a wide variety of medical patients. These measures are the Millon Behavioral Health Inventory (110) and the Symptom Checklist-90 (109). With regard to the MBHI, our research group has shown that the Somatic Anxiety and Gastrointestinal Susceptibility scales reliably differentiated patients with chronic noncardiac chest pain or the irritable bowel syndrome from patients with benign esophageal diseases and two groups of healthy control subjects (141). Among the chest pain patients, the prevalence rates of significant psychological disturbance identified by the MBHI and the more complex Diagnostic Interview Schedule were nearly equivalent. Other investigators have demonstrated that various MBHI scales are associated with chronic pain patients' responses to multidisciplinary pain clinic treatment (142, 143). Unfortunately, both of the studies cited above failed to show consistently strong relationships between the MBHI Pain Treatment Responsivity scale and patients' changes on subjective and objective outcome measures across assessment periods. Similar results also have been reported for patients treated by a behavioral program for headache reduction (144).

The SCL-90 has received little attention from investigators relative to the MBHI. Shutty, DeGood, and Schwartz (145) recently have demonstrated that three reliable second-order factors, Somatic Distress, Cognitive Distress, and Distrust, accounted for the majority of the variance in chronic pain patients' responses to the SCL-90. In addition, Duckro and his colleagues (146) have shown that the SCL-90 anxiety and depression scores generally were more highly related with chronic pain patients' pain ratings than were the MMPI Depression, Hysteria, and Psychasthenia scales.

Summary

In summary, the recent literature on chronic pain patients' affective responses has remained devoted primarily to studies employing the MMPI. This research has documented clearly that the interpretation of patients' MMPI profiles is confounded by factors such as functional disability, norms dating back to the 1940s, and heterogeneous item content of clinical scales. Nevertheless, the derivation of MMPI profile subgroups and their behavioral correlates continues to serve as a promising source of research with clinical utility. It will be necessary, however, to improve the predictive validity of the derived profile subgroups, perhaps by using more stringent criteria to determine subgroup membership, before this technique is adopted by a large number of investigators and health care providers.

Given the problems described above, it is recommended that health care providers use instruments in addition to the MMPI to evaluate the affective responses of chronic pain patients. The IBQ and the MBHI appear to be the most clinically useful alternatives to the MMPI. Nonetheless, health care providers should be aware that important questions exist concerning (a) whether the IBQ measures abnormal illness behavior or neuroticism, and (b) the predictive validity of the MBHI Pain Treatment Responsivity scale.

Given the paucity of data regarding the utility of the BPCS, pain drawing, and SCL-90 in making clinical decisions about patients, it is recommended at the present time that these instruments be employed only as research or clinical screening devices. Particular caution is urged concerning the BPCS since the prediction of physicians' attempts to differentiate psychogenic from organic pain has little clinical utility (4) and the reliability of these predictions has not been established.

COGNITIVE DISTORTION AND COPING STRATEGIES

Melzack and Wall's (147) gate control theory posits that cognitive factors interact with sensory and emotional factors in perceptions of pain. However, it was not until the late 1970s that clinical investigators began to develop techniques for assessing the cognitive activity of chronic pain patients (cf. refs. 148, 149). Early attempts at cognitive assessment consisted primarily of "think aloud" approaches in which patients described their pain-related thoughts and images as they were exposed to noxious stimulation, experienced exacerbations of their pain perceptions, or imagined episodes of increased pain (37). Subsequent cognitive assessment strategies have included the use of interviews (150), questionnaires (151, 152), multidimensional scaling of "think-aloud" responses (153), and modifications of coping strategy questionnaires originally developed for the healthy adult population (154, 155).

There has been a great deal of recent interest in developing cognitive assessment instruments specifically for use with chronic pain patients. This section examines the literature concerning the measurement of (a) cognitive distortions related to depression and (b) coping strategies among chronic pain patients.

Cognitive Distortions

Depression is commonly found among chronic pain patients (42, 156, 157) although there is disagreement regarding whether depression is primary (e.g., ref. 158) or secondary (e.g., ref. 159) to chronic pain. Beck's (160) cognitive model of depression suggests that depressed individuals systematically distort the meaning of events in order to perceive themselves and their experiences in a consistently negative fashion. Accordingly, Lefebvre (161) developed two questionnaires that measure cognitive distortions concerning general life experiences and low back pain–related problems. He then compared the responses of four groups to both questionnaires. These groups were: (a) depressed low back pain patients, (b) nondepressed low back pain patients, (c) depressed persons without low back pain, and (d) nondepressed persons without low back pain. It was found that both groups of depressed persons showed significantly higher levels of cognitive distortion than the nondepressed groups on the general and the low back pain questionnaire. However, the depressed pain patients showed greater cognitive distortion than the depressed persons without pain only on the low back pain questionnaire. Specific cognitive distortions that differentiated the two groups of depressed individuals were *catastrophizing* (misinterpreting an event as a catastrophe), *overgeneralization* (assuming that the outcome of one experience applies to the same or similar future experience), and *selective abstraction* (selectively attending to negative aspects of experiences). These results suggest, then, that cognitive distortions are common among depressed back pain patients, particularly with regard to pain-related situations.

Smith and his colleagues (162, 163) have clarified some of the clinical implications of the findings described above. These investigators demonstrated that low back pain patients' cognitive distortion scores on both the general and the low back pain questionnaires were more closely associated with MMPI measures of general distress (i.e., Depression, Psychasthenia, and Schizophrenia) than with measures of somatization (i.e., Hypochondriasis and Hysteria) (162). Cognitive distortion in pain-related situations, especially overgeneralization, also was associated with functional disability as measured by the SIP even after controlling for depression, pain severity, and number of pain treatments (163). Thus, treatment of chronic back pain patients may be hindered by patients' erroneous beliefs that their functional disabilities will remain stable in all future situations or that they do not have the skills necessary to benefit from rehabilitation training.

Measurement of Coping Strategies for Chronic Pain

Rosenstiel and Keefe (164) recently developed a questionnaire for the assessment of chronic pain patients' cognitive and behavioral coping strategies. A factor analysis of chronic low back pain patients' responses to the Coping Strategies Questionnaire produced three related underlying dimensions: (a) Cognitive Coping and Suppression (e.g., reinterpreting pain sensations); (b) Helplessness (e.g., catastrophizing); and (c) Diverting Attention and Praying (e.g., praying or hoping). It also was found that patients with high scores on the Cognitive Coping and Suppression or the Diverting Attention and Praying Factors tended to show high levels of functional impairment. Those who produced high Helplessness scores tended to display high levels of anxiety and depression.

Although the factor structure of the Coping Strategies Questionnaire may have been negatively influenced by a low ratio of subjects to items in the original analysis (8), Turner and Clancy (165) have replicated the factor structure among an independent sample of chronic back pain patients. These investigators also have demonstrated relationships among the three factors and measures of psychological and physical disability as well as pain similar to those found by Rosenstiel and Keefe (164). Moreover, it was shown that during a cognitive-behavioral or operant conditioning treatment program (a) decreased usage of praying and hoping strategies was associated with decreased self-reports of pain intensity, and (b) decreased use of catastrophizing strategies was correlated with decreased pain intensity ratings and SIP functional impairment scores.

Factor analyses of Coping Strategies Questionnaire responses produced by patients with relatively acute back pain (166) and chronic osteoarthritis of the knee (167) have revealed different underlying dimensions than those found with chronic back pain patients. With respect to osteoarthritis pain, Keefe and his colleagues (167) reported that the majority of the variance in patients' questionnaire responses was accounted for by a Coping Attempts (e.g., reinterpreting pain sensations, praying and hoping, increasing activity level) and a Self-Control and Rational Thinking (e.g., low levels of catastrophizing, ability to control pain) factor. It also was found that Self-Control and Rational Thinking predicted patients' ratings of pain intensity, functional impairment, and psychological distress on the Arthritis Impact Measurement Scales (AIMS) and the SCL-90 even after controlling for the influence of demographic and medical status variables. A follow-up study (20) replicated the factor structure of the Coping Strategies Questionnaire. Predictive relationships also were found between Self-Control and Rational Thinking and direct observations of patients' pain behavior and patients' scores on the AIMS measures of pain intensity, depression, anxiety, household activities, mobility, and dexterity.

In summary, since 1981 there has been a great deal of interest in developing measures of chronic pain patients' cognitive activity. Studies of low back pain patients' cognitive distortions and coping strategies have demonstrated that several distinct cognitive processes are associated with psychological distress and functional disability after controlling for the influence of various confounding variables. Catastrophizing appears to be an especially powerful and negative cognitive activity since it has been identified among chronic low back pain and arthritic knee pain patients using different measurement techniques (20, 161, 164, 167).

There are two major limitations associated with the cognitive assessment literature. First, all of the studies performed to date have been correlational. It is not known, then, to what extent patients' cognitive distortions and coping strategies actually produce psychological and functional impairments or result from these impairments. Furthermore, although it has been found that decreases in catastrophizing as well as praying and hoping strategies are associated with improved ratings of pain intensity and functional disability among chronic back pain patients (165), there is no information available concerning whether changes in certain cognitive activities might pro-

duce improved coping. This is a very important subject for future research given the emphasis of cognitive-behavioral therapists upon promoting adaptive cognitive activity among chronic pain patients (168, 169).

PAIN PERCEPTIONS

One of the most difficult tasks facing investigators and health care providers is the measurement of patients' subjective experiences of pain (37). Brief reviews of clinical pain assessment have been produced by Chapman and his colleagues (170–172). However, this section examines in detail pain assessment techniques that rely upon subjective judgments, including numerical or verbal category scales, visual analogue scales, the McGill Pain Questionnaire, and ratio scales developed with psychophysical scaling techniques.

Category Scales

One of the most frequently used pain assessment methods requires patients to rate the intensity of their pain along a numerical (e.g., 0 to 10) or verbal [e.g., "mild, discomforting, distressing, horrible, excruciating" (130)] scale. Although these scales are easily administered and scored, there are two major problems associated with the quantification of patients' category scale responses. First, numerical and verbal category scales suffer from a lack of sensitivity (173, 174). This lack of sensitivity is due to the fact that the number of categories must be limited (e.g., 0 to 6) since human sensory information processing is restricted to effective discrimination of approximately seven categories (4). Furthermore, it is not appropriate to treat category scales as interval scales unless one has evidence that patients respond as if the differences between the categories are equal to one another. Indeed, Heft and Parker (175) have shown that healthy volunteers do not respond to commonly used verbal categories (e.g., "faint, weak, mild, moderate, strong, intense, severe") as if they were equally spaced.

Visual Analogue Scales

Visual analogue scales require patients to indicate their perceptions of pain intensity by placing a perpendicular mark along a 10-cm horizontal line labeled "no pain" at one end and "unbearable pain" at the other (176). The evidence suggests that patients' responses to visual analogue scales are highly correlated with their responses to verbal category (177, 178) and numerical category scales (177, 179). However, during the 1970s and early 1980s, several advantages were associated with the use of visual analogue relative to category scales. First, given the infinite number of points between the scale endpoints, visual analogue scales were thought to be sensitive to small changes in perceived pain intensity following analgesic treatment (178, 180). Second, there was evidence that visual analogue scales, particularly those graded into 1-cm intervals with small markings along the horizontal line, were more reliable and judged by healthy volunteers as more preferable than verbal category scales (181). Third, the simplicity of the visual analogue scale procedure allowed it to be used with children as young as 5 with no greater incidence of failure than that associated with adults (182). Finally, one study (183) demonstrated that visual analogue scales of both the intensity and affective dimensions of chronic pain as well as experimentally produced pain have the properties of ratio scales. This report, however, has not been replicated by other investigators.

Unfortunately, the recent pain assessment literature has identified three important problems with visual analogue scales. First, several investigators have questioned the sensitivity of visual analogue scales to treatment-induced change in the subjective pain experience (170, 184). Second, there appear to be great differences between persons in their abilities to use visual analogue scales in a reliable manner (185–187). Moreover, it has been shown that age is positively associated with difficulty in using visual analogue scales (177, 185, 188). Heft and Parker (175) have suggested that visual analogue scales might be improved by adding verbal category designations along the horizontal line. Psychophysical scaling methods could be used to determine the spacings between verbal categories that are perceived by patients. This method, however, has not been used by other investigators. Rather, despite the problems associated with visual analogue scales, they continue to be employed by numerous investigators and health care providers in the evaluation of pain intensity, affect, and other experiences associated with pain (e.g., stiffness, interference with work) (189).

McGill Pain Questionnaire

The McGill Pain Questionnaire (MPQ; 130, 190) represents the first attempt to develop an assessment device that measures persons' perceptions of the sensory (e.g., temporal, spatial), affective (e.g., tension, fear), and evaluative or intensity dimensions of the pain experience. The MPQ also encompasses four miscellaneous dimensions of pain that are not easily classified in any one of the three categories noted above. The MPQ consists of 20 category scales of verbal descriptors; the descriptors within each category scale are rank ordered in terms of pain intensity. The patient is required to examine each category scale and choose one descriptor from each relevant scale that best describes his or her subjective pain experience at that moment. The MPQ administrator then may score the Number of Words Chosen (NWC) from among the 20 category scales or sum the rank values of the descriptors chosen from each of the four pain dimensions or across all dimensions to form a Pain Rating Index (PRI).

The MPQ rapidly has gained wide acceptance among health care providers and investigators (8) both in English-speaking countries and in countries such as Norway (191), Finland (192), Italy (193), and Germany (194) in which translated versions of the measure have been produced. It also has served as the basis for the development of other assessment instruments such as the BPCS and the Heacache Scale (195, 196). Only two studies have examined the reliability of patients' choices of category scales (130, 197) but both have produced positive results. However, the validity of the MPQ has been examined by numerous investigators using a wide variety of methods. Some investigators, for example, have shown that the NWC and PRI measures are positively associated with visual analogue scale ratings of pain intensity (e.g., refs. 198, 199).

A large number of investigators have examined the construct validity of the MPQ by performing factor analyses of patients' responses to the instrument. These investigators have attempted to determine whether the majority of variance in patients' MPQ responses is accounted for by the three major underlying dimensions (i.e., sensory, affective, evaluative or intensity) posited by Melzack and Torgerson (190). Investigators who have exposed healthy volunteers to noxious stimulation (e.g., refs. 200, 201) or who have used patients with relatively acute pain (e.g., ref. 202) have extracted five or more MPQ factors. Stronger support for the tripartite MPQ model has been generated, however, by studies that have factor analyzed the responses of chronic pain patients. Three investigations (203–205) have generated four-factor solutions, each of which included factors comprised solely of sensory and affective category scales, respectively. Prieto and his colleagues (204) produced a particularly significant study in that the analysis generated three factors composed entirely of sensory, affective, and evaluative category scales, respectively, as well as a fourth factor that was defined by both sensory and affective scales. Similarly, Burckhardt (206) derived four sensory, one affective, and one evaluative factor from the MPQ responses of a heterogeneous sample of arthritis patients.

Two independent groups of investigators have successfully cross-validated Prieto et al.'s findings. Byrne and her colleagues (207) derived three factors from the MPQ responses of an independent sample that were highly associated with the sensory, evaluative, and affective-sensory factors found by Prieto's group. The affective factor, however, was not successfully cross-validated. Turk et al. (208) recently used confirmatory factor analytic techniques to test the validity of the tripartite MPQ model with the sample drawn by Byrne et al. from an orthopedic hospital and another sample drawn from a Veterans' Administration hospital. The model was supported in both samples. However, the high levels of association among the sensory, affective, and evaluative factors (r's = .64–.81) led Turk and his colleagues to suggest that it was not appropriate to compute separate PRI scores for each MPQ dimension. Rather, only the total PRI should be used as a measure of general pain severity.

Three other paradigms for evaluating the construct validity of the MPQ should be noted. First, several investigators have correlated affective PRI scores with measures of affective disturbance such as the Brief Symptom Inventory (209), MMPI (203), and the Wakefield Depression Scale (210). All of these studies have produced positive findings, as have other investigations using modified MPQ scoring systems (211, 212).

The second paradigm has consisted of using multivariate procedures such as discriminant function analysis to differentiate various diagnostic patient groups on the basis of their MPQ descriptor choices. Several investigators have produced both positive (e.g., refs. 213–216) and negative (e.g., refs. 217, 218) evidence regarding the discriminative validity of the MPQ. It should be noted that the hit rates among the positive studies generally have been moderate (61–91%). Thus, the use of the MPQ for making clinical diagnoses should be restricted to generating hypotheses.

Reading and his colleagues (219) have used a third ambitious paradigm for evaluating the MPQ's construct validity. This paradigm involved the use of cluster analysis in an attempt to replicate the 20-category scale structure of the MPQ. Although a 20-category solution showed "considerable similarity" (ref. 219, p. 343) to the MPQ structure, a 16-category solution (13 sensory and 3 affective) appeared to be most appropriate. Thus, Reading and his colleagues (219) provided positive evidence concerning the construct validity of the sensory and affective dimensions of the MPQ.

The evidence reviewed above suggests that the reliability and validity of the MPQ are acceptable even though there continues to be disagreement regarding the accuracy of the MPQ in discriminating among diagnostic groups and whether it is appropriate to calculate PRI scores for each pain dimension. It should be noted, however, that several investigators have commented on the fact that patients who are unfamiliar with the English language or who come from low socioeconomic backgrounds have difficulty responding to the MPQ (4, 170). In addition, the scoring of the MPQ has been criticized on the grounds that PRI scores are confounded by differences in the number of descriptors that comprise each category scale. Charter and Nehemkis (220) and Melzack and coworkers (221) have developed new scoring systems for the MPQ, although these systems have been used only in a small number of studies (e.g., ref. 222). It is recommended that investigators and health care providers who wish to use an alternative to the current PRI scoring methods employ the weighted-rank method devised by Melzack and his colleagues (221). This recommendation is based upon the evidence that the sensitivity of the MPQ is increased when the weighted-rank method is used (221).

Ratio Scales of Verbal Pain Descriptors

Although the MPQ represents a major advance in the assessment of pain, the scaling procedures used in its development yield only ordinal data. A small number of investigators, therefore, have employed cross-modality matching to develop relatively bias-free ratio scales of verbal pain descriptors. This procedure requires individuals to use adjustable measures such as line length or handgrip force, rather than a finite set of numbers, to rate repeatedly the verbal descriptors. Gracely and his colleagues have presented impressive evidence concerning the reliability, objectivity (223), and validity (224) of sensory and affective verbal descriptor scales developed using the cross-modality matching procedure. They also have provided evidence that the scales may provide valid evaluations of clinical as well as experimental pain (225, 226).

It should be noted that all of the studies described above used a small number of well-educated and highly motivated subjects. Indeed, cross-modality matching and other psychophysical scaling procedures require the use of subjects who are familiar with the verbal descriptors and are homogeneous in background (170). Although dental patients have used these scaling procedures without great difficulty (e.g., refs. 225, 227), chronic low back pain patients, especially those with relatively low levels of psychological distress, have shown great impairment in scaling affective verbal pain descriptors (228). Thus, although some investigators have advocated the use of psychophysical scaling procedures with chronic pain patients (e.g., ref 229), our research group believes that further investigation with large samples of patients is necessary before these methods may be adopted for use outside of the laboratory setting.

Summary

In summary, there are several techniques available for the measurement of patients' pain perceptions. The evidence reviewed above suggests that visual analogue scales of pain intensity or affect and the McGill Pain Questionnaire may be superior to numerical or verbal category scales. However, health care providers and investigators should be aware that the sensitivity of both visual analogue scales and the MPQ has been questioned (184, 221). There also are unresolved issues regarding whether one of these measures might be superior to the other with certain populations. It has been established that older persons tend to have some difficulty completing visual analogue scales and that persons who are unfamiliar with the English language may not be able to respond accurately to the MPQ. Unfortunately, no investigation has compared the utility of visual analogue scales and the MPQ with these two patient populations.

Although the development of ratio scales of verbal pain descriptors represents a promising approach to pain measurement, their utility with chronic pain patients is limited at the present time by the technical complexities of psychophysical scaling procedures and the verbal sophistication required to scale the descriptors (170). It is anticipated that during the next several years significant effort will be devoted to the development of psychophysical scaling procedures for use in clinical settings.

Finally, it should be noted that numerous studies recently have shown that chronic pain patients find it very difficult to accurately rate prior pain experiences with category scales, visual analogue scales, and the MPQ (230–235). It is recommended, therefore, that these measures be used to evaluate patients' perceptions of their current pain states rather than retrospective perceptions of change in pain experiences.

PATIENTS' INTERACTIONS WITH FAMILY MEMBERS

Although Fordyce (12) and Sternbach (1) have emphasized the importance of family members in the maintenance of patients' chronic pain problems, only a small number of investigators have devoted attention to the assessment of these family members. Payne and Norfleet (236) have provided a comprehensive review of this literature. Briefly, however, it should be noted that two areas have emerged that are of interest to both investigators and health care providers. These are the effects of: (a) chronic pain on the marital relationship or spouse, and (b) family interactions upon patients' pain behaviors. The recent literature in these two areas is examined below.

Effects of Chronic Pain on the Marital Relationship or Spouse

It has been found repeatedly that chronic pain patients tend to have poor relationships with their spouses and show poor sexual adjustment (e.g., 237–239). A few investigators also have focused attention specifically on the spouses of chronic pain patients. For example, Ahern and his colleagues (240) found that 20% of 117 pain patient spouses reported clinically significant symptoms of depression and over 35% rated their marriages as maladjusted. It was particularly significant that spouses' marital maladjustment ratings were positively associated with the patients' levels of functional impairment, especially social interaction deficits as measured by the SIP. Similar findings regarding emotional distress and marital dissatisfaction of pain patient spouses have been reported by Flor et al. (241). However, there appears to be a subgroup of pain patients and spouses who share painful symptoms or beliefs regarding pain (239, 241–243). There also is some evidence that greater congruence between patients' and spouses' attitudes is associated with poorer treatment outcomes (243). Unfortunately, no one yet has attempted to replicate the relationship between patient and spouse congruence and treatment outcome.

Effects of Family Interactions Upon Patients' Pain Behaviors

It has been found in the laboratory that the reactions of models to noxious stimulation reliably affects the verbal and nonverbal pain behavior of healthy volunteers (e.g., refs. 244, 245). In addition, there is evidence that chronic pain patients report having more pain patient models in their families than do control individuals (e.g., refs. 239, 246, 247). Thus, observational learning may be related to the development of chronic benign pain or other forms of abnormal illness behavior.

Several investigators also have attempted to test Fordyce's (12) hypothesis that spouses are important sources of reinforcement for patients' pain behaviors. For example, Flor and associates (248) recently showed that patients' perceptions of reinforcement from spouses and spouses' self-reported reinforcement of pain behavior predicted a significant proportion of variance in patients' self-reports of pain intensity and activity levels. As Fordyce's operant model would predict, high levels of spouse reinforcement were associated with high levels of pain and low activity levels. Spouses' reports of reinforcement also were associated with longer duration of pain, high levels of patients' satisfaction with marriage, and spouses' ratings of (a) high interference of patients' pain with spouses' lives, (b) positive mood, and (c) high life control. Thus, spouses who tended to reinforce patients' pain behaviors experienced high levels of interference in their lives but they also may have been rewarded for their actions by positive mood, perceived life control, and patients' expressions of marital satisfaction.

The positive relationship between patients' perceptions of spouse reinforcement and pain intensity also has been reported by Anderson and Rehm (249). In addition, Block and his colleagues have attempted to examine the relationship between spouse and patient behavior with measurement techniques that are more objective than self-reports. Block et al. (250), for example, found that chronic pain patients who rated their spouses as relatively nonresponsive toward their pain complaints reported lower pain intensity levels when they believed they were being observed by their spouses rather than by a ward clerk. This demonstrated that spouses may serve as discriminative cues to some patients for pain behavior. Block (251) also has demonstrated that chronic pain patient spouses who reported relatively high levels of marital satisfaction showed greater skin conductance responses when they viewed facial pain displays of their marital partners than did spouses who reported relatively low levels of marital satisfaction. The two groups of spouses did not differ with respect to their ratings of the intensity of their partners' pain displays and did not show different skin conductance responses when they observed the pain displays of unfamiliar persons who were described as chronic pain patients.

Summary

In summary, the small literature concerning patients' interactions with family members indicates that there is a high level of marital dissatisfaction among chronic pain patients and their spouses. It is important, however, to examine individual differences among both patients and spouses. There are some couples, for example, who share very similar symptoms or beliefs regarding pain; patients within these couples may have poor prognoses for improvement. There also are patients whose pain appears to be influenced by observational or operant learning. However, it is not known to what extent these patients and their spouses may share pain-related attitudes or symptoms. It also is not known to what extent these patients' learning histories may be related to their use of various coping strategies or treatment outcomes. Thus, future investigators should attempt to further examine how individual difference variables affect the *interactions* between chronic pain patients and their spouses and how these interactions may be correlated with spouses' and patients' cognitive activities, as well as patients' functional status and outcomes. The results of this work then could be used to aid treatment planning. For example, it might prove useful early in treatment to identify spouses who are especially responsive to patients' displays of pain. These spouses may require very intensive training to change their reinforcement patterns and yet maintain their positive moods or perceptions of control over their lives. If attention is not devoted to the latter two variables, efforts to change the interactions between the patients and spouses as well as to change patients' behavior may fail.

DISCUSSION

The major portion of the chronic pain assessment literature has been devoted to studies of patients' cognitive and verbal responses. Three very important advances have been made in the evaluation of these responses. First, it has been shown consistently that there are reliable behavioral and affective differences among empirically derived MMPI profile subgroups. However, it is necessary to reduce the sources of error in current outcome prediction studies (e.g., use of heterogeneous outcome criteria, treatments, and subgroup members) in order to determine the predictive power of the MMPI profile subgroups.

The second major advance has been the development of reliable and valid measures of patients' cognitive distortions and coping strategies. Measures such as Keefe's Coping Strategies Questionnaire are far superior to the "think-aloud" methods upon which investigators and health care providers had to rely during the 1970s. Although it has been demonstrated that patients' cognitive activities are associated with their reports of pain intensity and functional impairment, it now is necessary to determine whether altering specific cognitions produces positive patient change and what interventions might best alter patients' cognitions.

The third major advance has been the acknowledgment among investigators and many health care providers that the use of unidimensional category scales is not sufficient to measure adequately patients' pain perceptions. The development of the MPQ, a verbal descriptor scale that evaluates three pain dimensions, has generated a great deal of clinical and research activity. The development of revised scoring systems for the MPQ may help investigators to determine better the extent to which the instrument actually measures the three relatively distinct dimensions of sensory, affective, and evaluative pain qualities. The

MPQ also has led to the use of psychophysical scaling methods to develop ratio scales of sensory and affective verbal pain descriptors. Although these verbal descriptor scales provide reliable and valid measures of pain perceptions, their use with chronic pain patients may be limited by the level of verbal sophistication and cognitive ability required by psychophysical scaling methods.

The remainder of the literature regarding patients' cognitive and affective responses has been devoted to the development of self-report measures that might complement the MMPI and to the investigation of chronic pain patients' interactions with family members. At present, it appears that the IBQ and the MBHI are the most clinically useful of the recently developed self-report measures. Nevertheless, the SCL-90 has been used in several recent research investigations (e.g., refs. 167, 240) and its clinical utility may be documented soon. It also is anticipated that investigators will extend their studies of the interactions among chronic pain patients and their spouses that may influence both spouses and patients. A great amount of research is necessary in order to delineate the complex relationships among marital interactions as well as the cognitive activity and behavior of patients and spouses.

MEASUREMENT OF PHYSIOLOGIC VARIABLES

The assessment of physiologic responses represents an attempt to find objective evidence of the experience of pain (170). However, no one yet has demonstrated a specific physiologic response that covaries reliably with reports of pain or is free from the effects of extraneous variables such as expectancy or attention. Nevertheless, assessment of physiologic responses is important because these variables may be (a) related to maladaptive behavior patterns (e.g., restricted activity or distorted gait); (b) related to specific pain syndromes (e.g., tension headaches); and (c) modified by behavioral interventions such as relaxation or biofeedback training (5).

The majority of the physiologic assessment studies in the chronic pain literature has been devoted to measurement of electromyographic (EMG) activity. Some investigators have examined variables such as evoked potentials (e.g., ref. 252) and cerebrospinal fluid levels of endorphins (e.g., ref. 253) and related physiologic measures as biologic markers of patients' pain experiences. However, none of the physiologic variables except EMG activity has shown good clinical utility. Thus, the following section examines recent studies of EMG response and a related measure of muscular activity, myofascial trigger point sensitivity. Reviews of research concerning other physiologic measures have been produced by Chapman et al. (170), Hoon et al. (67), White et al. (8), and Terenius (254, 255).

EMG ACTIVITY

It generally is believed that many patients who experience chronic pain tend to restrict their spinal motion and other movements and, thus, increase their muscle tension levels for prolonged periods. These changes, in turn, lead to a vicious cycle in which normal activities of daily living evoke increased muscle pain, which leads to further restriction of motion (5, 256). Therefore, many investigators have evaluated surface EMG recordings at patients' painful body sites. It should be noted, however, that there is some disagreement regarding whether these EMG data can be measured reliably (e.g., 257, 258).

A large number of investigators have examined the absolute levels of patients' EMG activity during conditions of rest and stress. Some investigators have reported that chronic back pain patients show elevated EMG levels at rest (e.g., ref 259) and during emotional stress or physical maneuvers (e.g., ref 260). However, investigators also have produced negative findings concerning patients' EMG levels (e.g., refs. 261, 262). Similar inconsistencies regarding the relationship between pain and elevated EMG activity have been reported in the tension headache literature (263). It is not surprising, then, that investigators have produced both positive (264–266) and negative (267–270) evidence regarding the effects of EMG reductions on patients' reports of pain.

Some investigators have attempted to resolve the inconsistencies in the literature by using novel assessment strategies. For example, Wolf and his colleagues (271, 272) have studied the patterns rather than the absolute levels of EMG activity in lumbar muscle sites among chronic back pain patients. These investigators have found that, during static and dynamic activities, normal individuals tend to produce low and symmetric levels of EMG activity from electrode placements on both sides of the lumbar spine. Chronic back pain patients, however, tend to produce abnormal EMG patterns (e.g., asymmetry of right and left lumbar spine EMG levels) during both static and dynamic activities. Similar findings have been reported by Cram and Steger (273). In addition, Wolf and his colleagues (272, 274) have demonstrated that patients who are trained to produce more normal EMG patterns tend to report reduced pain perceptions and to display increased activity levels.

A second novel approach to EMG assessment has consisted of comparing the EMG responses of back pain patients during conditions of rest, general stress, and *personally relevant stress*. The latter form of stress is induced by asking the patient to "recall a recent stressful event or a recent pain episode and describe it for 1 min" (ref. 275, p. 357). Flor and her colleagues have reported that chronic back pain patients, relative to healthy controls and patients with pain unrelated to the back, produced elevated right and left paraspinal EMG responses only during personally relevant stress. In addition, the back pain patients showed delays in return to baseline of paraspinal EMG activity following personally relevant stress. This effect, however, was strongest for the left paraspinal musculature.

MYOFASCIAL TRIGGER POINT SENSITIVITY

Myofascial trigger points are "discrete points of focal tenderness within tight bands of muscle that may refer pain, tenderness, and autonomic changes to distant locations in patterns characteristic for each muscle" (ref. 276, p. 203). These trigger points have been implicated in a variety of chronic pain syndromes, including primary fibromyalgia, (277) and both tension and migraine headaches (278, 279). In the case of fibromyalgia, trigger point activity has been associated with pathologic changes in muscle tissue such as degeneration, inflammatory infiltrates, and "moth-eaten" fibers (280). However, identification of trigger points has been dependent upon manual palpation of the muscles. Although skilled palpation might reliably and accurately identify trigger point location, it cannot quantify the sensitivity of various trigger points and thereby provide information relevant for assessment and treatment outcome evaluation. Thus, Reeves and his colleagues (281) recently evaluated a pressure algometer that allows the investigator or health care provider to measure the amount of pressure applied to a trigger point that evokes threshold reports of pain.

The pressure algometer, which has been used in pain research for many years (282), consists of a plunger mounted on a calibrated spring. However, it primarily has been used to evoke and to quantify pain rather than to assess the sensitivity of myofascial trigger points. Reeves and his colleagues (281) have demonstrated the reliability of the pressure algometer both between and within experimenters and the discriminative validity of the instrument. Similar findings have been reported by independent Swedish investigators (282). In addition, Jaeger and Reeves (276) have shown that the pressure algometer measure is sensitive to change following passive stretching and Fluori-Methane spraying of trigger points. These investigators also have shown that reliable decreases in trigger point sensitivity following "spray-and-stretch" treatment are accompanied by reliable decreases in reports of pain as measured by visual analogue scales.

The research described above suggests that the pressure algometer provides a reliable and valid measure of myofascial trigger point sensitivity. It should be noted, however, that the pressure algometer has been used thus far only with a small number of patients suffering from head and neck pain. It also should be noted that Jaeger and Reeves (276) did not find significant correlations between changes in pressure algometer readings and patients' reports of pain intensity. The low correlations, however, may have been due to the use of a 20-patient sample. Thus, the pressure algometer must be tested with larger patient samples, particularly those with patients who suffer from fibromyalgia and who often have numerous trigger points in many body areas.

DISCUSSION

It has been very difficult for investigators to identify physiologic variables that may serve as reliable markers of patients' pain experiences. However, three promising methods of evaluating abnormal muscle activity have been identified. These are measurement of paraspinal EMG patterns during static and dynamic activities, measurement of absolute EMG levels during periods of personally relevant stress, and assessment of myofascial trigger point sensitivity with the pressure algometer. These methods have appeared only in the recent assessment literature and represent attempts to resolve the many problems that have slowed the development of reliable and clinically useful physiologic pain markers. Nevertheless, several reviews have concluded that paraspinal EMG patterns should be evaluated routinely (5, 256). Our research group concurs with this conclusion, although health care providers and investigators should be aware that paraspinal EMG asymmetries among some individuals may be artifacts of postural factors such as unequal weight bearing during standing (256). Assessment of EMG activity with personally relevant stressors and evaluation of trigger point sensitivity with the pressure algometer require further study in multiple settings before they may be routinely used for clinical purposes.

CONCLUSIONS

This chapter has presented a critical review of the recent empirical literature regarding psychological testing of chronic pain patients. The review included discussion of the evaluation of overt motor behaviors, cognitive-verbal responses, and physiologic responses. A few investigators have attempted to study the relationships among two or more of these evaluation areas (e.g., refs. 17–19, 23, 129, 168). Nevertheless, the chronic pain assessment literature is best described as consisting of three relatively independent content areas, each of which is associated with various strengths and weaknesses.

The literature regarding the assessment of overt motor behaviors has advanced rapidly since 1980. There now exist standardized protocols for evaluating motor behaviors associated with several disorders, such as low back pain (16), rheumatoid arthritis (17), osteoarthritis (20), and head and neck cancer (21). These direct observation protocols or automated recording devices (e.g., 29, 31) may be used to supplement or validate self-report measures such as patient diaries or functional disability questionnaires. In addition, information is becoming available regarding how motor behaviors are associated with cognitive-verbal and physiologic responses. For example, the pain behavior of rheumatoid arthritis and low back pain patients is associated with physiologic measures of disease activity (18, 23); however, depression is an independent predictor of pain behavior only among low back pain patients (17, 19).

There are reliability and reactivity problems associated with the use of direct observation methods, automated recording devices, and self-monitoring. Functional disability questionnaires, such as the SIP, generally do not pose as many problems for health care providers and investigators as the other measures of motor behavior. These questionnaires also generate information regarding patient functioning in several areas that can provide targets for behavioral interventions and measures of treatment outcome. It should be emphasized, however, that several of the functional disability questionnaires (49–54) require further validation before they may be accepted for both clinical and research purposes.

There clearly are advantages and sources of error associated with each of the overt motor behavior measures. The advantages of these measures, however, far outweigh the difficulties associated with them. Thus, it is recommended that health care providers and investigators use at least one measure of overt motor behavior on a routine basis.

It was noted earlier that the three most important advances in the assessment of patients' cognitive-verbal responses were the development of (a) replicable, empirically derived MMPI profile subgroups and their behavioral and affective correlates; (b) reliable and valid measures of patients' cognitive distortions and coping strategies; and (c) measures of the sensory and affective dimensions of patients' pain experiences. Some effort already has been devoted to determining the relationships between the various MMPI subgroups and McGill Pain Questionnaire responses (e.g., ref. 86). However, it would be worthwhile to determine if the subgroups also differ with respect to cognitive variables, overt motor behavior, physiologic responses, and interactions with spouses or other family members.

Several of the cognitive-verbal assessment methods have been studied intensively while others have received relatively little attention. Our research group suggests that only the MMPI, Illness Behavior Questionnaire, and Millon Behavioral Health Inventory may be used with confidence to evaluate patients' affective responses in both clinical and research settings. The SCL-90 is appropriate for research purposes but there is little information available regarding its clinical utility with chronic pain patients.

With respect to patients' cognitive activities, our group encourages health care providers and investigators to employ Lefebvre's cognitive distortion questionnaire (161) and the Coping Strategies Questionnaire (164). It should be stressed, however, that there is a great need to determine whether changes in specific cognitive activities measured by these instruments reliably lead to improved coping.

The literature regarding measurement of patients' pain perceptions suggests that visual analogue scales and the McGill Pain Questionnaire are most appropriate for both clinical and research purposes. Our research group suggests that health care providers and investigators use both of these measures on a routine basis given the concerns that have been raised regarding the reliability and sensitivity of visual analogue scales and the language problems associated with the McGill Pain Questionnaire. The use of psychophysical scaling methods for clinical purposes is not recommended at the present time given the difficulty chronic pain patients may have in properly scaling affective verbal descriptors (228).

Based on the available literature and personal experience, our research group believes it is essential to attempt to evaluate family members' responses to chronic pain patients. Interviews with the patients and families together and separated from one another often provide highly valuable information. In addition, some information regarding pain-reinforcing responses generated by family members may be acquired using self-report measures described by Flor and her colleagues (248) and Block and his associates (250).

Our research group advocates the routine assessment of patients' physiologic responses for both clinical and research purposes. It should be emphasized, however, that current evidence does not support the use of any single physiologic measure as a marker of the pain experience. Even very promising measures, such as patterns of paraspinal EMG activity, may be subject to error due to extraneous factors. Thus, the evaluation of physiologic responses in both research and clinical settings must be performed carefully. Moreover, treatment decisions and interpretation of research findings based on physiologic response evaluation should be made with caution given the inconsistent relationships between physiologic measures and patients' reports of pain.

The preceding discussion indicates that none of the assessment methods described in this chapter provides a complete assessment of patients' pain experiences. As a result, it is necessary for both health care providers and investigators to use multiple measures of overt motor behavior, cognitive-verbal responses, and physiologic variables to fully evaluate chronic pain patients and their treatment outcomes. For example, our research group (283) recently published an evaluation of the efficacy of a cognitive-behavioral treatment program for rheumatoid arthritis patients that reported changes with respect to (a) direct observations of overt motor behavior, (b) visual analogue scale ratings of pain intensity and unpleasantness, (c) self-reports of depression and anxiety, (d) perceptions of control over general health outcomes and effects of rheumatoid arthritis (cognitive activity), and (e) peripheral skin temperature levels at the most painful joints as well as several clinical and laboratory measures of disease activity (physiologic variables). As is often the case with psychological interventions, significant treatment effects were found on overt motor behavior, anxiety, and several of the physiologic variables but not on the other outcome measures. This example illustrates the need for comprehensive testing of chronic pain patients in order to fully assess their pain-related difficulties and the effects of treatment.

References

1. Sternbach RA: *Pain Patients: Traits and Treatments.* New York, Academic Press, 1974.
2. Fordyce WE, Fowler RS, DeLateur BJ, Sand PL, Trieschmann RB: Operant conditioning in the treatment of chronic pain. *Arch Phys Med Rehabil* 54:399–408, 1973.
3. Fordyce WE, Fowler RS, Lehmann JF, DeLateur BJ: Some implications of learning in problems of chronic pain. *J Chron Dis* 21:179–190, 1968.
4. Bradley LA, Prokop CK, Gentry WD, Van der Heide LH, Prieto EJ: Assessment of chronic pain. In Prokop CK, Bradley LA (eds): *Medical Psychology: Contributions to Behavioral Medicine.* New York, Academic Press, 1981, pp 91–117.
5. Keefe FJ: Behavioral assessment and treatment of chronic pain: current status and future directions. *J Consult Clin Psychol* 50:896–911, 1982.
6. Keefe FJ, Bradley LA: Behavioral and psychological approaches to the assessment and treatment of chronic pain. *Gen Hosp Psychiatry* 6:49–54, 1984.
7. Keefe FJ, Gil KM: Behavioral concepts in the analysis of chronic pain syndromes. *J Consult Clin Psychol* 54:776–783, 1986.
8. White MC, Bradley LA, Prokop CK: Behavioral assessment of chronic pain. In Tryon WW (ed): *Behavioral Assessment in Behavioral Medicine.* New York, Springer, 1985, pp 166–199.
9. International Association for the Study of Pain Subcommittee on Taxonomy: Pain terms: a list with definitions and notes on usage. *Pain* 6:249–252, 1979.
10. Sanders SH: Behavioral assessment and treatment of clinical pain: appraisal of current status. In Hersen M, Eisler RM, Miller PM (eds): *Progress in Behavior Modification.* New York, Academic Press, 1979, vol 8, pp 249–291.
11. Fordyce WE: An operant conditioning method for managing chronic pain. *Postgrad Med* 53:123–128, 1973.
12. Fordyce WE: *Behavioral Methods for Chronic Pain and Illness.* St. Louis, CV Mosby, 1976.
13. Fordyce WE: Learning processes in pain. In Sternbach RA (ed): *The Psychology of Pain,* ed 1. New York, Raven Press, 1978, pp 49–72.
14. Fordyce WE, McMahon R, Rainwater G, Jackins S, Questal K, Murphy T, DeLateur B: Pain complaint: exercise performance relationship in chronic pain. *Pain* 10:311–321, 1981.
15. Fordyce WE, Lansky D, Calsyn DA, Shelton JL, Stolov WC, Rock DL: Pain measurement and pain behavior. *Pain* 18:53–69, 1984.
16. Keefe FJ, Block AR: Development of an observation method for assessing pain behavior in chronic low back pain patients. *Behav Ther* 13:363–375, 1982.
17. McDaniel LK, Anderson KO, Bradley LA, Young LD, Turner RA, Agudelo CA, Keefe FJ: Development of an observation method for assessing pain behavior in rheumatoid arthritis patients. *Pain* 24:165–184, 1986.
18. Anderson KO, Bradley LA, McDaniel LK, Young LD, Turner RA, Agudelo CA, Keefe FJ, Pisko RJ, Snyder RM, Semble EL: The assessment of pain in rheumatoid arthritis: validity of a behavioral observation method. *Arthritis Rheum* 30:36–43, 1987.
19. Anderson KO, Bradley LA, McDaniel LK, Young LD, Turner RA, Agudelo CA, Gaby NS, Keefe FJ, Pisko EJ, Snyder RM, Semble RL: The assessment of pain in rheumatoid arthritis: disease differentiation and temporal stability of a behavioral observation method. *J Rheumatol* 14:700–704, 1987.
20. Keefe FJ, Caldwell DS, Queen K, Gil KM, Martinez S, Crisson JE, Ogden W, Nunley J: Osteoarthritic knee pain: a behavioral analysis. *Pain* 28:309–321, 1987.
21. Keefe FJ, Brantley A, Manuel G, Crisson JE: Behavioral assessment of head and neck cancer pain. *Pain* 23:327–336, 1985.
22. Keefe FJ, Wilkins RH, Cook WA: Direct observation of pain behavior in low back pain patients during physical examination. *Pain* 20:59–68, 1984.
23. Keefe FJ, Wilkins RH, Cook WA, Crisson JE, Muhlbaier LH: Depression, pain, and pain behavior. *J Consult Clin Psychol* 54:665–669, 1986.
24. Follick MJ, Ahern DK, Aberger EW: Development of an audiovisual taxonomy of pain behavior: reliability and discriminant validity. *Health Psychol* 4:555–568, 1985.
25. Richards JS, Nepomuceno C, Riles M, Suer Z: Assessing pain behavior: the UAB pain behavior scale. *Pain* 14:393–398, 1982.
26. Cinciripini PM, Floreen A: An assessment of chronic pain behavior in a structured interview. *J Psychosom Res* 27:117–123, 1983.
27. Mayer TG, Gatchel RJ, Kishino N, Keeley J, Capra P, Mayer H, Barnett J, Mooney V: Objective assessment of spine function following industrial injury: a prospective study with comparison group and one-year follow-up. *Spine* 10:482–493, 1985.
28. Mayer TG, Gatchel RJ, Kishino N, Keeley J, Mayer H, Capra P, Mooney V: A prospective short-term study of chronic low back pain patients utilizing novel objective functional measurement. *Pain* 25:53–68, 1986.
29. Naliboff BD, Cohen MJ, Swanson GA, Bonebakker AD, McArthur DL: Comprehensive assessment of chronic low back pain patients and controls: physical abilities, level of activity, psychological adjustment and pain perception. *Pain* 23:121–134, 1985.
30. Report of the Commission on the Evaluation of Pain. *Soc Secur Bull* 50:13–44, 1987.
31. Cohen JA: A coefficient of agreement for nominal scales. *Educ Psychol Measure* 20:37–46, 1960.
32. Conger AJ: Integration and generalization of kappas for multiple raters. *Psychol Bull* 88:322–328, 1980.
33. Cairns D, Thomas L, Mooney V, Pace JB: A comprehensive treatment approach to chronic low back pain. *Pain* 2:301–308, 1976.
34. Sanders SH: Toward a practical instrument system for the automatic measurement of "uptime" in chronic pain patients. *Pain* 9:103–109, 1980.
35. Follick MJ, Ahern DK, Laser-Wolston N, Adams AE, Molloy AJ: Chronic pain: electromechanical recording device for measuring patients' activity patterns. *Arch Phys Med Rehabil* 66:75–79, 1985.
36. Keefe FJ, Hill RW: An objective approach to quantifying pain behavior and gait patterns in low back pain patients. *Pain* 21:153–161, 1985.
37. Bradley LA, Prokop CK: Research methods in contemporary medical psychology. In Kendall PC, Butcher JN (eds): *Handbook of Research Methods in Clinical Psychology.* New York, John Wiley, 1982, pp 591–649.
38. Taylor CB, Zlutnick SI, Corley MJ, Flora J: The effects of detoxification, relaxation, and brief supportive therapy on chronic pain. *Pain* 8:319–329, 1980.

39. Ready LB, Sarkis E, Turner JA: Self-reported vs. actual use of medications in chronic pain patients. *Pain* 12:285–294, 1982.
40. Kremer EF, Block A, Gaylor MS: Behavioral approaches to treatment of chronic pain: the inaccuracy of patient self-report measures. *Arch Phys Med Rehabil* 61:188–191, 1981.
41. Sanders SH: Automated versus self-monitoring of "up-time" in chronic low-back pain patients: a comparative study. *Pain* 15:399–405, 1983.
42. Ramano JM, Turner JA: Chronic pain and depression: does the evidence support a relationship? *Psychol Bull* 97:18–34, 1985.
43. McNairy SL, Maruta T, Ivnik RJ, Swanson DW, Ilstrup DM: Prescription medication dependence and neuropsychologic function. *Pain* 18:169–177, 1984.
44. Schwartz DP, Barth JT, Dane JR, Drenan SE, DeGood DE, Rowlingson JC: Cognitive deficits in chronic pain patients with and without history of head/neck injury: development of a brief screening battery. *Clin J Pain* 3:94–101, 1987.
45. Follick MJ, Ahern DK, Laser-Wolston N: Evaluation of a daily activity diary for chronic pain patients. *Pain* 19:373–382, 1984.
46. Bergner M, Bobbitt RA, Carter WB, Gibson BS: The Sickness Impact Profile: development and final revision of a health status measure. *Med Care* 19:787–805, 1981.
47. Bradley LA, Anderson KO, Young LD, McDaniel LK, Turner RA, Agudelo CA, Salinger MC: Psychological aspects of arthritis. *Bull Rheum Dis* 35:1–12, 1985.
48. Liang MH, Larson MG, Cullen KE, Schwartz JA: Comparative measurement efficiency and sensitivity of five health status instruments for arthritis research. *Arthritis Rheum* 28:542–547, 1985.
49. Follick MJ, Smith TW, Ahern DK: The Sickness Impact Profile: a global measure of disability in chronic low back pain. *Pain* 21:67–76, 1985.
50. Roland M, Morris R: A study of the natural history of back pain. Part I: Development of a reliable and sensitive measure of disability in low-back pain. *Spine* 8:141–144, 1983.
51. Deyo RA: Comparative validity of the Sickness Impact Profile and shorter scales for functional assessment in low-back pain. *Spine* 11:951–954, 1986.
52. Rock DL, Fordyce WE, Brockway JA, Bergman JJ, Spengler DM: Measuring functional impairment associated with pain: psychometric analysis of an exploratory scoring protocol for activity pattern indicators. *Arch Phys Med Rehabil* 65:295–300, 1984.
53. Feuerstein M, Greenwald M, Gamache MP, Papciak AS, Cook EW: The Pain Behavior Scale: modification and validation for outpatient use. *J Psychopathol Behav Assess* 7:301–315, 1985.
54. Kames LD, Naliboff BD, Heinrich RL, Coscarelli-Schag C: The Chronic Illness Problem Inventory: problem-oriented psychosocial assessment of patients with chronic illness. *Int J Psychiatry Med* 14:65–75, 1984.
55. Corson JA, Schneider MJ: The Dartmouth Pain Questionnaire: an adjunct to the McGill Pain Questionnaire. *Pain* 19:59–69, 1984.
56. Kerns RD, Turk DC, Rudy TE: The West Haven-Yale Multidimensional Pain Inventory (WHYMPI). *Pain* 23:345–356, 1985.
57. Sternbach RA; Clinical aspects of pain. In Sternbach RA (ed): *The Psychology of Pain.* New York, Raven Press, 1978, vol 1, pp 241–264.
58. Elkins GR, Barrett ET: The MMPI in evaluation of functional versus organic low back pain. *J Personal Assess* 48:259–264, 1984.
59. Love AW, Peck CL: The MMPI and psychological factors in chronic low back pain: a review. *Pain* 28:1–12, 1987.
60. Hanvik LJ: MMPI profiles in patients with low back pain. *J Consult Psychol* 15:350–353, 1951.
61. Fordyce WE, Brena SF, Holcomb RF, DeLateur BJ, Loeser JD: Relationship of patient semantic pain descriptions to physicians' diagnostic judgments, activity level measures, and MMPI. *Pain* 5:293–303, 1978.
62. McCreary C, Turner J, Dawson E: Differences between functional versus organic low back pain patients. *Pain* 4:73–78, 1977.
63. Sternbach RA, Wolf SR, Murphy RW, Akeson WH: Traits of pain patients: the low-back "loser." *Psychosomatics* 14:52–56, 1973.
64. Cox GB, Chapman CR, Black, RG: The MMPI and chronic pain: the diagnosis of psychogenic pain. *J Behav Med* 1:437–443, 1978.
65. Rook JC, Pesch RN, Keeler EC: Chronic pain and the questionable use of the Minnesota Multiphasic Personality Inventory. *Arch Phys Med Rehabil* 62:373–376, 1981.
66. Rosen JC, Frymoyer JW, Clements JH: A further look at the validity of the MMPI with low back pain patients. *J Clin Psychol* 36:994–1000, 1980.
67. Hoon PW, Feuerstein M, Papciak AS: Evaluation of the chronic low back pain patient: conceptual and clinical considerations. *Clin Psychol Rev* 5:377–401, 1985.
68. Naliboff BD, Cohen MJ, Yellin AN: Does the MMPI differentiate chronic illness from chronic pain: *Pain* 13:333–341, 1982.
69. Naliboff BD, Cohen MJ, Yellin AN: Frequency of MMPI profile types in three chronic illness populations. *J Clin Psychol* 39:843–847, 1983.
70. Watson D: Neurotic tendencies among chronic pain patients: an MMPI item analysis. *Pain* 14:365–385, 1982.
71. Pincus T, Callahn LF, Bradley LA, Vaughn WK, Wolfe F: Elevated MMPI scores for hypochondriasis, depression, and hysteria in patients with rheumatoid arthritis reflect disease rather than psychological status. *Arthritis Rheum* 29:1456–1466, 1986.
72. Ahles TA, Yunus MB, Gaulier B, Riley SD, Masi AT: The use of contemporary MMPI norms in the study of chronic pain patients. *Pain* 24:159–163, 1986.
73. Colligan RC, Osbourne D, Swenson WM, Offord KP: The ageing MMPI: development of contemporary norms. *Mayo Clin Proc* 59:377–390, 1984.
74. Hsu LM, Betman JA: Minnesota Multiphasic Personality Inventory T score conversion tables, 1957–1983. *J Consult Clin Psychol* 54:497–501, 1986.
75. Prokop CK: Hysteria scale elevations in low back pain patients: a risk factor for misdiagnosis? *J Consult Clin Psychol* 54:558–562, 1986.
76. Moore JE, McFall ME, Kivlahan DR, Capestany F: Risk of misinterpretation of MMPI Schizophrenia scale elevations in chronic pain patients. *Pain* 32:207–213, 1988.
77. Greene RL: *The MMPI: An Interpretive Manual.* New York, Grune & Stratton, 1980.
78. Bradley LA, Prokop CK, Margolis R, Gentry WD: Multivariate analyses of the MMPI profiles of low back pain patients. *J Behav Med* 1:253–272, 1978.
79. Prokop CK, Bradley LA, Margolis R, Gentry WD: Multi-

variate analyses of the MMPI profiles of multiple pain patients. *J Personal Assess* 44:246–252, 1980.
80. Chapman CR, Sola AE, Bonica JJ: Illness behavior and depression compared in pain center and private practice patients. *Pain* 6:1–7, 1979.
81. Holzman AD, Rudy TE, Gerber KE, Turk DC, Sanders SH, Zimmerman J, Kerns RD: Chronic pain: a multiple setting comparison of patient characteristics. *J Behav Med* 8:411–422, 1985.
82. Bernstein IH, Garbin CP: Hierarchical clustering of pain patients' MMPI profiles: a replication note. *J Personal Assess* 47:171–172, 1983.
83. Armentrout DP, Moore JE, Parker JC, Hewett JE, Feltz C: Pain patient MMPI subgroups: the psychological dimensions of pain. *J Behav Med* 5:201–211, 1982.
84. McGill JC, Lawlis GF, Selby D, Mooney V, McCoy CE: The relationship of Minnesota Multiphasic Personality Inventory (MMPI) profile clusters to pain behaviors. *J Behav Med* 6:77–92, 1983.
85. Hart RR: Chronic pain: replicated multivariate clustering of personality profiles. *J Clin Psychol* 40:129–133, 1984.
86. Bradley LA, Van der Heide LH: Pain-related correlates of MMPI profile subgroups among back pain patients. *Health Psychol* 3:157–174, 1984.
87. McCreary C: Empirically derived MMPI profile clusters and characteristics of low back pain patients. *J Consult Clin Psychol* 53:558–560, 1985.
88. Rappaport NB, McAnulty DP, Waggoner CD, Brantley PJ: Cluster analysis of Minnesota Multiphasic Personality Inventory (MMPI) profiles in a chronic headache population. *J Behav Med* 10:49–60, 1987.
89. Spitzer RL, Endicott J, Robins E: *Research Diagnostic Criteria (RDC) for a Selected Group of Functional Disorders*, ed 3. New York: Biometrics Research, New York State Psychiatric Institute, 1978.
90. Atkinson JH, Ingram RE, Kremer EF, Saccuzzo DP: MMPI subgroups and affective disorder in chronic pain patients. *J Nerv Ment Dis* 174:408–413, 1986.
91. Moore JE, Armentrout DP, Parker JC, Kivlahan DR: Empirically derived pain-patient MMPI subgroups: prediction of treatment outcome. *J Behav Med* 9:51–63, 1986.
92. Wilfling FJ, Klonoff H, Kokan P: Psychological, demographic, and orthopedic factors associated with prediction and outcome of spinal fusion. *Clin Orthoped Rel Res* 90:153–160, 1973.
93. Wiltse LL, Rocchio PD: Preoperative psychological tests as predictors of success of chemonucleolysis in the treatment of low back syndrome. *J Bone Joint Surg* 57A:478–483, 1975.
94. McCreary C, Turner J, Dawson E: The MMPI as a predictor of response to conservative treatment for low back pain. *J Clin Psychol* 35:278–284, 1979.
95. Strassberg DS, Reimherr F, Ward M, Russell S, Cole A: The MMPI and chronic pain. *J Consult Clin Psychol* 49:220–226, 1981.
96. Turner JA, Herron L, Weiner P: Utility of the MMPI pain assessment index in predicting outcome after lumbar surgery. *J Clin Psychol* 42:764–769, 1986.
97. Trief PM, Yuan HA: The use of the MMPI in a chronic back pain rehabilitation program. *J Clin Psychol* 39:46–53, 1983.
98. Waring EM, Weisz GM, Bailey SI: Predictive factors in the treatment of low back pain by surgical intervention. In Bonica JJ, Albe-Fessard D (eds): *Advances in Pain Research and Therapy*. New York, Raven Press, 1976, vol 1, pp 939–942.
99. Herron LD, Pheasant HC: Changes in MMPI profiles after low-back surgery. *Spine* 7:591–597, 1982.
100. Watkins RG, O'Brien JP, Draugelis R, Jones D: Comparisons of preoperative and postoperative MMPI data in chronic back patients. *Spine* 11:385–390, 1986.
101. Brennan AF, Barrett CL, Garretson HD: The prediction of chronic pain outcome by psychological variables. *Int J Psychiatry Med* 16:373–387, 1986–87.
102. Henrichs TF: MMPI profiles of chronic pain patients: some methodological considerations that concern clusters and descriptors. *J Clin Psychol* 43:650–660, 1987.
103. Sines JO: Actuarial methods as appropriate strategy for the validation of diagnostic tests. *Psychol Rev* 71:517–523, 1964.
104. Dolce JJ, Crocker MF, Dolesy DM: Prediction of outcome among chronic pain patients. *Behav Res Ther* 24:313–319, 1986.
105. Pilowsky I, Spence ND: Patterns of illness behavior in patients with intractable pain. *J Psychosom Res* 19:279–287, 1975.
106. Pilowsky I, Spence ND: Illness behavior syndromes associated with intractable pain. *Pain* 2:61–71, 1976.
107. Ransford AO, Cairns D, Mooney V: The pain drawing as an aid to the psychologic evaluation of patients with low-back pain. *Spine* 1:127–134, 1976.
108. Leavitt F, Garron DC: Detection of psychological disturbance in patients with low back pain. *J Psychosom Res* 23:149–154, 1979.
109. Derogatis LR: *SCL-90 Administration and Scoring Procedures Manual*. Baltimore, Johns Hopkins University Press, 1977.
110. Millon T, Green C, Meagher R: *Millon Behavioral Health Inventory Manual*, ed 3. Minneapolis, National Computer Systems, 1982.
111. Pilowsky I: Pain as abnormal illness behavior. *J Hum Stress* 4:22–27, 1978.
112. Pilowsky I: Psychodynamic aspects of the pain experience. In Sternbach RA (ed): *The Psychology of Pain*, ed 1. New York, Raven Press, 1979, pp 203–217.
113. Mechanic D: Effects of psychological stress on perceptions of physical health and use of medical and psychiatric facilities. *J Hum Stress* 4:26–32, 1978.
114. Pilowsky I, Spence ND: Is illness behavior related to chronicity in patients with intractable pain: *Pain* 2:167–173, 1976.
115. Pilowsky I, Spence ND: Pain and illness behaviour: a comparative study. *J Psychosom Res* 20:131–134, 1976.
116. Pilowsky I, Spence ND: Pain, anger, and illness behaviour. *J Psychosom Res* 20:411–416, 1976.
117. Pilowsky I, Smith QP, Katsikitis M: Illness behaviour and general practice utilisation: a prospective study. *J Psychosom Res* 31:177–183, 1987.
118. Pilowsky I, Chapman CR, Bonica JJ: Pain, depression, and illness behavior in a pain clinic population. *Pain* 4:183–192, 1977.
119. Speculand B, Goss AN, Spence ND, Pilowsky I: Intractable facial pain and illness behaviour. *Pain* 11:213–219, 1981.
120. Speculand B, Goss AN, Hughes A, Spence ND, Pilowsky I: Temporo-mandibular joint dysfunction: pain and illness behaviour. *Pain* 17:139–150, 1983.
121. Clayer JR, Bookless C, Roso MW: Neurosis and conscious

symptom exaggeration: its differentiation by the Illness Behaviour Questionnaire. *J Psychosom Res* 28:237–241, 1984.
122. Large RG, Mullins PR: Illness behaviour profiles in chronic pain: the Auckland experience. *Pain* 10:231–239, 1981.
123. Byrne DG, White HM: Dimensions of illness behavior in survivors of myocardial infarction. *J Psychosom Res* 22:485–491, 1978.
124. Pilowsky I, Spence ND, Waddy JL: Illness behaviour and coronary artery bypass surgery. *J Psychosom Res* 23:39–44, 1979.
125. Main CJ, Waddell G: Psychometric construction and validity of the Pilowsky Illness Behaviour Questionnaire in British patients with chronic low back pain. *Pain* 28:13–25, 1987.
126. Zonderman AB, Heft MW, Costa PT: Does the Illness Behavior Questionnaire measure abnormal illness behavior? *Health Psychol* 4:425–436, 1985.
127. Pilowsky I, Spence ND: *Manual for the Illness Behaviour Questionnaire*, ed 2. Adelaide, South Australia, Department of Psychiatry, Royal Adelaide Hospital, University of Adelaide, 1983.
128. Eysenck HJ, Eysenck SBG: *The Manual of the Eysenck Personality Inventory*. San Diego, CA, Educational and Industrial Testing Service, 1968.
129. Keefe FJ, Crisson JE, Maltbie A, Bradley L, Gil KM: Illness behavior as a predictor of pain and overt behavior patterns in chronic low back pain patients. *J Psychosom Res* 30:543–551, 1986.
130. Melzack R: The McGill Pain Questionnaire: major properties and scoring methods. *Pain* 1:277–299, 1975.
131. Schwartz DP, DeGood DE: Global appropriateness of pain drawings: blind ratings predict patterns of psychological distress and litigation status. *Pain* 19:383–388, 1984.
132. Margolis RB, Tait RC, Krause SJ: A rating system for use with patient pain drawings. *Pain* 24:57–65, 1986.
133. McNeill TW, Sinkora G, Leavitt F: Psychologic classification of low-back pain patients: a prognostic tool. *Spine* 11:955–959, 1986.
134. Von Baeyer CL, Bergstrom KJ, Brodwin MG, Brodwin SK: Invalid use of pain drawings in psychological screening of back pain patients. *Pain* 16:103–107, 1983.
135. Toomey TC, Gover VF, Jones BN: Spatial distribution of pain: a descriptive characteristic of chronic pain. *Pain* 17:289–300, 1983.
136. Leavitt F, Garron DC: Validity of a back pain classification scale among patients with low back pain not associated with demonstrable organic disease. *J Psychosom Res* 23:301–306, 1979.
137. Leavitt F, Garron DC: Validity of a back pain classification scale for detecting psychological disturbance as measured by the MMPI. *J Clin Psychol* 36:186–189, 1980.
138. Leavitt F: Comparison of three measures for detecting psychological disturbance in patients with low back pain. *Pain* 13:299–305, 1982.
139. Sanders SH: Cross-validation of the Back Pain Classification Scale with chronic, intractable pain patients. *Pain* 22:271–277, 1985.
140. Biedermann HJ, Monga TN, Shanks GL, McGhie A: The classification of back pain patients: functional versus organic. *J Psychosom Res* 30:273–276, 1986.
141. Richter JE, Obrecht WF, Bradley LA, Young LD, Anderson KO, Castell DO: Psychological profiles of patients with the nutcracker esophagus. *Dig Dis Sci* 31:131–138, 1986.

142. Gatchel RJ, Mayer TG, Capra P, Barnett J, Diamond P: Millon Behavioral Health Inventory: its utility in predicting physical function in patients with low back pain. *Arch Phys Med Rehabil* 67:878–882, 1986.
143. Sweet JJ, Breuer SR, Hazlewood LA, Toye R, Pawl RP: The Millon Behavioral Health Inventory: concurrent and predictive validity in a pain treatment center. *J Behav Med* 8:215–226, 1985.
144. Gatchel RJ, Deckel AW, Weinberg N, Smith JE: The utility of the Millon Behavioral Health Inventory in the study of chronic headaches. *Headache* 25:49–54, 1985.
145. Shutty MS, DeGood DE, Schwartz DP: Psychological dimensions of distress in chronic pain patients: a factor analytic study of Symptom Checklist-90 responses. *J Consult Clin Psychol* 54:836–842, 1986.
146. Duckro PN, Margolis RB, Tait RC: Psychological assessment in chronic pain. *J Clin Psychol* 41:499–504, 1985.
147. Melzack R, Wall PD: Pain mechanisms: a new theory. *Science* 50:971–979, 1965.
148. Fernandez E: A classification system of cognitive coping strategies for pain. *Pain* 26:141–151, 1986.
149. Turk DC, Rudy TE: Assessment of cognitive factors in chronic pain: a worthwhile enterprise? *J Consult Clin Psychol* 54:760–768, 1986.
150. Gray D: The treatment strategies of arthritis sufferers. *Soc Sci Med* 21:507–515, 1985.
151. Schwartz DP, DeGood DE, Shutty MS: Direct assessment of beliefs and attitudes of chronic pain patients. *Arch Phys Med Rehabil* 66:806–809, 1985.
152. Sternbach RA: Pain and "hassles" in the United States: findings of the Nuprin Pain Report. *Pain* 27:69–80, 1986.
153. Wack JT, Turk DC: Latent structure of strategies used to cope with nociceptive stimulation. *Health Psychol* 3:27–43, 1984.
154. Felton BJ, Revenson TA: Coping with chronic illness: a study of illness controllability and the influence of coping strategies on psychological adjustment. *J Consult Clin Psychol* 52:343–353, 1984.
155. Felton BJ, Revenson TA, Hinrichsen GA: Coping and adjustment in chronically ill adults. *Soc Sci Med* 18:889–898, 1984.
156. Crisson J, Keefe FJ, Wilkins RH, Cook WA, Muhlbaier LH: Self-report of depressive symptoms in low back pain patients. *J Clin Psychol* 42:425–430, 1986.
157. Krishnan KRR, France RD, Pelton S, McCann UD, Davidson J, Urban BJ: Chronic pain and depression. I. Classification of depression in chronic low back pain patients. *Pain* 22:279–287, 1985.
158. Blumer D, Heilbronn M: Chronic pain as a variant of depressive disease: the pain-prone disorder. *J Nerv Ment Dis* 170:381–406, 1982.
159. Ahles TA, Yunus MB, Masi AT: Is chronic pain a variant of depressive disease? The case of primary fibromyalgia syndrome. *Pain* 29:105–111, 1987.
160. Beck AT: *Depression: Clinical, Experimental and Theoretical Aspects*. York, PA, University of Pennsylvania Press, 1967.
161. Lefebvre MF: Cognitive distortion and cognitive errors in depressed psychiatric and low back pain patients. *J Consult Clin Psychol* 49:517–525, 1981.
162. Smith TW, Aberger EW, Follick MJ, Ahern DK: Cognitive distortion and psychological distress in chronic low back pain. *J Consult Clin Psychol* 54:573–575, 1986.

163. Smith TW, Follick MJ, Ahern DK, Adams A: Cognitive distortion and disability in chronic low back pain. *Cogn Ther Res* 10:201–210, 1986.
164. Rosenstiel AK, Keefe FJ: The use of coping strategies in chronic low back pain patients: relationship to patient characteristics and current adjustment. *Pain* 17:33–44, 1983.
165. Turner JA, Clancy S: Strategies for coping with chronic low back pain: relationship to pain and disability. *Pain* 24:355–364, 1986.
166. Gross AR: The effect of coping strategies on the relief of pain following surgical intervention for lower back pain. *Psychosom Med* 48:229–241, 1986.
167. Keefe FJ, Caldwell DS, Queen KT, Gil KM, Martinez S, Crosson JE, Ogden W, Nunley J: Pain coping strategies in osteoarthritis patients. *J Consult Clin Psychol* 55:208–212, 1987.
168. Turk DC: Cognitive behavioral techniques in the management of pain. In Foreyt JP, Rathjen DP (eds): *Cognitive Behavior Therapy*. New York, Plenum Press, 1978, pp 199–232.
169. Turk DC, Meichenbaum DH, Genest M: *Pain and Behavioral Medicine: A Cognitive-Behavioral Perspective*. New York, Guilford Press, 1983.
170. Chapman CR, Casey KL, Dubner R, Foley KM, Gracely RH, Reading AE: Pain measurement: an overview. *Pain* 22:1–31, 1985.
171. Syrjala KL, Chapman CR: Measurement of clinical pain: a review and integration of research findings. In Benedetti C, Chapman CR, Moricca G (eds): *Advances in Pain Research and Therapy*. New York, Raven Press, 1984, vol 7, pp 71–101.
172. Chapman CR: Measurement of pain: problems and issues. In Bonica JJ, Albe-Fessard D (eds): *Advances in Pain Research and Therapy*. New York, Raven Press, 1976, vol 1, pp 345–353.
173. Huskisson EC: Measurement of pain. *Lancet* 2:1127–1131, 1974.
174. Wolff BB: Behavioral measurement of human pain. In Sternbach RA (ed): *The Psychology of Pain*, ed 1. New York, Raven Press, 1978, pp 129–168.
175. Heft MW, Parker SR: An experimental basis for revising the graphic rating scale for pain. *Pain* 19:153–161, 1984.
176. Merskey H: The perception and measurement of pain. *J Psychosom Res* 17:251–255, 1973.
177. Kremer E, Atkinson JH, Ignelzi RJ: Measurement of pain: patient preference does not confound pain measurement. *Pain* 10:241–248, 1981.
178. Scott PJ, Huskisson EC: Graphic representation of pain. *Pain* 2:175–184, 1976.
179. Reading AE: A comparison of pain rating scales. *J Psychosom Res* 24:119–124, 1979.
180. Twycross RG: The measurement of pain in terminal carcinoma. *J Int Med Res* 4:58–67, 1976.
181. Sriwatanakul K, Kelvie W, Lasagna L, Calimlim JF, Weis OF, Mehta G: Studies with different types of visual analog scales for measurement of pain. *Clin Pharmacol Ther* 34:234–239, 1983.
182. Scott PJ, Ansell BM, Huskisson EC: Measurement of pain in juvenile chronic polyarthritis. *Ann Rheum Dis* 36:186–187, 1977.
183. Price DD, McGrath PA, Rafii A, Buckingham B: The validation of visual analogue scales as ratio scale measures for chronic and experimental pain. *Pain* 17:45–56, 1983.
184. Gracely RH: Psychophysical assessment of human pain. In Bonica JJ, Liebeskind JC, Albe-Fessard, D (eds): *Advances in Pain Research and Therapy*. New York, Raven Press, 1979, vol 3, pp 805–824.
185. Carlsson AM: Assessment of chronic pain. I. Aspects of the reliability and validity of the visual analogue scale. *Pain* 16:87–101, 1983.
186. Dixon JS, Bird HA: Reproducibility along a 10 cm vertical visual analogue scale. *Ann Rheum Dis* 40:87–89, 1981.
187. Scott PJ, Huskisson EC: Accuracy of subjective measurements made with or without previous scores: an important source of error in serial measurement of subjective states. *Ann Rheum Dis* 38:558–559, 1979.
188. Aun C, Lam YM, Collett B: Evaluation of the use of visual analogue scale in Chinese patients. *Pain* 25:215–221, 1986.
189. Million R, Hall W, Nilsen KH, Baker RD, Jayson IV: Assessment of the progress of the back-pain patient. *Spine* 7:204–212, 1982.
190. Melzack R, Torgerson WS: On the language of pain. *Anesthesiology* 34:50–59, 1971.
191. Ljunggren AE: Descriptions of pain and other sensory modalities in patients with lumbago-sciatica and herniated intervertebral discs. Interview administration of an adapted McGill Pain Questionnaire. *Pain* 16:265–276, 1983.
192. Ketovuouri H, Pöntinen PJ: A pain vocabulary in Finnish: the Finnish Pain Questionnaire. *Pain* 11:247–253, 1981.
193. Maiani G, Sanavio E: Semantics of pain in Italy: the Italian version of the McGill Pain Questionnaire. *Pain* 22:399–405, 1985.
194. Radvila A, Adler RH, Galeazzi RL, Vorkauf H: The development of a German language (Berne) pain questionnaire and its application in a situation causing acute pain. *Pain* 28:185–195, 1987.
195. Hunter M: The Headache Scale: a new approach to the assessment of headache pain based on pain descriptions. *Pain* 16:361–373, 1983.
196. Johanshahi M, Hunter M, Philips C: The Headache Scale: an examination of its reliability and validity. *Headache* 26:76–82, 1986.
197. Graham C, Bond S, Gerkovich MN, Cook MR: Use of the McGill Pain Quesionnaire in the assessment of cancer pain: replicability and consistency. *Pain* 8:377–387, 1980.
198. Walsh TD, Leber B: Measurement of chronic pain: Visual analog scales and McGill Melzack Pain Questionnaire compared. In Bonica JJ, Lindblom U, Iggo A (eds): *Advances in Pain Research and Therapy*. New York, Raven Press, 1983, vol 5, pp 897–899.
199. Mendelson G, Selwood TS: Measurement of chronic pain: a correlation study of verbal and nonverbal scales. *J Behav Assess* 3:263–269, 1981.
200. Crockett DJ, Prkachin KM, Craig KD: Factors of the language of pain in patient and volunteer groups. *Pain* 4:175–183, 1977.
201. Crockett DJ, Prkachin KM, Craig KD, Greenstein H: Social influences on factored dimensions of the McGill Pain Questionnaire. *J Psychosom Res* 30:461–469, 1986.
202. Reading AE: A comparison of the McGill Pain Questionnaire in chronic and acute pain. *Pain* 13:185–192, 1982.
203. McCreary C, Turner J, Dawson E: Principal dimensions of the pain experience and psychological disturbance in chronic low back pain patients. *Pain* 11:85–92, 1981.

204. Prieto EJ, Hopson L, Bradley LA, Byrne M, Geisinger KF, Midax D, Marchisello PJ: The language of the low back pain: factor structure of the McGill Pain Questionnaire. *Pain* 8:11–19, 1980.
205. Reading AE: The internal structure of the McGill Pain Questionnaire in dysmenorrhea patients. *Pain* 7:353–358, 1979.
206. Burckhardt CS: The use of the McGill Pain Questionnaire in assessing arthritis pain. *Pain* 19:305–314, 1984.
207. Byrne M, Troy A, Bradley LA, Marchisello PJ, Geisinger KF, Van der Heide LH, Prieto EJ: Cross-validation of the factor structure of the McGill Pain Questionnaire. *Pain* 13:193–201, 1982.
208. Turk DC, Rudy TE, Salovey P: The McGill Pain Questionnaire reconsidered: confirming the factor structure and examining appropriate uses. *Pain* 21:385–397, 1985.
209. Kremer E, Atkinson JH: Pain measurement: construct validity of the affective dimension of the McGill Pain Questionnaire with chronic benign pain patients. *Pain* 11:93–100, 1981.
210. Hunter M, Philips C: The experience of headache: an assessment of the qualities of tension headache pain. *Pain* 10:209–219, 1981.
211. Kremer EF, Atkinson JH, Kremer AM: The language of pain: affective descriptors of pain are a better predictor of psychological disturbance than pattern of sensory and affective descriptors. *Pain* 16:185–192, 1983.
212. McCreary C, Turner J: Psychological disorder and pain perception. *Health Psychol* 2:1–10, 1983.
213. Dubuisson D, Melzack R: Classification of clinical pain descriptions by multiple group discriminant analysis. *Exp Neurol* 51:480–487, 1976.
214. Grushka M, Sessle BJ: Applicability of the McGill Pain Questionnaire to the differentiation of "toothache" pain. *Pain* 19:49–57, 1984.
215. Wagstaff S, Smith OV, Wood PHN: Verbal pain descriptors used by patients with arthritis. *Ann Rheum Dis* 44:262–265, 1985.
216. Melzack R, Terrence C, Fromm G, Amsel R: Trigeminal neuralgia and atypical facial pain: use of the McGill Pain Questionnaire for discrimination and diagnosis. *Pain* 27:297–302, 1986.
217. Kremer EF, Atkinson JH: Pain language: affect. *J Psychosom Res* 28:125–132, 1984.
218. Atkinson JH, Kremer EF, Ignelzi RJ: Diffusion of pain language with affective disturbance confounds differential diagnosis. *Pain* 12:375–384, 1982.
219. Reading AE, Everitt BS, Sledmere CM: The McGill Pain Questionnaire: a replication of its construction. *Br J Clin Psychol* 21:339–349, 1982.
220. Charter RA, Nehemkis AM: The language of pain intensity and complexity: new methods of scoring the McGill Pain Questionnaire. *Percept Motor Skills* 56:519–537, 1983.
221. Melzack R, Katz J, Jeans ME: The role of compensation in chronic pain: analysis using a new method of scoring the McGill Pain Questionnaire. *Pain* 23:101–112, 1985.
222. Lahuerta J, Campbell J: Assessment of cancer pain by the McGill Pain Questionnaire: results of two scoring methods in a sample of British patients and comparison with previous studies. *Br J Med Psychol* 59:89–95, 1986.
223. Gracely RH, McGrath P, Dubner R: Ratio scales of sensory and affective pain descriptors. *Pain* 5:5–18, 1978.
224. Gracely RH, McGrath P, Dubner R: Validity and sensitivity of ratio scales of sensory and affective verbal pain descriptors: manipulation of affect by diazepam. *Pain* 5:19–29, 1978.
225. Gracely RH, Dubner R, McGrath P, Heft M: New methods of pain measurement and their application to pain control. *Int Dental J* 28:52–65, 1978.
226. Heft MW, Gracely RH, Dubner R, McGrath PA: A validation model for verbal descriptor scaling of human clinical pain. *Pain* 9:363–373, 1980.
227. Gracely RH, Wolskee PJ: Semantic functional measurement of pain: integrating perception and language. *Pain* 15:389–398, 1983.
228. Urban BJ, Keefe FJ, France RD: A study of psychophysical scaling in chronic pain patients. *Pain* 20:157–168, 1984.
229. Tursky B, Jammer LD, Friedman R: The Pain Perception Profile: a psychophysical approach to the assessment of pain report. *Behav Ther* 13:376–394, 1982.
230. Hunter M, Philips C, Rachman S: Memory for pain. *Pain* 6:35–46, 1979.
231. Linton SJ, Melin L: The accuracy of remembering chronic pain. *Pain* 13:281–285, 1982.
232. Linton SJ, Götestam KG: A clinical comparison of two pain scales: correlation, remembering chronic pain, and a measure of compliance. *Pain* 17:57–65, 1983.
233. Kent G: Memory of dental pain. *Pain* 21:187–194, 1985.
234. Roche PA, Gijsbers K: A comparison of memory for induced ischaemic pain and chronic rheumatoid pain. *Pain* 25:337–343, 1986.
235. Eich E, Reeves JL, Jaeger B, Graff-Radford SB: Memory for pain: relation between past and present pain intensity. *Pain* 23:375–379, 1985.
236. Payne B, Norfleet MA: Chronic pain and the family: a review. *Pain* 26:1–22, 1986.
237. Maruta T, Osborne D: Sexual activity in chronic pain patients. *Psychosomatics* 19:531–537, 1978.
238. Maruta T, Osborne D, Swanson DW, Halling JM: Chronic pain patients and spouses: marital and sexual adjustment. *Mayo Clin Proc* 56:307–310, 1981.
239. Mohamed SN, Weisz GM, Waring EM: The relationship of chronic pain to depression, marital adjustment, and family dynamics. *Pain* 5:285–292, 1978.
240. Ahern DK, Adams AE, Follick MJ: Emotional and marital disturbance in spouses of chronic low back pain patients. *Clin J Pain* 1:69–74, 1985.
241. Flor H, Turk DC, Scholz OB: Impact of chronic pain on the spouse: marital, emotional and physical consequences. *J Psychosom Res* 31:63–71, 1987.
242. Shanfield SB, Heiman EM, Cope DN, Jones JR: Pain and the marital relationship: psychiatric distress. *Pain* 7:343–351, 1979.
243. Swanson DW, Maruta T: The family's viewpoint of chronic pain. *Pain* 8:163–166, 1980.
244. Prkachin KM, Craig KD: Influencing non-verbal expressions of pain: signal detection analyses. *Pain* 21:399–409, 1985.
245. Craig KD: Social modeling influences: pain in context. In Sternbach RA (ed): *The Psychology of Pain*, ed 2. New York, Raven Press, 1986, pp 67–95.
246. Gentry WD, Shows WD, Thomas M: Chronic low-back pain: a psychological profile. *Psychosomatics* 15:174–177, 1974.
247. Violon A, Giurgea D: Familial models for chronic pain. *Pain* 18:199–203, 1984.
248. Flor H, Kerns RD, Turk DC: The role of spouse reinforce-

ment, perceived pain, and activity levels of chronic pain patients. *J Psychosom Res* 31:251–259, 1987.
249. Anderson LP, Rehm LP: The relationship between strategies of coping and perception of pain in three chronic pain groups. *J Clin Psychol* 40:1170–1177, 1984.
250. Block AR, Kremer EF, Gaylor M: Behavioral treatment of chronic pain: the spouse as a discriminative cue for pain behavior. *Pain* 9:243–252, 1980.
251. Block AR: An investigation of the response of the spouse to chronic pain behavior. *Psychosom Med* 43:415–422, 1981.
252. Benedetti C, Chapman CR, Colpitts YH, Chen AC: Effect of nitrous oxide concentration on event-related potentials during painful tooth stimulation. *Anesthesiology* 56:360–364, 1982.
253. Cleeland CS, Shacham S, Dahl JL, Orrison W: CSF β-endorphin and the severity of pain. *Neurology* 34:378–380, 1984.
254. Terenius L: Endorphins in chronic pain. In Bonica JJ, Liebeskind JC, Albe-Fessard D (eds): *Advances in Pain Research and Therapy*. New York, Raven Press, 1979, vol 3, pp 459–471.
255. Terenius L: Families of opioid peptides and classes of opioid receptors. In Fields HL, Dubner R, Cervero F (eds): *Advances in Pain Research and Therapy*. New York, Raven Press, 1985, vol 9, pp 463–477.
256. Dolce JJ, Raczynski JM: Neuromuscular activity and electromyography in painful backs: psychological and biomechanical models in assessment and treatment. *Psychol Bull* 97:502–520, 1985.
257. Ahern DK, Follick MJ, Council JR, Laser-Wolston N: Reliability of lumbar paravertebral EMG assessment in chronic low back pain. *Arch Phys Med Rehabil* 67:762–765, 1986.
258. Biedermann H-J: Comments on the reliability of muscle activity comparisons in EMG biofeedback research with back pain patients. *Biofeedback Self Regul* 9:451–458, 1984.
259. Cobb CR, deVries HA, Urban RT, Luekens CA, Bagg RJ: Electrical activity in muscle pain. *Am J Phys Med* 54:80–87, 1975.
260. Holmes TH, Wolff HG: Life situations, emotions and backache. *Psychosom Med* 14:18–33, 1952.
261. Cohen MJ, Swanson GA, Naliboff BD, Schandler SL, McArthur DL: Comparison of electromyographic response patterns during posture and stress tasks in chronic low back pain patterns and control. *J Psychosom Res* 30:135–141, 1986.
262. Collins GA, Cohen MJ, Naliboff BD, Schandler SL: Comparative analysis of paraspinal and frontal EMG, heart rate and skin conductance in chronic low back pain patients and normals to various postures and stress. *Scand J Rehab Med* 14:36–46, 1982.
263. Burish TG: EMG biofeedback in the treatment of stress-related disorders. In Prokop CK, Bradley LA (eds): *Medical Psychology: Contributions to Behavioral Medicine*. New York, Academic Press, 1981, pp 395–421.
264. Flor H, Turk DC, Koehler H: Efficacy of EMG biofeedback, pseudotherapy and conventional medical treatment for chronic rheumatic low back pain. *Pain* 17:21–31, 1983.
265. Belar CD, Cohen JL: The use of EMG feedback and progressive relaxation in the treatment of a woman with chronic back pain. *Biofeedback Self Regul* 4:345–353, 1979.
266. Nigel AJ, Fioscher-Williams M: Treatment of low back strain with electromyographic biofeedback and relaxation training. *Psychosomatics* 21:495–499, 1980.
267. Nouwen A: EMG biofeedback used to reduce standing levels of paraspinal muscle tension in chronic low back pain. *Pain* 17:353–360, 1983.
268. Peck CL, Kraft GH: Electromyographic biofeedback for pain related to muscle tension. *Arch Surg* 112:889–895, 1977.
269. Bush C, Ditto B, Feuerstein M: A controlled evaluation of paraspinal EMG biofeedback in the treatment of chronic low back pain. *Health Psychol* 4:307–321, 1985.
270. Biedermann HJ, McGhie A, Monya TN, Shanks GL: Perceived and actual control in EMG treatment of back pain. *Behav Res Ther* 25:137–147, 1987.
271. Wolf SL, Basmajian JV, Russ TC, Kutner M: Normative data on low back mobility and activity levels. *Am J Phys Med* 58:217–229, 1979.
272. Wolf SL, Nacht M, Kelly JL: EMG biofeedback training during dynamic movement for low back pain patients. *Behav Ther* 13:395–406, 1982.
273. Cram JR, Steger JC: EMG scanning in the diagnosis of chronic pain. *Biofeedback Self Regul* 8:229–241, 1983.
274. Jones AL, Wolf SL: Treating chronic low back pain—EMG biofeedback training during movement. *Phys Ther* 60:58–63, 1980.
275. Flor H, Turk DC, Birbaumer N: Assessment of stress-related psychophysiological reactions in chronic back pain patients. *J Consult Clin Psychol* 53:354–364, 1985.
276. Jaeger B, Reeves JL: Quantification of changes in myofascial trigger point sensitivity with the pressure algometer following passive stretch. *Pain* 27:203–210, 1986.
277. Wolfe F, Hawley DJ, Cathey MA, Caro X, Russell IJ: Fibrositis: symptom frequency and criteria for diagnosis. An evaluation of 291 rheumatic disease patients and 58 normal individuals. *J Rheumatol* 12:1159–1163, 1985.
278. Boxtel AV, Goudsward P, Janssen K: Absolute and proportional resting EMG levels in muscle contraction and migraine headache patients. *Headache* 23:215–222, 1983.
279. Tfelt-Hansen P, Lous I, Olesen J: Prevalence and significance of muscle tenderness during common migraine attacks. *Headache* 21:49–54, 1981.
280. Bengtsson A, Henriksson K-G, Larsson JL: Muscle biopsy in primary fibromyalgia: light-microscopical and histochemical findings. *Scand J Rheumatol* 15:1–6, 1986.
281. Reeves JL, Jaeger B, Graff-Radford SB: Reliability of the pressure algometer as a measure of myofascial trigger point sensitivity. *Pain* 24:313–321, 1986.
282. Jensen K, Andersen HO, Olesen J, Lindblom U: Pressure-pain threshold in human temporal region. Evaluation of a new pressure algometer. *Pain* 25:313–323, 1986.
283. Bradley LA, Young LD, Anderson KO, Turner RA, Agudelo CA, McDaniel LK, Pisko EJ, Semble EL: Effects of psychological therapy on pain behavior of rheumatoid arthritis patients: treatment outcome and six-month follow-up. *Arthritis Rheum* 30:1105–1114, 1987.

chapter 46
Early Recognition

Marc Hertzman, M.D.
Bruce M. Smoller, M.D.

The ideas of prevention and early intervention are among the cornerstones of public health work, under the names "primary" and "secondary prevention." They assume that disease is best deterred from happening altogether, or, failing this possibility, detected as early in the course of illness as possible, and arrested or retarded. Prevention/early intervention (hereafter designated P/I unless clearly one or the other is intended solely) subsumes a number of other propositions about our ability to intervene successfully, such as:

Without P/I the course of illness would be inevitably downhill, and/or

Even if the illness is self-limited, significant harm can occur while the course is being run, and this weakens the organism (patient) in harmful ways, which may make future episodes of illness more likely, or more damaging. In other words, tissue damage may be cumulative.

The earlier detection occurs, the greater the likelihood that an illness can be arrested, reversed, or retarded in the rate of its progression.

We have the appropriate tools of detection available, or,

We can effectively prevent a disease, whether or not we know its exact cause, or,

An effective intervention to retard the rate of progress, or ameliorate an illness exists.

P/I is likely to accomplish significantly more good than the potential harm of which it is capable.

The elaboration of this list of assumptions contained in the notion of P/I should be considered the public health advocate's Koch's postulates. That is, unless a reasonable minimum set of them is fulfilled, P/I may be worthless, or actually hazardous to one's health.

In this chapter we attempt to explore the idea of P/I as it may apply to pain, and especially the prevention of, or early intervention in, the chronic pain syndrome (CPS). For present purposes, generally CPS means the most widely accepted definition thereof: unremitting experience of pain that persists more than 6 months, and may not be consonant with the extent of the original injury, or the anatomic distribution of the pain described. As this book amply documents, CPS is one of the main unconquered territories in medicine generally, and particularly in industrial and compensation forensic medicine. One recent innovation in the pain field is an attempt at classification. How well does this suit P/I? We attempt to discuss the question from several different vantage points.

It is also clear that there are some grounds for cynicism about the subject of P/I generally, and particularly as it applies to CPS. We feel duty bound to let the reader know from the outset what our prejudices are: mainly, that much of the enthusiasm demonstrated for aggressive early identification of CPS and intervention is founded upon shaky evidence, or none at all. This assessment emerges repeatedly from our review in this chapter. However, in fairness to the reader, we attempt to present as balanced a point of view as possible, in hopes that the material will stimulate readers to make up their own minds, perhaps by pursuing the evidence to its original sources, and not simply relying upon our summary (but, we hope, thoughtful) judgments. After all, it is much easier to be a critic than it is to be a synthesizer. We recognize that clinicians must function in a world where diagnostic and treatment decisions are made every day, without the luxury of scientific backing, or perhaps the resources or time to weigh them at each step of a treatment regimen. To the busy clinician we hope to offer some guide for the perplexed, although no substitute for continuing scholarship.

PRIMARY PREVENTION, EDUCATION, AND EFFECTIVENESS

Education, according to a despairing, waggish educator, is what we throw at a social problem when we do not have any solution to it. This somewhat irreverent quip may, in fact, aptly characterize much of education in socially significant health and mental health problems. The idea of education before the fact, or education to prevent recurrence or worsening of a problem, is seductively attractive, often in naive ways. For prevention education to have a chance of succeeding, however, a number of conditions have to apply.

For one, there must be some reason to think that there is really a body of knowledge that, if mastered, will shed genuine enlightenment upon behavior. An example may be taken from the field of drug abuse prevention, the analogies to which are in some respects quite similar to CPS. When drug abuse education was first instituted in secondary and elementary schools, the flair of interest in it quickly turned to dismay. Even where teachers were prepared to convey information about the physiology of drugs—information often better known to the student users than to the teachers—the teaching appeared to have little impact upon students. At times it even had a negative impact: students who may not have previously been attracted to drugs, or who had limited their usage, had possible new experiences brought to their attention.

How could this happen? Perhaps the idea of what constitutes learning was somewhat narrowly conceptualized. In order for learning to change behavior, clearly more than the knowledge base must be affected. At a minimum, learning also includes motivations and behavioral responses. These, in turn, are conditioned by culture, previous experience, and social system influences.

The consequences of unidimensional thinking are, as one might expect, to handicap a program before it ever begins. Thus, in the recent revival of concern and interest in doing something constructive about drug abuse, there seems to be greater thought about the impact of education programs on drug abuse.

Public service announcements are noble, and difficult to oppose but for their expense. However, do they work? There are few data on the subject. A reasonable guess is that public service announcements and media advertisements may increase public consciousness. However, there is little reason to think that they convey even slightly complex information, or otherwise change behavior.

Of course, in P/I campaigns, the idea is to change public attitudes. How effective are they? Public images, as of popular figures, are notoriously fickle. On the other hand, given that attitudes are difficult to move and that fundamental switches in attitude are glacial, once attitudes do begin to shift, their new formations are likely to last a long time. It is every nonprofit agency public affairs specialist's dream to be able to achieve the latter. In fact, it rarely occurs.

In the classroom it is probably not unreasonable to be able to expect to demonstrate differences in information absorption on a short-term basis. Most assessments of educational programs are heavily weighted on short-term evaluations. Even getting children and adults to think in new ways can probably be considered a reasonable expectation in the short run from a P/I educational program.

This, however, begs the questions: how long-lasting is the effect, how widespread, and to what extent does it generalize to "real life" situations outside the classroom? These questions are much more difficult to address. Also, assuming that periodic reenforcement ("refresher courses") might maintain hard won gains is risky at best.

There are very few readily available data on this subject when it comes to chronic pain. This is of some interest, in that there are at least two types of P/I education programs, and a third that appears to be gaining credibility. The first is that of industrial accident prevention—"This is a hard hat area" publicity, as well as more formal didactic sessions and supervision for employees working in situations at risk. Elsewhere in this chapter we comment on the material that Strang has reviewed (1). It generally shows fairly limited benefits demonstrated to date for such programs, with no good fix on the cost/benefit ratio of mounting a campaign. In addition to these limitations, which seem somewhat more restrictive than in some other types of health P/I efforts, we also note that there is little or no information available on the longer term sustainability questions, the core evaluation issues upon which the advisability of P/I as a positive course should be measured.

The second type of educational program is that embodied in so-called back schools, which have shown a modest proliferation. Typically, they may be attached to a chronic pain clinic treatment operation, and may be prescribed as part of the rehabilitation program. Physical therapists (PTs) are the usual practitioners in them. The material is not just lectures and reading, although this may be part of the curriculum. Rather, PTs do what they know how to do best, which is to manipulate and demonstrate first passively, moving the patient's body, and soon actively, getting the patient to follow by small increments in doing motions themselves in the least hurtful ways.

This approach shows more promise. For one thing, it is literally "hands on." Theoretically, at least, it appears to incorporate several different elements of behavioral learning theory from the outset. Learning is active, not just passive. There is an emotional component, not only in the physical aspects of touching, but also in the informal talking that surrounds the instructional, supervised exercise parts of the curriculum. If thoughtfully conceived and constructed, such back schools are coordinated with other aspects of the treatment program, so that the physicians, PTs, and others are making use of their mutual findings for the patient's benefit.

It would be notable if we could say that evaluation data and follow-ups of back schools support this encouraging beginning. However, to the best of our knowledge, this has not been done. Clearly, it is a fruitful potential subject to pursue, either alone or in connection with other modalities of treatment.

Lately the fashion in industrial prevention programs has swung toward the mounting of "wellness" programs. These vary substantially. What may distinguish them from other generations of corporate health plans, or industrial accident prevention and containment campaigns, is:

1. They attempt to emphasize a variety of regular, health-promoting behaviors. These range from exercise and physical fitness training to "Smoke-enders" groups in the work place.
2. Wellness programs employ a range of therapies, and, although they may incorporate some psychotherapy, they tend to use biofeedback, relaxation techniques, and even behavioral modification.

Much the same assessment could be made concerning data on the efficacy of wellness programs as was done about back schools. They are relatively new, although not so much so that study has been impossible. Their promoters (fortunately) do seem to be at least somewhat more modest in public claims of their usefulness than some other P/I specialists have been. However, they are basically in the position of promoting approaches of uncertain efficacy and sustainability.

P/EARLY I WITH THE CPS-PRONE PATIENT

Although P/I is hard to study, and worthwhile studies in CPS are few and far between, there are several areas in which scientific work both is promising and offers some clinically practical applications. Probably the most energy has gone into the effort to identify which surgical patients will do well or poorly following surgery. A related, but somewhat independent subject is consideration of psychological predispositions to postsurgical depression, and the persistence of psychologically linked symptomatology.

The majority of work on surgical prediction is partially retrospective. That is, outcomes are rated on some scheme, usually combining measures of function (motor, social, and even work related) with decrease in pain and other subjective symptomatology. The basic strategy is to take general predictive measures, and see if they (more or less independently) corrolate later with the treatment outcome assessments.

By far the most common instrument to use for this purpose is the Minnesota Multiphasic Personality Inventory (MMPI). It is unclear exactly why this should be, although perhaps it is simply because the MMPI is one of the most widely used and studied psychological screening instruments, and clinical psychologists, who tend to do such work for pain treatment programs, are well-versed in MMPI scoring and interpretation. The so-called classic pain triad on the MMPI consists of high scores on the Hysteria and Hypochondriasis scales and low Depression scale scores (2). However, the presence of this triad has not been shown to have significant predictive value, either alone or with other parameters, for the outcome of treatment. [For a negative critique of the limits of the MMPI in CPS measurement, see Hall (3).] In recent work Moore et al. (4) have suggested a revised view of the MMPI, in which some subvariables may make a contribution to prediction, although not the "pain triad" per se, which can be present or absent in patients responsive to therapy.

A variety of psychological instruments for assessing the degree of pain have been developed. Analogue scales are widely used, and simple to apply, but of little demonstrated value. The McGill Pain Inventory is the most widely accepted adjective checklist for descriptors of pain (5). Recent studies by Gracely and coworkers suggest that, with some modifications, the McGill Pain Inventory probably can be an item of measurement, at least in well-controlled studies, for example, of oral pain in dental surgery (6).

The problem with single variables, or small numbers of variables, is that they are likely to have limited predictive power. This should not be surprising, considering the large and usually uncontrollable number of factors that influence health and social interventions generally. The implication of this principle is that it makes sense to examine multiple measures any time the question of prediction is being examined. Another principle, which is often violated or ignored in practice, is that the prediction should be made *in advance*, and as specifically as possible in order to make the result strongly believable. Many social outcome studies are either retrospective cullings of small numbers of predictive variables from large numbers of measurements or claims of confirmation of hypotheses, when, in fact, the "predictor" variables have only been discovered after the fact, thus running the risk of rationalizing findings. Replications of findings, especially with truly comparable measurements, are also uncommon. All of this makes clinicians—and public policymakers—understandably jaundiced about the claims for the results.

The overuse of the MMPI may be a case in point. Long has commented that "there is no single score or profile that reliably discriminates between groups of pain patients classified on the basis of organic signs" (7). Thus, not only is the MMPI by itself inadequate to predict outcome, it also does not clearly differentiate demonstrably organically based pain from that for which no reasonable objectified basis can be found. Indeed, no known test, or combination of tests will accomplish this.

From the point of view of prevention, thought must be focused on errors of commission, which are surely vastly more common than errors of omission. Doctors are always worried about overlooking something. As a result, garden variety and even exotic, dangerous, and invasive tests and procedures are repeatedly perpetrated upon CPS patients. Whereas no tissue damage may have existed when the testing and surgical procedures began, by the time one of more of the major ones are completed, scarring makes it impossible to tell any more.

One might well argue that expenditure of time and effort on structured interview schedules and the like becomes prohibitive in an evaluation. However, most pain patients do not necessarily have a heavy, crowded schedule to their day. Indeed, for many leisure is productive only of boredom, and the opportunity to concentrate more upon their symptoms and pain. Thus, it is hardly an imposition, even in a busy practice, to take patients aside and sit them down—perhaps over several sessions, in order to avoid fatigue and the negative consequences of it upon responding—to complete comprehensive testing.

Another device that has been found to be helpful is the use of diaries. Diaries have a respectable history in psychology, and particularly in cognitive-behavioral and similar psychotherapies. They have the advantages of focusing the patient upon rational, presumably healthy measures; they mobilize a patient's own inner resources; they are autogenic reinforcement measures; and they provide direct, or at least indirect (assuming they are completed diligently and honestly) measures of motivation. The pain diary is essentially "prescribing the symptom," telling the patient to obsess about his symptoms when you already know he is doing exactly that.

So, why do it? In telling him to do more of what he is already doing, you are getting him to examine his own behavior. Also, at the same time you are obtaining important information about the patient. Some examples of actual pain diaries are included in Tables 46.1 and 46.2. In the first (Table 46.1), the patient has been asked to indicate every waking hour what he was doing, and in what position; the degree of his pain (on an analogue equivalent scale); and what medication he took. Some patterns are apparent even at a glance. Like most pain patients, he is automatically scoring his pain all "10's out of 10." The question is not whether his pain really varies less than this. With this kind of record, it should not be hard to achieve a noticeable (to him) reduction in scores, no matter what the intervention.

Still another pattern is the consumption of medication. Over the week, he is taking his medication irregularly, of a variety of types, and with no subjective, reported impact upon his pain. Since the therapist is about to tell him that his pain medications are doing him little good, and possible harm, and should therefore be reduced or removed, this provides potent ammunition in the patient's own observations that the medicine is doing little to aid him in reducing pain. (The counterargument is, "But I'm afraid how much worse it would be if I stopped them." Of course, then "10" is not the correct score in the diary.)

Table 46.1
Pain Diary

Hour	Activities	Medications	Pain Rating
1–7 AM	Sleep		
7–8	Chair—walk	Percocet	10
8–9	Bed		10
9–10	Bed		10
10–11	Chair		10
11–12 PM	Chair		10
12–1	Lunch	Percocet	10
1–3	Bed		10
3–5	Chair	Valium	10
5–6	Stand, make dinner		10
6–7	Chair	Tylenol-III	10
7–9	Bed		10
9–10	Chair	Sleeping pill	10
10–1 AM	Bed	Percocet	10

In Table 46.2 a patient, now on a prescribed regimen of treatment, is recording the same items. Since the instructions are, "Record *exactly* what you were doing during the last hour," the absence of information may be quite revealing. In this example, which is quite typical, one or only a few words are all that is typically recorded. The responses tend to be repetitive, and give little hint of the degree to which the patient may actually have engaged in activity. Looking at the diary, it would appear that he was hardly even leaving the bed to eat or go to the bathroom. By actual observation in inpatient pain treatment, patients probably substantially underestimate their actual movements, and capacity therefor; just as they tend to underestimate the success of their outpatient treatment, compared to therapists estimates. (This should be contrasted to general mental health treatment, where exactly the opposite is the case: patients are consistently more optimistic than their caregivers.) It is also true that each patient's report in part reflect his (probably unconsciously) per-

Table 46.2
Pain Diary

Hour	Activities	Medications	Pain Rating
8–9 AM	Breakfast	Pill	10
9–10	Bed		10
10–11	Chair		9
11–12 PM	Bed		10
12–1	Lunch		10
1–3	Bed	Pill	10

ceived self-interest, as well. Nonetheless, these findings make for interesting discussions with the patients.

Although it has not been studied for results, it probably makes sense to administer a systematic, although semi-structured, interview as part of the initial examination. By "semi-structured" we mean that the areas to be covered, and even the basic questions, are specified. However, the interviewer is allowed room to pursue other leads, get more detail, proceed in a different order, or do whatever is required in order to put the patient at ease initially. In other areas besides treatment of CPS it is generally the case that semi-structured interviews have been shown to be somewhat superior to free-form interviews. The reasons include the likelihood of being complete and not forgetting important areas to cover, the opportunity to think through the wording of questions beforehand, and the enhancement of confidence that probes can be undertaken, without going so far afield that the main areas will be neglected.

In Table 46.3 we have presented such an interview instrument. It is not our purpose here to belabor the assessment. (For more on this subject, see Chapters 6 and 45.) However, we wish to underscore that the format encourages asking about areas that we have found that less experienced or even mature colleagues will sometimes shy away from, notably sexual functions, monetary affairs, and details of compensation and litigation. Elsewhere in this chapter we discuss the impact of such information, incentives, and disincentives for treatment.

Strang has discussed various aspects of primary, secondary, and tertiary prevention (1). As one might expect, tertiary prevention (treatment) takes up more text in the article than the other two combined. However, Strang does suggest both some clinical predictors that have proven unhelpful, and should therefore be avoided, and others that may yet yield some primary prevention value. Routine x-rays, especially of the lumbar back, fall in the "no proven utility for prevention" category (although a case might still be made for liability protection in high-risk jobs). Preemployment strength testing is one possible preventive: if the employee is straining near his limit to do the work, he probably should not be doing the job.

Education about lifting and fitness sounds like a good idea, but results have not been really well demonstrated to prevent back strain. Some effort has gone into mechanical aids and modification of work procedures for prevention. In terms of secondary prevention, Strang has drawn attention to the value of "an early and systematic case management program" as a claims limitation or prevention mechanism for insurers. Also, ergonomics may be useful in early impairment evaluation.

To these might be added certain key points about tertiary prevention. Often, patients could be returned to work if they were not required to do their old jobs, or were required only to do a fraction thereof. This is obviously an enormous problem for employers, who want to have able-bodied employees, and have them return to work. However, when the choice is paying—often for years—enormous sums of money for disability or finding less strenuous work that these partially disabled employees can do, it may pay to try to be innovative. Certainly this has worked for some companies. It may be realistic self-interest for companies under the compulsion of further payments.

THE HISTORY AND EXAMINATION OF PATIENTS: PREVENTING CHRONICITY

CPS has long eluded attempts to codify those factors that can be deemed responsible for promoting chronicity and disability. Variables as diffuse as age, amount of compensation, educational level, use of psychotropic medications, number of surgeries, psychological adaptation, and previous work history have been cited in various retrospective and prospective studies as items in the history and physical examination that will lead to chronic disability. It may be ventured that a comprehensive set of predictors that would be useful to the clinician who wishes to intervene in the early stages of a CPS must cut

Table 46.3.
Brief Pain Assessment Interview

What is the recent history of your pain? How did your pain begin? Tell me in detail what makes your pain worse? Better?
Describe the quality of your pain. (Probe.) What operations have you had?
Tell me in detail about your present medication; past medication:

  For sleep? "Nerves"?
  Coffee, tea, colas? Beer, wine, hard liquor? Past drinking?
  Illegal drugs, including marijuana?

Describe your sleeping patterns in detail; eating pattern; weight change. (Probe other depressive signs, symptoms.)
Tell me about others in your family. (Probe: marital difficulties and role changes; sexual problems; problems with children.)
Tell me about your other medical problems.
Tell me about your past. (Probe: previous episodes of pain, mental health problems, alcohol and drug abuse.)
When was the last time you worked? (Probe: Types of work, work history, physical requirements of jobs.)
Who is your attorney? (Probe: legal actions pending or past, disability or compensation actions.)
Now, tell me about how much of the following you can do, even though you may be greatly in pain:

  How far can you walk?
  How many pounds can you lift?
  What activities can you do around the house?

Please tell me what you expect from treatment.

across biologic, sociologic, and psychological antecedents to be of any use.

In any thoughtful history and physical, we look for the signs and symptoms that trigger the possibility that we are dealing with a syndrome that will become prolonged and dysfunctional. Factors that have been deemed to be correlated with long-term disability may include:

1. Nonspecificity of diagnosis
2. Inconsistency on physical examination, but without a clear-cut psychiatric diagnosis of conversion reaction
3. History of maladaptive behavior
4. Concrete, magical thinking (e.g., "If the doctor could only find the right drug . . .")
5. Passive dependent personality
6. Poor work history, with multiple job changes over a short span
7. Somatically focused and alexithymic disposition
8. Resistance to conservative treatment
9. A protracted psychological course
10. A protracted physical course

Often the history is notable for disagreement among physicians. The patient stimulates disputes among doctors, and between himself and the caregivers. He expects cure, not palliation, and demands no less.

Complete examination of the patient suspected of having CPS, which may lead to long-term disability, must include an evaluation of all of the topics mentioned (8). A clear and concise formulation based on the answers is extremely difficult to synthesize, given the multimodal nature of the contributing causality. However, the extra effort at times suggests avenues of treatment that might otherwise remain obscured (9).

Early recognition and intervention into pain states also require a certain boldness on the part of the clinician in telling the patient that he is at risk for developing chronic pain. That tag carries with it at present the stigmata of "weakness" or "differentness." Many physicians are surprised when patients themselves recognize that there is a growing difficulty in their ability to cope. The patients are reluctant to bring this to the attention of their physician for fear of being labeled "unusual."

For example, Mrs. C.L., who, after one laminectomy, was still disabled and complaining of low back pain, was anxious and depressed. It had been suggested to her by her physician that further surgery and a nuclear magnetic resonance scan were necessary to diagnose what must have been a residual of surgery or a new disk problem. When questioned closely, the patient herself recognized that further intervention was pointless. Her doctor, with the best of all intentions, had disabled her for work, cutting off a source of gratification this patient needed in an otherwise somewhat empty life. Mrs. C.L. recognized this, and declared not only her willingness but her desire to return to work as soon as possible, understanding that the pain would remain whether she worked or not. It was only through the intervention of an independent examining physician that the patient was able to verbalize her antipathy toward the diagnosis of disability and to state with some certainty that she was ready to resume a functional life.

A careful history will elicit whether the patient's symptoms fall into a psychiatric category that may be primary in producing them. There are only three syndromes that produce pain on a "purely" psychiatric basis. The first is psychosis with delusions of pain, a rare occurrence. The second is depression with somatization, a common enough syndrome and one that must be recognized because the depression must be treated directly, rather than the pain per se. The third is true conversion syndrome, which is limited to those patients experiencing hysterical paralysis or blindness or paresis of an extremity.

The clinician working up the chronic pain patient must be attuned to those psychiatric dilemmas that are "binding" great amounts of psychiatric problems into pain states. In contradistinction to the CPS patient, where psychological factors seem to be most important in promoting long-term disability, in the "binding" syndromes physical factors seem to be responsible for promoting and perpetuating mixed psychological/physical symptoms. An illustration will serve to differentiate binding syndromes from the early development of chronic disability syndromes.

Dorothy, a 62-year-old spinster, developed phantom limb symptoms 7 years after a four-quarter amputation of her left upper extremity. Lonely, unmarried, and working in an isolated fashion for a legal firm, the patient felt the fingers of her left, amputated arm helping her right arm in driving and sewing. After careful examination, it was determined that this phantom limb pain was in no way related to stump pain or neuromata and, indeed, had no demonstrable central pain representations. The physical symptoms were perpetuating a depression that had existed for many years and kept Dorothy from feeling alone, rejected, and crippled. Subsequent treatment of her depression, although not one of the primary psychiatric syndromes listed above, resulted in symptom amelioration after 6 weeks.

In contradistinction to the case of Dorothy, a CPS patient presented to a new physician with a 1-year history and a diagnosis of "chronic strain, refractory to all conservative therapies." The patient had had four jobs in the last 2 years. The family appeared oversolicitous and infantilizing. Passive, dependent features appeared in the patient's psychological testing and psychiatric evaluation. Perhaps most important, the transferential relationship with her previous doctor, who with all good intentions had emphasized her dysfunctioning, perpetuated this patient's disability. He had kept the patient off of work status. This served to reinforce the patient's disability, as did a solicitous family—all consonant with dependency needs in the patient (10).

In the first example of the binding syndrome, a clearly identifiable set of physical circumstances and a psychological syndrome combined to promote a serious depression, with pain syndromes a concomitant to that depression. In the second example, an alexithymic, concrete patient, aided and abetted by overprotective family members and physician, was well on her way to developing a chronic syndrome. This same patient 5 years later might have had a rigid, immovable CPS. The factors picked up on an initial history and examination should have served to alert those involved in the care of this patient that a potential long-term disability syndrome was being produced. Interventional steps needed to be taken immediately to prevent that syndrome from becoming fixed.

Physical examination of the chronic pain patient involves different types of testing depending on the locus of the syndrome. It is not true that nonanatomic pain distributions, hypersensitivity to examination, or a positive straight leg raising test while lying but not while sitting with the leg bent at 90° always indicate the presence of a CPS in the making. However, the presence of several such factors in combination with certain historic data are highly suggestive of the potential development of CPS (11). They indicate that intervention should be begun immediately to prevent the encrustation of a simple injury with all the factors leading to an intractable CPS. The presence of three such anomalous physical findings, in combination with three of the tagged historic features noted above, may be sufficient evidence for a diagnosis of incipient CPS, and vigorous steps should be called for at this stage. Early intervention with consistency by all physicians involved, based on the appropriate examinations, can lead to early termination of a progressively debilitating chronic syndrome.

The non–pain specialist can become quite adept at recognizing an incipient CPS (12). The red flags noted above should be considered potential harbingers of this most insidious of syndromes. A history of disability in the family, previous disability of the patient, or litigation for personal injury are particularly worrisome.

The goal is for early prevention of disability syndromes and adaptation to environmental adversity, which otherwise would tend to perpetuate obsessional concentration on pain. What should be done once the elements of a CPS have been detected? It is the responsibility of the assessing physician to demonstrate to the patient that a syndrome exists that is every bit as insidious as a purely physical chronic illness. Many patients will respond at least with acknowledgement and (later) acceptance, if the physician is forthright and open in explaining the peculiar set of circumstances that may lead to total dysfunction.

At the current state of knowledge, P/I in the clinic is limited. Laboratory techniques have been sought for years to aid in the early diagnosis of potential CPS. Endorphin levels, neuroamine transmitter levels, 3-methoxy-4-hydroxyphenylethyleneglycol levels, and many other tests have all been used to predict chronicity in early pain states. No consistently reliable indicators have generally been found for CPS. As noted above, the use of the MMPI and other psychological test variables has been inconclusive at best. In an extensive study by Moore et al., the MMPI, Profile of Mood States, Pain Severity Index, Sexual Functioning, activity diaries, MMPI subgrouping—all were nonpredictive of differential treatment outcomes (4).

Sometimes patients are so angry, presumably in part because their basic dependency needs are not being met, or because paranoid ideation plays a significant role in their thinking, that they will seek another opinion. Sometimes they will find physicians who concur that there are physical problems and enter into extensive therapy. This is a seduction, the promise to the patient of a pain-free existence through the use of either surgery or medical therapy. The outcome of such treatment is, too often, prolongation and worsening of the underlying CPS.

MYOFASCIAL SYNDROMES AS A PARADIGM OF P/I

Recognition of CPS in clinical practice lags behind recognition of pain states found in basic research. There are a number of reasons for this. First, physicians in practice are loathe to tag a patient as having a chronic pain-related syndrome until a certain amount of time has passed. Because chronicity certainly plays a central part in CPS, both definitionally and practically, this is certainly understandable. However, the state of our knowledge has now progressed to the point where we are able in some cases to identify sociologic, biologic, familial, physical, and psychological parameters that put at risk certain patients who present with pain complaints. To some extent this frees the diagnosis from the epithet of "chronic." Perhaps a redefinition for present purposes might be "early manifestations of a potentially disability-related syndrome." Although this unwieldy and cumbersome term will not be used clinically, it serves to underscore that the essence of CPS lies not only in the word "chronic," but also in the multifactorial nature of the problems.

Second, physicians are trained as "doers." Presentation of a syndrome requiring potentially the use of conservative techniques for amelioration of pain is a challenge to most physicians. Many physicians are loathe to treat in unconventional ways, or to withhold treatment based on a putative CPS.

Third, most CPS is diagnosed when it becomes unyielding and unremitting, and fails to respond to the usual interventions. The research laboratory offers us controlled studies of pain transmission systems. Few such controlled situations exist outside the laboratory.

The myofascial syndromes may serve to illustrate the ability to intervene early in a potentially disabling syndrome. A biochemical propensity predisposes a certain proportion of the population to CPS. The early recognition of this syndrome may be enhanced by the use of accurate history and a laboratory test, specifically the dexamethasome suppression test (DST). In addition, a specific personality constellation may be associated with certain myofascial pain syndromes.

Antidepressants alone or in combination have been used for years in the treatment of pain. There are three main subgroupings of antidepressant use. The first is in the primary treatment of depression with somatization. The goal for use of antidepressants in this case is to eliminate the somatic complaints by lifting depression. The assumptions behind the approach to treatment are:

1. That depression rather than pain is the primary difficulty.
2. The use of the antidepressant is directed toward the biochemical underpinnings of depression rather than pain.

The second use is in the direct treatment of pain. This idea is of more recent origin. The syndromes include headache, postherpetic neuralgia, diabetic neuropathy, and a host of postoperative pain states. Antidepressants are employed alone, or in combination with other medications, such as fluphenazine.

The third subgrouping of antidepressant use is in the treatment of adjunctive symptoms, such as insomnia, dysphoria, and irritability. Use of antidepressants for adjunctive symptoms is at times effective. It is argued below that this may correlate with a specific monoamine transmitter deficit, notably a CNS serotonin-deficiency pain syndrome with concomitant insomnia, dysphoria, and other symptoms resembling depressive equivalents.

Review of the literature reveals a number of articles that both support and criticize the use of antidepressants for mixed pain, and depression and pain states (13). A study by Pilowsky and Bassett showed no difference after 6 weeks with the use of antidepressants in mixed pain and depressive states (14). Hosobuchi et al. demonstrated a positive effect of tryptophan loading on opiate production during open cannulization of the third ventricle (15). Ward et al. found little evidence of effective use of antidepressants except perhaps in mixed pain states (16). Blumer and Heilbron found little consistent effect from antidepressant therapy in mixed pain/depression states (17). Diamond and Bates noted that 10 mg of amitriptyline rather than the usual 50–75 mg/day, were effective for headache patients (18). Among the questions that these studies raise are:

1. Are antidepressants effective in pain states?
2. If antidepressants are effective, are depression and pain linked on a biochemical level?

A paradigm to address these questions might be an exploration of the use of the DST in myofascial pain disorder (MPD), which consists of the constellation of cervical pain; shoulder girdle pain; and headaches, sleep disturbances, fatigue, and some depression. (These have been, in the past, referred to as fibromyositis, fibrocytis with trigger points, and other diagnoses, and have been described for over 150 years. In the last several years, an organized syndrome has been delineated that generally consists of a stress-driven myoligamentous syndrome.) Although controversy exists in the acceptance of the DST as a predictor of response in pain states, there are a series of mixed syndromes in which it has been demonstrated to be of some significant predictive value (T. Wehr, personal communication, 1984).

In earlier anecdotal studies MPD was shown to be responsive to amitriptyline in doses one-half to one-third of those used for depression. It was hypothesized that patients susceptible to debilitating MPD had some alteration of the monoamine transmitter serotonin, and that this was related to their ability to show consistently elevated pain thresholds.

Eight-three patients were selected with MPD. Each was given a 2-week trial of amitriptyline (75 mg/day). A Hamilton B Visual Analog Scale and orthopedic examinations were administered to each patient. Each of the patients was depressed, according to clinical descriptions of depression generally accepted in the psychiatric community. The duration of the syndrome varied from 6 months to 10 years. The results can be summarized as follows: 67 patients reported relief. Of those, 60 had a DST that was positive, 7 negative. Sixteen patients reported no relief. Of those, 1 had a positive DST, 15 negative.

It has recently been found that serotonin plays a part in the ability of the body to inhibit pain. The newly discovered dorsolateral funiculus, which runs from the periaqueductal gray to the nucleus cordalis, is a doubly functional pathway. That is, it originates in the periaqueductal gray, which is rich in endorphins. It has also been found to use serotonin as a neuronal transmitter. Thus, this pathway is both hormonal and neuronal (19).

It should be further noted that according to some neuroanatomists, the central pain pathways involved with chronic pain include limbic forebrain connections, and these limbic forebrain connections are rich in serotonin (20). The DST may be a sensitive test in determining with some degree of success those patients who respond to amitriptyline therapy because of the high correlation of these patients with the serotonin metabolism deficit.

It is the author's observation (B.M.S.) that amitriptyline has been used not only in myofascial syndromes, but also in postherpetic neuralgias and diabetic neuropathies combined with the anxiolytic lorazepam. (However, amitriptyline has limited demonstrable use in low back pain.)

Four psychological factors show up frequently in those patients in whom MPD will become a chronic problem. These are (a) an obsessive personality, (b) perfectionistic behavioral traits, (c) sensitivity to multiple demands, and (d) sensitivity to multiple simultaneous deadlines. A positive family history for possibly serotonin-related illnesses is relevant. For example, there may be a parent who has been depressed or an alcoholic parent. Myofascial disease in parents or siblings is also an indication of the potential chronicity of the syndrome.

In our example of MPD, out of a meld of basic science,

good history-taking, and physical observation an early CPS can be recognized. This early CPS involves components of physical, emotional, familial, and behavioral types. In the study outlined above the time period for existence of this syndrome had ranged from 6 months to 10 years. In this instance "chronic pain syndrome" of MPD should be divorced from the conventional term "chronic," because this would imply that the syndrome could only be diagnosed after a specified amount of time had elapsed. It is possible that early recognition of CPS in MPS may be achievable, even before chronicity develops.

MERITS AND DRAWBACKS OF A CLASSIFICATION SYSTEM

Recently a blue ribbon committee has taken up the banner of providing a classification scheme for pain syndromes, largely for chronic pain (21). The given impetus for devising such a system is

> It is possible to define terms and develop a classification of pain syndromes which are acceptable to many, albeit not *all* readers and workers in the field; even if the adopted definitions and classification are not perfect, they are better than the tower of Babel conditions that currently exist; adoption of such classification does not mean that it is fixed for all time and cannot be modified as we acquire new knowledge; and the adoption of such taxonomy with the condition that it can be modified will encourage its use widely by those who may disagree with some part of the classification. This in fact has been the experience and chronology of such widely accepted classifications as those pertaining to heart disease, hypertension, diabetes, toxemia of pregnancy, psychiatric disorders, and a host of others . . . . (22)

In other words, according to Bonica, some explicit system, however faulty, is better than none at all.

MERITS

In fact, is a faulty scheme really superior to none at all? Our tentative answer is a very qualified "yes," dependent mainly upon the particular merits and drawbacks of the system proposed. The advantages of such a scheme include the following.

1. It Forces Being Explicit. In general, this is probably a virtue, and it is the same one that "thinking models" generally serve. Most clinicians in practice operate upon many assumptions that they have only partially articulated. Often various propositions that constitute motivations for purposive action—interventions—are internally self-contradictory, even tautologic. Laying them out for others to see if perhaps the surest way to get feedback, some of it by way of agreement, and some, because of adverse counterattack by critics. In either event the strengths and weaknesses of one's thinking will be elucidated.

2. A System of Classification is Perforce an Attempt to be Relatively Complete, or Comprehensive. Therefore, it must have some logic to it. At the lowest level this would consist of the random assignment of corresponding numbers. However, this is a simplistic example. Most systems in medicine consist of signs, symptoms, and historic items that appear to cluster together, have some diagnostic or prognostic value, or are associated with particular etiologic theories. In practice these items may be mingled beyond the ability of the reader to reconstruct the logic or relationships.

3. If the Logic of a System is Coherent, and can be Demonstrated to be Tied to the Real World (Validation), then such Schemes may Reveal where Hitherto Unfound Diseases Ought to Occur. An analogy might be the Periodic Table of the Elements. When this two-by-two matrix was first recognized for its fundamental properties in chemistry, it also became clear that certain elements ought to occur in nature, even though they had not been previously identified. In medicine, however, it is more difficult to think of clear examples that might fit this logic. Perhaps the closest we can come is the discovery of microorganisms without reference to disease, and the later linking of them to previously unknown illnesses (e.g., *Serratia marcescens*).

DRAWBACKS

On the other hand, the imposition of order where previously there had been many loose threads or disagreements also sports potential disadvantages. Among them might be the following.

1. No System is "Culture Free," or Unbiased. That is, although the stated purpose of a disease classification system may be to describe syndromes, illnesses, and diseases, without reference to etiology where such is not clearly established, even a broad committee of clinicians and researchers must take some stands that at least imply their inclinations about theories of illness. In fact, as a practical matter, it is very difficult to conceive of devising any system in medicine that did not carry rather substantial implications of bias about causality, and probably treatment as well.

2. A Classification System may also (Albeit, Unintentionally) Emphasize Certain Aspects of a Problem and Deemphasize Others. A common problem, for example, is that disease classification systems set up for elusive diseases, in which the tissue pathology is poorly defined or the categories potentially substantially overlapping, may emphasize the most severe cases. The worst cases usually have the most blatant signs and symptoms, and it is easier to obtain reliable agreement among clinicians who examine the patients.

However, for purposes of P/I, this type of classification may be problematic: the whole point of P/I is to develop ways of intervening as early on in the course of illness as possible. Also, the cutting points chosen for where diagnosis can be properly conferred are arbitrary. The pathology is on a spectrum that is more or less continuous from the mildest to the most severe forms of the disease. By contrast, a nomenclature assumes an "all-or-nothing" decision, in which a patient either has the illness or does not. This may be incompatible with the notion of attempting to increase sensitivity among clinicians to possible early forms of the illness.

It is, of course, possible to devise systems that specifically emphasize P/early I. This presents the converse difficulty, but probably in more exaggerated form. If the utility is limited to P/I, or leans in this direction, most practicing clinicians are likely to ignore it. Since even the pathologic schemes are often ignored, or poorly understood in practice, including even the most universal (ICDA-IX), a system constructed for such a narrow purpose is unlikely to gain acceptance beyond the small number of secondary specialists who follow the field.

3. *A Classification System may be Inherently Incorrect, Unsatisfying, or Even Misleading.* The selection of a model does not ensure that it is the best available model, that it accurately reflects the real world (external validity question), that it is consensual, or that it is useful. The fact that an expert committee may have composed it does not mean that the entire field has a high degree of similar understanding of a particular problem. For instance, in constructing and revising the *Diagnostic and Statistical Manual (DSM)—III*, the American Psychiatric Association (APA) has had to resort to votes of the membership upon a number of occasions in order to settle what purport to be "scientific" questions (23). Once a classification system is in place, it also may gain official credibility beyond its capabilities or its authors' intentions. It may become the official guide for purposes of insurance reimbursement, compensation, and even legal expertise on the subject. Laymen may presume that scientific standards underlie the work, when this may well not be the case.

THE CPS CLASSIFICATION SCHEME

Recently a scheme for CPS has been proposed and published (21). This system of nomenclature resembles the DSM-III in a number of major regards. Perhaps the construction of the CPS classification should not be surprising, considering the interest of at least some prominent psychiatrists in CPS, and the fact that the panel was chaired by Merskey, an English psychiatrist noted for his work upon psychosocial aspects of pain.

In particular, the CPS nomenclature uses a multiaxial system of classification for each diagnosis. The major component of the illness is along Axis I, much as in DSM-III. However, the axes do differ somewhat from DSM-III in a number of ways.

Axis I categorizes the anatomic region where the pain largely occurs (including a residual category, "More than three major sites"). Axis II catalogs the pain body system. Axis III is about duration, and Axis IV, intensity (from time of onset). Axis V makes some statement about etiology. Axis V includes residual categories for "Dysfunctional (including psychophysiological)," "Unknown or other," and "Psychological origin." Axis V is an innovation, in that it offers several alternatives for diseases or pain of unknown cause, intertwined with psychosocial factors, be they cause or effects.

There are a number of specific diagnoses under which difficult-to-diagnose pain occurs. We consider several examples here. Under "Pain of Psychological Origin: Muscle Tension Pain," the authors have included a definition, description of the "site" and "system" involved, and a short paragraph entitled "Main Features." This addresses epidemiology to an extent (e.g., age, sex, distributions), in much the same manner as DSM-III. It also describes the quality of symptoms and other features. It attempts to deal with a number of aspects of "Associated Symptoms," "Signs," forms of "Relief," disability-related parameters, and differential diagnosis. This format is also reminiscent of DSM-III.

The Disease heading "Pain of Psychological Origin" is further broken down by psychological type of symptamatology. Thus, a "Delusional or Hallucinatory Pain" is given a separate heading from pain that is "Hysterical or Hypochondriacal." These usages of the psychiatric terms are different from, and less rigorous than, those of DSM-III. However, the thrust of their argument appears to be roughly similar.

THE PAIN CLASSIFICATION SYSTEM: A CRITIQUE

As we have suggested in our general comments about classification systems, there are usually major advantages and disadvantages to any scheme. How does this particular scheme measure up to reasonable standards?

1. *It Certainly Attempts to be Comprehensive.* The skeleton is capable of accommodating new diseases, or shuffling up old, based upon new data, thinking, or even fashion. It is already extensive, and, although it is probably impossible even in principle to be sure whether a system is complete, this scheme is at least thoughtful, and it is clear that a prodigious amount of work has gone into producing it. Whether one agrees with its premises or not, they are generally stated sufficiently clearly that at least there is basis for argument, and confirmation or refutation.

2. *The Logic of the Scheme is Clear.* It is fundamentally based around the existing (largely body system–based) coding system, although it often uses different diagnoses than the extant ICDA-IX, or uses words in unusual ways, to which most physicians and other practitioners may not be accustomed.

However, beyond Axis I, the theoretical basis for the subcategories is less clear. It appears to be a division based upon a series of parameters that describe pain. Thus, duration and so on are reified into axes. This is a subtle but important departure from DSM-III, where the first two (and most important) axes are psychiatric diagnoses, the third relates to other medical illnesses, and the remaining two are rating schemes.

The Pain Nomenclature also employs ratings, but each one of the axes appears to be anchored, at least for certain diagnoses, largely around the patient's self-reports of pain. On the one hand, this is not surprising, since this may be the state of the art in terms of our understanding of much of clinically relevant pain. On the other hand, it also draws attention to a severe limitation of this scheme: mainly, that, in the absence of patient self-reports, there would be no classification scheme at all. Although the psychiatric nomenclature is also heavily dependent upon patient self-reports, it accommodates to other sources of information. It is not yet clear whether the pain scheme is capable of being useful without overwhelming reliance upon patient's self-reports. Although a number of studies now document the reliability of behavioral observations in CPS, they prove nothing about their validity.

3. *The Pain Classification Definitely Comes Down Heavily Upon the Side of the Severe Illness.* As we have suggested above, this is an ominous development from the point of view of the student concerned about P/I. Some attempt is made to catalog a range of factors that influence or modify the pain, psychosocial parameters in particular. However, this does not clearly aid in using the system to raise consciousness about P/I. When do the various factors involved in a given diagnosis become important? The course of the illness, by definition, does not become clear except in retrospect. This makes empirical confirmation very difficult, since prospective study is possible only in high-risk populations. Although it should be possible to identify such populations, little such empirical work has actually been done. The data on predictions of surgical outcome (see elsewhere in this chapter), at their best, leave substantial groups of false-positives and false-negatives incorrectly classified. The authors of the present scheme have not, to our knowledge, printed a "concordance" that would clearly indicate which assertions are based upon study, and which upon "expert opinion." (This is, if anything, even more true of DSM-III.)

What can be said, in sum, of the proposed classification system and its impact upon P/I? On the balance, it does not necessarily augur well for future developments in this area. It appears to lean fairly heavily in the direction of severe pathology, including psychopathology, possibly to the exclusion or at least deemphasis of early identification. The authors are undoubtedly sincere in wishing to advance the search for causes and cures in CPS. Indeed, the blue ribbon committee is filled with distinguished researchers. Why, then, this somewhat top-heavy pathologic presentation?

As we intimated, one of the major political issues for the chronic pain field is simply gaining respectability among professionals, especially practitioners. P/I is a relatively young, underdeveloped discipline in chronic pain and most similar fields. The effort to gain acceptance has quite properly taken precedence here. This is not a criticism of what, to us, appears to be a correct political judgment at this time: mainly, that a foot in the door of medicine may allow CPS treaters to have more access to and impact upon medicine generally. However, it is also an instance where a decision made results in a trade-off, and P/I may be lost in the shuffle.

In the last analysis, the value of a nomenclature is in the new work it generates. If this system stimulates thought and critical examination of the subject, then it will have been worthwhile, even were it eventually to be significantly modified or even abandoned. We must await those studies—hoped to be forthcoming in the next few years—before passing judgment.

COMPENSATION, DISABILITY, AND LEGAL IMPACTS UPON PREVENTION AND EARLY INTERVENTION

One of the central issues around which debate rages on the subject of CPS is that of the potential disincentives offered by compensation and disability programs, public and private. It is clear that CPS in its various forms is one of the largest contributors to our annual health payments in both the public and private insurance sectors (see elsewhere in this book), and has been identified by Bonica and others as adding costs of billions of dollars per year to manufacturing and service industries (24). For this reason, among others, it is commonly and widely assumed that CPS is only a disincentive to improvement in symptomatology, the compensation system working massively against motivation to improve in treatment.

A recently completed national Commission on Pain Evaluation of the Social Security Administration (SSA) wrestled mightily with this problem of how to deal with the potential disincentives of CPS (25). The Commission report concluded that powerful disincentives exist in the SSA for patients to get better. By implication, the report is also an indictment of Workers' Compensation, and even private insurance systems, which generally fail to return people to work.

After more than a year and a half of testimony and review of the subject, the Commission, however, substantially failed to consider any testimony or significant evidence that might suggest the possibility that disincentives are less important than generally thought, or that judiciously constructed compensation and treatment systems can at least partially overcome them when the concern is CPS. Indeed, the systematic evidence on the side of the power of the disincentive turns out to be disturbingly inadequate. There are at least some arguments and studies on the opposite side of the question, and these are worthy of mention.

In the general case, the answer to the questions of how powerful incentives and disincentives are can be hinged upon the character of the population being treated and studied, the nature of the incentives, and the timing of the interventions. Reviews of treatment outcome in chronic pain–specific treatment programs are relatively optimistic. These results are on selected populations. Although we do not detail these reviews extensively here, a number of comments about such studies are pertinent.

First, in general, the strength of the positive results from treatment is inversely proportional to the number and power of the outcome measures. For example, almost all studies report major reductions in unwanted medication usage, often approaching zero, at least during the time of the treatment itself. When other measures, such as assessment of mobilization, are added, "success" rates typically drop from the 70% range to the below-50% range. However, insurers and government are primarily interested in return to productive work. The figures in this area are typically quite discouraging, generally well below the 30% range. Those who are advocates of such programs argue that, without treatment, the figures would be closer to 0. This is a complex argument, which hinges upon the believability of cost/benefit studies, since the cost of treatment is certainly significant. Occasional studies do, nevertheless, tend to be optimistic, even upon this score.

Second, the nature of the incentives, what they are, and how to quantitate them is a thorny and elusive area to try to understand. Carron has argued forcefully that the entire compensation-disability system is structured to militate against incentives to return to work (26). His analysis of secondary data suggests that many workers are close to their previous level of pay and perquisites in compensation, and are ill-advised to go back to work, since they might not actually come close to breaking even, or even lose ground financially by doing so.

It is less clear that this analysis applies to the entire spectrum of disabled populations (as Carron would probably agree). The Pain Commission (vide supra) heard testimony from Social Security's Chief Statistician, Aaron Krute, Ph.D., about an in-house study of SSA-disabled lists. The data had many problems in terms of reliability, but this was partially balanced out by the large populations with which the government deals. It appeared that few of the disabled could reasonably qualify for an experiment to put them back to work, even though the numbers of the potentially totally disabled CPS population were large (perhaps upward of 10%).

In Social Security law, these people can only enter through a "back door" diagnosis at present, since chronic pain is not legally admissible as a diagnosis for purposes of this disability program. The reason for the small numbers who it appeared might qualify to be rehabilitated may have to do with the severe and pervasive nature of illness, poor education, low social status, and unskilled labor that go into the concoction that characterizes much of the SSA disability population. The Commission heard testimony that indicated the general failure of rehabilitation experiments of all kinds previously through SSA, generally attributable to the multiple handicaps that face most recipients of aid.

On the other hand, experiments in other countries may shed some light upon what constitute reasonable incentives and motivational factors, even if the populations are not precisely comparable. In a Canadian study, Catchlove and Cohen dramatically reoriented the nature of their treatment program for CPS (27). They found that, although they could not develop a cure-all, they could significantly improve their batting average for people going back to work. Basically, what they did was to announce to patients that they intended to get everyone back to work, and put teeth into this. Most patients and their families became vociferously angry, but a "working through" process generally occurred, and acceptance was manifested by greater effort put into the graded exercise program and vocationally directed rehabilitation.

Third, little is known about the timing of interventions, except that there is unanimity about the idea that sooner is better. The most widely accepted definition of CPS requires 6 months of pain without remission. Many industrial and other physicians believe that they can identify potential CPS victims within weeks of a reported accident on the job. Elsewhere in this chapter we mention the efforts to predict who make good surgical candidates. The present problem is more amorphous: predicting who will go on to develop chronic, unremitting pain, no matter what the intervention.

There may an ethical dilemma here. At the present state of the art, identification of the pain-prone individual is fraught with peril and uncertainty at best. But even if this were not the case, would there be a problem? Let us assume that we could predict who would become a victim of CPS early on with a high degree of certainty, say, 95% of the time. Does that mean that 1 out of 20 patients should be incorrectly denied an operation that they want? Should patients share in the risk and liability under such circumstances? And only if they are operated on, and the operation fails? Besides, most such patients have few resources in the first place. What is the social obligation to CPS victims, and how broad is it?

The same potential ethical dilemma applies to early identification of CPS. The various designations for this syndrome are not neutral. They carry negative connotations of judgment about the patient, the patient's motivation, and even his character. Is the gain from early identification sufficient to warrant the epithets? At this state of the art—our ignorance—it is hard to make such a case convincingly.

How, then, can liability be limited within economically reasonable bounds? The answers to the question are basically political, and probably most closely influenced by the self-interest of the group responding. The insurance industry supports tough measures. Their assertion is that smart investigations can uncover dissembling and malingering, and that such measures, if adopted wholesale by government sanction, would go a long way toward containing spiraling costs and protecting the public interest. On the other hand, physicians expert in CPS who testified before the Pain Commission repeatedly asserted that malingering was rare, and could be detected relatively easily by examination. The insurance executives on the panel did not vigorously dispute this point, and it became a finding of the Commission.

Findings and fact, however, are not necessarily the same. We can detect little evidence that bears upon this point one way or another. Is it really possible to distinguish clearly between malingering and limited effort at recovery? Or, is it a continuum, where only the extremes can be defined satisfactorily? The latter seems more likely. Would it be possible to test this proposition, experimentally or statistically? The answer seems to be a qualified "yes." In that case, the fact that essentially no research has gone into answering the question may speak for how much investment anyone has in knowing the answer.

P/I AND LEGAL DISINCENTIVES

All of this brings us to the practical question of the circumstances under which P/I may or may not be possible in the face of legal disincentives, and how the likelihood of success can be maximized, even under adversity.

First, as a practical matter, the majority of patients who enter CPS treatment are under some kind of compensation disincentive, often one that compels their entry into the treatment. Given this fact, it is surprising that many are able to use the treatment to some advantage. In short, it pays to try.

Second, it probably clears the air to have as much in detail about the compensation aspects of a case up front as possible. If the patient is self-referred, or the issues have not been addressed directly, they should be so, and frankly, even over the telephone, before a potential patient is seen the first time (Table 46.3).

Third, caregivers need to be absolutely clear about the limits to which they are willing to go in rendering care in the face of disincentives. Self-interest is hardly sufficient rationalization for rendering care, especially extended, supportive care, if there is little reason to think it will help, or if the gain is prognosticated to be small and the cost large.

Fourth, in the initial interviews, certain questions help lead into frank discussions of compensation issues. When patients come for admission to the hospital, especially those who have "tickets of admission," say, to a psychiatry service (and CPS is one of them), they need to be questioned in a friendly but probing way. Our first question is sometimes, "Now, please tell me the name of your attorney." People without potential litigation rarely can name one. Next, details of cases determined or pending are relevant. The work history needs to be included in the preliminary history taking.

Fifth, if disability or compensation issues are raised by patients after treatment has already begun, the "treatment contract" should be renegotiated. When the patient has not been candid in the first place about the hidden motives for his engaging the caregiver, it is not clear that the original contract is still in force.

Whether the professional is legally obligated, for example, to provide an opinion to an insurer or government agency is murky at best. Certainly, it is a foolish patient who acts in this way, since the therapist feels betrayed, lied to, and angry. However, once the patient is engaged in treatment, it is also hard to ignore the professional's potential self-interest, which is to say, guaranteed payment.

One way around this dilemma is to insist that the treatment and the disability evaluation be performed by separate, unconnected professional parties. Ideally, this means that the evaluator has no stake in recommending treatment, or being optimistic about it. In practice, however, it is common (*a*) for such evaluators to honor the opinion of the treating physician, or (*b*) for companies to send patients for evaluations where they can guess the opinion in advance (thereby inviting litigation), or (*c*) for the insuror to insist upon the "treating physician's" records, and refuse to accept another opinion.

For example, a 34-year-old statistical analyst was in pain, and claimed to be phobic of his work place. The treating psychiatrist instituted a behavioral desensitization program for return to work. Although this seemed to be working up to a point, as the patient actually took steps to get in the door of his workplace, he reported suicidal thoughts and actions behind the wheel of his car. Shortly after this, the patient's Workers' Compensation carrier contacted the psychiatrist, the first that the psychiatrist knew of the claim. After some discussion with his peers, the psychiatrist attempted to insist upon an independent evaluation. The patient, the patient's wife, and the insuror together then began to pressure the treating doctor to render an opinion. When he stood firm, the patient angrily left treatment, threatening suit—which, however did not materialize.

Finally, limited hope should be offered to both carriers and patients about success rates for treatment of CPS in the face of continuing compensation issues. Insurors have become understandably cynical. Perhaps partly in response to this, the claims for success of treatment in CPS have become more and more extravagant and unreasonable. Treatment does have something to offer, but optimistic projections can only lead to dashed hopes and further cynicism.

REHABILITATION OF THE CPS PATIENT, AND TERTIARY PREVENTION

Tertiary prevention involves recognition that illness has taken its toll, and yet measures of treatment may either prevent recurrence or at least lessen its impact. In some cases tertiary prevention is conceived of as retarding the inevitable progression of disease, or attempting to lessen pain and suffering. This, of course, is a tautology when speaking of CPS, since reported pain and suffering are central, and (by definition) are not improving, or there would not be a tertiary problem. There is also the constant uphill task of working against the patient's—and often the family's and the doctor's—hopes that somehow a "cure" will be found, and hard work on rehabilitation will not be a necessity. Regrettably, the latter hopes often work strongly against optimal coping with the existing illness.

The heart of tertiary prevention is generally a behavioral approach. The theoretical as well as practical basis for this approach has generally been associated with Fordyce (28). It is not our purpose to detail this approach here, but to examine enough of its bases to comment upon its P/I value and limitations. First of all, it assumes at least a modicum of cooperation and motivation upon the part of the patient. It postulates that an incremental, goal-oriented system of rewards (and deterrants) will be additive, in a reasonable time period.

The goal is to be as functional as possible, given that pain may persist, or even worsen. In other words, it deemphasizes the communications about pain and suffering, on the theory that they are counterproductive to functionality.

This approach has been reviewed in detail by Keefe (29) and by Linton (30). The main questions for present purposes have to do with the following considerations:

1. What is the evidence that behavioral change is sustained over time?
2. What is necessary in order to sustain gains from a behavioral modification approach, assuming that they do occur?
3. What are the costs in time and resources to optimize sustained functionality?

There are now some relatively long-term studies of outcome of treatment. Most CPS treatment programs have behavioral approaches at their core, although it is fair to say that most also take a variety of approaches simultaneously, and this makes it difficult to single out one for special consideration. In fact, it is generally true that multimodality treatment programs have generally been demonstrated to be the most consistently successful (31). Analysis is presently going on of over 5 years of follow-up of patients in the University of Virginia program, and the initial results appear to be more promising in terms of patient functionality than the very ominous predictions usually made for this group (H. Carron, personal communication, 1986).

Perhaps the most difficult task is sustaining outpatient regimens that are roughly consistent with the intensive phase of treatment, be it originally inpatient or outpatient. Certain principles may have some practical value in bringing this about.

First, every effort needs to be made to concentrate care in one treatment coordinator's hands. Since the CPS patient is particularly prone to have multiple doctors, this is essential.

Second, innovative and strenous efforts may need to be undertaken in order to bring about this coordination. This is an example of where spouses and other family members may be essential in order to augment or correct communications between doctor and patient. Pharmacists may need to have detailed knowledge of the patients and their needs.

Third, at the present state of the art, if in doubt, a whole series of concurrent therapies should be directed at patients, including them as maintenance treatment after the intensive initial push. Although, as indicated above in this chapter, the evidence for multimodality treatment is not so clear as one would like, the "grapeshot" approach to treatment can be justified on a number of grounds. Since our ability to predict who will respond to a given treatment is minimal, but we know that a group of CPS patients will respond to some treatment, all bases being covered may heighten the likelihood of success. Also, there is a tendency in practice to reify those treatments that the caregiver knows how to render best. This is not better personified than in the liberal overuse of medications, at the expense of behavioral and cognitive treatments that may be quite important or even essential.

Fourth, since compliance is a notorious problem with outpatient treatments, any simple measures that will enhance the likelihood of following a treatment regimen have the promise of high payoff. A doctor's office can schedule telephone calls at intervals in order to provide a friendly reminder. Since intermittent reinforcement schedules tend to be more effective at maintaining established operant behavior, the calls should not be at regular, expectable intervals, but spaced out at close enough intervals in order that compliance will not necessarily have strayed too far off of prescription between calls. Postcards and newsletters, although less effective, are cheap, simple, and may have some value in this regard.

Other innovative devices should be employed without hesitation. For example, patients may continue their plan diaries at home, and have their entries checked at interval by treaters.

Although devices as reinforcers have not been studied extensively, some are known to be effective in certain patients. The paradigm for this is the TNS unit. How TNS works—when it works—is not well established. However, at least one function it serves is to remind the patient of the caregiver's expectations. The same thing may be true of programmable timers, which can be purchased inexpensively at radio discount stores and preset for the appropriate intervals to sound an alarm, and remind the patient to carry out a particular set of tasks.

Fifth, visits to homes and work places may provide surprising diagnostic vignettes that require the caregiver to adjust his judgments of the patient's goodness of fit with his environment. Although it may be unrealistic for a doctor in practice to do this, there is now a cadre of enterprising vocational rehabilitation specialists, including public workers and private firms, who have particular interest in job and task analysis. Some are also experienced in negotiating job redefinition for workers who must be either returned to partial duty or retired at full pay.

Hertzman et al., have described an augmented operant/multimodality treatment process (unpublished paper). The treatment is both educational, and behavioral-psychological. The inducements to the families to assist are multiple. For one, they are often at their wits' end as to how to help a family member who may be not merely noncontributory, but actually a tremendous drain on family resources of patience, affection, and even money. Dramatic role changes in families surrounding one person's becoming a CPS victim upset the family's equilibrium dynamics. A wife who was a homebody is forced to go out and become the principal wage earner, while a hitherto macho construction worker is reduced to housework. Often the children are caught in between them, and everyone suffers.

Certainly family participation in treatment seems to bode better for good outcome. Although there are few systematic studies of the question, those that exist generally reflect the commonsense wisdom on the subject. Khatami and Rush (32) studied the impact of family participation in a multimodality CPS treatment program. They were able to show strongly suggestive evidence that family work enhanced positive outcomes. Also, these effects were persistent upon follow-up. Hertzman et al., in another open study, obtained results that suggested the superiority of outcome when families participated in treatment (unpublished data). However, in this study "preselection" may have occurred: for example, the results could alternatively be explained in that families willing to cooperate may have been positive risk factor families before the study started.

What is it about family participation that maximizes its usefulness? Many family members, usually inadvertently, are reinforcing pain and suffering communicative behavior. By observing the families directly, preferably even in a naturalistic setting (e.g., at home), it may be determined that they are enabling the dysfunctional behavior to continue. The analogy to the "enabler" in the alcoholic family is possibly more than coincidental: alcohol and drug abuse is rife in these families, in both patients and relatives, and often precedes the CPS (and may continue during it).

It is also the case that families are generally the best supporters that the CPS patient is going to have. Thus, if these family members can be bolstered in their own most functional roles, it is often also of assistance to the patient. Of course, this is easy to assert, but not necessarily easy to do in practice. For instance, some research suggests that families in which spouses are in the most agreement about their analysis of the "pain problem" are also the most closed to changing it (33). Conversely, when marital (or other family) disagreement exists about what the CPS patient should be doing, what roles family members should be assuming, and what treatment the patient should be getting are discordant, this may predict greater likelihood of willingness to change within the family.

Perhaps the most valuable piece of advice to the office clinician would be to take a healthy, skeptical attitude toward very optimistic, or global claims to success in treatment. For example, flying in the face of most other opinion, one respected researcher suggested that multimodality treatment is poorly established as effective, and that relaxation techniques have a much more solid body of evidence behind them (30). This is contrary to our reading of the scientific literature on the subject, and also to common sense.

Today much research is focused upon isolating out the value of particular treatment components, such as relaxation techniques. However, the state of the art of treatment outcome research remains crude, and the suggestion that single treatments with some demonstrated efficacy may be superior to "grapeshot" approaches confuses the value of partialing out treatments for research purposes, and maximizing outcome by attempting a number of different strategies simultaneously, any combination of which may work.

References

1. Strang JP: The chronic disability syndrome. In Aronoff GM (ed): *Evaluation and Treatment of Chronic Pain*. Baltimore, Urban & Schwarzenberg, 1985, pp 603–623.
2. McCreary C, Turner J, Dawson E: The MMPI as a predictor of response to conservative treatment for low back pain. *J Clin Psychol* 35:278–284, 1976.
3. Hall W: Review: psychological approaches to the evaluation of chronic pain patients. *Aust NZ J Psychiatry* 16:3–9, 1982.
4. Moore JE, Armentrout DP, Parker JC, Kivlahan DR: Empirically derived pain—patient MMPI subgroups, prediction of treatment outcome. *J Behav Med* 9:51–63, 1986.
5. Melzack R: The McGill Pain Questionnaire: major properties and scoring methods. *Pain* 1:277–299, 1975.
6. Gracely RH: Pain measurement in man. In Ng LKY, Bonica JJ (eds): *Pain, Discomfort and Humanitarian Care*. Amsterdam, Elsevier/North-Holland, 1980, pp 111–138.
7. Long CJ: The relationship between surgical outcome and MMPI profiles in chronic pain patients. *J Clin Psychol* 37:744–749, 1981.
8. Reich J, Steward M, Tupin J, Rosenblatt RM: Prediction of responses to treatment in chronic pain patients. *J Clin Psychiatry* 46:425–427, 1985.
9. McCreary C, Turner J, Dawson E: Principal dimensions of the pain experience and psychological disturbance in chronic low back pain patients. *Pain* 11:85–92, 1981.
10. Feuerstein M, Sults S, Hocke M: Environmental stressors and chronic low back pain—life events, family and work environments. *Pain* 22:295–307, 1985.
11. Guck TP, Meilman PW, Skultety FM, Dowd ET: Prediction of long-term outcome of multidisciplinary pain treatment. *Arch Phys Med Rehabil* 67:293–296, 1986.
12. Chapman CR, Case KL, Dubner R, Foley KM, Gracely RH, Reading AE: Pain measurement: an overview. *Pain* 22:1–31, 1985.
13. France RD, Krishnan KR: The dexamethasome suppression test as a biologic marker of depression in chronic pain. *Pain* 21:49–55, 1985.
14. Pilowsky F, Bassett D: Pain and depression. *Br J Psychiatry* 141:30–36, 1982.

15. Hosobuchi Y, Lamb S, Baskin D: Tryptopham loading may reverse tolerance to opiate analgesic in humans: a preliminary report. *Pain* 9:161–169, 1980.
16. Ward N, Bloom V, Friedel R: Effectiveness of tricyclic antidepressants in the treatment of coexisting pain and depression. *Pain* 7:331–341, 1979.
17. Blumer D, Heilbron M: Chronic pain as a variant of depressive disease—the pain prone disorder. *J Nerv Ment Dis* 170:381–406, 1982.
18. Diamond S, Bates D: Chronic tension headache—treatment with amitriptylene. *Headache* 110–115, 1971.
19. Basbaum A, Marley N, O'Keefe K, Clanton C: Reversal of morphine and stimulus—produced analgesic by sub-total spinal cord lesions. *Pain* 3:43–56, 1977.
20. de Montigny L, Aghajanian GK: Tricyclic antidepressants; long-term treatment increases responsivity of rat forebrain nerves to serotonin. *Science* 202:1303–1306, 1978.
21. International Association for the Study of Pain: Classification of chronic pain. *Pain Suppl* 3:S3–S226, 1986.
22. Bonica JJ, quoted in: Classification of chronic pain. *Pain Suppl* 3:S3, 1986.
23. American Psychiatric Association: *Diagnostic and Statistical Manual of Mental Disorders*, ed 3. Washington, DC, Author, 1980.
24. Bonica JJ: Importance of the problem. In Aronoff GM (ed): *Evaluation and Treatment of Chronic Pain*. Baltimore, Urban & Schwarzenberg, 1985, pp xxxi–xliv.
25. Social Security Administration: *Report of the Commission on the Evaluation of Pain*. Washington, DC, US Government Printing Office, 1986.
26. Carron H: Compensation aspects of low back claims. In Carron H, McLaughlin RE (eds): *Management of Low Back Pain*. Littleton, MA, John Wright–PSG, 1982, pp 17–26.
27. Catchlove R, Cohen K: Effects of a directive return to work approach in the treatment of workman's compensation patients with chronic pain. *Pain* 14:181–191, 1982.
28. Fordyce W: *Behavioral Methods for Chronic Pain and Illness*. St. Louis, CV Mosby, 1976.
29. Keefe FJ: Behavioral assessment and treatment of chronic pain: current status and future directions. *Psychology* 50:896–911, 1982.
30. Linton SJ: Behavioral remediation of chronic pain: a status report. *Pain* 24:125–141, 1986.
31. Hertzman MP: Pain as stress. In American Psychiatric Association: *Methods of Psychiatric Treatment*. Washington, DC, American Psychiatric Association, (in press).
32. Khatami M, Rush AJ: A one-year follow-up of the multimodel treatment for chronic pain. *Pain* 14:45–52, 1982.
33. Bloch AR, Kremer EF, Gaylor M: Behavioral treatment of chronic pain: the spouse as a discriminative cue for pain behavior. *Pain* 9:243–252, 1980.

chapter 47
Ergonomic Considerations in the Workplace

Mahmoud A. Ayoub, Ph.D.

ERGONOMICS

Ergonomics, derived from two Greek words, *ergon* and *nomikos*, means literally the "laws of work." It seeks to design jobs, workplace, and products for people to reduce physical discomfort, to enhance safety and well-being, to improve job effectiveness and productivity—at home, on the road, and at work. Other labels are used to describe the field of ergonomics: human factors, human ergology, human performance, and the like. In the United States human factors is the well-known and heavily referenced label. However, ergonomics is the label recognized and used worldwide. Biomechanics, work physiology, and man-machine systems are special areas of study within the field of ergonomics. For example, biomechanics is concerned with the interaction between people and their environments; it considers various aspects of energy exchange between people and the physical entities of the workplace: tools, seats, materials, and the like. It measures and assesses the internal and external forces generated by and acting upon the human body.

Ergonomics, as a discipline, is concerned with the design of jobs, workplace, and products as well as employee selection and training. In this context, ergonomics is closely allied with industrial engineering, for both seek efficiency and productivity. The point of departure between the two is in the consideration given to human capabilities and limitations. While seeking high levels of productivity, ergonomics attempts to assure that job stresses (physical, physiologic, and psychological) can be tolerated by the human body and its systems. It minimizes job stress through design and integration (interfacing) of workplace hardware (seating, work surface, etc.), and elimination of motion elements and associated forces that might cause excessive muscular loading.

Ergonomics bases its principles and recommendations on knowledge and data taken from a wide cross-section of disciplines: engineering, physiology, anatomy, psychology, medicine, mathematics, and statistics. To this end, ergonomics offers a philosophy and approach for dealing with people's characteristics and limitations; it accepts people as they are, as individuals having various abilities that are neither constant nor completely measurable. It attempts to effect a match between people and their working environment, their products. In so doing, it considers the whole of the person: behavioral, physical, and physiologic attributes.

The key to a successful ergonomic effort lies in the integration of people's abilities and the demands of their environment (Fig. 47.1). Successful integration is achieved when people are not exposed to safety or health risks; when the job demands do not tax human work capacity, or can be met only by selected few individuals; when people are in control of their environment and machines; and when jobs promote the social interactions and well-being of those who perform them.

The literature of ergonomics contains numerous examples of how the interface between man and machine, if not controlled, can be hazardous to one's safety and health. In most instances, the interface may subject both man's

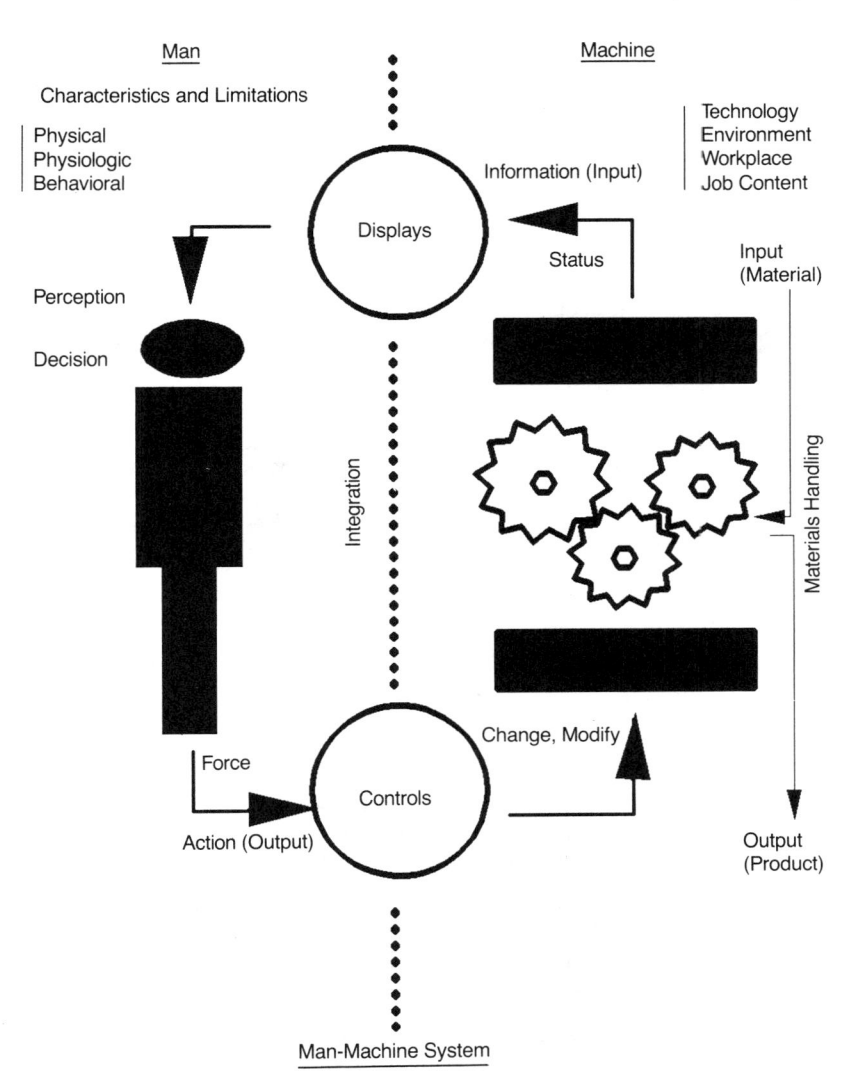

Figure 47.1. A man-machine system.

anatomy and physiology to excessive and highly concentrated stresses and strains. Persistence of these stresses can lead to the occurrence of an array of health disorders and occupational diseases.

For example, the task in some occupations might force the individual to maintain an awkward posture during extended periods. Such awkward postures, when imposed (through faulty equipment design or workplace arrangement) over a number of years, are apt to deform the anatomic system of the human body and ultimately lead to permanent occupational deformities—a case that is not uncommon in dentistry. Furthermore, there is a correlation between diseases of the musculoskeletal system (muscles, tendons, joints, and bones) and work postures. For instance, static loading of the cervical vertebrae—a posture prone to the meat-packing industry—has been found to be conducive to lesions of the spine. After surveying many females (weavers, spinners, and office clerks) of a silk spinning and weaving mill, it was concluded that most of the workers' complaints stemmed from static loading of the legs and feet. This static loading was aggravated by wearing unsuitable shoes. The problem was solved by providing the workers with specially designed shoes and allowing for periods of exercise. Many studies attribute to faulty postures the dissatisfaction and failure of workers to adapt to work on assembly lines.

In man-machine systems, physiologic stress damage is known to occur. This is common to tasks and situations where overloading, ranging from strained muscles to complete exhaustion, takes place. It has also been shown that great mental stress affects the flexibility of the muscular system adversely, thereby setting the stage for backache episodes. Physical problems resulting from the poor design and misuse of handtools are a reality in industry. Injuries associated with the use of handtools may not be as severe or as well pronounced as those from other hazards (e.g., noise and toxic gases), yet handtool ailments do exist. To this extent, a person who is crippled by repeated long-term usage of a poorly designed tool has just as much right to receive protection (as well as compensation) as the worker who is adversely affected by the breathing of toxic gases. Recent rulings by the courts in liability cases consider handtool ailments and disorders of the spine as occupational diseases for which compensation claims may be awarded.

Health disorders may result from improperly designed seating devices. Women performing repetitive hand motions while maintaining static postures (sitting or standing) in noisy environments incur cardiovascular disorders and disturbance of the locomotor system. A survey of sewing machine operators disclosed that incorrect postures, resulting mainly from poor seating arrangement, led to tiredness and localized aches in different parts of the body. Vibration, prolonged sitting, and continuous spells of nervous and muscular tension are all possible causes of circulatory disorders in the lower limbs of truck drivers.

Manual materials-handling activities (lifting, carrying, pushing, and pulling) constitute a major source of spinal disorders and back problems.

The preceding are few examples of harmful effects of excessive stress and strain that may result from a man-machine interface imposed for extended periods of time. However, keeping these stresses to a minimum will not eliminate or control disorders of the man-machine system; it has been shown that maintaining the body under minimum stresses and strains will adversely affect the cardiovascular dynamics and metabolic processes. In addition, reduction in stresses may lead people to lose interest in their jobs and to become discontented and bored.

THE APPROACH

The ergonomic approach to job design considers human capabilities, task demand, and workplace (equipment) characteristics. It attempts to determine the optimum interface (physical) between man and his machine—the interface that will protect the human structure from excessive stresses and strains without compromising productivity and efficiency. This optimum interface can be realized if industrial tasks are designed so as to achieve maximum adjustments between human physiologic capacity and job demands.

A body responds to job demands by exerting a muscular force. If the muscle is in shape, having sufficient strength, the force is delivered. When delivering this force over time, the body calls on the heart and the lungs to provide oxygen to the working muscle, and rid the muscle of waste products being produced. A complication of this scenario is the addition of a heat component to the job. When a body gains heat, it must face the problem of maintaining a constant core temperature. To accomplish this, the body must lose the heat gained from the environment; here sweating becomes a factor.

The term *physiologic capacity* refers to man's physical capabilities in performing his tasks. These capabilities can be divided into: (a) physical reach capabilities, (b) muscular strength capabilities, (c) metabolic energy output capabilities, and (d) cardiac output capabilities. Man's physiologic capacity varies considerably during his life cycle. It is influenced by factors such as age, exercise, environment, and occupation. In some occupations, such as heavy industry and agriculture, physiologic demands predominate and thereby mask psychological requirements imposed upon workers. On the other hand, sedentary occupations (e.g., bank clerks and drivers) involve a relatively small physical load, but by nature utilize a large portion of man's mental capacity. Finally, tasks that require sizable amounts of both physiologic and mental capacities are not uncommon in occupational settings. For example, in the medical field the work of nurses is often characterized by physical exertion as well as by a high degree of responsibility (i.e., large mental load).

ERGONOMIC ANALYSIS

A worthwhile and trustworthy ergonomic design or assessment has to commence with the definition of the characteristics and attributes of the man-machine system under evaluation. Here, we would be interested in evaluating the strength/weakness of each of nine specific areas of ergonomic concern: management, job, workplace, machine, method, materials handling, environment, health care programs, and employee fitness/awareness. An ergonomic checklist (such as shown in Appendix 47.A) may be used for gathering data and documenting the observed conditions. In addition, employees should be interviewed concerning the demands of their jobs. When possible, employees should complete a pain questionnaire.

Following the initial survey, a set of objective data would be collected for the purpose of profiling job demands and the corresponding human responses (physical and physiologic).

This is carried out in two steps: first, the determination of data profiles for (a) anthropometric characteristics (static and dynamic), (b) motion characteristics (force and moment profiles), and (c) physiologic responses to stress (heart rate, energy expenditure, myograms, etc.); and second, the objective assessment of the data profiles for either establishing work tolerance or defining effects of stresses and strains of a given situation on the human body. Based on this, a conclusion can be reached as to whether the task, as presented, constitutes an unreasonable demand on man's capabilities; also, the "best" method for performing the task can be established.

Some of the techniques used for this phase include: (a) motion recording and analysis, (b) electromyography, (c) posture targeting, and (d) physiologic responses.

Motion Recording and Analysis

Displacement, velocity, and acceleration (also known as kinematic data) can be obtained by photographic methods, electromechanical methods (e.g., accelerometer), or electronic methods. As must be obvious, the differences among these methods are due to (a) the initial parameter recorded and (b) the medium used for recording. For photographic methods, displacement versus time is obtained as the initial parameter. Through successive differentiation, velocity and acceleration profiles are obtained. This is done for all body segments. On the other hand, by using accelerometers, the parameter measured is acceleration. By integrating two times, velocity and displacement profiles are obtained, respectively. Changing from cinematography to video is an example of how the medium can change the method of data recording and subsequent analysis. Using a combination of video cameras and image digitization by computers is an example of how the recording medium can influence the speed and ease of recording, as well as the accuracy of the results.

Electromyography

Dynamic analysis yields information on the forces and moments to which the body and musculoskeletal system respond. As is known, motion recording and the corresponding analysis are cumbersome and may be of little interest to most practitioners. Electromyography (EMG) offers a reasonable alternative to dynamic analysis. It is a technique for measuring the tension (force) developed as the muscle is shortened or put to work. The action potential that accompanies muscle tension is measured in terms of microvolts. Monitoring a specific muscle consists of placing a pair of electrodes on the muscle "belly." The signal from the electrodes is picked up and then "conditioned" before it is displayed on a meter or chart. For some applications, the raw EMG signals are integrated or averaged over a specific period of time. Muscle action potential (EMG data) varies as a function of several task, person, and workplace variables. The list of variables includes: posture, speed, force (weight handled), range of motion, muscle mass used, work/rest schedule, initial muscle length, individual degree of fitness, clothing, and static loading.

Electromyography can be used to objectively express job muscular loading as a percentage of monitored muscle maximum. If the computed percentage is less than 20% (or even 30%) then we may conclude that task loading is acceptable. For higher percentages, the task must be examined closely for possible redesign or adjustments.

Posture Targeting and Analysis

Posture analysis may be used as a substitute for both dynamic analysis and EMG measurements. Describing the posture of various body segments versus time does provide much information concerning (a) static loading, (b) concentration of job motion, and (c) extreme motions of various body joints. This information is very important when a job/workplace is evaluated or redesigned. The advantage of posture analysis over other methods rests with the ease with which the assessment/evaluation can be carried out. The procedure involves the following steps. First, the person is filmed (videotaped) while performing the job. Filming is done from two different angles in order to record body segment motions in all planes. It should continue until several job cycles are covered. For repetitive jobs, this is usually accomplished in a few minutes. For most jobs, 5 min of recording would be long enough to cover hundreds of cycles or more. Recordings should be made for a representative sample of the persons assigned to the job being evaluated.

Following recording, the film or videotape is viewed in a systematic manner to sample for the occurrences of certain segment positions. The standard posture descriptors, such as flexion and extension, are used to categorize observed postures. The films or tapes are sampled for these positions for each body segment. The analysis goes through a frame-by-frame sampling until sufficient data are obtained to profile the various body segments on an 8-hr basis. Again, such information can be very useful when the redesign of jobs/workplaces is contemplated.

Physiologic Responses

Physiologic responses are assessed in terms of changes of some specific and measurable parameters such as heart rate, blood pressure, skin temperature, rectal temperature, oxygen consumption, ventilation rate, respiration rate, and concentration of metabolites in blood and urine. These physical responses can be measured using a number of well-established techniques and methods. For example, in case of oxygen consumption, the Douglas bag method involves collecting the expired air in a bag. Collecting the air over a specified period of time and emptying the bag through a meter will yield the volume per unit time. This volume is then corrected to a standard temperature and pressure to give ventilation rate expressed in liters per minute. If a sample of the expired air is analyzed for oxygen content, the oxygen consumption can be estimated. If we assume that each liter of oxygen would yield 4.8–5.0 kcal, energy expenditure can be estimated directly from oxygen consumption. There are devices and instruments that can be used to obtain this information without too much input or manipulation. An example of these is the Oxylog. The Oxylog (manufactured in England and commercially available in this country) is used for gas collection and analysis. It is a small, lightweight unit, easily transported by the subject, and connected directly to a face mask via hosing. It provides digital readings of oxygen consumption and ventilation rates.

There exist definitive linear relationships among all of the response measures. In other words, monitoring heart rate will be sufficient for all practical purposes to categorize the other measures.

Maximum (limiting) values of the physiologic responses can be determined by using standard tests utilizing bicycle ergometers, treadmills, or other physical demand simulators. These tests can be carried out either under maximum or submaximum conditions (protocol). In absence of actual testing, the maximum values for some responses can be obtained by using well-defined empirical relationships. For example, in the case of heart rate, the maximum value (for both males and females, and in the absence of disease) is given by:

$$\text{Max heart rate (beats/min)} = 210 - \text{age (years)} \times .65$$

For oxygen consumption (oxygen uptake), the limit for males is:

$$60 - .55 \times \text{age (years)} \text{ (ml/kg/min) (SD = 7.5)}$$

The limit for females is:

$$48 - .73 \times \text{age (years)} \text{ (ml/kg/min) (SD = 7.0)}$$

The above expressions do serve as a means for predicting the limiting responses for individuals. Therefore, individual differences may not be reflected in the limits computed. To avoid this pitfall, and if the situation warrants, the limits should be established based on direct testing of the individuals concerned.

Response-Time Curve Each of the body physiologic responses (e.g., heart rate and oxygen consumption) follows a specific pattern. At rest, the response, say heart rate, is at a minimum. When work commences it will be a brief time before it is elevated to a level compatible with the workload. If the response level maintained by the body is sufficient to meet the demand imposed by the workload on the muscles, a steady state is achieved. On the other hand, if the demand is such that it requires a maximum response, then a steady state will not be realized. Instead, a steady climbing of the response level will be observed until the work is stopped, due to either its completion or reaching complete exhaustion. Upon termination of work, the level will start to drop down gradually until it reaches the resting value. Rest-work-rest gives a cyclic pattern that may be repeated hundreds of times in the course of an 8-hr day. It should be obvious that work/rest periods depend, to a large extent, on the workload.

For light to moderate levels, the length of work cycle could last for 2 hr or so without an outright need for rest. However, for heavy and highly demanding work, the work cycle will, by necessity, have to be short and should be followed by a rest period of proper duration. Another alternative to this would be to enlarge the job to encompass tasks with varying levels of demand. Job rotation (assigning two or more tasks, different in demands but related otherwise) will tend to bring the overall demand to a managing level.

Contributing Factors Job demands and the subsequent responses depend on several contributing variables, such as:

1. Age, sex
2. Fitness
3. Posture
4. Workload
5. Rest schedule
6. Environment

Variables 1 and 2 reference the person as is, variables 3 and 4 reference the job itself, and variables 5 and 6 reference the job content—how it is structured.

The following are some observations concerning the influence of some of these variables on the physiologic responses.

1. In general, females pay a higher price (physiologic cost) by approximately 20% above that for the males.
2. With age, maximum capacity declines. For example, with every decade, maximum heart rate decreases by 10 beats. As age increases, in absence of other conditions, recovery time increases; that is, for the same level of demand, older persons are taxed at a higher level.
3. Training can change the level of taxation and the corresponding recovery time. With training, a high improvement in recovery capabilities occurs after 30–60 days. The opposite is also true; if one stops exercising, the degree of fitness is lost quickly. For example, upon return to work from a holiday or vacation, a person may not resume work at the same fitness level exhibited prior to going away.
4. Posture contributes to the overall response level. If extreme reach is combined with maximum exertions (e.g., using a power tool) the response will be high. A reduction in the extent of reach can reduce the corresponding heart rate; a simple solution that often provides good results.
5. Temperature influences the response to a given workload. If the temperature is elevated, the heart rate will be elevated because of the additional strain placed upon the heart in the course of pumping more blood to the surface to maintain heat balance. Temperature also increases recovery time.
6. Without a proper work/rest schedule, a person will pay a price. If one task is performed and then followed by a rest period, the heart rate will be somewhat low and steady. If the person does two exertions (two tasks) without sufficient rest in between, it will take longer to recover from this double duty. Thus, one can predict a trend, so planning a job is important. Comparing the recovery curves for a job with no rest given, the same job with rest periods every hour, and the same job with rest periods every 30 min would show that a person who is allowed to rest every 30 min achieves complete recovery. Accordingly, no cumulative fatigue effect will be experienced.
7. Crew size also has an effect. The more members on a crew the lower the heart rate response to a job. Proper sharing of the scheduled work can therefore increase productivity at a decreased level of response.

8. When considering clothing in hot environments, one can compare shorts to a pair of coveralls. Shorts allow for air circulation, evaporation, and convection to occur. Coveralls decrease the area of skin exposed to the air, therefore the level of evaporation and convection decreases. With less air circulation, increased body temperature results in higher heart rate.
9. The quality of the environment in which rest is taken becomes an important factor if the job is performed in the presence of heat. Resting in a cool environment will improve recovery time (i.e., less time) and eliminate the potential for cumulative effects. Accordingly, the response level will remain basically low across all work periods.
10. Muscle mass used in task performance affects levels of physiologic responses. Tasks with predominant arm movements tend to tax the heart higher than those performed by the powerful muscles of the lower extremity. This is attributed to the size differences between blood vessels of the arms and those of lower extremity. Small blood vessels in the arms cause increase in blood pressure, hence higher heart rate.
11. Fatigue plays a large role in the development of musculoskeletal trauma. Overexertion (resulting from excessive force, extreme reach, and repetition of specific task) is a direct cause of fatigue. With repetitive use and high levels of loading, a muscle's energy reserve decreases as the amount of waste products increase. This results in impaired muscular coordination, leading to injury, errors, and accidents.
12. Standing jobs that do not allow the person to move around or utilize the feet much of the time impede return of the venous blood to the heart. In other words, the phenomenon known as "muscle pump" will be drastically reduced, if not lost. Slowing venous blood return results in blood pooling in the lower extremities, causing an increase in heart rate. This increase compensates for the lower stroke volume caused by blood pooling.
13. Wearing tight clothing may place an added stress on the cardiovascular system. For example, tight pants impede blood flow to and from the lower extremity. This causes an increase in heart rate.
14. Smoking does influence the responses. It increases breathing resistance, which may become a limiting factor during exercise. Two cigarettes may raise the heart rate by 20–30 beats above normal level. Smoking lowers the oxygen-carrying capacity of the blood as a result of combining of carbon monoxide and red blood cells. This means that for the same level of effort, more blood must be pumped to the working muscles in order to compensate for loss of oxygen supply.
15. Alcohol affects the body in a number of well-defined ways: impaired judgment, loss of coordination, speech disturbances, memory loss, and loss of manual dexterity. In addition, alcohol causes change in blood circulation, which in turn increases the workload on the heart.
16. A person handling a highly intense task for extended periods of time will undoubtedly exhibit some signs of fatigue. This fatigue will take the form of higher levels of physiologic responses. In this case as time goes on, heart rate, oxygen consumption, and other physiologic responses will increase even though the work load has remained the same. Introduction of proper rest periods (duration and timing) will tend to control or moderate the onset of fatigue.

ERGONOMIC DEFICIENCIES

Absence of ergonomics will bring inefficiency and pain to the workplace. An ergonomically deficient workplace will not cause immediate pain, because the human body has a great capacity for adapting to a poorly designed workplace or structured job. However, in time the compounding effect of the job/workplace deficiencies will surpass the body coping mechanisms, causing the inevitable—occupational disease, emotional scars, low productivity, and poor quality of work.

Ergonomic deficiencies are manifested by a number of well-defined and well-recognzied symptoms: extreme posture, excessive force, concentration of stress, static loading, pain/discomfort, and high incidence of occupational diseases/disorders. The first four symptoms can be considered as early warnings; the remaining two are the final outcome, occurring only when nothing is done to correct the existing deficiencies.

Extreme Posture

Posture refers to alignment of body segments. Placing one or more body segments in extreme position or out of alignment with other segments will produce extreme posture. Such posture places much strain on the body, including joints, tendons, and muscles. Alternating between extreme postures is also stressful. In most cases, extreme postures are the result of improper reach. Any reaches made with the arms fully extended and to points above shoulders or below waist are typical causes of extreme postures. Another cause of extreme posture is improperly designed hand-held tools, products, and machine controls. For many of these either the object is too bulky to hold with ease or it is hard to get to without adapting an extreme posture, especially for the wrist and arm. In general, any posture (body alignments) that does not look right or looks difficult to maintain can safely be labeled as extreme.

Excessive Force

Materials handling and use of hand and power tools require exertion of force. The force required will depend on the weight and bulk of the object handled/manipulated as well as body posture. If any of these parameters is improper, a condition for exerting too much force develops. The following are examples of jobs/situations that lead to overexertion:

1. Picking a bulky and heavy box off a shelf with the arms fully extended.
2. Assignment of a relatively short person (5'0") to the task described in (1) above, making it extremely taxing.
3. Retrieving bulky and heavy items from underneath shelves or work surface with the back fully bent and arms stretched.
4. Handling items or objects that have little or no rigidity, not equipped with handles.
5. Placing objects in deep containers. This is most difficult when the object is bulky and the container is deep (waist high).
6. Asiding work pieces by throwing them to the front or the side. The amount of force will depend on the object weight and speed. The faster the action, the higher the force exerted; a force of 5 to 10 times the weight of the object may be encountered in such actions.
7. Use of power tools, which are typically heavy or in some cases bulky. Their use is always accompanied by exertion of high force. To this we may add the effects of vibration and noise resulting from improperly designed handles and mechanisms.

In all the above examples, the level of stress on the body will depend on the person's fitness level. Individuals who are out of shape, overweight, or perhaps suffering from musculoskeletal diseases (limitations) will find any of those situations very stressful.

Concentration of Stress

By definition, stress is a force divided by the area over which it is applied. For a given force, the larger the area, the less the stress; the opposite is also true. Putting it in the context of the human body, the fewer the muscles used to deliver force, the higher the stress placed on the body. Any task that utilizes few muscles or relatively weak muscles constitutes a troublesome concern and results in inefficient loading of the musculoskeletal system.

Repetitive jobs characterized by short and fast motions are prone to causing stress concentration. Miniature hand-tools or tools that tend to be buried within the palms are another example. As a rule, level of stress concentration is inversely related to the number of body segments engaged in the task motion/force application. That is, the fewer the segments, the higher the potential for stress concentration.

Time is an important consideration in developing stress concentration. That is, stress applied infrequently may not be as harmful as stress that dominates throughout the working day.

Static Loading

This is a label given to a host of situations where one or more body segments are kept motionless or allowed to change positions very infrequently. Static loading interferes with muscle/tendon functions and if allowed to persist over time will eventually cause damage to the body and the occurrence of cumulative trauma disorders. A comparable situation to static loading can be realized when the body performs repetitive and forceful motions with little or no chance for rest. In this case, although the body is kept in motion, speed and repetitiveness of the activity will make it equivalent to maintaining static posture.

The following is a list of some examples of situations prone to producing static loading:

1. Tasks that are dominated by one activity (element) such as reach, grasp, move, and position.
2. Jobs consisting of one primary task that loads the same muscle or groups of muscles with no opportunity for their relief.
3. Tasks performed by hand/wrist motions while the rest of the body is maintained in a fixed position throughout the repeating job cycles.
4. Jobs that have improper rest periods (number, duration, and schedule) or having rest periods that are skipped at will by employees.
5. Workplaces lacking sufficient space to allow for balanced moves and frequent change in posture.
6. Jobs in which the body is used to support material/tools while performing the job activity.
7. Jobs requiring the person to look through optical aids such as microscopes for long periods.
8. Data entry operations, VDT tasks.

Most situations of static loading can be attributed to method/job designs and fair number could be attributed to workplace/machine interfacing with the individuals performing the tasks.

Pain-Discomfort

Frequent complaints of discomfort, fatigue, and outright pain are positive indications of the existence of ergonomic deficiencies. When the complaints increase in frequency or start to interfere with job performance, one can conclude that the need for ergonomic intervention is urgent. If management fails to recognize the meaning of the reported pain, the situation will worsen, consequently setting the stage for developing cumulative trauma disorders.

Cumulative Trauma Disorders

When management lacks awareness of how its practices and policies are creating a deficient workplace, when it absolves itself from close monitoring of work practices, when it does not share with the employees the responsibility of defining practical job standards, then cumulative trauma disorders are a certain outcome. This may take a number of forms: sudden and unexpected increase in the number of reported cases of the disorders; increase in the number of employees out of work because of disability; high number of employees seeking treatment from the company medical department or from outside physicians; and increasing rate of turnover or transfers from some jobs.

CUMULATIVE TRAUMA DISORDERS

Tendinitis, tenosynovitis, and carpal tunnel syndrome are new words in today's workplace, replacing more descriptive titles such as housemaid's knee, telegraphist's wrist, tennis elbow, golfer's shoulder, and baseball player's glass arm. Each describes a disorder characteristic of the occupation it typifies. All names indicate an injury or disorder of the tendon and related anatomic structure (sheaths and nerves). Tendon injuries are found in labor-intensive industries (textiles, apparel), highly mechanized assembly-type industries (electronics), heavy industry, data processing, and jobs requiring use of vibrating tools and awkward postures coupled with repetitive motions. Cumulative trauma disorders (CTDs) is the label used to define tendon- or nerve-related disorders resulting from repetitive motions (usage), mechanical trauma (injury), and excessive forceful exertion.

To industry, CTDs mean low productivity, poor quality, and high medical and health maintenance costs. To the injured employee, the disorders spell pain, suffering, and low morale. In both cases, it is an undesirable outcome. Most states recognize cumulative trauma disorders as compensable work-related injuries/diseases. Current industry data show that a typical case would carry a cost tag of $5,000–$15,000, excluding indirect costs. Medical and legal costs constitute the major expense associated with CTDs trauma disorders. Such costs are expected to continue to increase. In recent years, the Occupational Safety and Health Administration (OSHA) has issued several well-publicized citations to various industries because of problems stemming from excessive cumulative trauma. Therefore, it is imperative that industry moves toward the recognition and elimination of ergonomic deficiencies in the workplace. *Ergonomics "done right, on time" would put a lid on the disorders.*

CAUSATIVE FACTORS

The primary causes of CTDs are excessive physical stress, anatomic/physiologic predisposition, and mental stress. Although the role each plays in the production of CTDs has yet to be established or delineated, it appears that a mix of the three is necessary.

Physical Stress

Excessive physical stress can result from the performance of highly repetitive tasks on or off the job. Repetitive motions coupled with work postures that force body segments to assume extreme positions (flexion, extension, deviation) may cause stretching of the tendons involved and deliver pinching forces to neighboring soft tissues. When applied over time (static loading), inflammation of tendon sheaths and pressuring of nerves may result.

Poor posture associated with physical stress may be manifested in situations including work with elevated arms, prolonged overhead work, carrying heavy shoulder loads, and force applications accompanied with extreme posture (grasping with fingers wide open, forceful exertion with elbow in extension). Certain motions linked to CTDs are rapid and repetitive arm and hand motions, repetitive abduction-rotation movements, repeated dorsiflexions of wrist, alternating pronation and supination, and use of forearm extensors in a forceful and monotonous way. Mechanical trauma and forceful exertions by unaccustomed workers are considered important contributors. Mechanical trauma may be due to direct (blunt force) or indirect (strain/sprain) causes.

For persons engaged in activities that require repetitive motions on and off the job, pinpointing the cause of the manifested disorder is difficult. This is precisely the reason for emphasizing that rehabilitation programs consider both types of activities.

Anatomic/Physiologic Disposition

Age, sex, anatomic difference, and disease have been repeatedly cited as contributing factors in the causation of tendinitis and related disorders. The contribution of each has not been well ascertained; however, they can be viewed as factors that predispose to rather than initiate CTDs.

The Environment

Noise, illumination, vibration, and cold can play a role in the causation of CTDs. Noise, considered a source of annoyance, may contribute to mental stress. Poor or inadequate levels of illumination causing visual strain (eye fatigue) may force the individual to assume and maintain a poor posture. For tasks where close visual contact is required, the contrast levels become extremely important. Poor contrast (white object on a white background) yields eye strain that forces the individual to concentrate more, resulting in mental and physiologic fatigue. Vibration contributes to the problem by acting as a direct physical stressor disturbing anatomic and physiologic characteristics of the soft tissues and by forcing an individual to develop and maintain awkward postures. A cold environment may affect the physiology of muscular actions, resulting in excessive physical loading.

Mental Stres

Mental stress is due to many causes, such as depression, mental fatigue (information overload), monotonous work, excess responsibility, and tension. Mental stress alone does not cause CTDs, but does sensitize individuals to pain, real or imagined. With mental stress, an individual may become susceptible to suggestions and experience decreased tolerance to pain.

Performance Rates

High achievers and low achievers have the same probability of contracting CTDs since the amount of static loading will be the same for both. High achievers (exceeding the standard rate) end up with shorter work cycles and a higher number of work cycles per shift. Low achievers (falling below the standard) use a longer cycle coupled with proportionately fewer cycles per shift. Combining cycle time and total number of cycles per shift yields the exposure time during which static loading occurs. This time of static loading will be the same for those who fall below or exceed the standard by the same amount. Thus, low and high achievers following the same method are subject to the same risk of CTDs.

Rate of Occurrence

Management style, quality of supervision, and a host of behavioral factors play an important role in controlling the onset and spread of CTDs in a given plant. A workplace that nurses conflict either between management and employees or among employees may influence the prevalence and incidence rate of CTDs. Many industrial experiences support the contention that tendinitis cases seem to spread like a "rash," often developing without substantial forewarning. Case studies show that a plant without a significant history of CTDs may suddenly experience an overwhelming and alarming incidence rate. Two plants similar in every respect (work method, performance standards, equipment, management) may exhibit quite different CTD history. In most cases, the differences may be attributed to management practices and communication between management and employees.

THE CTD PROCESS

Cumulative trauma disorders do not happen instantaneously or overnight; rather these disorders mark the end of a process that spans several stages of development. A person may go through four stages of pain prior to receiving a piece of paper from a physician designating the presence of a specific disorder such as tendinitis.

In *Stage 1*, the beginning, the person feels discomfort that usually disappears at the end of the day or with some extended rest. If the job and workplace characteristics are left unchanged, the discomfort will then turn into pain that is localized at some specific areas in the body such as the wrist or shoulder. Again, if nothing is done to address the root cause of this pain, it will become chronic. The pain then progresses to a point at which it starts to interfere with job performance. This is *Stage 2*.

During the second stage of chronic pain, the person shows no specific signs such as warmth, tenderness, or redness. In many cases, the specificity of the cause of the pain may not be too apparent to the treating physician. More often than not, the situation is one of frustration for both the patient and the physician. Given time to run its full course, the pain will be present along with some specific signs (*Stage 3*). The presence of such signs will help the physician in reaching a definitive diagnosis. At this point, *Stage 4* is reached. To this end, standard clinical tests (such as Phalen's test for carpal tunnel syndrome) would yield reliable conclusions.

During the first two stages of the process, ergonomics can make its biggest contribution, and if done right, it will eliminate the undesirable outcome—diagnosed cases. In contrast, if nothing is done about the early symptoms of pain, the condition will become progressively worse—changing from discomfort to a specific diagnosis. Consider the following case history.

ANATOMY OF A CTD CASE

January Mrs. X is 44 years old. Since her early twenties, she was diagnosed as diabetic and has been on insulin ever since. She works on an incentive job in an electronic assembly plant. She has been with her company for approximately 6 years. She is slightly overweight and has been complaining about numbness in her right hand for about 3 months, which initially would come and go. However, recently, her condition has worsened and the numbness is present at all times. Her job performance has been affected. She is having much difficulty meeting the new production standard that was established a few months ago.

February The plant nurse arranges for Mrs. X to see an orthopedic surgeon. Following detailed clinical examination and various tests, including nerve conduction, it was decided to perform a carpal tunnel release on the right wrist.

One Week Later Following the operation, Mrs. X started to feel better. The numbness in her hand is now gone. She and her doctor are quite pleased with the outcome. The doctor assures Mrs. X that it will not be long before she can go back to work.

Four Weeks following the Operation Mrs. X is back at work. She started to feel some discomfort and occasional pain in the right wrist, the site of her old wound. She went back to see the doctor. He recommended that she should start wearing a wrist splint while at work.

Two Months following the Operation Mrs. X. is very concerned about her performance on the job. She is having a hard time meeting her production quota. The pain in her wrist is getting worse. She fears that the old problem will start all over again. She makes an appointment to see the doctor.

Three Months following the Operation Mrs. X is in pain; things are not going well for her. She has become very emotional about the whole thing. She has started to doubt the value of the operation. She blames the company and the job for all her problems. She is overcome with fears.

From the Doctor Mrs. X's case is extremly frustrating. Her wound healed satisfactorily. She has a good range of motion in her wrist. Her return to work was uneventful at the beginning. However, as she started trying to reach the target performance level for her job, things got worse. Her wrist started to hurt all over again. She has become very emotional. She talks about having the company to blame for all her troubles. It is quite difficult for me to advise her or answer the questions she raises about her job and the responsibility of the company.

There is nothing more to do for Mrs. X except to ask her to return to work. She qualifies for 5% permanent disability.

The End Mrs. X does not return to work. Rather, she goes straight to see her attorneys. A suit is filed . . . well, the rest of the story should be familiar to everyone!

What Went Wrong?

Mrs. X's case is rather typical and is seen quite often in industry. The facts of the case are:

1. Predisposed person assigned to unsuitable job.
2. Management failed to recognize the early warning signs of Mrs. X's condition—she experienced pain and numbness on and off for a period of time.
3. Following her surgery, no attempt was made to improve her workplace, method, or job content. That is, no effort was made to eliminate possible causative or aggravating factors that may retrigger the problem.
4. The doctor did not communicate to management what Mrs. X can or cannot do. Furthermore, the doctor did not attempt to learn much about Mrs. X's job demands.
5. From beginning to end, it is very obvious that the involved parties (Mrs. X, management, and the doctor) did not communicate with each other. Mrs. X worked in pain for as long as she could tolerate it; management considered its job done when Mrs. X was sent to the doctor. The doctor's main concern was treatment of Mrs. X's condition and very little else mattered.

The unhappy and emotional ending for Mrs. X was not warranted and certainly could have been avoided. Again, this shows the need to have ergonomics utilized early in making a job fit a person with or without limitation.

CTD CONTROL PROGRAM

A reliable and practical CTD control program would encompass: (*a*) improvement and redesign of the workplace, materials handling, method, and job structure; (*b*) education of employees and management; (*c*) monitoring employees at risk; (*d*) rehabilitation (return to work programs); and (*e*) preemployment screening.

Improvement and Redesign

Workplace Modification Static loading has been implicated as the primary cause of tendinitis and related disorders. It is caused by coupling and sequencing of motion elements and is intensified by factors attributable to seating, work surface, handtools, and machine controls. Rearrangement of all the workplace components (to assure proper integration) most often eliminates much of the problem. In some cases, redesign of machines, tools, and support surfaces may be required to achieve an acceptable solution.

Materials Handling Materials handling within and among work stations should be improved through the use of appropriate handling aids (e.g., gravity feed devices, conveyors). Product flow and workplace layout dictate the extent of any improvements.

Method Improvement From an evaluation of time standards and work postures, a content profile of each task can be developed and used to illustrate coupling among various motion elements. From the element profile, specific task posture versus time can be estimated. Careful review of content profiles should reveal work elements where posture improvement and streamlining can be made.

Education

An introductory presentation defining CTDs (symptoms, their causes, diagnosis and treatment) should be prepared and used for training new and current employees. Specific presentations should focus on causative factors of CTDs.

Monitoring

Employees should be encouraged to report symptoms of pain, swelling, and the like immediately to the medical department. Those involved with the "early symptom recognition and reporting program" should receive attention from medical staff, supervisors, and engineers until the reported symptoms disappear and the posture/work method becomes acceptable.

Individuals identified as potential risks should be monitored closely. If warranted, a review of individual method and work posture should be made and corrective actions instituted.

Rehabilitation

Upon return from medical leave following a CTD incident, the employee should be retrained to perform the job according to an ergonomically sound method. Emphasis should be on performance of tasks without assuming extreme postures or forceful exertions and unnecessary motions. The employee's supervisor and engineering and the medical staff should work together in planning and developing the retraining program.

Preemployment Screening

It is advisable to modify preemployment physicals to include screening for joint disorders (diseases) by obtaining a comprehensive medical history of past incidents, range of motion tests, and other information deemed appropriate by the plant physician.

AN EXPERT SYSTEM FOR CTDs

An expert system for aiding in the detection of trauma-causing situations would ideally encompass the following:

1. The detection of ergonomic deficiencies in the workplace and the work method that could cause cumulative trauma disorders.
2. The prediction of possible disorders resulting from

recognized deficiencies in order that the seriousness of the situation can be assessed.

3. The interrelation of symptoms and deficiencies to a specific disorder in order to aid the treating physician in the diagnosis of specific disorders, and to link such disorders with specific ergonomic deficiencies.

The system, using artificial intelligence, would query the user about disease symptoms, workplace, and work method characteristics. Based on these responses and its knowledge domain, the system would then produce lists of possible disorders, relevant deficiencies, and suggestions for improvements (see Fig. 47.2).

We developed a prototype of such a system using artificial intelligence. Artificial intelligence expert systems are computer-based systems that make judgments and decisions of a complex nature similar to those rendered by an expert in a given field. They are used when the shear magnitude of a problem involves an enormous amount of data for building the knowledge base of the system, coupled with the availability of few experts in the field. Such was the case concerning the many facets of CTDs and their causes.

Applications of expert systems already exist in several fields, ranging from agriculture to space technology, from engineering to medicine, from meteorology to information management, from electronics to law.

Illustrative Examples

The intended uses and internal functioning of this prototype system can best be illustrated by considering three different application scenarios. All three scenarios deal with a female operator who assembles a variety of electronic parts. She performs her job sitting down. She is provided with a plastic chair that is fixed in height. The job method consists of reaching for parts placed in angled bins at eye level, and then attaching the parts at approximately shoulder level with a screwdriver to a board held in a vertical fixture (see Figure 47.3).

Scenario 1: Ergonomic Deficiencies The plant industrial engineer decides to use the expert system to evaluate the deficiencies of the work station and the work method. Categories chosen to be evaluated are tools, seat, and work surface. Approximately 60 questions are asked by the expert system while searching for deficiencies. A condensed version of the session is presented below.

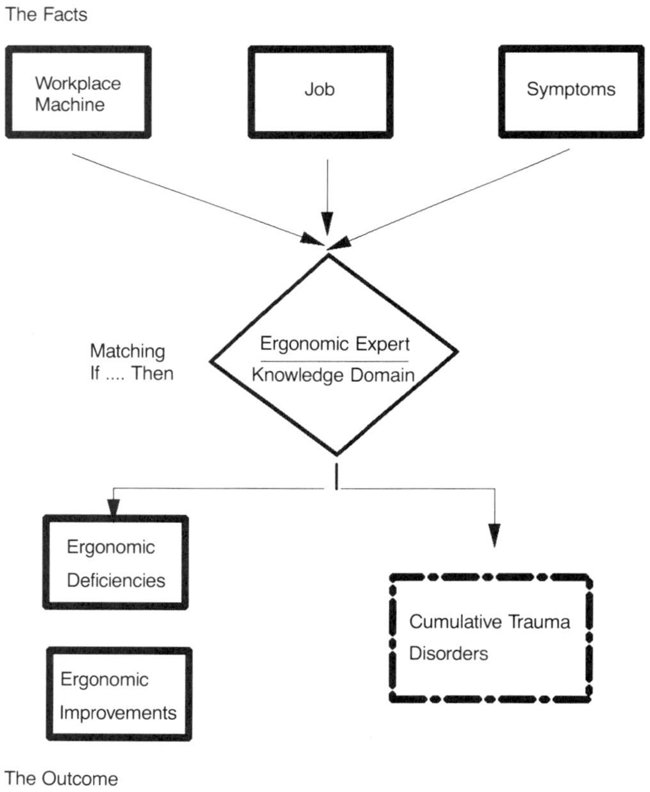

Figure 47.2. A CTD expert system.

How many tasks or operations do you perform (type an integer)?	1
Is the cycle time of your task less than 1 minute?	yes
Is your task performed mostly with arm-hand motions?	yes
Is your task equally shared by both arms? [Options = yes, left-dominated, right-dominated]	right
Do you remain stationary during the entire task?	yes
Do you follow the standard method for performing your task?	yes
Is your tool a standard one?	yes
Do you support your tool yourself while using it?	yes
Does your tool pressure any part of your body?	yes
Which body part receives the pressure?	hand
Is your wrist extremely bent up or down during most of the processing?	yes

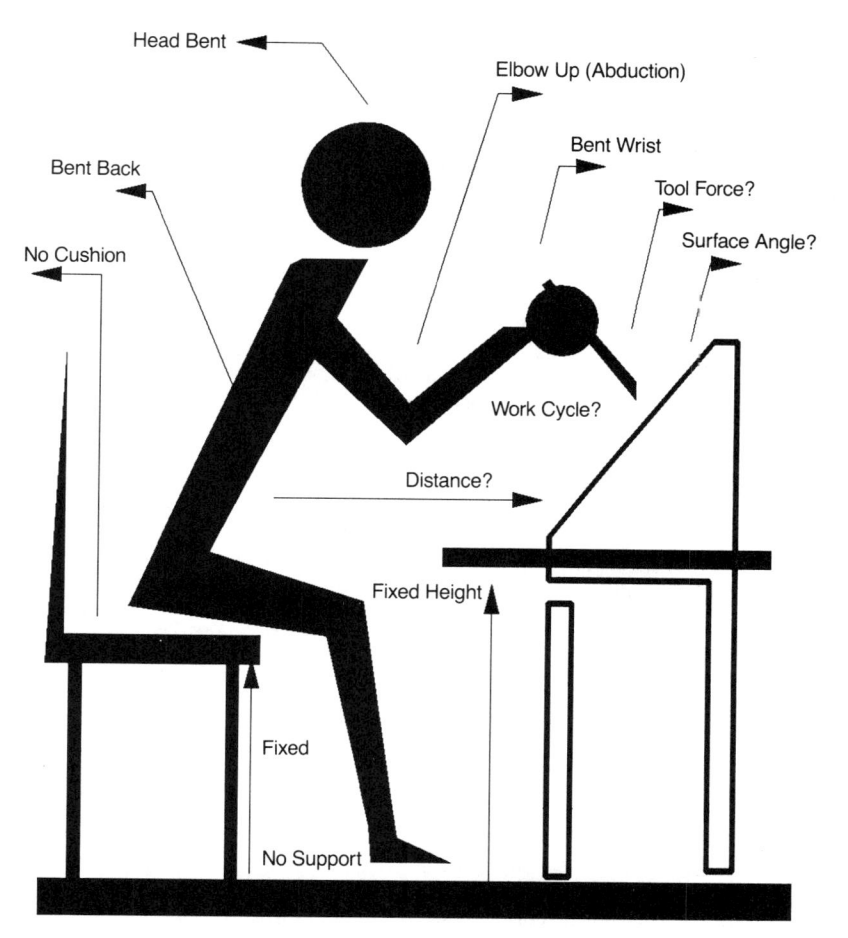

Figure 47.3. Workplace assembly task.

Are your wrist motions accompanied with the use of twisting or force?	yes
Is your elbow held up in the air when you use your tool?	yes
Is your seat adjustable in height?	no
Do you have sufficient space for your legs and knees?	yes
Do you usually sit forward on the front edge of your seat?	yes
Is your work surface height adjustable?	no

After asking the user the above questions, the system returns the following conclusion(s):

I have determined that
  Possible workplace deficiencies are:
    Nonadjustable seat causing static loading on legs or lower back from not being able to change postures in chair; consider chair replacement with adjustable-type chair

    Unadjustability of work surface height or angle causing possible eventual trauma to shoulder, head, lower back, or upper arms

  Possible work method deficiencies are:
    Use of tool with extreme wrist deviation accompanied with use of force; suggest changing angle of tool so that wrist is kept straight

    Standard tool is being used; investigate using tool more suitable for the job (possibly with ergonomically designed handle)

Short, concentrated task causing the likelihood of static loadings on muscles used; suggest enlarging job to include more tasks (such as obtaining materials—tasks having motions that would use a different set of muscles)

Scenario Two: Possible Disorders If the above operator is actually experiencing aches and pains, or other symptoms, the operation of the system can be switched to the disease mode. If the operator states that her current pain areas involve the wrist and shoulder, the system will attempt to match symptoms to diseases by asking questions such as:

Is it true that symptoms = numbness and night-pain?	yes
Is the affected trauma area stiff in the morning?	yes
Can you make a strong fist?	no

etc.

Once all the questions have been answered, the system then concludes:

Possible diseases:
   carpal tunnel syndrome or pre–carpal tunnel nerve entrapment damage to the wrist and hand

Scenario Three: Potential Disorders If the operator is not yet experiencing any symptoms, but wishes to receive an evaluation of possible diseases that may develop in the future, the system will first search for a body part that is being currently traumatized by work methods and/or the workplace. Once a body part has been matched with a workplace deficiency, possible diseases can be presented.

The preceding scenarios examining the same task from three different points of view show how the system data base is cross-linked among several categories. In other words, many of the queries are used in several categories with different rules. Accordingly, the expert system can take a minimal amount of information and apply it either to a disease or to work method/workplace deficiencies. This is how a CTD expert system incorporates the flexibility of a true expert into its program. The system, as presented and illustrated, can be considered a unique contribution to the field of artificial intelligence. Almost all medical expert systems in existence have dealt solely with matching symptoms with diseases in a diagnostic capacity. For instance, AI/Rheum diagnoses connective tissue rheumatology-related disorders. Succeeding in relating symptoms not only with diseases but also with actual causal element takes expert systems a step further into the realms of occupational preventive medicine and ergonomics.

CASE STUDY; ERGONOMICS OF BOARDING

Boarding is a process whereby a hose is shaped into a leg form. This gives it the elegant look some hosiery is known for. Boarding can thus be viewed as an ironing process. It is accomplished by placing the hose on a leg-shaped form that is mounted upside down on a movable platform. The operator has to reach to the top of the form for hose placement. Then he or she pulls down the hose to stretch it over the entire length of the form. This stretching involves considerable back bending (flexion) in the process of reaching the bottom of the form. Operators' earnings are based on incentive pay.

Three machines are used for the boarding process. The machines represent three generations of changes in technology and job design. The first machine (A; Fig. 47.4) is the oldest and requires the operator to load the hose on one side and then walk to the other side to remove it after boarding has been completed. In addition to loading and unloading, the operator does the necessary folding and bagging. The boards on the machine can be angled from a vertical position to allow for easy reach by the operator during handling of the hose. Two operators are usually assigned to the machine. It is possible for one operator to work alone on one side of the machine. The work is machine paced; however, the operator can stop the machine without affecting the work of others. The environment around the machine is hot and humid from the steam (used for boarding) released between loading and unloading. Operators are given two 10-min breaks (in the morning and afternoon) in addition to a 30-min lunch.

The second machine (B; Fig. 47.5), is a newer version of the first machine. The basic differences are: (a) the boards are no longer adjustable in position, (b) two operators are teamed together, and (c) the pace is closely controlled by the machine. Gone is the walking between the loading and unloading points of the first machine. Instead, the operator stands in one position during both hose loading and unloading. Because the board is fixed on its base, extreme reach and back bending are observed for the majority of the operators. Closeness to the machines causes the operator to be exposed to a hot and humid environment almost continuously. Again, the stationary nature of the job does not help. Both operators on the machine have to fold and bag their work. The two operators are paid as a team (i.e., group incentive).

The third machine (C; Fig. 47.6), is the newest addition to the plant, and it marks a major design change from its two predecessors, A and B. First, four operators are assigned to the machine. They work together as a team and are paid as a team (incentive pay). The job is divided, although not equally, among its four operators. Second, the boards are arranged to simulate the concept of an assembly line. Three of the operators work together, in front of the line, while the fourth handles the folding of boarded hose as well as supplying the first operator with

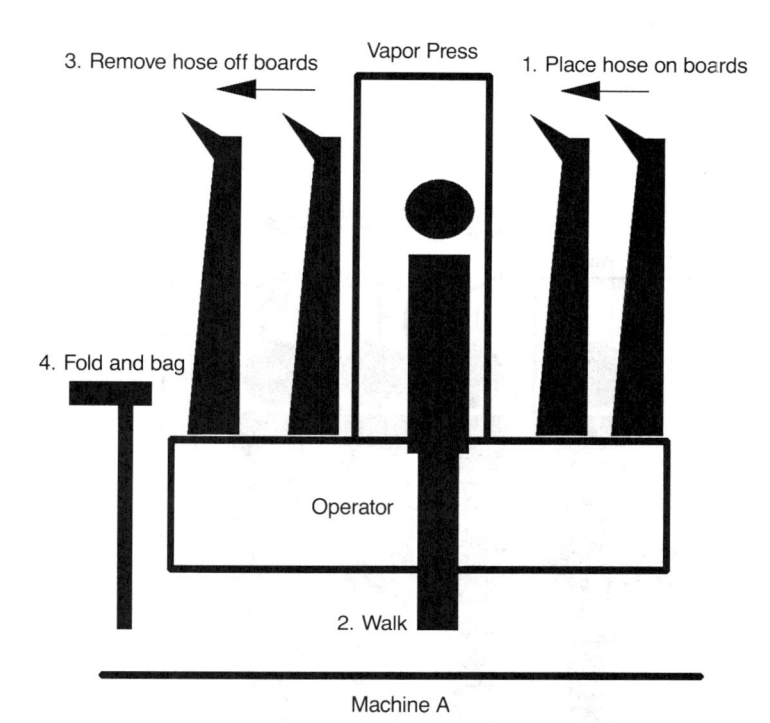

Figure 47.4. Boarding machine A.

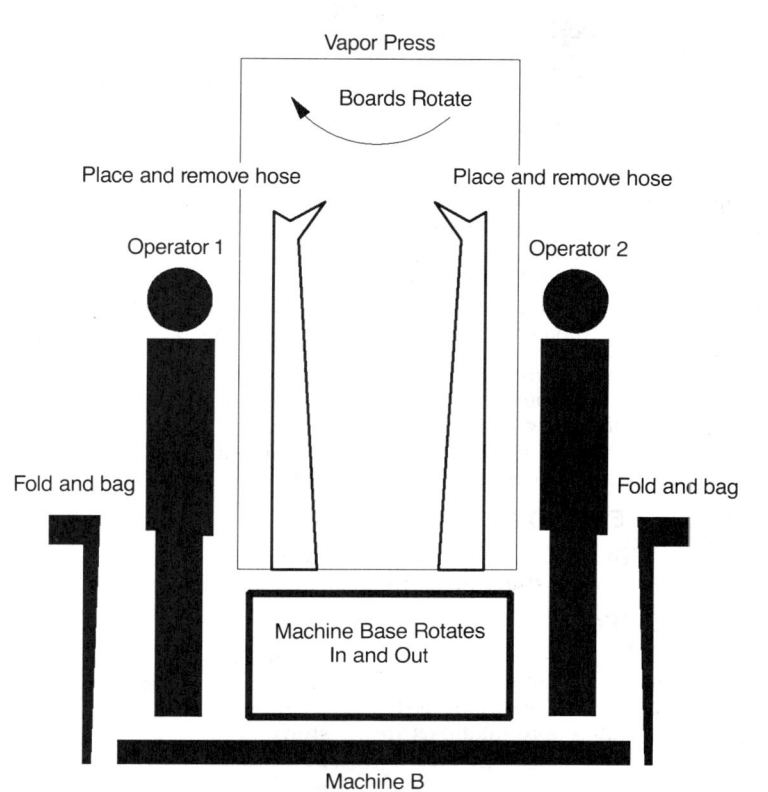

Figure 47.5. Boarding machine B.

Figure 47.6. Boarding machine C.

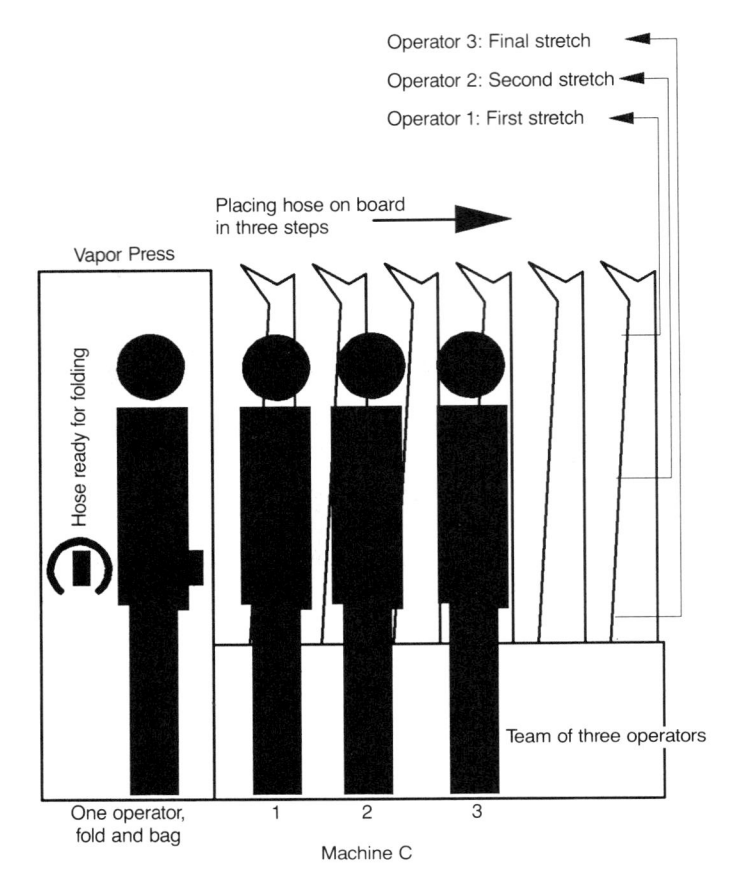

fresh hose. The first three operators work in unison. The first operator places the hose on the form; the second and third operators stretch each hose down the form. They do this by each stretching every other hose. The entire process is machine paced and very little chance exists for accommodating individual differences. The four operators are allowed the customary breaks, similar to those given to the others on the first two machines. Operators are encouraged to change positions (i.e., rotate). However, the practice is not enforced, and many teams do not follow it. The environment is not as humid because the operators are well shielded from the released steam.

In comparison with the first and second machines, the job on machine C is highly concentrated, a feature that is typical of many assembly lines. The arm reach is not as extreme as in the case of machine B. However, this is offset by extreme and concentrated back flexion (bends) occurring during hose stretching. The stationary feature observed for the second machine is the same for this machine, if not worse.

OBJECTIVES

Boarding was recognized by management as the job with a high prevalence rate of tendinitis and related disorders. It has a rate that is above all other jobs in the plant. Alarmed by the potential gravity of the situation, management requested an in-depth ergonomic evaluation and subsequent improvements of the boarding job.

To this end, management composed a list of key questions to be addressed by the study design. These include:

Is the job physically demanding?
Is the job perceived by the operators as demanding?
Is job content (mix of tasks) acceptable?
Is the pain reported by the operators job related?
Are some operators not fit for this type of work?

THE STUDY

To answer these questions as well as others, we initiated a detailed study of all the boarding machines.

Subjects

First, we met with all the boarding operators on both shifts. We explained to them the study objectives and the procedure planned for data collection. We asked for 50–60 volunteers to take part in the study.

Following the briefings, approximately 70 operators agreed to participate in the study. However, we were able to use only 53 operators.

The operators were distributed among the three machines (not in equal proportions) and the two shifts. Females were the majority in the sample. Only six males participated. Females are the dominant sex on the job.

Data

For each operator that participated in the study, we collected several pieces of data. First, we measured heart rate and skin temperature (while the person was performing the job). This was done for 1 hr during the shift. Forty-one operators were monitored in this fashion. In addition, 12 operators were monitored continuously for the entire shift. State-of-the-art equipment (Vitalog) that utilizes computers for data collection and analysis was used.

Second, each operator was videotaped for posture targeting and analysis. Posture evaluation was performed for the purpose of determining the degree of static loading and range of joint motions associated with each of the machines.

Third, the degree of muscle loading on each machine was measured using electromyography. Finger flexors, deltoid, and trapezius muscles for both right and left arms were monitored as the operator performed the various job elements, such as loading and stretching the hose, stripping hose, and then folding and bagging.

Finally each operator was asked to complete two questionnaires. The first attempted to find how difficult the job is. The second was a pain survey (pain drawing). Each operator was asked to indicate areas of discomfort and/or pain and to state their relative severity.

Additional information relative to past incidence of tendinitis and related disorders was obtained from the files of the medical department. Each of the employees signed a consent form prior to the start of data collection.

Findings

A large number of data were collected, and a detailed coverage of all the results is beyond our purposes here. However, some general findings are readily useful.

Job Difficulty and Pain When asked about job difficulty, the operators placed boarding using machine A on top of the scale as the most demanding. In contrast, in their opinions, knitting is viewed as the least demanding (Fig. 47.7). As to the most painful body area, the operators placed the back on top of the scale; elbows were a distant last (Fig. 47.8).

In considering their responses in terms of some individual and job characteristics, we observed a number of relationships. For example, the data show that those who reported the most pain tended to be slow performers (Fig. 47.9). A tall person reports more back pain than short persons. The reverse is true for shoulder pain. That is, a short person will tend to report more shoulder pain (Fig. 47.9). These two relationships should be expected. Back pain for tall persons comes about because extreme flexion (bending) that accompanies hose stretching on the form. For short persons, shoulder pain is the result of extreme reach that occurs while placing the hose on the form.

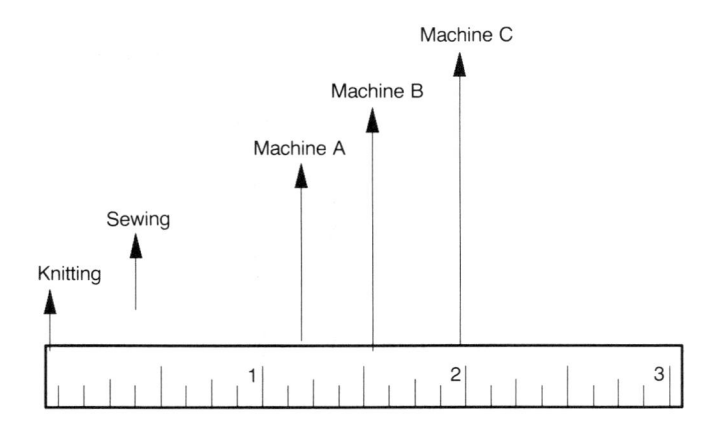

Figure 47.7. Relative pain in body areas.

Neck pain, as expected, is more pronounced for the older operators. This means that as the person gets older, the potential for reporting neck pain increases.

There is a general correspondence between current pain/discomfort and the problems reported previously to the medical department (Table 47.1). This may indicate that the causes of pain continue to be present in the job situation.

Heart Rate during Work Monitoring of physiologic responses showed that machine C is the most demanding in terms of average and maximum heart rates. Although all the operators started at relatively the same level of heart rate, within an hour of continuous work the rate for those on machine C steadily climbed to a level of 15–20 beats/min above the initial value (Fig. 47.11). This climb is not as significant for the first machine (A) and moderately less for the second machine (B). We attribute this steady and steep increase in heart rate to the highly concentrated nature of the job. The same conclusion can be reached based on the 8-hr studies.

When all the data from all the machines are pooled, we see that 60% of the operators maintain an average heart

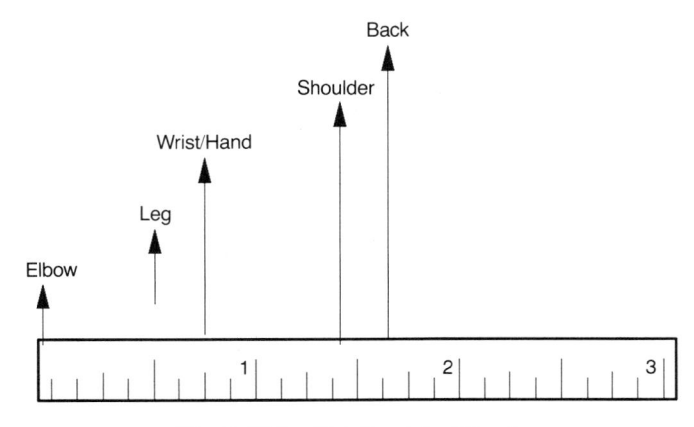

Figure 47.8. Relative job difficulty.

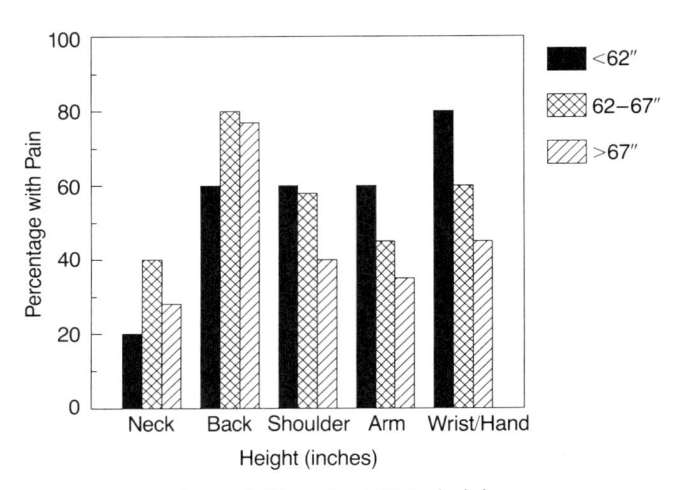

Figure 47.9. Pain versus height.

Table 47.1.
Pain versus Performance Based on Medical Records

	Correlation (r)
Age	−.50
Tenure	−.64
Back Pain	−.94
Neck Pain	−.52
Shoulder Pain	−.55
Arm Pain	−.55
Wrist/Hand Pain	−.60
Foot Pain	−.69

rate between 100 and 135 beats/min. This can be considered marginal for 8-hr jobs. On the other hand, 17% of the operators averaged heart rates in excess of 135 beats/min. This last figure is too high and is of concern.

In general, no person should work at a heart rate that exceeds 70–75% of the maximum value. Having such a high rate may be due (a) to demanding job activities or (b) to the fact that some operators lack the degree of fitness appropriate for the job.

Muscle Loading Electromyography was used to measure muscle loading for three specific muscle groups utilized in handling the hose. We monitored the flexors of the fingers, muscles that are involved in picking, stretching, and stripping (removing) the hose before and after boarding.

The deltoid and trapezius muscles were monitored to measure the degree of shoulder involvement through the boarding process. The data show that most of the operators work at about 60% of the limits for the three muscle groups (Fig. 47.12). Certain job elements tend to increase the level of muscle loading. Elements such as stripping, folding, and bagging exhibit higher values across all muscle groups.

A closer look at the data reveals two phenomena associated with machine B:

1. Much force is required to pack the hose tightly in the bag. In this case, the corresponding muscle activity (as measured by EMG) will increase as performance goes on.
2. A phenomenon occurs when the hose is removed from the board (stripping). The EMG levels for this activity actually decline as time goes on. This change in the values is attributed to the combined effect of static loading and muscle fatigue.

The reported high percentage of utilization of maximum muscle forces would indicate that all three machines tax the operators beyond reasonable levels. Sound ergonomics

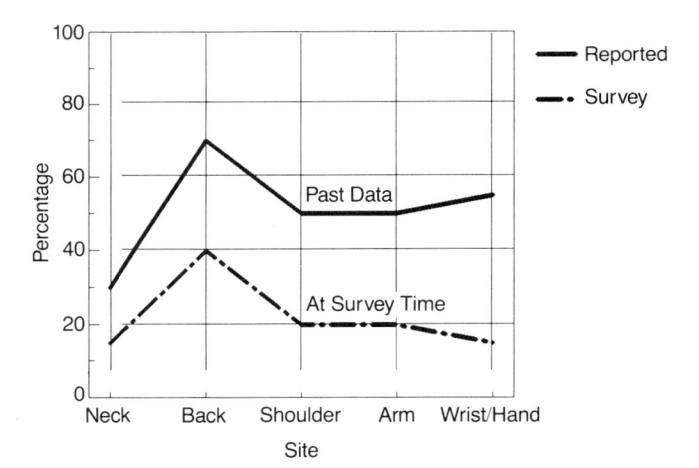

Figure 47.10. Reported pain.

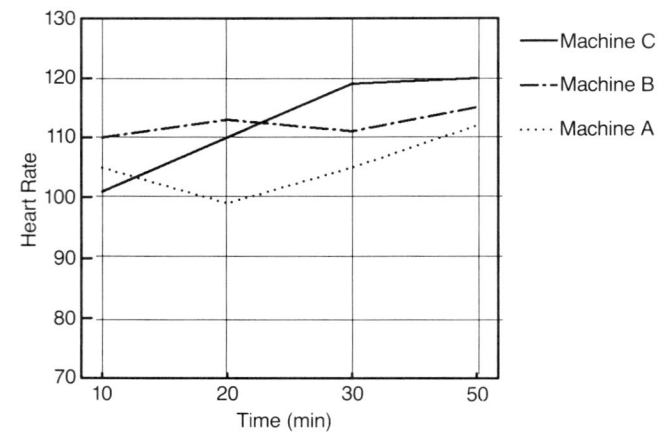

Figure 47.11. Heart rate versus machine.

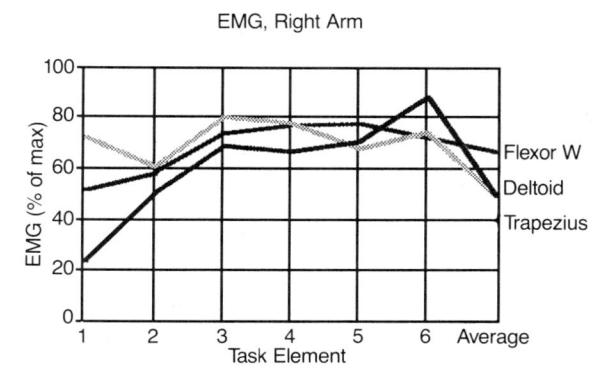

Figure 47.12. Muscle loading, machine B.

means that for repetitive work, muscle loading should be within 20–30% of maximum values. Observed values for most operators far exceed this recommendation.

Posture Analysis Posture recording and analysis were made to determine the positions assumed by various body segments over time. All operators were videotaped from two angles for 5–10 min, long enough to capture several job cycles on tape. Frame-by-frame analysis permitted various body postures to be categorized.

Posture of each body segment was described using the standard anatomic positions, such as flexion and extension. The relative position of each body segment was in turn described using "moderate," "extreme," and "very extreme" labels. An aggregate profile of each of the body segments was thus obtained.

Correlating observed postures with reported pain demonstrates that there is a definitive relationship between the two (Fig. 47.13). That is, operators who exhibit extreme posture also report more pain. The lesson to be learned here is rather simple and straightforward: Following an ergonomically sound method is an important step toward the control of CTDs. This supports our placing much emphasis on the need for the operators to follow good methods.

SUMMARY

Reflecting upon what has been presented so far and the data available to us, it is not difficult to answer the questions posed by management.

Yes, the job is demanding.
Yes, the job is perceived as demanding.
Yes, job content (standard) is not acceptable.
Yes, pain is related to the job (content and machine).
Yes, some operators may not be fit for this type of work (as currently structured).

RECOMMENDATIONS

In view of the study findings and the basic characteristics of boarding, we made several recommendations to management.

1. Modify Job Content to Reduce Concentration of Stress

Modifying the job content may be accomplished through (a) changing the manufacturing process; (b) enlarging the boarding job by incorporating materials handling with the existing boarding tasks (this is feasible for both machines A and B); and (c) introducing a carefully balanced job rotation for machine C teams (the rotation should be every 2 hr for the four machine positions).

2. Reduce Job Demands

Reducing job demands can be accomplished through the development and enforcement of appropriate breaks. Traditional use of fatigue allowances is not adequate for boarding. Breaks of the right duration and scheduled at the right time will reduce the overall level of physiologic response (heart rate) and muscle fatigue.

3. Improve Operator's Fitness for the Job

The following changes can be made to improve operator fitness: (a) achieve better matching and assignments of individuals to machines and teams; (b) increase operators' awareness relative to proper posture, method, clothing, and fitness; (c) effectively monitor job postures and methods (to be done by supervisors).

4. Modify/Redesign the Machine

Changes and modifications in the machine should eliminate (or at least minimize): (a) excessive reach (through adjustability of platforms); (b) static loading by a combination of machine and method changes (the use of rods for hose support may provide an answer for machine B); and (c) excessive pinch forces (through the use of collapsible boards).

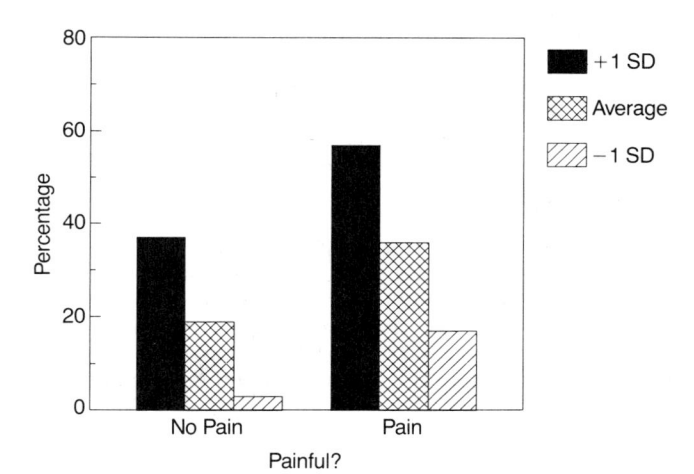

Figure 47.13. Posture and pain.

5. Reduce Thermal Stress

To reduce thermal stress, consider the following: (a) improving air distribution and circulation through the boarding department; (b) providing shields to protect operators from the steam released by the machine (B); and (c) providing protective clothing to guard against burns by the "hot" boards.

NEW DESIGN

In concert with the study findings and recommendations (discussed above), management decided on prototyping a new design for the boarding machine (Fig. 47.14). The new design marks a major departure from all existing machines in the manner by which the hose is placed on the boards. Specifically, the following features are exhibited by the new design:

1. *Use of collapsible boards.* During hose placement, the board width is kept at a minimum. This allows the hose to simply fall down on the board under its own weight, with little effort on the part of the operator. As the board clears the operator's position, it is automatically spread out to simulate a tight fit of the hose.
2. *Use of vacuum system.* Placement of the hose on top of the board is aided by a suction action. As the operator takes the hose to the board, the vacuum system helps by picking it up toward the board. This tends to minimize overhead reach and facilitates hose placement.
3. *Automatic stripping.* Upon completion of boarding, hoses are stripped off their boards and placed on special arms located on the left side of the operator. Hoses are allowed to accumulate on the arms prior to removing them for folding and bagging.

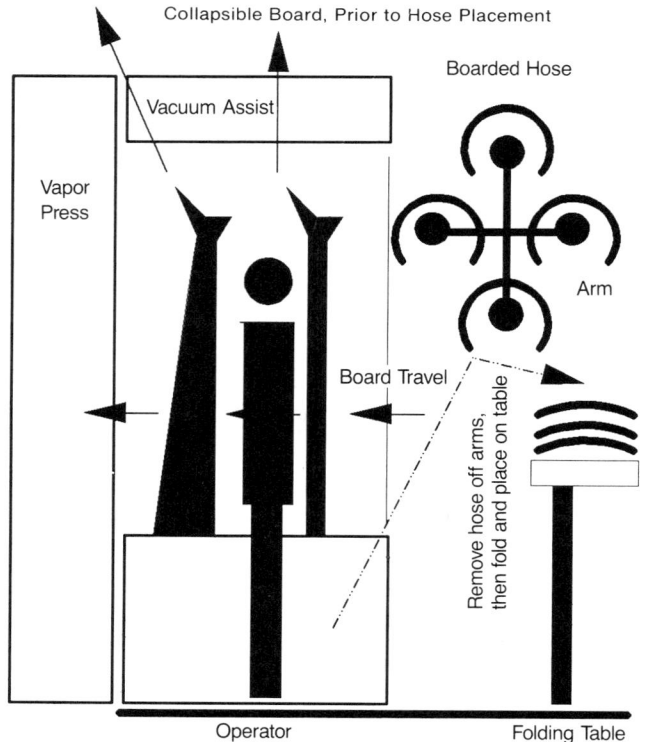

Evaluation

Three operators were evaluated on the new machine. Following 2 months of practice by the operators, we carried out a detailed ergonomic evaluation of their performance on the new machine. As with the previous evaluations, this involved the following:

1. Heart rate monitoring using the Vitalog
2. Assessment of muscle loading using electromyography (Cybord Biolab)
3. Muscle force output (pinch force) using electrodynagram
4. Subjective assessment by the three operators

At the time of this second evaluation, EDG was a new addition to our data collection equipment. We used it with the new machine to assess pinch forces associated with the placement and stretching of the hoses over the boards. EDG collects pressure data (kg/cm^2) delivered by the fingers using a total of 14 sensors (strain gauges). Pressure data collected over time are logged and analyzed using an IBM PC.

The evaluation confirmed the value of the design changes incorporated in the new machine. Physiologic responses (while working) are now within acceptable or tolerable limits. Heart rate averaged between 110 and 120 beats/min for most of the shift. Muscle loading levels (deltoid, wrist flexors, and extensors) were within 20–30% of maximum for the three operators. Although above-head reach remains a source of concern, the presence of a vacuum system provides some relief. In addition, by having the operators do their own folding and bagging, a rest is taken frequently and regularly. Pinch forces were low (less than 10% of measured maximum) and occurred for a brief period during each cycle.

CONCLUSION

Encouraged by the findings of the ergonomic evaluation and the assessment by the operators, management decided to adopt the new design (with some additional refinements) for plant-wide implementation. In addition to having the new machine, management made provisions to improve job content through rotation and mixing of tasks.

Suggested Readings

Ergonomics

Alexander DC, Pulat BM: *Industrial Ergonomics: A Practitioner's Guide.* Norcross, GA, Industrial Engineering & Management Press, 1985.

Figure 47.14. New design for boarding machine.

Drury C, Czaja S: *Ergonomics in Manufacturing.* Philadelphia, Taylor and Francis, 1987.
Ergonomics Group, Eastman Kodak: *Ergonomic Design for People at Work, Volume II.* New York, Van Nostrand Reinhold, 1986.
Grandjean E: *Fitting the Task to the Man: An Ergonomic Approach.* Philadelphia, Taylor & Francis, 1980.
Human Factors Section, Eastman Kodak: *Ergonomic Design for People at Work.* Lifetime Learning Publications, 1983, vol. I.
McCormick EJ, Sanders MS: *Human Factors in Engineering and Design,* ed 5. New York, McGraw-Hill, 1982.
Murrell KFH: *Ergonomics: Man in His Working Environment.* London, Chapman & Hall, 1965.
Shephard, Roy J. *Men at Work: Applications of Ergonomics to Performance and Design.* Springfield, IL, Charles C Thomas, 1974.
Singleton WT: *Introduction to Ergonomics.* Geneva, World Health Organization, 1972.
Singleton WT: *Man-Machine Systems.* London, Penguin, 1974.

Biomechanics/Work Physiology
Astrand PO, Rodahl K: *Textbook of Work Physiology,* ed 3. New York, McGraw-Hill, 1986.
Brouha L: *Physiology in Industry* ed 2. Elmsford, NY, Pergamon Press, 1967.
Chaffin DB, Andersson G: *Occupational Biomechanics.* New York, John Wiley & Sons, 1984.
Ghista DN (ed): *Human Body Dynamics.* Oxford, England, Clarendon Press, 1982.
Greenberg L, Chaffin DB: *Workers and Their Tools.* Midland, MI, Pendell Publishing Co., 1977.
Kroemer KHE, Kroemer HJ, Kroemer-Elbert KE: *Physiologic Bases of Human Factors/Ergonomics.* New York, Elsevier Science Publishers, 1986.
Pheasant, S: *Bodyspace: Anthropometry, Ergonomics and Design.* Philadelphia, Taylor & Francis, 1986.
Ricci, B: *Physiological Basis of Human Performance.* Philadelphia, Lea & Febiger, 1967.
Simonson E (ed): *Physiology of Work Capacity and Fatigue.* Springfield, IL, Charles C Thomas, 1971.
Singleton WT (ed): *The Body at Work: Biological Ergonomics.* Cambridge, England, Cambridge University Press, 1982.
Tichauer ER: *The Biomechanical Basis of Ergonomics.* New York, John Wiley & Sons, 1978.
Winter D: *Biomechanics of Human Movement.* New York, John Wiley & Sons, 1979.

Environment
Boyce PR: *Human Factors in Lighting.* New York, Macmillan, 1981.
Edholm OG, Bacharach AL (eds): *The Physiology of Human Survival.* New York, Academic Press, 1965.
Fanger PO: *Thermal Comfort.* New York, McGraw-Hill, 1973.
Hopkinson RG, Collins JB: *The Ergonomics of Lighting.* London, MacDonald & Co., 1970.
Horvath SM, Yousef MK (eds): *Environmental Physiology: Aging, Heat, and Altitude.* New York, Elsevier, 1981.
Huchingson RD: *New Horizons for Human Factors in Design.* New York, McGraw-Hill, 1981.
Osborne DJ, Gruneberg MM (eds): *The Physical Environment at Work.* New York, John Wiley & Sons, 1983.

Special Topics
Buckle P (ed): *Musculoskeletal Disorders at Work.* Philadelphia, Taylor & Francis, 1987.
Colguhoun WP, Rutenfranz J (eds): *Studies of Shiftwork.* Philadelphia, Taylor & Francis, 1980.

Grandjean E (ed): *Sitting Posture.* Philadelphia, Taylor & Francis, 1976.
Hockey R (ed): *Stress & Fatigue in Human Performance.* New York, John Wiley & Sons, 1983.
Ivergard T: *Information Ergonomics.* Kent, England, Chartwell-Bratt Ltd., 1982.
Noro K (ed): *Occupational Health and Safety in Automation and Robotics.* Philadelphia, Taylor & Francis, 1987.
Polk EJ: *Methods Analysis and Work Measurement.* New York, McGraw-Hill, 1984.
Pope MH, Frymoyer JW, Andersson G (eds): *Occupational Low Back Pain.* New York, Praeger, 1984.
Salvendy G (ed): *Handbook of Industrial Engineering.* New York, John Wiley & Sons, 1982.
Sell RG, Shipley P (eds): *Satisfactions in Work Design: Ergonomics and Other Approaches.* Philadelphia, Taylor & Francis, 1979.
Sheridan TB, Ferrell WR: *Man-Machine Systems.* Cambridge, MA, MIT Press, 1974.
Taylor W, Pelmear PC (eds): *Vibration White Finger in Industry.* New York, Academic Press, 1975.
Welford AT (ed): *Man Under Stress.* Philadelphia, Taylor & Francis, 1974.

Design
Clark TS, Corlett EN: *The Ergonomics of Workspaces and Machines: A Design Manual.* Philadelphia, Taylor & Francis, 1984.
Corlett EN, Richardson J (eds): *Stress, Work Design and Productivity.* New York, John Wiley & Sons, 1981.
Fallik F: *Managing Organizational Change: Case Studies in Ergonomics Practice* (Vol 3). Philadelphia, Taylor & Francis, 1987.
Flurscheim CH (ed): *Industrial Design in Engineering.* New York, Springer-Verlag, 1983.
Harker S, Eason K (eds): *The Application of Information Technology: Case Studies in Ergonomics Practice* (Vol 4). Philadelphia, Taylor & Francis, 1987.
Konz S: *Work Design: Industrial Ergonomics* ed 2. Columbus, OH, Grid Publishing, Inc., 1979.
Kvalseth TO (eds): *Ergonomics of Workstation Design.* Stoneham, MA, Butterworth, 1983.
Maule HG, Weiner JS (eds): *Design for Work and Use: Case Studies in Ergonomics Practice* (Vol 2). Philadelphia, Taylor & Francis, 1981.
Nadler G: *Work Design: A Systems Concept.* Homewood, IL, Richard D. Irwin, 1970.
VanCott HP, Kinkade RG (eds): *Human Engineering Guide to Equipment Design.* Washington, DC, US Government Printing Office, 1972.
Weiner JS, Maule HG (eds): *Human Factors in Work, Design & Production: Case Studies in Ergonomics Practice* (Vol 1). Philadelphia, Taylor & Francis, 1977.

Applications
Grandjean E: *Ergonomics of the Home.* Philadelphia, Taylor & Francis, 1978.
Grandjean E: (ed): *Ergonomics and Health in Modern Offices.* Philadelphia, Taylor & Francis, 1984.
Grandjean E: *Ergonomics in the Computerized Office.* Philadelphia, Taylor & Francis, 1987.
Grandjean E, Vigliani E (eds): *Ergonomics Aspects of Visual Display Terminals.* Philadelphia, Taylor & Francis, 1983.
Salvendy G, Smith MJ (eds): *Machine Pacing and Occupational Stress.* Philadelphia, Taylor & Francis, 1981.

Methods

Basmajian JV: *Muscles Alive: Their Functions Revealed by Electromyography* ed 4. Baltimore, Williams & Wilkins, 1979.
Chapanis A: *Research Techniques in Human Engineering.* Baltimore, Johns Hopkins Press, 1959.
Corlett EN, Wilson J (eds): *The Ergonomics of Working Postures.* Philadelphia, Taylor & Francis, 1986.
Corlett EN, Wilson J (eds): *Methods in Applied Ergonomics.* Philadelphia, Taylor & Francis, 1987.
Hashimoto K, Kogi K, Grandjean E: *Methodology in Human Fatigue Assessment.* Philadelphia, Taylor & Francis, 1971.
Meister D: *Behavioral Analysis and Measurement Methods.* New York, John Wiley & Sons, 1985.
Meister D: *Human Factors Testing and Evaluation.* New York, Elsevier Science Publishers, 1986.
Roebuck JA, Kroemer KHE, Thomson WG: *Engineering Anthropometry Methods.* New York, John Wiley & Sons, 1975.
Rohgmert W, Landau K: *A New Technique for Job Analysis.* Philadelphia, Taylor & Francis, 1983.
Singleton WT, Spurgeon P: *Measurement of Human Resources.* Philadelphia, Taylor & Francis, 1975.

Journals

American Industrial Hygiene Association Journal. Akron, OH, American Industrial Hygiene Association (monthly).
Applied Ergonomics. Surrey, England, IPC Science and Technology Press.
Behaviour and Information Technology. Philadelphia, Taylor & Francis (quarterly).
Ergonomics. Philadelphia, Taylor & Francis (monthly).
Ergonomics Abstracts. Philadelphia, Taylor & Francis (quarterly).
Human Factors. Santa Monica, CA, Human Factors Society (monthly).
IIE Transactions. Norcross, GA, Institute of Industrial Engineers (bimonthly).
International Journal of Industrial Ergonomics. New York, Elsevier (quarterly).
International Reviews of Ergonomics. Philadelphia, Taylor & Francis (annual).
Journal of Human Ergology. Tokyo Japan (semiannually).
Journal of Occupational Medicine. Arlington Heights, IL, American Occupational Medical Association (monthly).
Work & Stress. Philadelphia, Taylor & Francis (quarterly).

Expert Systems/Artificial Intelligence

Andriole SJ (ed): *Applications in Artificial Intelligence.* Princeton, NJ, Petrocelli Books, Inc., 1985.
Waterman DA: *A Guide to Expert Systems.* Boston, Addison-Wesley, 1986.

Data

Diffrient N, et al: *Human Scale 1/2/3, 4/5/6/, 7/8/9.* Cambridge, MA, MIT Press, 1978.
National Aeronautics and Space Administration: *Anthropometric Source Book, Volumes I, II, and III.* NASA Reference Publication 1024. Washington, DC, Scientific and Technical Information Office, 1978.
National Aeronautics and Space Administration. *Bioastronautics Data Book* ed 2. Washington DC, U.S. Government Printing Office, 1973.
University of Surrey: *Force Limits in Manual Work.* Surrey, England, IPC Science and Technology Press, 1980.
Woodson WE: *Human Factors Design Handbook.* New York, McGraw-Hill, 1981.

Appendix A
Ergonomic Survey

The purpose of an ergonomic survey is to locate areas where the worker and his/her environment have been mismatched. This mismatch frequently results in employee discomfort, the occurrence of cumulative trauma disorders, and degradation of efficiency and product quality. Identification of ergonomic deficiencies and their probable causes at the outset of the study allows the investigator to proceed in a systematic, goal-oriented manner. That is, the survey results provide a guideline for an approach to solving the problems.

Ergonomic deficiencies are typically found in nine specific areas:

Management
Workplace
Method
Job content/structure
Machine design/technology
Materials handling
Environment
Employee fitness/awareness
Health care programs

It is important to begin an evaluation with an open mind and avoid making "snap" decisions. Follow a systematic method of evaluation that can support findings and conclusions.

The following steps are guidelines that can be used when conducting an ergonomic evaluation; they may serve as a reference for future evaluations.

PHASE 1: INITIAL TOUR OBSERVATIONS

The first step is to meet with management, identify specifically what requires improvement or change, and obtain all the necessary background data. It is critical to pinpoint the purpose of the study and identify a starting point.

Tour the plant in a systematic fashion; begin with the receiving area, follow the process flow, and finally finish with the shipping department. In each department make note of the equipment and layout of the work stations. For each work station document what each person does. Record how the operators load and unload machinery and note the amount of weight handled. Determine what material preparation is required. Take measurements that show the extent of reaching and walking. Take note of environmental factors such as noise, vibration, temperature, air circulation, and lighting at each work station. It is important to record the amount of space allowed for each operator.

Upon completion of the initial tour, review the information you have observed and your overall impressions concerning the various jobs. It is important to summarize the overall flow by sketching the areas observed. Make a list of measurements to be taken at the primary work stations and any additional data you would like management to provide, such as detailed work method documents, work standards, performance ratings, or a list of health problems encountered in the past year. Always obtain a copy of the OSHA log and any compensation forms that may be in the files. After this brief assessment of the situation, go back to the plant floor and conduct the second phase of the ergonomic survey.

PHASE 2: DATA COLLECTION

The data collection phase will involve videotaping several operators in the suspected problem jobs while they perform their tasks. Each operator should be filmed long enough to record several task cycles on tape. If deemed important you may want to make an EMG (electromyographic) study of certain task elements (this requires special equipment and data forms).

Interview operators in the suspected job categories, and give them a chance to reflect on what they consider to be the most demanding part of their job, and what type of improvements they might like to see. Operator interviews can be enhanced considerably by using a pain questionnaire. The questionnaire should have drawings of the body (front and back) so that each operator may simply mark the body areas he/she considers to be the source of pain and discomfort. If an operator indicates the presence of pain, pursue the matter and determine the circumstances that lead to such pain. Ask questions such as: When does it start? How long does it last? What makes it worse? What makes it better? What kind of medication or treatment do you use for pain relief? Are you under medical care? If the operator is under medical care you may want to ask for reports from the treating physician(s).

PHASE 3: CLOSING CONFERENCE

After the second detailed tour of the plant, schedule a conference with plant management. Ask questions about the situations you encountered on the plant floor and request additional information that was not obtained at the first meeting. Resist the temptation of providing instant answers and conclusions concerning the ergonomic health of the plant. You need time away from the situation to digest what you have observed and measured. Providing quick responses based on instinct cannot be erased later when the data support other conclusions.

Determine any general constraints placed on any improvements you might propose. For isntance, would it be feasible to modify existing machines and work stations or are they restricted with the existing technology for the manufacturing process? Are funds available to finance appropriate changes? Can the jobs be restructured without violating labor contracts?

If the plant has a history of cumulative trauma disorders, pay close attention to health care programs and the availability of in-house medical care.

PHASE 4: ANALYSIS OF OBSERVATIONS

Following your investigation and examination of notes and data collected, you are ready to report your observations.

> Begin with an introduction about the purpose of the investigation and the goals previously identified. In addition, describe the steps involved in your analysis.
>
> The second section should focus on the existing conditions in the plant. Summarize plant characteristics and highlight strength and/or weakness of each work station, method, environment, material handling, job content, training, health care, and management. Support comments with appropriate diagrams, charts, and data (see Checklist below).
>
> The third section is simply an itemized list of the major deficiencies that exist in the plant (see Summary of Deficiencies below). Again this determination should be based on objective and reproducible data, thus providing support to the report.

PHASE 5: RECOMMENDATIONS

Provide some recommendations to be considered. These recommendations should be specific and address the root cause of the deficiencies described in the third section of the report. Each proposed improvement should assure the following:

It will improve the ergonomics of the area in question.
It will be feasible for management to implement the recommended change (or modification) within the plant.
It is based on sound ergonomic principles.

Describe the overall impact of your recommendations on the plant operations, jobs, employees, and productivity. Include a time table for implementing your recommendations as well as general cost estimates. When making several alternate improvement proposals, indicate the strength and weakness of each and schedule a meeting to discuss the options.

PHASE 6: CONCLUSION

Conclude the report by restating the main deficiencies observed, their root causes and your prognosis for eliminating or treating the problems. State your availability to meet with management to answer questions. If applicable, include an appendix containing all relevant data that were not included in the main section.

CHECKLIST

MANAGMENT (General)   COMMENTS

A M C N	1.	Communication
A M C N	2.	Awareness
A M C N	3.	Safety committee
A M C N	4.	Working hours
A M C N	5.	Shiftwork
A M C N	6.	Overtime
A M C N	7.	Breaks
A M C N	8.	Pay system
A M C N	9.	Standards
A M C N	10.	Training
A M C N	11.	Supervision
A M C N	12.	Safety/health problems

THE REMAINDER OF THE CHECKLIST SHOULD BE COMPLETED FOR EACH JOB.
SEAT   COMMENTS

A M C N	1.	Type
A M C N	2.	Adjustable
A M C N	3.	Dimensions
A M C N	4.	Padding
A M C N	5.	Footrest
A M C N	6.	Backrest
A M C N	7.	Armrest
A M C N	8.	Interface
A M C N	9.	Posture
A M C N	10.	Proper use
A M C N	11.	Maintenance

WORK SURFACE   COMMENTS

A M C N	1.	Dimension
A M C N	2.	Orientation
A M C N	3.	Properties
A M C N	4.	Pressure points
A M C N	5.	Adjustable

WORK SPACE   COMMENTS

A M C N	1.	Fixed/defined
A M C N	2.	Amount of space
A M C N	3.	In-process storage
A M C N	4.	Floor type
A M C N	5.	Isolation
A M C N	6.	Shared with others

A = Acceptable; M = Marginal; C = Critical; N = Not Applicable

MACHINE   COMMENTS

    A   M   C   N   1. Control of pace
    A   M   C   N   2. Interface
    A   M   C   N   3. Loading/unloading
    A   M   C   N   4. Posture
    A   M   C   N   5. Pressure points
    A   M   C   N   6. Vibration/noise
    A   M   C   N   7. Safety/health hazards
    A   M   C   N   8. Isolation

CONTROLS   COMMENTS

    A   M   C   N   1. Type
    A   M   C   N   2. Location
    A   M   C   N   3. Force
    A   M   C   N   4. Posture
    A   M   C   N   5. Coding
    A   M   C   N   6. Labeling
    A   M   C   N   7. Sequencing
    A   M   C   N   8. Grouping

DISPLAYS   COMMENTS

    A   M   C   N   1. Type
    A   M   C   N   2. Location
    A   M   C   N   3. Size
    A   M   C   N   4. Labels
    A   M   C   N   5. Light
    A   M   C   N   6. Grouping
    A   M   C   N   7. Control association

INSTRUCTION   COMMENTS

    A   M   C   N   1. Form
    A   M   C   N   2. Amount
    A   M   C   N   3. Location
    A   M   C   N   4. Visibility

HAND TOOLS   COMMENTS

    A   M   C   N   1. Weight
    A   M   C   N   2. Handle
    A   M   C   N   3. Dimensions
    A   M   C   N   4. Location
    A   M   C   N   5. Posture
    A   M   C   N   6. Muscles used
    A   M   C   N   7. Proper use
    A   M   C   N   8. Force
    A   M   C   N   9. Support

A = Acceptable; M = Marginal; C = Critical; N = Not Applicable

MATERIALS HANDLING   COMMENTS

A	M	C	N	1. Manual (lifting, carrying, pushing/pulling)
A	M	C	N	Weight
A	M	C	N	Starting points
A	M	C	N	Distance
A	M	C	N	Frequency
A	M	C	N	2. Conveyors
A	M	C	N	3. Buggies, trucks, etc.
A	M	C	N	4. Containers

METHOD   COMMENTS

A	M	C	N	1. Standard method
		Reach		
A	M	C	N	2. Motion
A	M	C	N	3. Force
A	M	C	N	4. Muscle loading
A	M	C	N	5. Frequency
		Process		
A	M	C	N	6. Motion
A	M	C	N	7. Force
A	M	C	N	8. Posture
A	M	C	N	9. Muscle loading
		Aside		
A	M	C	N	10. Motion
A	M	C	N	11. Force
A	M	C	N	12. Muscle loading

JOB   COMMENTS

A	M	C	N	1. Number of tasks
A	M	C	N	2. Mix of tasks
A	M	C	N	3. Minimum task time
A	M	C	N	4. Break
A	M	C	N	5. Team work
A	M	C	N	6. Physical demand
A	M	C	N	7. Visual demand
A	M	C	N	8. Mental demand

CLIMATE   COMMENTS

A	M	C	N	1. Temperature
A	M	C	N	2. Humidity
A	M	C	N	3. Air movement
A	M	C	N	4. Clothing
A	M	C	N	5. Workload
A	M	C	N	6. Control measures

A = Acceptable; M = Marginal; C = Critical; N = Not Applicable

NOISE — COMMENTS

A	M	C	N	1.	Intensity
A	M	C	N	2.	Quality
A	M	C	N	3.	Exposure time
A	M	C	N	4.	Control measures

VIBRATION — COMMENTS

A	M	C	N	1.	Source
A	M	C	N	2.	Frequency
A	M	C	N	3.	Exposure time
A	M	C	N	4.	Control measures

LIGHTING — COMMENTS

A	M	C	N	1.	Intensity
A	M	C	N	2.	Distribution
A	M	C	N	3.	Contrast
A	M	C	N	4.	Glare
A	M	C	N	5.	Flickering/stroboscopic effects
A	M	C	N	6.	Optical aids
A	M	C	N	8.	Viewing distance

EMPLOYEE — COMMENTS

A	M	C	N	1.	Physical limitations
A	M	C	N	2.	Awareness/training
A	M	C	N	3.	Quality of work life
A	M	C	N	4.	Diet/exercise
A	M	C	N	5.	Smoking

MEDICAL PROGRAMS — COMMENTS

A	M	C	N	1.	Pain recognition
A	M	C	N	2.	Treatment, first visit
A	M	C	N	3.	Referral
A	M	C	N	4.	Job reviews
A	M	C	N	5.	Follow-up and tracking
A	M	C	N	6.	Rehabilitation programs
A	M	C	N	7.	Wellness program

A = Acceptable; M = Marginal; C = Critical; N = Not Applicable

SUMMARY OF DEFICIENCIES

Category	Deficiency	Seriousness[a]	Job(s)	Recommendation[b]

---

[a] 1 = Critical; 2 = Serious; 3 = Moderate; 4 = Other.
[b] AT = Awareness Training   MH = Material Handling Improv.
ET = Environmental Improvement   MI = Method Improvement
(noise, light, etc.)   MT = Machine/Tool Redesign
JR = Job Restructure   WI = Workplace Improvement

chapter 48
Legal Aspects of Pain and Social Security Disability

G. Wayne McCall, M.Ed., CRC

"Disability has been defined for the purpose of claims adjudication under the Social Security Act as an "inability to engage in any substantial gainful activity by reason of a medically determinable physical or mental impairment which can be expected to result in death or has lasted or can be expected to last for a continuous period of not less than 12 months" (1). The adjudication of claim for disability benefits under Title II (Social Security Disability benefits) and Title XVI (Supplemental Security Disability Income) of the Social Security Act is based upon the use of well-established, objectively demonstrable medical criteria described in the Listing of Impairments, Appendix to Subpart P of Regulations Number 4 and Subpart 1 of Regulations Number 16 of the Social Security Act. However, clear differences exist between what constitutes an "impairment" and what constitutes a "disability" within the context of the Social Security regulations, and it is within the interpretation of these differences that the Social Security Administration has placed considerable focus in the past several years.

The very definition of "disability" for Social Security purposes is based upon the claimant's ability (or inability) to "engage in substantial gainful activity," or to work. Thus, the adjudication of Social Security Act claims for disability is fundamentally a vocational issue rather than a medical one, according to Nadolsky (2). Nadolsky's position has been supported as far back as 1958, when the American Medical Association Committee on the Rating of Mental and Physical Impairment wrote in their "Guide to the Evaluation of Permanent Impairment, the Extremities and Back" that the determination of permanent impairment is purely a medical decision, and that whether or not a given impairment represented a disability was an administrative responsibility and function, rather than a medical one (3).

THE SEQUENTIAL EVALUATION PROCESS

The Social Security Administration (SSA) uses a process of "sequential evaluation" in determining eligibility for Title II and Title XVI disability benefits, and the first criterion of eligibility is a vocational, rather than a medical one, and involves determining whether a claimant is "engaging in substantial gainful activity," or working for a specific monetary amount in a specific period of time. These amounts may change from time to time based on changes in the national economy. Regardless of a claimant's medical or psychological status, he/she are not considered "disabled" for benefit purposes if he/she is working at a substantial gainful activity level.

If a claimant is not working, the next step in the sequential evaluation process is to determine whether the claimant has a "severe" impairment, or one that "has more than a minimal effect on the individual's ability to perform basic work activities" (4). Thus, a client's ability to work is the critical operational definition of disability, rather than the degree of medical impairment per se. In this step of the sequential evaluation process, the claimant's eligibility for benefits is presumed if functional restrictions in performing work-related activities are alleged by the claimant and supported by appropriate medical documentation. In the absence of medical support, however, a decision may be made that the claimant has a "slight" or "nonsevere" impairment. This step provides for the evaluation of the claimant's medical status to determine the extent to which objective medical findings support the alleged functional restrictions. This process uses the Listing of Impairments criteria referred to above and represents a statutory delineation of required medical signs, symptoms, and findings, broken down by body systems, that must be either "met" or "equaled" if an award is granted on a purely medical basis. If the criteria described in the Listing of Impairments are met or equaled, then the medical impairment becomes a legal definition of "disability," and an award is made based upon the statutory presumption that clients who "meet or equal" the Listings are incapable of engaging in substantial gainful activity.

The last step in the sequential evaluation process requires the evaluation of the client's vocational prognosis to engage in work activity despite any functional restrictions that may be associated with his/her impairment or impairments. The determination of vocational prognosis is in itself a sequential process that requires evaluation of medical and psychological variables, along with evaluating the claimant's age, education, and prior work experience.

RESIDUAL FUNCTIONAL CAPACITY

The first step in determining the vocational prognosis of the client requires a medical determination of the client's residual functional capacity in terms of the work-related functions as described in the *Dictionary of Occupational Titles* (5), and at this point the objective determination of "disability" is based upon a physician's subjective interpretation of the impact of the claimant's medical impairments on his/her ability to perform work-related functions. The residual functional capacity assessment made by the physician requires evaluation of both exertional and nonexertional factors that may impact on the client's ability to work.

EVALUATING EXERTIONAL FACTORS

The evaluation of functional capacity based on exertional factors involves the physician's evaluation of the claimant's ability to function in six physical demand areas under seven different kinds of working conditions, as described in Supplement 2 to the *Dictionary of Occupational Titles* (DOT, 3rd edition, 1968) (see Appendices 48.A and 48.B).

In making judgments regarding a claimant's residual functional capacity, the factors of strength, exertional capabilities, and endurance must be considered. Review of the DOT Appendices suggests that a significant volume of data regarding vocational factors must be processed by the physician when making residual functional capacity judgments based on exertional factors alone, but the process may become more subjective when nonexertional factors are considered.

EVALUATING NONEXERTIONAL FACTORS

Nonexertional factors include the claimant's cognitive capabilities to perform behaviors related to understanding and remembering instructions, responding appropriately to supervision in the workplace, and relating to coworkers and responding to customary work pressures in the work environment. It is in this area, where objective documentation is most often lacking, that the physician must make "educated guesses" based upon available psychological evaluation data or data from observations made in the workplace.

THE CONCEPT OF VOCATIONAL RELEVANCE

The concept of vocational relevance in establishing a vocational prognosis for a claimant is based upon not only the claimant's residual functional capacity but upon his/her age, educational background, and previous work history. This triad of factors is considered in the following general terms: (a) younger workers are presumed to be more employable than older workers, (b) skilled workers are presumed to be more employable than unskilled workers, and (c) claimants with higher education are presumed to be more employable than undereducated workers. Vocational relevance in establishing a vocational prognosis for the adjudication of SSA disability claims is further dependent upon the temporal concept of vocational recency and the concept of transferability of skills: (a) the longer a person is unable to work, the higher the probability that skill level will diminish, and (b) unskilled workers will remain unskilled workers regardless of time away from the job.

TRANSFERABILITY OF SKILLS

The sequential evaluation process for determining a vocational prognosis must consider whether the claimant possesses skills that will enable him/her to be more readily employable. Given two workers with the same residual functional capacity profile, a worker with transferable skills would have a better vocational prognosis than one who did not. The determination of a claimant's skills is based upon two variables defined in the DOT: general educational development level and specific vocational preparation time (see Appendix 48.C). As may be seen from these descriptions, the level of cognitive capability and general educational development level required for jobs described in the DOT has been well defined functionally in the reasoning, mathematical, and language spheres through the use of a 1 to 6 rating scale, and the specific vocational preparation time required to perform the job within industrially established norms is defined by a 1 to 9 rating scale.

The SSA has described in Section 404, Appendix 2 of the Social Security Regulations specific guidelines for the use of vocational factors in the adjudication of claims that evaluate a client's vocational prognosis by functional capacity level, based on the interrelationship between the vocational factors of age, education, and previous work experience. Each general vocational factor is divided into subcategories: age into specific age ranges; education into categories of illiteracy, limited or less education, and high school or more; and previous work experience into unskilled, semi-skilled, and skilled workers with transferable skills, and semiskilled and skilled workers without transferable skills. These subgroupings provide a structured mechanism for making vocational decisions and represent an attempt to objectify the decision-making process as it relates to the vocational arena.

OVERVIEW OF THE DISABILITY ADJUDICATION PROCESS

The process of sequentially evaluating medical, psychological, and vocational data provides an orderly process of disability claim adjudication in the Social Security system, and the statutory requirements of the law provide a mechanism for obtaining the necessary objective information to make an informed adjudication on a claim. The law also provides a mechanism of appeals if the claimant disagrees with the decision made on his/her claim. If a claim is denied initially, the claimant may ask that a reconsideration be made, and a reevaluation of the medical, psychological, and vocational evidence is performed by another disability adjudicator employed by the state agency performing the claims adjudication for the SSA. If the reconsideration results in a continued denial of benefits, the mechanism is available for the claimant to appeal his/her case to an administrative law judge.

SOCIAL SECURITY AND CHRONIC PAIN

The use of objectively demonstrable signs, symptoms, and medical findings as a basis for disability adjudication has served the intent of the law relatively well in problems related to acute medical conditions, but the law does not provide an objective mechanism for evaluating the chronic pain patient. Because the pain experience is a perception and because perceptions are not directly objectively quantifiable, pain was considered in the evaluation of disability only as a secondary factor associated with a medically determinable impairment. The SSA has had increasing numbers of court cases challenging this policy regarding the evaluation of pain since chronic pain sufferers often present with allegations of pain that are not consistent with medically determinable impairment(s). As a consequence of an increasing number of cases within the courts, the Social Security Disability Benefits Reform Act of 1984 (Public Law 98-460) directed the Secretary of Health and Human Services to appoint a Commission on the Evaluation of Pain to conduct a joint study with the National Academy of Sciences on the evaluation of pain as it pertains to claims adjudication under Titles II and XVI of the Social Security Act.

CLASSIFICATION OF CHRONIC PAIN PATIENTS

The Social Security Commission on the Evaluation of Chronic Pain recognized the pain experience as a multifaceted physical, mental, social, and behavioral process that may impact on the patient's behavior in all areas of his/her life, and recognized that chronic pain patients often experience similar behavioral consequences as they attempt to adjust to the perception of pain. The typical pain patient is one who develops a preoccupation with the pain that causes an increase in his/her use of the health care system, experiences a decrease in level of functional activity, has an increase in pain behavior as he/she becomes physiologically deconditioned, and has a decrease in vocational productivity with a correspondent decrease in ability to earn a living. The chronic pain patient syndrome represents a well-recognized symptom complex in which allegations of pain persist far beyond the expected healing time for an acute injury and most often are not supported by an objectively demonstrable medical etiology for said pain. Numerous psychological, social, and environmental factors have been demonstrated to affect the chronic pain experience (6, 7). The effects of chronic pain on economic considerations related to social disability systems are well described by Chapman and Brena (8).

The Commission defined four groups of chronic pain patients: (*a*) chronic pain, inability to cope, insufficiently documented impairment; (*b*) chronic pain, competent coping, insufficiently documented impairment; (*c*) chronic pain, inability to cope, sufficiently documented impairment; and (*d*) chronic pain, competent coping, sufficiently documented impairment. The Commission determined that groups c and d posed no problems in disability adjudication according to the current law, and recommended protocols for the evaluation of patients within groups a and b. The Commission specifically recommended interdisciplinary evaluation by appropriately trained medical, psychological, functional, social, and vocational specialists, and recommended the development of quantitative measurement of functional capacity and the establishment of rehabilitation goals within each disciplinary specialty. The Commission further recommended periodic reevaluation of the chronic pain patient as a measure of his/her compliance with the prescribed pain rehabilitation program and recommended vocational and avocational counseling to increase the patient's productivity level after completion of pain rehabilitation.

LEGAL IMPLICATIONS

The fact that the determination of disability for SSA purposes is an administrative function controlled by the statues within the Social Security law makes the Social Security disability adjudication essentially a legal decision based upon well-defined findings of fact. The recommendations of the Commission represent a positive advance in the SSA's perception of the need for interdisciplinary evaluation of chronic pain paients, and the need for regulatory criteria for establishing minimum standards for centers that provide these evaluations.

The utilization of psychometric evaluation tools, behavioral observation, and behavioral rating scales of pain behavior have been well described by numerous references in the literature and represent current advances in the sophistication of mechanisms for quantifying pain behavior. However, because of the differences between the medical determination of impairment and the legal determination of disability that follows, the critical operational definition that defines the differences between impairment and disability is the vocational prognosis for engaging in substantial gainful activity.

Brena, McCall, and Franco have addressed the need for standardized vocational evaluation protocols in the interdisciplinary evaluation of chronic pain patients and described the use of the vocational evaluation process and the data derived from same as a critical part of the objective documentation process (9). The use of vocational evaluation methodologies provides a common point of reference between the medical (impairment rating) professions and the administrative/legal (disability rating) professions, and the process of vocationally evaluating a patient affords the vocational evaluator an extended opportunity to observe the patient's level of motivation, endurance, attention span, concentration, and pain behavior, all of which assist in the developing of a functional diagnosis, which impacts directly on the resulting vocational prognosis.

The results of the vocational evaluation proper also yields important information relative to the establishment of a vocational prognosis if the claimant is prevented from returning to relevant past work by virtue of the functional restrictions placed upon him/her by the impairment rating physician. Botterbusch (10) gave an excellent overview and comparison of commercially available vocational evaluation systems, but the Career Evaluation System offers several advantages in evaluating patients impaired by chronic pain; a comprehensive vocational evaluation can be obtained in one extended session of 4–6 hr, which causes minimal disruption in the provision of therapeutic services; and the specific subtests yields a comprehensive profile of the patient's level of function in terms of nonverbal IQ and abstract reasoning, verbal and numerical aptitudes, and several measures of strength, reaction time, and visuospatial and perceptual-motor coordination. After computer processing of the raw data, including the functional restrictions imposed on the patient by the impairment rating physician, the resulting printout yields jobs within the patient's functional profile that the patient has demonstrated in evaluation to have the abilities to perform, and gives the pain treatment team valuable information with which to develop task-specific rehabilitation plans that are most cost-effective and oriented toward returning the pain-impaired patient back to vocational productivity.

The utilization of commercially available job-matching software is another technological advancement that has improved the provision of comprehensive vocational services in chronic pain rehabilitation centers. The Occupational Access System (OASYS) is but one example of job-matching software, but it has particular advantages in Social Security disability evaluations of vocational prognosis in pain centers because it allows for maximum flexibility in adjusting both worker traits and worker ability profiles across medical, vocational, aptitude, vocational interest, and temperament variables. The resulting transferability of skills profile documents the presence (or absence) of jobs into which the pain patient could transfer within his/her medically established functional capacity, and offers the advantage of addressing the need for job modification strategies and on-the-job training. A recent overview by Botterbusch provides a detailed comparison of job-matching systems (11).

SUMMARY

In summary, the adjudication of Social Security disability claims under Title II and Title XVI of the Social Security Act is based upon objectively demonstrable evidence of medical impairments that may or may not constitute a legal definition of disability. The recommendations of the Commission on the Evaluation of Pain support the need for comprehensive, multidisciplinary evaluation of chronic pain patients, including the provision of comprehensive vocational counseling and evaluation services. The necessary objective data base for closing the gap between impairment and disability exists within the vocational rehabilitation profession, whose standardized vocational evaluation and transferability of skills technologies can offer objective vocational prognoses that are cost-effective and time-efficient applications of the sequential evaluation process that will meet the needs of both the medical and legal professions.

References

1. US Department of Health and Human Services, Social Security Administration, Office of Operational Policy and Procedures: *Social Security Regulations: Rules for Determining Disability and Blindness*, 4.04.1505. SSA Pub. No. 64-014. Washington, DC, US Government Printing Office, 1981, p 2.
2. Nadolsky JM: Social security: in need of rehabilitation. *J Rehabil* 50:6–8, 1984.
3. AMA Council on Rating Mental and Physical Impairment: Guides to the evaluation of permanent impairment—the extremities and back. *JAMA* 166:1958.
4. US Department of Health and Human Services, Social Security Administration. Office of Operational Policy and Procedures: *Social Security Regulations: Rules for Determining Disability and Blindness*. 4.04.1521. SSA Pub. No. 64-014, Washington, DC, US Government Printing Office, 1981, p 5.
5. US Department of Labor, Bureau of Employment Security:

Supplement 2 to the Dictionary of Occupational Titles, ed 3. Washington, DC, US Government Printing Office, 1968.
6. Fordyce WE: *Behavioral Methods for Chronic Pain and Illness*. St. Louis, CV Mosby, 1976.
7. Brena SF, Chapman SL: The "learned pain syndrome": decoding a patient's signals. *Postgrad Med* 69:53–64, 1981.
8. Chapman SL, Brena SF: Pain and society. *Ann Behav Med* 7:21–23, 1985.
9. Brena SF, McCall GW, Franco AM: Functional diagnosis: vocational and disability evaluation. In Bonica JJ (ed): *The Management of Pain in Clinical Practice*, ed 2. (in press).
10. Botterbusch KF: *A Comparison of Commercial Evaluation Systems*. Menomonie, WI, University of Wisconsin–Stout, Material Development Center, 1987.
11. Botterbusch KF: *A Comparison of Computerized Job Matching Systems*. Menomonie, WI, University of Wisconsin–Stout, Material Development Center, 1987.

Appendix A
Physical Demands*

Physical demands are those physical activities required of a worker in a job.

The physical demands listed in this publication serve as a means of expressing both the physical requirements of the job and the physical capacities (specific physical traits) a worker must have to meet the requirements. For example, "seeing" is the name of a physical demand required by many jobs (perceiving by the sense of vision), and also the name of a specific capacity possessed by many people (having the power of sight). The worker must possess physical capacities at least in an amount equal to the physical demands made by the job.

The Factors

1 **Lifting, Carrying, Pushing, and/or Pulling (Strength):** These are the primary "strength" physical requirements, and, generally speaking, a person who engages in one of these activities can engage in all.

Specifically, each of these activities can be described as:
(1) Lifting: Raising or lowering an object from one level to another (includes upward pulling).
(2) Carrying: Transporting an object, usually holding it in the hands or arms or on the shoulder.
(3) Pushing: Exerting force upon an object so that the object moves away from the force (includes slapping, striking, kicking, and treadle actions).
(4) Pulling: Exerting force upon an object so that the object moves toward the force (includes jerking).

The five degrees of Physical Demands Factor No. 1 (Lifting, Carrying, Pushing, and/or Pulling), are as follows.

S Sedentary Work

Lifting 10 lbs. maximum and occasionally lifting and/or carrying such articles as dockets, ledgers, and small tools. Although a sedentary job is defined as one which involves sitting, a certain amount of walking and standing is often necessary in carrying out job duties. Jobs are sedentary if walking and standing are required only occasionally and other sedentary criteria are met.

L Light Work

Lifting 20 lbs. maximum with frequent lifting and/or carrying of objects weighing up to 10 lbs. Even though the weight lifted may be only a negligible amount, a job is in this category when it requires walking or standing to a significant degree, or when it involves sitting most of the time with a degree of pushing and pulling of arm and/or leg controls.

M Medium Work

Lifting 50 lbs. maximum with frequent lifting and/or carrying of objects weighing up to 25 lbs.

H Heavy Work

Lifting 100 lbs. maximum with frequent lifting and/or carrying of objects weighing up to 50 lbs.

V Very Heavy Work

Lifting objects in excess of 100 lbs. with frequent lifting and/or carrying of objects weighing 50 lbs. or more.

2 **Climbing and/or Balancing:**
(1) Climbing: Ascending or descending ladders, stairs, scaffolding, ramps, poles, ropes, and the like, using the feet and legs and/or hands and arms.
(2) Balancing: Maintaining body equilibrium to prevent falling when walking, standing, crouching, or running on narrow, slippery, or erratically moving surfaces; or maintaining body equilibrium when performing gymnastic feats.

3 **Stooping, Kneeling, Crouching, and/or Crawling:**
(1) Stooping: Bending the body downward and forward by bending the spine at the waist.
(2) Kneeling: Bending the legs at the knees to come to rest on the knee or knees.
(3) Crouching: Bending the body downward and forward by bending the legs and spine.
(4) Crawling: Moving about on the hands and knees or hands and feet.

4 **Reaching, Handling, Fingering, and/or Feeling:**
(1) Reaching: Extending the hands and arms in any direction.
(2) Handling: Seizing, holding, grasping, turning, or otherwise working with the hand or hands (fingering not involved).

640 Selected Topics/Section 4

(3) Fingering: Picking, pinching, or otherwise working with the fingers primarily (rather than with the whole hand or arm as in handling).

(4) Feeling: Perceiving such attributes of objects and materials as size, shape, temperature, or texture, by means of receptors in the skin, particularly those of the finger tips.

5 **Talking and/or Hearing:**
  (1) Talking: Expressing or exchanging ideas by means of the spoken word.
  (2) Hearing: Perceiving the nature of sounds by the ear.

6 **Seeing:** Obtaining impressions through the eyes of the shape, size, distance, motion, color, or other characteristics of objects. The major visual functions are: (1) acuity, far and near, (2) depth perception, (3) field of vision, (4) accommodation, (5) color vision. The functions are defined as followed:

(1) Acuity, far—clarity of vision at 20 feet or more. Acuity, near—clarity of vision at 20 inches or less.

(2) Depth perception—three-dimensional vision. The ability to judge distance and space relationships so as to see objects where and as they actually are.

(3) Field of vision—the area that can be seen up and down or to the right or left while the eyes are fixed on a given point.

(4) Accommodation—adjustment of the lens of the eye to bring an object into sharp focus. This item is especially important when doing near-point work at varying distances from the eye.

(5) Color vision—the ability to identify and distinguish colors.

Appendix B
Working Conditions*

Working conditions are the physical surroundings of a worker in a specific job.

1 **Inside, Outside, or Both:**
  I Inside: Protection from weather conditions but not necessarily from temperature changes.
  O Outside: No effective protection from weather.
  B Both: Inside and outside.

A job is considered "inside" if the worker spends approximately 75 percent or more of his time inside, and "outside" if he spends approximately 75 percent or more of his time outside. A job is considered "both" if the activities occur inside or outside in approximately equal amounts.

2 **Extremes of Cold Plus Temperature Changes:**
  (1) Extremes of Cold: Temperature sufficiently low to cause marked bodily discomfort unless the worker is provided with exceptional protection.
  (2) Temperature Changes: Variations in temperature which are sufficiently marked and abrupt to cause noticeable bodily reactions.

3 **Extremes of Heat Plus Temperature Changes:**
  (1) Extremes of Heat: Temperature sufficiently high to cause marked bodily discomfort unless the worker is provided with exceptional protection.
  (2) Temperature Changes: Same as 2(2).

4 **Wet and Humid:**
  (1) Wet: Contact with water or other liquids.
  (2) Humid: Atmospheric condition with moisture content sufficiently high to cause marked bodily discomfort.

5 **Noise and Vibration:** Sufficient noise, either constant or intermittent, to cause marked distraction or possible injury to the sense of hearing, and/or sufficient vibration (production of an oscillating movement or strain on the body or its extremities from repeated motion or shock) to cause bodily harm if endured day after day.

6 **Hazards:** Situations in which the individual is exposed to the definite risk of bodily injury.

7 **Fumes, Odors, Toxic Conditions, Dust, and Poor Ventilation:**
  (1) Fumes: Smoky or vaporous exhalations, usually odorous, thrown off as the result of combustion or chemical reaction.
  (2) Odors: Noxious smells, either toxic or nontoxic.
  (3) Toxic Conditions: Exposure to toxic dust, fumes, gases, vapors, mists, or liquids which cause general or localized disabling conditions as a result of inhalation or action on the skin.
  (4) Dust: Air filled with small particles of any kind, such as textile dust, flour, wood, leather, feathers, etc., and inorganic dust, including silica and asbestos, which make the workplace unpleasant or are the source of occupational diseases.
  (5) Poor Ventilation: Insufficient movement of air causing a feeling of suffocation; or exposure to drafts.

Appendix C
Training Time*

The amount of general educational development and specific vocational preparation required for a worker to acquire the knowledge and abilities necessary for average performance in a particular job.

General Educational Development: This embraces those aspects of education (formal and informal) which contribute to the worker's (a) reasoning development and ability to follow instructions, and (b) acquisition of "tool" knowledges, such as language and mathematical skills. It is education of a general nature which does not have a recognized, fairly specific, occupational objective. Ordinarily such education is obtained in elementary school, high school, or college. It also derives from experience and individual study.

A table explaining the various levels of general educational development appears below.

Specific Vocational Preparation: The amount of time required to learn the techniques, acquire information, and develop the facility needed for average performance in a specific job-worker situation. This training may be acquired in a school, work, military, institutional, or avocational environment. It does not include orientation training required of even every fully qualified worker to become accustomed to the special conditions of any new job. Specific vocational training includes training given in any of the following circumstances:

a. Vocational education (such as high school commercial or shop training, technical school, art school, and that part of college training which is organized around a specific vocational objective);
b. Apprentice training (for apprenticeable jobs only);
c. In-plant training (given by an employer in the form of organized classroom study);
d. On-the-job training (serving as learner or trainee on the job under the instruction of a qualified worker);
e. Essential experience in other jobs (serving in less responsible jobs which lead to the higher grade job or serving in other jobs which qualify).

The following is an explanation of the various levels of specific vocational preparation.

Level
1. Short demonstration only.
2. Anything beyond short demonstration up to and including 30 days.
3. Over 30 days up to and including 3 months.
4. Over 3 months up to and including 6 months.
5. Over 6 months up to and including 1 year.
6. Over 1 year up to and including 2 years.
7. Over 2 years up to and including 4 years.
8. Over 4 years up to and including 10 years.
9. Over 10 years.

---

* From US Department of Labor, Bureau of Employment Security: *Supplement 2 to the Dictionary of Occupational Titles*, ed 3. Washington, DC, US Government Printing Office, 1968, by permission of Mr. John Hawk, US Employment Service, Washington, DC 30210.

General Educational Development

Level	Reasoning Development	Mathematical Development	Language Development
6	Apply principles of logical or scientific thinking to a wide range of intellectual and practical problems. Deal with nonverbal symbolism (formulas, scientific equations, graphs, musical notes, etc.) in its most difficult phases. Deal with a variety of abstract and concrete variables. Apprehend the most abstruse classes of concepts.	Apply knowledge of advanced mathematical and statistical techniques such as differential and integral calculus, factor analysis, and probability determination, or work with a wide variety of theoretical mathematical concepts and make original applications of mathematical procedures, as in empirical and differential equations.	Comprehension and expression of a level to— —Report, write, or edit articles for such publications as newspapers, magazines, and technical or scientific journals. Prepare and draw up deeds, leases, wills, mortgages, and contracts. —Prepare and deliver lectures on politics, economics, education, or science. —Interview, counsel, or advise such people as students, clients, or patients, in such matters as welfare eligibility, vocational rehabilitation, mental hygiene, or marital relations. —Evaluate engineering technical data to design buildings and bridges.
5	Apply principles of logical or scientific thinking to define problems, collect data, establish facts, and draw valid conclusions. Interpret an extensive variety of technical instructions, in books, manuals, and mathematical or diagrammatic form. Deal with several abstract and concrete variables.		
4	Apply principles of rational systems[1] to solve practical problems and deal with a variety of concrete variables in situations where only limited standardization exists. Interpret a variety of instructions furnished in written, oral, diagrammatic, or schedule form.	Perform ordinary arithmetic, algebraic, and geometric procedures in standard, practical applications.	Comprehension and expression of a level to— —Transcribe dictation, make appointments for executive and handle his personal mail, interview and screen people wishing to speak to him, and write routine correspondence on own initiative. —Interview job applicants to determine work best suited for their abilities and experience, and contact employers to interest them in services of agency. —Interpret technical manuals as well as drawings and specifications, such as layouts, blueprints, and schematics.
3	Apply common sense understanding to carry out instructions furnished in written, oral, or diagrammatic form. Deal with problems involving several concrete variables in or from standardized situations.	Make arithmetic calculations involving fractions, decimals, and percentages.	Comprehension and expression of a level to— —File, post, and mail such material as forms, checks, receipts, and bills. —Copy data from one record to another, fill in report forms, and type all work from rough draft or corrected copy.
2	Apply common sense understanding to carry out detailed but uninvolved written or oral instructions. Deal with problems involving a few concrete variables in or from standardized situations.	Use arithmetic to add, subtract, multiply, and divide whole numbers.	—Interview members of household to obtain such information as age, occupation, and number of children, to be used as data for surveys or economic studies. —Guide people on tours through historical or public buildings, describing such features as size, value, and points of interest.

General Educational Development (continued)

Level	Reasoning Development	Mathematical Development	Language Development
1	Apply common sense understanding to carry out simple one- or two-step instructions. Deal with standardized situations with occasional or no variables in or from these situations encountered on the job.	Perform simple addition and subtraction, reading and copying of figures, or counting and recording.	Comprehension and expression of a level to— —Learn job duties from oral instructions or demonstration. —Write identifying information, such as name and address of customer, weight, number, or type of product, on tags or slips. —Request orally, or in writing, such supplies as linen, soap, or work materials.

[1] Examples of "principles of rational systems" are: Bookkeeping, internal combustion engines, electric wiring systems, house building, nursing, farm management, ship sailing.

chapter 49
Workers' Compensation

Penny Lozon Crook, J.D.

Workers' compensation is, in the most general terms, a system of social legislation designed to protect workers from suffering undue financial hardship when they are unable to work as the result of an on-the-job injury. More specifically, workers' compensation is not a system, but a number of systems; there are separate workers' compensation laws in each state, the District of Columbia, and various U.S. territories. In addition, federal laws provide coverage for federal employees, and many maritime workers are covered under the federal Longshore and Harbor Workers Compensation Act. Despite the multiplicity of laws, however, they are for the most part sufficiently similar that we can, for the purposes of this chapter, discuss workers' compensation as though it were a single system, as first conceived by Larson (1).[a]

The definition of who is a covered worker varies from state to state. For the most part, however, the majority of "employees" are included in the system, while independent contractors are excluded. Certain classes of employees may also be excluded; some of the more prevalent exclusions are domestic employees, farm workers, executives and partners, and employees of very small employers (employers of fewer than the minimum number, e.g., two or five employees, are not required to have workers' compensation, although they may be able to affirmatively opt to be covered). In three states, workers' compensation coverage is extended only to employees in "hazardous" occupations, but in those states the term "hazardous" is broadly defined. In all but three states, workers' compensation coverage is mandatory for all employers and employees who fit within the statutory definition.

As noted in the general definition, workers' compensation is designed to protect injured workers from undue financial hardship; it is not designed to totally replace lost income. Thus, under the most typical benefit scheme, a totally disabled worker will receive only two-thirds of his average weekly wage, subject to a state maximum benefit. Also, unlike tort systems, under which an injured person can collect for pain and suffering and other intangible injuries, the workers' compensation system is designed only to compensate injured workers for medical expenses and lost wages.

WORKERS' COMPENSATION VERSUS TORT-BASED SYSTEMS

As noted in the previous section, workers' compensation differs from the tort system in that the workers' recovery is limited to medical costs and compensation for lost wages. Workers' compensation also differs from tort-based systems in another major way. Tort systems are designed to provide compensation (in the form of damages awards) from wrongdoers to those injured because of the wrongdoers' fault or negligence. Workers' compensation, however, is generally not concerned with questions of

---

[a] Dr. Arthur Larson first conceived of the idea of treating the 50-odd separate workers' compensation statutes in terms of their similarities in his 1952 treatise, *The Law of Workmen's Compensation*. During the ensuing 35 years, while that original 2-volume treatise has grown to 10 volumes, courts, compensation boards, and state legislatures have increasingly looked to Dr. Larson's wisdom in determining how issues should be handled.

fault or negligence.[b] The only main focus is on work connection—that is, was this injury sufficiently related to the injured person's working conditions or duties.

To illustrate the differences between tort systems and workers' compensation, consider two simple "slip and fall" cases, in which Mr. Smith and Ms. Jones are hurt when they slip in a puddle of water on the floor and fall. In a tort system, whether Mr. Smith could recover from someone else for his injuries would depend on how the water got on the floor (for instance, he would be unlikely to recover anything if he had spilled the water himself); whether the owner of the building knew, or should have known, that the water was there and that Mr. Smith or persons like him were likely to be walking in that area (i.e., the owner probably has no duty to protect against the possibility that a trespasser would slip in the puddle); and whether Mr. Smith should have been able to see the water in time to avoid stepping in it. If all of these issues were resolved in Smith's favor, he could recover for his medical expenses in treating the injury, his past and future lost wages attributable to the injury, and his pain and suffering. In addition, his wife could recover for loss of consortium, that is, the diminution in value of his services to her as a result of the injury. The Smiths might also recover punitive damages if the judge or jury found that the defendant's conduct was especially blameworthy; for instance, if the puddle had been on the floor in an area heavily frequented by the public for a long time and the building's owner had deliberately refused to clean it up.

In contrast, if Ms. Jones had slipped in the puddle while she was working, questions of whose fault the accident was and who knew or did not know about the puddle would be generally irrelevant. The only issues would be whether her injuries were sufficiently work connected (under the formula discussed below) and whether those injuries kept her from working. Her recovery, however, would be limited to payment of her medical bills, payment of compensation benefits for the weeks she was unable to work, and, in most states, a "schedule award" for her presumptive future loss of wages if, after reaching the maximum medical recovery, it was determined that she had a residual permanent loss of function attributable to her injuries.

There are two more facets that should be noted in connection with these examples. First, if Ms. Jones' injury had occurred off the employer's premises—as, for instance, if she were a salesperson who slipped while calling on a customer—she could still bring tort action (a "third-party action") against the owner of the premises. That action would proceed just like Mr. Smith's action, except that Ms. Jones would be obliged to reimburse her employer out of her damages award for any workers' compensation benefits she received. Second, as to the employer, Ms. Jones does not have the option of suing or receiving workers' compensation; except in very limited circumstances not present in this example, workers' compensation is the exclusive means of collecting from the employer for an employee's injuries.

Injured workers are increasingly attempting to bring third-party actions so as to recover for intangible injuries such as pain and suffering and punitive damages. In addition to bringing actions against manufacturers and distributors of products involved in the injury, employees often attempt to sue their employers on the ground that their injuries were caused by the employer's "intentional" misconduct. Although most workers' compensation acts do indeed allow workers to sue the employer for "intentional" acts, these exceptions are generally applied strictly so as to allow actions only in cases of deliberate assaults on the employee and the like. In virtually every state, actions will not be allowed on the basis that the employer "intentionally" failed to furnish a safe place to work. [The problems involved in third-party actions occupy an entire volume in Larson's 10-volume treatise (ref. 1, vol. 2A).]

MEDICAL WITNESSES IN THE WORKERS' COMPENSATION SYSTEM

As the examples in the preceding section show, the workers' compensation system avoids much of the protracted litigation present in the tort system over issues of fault and damages. Thus, in the majority of workers' compensation cases, the system functions almost automatically; upon receipt of notice that an employee has been injured, the employer arranges for payment of his medical expenses and begins making weekly payments of the workers' compensation benefits to which the employee is entitled until he is able to return to work. Nevertheless, there remain many cases in which there is disagreement between the parties as to whether the employee has sustained a compensable injury and, if so, what benefits he is entitled to receive. Before discussing these issues more specifically, however, it will be helpful to understand the context in which the issues are decided and the role physicians can and do play in the process.

In most states, the initial determination on contested proceedings is a hearing before a hearing officer (often called a referee, an administrative law judge, or a deputy commissioner), a quasi-judicial employee of the state labor department. Because the procedure is an administrative-type hearing rather than a court trial, the rules of evidence

---

[b] Fault considerations are a part of some workers' compensation statutes in the form of penalties to be assessed when the conduct of either the employer or the employee is particularly blameworthy. For instance, in many states an employee's compensation award may be reduced (and in some states, denied altogether) if his on-the-job accident was caused by his voluntary intoxication. Similarly, in many states an employee's award may be increased if the accident was caused by the employer's failure to follow state or federal safety rules. Since penalties are generally not favored in the law, both types of statutes are strictly construed and therefore of relatively little importance in the total workers' compensation scheme.

may be less strictly applied than they would be in a court action. For instance, medical evidence may be admitted not only in the form of live testimony and sworn depositions, but also in the form of unsworn medical reports and letters. It should also be remembered that the hearing officers rarely have any medical training. Although a long-time hearing officer may have acquired familiarity with medical terminology, a relatively new hearing officer is unlikely to have such familiarity, nor is he likely to understand more esoteric terms and relationships.

And yet, the issues that are often contested are those of the causation of an injury and the extent and duration of a workers' disability. The proper resolution of both these issues often depends on expert medical evidence. This evidence must be properly introduced at the initial hearing on the claim, since, in most states, the hearing officer's determination will be affirmed in appeals to higher levels of the workers' compensation commission and the courts unless it is "clearly wrong." Although the terminology for this standard of review varies from state to state, the general rule is that the hearing officer's decision is presumed correct as long as it comports with any substantial evidence (see ref. 1, vol. 3, 80.20 *et seq.* for a collection of literally hundreds of cases that were affirmed on this ground). A hearing officer who accepts the credible testimony of one physician is not likely to be overruled merely because two or three physicians expressed an opposite view, particularly if the physician whose testimony was accepted actually treated the worker and the other physicians' evidence is based on merely reviewing the medical records.

Of course, the hearing officer stage is reached only in contested cases—those in which the worker and the employer (or more accurately in most cases, the employer's workers' compensation insurance carrier) disagree as to the cause of the injury or the extent of the disability. Most cases are disposed of simply on the basis of the reports given by the treating physician(s), and perhaps those of physicians who are called upon, by either party, to give a second opinion. Determinations in these cases are made by insurance adjusters.

Thus, whether or not a case is contested, medical evidence is often accorded great weight by persons who may be untrained in medical terminology. Therefore, a physician who is called upon to give a report in a compensation case must remember to be clear in explaining his diagnosis and prognosis, particularly in cases involving more unusual injuries and diseases. One should be prepared to explain an official diagnosis in layman's terms and to spell out in detail the causal relationship between the events of the job and the employee's current disability. When it comes to rating the degree of permanent partial disability sustained by a claimant, the physician should be aware that insurance companies and workers' compensation hearing officers expect to have ratings based on standard AMA Guidelines. If a chronic pain specialist believes that these Guidelines do not accurately reflect the true extent of the worker's disability because they do not take into account the degree of pain, he should be prepared to spell out clearly how and why his rating departs from the Guidelines. (The issue of chronic pain as a factor in disability is discussed more fully later.)

Another rule the physician should be aware of when reporting or testifying in a workers' compensation case is the "speculation and conjecture rule." Simply stated, this rule means that the workers' compensation commissions cannot legally make an award based on "maybes." Although hearing officers are rarely as unsophisticated as to expect medical testimony to be phrased in terms of certainty, they are nonetheless liable to find their decisions overturned if they accept testimony that is too equivocal. Thus the physician should be prepared to state his conclusions in as positive terms as possible. Instead of "I think" and "I feel," he should be prepared to express his opinions in terms of "reasonable medical probability" or percentages of probability if he can conscientiously do so.

THE COMPENSATION FORMULA

The workers' compensation system is designed to provide benefits only for work-related injuries; it is not designed to handle all disability of employed persons. Therefore, it is incumbent on a workers' compensation claimant to show that his injury comes within the state's statutory definition of work relatedness. The relevant wording of this definition varies from state to state, but it generally requires the employee to show that he has sustained "a personal injury by accident arising out of and in the course of employment." This requirement thus has several subparts, which may be broken down as follows:

1. A personal injury
2. An injury by accident
3. An injury that arises out of the employment
4. An injury sustained during the course of employment

For purposes of this chapter, we may safely dispense with the fourth requirement, that of course of employment, since the issues there rarely involve medical questions, but rather are confined to legal and factual issues, such as whether injuries sustained on a lunch or coffee break or while engaged in horseplay can be said to have happened during the course of employment (see ref. 1, vols. 1–1A, sects. 14.00–29.00). However, the other three parts of the formula often involve not only legal and factual questions, but also questions that can be resolved only through expert medical testimony.

PERSONAL INJURY

It may be difficult for a physician to understand why the requirement that an employee sustained a personal injury should be at all controversial, let alone one of the most controversial areas in current workers' compensation law. It must be recalled that the workers' compensation system was originally geared toward dealing with problems like that of an assembly line worker who loses a finger or breaks a leg in a fall. To a compensation board or commission used to dealing with clearly observable physical injuries like cuts and broken bones, the term *injury* may not seem to include mental or nervous "injuries." Yet employees do develop mental and nervous injuries as the result of events that happen at work. In fact, there are apparently an increasing number of employees whose work causes them to undergo emotional injuries; at least the number of reported cases in which such "injuries" appear is growing, and much controversy has been engendered as workers' compensation commissions and the courts that hear appeals from those commissions try to deal with the problems of emotional injuries.

In order to understand the scope of the controversy, it is helpful to use Larson's breakdown of the three categories of mental injuries (ref. 1, vol. 1B, sect. 42.21–42.25). These categories are:

1. *Physical-mental.* This includes all injuries in which a worker who first receives some sort of physical trauma to the body (e.g., a blow or a cut) becomes disabled from the psychic repercussions of that trauma.
2. *Mental-physical.* This category is comprised of cases in which the initial trauma is emotional—perhaps a sudden shock or fright or perhaps merely the cumulative effect of job stress—but the result is a clearly observable physical injury, such as a heart attack or bleeding ulcers.
3. *Mental-mental.* These are the cases in which there is no "visible" injury at either end of the equation (e.g., a disabling neurosis caused solely by stress).

The courts almost invariably find that cases in the first category are compensable, even where the initial trauma was slight. In fact, even in states with an express provision that mental injuries are compensable only if preceded by a physical impact, the courts have been quite resourceful in finding an initial physical trauma sufficient to satisfy the statute.

Cases in the second category have become increasingly prevalent in workers' compensation literature in recent years, particularly those cases involving stress-related heart attacks. In the heart attack cases, the issue of compensability almost always depends on the degree of stress involved. A claimant can rarely recover unless he can show some unusual degree or type of work-related stress that led up to the debilitating attack. (And his case will be strengthened greatly if some degree of abnormal physical exertion was also present.)

As might be expected, it is the last category, that of "mental-mental" injuries, that is the most controversial. Even within this category, a distinction must be made between cases in which the initial emotional stress was a sudden fright or shock and cases in which the causative factor was merely the gradual buildup of stress. Compensation is more or less routinely awarded in cases involving a sudden stimulus, as for instance a worker who suffers an emotional breakdown after seeing a friend or coworker killed on the job. It is much more difficult, however, for a worker to recover when his breakdown is attributable merely to the cumulative stresses of the job. Although there have been recent awards in such cases, the courts in these cases have stressed that awards in this category are permissible only if the worker can show greater than ordinary stress leading up to the breakdown. There remains a very strong fear among courts and employers that allowing recovery for those debilitated by ordinary pressures and stress would turn the workers' compensation system into a general mental health insurance system that would favor those too emotionally "weak" to handle the normal pressures of life.

INJURY BY ACCIDENT

Because workers' compensation was not designed as insurance against the "wear and tear of ordinary life," most workers' compensation statutes protect only against "accidental" injuries. One obvious way that the accident requirement functions is to prevent recovery for deliberately self-inflicted injuries. This issue, which is currently usually handled by a specific statutory exclusion for intentional self-injuries, arises seldom and then usually only in the context of suicides. (As a general rule, suicide is noncompensable, but two major rules work so as to make many probable suicides compensable. First, there is a general civil law presumption that an unexplained death was not suicide, which, combined with the general rule that the workers' compensation acts are to be liberally construed in favor of the worker, serves to make the decision in many unexplained death cases one in favor of accident, rather than suicide. Second, most courts to have considered the issue have ruled that the suicide of a disabled worker is compensable if he was driven to commit the act by the pain caused by his work-related injury.)

Even though the self-injury question is of relatively little importance, there remain two primary areas of concern within the "by accident" requirement. The first, which is closely related to the preceding discussion of emotional injuries, is the unusualness requirement that has been read into the definition of an accidental injury. The second is the issue of disease as an accidental injury.

The Unusualness Requirement

Even though workers' compensation is supposed to be a no-fault system, the historic requirement that an accident must have been unusual in order to satisfy the "by accident" definition reminds one of the "assumption of risk" doctrine in traditional tort law. The assumption of risk doctrine may be easily illustrated by imagining a professional boxer attempting to sue his opponent for his injuries. The assumption of risk rule dictates that he cannot recover; when he agreed to engage in the fight he voluntarily chose to assume the risk that he would be injured. A similar rationale was applied in early workers' compensation cases when courts denied recovery to workers whose injuries arose from the normal incidents of their employment—for example, a night watchman who suffered frostbite while making his rounds on a wintery night. Although the courts did not phrase their denials in terms of assumption of risk, their use of the "accident" terminology revealed the same reasoning as the assumption of risk doctrine. Common sense tells us that the boxer should anticipate the risk of being injured when he steps into the ring; common sense also tells us that a man who walks around checking doors all night in freezing temperatures should anticipate the risk of being frostbitten. Since the watchman, like the boxer, should have expected the result that actually occurred, the result was not unusual and thus was not a compensable "accident" under this reasoning.

Although the refusals to recognize the effects of exposure to the elements as accidents are now almost entirely a historic anomaly, the unusualness requirement has taken over another entire field of workers' compensation cases, those involving "breakage" of the body from the routine exertions of the job, particularly in cases involving heart and back injuries. The paradigmatic example of how these cases arise is that of a worker at the end of an assembly line whose job is to remove 40-pound boxes from the line and stack them on pallets. After months or years of routinely performing this task, he picks up a box and feels a sharp pain in his back or, perhaps more typically, goes home one night and wakes up with back pain. His physician reports that he has a lumbar strain or, perhaps, a herniated disk. Has he sustained an "accidental" injury?

The traditional answer to this question was no; there was no accident because nothing unusual occurred during the work. Although the result—the back injury—was unusual, the cause was not; the worker was simply doing his regular job. But in some instances, the courts found that there was an "accident" if there was anything unusual about the day's work—the boxes weighed 50 pounds, rather than the regular 40 pounds, or the worker had to carry them 2 feet further that day. In some instances, it might be held that there was a compensable accident if the worker felt a sudden pain on the line, but not if he simply awoke one morning with a back problem—that is, an injury was considered "accidental" only if the worker could point to a definite time and place where it occurred.

A moment's reflection will show that these distinctions are not only arbitrary but are also liable to draw false distinctions between workers with identically caused injuries. Thus, many jurisdictions are gradually coming to drop their artificial unusualness requirements in favor of a simpler test of medical causation: did this worker's exertion, whether or not unusual, in fact cause this injury. The process of change is, however, not only slow but uneven; a particular jurisdiction may require only proof of medical causation for heart injuries, but require a showing of unusual effort for back injuries, and retain elaborate rules on showing a definite time and place of injury for hernia cases. (See ref. 1, vol. 1B, sects. 36.00–38.85 for a discussion of the "by accident" requirement and unusualness rules.)

Accident and Disease

The "by accident" requirement was originally thought to bar a workers' compensation recovery when the injury was due to a disease or allergy caused by exposure to conditions on the job, rather than to some sort of traumatic injury. However, recovery was generally allowed if the disease was a result of an initial trauma. Some cases also held the disease was compensable if it could be shown that the germs entered the body suddenly and unexpectedly, as where a tubercular coworker sneezed in the employee's face or where an employee was exposed to infection through an open cut or wound. Some occupational disease cases could also be brought within the accident requirement under the "repeated trauma" theory. This theory envisions each onslaught of germs or noxious particles as a small trauma—a "mini-accident"—and holds the resulting disease process compensable as the result of a series of accidents.

This sort of elaborate rationale is less frequently needed nowadays, since every state has some sort of occupational disease act, as part of, or as an adjunct to, its workers' compensation act. Difficulties may still arise, however, in states where the occupational disease statute is merely in the form of an exclusive schedule or list of covered occupational diseases.[c] In those states, it may be necessary to invoke the "repeated trauma theory" in order to attempt to fit an unlisted disease into the "accident" theory.

In states that do not have a schedule, or whose schedule is not exclusive, an occupational disease is usually defined as one "peculiar to" or "characteristic of" the type of employment, or at least one to which the employee had a greater exposure than that of the general public. Thus, an employee who seeks workers' compensation benefits for disability caused by a relatively common disease, such as pneumonia or hepatitis, must be prepared to show how the duties of his job exposed him to a greater risk of contracting this disease than he would have had in his everyday life. For example, in one Pennsylvania case, an employee was unable to convince either the commission or the

---

[c] The types of diseases included in these schedules are usually respiratory diseases, such as asbestosis and byssinosis, along with diseases caused by exposure to various heavy metals and toxic industrial chemicals. One major problem with both exclusive and nonexclusive schedules of covered diseases is the propensity of their drafters to include arbitrary time limits within the definitions. For instance, silicosis may be defined as a disease only if it results from exposure to certain forms of silica for a specified number of hours or workdays; or asbestosis may be defined as a covered disease only if it is diagnosed as such within a certain number of years after the employee's last on-the-job exposure to asbestos. These arbitrary limitations are criticized in Larson (ref. 1, vol. 1B, sect. 41.72).

reviewing court that distillery workers have a greater risk of developing alcoholism than does the general public. On the other hand, several recent cases have awarded workers' compensation benefits to assembly workers who developed tenosynovitis and/or carpal tunnel syndrome from the repetitive hand and arm movements required by their job, even though these diseases can also arise from nonoccupational causes (ref. 1, vol. 1B, sect. 41.00 passim).

INJURY "ARISING OUT OF" THE EMPLOYMENT

The "arising" requirement is a primary test for work connection of an injury. Like the course of employment test mentioned earlier, it has a strong factual and legal component. Among the legal-factual questions under the "arising" requirement are those dealing with positional or neutral risks—for instance, whether a worker who is injured by a sniper's bullet while on the job has sustained an injury arising out of the employment. One can argue that the worker was in no greater danger from the sniper than the members of the general public who were also in the area. On the other hand, however, one can argue in many cases that the general public had a choice over whether to be in that area, while the worker had no choice in the matter; the duties of his job required him to be in the "zone of danger." The latter view, which has been increasingly accepted by the courts, is the "positional risk" rule, under which risk is deemed to have arisen out of the employment if the worker's exposure to the risk was due to the fact that his employment required him to be in that place at that time. The positional risk rule is applied to a wide range of risks, not only to attacks by snipers and the like, but also to acts of God, such as tornados and lightning, as well as attacks by animals, such as bee stings, rat bites, and the like.[d]

In addition to these legal questions, the "arising" requirement also raises issues of medical causation, particularly in cases involving unexplained accidents, accidents arising from idiopathic causes, and the sequalae to on-the-job injuries.

Idiopathic and Unexplained Accidents

The controversy in both the unexplained accident and idiopathic causes cases centers around the rule that workers' compensation is not payable for an injury caused solely by the employee's own internal weakness. For instance, if a worker is disabled because high blood pressure (or low blood sugar, or any other idiopathic cause) causes him to collapse, the disability is not compensable merely because of the fortuity that the collapse happened while he was at work. However, even an idiopathically caused collapse may be compensable if the severity of the injury was enhanced because of the work environment. Thus, compensation would probably be awarded if an employee who fainted from an idiopathic cause sustained serious injuries when he landed on a piece of machinery or fell to the ground from a scaffolding on which he was working.

In summary then, the general rule is this: an injury caused solely by idiopathic causes is not compensable but even an idiopathically caused injury is compensable if it was exacerbated by the employment. With this principle in mind, we can turn our attention to another "arising" issue; that of unexplained accidents. A fairly easy unexplained fall case would be one where a worker was found on the floor under the scaffold on which he was working, having sustained injuries consistent with a fall from the scaffold, but with no memory of how he happened to fall. This case presents a clear case for compensability since, as we have seen, the danger involved in working on the scaffold brings even an idiopathically caused fall within the "arising" rule. But the case becomes more difficult if there was no evidence that the worker was even on the scaffold and if his injuries are such that they may have been caused merely by the faint. Of course, unexplained accidents are not limited to falls; they also include unexplained deaths due to assaults and automobile accidents, as well as a variety of accidents in which the employee is unable or unavailable to explain what happened. Although the claimants in these cases are often aided by a presumption that the accident was work connected, the establishment (or refutal) of work connection can be aided greatly by medical "detective work." To the extent that the physician can clearly pinpoint (or rule out) an idiopathic cause, the legal conclusion as to whether the accident arose out of the employment is made much easier.

Consequences of Compensable Accidents

As a general rule, the natural and proximate consequences of a compensable job-related accident are also compensable, even though the seriousness of those consequences may be attributable to the employee's own preexisting weakness or disease. For example, if a worker sustains a minor cut, which would normally be expected to heal without incident, but, because of his preexisting diabetes, develops an infection that requires extensive treatment and/or surgery, the entire course of treatment and any resulting permanent impairment would normally be compensable. Likewise, depression or anxiety suffered by an employee as the result of the original accident or his inability to return to work is generally considered a compensable consequence, even if the employee had a preexisting tendency toward depression. Of course, in either case, the causal connection between the original

---

[d] The "positional risk" rule, along with the other risk rules and their historic development, is discussed in Larson (ref. 1, vol. 1, sects. 6.00–12.20). The cases in those sections are among the most interesting in the workers' compensation field, including as they do issues such as assaults by jealous suitors and insane strangers, and buildings being attacked by all sorts of natural disasters, as well as the unexplained and idiopathic accidents discussed below.

injury and the consequences must be clearly established, usually through expert medical opinion.

If a worker's injury is exacerbated by medical malpractice or by a forseeable accident flowing from the original injury—as, for instance, an automobile accident while the worker is on the way to his physician's office—the resulting exacerbation is generally compensable. (In these instances, the worker may also be able to maintain a tort action against the malpracticing physician or the driver of the car responsible for the accident. If so, the employer will be entitled to reimbursement from the worker's third-party recovery for the extra compensation he was required to pay because of the consequences caused by the third party.) Here again, however, the causal relationship between the original injury and the consequences must be established; the employer will not be held responsible if the employee sustains a new and independent injury while he is disabled—for instance, an injury in an automobile accident while on the way to his sister's house. In fact, if the new injury is to the same part of the body as the original work-connected injury, the commission, with the help of medical experts, will be faced with the nightmarish task of trying to establish when the original disability would have ceased had it not been for the intervening noncompensable injury.

There are two major exceptions to the general rule that a worker may recover for the natural consequences of an initial injury: no recovery is available for exacerbation due to the employee's own rash acts or to his unreasonable refusal of treatment. The "rash acts" exception is usually applied on a fairly straightforward and commonsense basis. For example, if an employee with an injured knee breaks his arm when the knee gives way and causes him to fall to the ground, the broken arm would probably be treated as a compensable consequence of the original knee injury if the fall occurred while he was walking sedately to his mailbox, but not if it happened while he was engaging in a foot race.

The other major exception to the compensable consequences rule is that for consequences attributable to the employee's unreasonable refusal of surgery or other treatment. Two of the contexts in which this issue frequently arises are weight reduction and surgery. The weight reduction cases usually involve employees with back or leg injuries whose physicians state that their disability would be lessened if they were to lose weight. The courts generally take a tolerant attitude toward these employees and will not deprive them of benefits if they have been making any reasonable efforts to lose weight.

The courts are also usually quite tolerant toward employees in the surgery cases, particularly in cases involving back surgery (spinal fusion or laminectomy). Apparently, for every medical witness who asserts that a spinal fusion will clear up the employee's back problems, one can find another equally reputable physician who will testify that the operation is as likely to make matters worse as it is to cure the problem. Since even the medical experts disagree as to the efficacy of the proposed surgery, the court is unlikely to find the employee is unreasonable in refusing to undergo the risks. On the other hand, if the employee has refused to undergo a relatively risk-free surgery (e.g., one that can be performed under local anesthetic), which has a great probability of success, his refusal is likely to be deemed unreasonable and the continuing consequences attributable to his refusal to undergo the surgery will not be compensable. Likewise, refusal to take prescribed medications or to cooperate with a physical therapy program will almost invariably be deemed unreasonable, since the benefits of the treatment will clearly outweigh the risks. The range of compensable consequences and the exceptions are covered in Larson (ref. 1, vol. 1, sect. 13.00 *et seq*).

BENEFITS

DISABILITY BENEFITS

As noted earlier, worker's compensation benefits are paid only during the period in which the employee is disabled from returning to work (and, in some instances, for presumed future disability). Simply put, the benefits are a fractional proportion (most commonly two-thirds) of the worker's loss in earning capacity attributable to the work-related injury. The details of how workers' compensation commissions calculate a worker's pre-and postinjury "average weekly wage" in order to determine the amount of his benefits are far too complicated for this chapter (see ref. 1, vol. 2, sect. 60.00 *et seq*). Suffice it to say that issues such as whether certain items should be included in the calculation are often fiercely litigated. In fact, in one recent case, the propriety of including certain contributions made to union benefit funds on a worker's behalf was contested all the way up to the Supreme Court of the United States.

The disability for which benefits are payable can be either temporary or permanent and either partial or total, leading to four "classes" of disability benefits:

1. Temporary partial
2. Temporary total
3. Permanent partial
4. Permanent total

Of these classes, temporary partial is a category that appears more often in theory than in practice—in fact, the author has never encountered a reported case in which the issue of temporary partial disability was a litigated issue.

Typically, an injured worker will go through a period of temporary total disability following an on-the-job injury. If this period is very short, he may not be entitled to disability benefits. For purposes of administrative convenience, many states impose a "waiting period" of, for example, 5 days during which no disability benefits are payable. If the worker is disabled for longer than the waiting period, benefits will be paid from the date of injury, but it is considered to be too much of a burden on the system to go through all the benefit computations when an employee misses only a few days or less of work as a result of an on-the-job injury.

Assuming that there was a period of temporary total disability, it will be determined at some point that the injured worker has attained the maximum medical improvement (MMI) that can be expected. Once MMI has been reached, a determination must be made, with the assistance of medical opinion, as to whether the worker has sustained any permanent impairment and, if so, the extent of that impairment. If it appears that the worker will be unable to return to work at any time in the forseeable future, he will be classified as permanently and totally disabled and will be awarded benefits accordingly. In many states, this means that he will be entitled to receive his weekly benefit rate for the rest of his life or until circumstances change so that he can rejoin the workforce. However, in some states, even permanent total disability benefits are limited to a set time period of, for example, 400 weeks. Once that period has ended, the injured person will be totally without funds, unless he is able to qualify for some type of assistance such as welfare or Social Security disability. Also, in most states, the weekly benefit level determined at the outset of disability remains immutable throughout the period of disability—workers' compensation systems, unlike much other humanitarian legislation, rarely provide for cost-of-living adjustments.

If the worker is able to return to work, but has some residual physical disability attributable to the injury, he is likely to receive an award based on the state's "schedule" of injuries, combined with the medical ratings as to the degree of residual impairment. For instance, if the state's schedule provides that the loss of a leg is equal to 240 weeks of total disability, and the worker is rated as having impairment equivalent to a 15% loss of use of the leg, he would be given a permanent partial disability award equal to .15 × 240 × his weekly benefit rate. Depending on the rules of the state, this award might be for 240 weeks of payments at 15% of his previous weekly benefit, 36 weeks of full benefits, or a lump sum payment of the whole amount.

The alert practitioner will have already noted two points in this process where medical opinion is not only necessary, but almost always indispensable—determining when the worker has reached MMI and "rating" the degree of permanent disability, which includes diagnosing whether residual impairment will cause permanent total or merely permanent partial disability. Detailed discussion of these two points is deferred to the next section, after we complete the discussion of the other types of benefits available to workers' compensation claimants.

DEATH BENEFITS

If a compensable accident causes a worker's death, his dependents will generally be entitled to death benefits. In most states, they need only establish that they fit within the statutory definition of dependents[e] and that the worker's death was causally connected to an injury that comes within the state's coverage formula. In a handful of states, however, the dependents' claim will be barred if the worker was not considerate enough to expire from his injuries within an arbitrary time period, such as 2 years after the date of the accident.

The weekly death benefit available to the dependents is usually the same as the worker would have received for permanent total disability. Benefits for dependent children usually terminate when they reach the age of majority, and benefits for dependent spouses are almost always stopped when they remarry. Benefits for other dependents (e.g., spouses who do not remarry, and dependent parents or siblings) may be limited to a set period, such as 400 weeks, or may last until their deaths.

MEDICAL BENEFITS

A worker who sustains a job-related injury is entitled to medical benefits, whether or not he is also entitled to disability benefits. Even if a worker misses no time from work because of his injury, he is entitled to have his medical treatment for the injury paid for by the employer. State statutes vary on whether it is the employee or the employer who has the right to choose the treating physician; some states compromise by providing that the employer may furnish the employee with a list of acceptable physicians and the employee must choose from among those listed. The commission will also generally provide procedures for change of physician, referrals to specialists, and the procuring of additional opinions in contested cases (ref. 1, vol. 2, sect. 61.00 et seq).

Medical benefits generally cover not only the cost of physicians, hospitals, and prescribed medications, but also nursing services, prostheses, and other medically necessary forms of treatment. The treatment costs awarded have, on occasion, included items such as the cost of day care for a mother with an injured back whose physician prescribed that she not lift her small child, and the cost of swimming lessons for another employee with a back injury when his doctor prescribed swimming as therapy. Psychiatric treatment for injury-related depression is also included, under the compensable consequences rule.

An issue that has been addressed in several recent cases is the extent of medical benefits that can be awarded for

---

[e] Determining who are dependents can occasionally be quite complicated. It is not unheard of for a commission to be presented with the claims of two or more wives, each of whom contends she was never divorced from the deceased worker, along with children from both marriages, a handful of stepchildren, and, for good measure, one or two illegitimate children by a third woman. Or, in cases where the decedent left neither wives nor children, his parents, his grandparents, and his siblings may all present claims that they were actually dependent on his earnings. These issues are discussed in detail in Larson (ref. 1, vol. 2, sects. 62.00–63.00).

purely palliative treatment. Many workers' compensation statutes are worded in terms of supplying medical treatment to "cure" the employee's condition. Under such statutes, questions arise, particularly in cases involving workers who are permanently and totally disabled, as to whether the commission can order payment for treatment that merely relieves the claimant's pain, without effecting any change in the underlying condition. Most courts have been able to find a rationale that allows them to uphold such orders.

REHABILITATION BENEFITS

Nearly every state provides benefits for the costs of physical rehabilitation of injured workers; in fact, these costs may often be subsumed under the general medical benefits provisions. The majority of the states also have some sort of provision for vocational rehabilitation, although the availability of those rehabilitative services may be limited to those who would otherwise be considered permanently and totally disabled. The benefits available under these provisions are generally limited to furnishing the worker with "vocational training" (i.e., training in a trade or skilled labor field). College costs are almost invariably excluded, although some claimants have attempted to secure college training. In one recent case, a young man who had been injured on his summer job as a laborer sought to have that employer pay for the remainder of his college program as vocational retraining. Although the state supreme court correctly rejected his claim—since, after all, he was not really a laborer who needed retraining—it is the author's opinion that college training should not be foreclosed in all instances.

Vocational retraining benefits are often offered on a "carrot and stick" basis. The "carrot" in this instance is in the form of full payment for the costs of the training, in addition to the worker's normal disability benefit, and sometimes also an additional payment during the period of study. The stick takes the form of diminished weekly benefits for those who refuse to undergo training or make only minimal efforts to comply with their training programs.

Vocational rehabilitation benefits need not always be in the form of retraining. Benefits can also be directed toward reequipping the employee to perform his former job, as for instance by providing a specially designed work station to accommodate the employee's loss of physical function. Continued supervision and the ability to deal with changing conditions by the commission is indicated in these types of cases, however. If an employee who would otherwise be totally disabled is able to perform his old job with the help of special tools and the like, his disability benefits may be discontinued on the ground that he no longer has any loss in earning capacity. But if he loses that job as a result of economic conditions or other forces outside his control, he will again need the help of the workers' compensation system, either to again pay disability benefits or to help him find another job that is within his limitations.

DISABILITY, PAIN, AND THE CHRONIC PAIN SPECIALIST

Before discussing more specifically the role of the physician, and particularly that of the chronic pain specialist, in evaluating disability, we need a more exact definition of "disability" than we have used in preceding sections. Although we have spoken of disability as the employee's inability to return to the duties of his job, that definition is too narrow, because it would mean that an employee could be considered permanently and totally disabled merely because he could not perform his previous job, as for instance a typist who was perfectly healthy except for the loss of a finger. On the other hand, if we merely define disability as an inability to work, the definition becomes too broad; it is irrational to say that a skilled craftsman is not disabled because he is still able to do some kind of work, albeit as a dishwasher. Thus, disability in the workers' compensation sense can be defined as "inability, as the result of a work-connected injury, to perform or obtain work suitable to the claimant's qualifications and training" (ref. 1, vol. 2, sect. 57.00).

However, even that definition is somewhat ambiguous because it leaves open the question of what is the "inability to perform work"; must the worker be physically unable to make the necessary muscle movements or can he be said to be unable to do the work if he can make those movements only in great pain? The answer, in most cases, lies somewhere between those two extremes: pain will generally be considered as a factor in assessing the extent of the worker's disability, but pain alone will rarely be considered disabling. As to where the line will be drawn in any given case, much will depend on the medical witnesses and on how well they can evaluate the worker's pain and its effect on his ability to perform his job and then "educate" the hearing officer, so that their evaluation will be properly understood.

In this respect, the author would like to suggest that a primary duty of a pain specialist called upon to give an evaluation in a workers' compensation case is not only to evaluate the pain in relative terms but also to gain a clear understanding of the worker's job so that he can evaluate the pain in terms of the job duties. This suggestion is grounded in the author's own experience: A few years ago her husband sustained an accidental (although not work-related) cervical strain. The orthopedist who was treating him kept prematurely attempting to release him to return to work, in the belief that his continuing pain would not prevent him from working as an electrician. Those releases were apparently based on the physician's understanding of an electrician's job duties as installing lighting fixtures and switches and other light objects. He could not be made to understand that the patient was an industrial electrician, specializing in the installation of heavy pipes and metal trays that often weighed several hundred pounds and had to be carried a half-mile or more on the electrician's shoulders.

Similar misunderstandings could occur in almost any field of endeavor: leg pain that might not prevent a research physician or a trusts and estates attorney from working could render a busy clinician or a litigation attorney unable to perform normal duties. Thus, a full understanding of the worker's job duties would always seem to be indicated. Similarly, if it is contended that the employee is able to enter an alternative workfield, the duties of that field should be carefully considered in light of the worker's pain.

The pain specialist called upon to report or testify in a workers' compensation case should also remember that there is often a suspicion on the part of the employer that the injured worker is shirking and exaggerating his symptoms, particulary if there is no observable evidence of injury (i.e., "we can't see a thing on the x-ray"). In those cases, the specialist should be prepared to explain, and demonstrate if necessary, to the employer and the hearing officer how he can measure the pain. The more that the worker's pain can be objectified, the more likely it is to be believed. Of course, if the specialist has been called upon by the employer, an equally strong and objective showing should be made to demonstrate why the specialist believes that the worker's pain is nonexistent or less acute than the worker claims.

Acknowledgments The author acknowledges with gratitude the support and encouragement of her husband, Jim, her daughter, Dawn, and her law partner, MaryEllen McDonald. A special thanks is due to the author's mother, Doris A. Lozon, who not only offered encouragement but also helped with the typing of the manuscript. Finally, the author cannot adequately express the gratitude that she personally owes to Dr. Arthur Larson, not only for encouraging her to write this chapter, but in teaching her, during the years she worked for and with him, this fascinating field of law.

Reference

1. Larson A: *The Law of Workmen's Compensation.* New York, Mathew Bender & Co, 1952–1987.

pain clinics
section 5

chapter 50
Assessment and Treatment at Pain Therapy Centers[a] Programs

C. David Tollison, Ph.D.

The assessment and treatment of chronic nonmalignant pain have received considerable attention over the past decade, and their prominence has been reflected in Sunday newspaper supplements as well as in the scientific and medical literature. Today, pain management has truly moved into the mainstream of health care delivery as a viable alternative to the human suffering and socioeconomic costs of chronic pain. This trend has spawned a virtual explosion in the number of programs, clinics, and centers exclusively or in part targeted toward pain management. Although such clinics and programs can run the gamut from an "acupuncturist practicing in the back of a shoe store" (1) to a comprehensive hospital-based interdisciplinary program, most legitimate programs have been influenced by Fordyce (2), Bonica (3), and Sternbach (4). Each author has promoted a unique approach to conceptualizing, assessing, and treating complex intractable pain, yet each proposes a psychophysiologic model and warns against dichotomizing chronic pain into physiologic and psychological components.

This approach is in sharp contrast to conventional medical care. By training, physicians generally isolate symptoms and focus treatment on identified or organic systems within a stimulus-response model. The same may be said of patients seeking medical assistance, workers' compensation carriers seeking an equitable solution to pending litigation, and insurance companies seeking to resolve mounting medical bills. For the great majority of medical disorders the organic system stimulus-response model of practice is appropriate and effective.

However, there is an increasing body of scientific research suggesting that chronic benign pain is far more than the sum of its parts. Today we recognize pain as a multidimensional phenomenon composed of physiologic, psychological, social, economic, cultural, motivational, and, likely, other components, and recognition is also given to the limitations of isolated treatment approaches.

PAIN THERAPY CENTERS

Pain Therapy Centers was developed in 1980 as part of the Greenville (South Carolina) Hospital System, with three beds tucked away in a remote corner of a 50-bed rehabilitation wing. Full-time staffing included a clinical psychologist specializing in pain management and behavioral medicine, and a secretary. Part-time clinical services were borrowed from the departments of physical therapy, nursing, social services, vocational therapy, vocational rehabilitation, and medicine.

Pain Therapy Centers is today a growing network of both outpatient and inpatient facilities available at numerous hospital-based Centers located in the southeastern and eastern United States. An interdisciplinary staff of health care professionals—including physicians, psychologists, physical therapists, behavior therapists, recreational therapists, vocational rehabilitation specialists, and nurses—devote their total time and attention to pain management. Consultants representing neurology, neurosurgery, rheumatology, orthopedic surgery, internal medicine, and fam-

---

[a] Pain Therapy Centers is a registered trademark.

ily medicine are actively involved. Although the duration and details of pain management are individualized for every patient, the general approach is consistent. Patients are actively involved in a 21- to 28-day (average 25 days) inpatient or outpatient interdisciplinary program emphasizing a nonsurgical behavioral approach to the physical, vocational, and psychological rehabilitation of patients with chronic pain. This effort consists of an active "sports medicine" functional restoration approach, as opposed to passive physical therapy. Body mechanics classes, medical rounds, vocational counseling and assistance, recreational therapy, relaxation training, behavioral modification, individual and group psychotherapy, and educational classes and discussions are conducted in a behavioral therapeutic setting. Active patient participation in a highly structured, intensive, graded program of comprehensive rehabilitation is emphasized. The goals of pain management treatment include (a) increased physical activity, (b) decreased intake of analgesic agents, (c) decreased subjective estimates of pain, (d) decreased use of health care facilities, and (e) return to employment and productivity.

Since 1980, Pain Therapy Centers[a] has conducted evaluations and treated approximately 6000 patients, all by referral. Table 50.1 shows descriptive characteristics from a recent sample of patients (5). Historically, 69% of all patients are referred by orthopedic and neurosurgeons while internal medicine and family medicine physicians collectively refer the majority of the remainder. Approximately 80% of the patients referred complain of back pain, 9% of headaches, and the remainder are diagnosed as suffering a variety of pain complaints.

ASSESSMENT

PREADMISSION EVALUATION

Each patient referred to our Centers is first scheduled for an outpatient preadmission evaluation to determine his/her potential for specialized pain management and restorative treatment. Admissions criteria include the following:

1. No clinical evidence of pain etiology likely to respond to conventional medical or surgical interventions.
2. Referral by physician with medical records of appropriate diagnostics.
3. Patient's cooperation and participation in an interdisciplinary program of comprehensive examination and testing.
4. Cooperation and active participation of the patient's spouse and family.
5. Clinical staff agreement that the patient is motivated to reduce pain and disability.
6. No evidence of severe psychological/psychiatric disturbance.

During the preadmission evaluation, every patient is examined by a physician, clinical psychologist, physical therapist, and vocational specialist, and family members are interviewed by a social worker. Each staff member reviews the medical records on every patient prior to the evaluation.

The medical and physical therapy components of the preadmission evaluation include an interview, physical examination, and functional assessment. Particular attention is given to measurement of range of motion and discrepancies between pain behavior and observed or inferred abnormality. A discrepancy is not a requirement of psychophysiologic pain but does facilitate the likelihood that pain behavior is influenced by factors other than pure tissue disease. The medical and physical therapy examinations also serve to define physical limitations and to better identify specific amounts, types, and rates of physical activities indicated as medically advisable at the outset and at subsequent points throughout the treatment program.

The psychological evaluation is intended to determine the general psychological and personality status of every patient and to explore for systematic relationships between pain behavior and reinforcing consequences. In addition to the clinical interview, psychological testing in the form of the Minnesota Multiphasic Personality Inventory (MMPI) is administered with interpretation based on standards consistent with the population of patients in pain (5, 6). In selected cases, additional testing is administered utilizing the Millon Behavioral Health Inventory and Hendler Back Pain Scale.

A vocational history and interview are conducted by a certified vocational evaluator in order to identify vocational experience, skills, and interests of patients who may require vocational assistance in returning to or modifying employment. Since appropriate employment is considered within our philosophy to be physically and psychologically therapeutic, considerable emphasis is placed on identifying and satisfying those factors that may otherwise prohibit a return to a level of employment consistent with any physical or psychological limitations.

Table 50.1.
Characteristics of 100 Patients with Chronic Back Pain

	No.	Mean	Range
Men	56		
Women	44		
Workers' compensation	72		
Age		42.6 years	19–66 years
Education		10.3 years	3–17 years
Time since onset of pain		32 months	5–96 months
Medications for pain		2.2	0–7
Major back operations		2.1	0–6
Time since last employment[a]		22 months	1–77

[a] For housewives, months since beginning to require help with housework.

While referred patients participate in the structured preadmission evaluation, our social worker interviews family members who are required to accompany the patient to the initial examination. The social work interview is intended to investigate family response and reinforcement of pain behavior and to identify the impact of every patient's pain on his or her family. During the interview a determination is also made as to whether the family is agreeable to participating in required family training sessions.

PREADMISSION STAFFING

Following the preadmission evaluation, the professional staff meets and formally presents clinical findings and opinions. With the admissions criteria as a guide, each staff member is allowed one vote for or against an offer of program admission. Those patients judged as not meeting the admissions criteria receive particular attention since it is our policy to forward to the referring physician a summary of formal treatment and management recommendations on all patients not offered program admission.

Since 1981, approximately 28% of referred patients examined in the preadmission evaluation have been rejected for program admission. Historically, newly opened Pain Therapy Centers programs will average a rejection rate closer to 50% during the first year or two of operation, whereas our Centers, in operation for several years, demonstrate a gradual reduction in the percentage of patients not offered admission. It is our belief that as a specialized elective pain management and restoration program, accountability to patients, referring physicians, insurance carriers, and employers with a financial and/or personal interest in treatment success is critically important. As a result, admissions criteria are relatively stringent and we attempt to offer admission only to those individuals demonstrating adequate motivation and potential for success. In opening our Centers, it generally takes a year or so to educate referring physicians in the value of this philosophy and to allow each new medical community the opportunity to determine what constitutes an appropriate referral. Of the 28% rejected for program admission, 63% have been judged as demonstrating inadequate motivation to reduce pain and disability, 28% were judged as suffering severe psychological/psychiatric disturbance requiring traditional psychological/psychiatric referral, and the remaining 9% were rejected for a variety of reasons, including lack of cooperation in the preadmission evaluation or a belief on the part of our staff that further traditional medical diagnostics and/or treatments were indicated.

TREATMENT

At Pain Therapy Centers programs, we have a motto that so accurately describes our philosophy and beliefs that it frequently appears as both a verbal and printed descriptive. The motto is this—"It's not just WHAT we do, but HOW we do it. . ." Simple, yes, but it is an effective and accurate philosophy that serves as the foundation for our clinical delivery and operations. The reasoning is straightforward. As can be determined in the description of the treatment modalities that follows, there is little in the way of clinical techniques that is not abundantly available in the literature and at numerous hospitals and health care facilities. As those of us in pain management realize only too well, treatment is far more "blood, sweat, and tears" than "whistles, magic, and novel clinical techniques." So if the "what" is readily available and relatively standard, then we must attend to the "how" in an effort to facilitate clinical effectiveness.

At our Pain Therapy Centers programs, we have attempted to address the "how" by developing a network of treatment programs based on a clinical model that remains under constant research revision. As the model program is frequently modified, details of the revision are forwarded to the program directors and staffs of our satellite programs for similar modification. The vehicles for communicating the frequent modifications in clinical delivery to satellite Pain Therapy Centers programs include revision of the policies and operations manuals, publication of monthly newsletters and quarterly educational updates, distribution of audiovisual training films, and frequent on-site visits by our training and supervisory personnel. All Pain Therapy Centers programs are linked by computer, and our model program serves as a data bank where quality assurance information from every Center is received and reviewed on a daily basis. Furthermore, in addition to the minimum 700-hr intensive and highly structured residency training program in pain management required of all program directors and frequent on-site visits by supervisory professionals, program directors are required to return to our model program at least once a year for further training and supervised clinical practice.

The treatment program at Pain Therapy Centers is highly structured and targeted toward accomplishing three primary goals: physical, psychological, and vocational restoration. Clinical delivery is not the servicing of "sick" individuals; rather, it is active and goal oriented, and attempts to foster independence. Every effort is made to make each patient responsible for his own treatment and for managing his pain. Treatment is delivered in an upbeat, enthusiastic style and a behavioral orientation blankets delivery of all clinical services. A partial listing of program components is presented below.

PHYSICAL REACTIVATION

Research has indicated that a program of regular stretching, strengthening, endurance, stamina, and physical conditioning exercises is an important part of chronic benign pain rehabilitation, particularly in cases of low back pain (5). Flexion, general conditioning, and range of motion exercises have been proven to be important in reducing the amount of pain that patients report (7), and, when introduced as part of a multimodal behavioral program as early as within 2 days of pain onset, results in a superior clinical outcome when compared to traditional conservative medical management (8).

At Pain Therapy Centers programs, patients are routinely scheduled for two daily classes of physical reactivation exercises totaling more than 2½ hr each day. No passive physical therapy is offered; all exercising is active, using a work-to-quota approach to increasing strength, walking distances, sitting and standing tolerance, bicycle riding, range of motion, and physical endurance (9).

Patients are introduced to physical reactivation by explaining the rationale of a graded program of physical reconditioning and through a 2-day program of establishing appropriate baseline measures on a sampling of physical exertional stations (9). During this time, an individualized program of morning and afternoon stretching exercises is outlined for every patient from a general collection of appropriate and effective exercises designed by Center staff (9).

Following baseline measurement, a daily work-to-quota system is implemented that is maintained throughout each patient's hospitalization and follow-up (10). Increased physical activity is also encouraged outside the scheduled reactivation classes. Patients are required to walk stairs rather than use the elevator, go through the hospital cafeteria line for meals, make their own beds, and clean their rooms. Treatment is goal oriented and emphasizes each patient's responsibility for his own treatment program, as well as increased physical strength, stamina, endurance, and independence.

MEDICATION REGULATION

Most patients referred to Pain Therapy Centers programs have a lengthy history of consuming multiple analgesics, including narcotics, in an effort to control pain (10). Analgesic medications are typically given to patients on an as-needed basis with restrictions as to the total amount to be taken each day. A frequent scenario encountered is that the patient hurts and then asks for or takes medications. In that sequence, the immediate and systematic consequences of asking for or taking medications are chemotherapeutic relief and, if it is given by another, the attention of the person giving it. Relief and attention are both powerful reinforcers of pain behavior (2).

At Pain Therapy Centers programs, medications are shifted from a pain-contingent to a time-contingent basis to encourage extinction of unnecessary analgesic drugs. This procedure is used with inpatients only, since medical complications may occur during detoxification. Medications are given at fixed intervals, regardless of whether or not the patient expresses a need for it. Medications are also administered by means of a "pain cocktail" (5). Pain cocktails consist of analgesic medications mixed in a liquid vehicle that masks color and taste, and the active ingredients are systematically reduced until none, or almost none, are being given (Table 50.2).

References to "chronic pain syndrome" generally identify syndrome components as pain, depression, insomnia,

Table 50.2.
Pain Therapy Centers Pain Cocktail Formulas for Reduction of Analgesics

Cocktail	Components	Dosage
A	Cherry syrup Elixir Gevrabon[a] Demerol (100 mg)	15 ml, q 4 h
B	Cherry syrup Elixir Gevrabon Demerol (50 mg)	15 ml, q 4 h
C	Cherry syrup Elixir Gevrabon Codeine (60 mg)	15 ml, q 4 h
D	Cherry syrup Elixir Gevrabon Codeine (30 mg)	15 ml, q 4 h
E	Cherry syrup Elixir Gevrabon	15 ml, q 4 h

[a] Vitamin-mineral supplement.

and anxiety (11). The incidence of pain in depression has been reported to average 65%, and the incidence of depression in chronic pain has been reported to be as high as 87% (12). A significant majority of patients treated at Pain Therapy Centers programs are judged to be clinically depressed by means of psychological testing and clinical interviews (5). Therefore, depression and pain may share common pathophysiology and potentiate negative effects on patients' coping and pain tolerance. Accordingly, tricyclic antidepressants are commonly prescribed for individuals suffering the combination of symptoms associated with chronic pain.

Of the two general groupings of tricyclic antidepressants, the tertiary amines, including doxepin and amitriptyline, have received the greatest attention in pain and symptom management (12). This is primarily due to research suggesting the effectiveness of doxepin and amitriptyline in blocking the reuptake of serotonin in excess of norepinephrine blockage and to research suggesting that serotonic enhancement helps raise the pain threshold, improve sleep, and relieve depression (11, 13).

At Pain Therapy Centers programs, doxepin and amitriptyline are frequently utilized as temporary adjuncts in our multimodal program. At present, a large-scale research investigation is underway to better determine the clinical effectiveness of doxepine, amitriptyline, trazodone, and other antidepressant medications in the management of chronic benign pain.

RELAXATION TRAINING

Formalized relaxation training, as part of a multimodal interdisciplinary treatment program, has proven valuable in helping patients learn to modify physiologic and psychological tension associated with chronic pain (9). Our typical patient does not know which of his muscles are tense, cannot accurately judge whether he is relaxed, does not realize any connection between prolonged muscle tension and pain, and does not know how to relax (9). Relaxation training has proven helpful in breaking the "pain-tension cycle" of chronic pain and in teaching patients to gain control over both physiologic and psychological functioning (14) (Fig. 50.1).

At Pain Therapy Centers programs, progressive muscular relaxation instruction takes place in a dimly lit, quiet room specifically designated for relaxation training. Patients are encouraged to visit the relaxation room on their own during unscheduled times, and audio recordings of the relaxation technique along with portable tape players are available for use in every patient's room. In addition, formalized relaxation therapy is scheduled daily. Patients are instructed in a specialized relaxation technique designed by Center staff based, in part, on combining imagery and muscle-tensing techniques (9).

Learning to relax can be a powerful tool in combating chronic pain, and is frequently cited by our patients as one of the more beneficial aspects of the total treatment program (7). Furthermore, pain control, anxiety relief, and improved sleep through instruction in relaxation therapy facilitates the transfer of responsibility of pain management to the patient.

PSYCHOLOGICAL REHABILITATION

The patient with intractable pain and altered life-style almost always becomes depressed, frustrated, irritated, and helpless in the course of the disabling illness, and chronic anxiety and sleep disturbances also frequently accompany chronic pain (11). This is generally considered to be a "normal" response to chronic pain, although a reaction that is believed to greatly complicate, hinder, and confuse treatment and rehabilitation (15).

At Pain Therapy Centers programs, daily individual psychotherapy is intended to allow patients an opportunity to verbalize pain and psychological complaints in a private environment where reinforcement for such complaints may be controlled by the therapist. Although individual counseling may, on rare occasion, allow a reflective, open type of therapeutic exchange, we have found that daily group therapy requires a consistently direct and structured therapeutic format to avoid deterioration to a competition among patients as to "who hurts worse." As a result, every effort is extended to maintain a goal-oriented approach to both individual and group treatment, which is geared toward maximizing existing skills and developing new skills for effectively coping with the physical discomfort and altered life-style as well as the depression, anxiety, and frustration associated with chronic pain. In individual and group psychological treatment, a positive and energetic effort is made to teach patients that they may elect to learn to control pain, or choose to allow pain to control them.

PATIENT EDUCATION

It is the philosophy of Pain Therapy Centers that patient education plays a valuable and unique role in effective pain management. We have found that an alarming number of our patients have previously consented to multiple spinal surgeries with no concept of the surgical procedure, what a disk or vertebra looks like, the function of the spine, or even what to expect after surgery (9).

Patient education in the form of didactic lectures and discussions is scheduled several times each day. Discussions led by psychologists, physicians, nurses, physical therapists, and vocational counselors are helpful in explaining to patients the continuing mechanism of chronic pain, the value of proper body mechanics and physical reactivation, and why surgery usually cannot simply "cut out" the cause of chronic benign pain.

A daily scheduled 1-hr educational class that is a particular favorite among our patients is termed "Pain School." Pain School incorporates over 50 prepared and outlined lectures and group discussions of specific topics frequently requested by our patients. Each of these specific topics falls under one of 11 general educational categories found to significantly impact effective pain management. Lectures and discussions of problems dealing with sexual functioning and physical disability as well as how chronic pain can affect an individual's behavior and personality are empirically judged as beneficial in allowing patients to more effectively deal with their pain problems. Lectures in basic anatomy and physiology, as well as presentations and discussions of the various types of medications, are particularly popular topics.

One class each week is devoted to dealing openly and honestly with how secondary gains, such as financial compensation and avoidance of responsibility, may occasionally be associated with chronic benign pain. Problems associated with workers' compensation claims and disability determination are thoroughly discussed in a nonjudgmental, educationally oriented fashion.

Finally, involvement of the spouse and family is con-

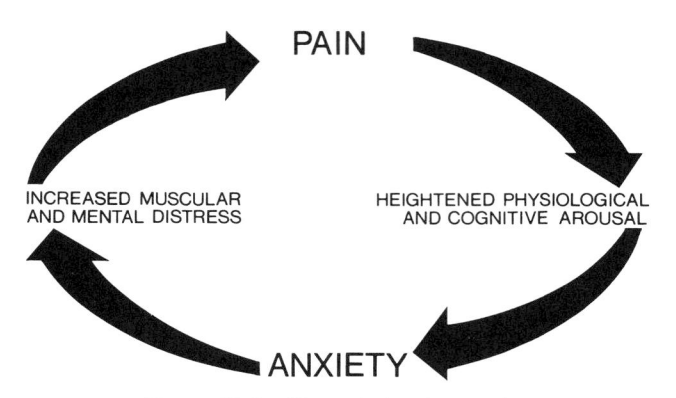

Figure 50.1. The pain-tension cycle.

sidered a critical aspect of behavioral treatment. Family members are considered "extenders" of behavioral therapists and are recognized as being capable of providing either potent reinforcement or extinction of the treatment program. Regular family group meetings are held during the course of treatment. Basics of behavior modification are taught and rehearsed, and family members are held responsible for practicing these principles at home.

BEHAVIOR MODIFICATION

The publication in 1968 of two papers describing applications of behavioral methods to the management of chronic pain, and in 1973 of a report of outcomes of a series of patients treated with those methods, has been followed by numerous studies and clinical programs applying this general approach (15–17). As Fordyce et al. have stated,

> Responses by others to overt pain behavior accompanying the subjective experience of pain may serve to reinforce or to extinguish aspects of that behavior. When the pain behavior occurs with some consistency over a protracted period of time, as in chronic pain problems, the environment may come to be shaped in such a way as to reinforce the pain behavior and thereby sustain it (16).

At Pain Therapy Centers programs, all treatment, classes, and activities are conducted with adherence to the principles of behavioral psychology. The following basic principles are employed:

1. Reinforcement of "well behavior," such as reduction of analgesic usage, increased physical activity, and increased exercise quotas.
2. Extinction of reinforcers for established maladaptive behaviors, such as complaining of pain, dependency behavior, and walking with an antalgic gait.
3. Reinforcement of behavior that is incompatible with pain behavior, such as investigating vocational alternatives consistent with any physical impairment, which is incompatible with chronic pain and viewing oneself as disabled.

We believe integration of staff into an interdisciplinary team is also an important part of the behavioral psychology program. Team meetings are scheduled daily, complemented by weekly interdisciplinary staffing conferences in which all treatment modalities are discussed. Each patient's progress is carefully monitored, and appropriate treatment plans are formulated. Thus, each member of the treatment team is aware of how a particular patient is responding in all aspects of the treatment program.

VOCATIONAL REHABILITATION

One of the Pain Therapy Centers treatment goals is to return vocationally disabled victims of chronic benign pain to productive employment. The decision to identify vocational return as a treatment goal is the primary result of both clinical and economic research data. First, research indicates that chronic pain victims who are employed suffer a decreased intensity of depression, are more physically active, and have fewer physician visits than pain patients who are not employed (9). Second, figures quoted in multiple sources indicate that the cost of chronic pain is staggering, in terms of human suffering, social costs, and general monetary loss. In addition to the spiraling cost of medical care, employee replacement costs, loss productivity, and the like, the personal economic loss to pain victims and society for disability is great. In a 1981 study by Brena et al., the loss of wages combined with social support systems could cost taxpayers from $15,000 to $24,000 per disabled individual per year (18).

As a result, we employ several full-time specialists in vocational evaluation and counseling who work exclusively in the areas of rehabilitation. Our vocational specialists meet with each patient within 24 hr of hospital admission to conduct a vocational history and interview designed to determine vocational goals. For patients whose pain problem precludes a return to a former occupation, vocational alternatives and job training are explored. For patients who wish to return to employment but have no job, interview skills teaching and assistance in job placement are provided. Many pain patients who wish to return to former jobs after a prolonged disability choose to allow our vocational specialist to serve as an effective and knowledgeable liaison between the patient and employer.

In addition to working with each patient several times weekly on an individual basis, our vocational specialists also regularly conduct group didactic lectures and discussion groups on a variety of employment-related topics. Applied "hands-on" information is emphasized. For example, patients rehearse how to complete a job application and résumé, role play job interviews, and may elect to participate in a vocational workshop where an individual's physical and psychological ability to sustain employment is assessed in a supportive and therapeutic environment.

RESULTS

A recent clinical outcome investigation was conducted to assess multimodal interdisciplinary treatment effectiveness (5). One hundred patients consecutively admitted to Pain Therapy Centers programs with a diagnosis of chronic low back pain served as subjects. All patients were adults, with a mean age of 42.6 years and a range of 19 to 66 years. Fifty-six per cent of the admissions were male, and 72% of the sample were injured in occupational injuries and admitted under workers' compensation. The mean time from pain onset to program admission was 32 months and the average length of vocational disability was 22 months. The mean number of major spinal surgeries for the group was 2.1 and the average number of medications taken for pain complaints was 2.2.

Each of the 100 patients in this sample had active and current low back pain that had not responded to multiple medical interventions and treatments in the past. All patients were admitted for program participation based on the following criteria:

1. Pain of at least 6 months' duration.
2. No significant clinical evidence of surgically or medically remediable pain.
3. Referral by a physician or service agency after appropriate medical workup.
4. Cooperation in psychological and physical examination and testing.
5. Cooperation and active involvement of the patient's spouse and family.
6. Staff agreement that the patient is motivated to reduce pain and disability.
7. No debilitating psychological/psychiatric disturbance.

The results of this clinical outcome investigation indicate that all 100 patients had increased physical strength, stamina, endurance, range of motion, and overall physical activity averaging 356%. These measurements were recorded daily, but statistical analysis compared physical measurements recorded at the time of admission (baseline) and at discharge. At 12-month follow-up, 83 patients were evaluated to determine maintenance of treatment gains. (Because Pain Therapy Centers are regional referral centers serving a number of southern states, 17 patients could not return for 1-year follow-up owing to excessive distances.) Of the 83 patients who returned for follow-up, 74 (89%) had successfully maintained the treatment gains as measured at discharge.

Eighty-four patients (84%) were taking an average of 2.2 medications for pain (including narcotics) at the time of program admission (16 patients were taking no medication for pain). At discharge 74 patients (88%) formerly taking medications were taking no medication for pain, and the average number of medications (1.0 medications, no narcotics) taken by the remaining 10 patients showed a 55% reduction. At 12-month follow-up, 63 patients (75%) who were taking medication at the time of admission were taking no medication for pain, and the average number of medications (1.1 medications, no narcotics) taken by the remaining patients indicated a reduction of 50%.

Subjective pain intensity was rated daily by each patient on a 5-point scale of intensity, but for purposes of analysis, significant decreases in subjective pain intensity were noted at discharge and at 1-year follow-up. Utilizing the daily rating scale, 69 patients (69%) reported subjective decreases in pain intensity and increased ability to cope with residual pain. At discharge, the average decrease in pain intensity was 31%. At 12-month follow-up, 61 patients reported decreases in pain intensity averaging 40%. Furthermore, the majority of patients also reported an increased ability to relax, improved sleep, and renewed confidence in their ability to function independently.

Overuse of medical care also sharply decreased after specialized treatment. At 1-year follow-up, 15 patients continued under active medical care, and 85 patients reported no additional visits to physicians or hospitalizations for pain except for appointments initiated by workers' compensation personnel. This represents an 85% reduction in use of health care and a significant reduction in health care expenditures.

At the time of admission to Pain Therapy Centers programs, three patients with low back pain were working daily. At the time of discharge, 37 additional patients (38%) returned to full-time employment or were attending school or vocational training. Twelve-month follow-up indicated that an additional 27 patients (28%), for a total of 67 patients, were working or attending school daily, an increase of 66% from admission. Of the remainder, 5 patients had taken early treatment and 28 had not returned to employment.

SUMMARY

Chronic benign pain is one of the most prevalent and resistant of all psychophysiologic disorders and creates severe medical, social, and economic problems for patients, medical personnel, hospitals, insurance companies, and industry.

Physicians have traditionally sought to remedy chronic pain through either conservative management such as bed rest, traction, braces, corsets, nerve blocks, and medication, or surgical procedures such as laminectomy, fusion, facet rhizotomy, and cordotomy. Although in some cases pain relief may result from such procedures, there is increasing research indicating that for many patients, procedures that involve surgical intervention may, in the long run, prove ineffective as a method of long-term pain relief (19).

As the facts are collected, the population with chronic pain appears to be one of the most highly refractory to medical care by either conservative management or surgical intervention. Despite quality medical treatment, many individuals with chronic benign pain eventually become physically and/or emotionally disabled. Recent research has attempted to explain the complexity of intractable benign pain and the frequent failure of conventional medical treatment by suggesting that chronic benign pain does not conform to the stimulus-response model of medicine.

We now know that chronic pain has the potential for being heavily influenced by psychological variables and the psychological laws of learning and conditioning. We all have seen such patients have emotional changes that impair interactions with family, friends, and environmental surroundings. Overt, or, more frequently, covert psychological factors significantly complicate the medical picture. Often the patient is unintentionally encouraged to engage in "chronic pain behavior" because of a perceived lack of reaction or overattentiveness by well-meaning individuals, including physicians. As a result, the patient can unconsciously become highly manipulative in terms of his environment and the people around him, including employers and medical personnel. In a constant search for a "cure," these patients often go from doctor to doctor, requesting more and stronger drugs as well as repeated operations and treatment. When the patient perceives that one physician is near completion of what is most always an unsuccessful treatment trial, the patient goes "doctor shopping" to locate a new physician who innocently starts the cycle all over again with more examinations, tests, and hospitalizations. As a result, most patients with chronic pain have been extensively treated with multiple operations, tranquilizers, sedatives, synthetic analgesics, and narcotics, frequently leading to habituation and dependence. During this time, patients engage in "pain behavior" such as moving with guarded motions, antalgic gaits, excessive bed rest, medication abuse, and retiring from normal activities. Patients may be worse after a prescribed period of bed rest because they try to return to full activity immediately rather than after an appropriate program of physical reconditioning. As a result, these individuals have not only a psychological deterioration but also a gradual deterioration of physical conditioning. The product of this endless cycle is the patient with chronic pain whose entire economic, social, and personal life revolves around disability and suffering.

As our data indicate, a multimodal interdisciplinary treatment regimen such as Pain Therapy Centers offer an alternative treatment approach for the patient refractory to conventional medical interventions. This comprehensive functional restoration approach, which is targeted at increasing physical and social activity, eliminating or reducing medication intake, reducing subjective pain intensity, and reducing the overuse of health care, can lead to vocational and physical rehabilitation and the patient's resumption of a more normal life-style. We suggest that where predictors of treatment failure from conventional interventions are evident, or when traditional medical care is not successful, the comprehensive functional restoration approach can offer to the physician, insurance carrier, and patient a relatively inexpensive and proven option to repeated operations, medications, learned helplessness, and adoption of the chronic invalid role.

Furthermore, the outcome of this clinical work supports the view that although physical repair of tissue damage for pain relief may be necessary in many cases, this approach does not always constitute a necessary or sufficient intervention for the relief of pain or the comprehensive functional restoration of the patient. It is known that the intensity, direction, and frequency of reactive pain behavior are not direct functions of the degree, locus, or amount of organic tissue damage associated with the patient's injury [19]. For a sizable number of patients with a medical diagnosis of chronic benign pain, the successful management of psychophysiologic factors (e.g., anxiety, muscle tension levels, depression) believed to strongly influence chronic pain should now be given careful attention as part of a comprehensive approach to the functional restoration of the chronic pain population.

References

1. Crue BL, Aronoff GM, Rosomoff HL: Pain clinics: which one for your patient? *Aches Pains* 2:8–12, 1981.
2. Fordyce WE: *Behavioral Methods for Chronic Pain and Illness.* St Louis, CV Mosby, 1976.
3. Bonica JJ: Organization and function of a pain clinic. *Adv Neurol* 4:433–443, 1974.
4. Sternbach RA: *Pain Patients: Tracts and Treatments.* New York, Academic Press, 1974.
5. Tollison CD, Kriegel ML, Downie GR: Chronic low back pain: results of treatment at the Pain Therapy Center. *South Med J* 78:1291–1295, 1986.
6. Tollison CD: Diagnosing and managing chronic pain syndrome. *SC Med J* 9:449–453, 1984.
7. Tollison CD: *Managing Chronic Pain: A Patient's Guide.* New York, Sterling Press, 1982.
8. Fordyce WE, Brockway JA, Bergman JA, Spengler D: Acute back pain: a control group comparison. *J Behav Med* 9:127–140, 1986.
9. Tollison CD: *Relief From Back Pain.* New York, Gardner Press, 1987.
10. Tollison CD: Chronic benign pain: an innovative program for South Carolina. *SC Med J* 7:379–383, 1982.
11. Hendler N: The anatomy and psychopharmacology of chronic pain. *J Clin Psychol* 8:15–21, 1982.
12. MacDonald-Scott WA: The relief of pain with an antidepressant. *Practitioner* 202:802–807, 1969.
13. Sulser F, Ventulani J, Mobley P: Mode of action of antidepressant drugs. *Biochem Pharmacol* 7:257–261, 1978.
14. Tollison CD, Tollison JW: *Headache: A Multimodal Program For Relief.* New York, Sterling Press, 1983.
15. Fordyce WE, Fowler R, Lehmann J, DeLateur B: Some implications of learning in problems of chronic pain. *J Chronic Dis* 21:179–190, 1968.
16. Fordyce WE, Fowler R. DeLateur B: An application of behavioral modification techniques to a problem of chronic pain. *Behav Res Ther* 6:105–107, 1968.
17. Fordyce WE, Fowler R, Lehmann J, DeLateur B, Sand P, Trieschmann R: Operant conditioning in the treatment of chronic clinical pain. *Arch Phys Med Rehabil* 54:399–408, 1973.
18. Brena SF, Chapman SL, Decker R: Chronic pain as a learned experience. In Ng LKY (ed): *New Approaches to Treatment of Chronic Pain.* Washington, DC, US Department of Health and Human Services, 1981.
19. Wilfing FJ, Klonoff H, Kogan P: Psychological, demographic and orthopaedic factors associated with prediction of outcome of spinal fusion. *Clin Orthop* 90:153–160, 1973.

chapter 51
Pain Centers: A Survey and Analysis of Past, Present, and Future Functioning

Crystal C. Dickerson, M.A.

The commonly accepted definition of algology among pain management professionals is that algology is the art and science of pain management. It is also commonly accepted that pain centers are organizations established with the purpose of practicing algology. These definitions have been formally established by the International Association for the Study of Pain. Yet Dennis Turk, Ph.D., of the Center for Pain Evaluation and Treatment, recently and humorously reminded the author that *Webster's Dictionary* defines algology as the study of algae and makes no mention of algology as the study of pain management. Despite their anonymity among the general public, for numerous reasons that are considered in this chapter, pain centers have become quite widespread. This advancement has not been achieved easily or quickly. Like any new idea or new venture, pain centers have had their share of difficulties along the way to acceptance. And like only the best of new ventures, pain centers have become a respected, growing, and financially profitable entity.

THE PAST

The historic generation of chronic pain treatment and of pain centers is by now a familiar and oft-repeated sequence of events (1). After World War II, F.A.D. Alexander noted that many veterans returning home to the states continued to complain of pain well after their battle wounds had healed. He thus undertook to treat the pain from which these veterans sought relief and in doing so is credited with offering the original treatment for chronic pain. Soon after, John Bonica established a similar treatment program at a private hospital in Washington State. Bonica's program was staffed by a coordinated group of professionals interested in treating chronic pain, and during the decade that followed the patient population expanded to include civilians.

In 1953, Bonica published a landmark text entitled *The Management of Pain* (2), in which he introduced the important role of emotions in the pain experience and introduced the concept of multidisciplinary pain treatment. His text was seemingly the impetus for the literal explosion of pain studies during the subsequent three decades. In 1961, Bonica, along with Lowell White, established the Pain Clinic at the University of Washington (1). Their efforts were so well organized and their multidisciplinary treatment so successful that this clinic has since become a model for numerous other pain centers.

The late 1950s and early 1960s spawned a great deal of interest and research in pain, in psychophysiology, and in the important role of emotions, cognitions, and learning in our physical responses. Jacobsen developed and popularized progressive muscle relaxation, Miller demonstrated parameters of autonomic activity, and Melzack and Wall introduced the "gate control theory" of pain (3). In 1968, Fordyce and his associates published two works (4, 5) that demonstrated successful applications of an aggressive decade of research in which chronic pain became recognized, defined, and considered treatable.

The International Association for the Study of Pain (ISAP) was incorporated in 1974 and serves as a worldwide base for the development of pain treatment and as a meeting ground for pain professionals (3). The American Pain Society (APS), founded in 1979 as a national chapter of the IASP, has helped to extend the study of pain on a national level (3).

The rapid development of pain treatment facilities is best demonstrated by simple statistics. In 1976 only 17 pain clinics were identified by a nationwide survey (3). A questionnaire administered and collected by the American Society of Anesthesiologists in 1979 identified 285 pain control facilities (6). In 1986 there were easily more than 1000 facilities calling themselves pain clinics. A 1986 survey of major U.S. hospitals revealed that 33% of responding hospitals operated at least a back pain clinic. The percentage was the greatest in the midwest, where 41.6% of responding hospitals operate a back pain clinic (7).

Statistics may be somewhat deceiving, however. Facilities claiming to be pain centers range from one-man, single-discipline operations to self-contained medical units employing a variety of professionals and utilizing many modalities and disciplines. This chapter considers those comprehensive and interdisciplinary centers who treat a variety of chronic painful conditions with more than one modality and/or professional specialty, and who have multiple goals for their patients. For the purpose of clarity in this chapter, unidisciplinary clinics such as those who offer only biofeedback or nerve blocks or only a Back School are excluded from discussion. The literature contains numerous discussions on what a viable pain treatment facility is and has also defined the terms *pain clinic* and *pain center* based upon the qualifications discussed here (number of professional disciplines and modalities employed, types of pain treated, organization, etc.) (1, 3, 8). From that perspective this chapter discusses pain centers and does not consider pain clinics.

Interdisciplinary and multidisciplinary treatment centers must also be distinguished at this point. A true pain center is interdisciplinary. That is, an effective center should have perpetual communication and cooperation between professionals and disciplines. At all times, each professional involved in a patient's treatment should be aware of and reinforce the treatment being administered by other involved professionals. In a multidisciplinary center, the patient is routed from one department to another for treatment by first one professional and then another. Treatment pursued in this manner can easily become fragmented and has few advantages over standard medical treatment with numerous consultations.

The number of existing comprehensive and interdisciplinary pain centers is small relative to the number of pain treatment facilities cited by the 1986 survey of hospitals (7) noted above. Although that survey identified more than 1000 pain treatment clinics, truly interdisciplinary centers that have enough visibility to be discovered by a moderately persistent consumer are quite difficult to locate. As of January 1987, the national Commission on Accreditation of Rehabilitation Facilities (CARF) (see Appendix 51.C) had accredited only 63 centers, including both inpatient and outpatient facilities, which it thought offered quality multidisciplinary or interdisciplinary treatment for chronic pain. Even so, to identify 63 comprehensive centers among a thousand or so clinics is indication of rapid growth and demonstrable success for a field as young as chronic pain treatment. A majority of the currently existing comprehensive centers first opened in the past 10 years.

FACTORS IN DEVELOPMENT OF PAIN CENTERS

What factors have spurred on the growth and development of pain centers, and what factors have limited or slowed their expansion? Growth and develpment has been stimulated by multiple factors:

1. Pain centers fill a gap in previously available medical services by treating chronic pain, which was once considered untreatable except by the psychiatrist or psychologist.
2. Pain centers allow for the simultaneous treatment of the physical, emotional, cognitive, behavioral, vocational, and social aspects of chronic pain.
3. Once a center is established, it can treat the multiple aspects of pain less expensively than can a series of individual practitioners.
4. The center can complete treatment with a pain patient more quickly than can a series of individual practitioners and can thus limit disability (which has been demonstrated to increase with increasing duration of pain).
5. From an administrative standpoint, the pain center concept is popular and is a good marketing tool for the hospitals and universities who sometimes sponsor the centers.
6. Operated effectively, pain centers can be large revenue-generating ventures.

Multiple factors have also been responsible for limiting the establishment and success of new pain centers:

1. The concept of interdisciplinary treatment has experienced slow acceptance by the medical community in general, although this has certainly improved over the past 10 years.
2. For some centers, especially free-standing proprietorships, set-up costs for staff and equipment can be prohibitive.
3. Clinics who have failed to establish good relationships with third-party payors have not experienced good reimbursement for services rendered.
4. Because of lack of training facilities, some centers have

been staffed by technically incompetent individuals and this has resulted in poor outcome for their patients.
5. Mismanagement has sometimes resulted in policy decisions that ignore the best interest of the patients in favor of financial gain, or the reverse.
6. Some established centers are reluctant to reveal "trade secrets for successful treatment" to other potentially competitive centers.
7. Definitive outcome research is lacking as proof positive of the value of services.
8. Public education has been limited, and potential consumers remain ignorant to the availability of treatment.

Pain centers originated because of an identified gap in available effective services for the growing population of individuals with chronic intractable pain. Despite the high cost of set-up and treatment, despite public ignorance, and despite the doubts of numerous medical, insurance, and legal professionals, pain centers have survived because they fill that gap.

The Clinical Perspective

Some negative commentary in the literature would lead naive readers to think that if the interdisciplinary facets of pain centers have not been statistically proven to be effective as individual parts then they should not be honored as an effective whole. Pure statisticians have often had difficulty conceptualizing the clinical whole as more than the sum of parts. The positive majority of such commentary, however, has repeatedly pointed out that it is the interdisciplinary nature of the pain center that makes it so effective (see ref. 9 for a review). The pain center, because of its interdisciplinary nature, is the optimal environment for the simultaneous treatment of the emotional and physical components of pain. In the traditional environment, the treatment of the medical and emotional components of pain are so separate, and sometimes disparate, that the patient may even have difficulty grasping the connection between the two.

The medical orientation of the pain center gives patients a familiar framework that engenders trust and a positive expectation for improvement. Many patients would not submit to treatment at a pain center without the obviously present medical components, because that might imply that the patient was being treated only for psychosocial problems and not for the physical pain. The endorsement of the physician often lends credence to psychosocial treatment in the eyes of the patient. This is especially true when the physician demonstrates understanding of and participates as an integral part in the psychosocial milieu. The interdisciplinary nature of the pain center also reinforces to the patient the necessity of the patient's participation in treatment of both the medical and emotional aspects of his pain. Without the patient's participation in both the medical and psychosocial aspects of treatment, the chances of treatment being effective are drastically reduced. The interactive relationship between the emotional orientation and cooperation of the patient and success of treatment has been demonstrated repeatedly. This may be noted best in Brena's 1985 commentary on "nocebo responses" to nerve blocking (10). A "nocebo response" is "an escalation of bizarre and dramatized complaints, with various alleged bodily impairments" inconsistent with anatomic patterns, that may last for weeks in reaction to a nerve block (p. 84). Brena considers the nocebo response to be a definite indication of the need for psychophysiologic rehabilitation.

Not only is the interdisciplinary pain center clinically effective with the symptom complex of chronic pain, it is cost-effective as well. Cost is an important factor, because the annual cost of chronic pain treatment has been conservatively estimated to be in excess of $80 billion (3). The pain center concept eliminates the need for repeated exams and costly diagnostic tests, by assuring that all disciplines have access to each others' information. In the same manner, the pain center also shortens the amount of time required for appropriate diagnosis, medical treatment, and psychosocial and vocational rehabilitation to take place. Time is important in two respects. First, for every year an individual is disabled by pain, the cost to taxpayers for lost wages and social support programs is estimated to be $15,000 to $24,000 (3). Second, the longer an individual is disabled by pain, the smaller are the odds that he will be successfully rehabilitated, returned to productive employment, and removed from the social support program rolls.

A further reason for the successful development of pain centers may be termed multivariate improvement. In traditional medical treatment, a patient is first treated physically until maximum medical improvement is reached. Then the patient may be referred to another professional for assistance with psychosocial issues. Only after the patient has resolved outstanding psychosocial issues is he generally steered with success toward resuming gainful employment. When treated in a pain center, the patient is admitted to an environment that concentrates rehabilitation efforts so that he may work simultaneously toward medical, psychosocial, and vocational improvement. The combined nature of treatment may in itself save a year or more of rehabilitation for the involved patient.

Until the advent of pain centers vocational rehabilitation was always saved for last, after the patient had achieved maximum medical and psychosocial improvement. It is now commonly noted that vocational rehabilitation is not an appropriate aftereffect of treatment, but is an appropriate treatment itself (11, 12). Return to gainful employment has been shown to decrease subjective and objective disability of the pain patient and also to decrease the chronicity of symptoms. Appropriate work does not increase pain. Instead, work can decrease pain by decreasing the subjective anxiety and depression experienced by the patient and therefore effecting a positive change in the psychophysiologic processes of the pain itself. This again demonstrates the logic of interdisciplinary treatment.

From a clinical perspective, then, pain centers have survived and grown because they meet a need unmet by any previously existing medical service—they treat chronic pain effectively. They do so by simultaneously treating the physical, emotional, cognitive, social, and vocational aspects of the pain experience.

The Administrative Perspective

From an administrative and economic perspective, pain centers have succeeded because they can be highly visible as marketing tools and can be quite lucrative. Marketing of pain center services has reached national proportions, as cover-story versions of pain treatment have been published in *Time*, *Newsweek*, and almost every major newspaper in the country. These cover stories have made pain centers a true "growth industry" in the 1980s. There are now franchise versions of well-established centers being marketed to hospital management organizations on a national basis.

Within established hospitals, a pain center may be set up with minimal extra space, minimal capital outlay, and minimal increases in staffing. Most hospitals already offer many of the clinical services included in the pain center, but simply do not coordinate the services effectively and appropriately. Organized properly, the pain center acts as a significant revenue generator for the hospital, increases utilization of inpatient beds (which is no small task with increasingly strict DRGs), and even attracts patients from outside established primary service areas. Because pain treatment is considered "elective" treatment and patients are screened before admission, it is often possible to secure approval for treatment from third-party payors prior to treatment and to thus guarantee reimbursement for services. Also, since many chronic pain patients are also Workers' Compensation recipients, reimbursement for services is further increased if appropriate channels are served prior to admission. Reimbursement to some centers has been cited to be as high as 90% (13). The Diamond Headache Clinic's reimbursement for outpatient services is 100% as a result their set up as a cash-basis center (S. Diamond, personal communication, 1986).

University-based pain centers may have a more difficult time with reimbursement and financial support because of their orientation toward research and sometimes fragmented administrative hierarchy, but they certainly maintain the benefit of high visibility and marketability (14). University-based centers have historically been excellent sources of scientific research on pain and treatment modalities and sources of training for new pain specialists. This is a necessary precursor to the enormous growth of pain centers and a source of increased visibility for the supporting institution. However, by virtue of this orientation to research and training the university-based centers have often relied heavily on federal funding and research grants to support their staff and capital expenditures. This has decreased their emphasis on reimbursement for services and they may not therefore be so financially lucrative as the hospital-based centers or the free-standing centers. Administration is usually a constraining factor for university-based centers because of the preestablished organization of universities. The same holds true of administration in some hospital-based centers.

Private-sector pain centers that operate as free-standing proprietorships experience their greatest difficulty with set-up cost. They have no preexisting capital equipment, space, or staff to organize as hospital-based or university-based centers often do. However, the private-sector pain centers have a much better chance of setting up an effective and unencumbered administrative hierarchy than do other pain centers, and therefore may be set up to run smoothly and to expect a good financial return.

PARAMETERS OF A QUALITY PAIN CENTER

With the growth of pain centers, an intensive effort at quality control necessarily needs to take place. Attempts at defining the parameters of a quality pain center have peppered pain research for the past 20 years. The IASP and APS have also contributed to the quality control process by defining parameters of pain treatment and by encouraging research and continuing study among pain professionals. However, because of several factors, including the youth of chronic pain treatment, the lack of formal governing practices, limited training resources, mismanagement, and lack of outcome research and quality assurance measures, pain centers continue to run the gamut from unidisciplinary to interdisciplinary, from barely effective to extremely effective, from clinically oriented to research oriented, and so on. Because of this diversity in type and quality of services offered, reputable and effective centers have sometimes had difficulty establishing their credibility with the public, the medical community, insurance providers, and the legal community. As conveyed by the literature, most pain specialists have definite and appropriate ideas of what a comprehensive, interdisciplinary pain center should be administratively, academically, economically, and clinically. They do not all have the same ideas, but there are some general parameters that emerge.

Administrative Parameters

1. The pain center should have a pain professional at its helm. The administrator must understand the clinical management of pain so that key decisions are made to benefit not just the organization but the patient and the science of pain management as well. The top administrative position may be held by a physician (specializing, for instance, in neurology or anesthesiology) or by a psychologist who has specialized in behavioral medicine and pain physiology. In some instances this may be a dually-held position with both a physician and a psychologist sharing the top administrative position.
2. The administrator should have a clearly defined position within the sponsoring organization, whether that be a hospital, free-standing proprietorship, or university. This parameter eliminates general confusion in day-to-day decisions of policy and procedure.
3. The center should preferably operate as an independent

entity or as a department unto itself if it is associated with a hospital or university. This circumvents dual roles and dual allegiances of staff.

Academic Parameters

1. Research within the pain center is desirable to further develop pain treatment, and is necessary to demonstrate quality of patient care and treatment outcome.
2. Many centers host residency programs and offer training for pain professionals.
3. Public education should be a priority academic activity of the pain center.
4. Clinical employees should be interested in furthering their knowledge by continued study and should spend the majority of their clinical time in pain treatment.
5. All staff should be trained through academics and experience in the management of chronic pain as a health care specialty.

Economic Parameters

1. The center should strive to contain cost of services so that it remains economically feasible for patients to obtain treatment, whether they are supported by third-party payors or self-supported.
2. The center should establish good relationships with third-party payors. This helps increase reimbursement percentages and makes it more likely that when precertification is needed it will be granted.
3. The center will likely spend some effort marketing services to referral sources, both to increase the number of referrals and to provide education to the referral sources.
4. To expect to market services successfully, the center must be able to demonstrate the effectiveness of their services, usually through quantified outcome research.

Clinical Parameters

The clinical parameters of a good pain center are many and varied, but they emerge clearly from the literature:

1. The center should be interdisciplinary, meaning that professionals from various disciplines should work conjointly in diagnosis, treatment, and follow-up of patients. These professionals should meet to discuss patients and not simply refer patients back and forth. The clinic staff should include specialists from nursing, social work, psychology, physical therapy and vocational rehabilitation in addition to specialty physicians.
2. Prior to treatment, each patient should undergo a thorough medical and psychosocial evaluation that is as objective and quantitative as possible.
3. Treatment for each patient should be individualized and based on diagnosis and the results of an initial clinical evaluation.
4. The primary goal of any pain center should be to assist each patient in regaining maximum physical and psychosocial functioning within the limits imposed by his/her pain.
5. Centers should attempt to reduce the patient's reliance on medication for pain relief.
6. Centers should offer vocational services and, when appropriate, include return to productive employment among their goals for the patient.
7. Centers should work with the family of the patient to increase the chances of generalization of treatment gains.
8. Every center should establish a follow-up program to help ensure maintenance of treatment gains.
9. All centers should stress patient education.
10. Centers should offer pharmacologic, psychotherapeutic, educational, and milieu treatment of the anxiety and depression that accompany the chronic pain syndrome.
11. Centers should offer a structured physical reconditioning program based on graduated physical exercise.
12. Most centers offer both inpatient and outpatient services.
13. Centers should apply the principles of learning (operant, respondent, and classical conditioning) to the modification of the patient's pain behaviors.

So, how do existing pain centers measure up?

THE PRESENT

At the time of the writing of this chapter, the literature contained much more conjecture on what a pain center should be doing than it did actual information on what the average pain center was in actuality doing. For this reason, the author set out to survey a number of pain centers that were thought to be interdisciplinary centers of high quality with good, documented reputations. A 31-question survey was composed (see Appendix 51.A), and 21 pain centers were asked to participate in telephone interviews that would last 35 min, in order to complete the survey. Thirteen centers who were asked agreed to do so. After the surveys were completed, it was determined that one center should be considered a unidisciplinary center and so this one center was eliminated from consideration when the data were compiled. Therefore, the final data cited in the present chapter have been obtained from 12 pain centers, all of whom are considered interdisciplinary centers (see Appendix 51.B). Percentages cited within this chapter are ballpark percentages, because interviewees often did not have actual percentages in front of them during the interview. However, all percentages should have a basis in fact, since the individuals interviewed were either the chief executive officers, directors, or program coordinators for the pain centers.

As an aside, it was somewhat interesting to note the lack of response to the survey by those programs who did not wish to participate. The reason generally cited for unwillingness to participate was lack of time. However, one also got the feeling that there was some territorialism and some reluctance to share "trade secrets" on the part of these centers as well. This is a sad commentary since part of the role of all competent pain centers is to add to public knowledge regarding the treatment of chronic pain.

Let us look at how the interviewed centers measured up against the parameters cited in the literature for effective pain center operation administratively, academically, economically, and clinically. The pain centers interviewed were affiliated variously with public hospitals, private hospitals, and medical schools, or were free-standing proprietorships. Of the total, six were associated with hospitals: three with public hospitals and three with private hospitals. Five were free-standing proprietorships, and only one was associated directly with a university medical school. In reviewing the data, it did not appear that any substantial differences emerged in the day-to-day operations of these centers as a result of their affiliation. Surprisingly, the university-associated pain center did not have any greater emphasis on research and training than did the other centers. As is discussed below, most centers put some degree of emphasis on research and training. Neither did the affiliation of the center readily correlate with the type of professional at the administrative helm of the center.

ADMINISTRATIVE PARAMETERS

Administratively, most programs surveyed were structured so that several professionals shared responsibility for day-to-day operations of the center. In fact, only one program was run by a single individual with no codirector or subdirector. That particular center was administered by a psychiatrist.

On an average, the programs divided executive responsibilities between 2.6 professionals, one of whom usually was a physician. In most centers, a physician was involved either as medical director or as executive director. Among the physicians involved in administration of the centers, the neurologist was found most commonly, in 6 of 12 centers. The neurologist served as CEO or executive director in 3 of the 12 centers. Psychiatrists were seen second most commonly, being involved in the administration of 4 of 12 centers and in the executive position in 2 centers. Family practice specialists were in administrative positions in 3 of 12 centers, but none were in the position of executive director. An orthopedic surgeon was involved in the administration of 1 of 12 centers, and in this case served as executive director. There was also one anesthesiologist and one physiatrist on the administrative staff of the polled centers, with neither of these being in the top executive position.

Psychologists were also well represented in leadership roles within the surveyed centers. Doctoral-level psychologists were involved in the leadership of 50% of the centers. Four of the centers had Ph.D.-level psychologists serving in the executive director position. Two individuals with master's degree training in psychology were also involved in program administration: one as program coordinator and one as director of biofeedback services.

One of the 12 centers had in their top administrative position a Ph.D.-level exercise physiologist. A registered nurse was found on the administrative staff of another center, and a master's level vocational counselor was also found on one administrative staff.

The administrative positions in most of the centers were generally held by professionals from medicine or psychology who were considered algologists (professionals trained in the treatment of chronic pain). Only two of the programs had individuals at their helm whose training was in business administration instead of a medical or psychosocial specialty. One of these individuals served as the chief executive officer, and the other served as program coordinator. In summary, the average program surveyed had 2.6 professionals sharing the administrative directorship of their program. Generally, programs had the combined leadership of a specialty physician along with at least one professional from another medical or psychosocial specialty.

ACADEMIC PARAMETERS

Academically, the centers polled appeared to be meeting at least the first parameter noted above, that research within the pain center is desirable to demonstrate quality of patient care and treatment outcome. As a group, the centers described themselves as clinical facilities that conduct related research. They report spending less than 50% of their time in research activities, but every center polled had at least one staff member conducting research part time. In fact, the average center had four individuals on staff conducting research part time, with actual numbers ranging from one to eight. Only two centers had staff members dedicated to full-time research. Most of the centers reported having at least some treatment outcome studies underway. Additionally, most centers focused on one or two major areas for intensive concentration in applied pain research. Examples of areas of research commonly cited include psychopharmacology in pain treatment, pain and depression, biofeedback, and ergonomics. Generally, the research appeared to be directed toward determining outcome and quality of care for the patient and toward determining the usefulness of specific modalities in the future.

It is vital that currently existing interdisciplinary pain centers offer training for other professionals interested in offering treatment to the pain patient. The centers polled seemed to be fulfilling this training role quite admirably. Every center polled offered at least informal training rotations for at least one professional specialty. As a whole, formal or informal training opportunities were available at over 50% of the centers for medical students, nursing students, medical residents, and psychology students. Five of the 12 centers offered a physical therapy rotation. Other training opportunities available included formal rotations in social work, occupational therapy, biofeedback, vocational rehabilitation, exercise physiology, chaplaincy, psychiatry, and a fellowship for physicians. Certainly if other interdisciplinary centers are offering as many training opportunities as the 12 centers who were polled, then we are adequately fulfilling our need to train future professionals.

The professional specialities of pain center employees were even more varied than the training opportunities available at these centers. As already noted in the section on administrative parameters above, most of the centers polled had at least one physician and many times more than one physician on staff. In fact 83% of the programs polled have at least one full-time physician on staff. Almost every center noted that it had available by consultation physicians from most appropriate specialities. Aside from those available on a consultative basis, no centers had any neurosurgeons, dentists, oral surgeons, or rheumatologists on their full-time staff. One center did have an orthopedic surgeon on its part-time staff. As already noted in the administrative section, the most common physician as a full-time staff member was the neurologist. Second to that was the family practice specialist, followed by psychiatry, physiatry, internal medicine, and anesthesiology.

In addition to the physician, all of the centers complemented their staff with professionals from various disciplines. Every center polled had on staff at least one part-time psychologist at the Ph.D. level. The average center employed 2.2 full-time psychologists and 0.5 part-time psychologists. Additionally, every center employed at least one part-time physical therapist. The average center employed 1.75 full-time physical therapists and 0.75 part-time physical therapists. Ten of 12 centers employed professional nurses, with the average center employing 4.75 full-time nurses and 0.50 part-time nurses. Eight centers employed at least a part-time vocational rehabilitation professional. Seven centers utilized technicians for biofeedback labs and relaxation instruction. Six centers employed occupational therapists at least part time, and six centers employed at least one part-time social worker. There were also other professional specialists employed by less than 50% of all centers. These specialists included pharmacists, dieticians, counselors, physician assistants, chaplains, music therapists, acupressurists, and exercise physiologists.

ECONOMIC PARAMETERS

Economically, one concern identified in the literature was that pain centers should strive to contain the cost of services to preserve the economic feasibility of treatment for patients, whether they are supported by third-party payors or self-supported. The cost of services among the programs polled would appear to be tied to program type (whether inpatient or outpatient), to program duration, and also perhaps to the utilization of available inpatient beds.

Type of Services

Among the centers polled, the percentage of clinical services that were provided on an inpatient basis varied from 0 to 100%. In the average center, 41% of the services provided were inpatient and 59% were outpatient. The free-standing proprietorships offered the least inpatient treatment. Three of the five free-standing centers offered no inpatient treatment and the remaining two provided 15% of their services on an inpatient basis. This makes sense in terms of the prohibitive additional cost involved in setting up a facility for inpatient services. Only one center among the 12 offered no outpatient services. This center is quite unusual considering the current pressure from insurance companies to decrease cost by increasing the percentage of services rendered on an outpatient basis. This center was associated with a private hospital.

Where inpatient programs were concerned, utilization of bed space was quite variable, ranging from near 0 to 100%. The average inpatient program had 16 beds available for occupancy, with a range from 6 to 35 beds. The average census among the programs with inpatient services was 12. This calculates to a 75% utilization of available inpatient beds. This increases to 84% utilization if the one program with 6 beds who stated that they rarely admit inpatients and would prefer to treat their patients on an outpatient basis is omitted.

Program Duration and Cost

The duration of the inpatient programs ranged from 10 to 26 days, with the average program having a duration of 19 days. The cost of the programs was also quite variable, generally paralleling the length of the program. The cost of the inpatient services ranged from a low of $4000 for a 10-day program up to $16,000 for a 26-day program. The average cost across all inpatient programs was $8500.

Among outpatient programs, duration of treatment and cost of services were somewhat difficult to calculate, because many outpatient programs are variable in length within each center. This makes it difficult to give accurate statistics on what is currently being offered in outpatient treatment. The notable lack of definitive treatment duration from center to center is a positive factor if it reflects individualization of treatment, but it is a negative factor if it reflects the lack of basic structure among outpatient treatment programs. The average duration, for those programs who had definitive lengths of treatment, was 16 days. This is 85% of the average treatment duration of inpatient programs. The average cost among outpatient programs is $3452, which is only 40% of inpatient program cost. Simple statistics may lead insurance providers and others to recommend outpatient treatment when possible, especially if other factors (e.g., the need to maintain reinforcement and medication procedures 24 hr/day; dependability of the patient for attending the pain center every day) are held constant or are subtly disregarded.

Reimbursement

From an economic perspective, the charges for services rendered do not alone determine the profitability of any center. Relationships between the center and third-party payors often determine reimbursement percentages. There is no better example of this than that of one interviewee who said that the center for which he was administrator was soon to change medical directors because of the current medical director's poor relationship to third-party payors. Their reimbursement percentages had been so low as a result of this poor relationship that they could not economically continue to exist in their present pattern. Another factor, of course, in determining reimbursement percentages is who the third-party payor is. Medicaid generally has a low reimbursement rate and, consequently, centers who treat many Medicaid patients have lower reimbursement rates. Private insurance also sometimes requires precertification, and if this precertification is not done then reimbursement rates for private insurance carriers can be low also.

The centers who were surveyed were asked to estimate the percentage of their patients funded by various payors. An overwhelming average of 41% of all patients were reported to be funded by Workers' Compensation insurance. Second in line were patients funded by standard insurance, which accounted for 33.5% of all patients. Personal injury compensation was the funding source for an estimated 9.5% of all patients, and 8% were funded under Medicaid and 3% under Medicare. Three per cent were funded by personal finances, and the remaining 2% of patients were funded by grants or research funds.

Each center was also asked to estimate the percentage of the fees for their services that are collected. Two of the 12 centers did not divulge this information. Of the remaining 10 centers, the collection rate ranged from 63 to 95%, with the average for the centers as a whole being 86%. One center reported 100% collection for outpatient services, because it was set up on a cash-only basis for outpatient services. The collection rate for this center's inpatient services was only 85%, however, so that the center's overall collection rate was 92.5%. Other centers did not subdivide their collection rates between inpatient and outpatient programs. The center with the 63% collection rate noted two reasons for this lower rate of return on services rendered. The first, as noted above, was the relationship of the center's medical director to third-party providers. The second reason cited for the low rate of return was the high volume of Medicare and Medicaid patients whom the center treats. Three centers noted a 95% collection rate. Considering all the possible hurdles to full collection on any service rendered, this 95% seems to be a quite phenomenal overall rate. There may be any number of reasons for this economic success, but those reasons certainly include attention to precertification requirements, relationships with insurance providers, treatment of a high percentage of Worker's Compensation patients, and definitive outcome research to demonstrate to third-party payors that treatment is worth the costs involved.

Marketing

Marketing to increase referral sources is also an economically important activity of pain centers. Overwhelmingly, it would appear that most of this marketing has been targeted toward physicians, because an estimated 72% of all patients were referred to the 12 centers by physicians. The second largest referral source, with 10% of patients, was Worker's Compensation. Coming in third with 7% were insurance companies and rehabilitation personnel. Four and one-half per cent of patients were reportedly referred by other patients or by word of mouth. Four per cent were referred by attorneys, and the remaining 2.5% were referred by other health agencies, which included mental health centers, private medical centers, the National Institutes of Health, and state agencies.

CLINICAL PARAMETERS

The information on clinical services that emerged from the current survey indicated that most of the centers polled are answering satisfactorily the concerns that have been addressed in the literature. All 12 of the centers specialize in treating chronic pain patients, and 2 of the centers additionally treat acute pain patients. Eight of the centers do not limit their treatment to pain of any specific origin or physical location. Two of the centers stated that they treat primarily spinal pain, and two of the centers stated that they treat primarily headache pain.

Concerning the clinical services offered, each center was asked to determine whether their services are behavioral and rehabilitation oriented, diagnostic and biologically oriented, or a mixture of both. An overwhelming majority (83%) stated that at least 50% of their emphasis is on behavioral treatment and rehabilitative services. Two centers said their total emphasis is on behavioral and rehabilitative treatment, and six centers said they also offer limited diagnostic or biological components in their treatment. Two centers said their treatment is divided equally between behavioral/rehabilitative services and diagnostic/biologic services. The only two centers whose primary treatment orientation was described as biologic and diagnostic were the two centers in the survey who specialize in headache treatment.

Pretreatment Evaluations

The clinical literature has emphasized the importance of pretreatment medical and psychosocial evaluations so that treatment for each patient can be individualized and made appropriate for the patient based on his/her diagnosis and the results of the initial clinical evaluation. As part of the survey, each center was asked to review with the interviewer the pretreatment evaluation process that they complete with the average inpatient and with the average outpatient at their center. The results of the survey would indicate that there are some discrepancies between the pretreatment evaluations given to inpatients and those given to outpatients.

The first segment of the pretreatment evaluation inquired about was the interview. It appears that if a patient walked into the average pain center for a pretreatment evaluation, the patient would be interviewed by a psychologist and a nurse and then the patient's family would also be interviewed, if the patient was to be treated on an inpatient basis. The typical outpatient would be interviewed only by a psychologist. Of the nine programs that offer inpatient services, seven of them include nursing interviews in their pretreatment evaluation, six include psychology interviews, five include an interview of the family, four include an interview by vocational rehabilitation, two include interviews by a social worker, and only one includes a psychiatric interview. Of the 11 centers who offer outpatient programs, 9 stated that outpatients would be interviewed by a psychologist prior to treatment, 5 would include a nursing interview, 4 would include a vocational rehabilitation interview, and 1 would include an interview by a social worker and by a psychiatrist, and would interview the family.

The next segment of the pretreatment evaluation inquired about was psychological testing. The Minnesota Multiphasic Personality Inventory (MMPI) continues to be the most popular psychometric evaluation for chronic pain patients, but it is used by only 56% of the centers polled prior to treatment with inpatients and by only 45% of the centers prior to outpatient treatment. No other psychometric tool came close to the MMPI in frequency of use. The McGill Pain Questionnaire ranked second, with two of the nine possible centers using this instrument as part of the pretreatment evaluation for inpatients. The Symptoms Checklist-90 (SCL-90) ranked third, with 2 of 11 centers using this scale prior to treatment of outpatients. A variety of other scales are used by single centers, including the Health Locus of Control Scale, the Beck Depression Scale, the Stress Audit, and the Psychosocial Adjustment to Illness Scale (PAIS). The statistics may indicate that either (a) there are no psychological tests that can effectively help determine the appropriateness of treatment for the chronic pain patient, or (b) very few centers are using the available psychometric assistance for determing treatment appropriateness.

The third segment of the pretreatment evaluation inquired about was the physician's examination. All but one center has a physician evaluate the majority of their inpatients prior to treatment. All but one center (not the same one) has a physician evaluate the majority of their outpatients prior to treatment. The physician is usually the staff physician for the center, and neurologists top this list.

Physical therapy evaluations are quite common as part of the pretreatment evaluation. Seven of 9 centers use physical therapy evaluations prior to treatment for their inpatients, and 7 of 11 centers include the physical therapy evaluations prior to treatment for outpatients.

Medical diagnostic testing is much less commonly used as part of a pretreatment evaluation. Most of the centers reported that they review records of diagnostic tests that are expected to be performed prior to treatment at the pain center. This is consistent with the orientation of the majority of centers toward behavioral and rehabilitative treatment. Among the centers who order their own diagnostics, the most popular diagnostic tests for pretreatment analysis are computed tomography scans (used by 3 of 12 centers), temporomandibular joint screening for headache sufferers (used by 5 of 12 centers), and lab work (urine and blood studies) (used by 2 of 12 centers). None of the centers reported routine use of myelograms or nuclear magnetic resonance imaging, and only one center uses thermography or a spinal capacity evaluation routinely. This may be related to economics as much as to other factors, since most of these procedures require very expensive equipment that may not be available routinely to the center.

Treatment Modalities

Once the pretreatment evaluation is complete, goals for the patient are set and treatment is begun. The clinical literature emphasizes that treatment for each patient should be individualized and should have as a primary goal assisting the patient in regaining maximum physical and psychosocial functioning within the limits imposed by his/her pain. A survey such as the present one cannot determine to what extent each program individualizes each patient's treatment, but certainly each of the programs surveyed offers substantial varieties of treatment so that they are able to individualize each patient's treatment if they choose to do so. Centers participating in the survey were asked to determine what approximate percentage of their inpatients and what approximate percentage of their outpatients receive each of 28 modalities available to the pain treatment center. It appears that most centers use a combination of pharmacologic, physical, psychotherapeutic, milieu, educational, and vocational modalities. Consistent with the orientation of most of these centers to rehabilitative and behavioral treatment, only one center stated that they perform any type of surgery. This was a center that specializes in treating headache patients and the specific type of surgery offered was occipital neurectomy. This surgery was reported as being used with only 2% of the center's patients. One other center reported that they refer out less than 1% of their patients for surgery. None of the centers reported performing any chymopapain injections, rhizotomies, chordotomies, diskectomies, temporomandibular joint replacements, or any other type of surgery.

The modality used most frequently by the centers surveyed is education. One hundred per cent of centers surveyed use patient education as a modality with an average of 94.2% of their patients. There was no difference in the frequency of use of patient education between inpatients and outpatients.

The second most frequently used modality among all 12 centers surveyed is physical exercise. One hundred per cent of the centers use physical exercise as a modality with an average of 86.8% of their patients. The frequency of use of exercise as a modality varied only 5% between inpatients and outpatients.

Medications comprised the third most popular modality. Antidepressants were reported as being used by 100% of participating centers. An average 51% of inpatients and 44% of outpatients receive antidepressant medications. Other pharmacologic therapies are not so readily used by the centers in the survey. Five centers use narcotic pain medications with just under 11% of inpatients and slightly less than 1% of outpatients. Eight centers use nonnarcotic pain medications with an average 21% of inpatients and 10% of outpatients. Benzodiazepines are reportedly used by seven of the centers but only with 5.3% of their patients. Phenothiazines are used by 8 of 12 centers, but only with 8.8% of their patients. Benzodiazepines and phenothiazines were often reported as being used to decrease nausea or to help with drug detoxification regimens.

Eleven of the centers surveyed reported using some form of drug detoxification or drug withdrawal with 50% of their patients overall. Of inpatients, 59.9% are put on some detoxification regimen; 42% of outpatients are detoxified. Most of the centers attempt to reduce the patient's reliance on medication for pain relief.

Concerning pharmacologic treatment, one center that specializes in treatment of headache patients reported that they use preventive pharmacotherapy (e.g., calcium channel blockers, beta blockers, and anti-inflammatories) with 8% of their patients.

Of the physical modalities, that is, those treatments designed primarily to alter musculoskeletal sources of pain or to interrupt pain pathways, exercise of course is the most commonly used. Second only to exercise among the physical modalities is training in progressive muscle relaxation. One hundred per cent of the centers surveyed train approximately 78.1% of their patients overall in progressive muscle relaxation.

Next on the hit parade of physical modalities is biofeedback, a modality used by 100% of the centers with approximately 59% of their inpatients and 33% of their outpatients. Physical therapy modalities such as electrical stimulation, heat, and ultrasound are used by 11 of the centers surveyed with a reported 32.5% of their patients. Several centers reported using physical therapy modalities only as a precursor to exercise. Transcutaneous electrical nerve stimulation (TENS) is a physical modality used by 11 of the 12 centers, but this modality is only used with an average 24% of all patients.

Among other physical modalities are some that seem to be less popular. Ice massage is reportedly used by eight of the centers surveyed, but with only 20% of their patients. Similarly, acupressure is used by eight of the centers with only 19.3% of all patients. Five of the 12 centers report administering nerve blocks to approximately 10% of their patients overall. Ten years ago, nerve blocks were almost the only nonsurgical modality used in pain clinics (15). The least popular of the physical modalities listed in the survey was acupuncture, used by only two centers. One of these, which only treats outpatients, uses acupuncture with 33% of the outpatients it treats. The other center, which treats both inpatients and outpatients, uses acupuncture with less than 1% of its inpatients and with less than 2% of its outpatients.

Of the psychological or psychotherapeutic modalities used, group psychotherapy is the most common, with 100% of the centers utilizing group therapy with approximately 69.3% of their patients. The distribution in use of group therapy between inpatients and outpatients, however, was quite disparate. Among inpatients, 92.8% reportedly receive group therapy, whereas 50.1% of outpatients receive group therapy. Second most popular among psychological therapies was individual psychotherapy. One hundred per cent of centers stated that they offer individual psychotherapy to 60.2% of their patients, with a breakdown of 72.2% of inpatients receiving individual psychotherapy while only 51.0% of outpatients are recipients. It is notable regarding the group and individual psychotherapies that one center reported individual psychotherapy being conducted by nurses and group psychotherapy being conducted by "various trained staff." Eleven centers stated that they use some form of behavior modification or behavior therapy with 78% of their patients overall. The distribution with inpatients and outpatients was not significant here. Eleven centers also reported offering some form of family therapy or family education designed to enhance the maintenance of treatment gains upon return home. Interestingly, 80.6% of inpatients receive some form of family therapy whereas only 50.9% of outpatients receive family therapy. Hypnosis is reportedly used by half of the centers surveyed, but not commonly. Overall, 13.4% of patients receive hypnosis. Least popular among the psychotherapeutic interventions listed in the survey were home visits by social work or psychology staff. Only 1 center out of the 12 offers home vists, and this is with less than 15% of inpatients and outpatients.

Vocational rehabilitation is also commonly offered, being an alternative treatment in 11 of the centers. However, only an average of 37.5% of all patients receive any intervention by vocational rehabilitation. It would be nice to think that only 37.5% of all chronic pain patients experience vocational difficulties as part of their chronic pain syndrome, but this of course is not the case. One center offers no vocational rehabilitation services, stating that most of the patients treated at that center are from out of state and would be referred back to Vocational Rehabilitation in their home state.

Recreational therapy is used fairly commonly by eight of the centers. The division between inpatients and outpatients was significant here, with 67.8% of inpatients and 28.6% of outpatients receiving recreational therapy.

The sparsely used therapies included occupational therapy, used by two centers with 15% of patients overall; swimming, used by one center with 10% of patients overall; and music therapy, also used by only one center with 5% of patients overall.

Goal Setting and Outcome

An important part of treatment with every patient is goal setting. Goals should be established prior to treatment, monitored throughout treatment, and evaluated after treatment. All of the 12 centers surveyed appeared to have appropriate and sufficiently varied goals for their patients. All 12 of the centers have as goals for their patients return to work (when appropriate), elimination of pain medication, increase in strength and stamina, and decreased utilization of unnecessary health care. Ten programs have as one of their goals decreased pain intensity, and nine of the programs have as a goal elimination of other medications. The medications generally targeted for elimination included sedating and dependency-producing medications. Specifically cited for elimination were benzodiazepines, phenothiazines, hypnotics, barbiturates, anxiolytics, and alcohol. Additionally, five centers listed improved mood or decreased depression as one of their major goals for patients. Other goals variously cited by centers included improved quality of overall life, smoking cessation, transfer of pain management skills to home, resolution of social issues such as legal suits, improved interpersonal skills, decreased pain behaviors, and improvement in structural abnormalities such as gait and posture.

Most of the centers stated that they keep statistics on the percentage of patients achieving each of the preset goals. Of the goals discussed above, it would appear that return to work is the most difficult goal for the centers to accomplish with their patients. The 12 centers on an average stated that 61.2% of their patients for whom this is a goal actually return to work when treatment is completed. Second most difficult to accomplish was a decrease in the patients' reported pain. Within the centers who kept statistics on decrease in pain reports, it appears that 72.1% of patients reported some decrease in their pain. The data concerning decreased utilization of health care are likely flawed, since utilization will often change between time of discharge and later follow-up. However, among the centers who kept such statistics, 86% of their patients did decrease their utilization of unnecessary health care. Of the patients monitored, 90.8% were reported to have experienced decreased depression as a result of treatment at a pain center. Elimination of pain medication was reportedly achieved by 91.2% of patients treated by the 12 centers. This statistic, too, may vary depending upon when the measure is taken (directly after treatment or at follow-up). The same percentage of patients, 91.2%, were stated to have increased their strength and stamina during treatment at a pain center. Elimination of other medications, when this was a goal, was reportedly achieved by 92.5% of targeted patients. The highest achievement rate was in improved quality of life. For the few centers who monitored this, 96% of patients reported that their quality of life was improved after treatment. This goal, however, is fairly nonspecific and may reflect many of the other measures noted above.

Quality assurance programs generally require pain centers to collect statistics on goal achievement as a measure of treatment effectiveness. In addition to serving as a quality assurance measure, the goal achievement data may be used as a marketing tool for referral sources and third-party payors. Eleven of the 12 programs surveyed have a quality assurance program, either self-administered or administered by the hospital where the center is located.

Impairment Ratings

In addition to goal achievement, another end product of treatment is sometimes a statement of the patient's limitations or an impairment rating. Formal statements of physical limitations are given to a majority of patients by 9 of 12 centers. This statement is sometimes associated with a physical capacities evaluation or with a work hardening type of program where simulated job requirements have been rehearsed. Additionally, this statement of limitations is sometimes requested by referral sources, by employers, or by rehabilitation counselors. Six of the 12 centers surveyed offer impairment ratings. This service is most often provided only when requested by physicians, rehabilitation counselors, or insurance personnel, and is not done routinely.

Follow-up

Follow-up is a part of treatment that takes place after the patient has completed the core program. The literature repeatedly emphasizes the necessity of establishing a follow-up program to help ensure maintenance of treatment gains. This maintenance of treatment gains appears in many cases to be the most difficult part of treatment, and is why not only follow-up but family education is so important. All but one center polled offers a follow-up program. The nature of the follow-up programs offered is quite variable, with most programs offering in-person follow-up and the others offering follow-up by mail or by phone. Time limits on follow-up are also quite variable.

Follow-up programs for *inpatients* are conducted in person except by one center. This center reported that most of its patients are from out of state, and stated that their follow-up is by letter only, at 3 months, 1 year, 2 years, and 3 years. This is quite different from the other programs, whose in-person follow-ups range from a time period of 8 weeks to more than 1 year. Most of the programs also have phone contact with patients that supplements the in-person visits. Where *outpatients* are concerned, two programs have either "variable" or phone-only contact for follow-ups, and the other programs have in-person contact, which again varies from 8 weeks to more than 1 year. Several of the programs have different follow-up regimens for inpatients and outpatients, usually requiring more frequent visits for a longer time from their inpatients.

SUMMARY

Administratively, academically, economically, and clinically, the 12 pain centers who were surveyed seemed to measure up quite well to the expectations presented within the literature on pain management. Each of the centers has strong points and weak points, but none of them emerges as being clearly superior or inferior overall. Each seems to have developed a fairly individualized program while keeping the standard expectations of quality pain management intact. The final question asked in the survey of each of the 12 centers was, "If you could influence the growth of pain centers in the next five years, what would you encourage your pain center and other centers to improve upon, move toward, or change?" Each center responded with very appropriate and also adamant answers, some of which were directed toward perceived weaknesses in other programs and some of which were directed toward aspirations within their own program. Taken as a whole, many of the suggestions for changes in the future of pain management address the few weaknesses that have been discussed thus far in this chapter.

THE FUTURE

Certainly, pain management and pain centers are not going to become stagnant in the next 5 years. They are still very young, and in some senses immature; although the changes in the next 5 years may not be as radical as those of the past 10 years, there are certain areas that show potential for future change. Let us take a look at some of the changes suggested by survey participants that may occur in the next 5 years.

ADMINISTRATIVE PARAMETERS

Improved quality control was the major administrative concern expressed by the persons interviewed for this chapter. The most frequently suggested change was for pain centers to develop more standardized and consistent care, and to have this care documented, before the centers are permitted to operate as accredited pain programs. In particular, the suggestion was made by several participants that CARF accreditation should be much more widespread among pain centers. It was even suggested that CARF accreditation be a required credential for facilities to call themselves pain centers. It was also suggested that pain centers should make sure that the product that they advertise is delivered. For instance, if a center is a unidisciplinary biofeedback clinic it should advertise itself as such, or, if the center is an interdisciplinary symptom management program, it should advertise itself as such.

From the administrative perspective, the second most frequently cited area of needed change was in the nature of individual clinics. It was stated several times that the number of interdisciplinary pain centers should be increased while unidisciplinary clinics should be decreased or eliminated. It was also suggested that multidisciplinary clinics should strive to become interdisciplinary to improve effectiveness of treatment.

Although several of the participants suggested that the pain center should offer a better variety of treatment modalities (in terms of being more interdisciplinary), one participant suggested that pain centers should increase their emphasis on specialization. This suggestion was not intended to limit the modalities used within each center, but to encourage centers to specialize in pain of a particular origin or physical location. For instance, it was suggested that centers should strive to treat only headaches, or musculoskeletal pain, or sports injury, or cancer, and so forth. On a personal note, the author believes that it might be counterproductive to limit the types of pain treated by each center, but we again come back to the above suggestion that the product that is delivered should be the product that is advertised. If a clinic does not have expertise in a particular type of pain, it should not advertise itself as being qualified to treat that type of pain. Accreditation by an organization such as CARF would certainly improve the quality control among pain centers as well as establish definitive guidelines for which facilities may call themselves a pain center.

ACADEMIC PARAMETERS

There was more concern among the centers polled over the academic future of pain centers than over their administrative futures. Most centers would agree that education of the public, of pain management professionals, of other health care providers, of insurance carriers, and of the legal professionals involved in the rehabilitation of pain patients is the key to better overall disability management. Pain management professionals need to be educated about the roles and the goals of the coplayers in the lives of their pain patients, such as other physicians, insurance carriers, and attorneys. This knowledge on the part of the pain management professional can help to decrease the mixed messages about rehabilitation given to the patient, and can improve the chance of rehabilitation overall if all parties work toward the same end or at least agree not to undo each others' treatment. The flip side of this is also true. It was stated emphatically by several centers that there is a need to increase their impact on the third-party payors and other health care providers so that patients are referred to pain centers sooner and avoid getting inappropriate analgesics and unnecessary treatments while being shuffled from one medical specialist to another. Pain centers can effectively increase their impact on these third parties through education, outcome research, and marketing.

In particular, education of physicians as to recognition of and appropriate treatment of the chronic pain syndrome should continue to be a primary objective of pain centers. This need is supported by several factors:

1. Chronic pain patients are frequently noted to have their pain increased by iatrogenic complications (16).

2. Patients with pain of less than 3 years' duration and work time loss of less than 1 year have significantly better outcomes in pain center treatment (17).
3. Patients with zero or one operation for pain have better treatment outcomes than those with three or more operations for pain (17).
4. Drug dependence is associated with poor prognosis in pain center treatment, and the frequency of drug dependency increases with increasing duration of disability (17).

In addition to educating physicians, pain centers should direct their efforts toward educating the public about the availability of pain center treatment and also about what a pain center does. Most of the public and also many medical specialists continue to be unaware of the existence of quality rehabilitative treatment for chronic pain. Some of the public who have read accounts of pain treatment in such periodicals as *Newsweek* and *Parade* may be aware that some rehabilitative treatments exist but are not aware that they exist close enough to home to be easily utilized. Although not widely advertised, the CARF has available a list of the 63 pain programs that they have accredited for either inpatient or outpatient treatment, and will mail this list free of charge to interested parties (see Appendix 51.C for CARF's address). The American Academy of Pain Medicine, in conjunction with the APS, is also currently compiling a list of pain centers for a Pain Clinic Registry (see Appendix 51.C for the Academy's address).

Also adamantly stated as a future educational need for pain management centers is improved outcome research and quality assurance–type research. It is well accepted that treatment, if it is to be effective, should be outcome oriented. This requires that centers be able to document the effectiveness of the individual modalities as well as the combination of modalities that they offer to their patients. Traditionally, this has been done in a less than systematic way across pain centers. There is a need for better defined outcome measures to allow increased understanding between pain centers of the effectiveness of various modalities and treatment approaches. There is also a need for increased sharing among programs of their outcome research. An appropriate forum for these issues may be the clinically oriented pain management journals such as the new *Journal of Pain Management* or the IASP journal, *Pain*.

In addition to documentation regarding immediate treatment outcome, there is a recognized need for increased documentation of long-term clinical effectiveness. This is important not only in regard to the value of treatment, but as a marketing tool directed toward third-party payors and referral sources. Without documentation of long-term clinical effectiveness, it is extremely difficult to demonstrate cost-effectiveness of the pain center concept.

Regarding the need for documentation of treatment effectiveness, it is noted from the survey results that, across modalities, there was often a difference between the frequency of the use of particular modalities with inpatients and outpatients. Take, for example, group therapy, which was shown in the survey to be offered to 92.8% of inpatients while it was offered to only 50.1% of outpatients. Is this treatment difference due to differences in the patients being treated on inpatient and outpatient bases? If so, then there should be some documentation regarding the noted differences in patients and the treatment parameters that are affected. There are many areas in which clinical documentation is either lacking or is so specific to a particular center that it cannot be used for comparison by other centers.

Research should also continue on patient selection criteria to determine which patients respond best to which treatment. Patients should be selected for treatment based on the likelihood that the pain center can help them. However, patient selection criteria should not be so stringent as to eliminate patients who can get partial benefit from the center, even though such patients may lower the center's statistics on treatment success (18).

It was also suggested by the survey participants that research should continue toward the understanding of the physiologic and behavioral management of pain. Specifically cited was the importance of brain mechanisms to understanding the physiologic and behavioral aspects of pain. Research on endorphins is a particular area that may prove to be pivotal in advancing both our understanding and treatment of pain. Such controversial procedures as subcortical electrical stimulation have also been shown by some centers to have positive effects on pain of both peripheral and central origins (19). In addition to these areas, which are extremely difficult to research, there is ample opportunity to expand our technology in less difficult areas. For instance, an immediate need is for a more accurate means of measuring physical capacities.

All of these areas of potential development in pain treatment will be achieved much more quickly if pain center staff professionals make the effort to join and participate in the scientific organizations that study pain. The purpose of joining these organizations, of course, would be to continue to educate themselves and also to share information with other professionals and to promote the science of pain management as a whole. Among the organizations that have been established for this purpose are the IASP, the APS, the American Academy of Pain Medicine, and the American Society of Anesthesiologists (see Appendix 51.C for addresses).

ECONOMIC PARAMETERS

Several of the centers polled were concerned about one particular economic parameter of pain center operation, that of cost containment. Cost containment will be necessary on a long-term basis if third-party payors are going to continue to reimburse the pain center for services rendered. Costs must be contained if pain centers are to remain competitive with the standard procedure of medical intervention by one professional at a time. Survey participants suggested that cost containment may be achieved by decreasing the use of "routine" diagnostic testing and by decreasing the overutilization of testing for economic gain. As demonstrated by the survey above, it is also possible to contain cost by increasing the use, when appropriate, of outpatient services.

Closely related to general cost containment is the need for increased documentation of the cost-effectiveness of pain center treatment. As yet, there has been very little demonstration statistically of the cost-effectiveness of the pain center concept despite the fact that many writers have referred to the same. In statistical documentation, it would be quite important to relate the cost-effectiveness of pain center treatment to long-term clinical effectiveness and to the decreased length of disability that is often seen with pain center intervention. A massive investment in research now to demonstrate the cost-effectiveness of pain center treatment would certainly work to our financial advantage in the future because of the potential for increasing both referrals and reimbursement rates.

CLINICAL PARAMETERS

There were numerous comments from the persons interviewed regarding the directions in which clinical treatment needs to progress in the coming 5 years. The overall assessment was that clinical treatment should be: (a) better defined, (b) criteria based, (c) individualized, and (d) outcome oriented. In terms of being better defined, it was suggested that medical workups and biologic treatments should be completed prior to a patient's being treated for a chronic pain syndrome. This was suggested as a way to decrease the proverbial mixed message that patients are sometimes given when told that they have a chronic pain syndrome but when various medical treatments are continued in hopes of eliminating their pain. Treatment should be defined in terms of medical intervention for physical abnormalities versus rehabilitation and psychosocial intervention for chronic pain and associated psychosocial abnormalities. Still other individuals in the survey suggested that the biologic and psychological treatments offered within individual clinics should be balanced and used concurrently.

Nearly half of the persons interviewed made some reference to the need to increase the individualization of treatment. Variously, the participants suggested that there should be increased emphasis placed on getting patients off of medication; on increasing the activity level of patients; on cognitive variables such as the patient's perceptions, beliefs, and expectations about their pain; on family involvement; and on vocational evaluation as a part of consideration in treatment planning. Each of these suggestions should be taken seriously, because each of them are vital parts of an interdisciplinary pain treatment program. One does not need to consider which of the suggestions is correct because all of them are. One participant summed it up fairly well by saying that each patient is a person and not just an embodiment of a chronic pain syndrome. Therefore, for each patient, there may need to be increased emphasis on any of a variety of areas of treatment.

Where particular modalities are concerned, one area that is beginning to get attention, but that in the past has been too often ignored, is the area of vocational evaluation and work hardening. The survey conducted for this chapter revealed that only 37.5% of the patients in the centers polled were receiving vocational therapy services. Yet the literature has been very clear in stating the advantage in decreased rehabilitation time for patients who are returned to work. Many chronic pain patients are in need of vocational services. Not all of them can be expected to return to work because of their age or physical limitations, but many of them with appropriate evaluation, vocational counseling, and work hardening can return to a more productive life-style, to include some type of paid employment. One factor that seems to inhibit speedy return to a productive life-style is the patients' frequent involvement in the Worker's Compensation system. Patients who are involved in the worker's compensation system of any state should receive education about the legal parameters of that system. That is, they should know what they are entitled to under the Worker's Compensation law and also what the limits of the system are (11, 12). This education about the Worker's Compensation system should serve two purposes: (a) to alleviate the anxiety that comes with being involved in a legal matter that one does not understand and (b) to decrease the negative effects of compensation issues on treatment outcome (15).

Clinical services may expand dramatically in the future based on the results of the research that is discussed above. There is room in the young field of pain management for extensive and innovative additions to current treatment regimens. Potential areas of exploration may include nutrition therapies, experimental nonnarcotic medications, or the area of bradykinins and endorphins.

It is frequently and importantly stated that all clinical treatment should be outcome oriented and based on the documented usefulness of a particular set of modalities. In addition to documenting the success or failure of particular modalities, it is important that we remember to provide adequate follow-up management for our patients. Without appropriate continuity of care, treatment gains are not likely to generalize or to be maintained. So without adequate follow-up, the original success of any particular treatment modality may be negated. It was suggested by many of the participants that more personal contact either by phone or in person with clinic staff is needed after discharge for each patient.

Not only is it important that the patient have contact with pain management professionals after treatment, but the patient should also be supported in his/her own environment by supportive family members. For outcome to be lasting and positive, family education and/or family therapy should be considered a primary treatment modality. If no family is avilable to participate in the patient's treatment, perhaps a close friend would be a good substitute. No patient should complete pain treatment without one-to-one support from someone other than a center staff member. In some cases it may even be helpful to establish support circles among patients who have been in treatment together.

CONCLUDING COMMENTS

The future of pain management centers not only lies in improving already available services, establishing documentation of treatment success, marketing referral sources, or establishing accreditation criteria for chronic pain treatment. The future of pain centers may also lie in extending our present knowledge to provide primary prevention services for potential victims of chronic pain syndromes. In the survey conducted for this chapter it was noted that two of the centers that were polled stated that, in addition to treating chronic pain patients, they also treat acute pain patients. This may be a quite appropriate avenue of expansion for pain centers, not only because the modalities in use are also effective with acute pain patients, but because early intervention can reduce the rehabilitation time for acute pain patients as well. Even in 1974, Shealy (16) recognized that patients with acute pain, especially back and neck pain, might beneficially be treated in an interdisciplinary setting much like chronic pain patients. He found this was true especially if the acute pain patients were treated prior to their first surgery. By his count, 60% of the chronic pain patients whom he saw had increased levels of pain due to iatrogenic sources, particularly failed surgery.

It has taken many years for the basic concept of the interdisciplinary pain center to become reasonably well accepted among medical professionals, third-party payors, scholars, attorneys, and patients. Yet pain centers are miles ahead of where they were in the late 1960s and early 1970s when only a handful of centers existed and only a handful of professionals in medicine could even define the chronic pain syndrome. The pain center is still somewhat imperfect, but it is no longer just an accumulation of ideas and experiments. It has at least become an accepted part of available medical services for patients who suffer from chronic pain. As scientists, the energy to improve services to patients and to expand the pain knowledge base should be fueled by the errors and by the flaws that are pointed out in examination of one's own and others' work. It is very important for the future of pain management that pain professionals not act in a territorial manner, try to outdo each other, and see who can be "the best." Instead of one-upmanship the pain professional must practice cooperation and unite efforts at research and at treatment if the current weaknesses within pain centers are to be addressed appropriately. The suggestions made by the participants in the survey conducted for this chapter are appropriate beginning guidelines to address weaknesses in the field. It is especially important that as the volume of outcome research increases, the knowledge gained is used to tailor our treatments. It is always very tempting to hang onto the old way of doing things just because it has worked before and to be somewhat reluctant to explore the advantages of change. The pain center concept is much too young to be approached narrow-mindedly. If the 10 or 15 years that have just passed are any indication of what there is to come, there should be many changes, many surprises, and much innovation and fine tuning in the 5 years to come. Pain centers are at a pivotal point in acceptance by the medical community and by many other individuals who come into contact with pain patients. It is important that the pain center not become complacent with its responsibility.

References

1. Bonica JJ: Organization and function of a pain clinic. In Bonica JJ (ed): *Advances in Neurology.* New York, Raven Press, 1974, vol 4, pp 433–443.
2. Bonica JJ: *The Management of Pain.* Philadelphia, Lea & Febiger, 1953.
3. Brena SF: Pain control facilities: roots, organization and function. In Brena SF, Chapman SL (eds): *Management of Patients with Chronic Pain.* New York, Spectrum Publications, 1983, pp 11–20.
4. Fordyce W, Fowler R, DeLateur B: An application of behavior modification techniques to a problem of chronic pain. *Behav Res Ther* 6:105–107, 1968.
5. Fordyce W, Fowler R, Lehmann J, et al: Some implications of learning in problems of chronic pain. *J Chronic Dis* 21:179–190, 1968.
6. Carron H, Committee on Pain Therapy, American Society of Anesthesiologists: *Pain Center/Clinic Directory, 1979.* Park Ridge, IL, American Society of Anesthesiologists, 1979.
7. JR: Programs target chronic back pain. *Hospitals* 60:87, 1986.
8. Cure BL, Pinsky JJ, Agnew DC, et al: What is a pain center? *Bull Los Angeles Neurol Soc* 41:160–167, 1976.
9. Fordyce WE, Roberts AH, Sternbach RA: Behavioral management of chronic pain: a response to critics. *Pain* 22:113–125, 1985.
10. Brena SF: Nerve blocks and chronic pain states—an update. 2. Clinical indications. *Postgrad Med* 78:77–86, 1985.
11. Mendelson G: Chronic pain and compensation: a review. *J Pain Symptom Manage* 1:135–144, 1986.
12. Goldberg RT: The social and vocational rehabilitation of persons with chronic pain: a critical evaluation. *Rehabil Lit* 43:274–283, 1982.
13. Hassett III TE: Pain therapy centers: just what the doctor ordered. *Healthcare Executive* 1(4):54–57, 1986.
14. Ghia JN, Sugioka K: Are pain centers viable: *NC Med J* 43:493–495, 1982.
15. Brena SF: Nerve blocks and chronic pain states—an update. 1. Basic considerations. *Postgrad Med* 78:62–71, 1985.
16. Fordyce WE: Floor discussion: psychologic and psychiatric techniques. In Bonica JJ (ed): *Advances in Neurology.* New York, Raven Press, 1974, vol 4, pp 611–613.
17. Flinn D, Yung C: Recent clinical approaches to pain treatment. *Psychosomatics* 23:33–40, 1982.
18. Fordyce WE: Treating chronic pain by contingency management. In Bonica JJ (ed): *Advances in Neurology.* New York, Raven Press, 1974, vol 4, pp 583–589.
19. Hosobuchi Y: Subcortical electrical stimulation for control of intractable pain in humans. *J Neurosurg* 64:543–553, 1986.

Appendix A
The Survey for Pain Centers

1. Name and mailing address of pain management facility

2. Person interviewed/specialty _____.
3. Title _____.
4. Pain clinic is affiliated with: public hospital ( ), private hospital ( ), VA ( ), university or medical school ( ), free-standing proprietorship ( ), other ( ).
5. What percentage of clinical services are inpatient _____; outpatient _____.
6. Number of inpatient beds _____.
7. Average inpatient census _____.
8. Average duration of inpatient program _____.
9. Average cost of inpatient program _____.
10. Average number of outpatient visits per month _____.
11. Average cost of outpatient pain program _____.
12. Following is a list of professional specialists often employed by pain clinics. Please tell me how many individuals from each specialty area are employed by your facility. I would like to break this down into full-time and part-time employees (e.g., Anesthesiology: 5 total—3 full-time, 2 part-time).

Specialty	Total No.	Full-time	Part-time
Anesthesiology			
Family Practice			
Orthopedic Surgery			
Neurosurgery			
Dentistry			
Oral Surgery			
Neurology			
Rheumatology			
Physiatry			
Internal Medicine			
Psychiatry			
Psychology			
Physical Therapy			
Nursing			
Occupational Therapy			
Recreational Therapy			
Vocational Rehabilitation			
Social Work			
Other (Identify)			
Other (Identify)			
Other (Identify)			

13. Training opportunities available at your pain facility:
    Medical student rotation _____
    Nursing student rotation _____
    Medical resident rotation _____
    Psychology student rotation _____
    Physical therapy rotation _____
    Other (identify) _____
    Other (identify) _____
    Other (identify) _____

14. How many people on your staff conduct research full-time? _____
    part-time? _____

15. Research interests of staff:
    1. _____
    2. _____
    3. _____
    4. _____
    5. _____

16. REFERRALS: Please list estimated percentages of patients referred to you by the following sources:
    Physician referred _____   Health agency referred _____
    Insurance referred _____   Worker's Compensation _____
    Attorney referred _____   Other _____

17. FUNDING: Please list estimated percentages of patients funded under each category:
    Standard health insurance _____   Personal finances _____
    Medicare _____   Medicaid _____
    Personal injury case _____ Grants or research funding _____
    Worker's compensation _____ Other _____

18. What percentage of the fees for your services are collected? _____

19. Please tell me the names, titles, and trained specialties of your clinic directors or of the persons who head your organizations
    1. _____   2. _____   3. _____
       _____   _____   _____

20. Does your facility specialize in treatment of specific types of pain? (yes/no)
    Types _____

21. I am going to read you five statements that characterize various types of pain clinics. Please listen carefully, then decide which statement best characterizes your clinic.
    (a) A research facility that offers associated clinical services.
    (b) A clinical facility that conducts associated research.
    (c) Strictly a research facility.
    (d) Strictly a clinical facility.
    (e) 50% clinical, 50% research.

22. Which of the following statements best characterizes your clinical services?
    (a) Primarily diagnostic and surgical, with behavioral components
    (b) Primarily behavioral, with diagnostic and/or surgical services available
    (c) Totally behavioral
    (d) Totally diagnostic or surgical

23. I'm interested in finding out what type of evaluation process you go through with your inpatients and outpatients prior to admitting them to treatment. As I read a list of diagnostic procedures, please tell me whether the average inpatient, and then whether the average outpatient, is evaluated with each procedure prior to treatment.

    Interviews by:
       Social work _____ / _____
       Psychology _____ / _____
       Psychiatry _____ / _____
       Nursing _____ / _____
       Vocational rehab. _____ / _____
       Family interviewed _____ / _____
    Psychological testing
       MMPI _____ / _____   Millon _____ / _____
       McGill _____ / _____ Other _____ / _____

Physician's exam _____ / _____
    What specialty? _____
Physical therapy _____ / _____
Diagnostic tests:
    Computed tomography _____ / _____
    Nuclear magnetic resonance imaging _____ / _____
    Myelogram _____ / _____
    X-rays _____ / _____
    Other (identify) _____ / _____ / _____
    Other _____ / _____ (_____)
    Other _____ / _____ (_____)
    Other _____ / _____ (_____)
TMJ screening (for headache sufferers) _____ / _____

24. What approximate percentage of your inpatients, and what percentage of your outpatients, receive the following treatment modalities?
Nerve blocks _____ / _____
TENS _____ / _____
Narcotic pain meds _____ / _____
Nonnarcotic pain meds _____ / _____
Antidepressant meds _____ / _____
Benzodiazepines _____ / _____
Phenothiazines _____ / _____
Drug detoxification _____ / _____
Surgery (laminectomy, diskectomy, fusion, TMJ replacement) _____ / _____
Rhizotomy/cordotomy _____ / _____
Chymopapain injection _____ / _____
Acupuncture _____ / _____
Acupressure _____ / _____
Biofeedback _____ / _____
Physical exercise _____ / _____
Physical therapy modalities (elec. stim., heat, ultrasound) _____ / _____
Ice massage _____ / _____
Relaxation training (progressive) _____ / _____
Hypnotherapy _____ / _____
Behavior modification/behavior therapy _____ / _____
Individual psychotherapy _____ / _____
Group psychotherapy _____ / _____
Family therapy _____ / _____
Home visits by social work or psychology staff _____ / _____
Recreational therapy _____ / _____
Education (i.e., back care, stress mgt.) _____ / _____
Vocational rehabilitation _____ / _____
Other (identity) _____ / _____ / _____
Other _____ / _____ / _____
Other _____ / _____ / _____

25. Do you consider your program interdisciplinary or multidisciplinary? _____

26. (a) Do major goals for patients include the following? (√)
    (b) What percent of patients achieve the goal? (%)

	(√)	(%)
Return to work	_____	_____
Eliminate pain meds	_____	_____
Eliminate other meds (specify _____)	_____	_____
Increase in physical capabilities (strength & stamina)	_____	_____
Decreased utilization of health care	_____	_____
Decreased intensity of pain	_____	_____
Other (_____)	_____	_____
Other (_____)	_____	_____
Other (_____)	_____	_____

27. Do you have a formal quality assurance program? (yes/no)
28. Do your patients leave with
    (a) formal statements of limitations (yes/no)
    (b) formal impairment rating (yes/no)
29. Do you have a formal follow-up program? (yes/no)
30. How long do you follow up with:
    (a) inpatients: in person _____   by phone _____
    (b) outpatients: in person _____   by phone _____
31. Future directions
    If you could influence the growth of pain centers in the next five years, what would you encourage your pain center and other centers to improve upon, move toward, or change?

Appendix B
Survey Participants Used in Final Data Compilation

Boston Pain Center at Spalding Rehabilitation Hospital
125 Nashua Street
Boston, MA 02114
(617) 720-6400
Gerald Aronoff, M.D., Administrative and Clinical Director

Center for Pain Evaluation and Treatment
University of Pittsburgh School of Medicine
230 Lothrop Street
Pittsburgh, PA 15213
(412) 647-2096
Dennis Turk, Ph.D., Director

Chronic Pain Rehabilitation Program of
  Sister Kenny Institute
Division of Abbot Northwestern Hospital
800 East 28th Street
Minneapolis, MN 55407
(612) 874-5023
Dave Jones, Ph.D., Director

Colorado Rehabilitation Institute
12061 Tejon Street
Denver, CO 80234
(303) 444-7400
Richard L. Stieg, M.D., Medical Director

Diamond Headache Clinic
5252 North Western Avenue
Chicago, IL 60625
(312) 878-5558
Seymour Diamond, M.D., Director

Michigan Headache and Neurological Institute
3120 Professional Drive
Ann Arbor, MI 48104
(313) 973-1155
Joel Saper, M.D., Director

Pain Control and Rehabilitation Institute of Georgia
350 Winn Way
Decatur, GA 30030
(404) 297-1400
Steven H. Sanders, Ph.D., Executive Director

Pain Management and Behavioral Medicine Center
270 Farmington Avenue
Farmington, CN 06032
(203) 674-0084
Bruce Gottlieb, Ph.D., Clinical Director

Pain Management Center
Mayo Clinic
St. Mary's Hospital
Rochester, MN 55902
(507) 285-5921
Mary Jane MacHardy, M.S., Program Coordinator

Pain Therapy Center
Greenville General Hospital
100 Mallard Street
Greenville, SC 29601
(803) 242-8088
C. David Tollison, Ph.D., Director

Rehabilitation Institute of Chicago
Center for Pain Studies
345 East Superior Street
Chicago, IL 60611
(312) 908-2845
Jean Butler, M.S., Program Coordinator

Washington Pain and Rehabilitation Center, Inc.
2100 M Street, NW, Suite 311
Washington, DC 20037
(202) 429-0990
Lorenz Ng, M.D., Director of Medical Services, President,
  and Chief Executive Officer

Appendix C
Organizations Involved in the Advancement of Pain Treatment

American Academy of Pain Medicine
43 East Ohio
Suite 914
Chicago, IL 60611
(312) 645-0083
Robert Addison, President
Ellis Murphy, Executive Director

American Pain Society
340 Kingsland Street
Nutley, NJ 07110
(201) 235-0587
Diane T. Chen, M.D., Administrative Officer

American Society of Anesthesiologists
515 Busse Highway
Park Ridge, IL 60068
(312) 825-5586
John W. Andes, Executive Secretary

Commission on Accreditation of Rehabilitation Facilities
101 North Wilmot Road
Suite 500
Tucson, AZ 85711
(602) 748-1212
Alan H. Toppel, Executive Director

International Association for the Study of Pain
Westlund Building
1309 Summit Avenue
Seattle, WA 98101
(206) 292-7521
Ainsley Iggo, President

Index

Page numbers followed by *italic* "t" denote tables.

A fibers, 10, 537. *See also* A-delta fibers
Abdominal muscle pain, 503
Abdominal pregnancies, 374
Aberrant movement subluxation, 165
Ablative neurosurgery, 397–398, 417–420. *See also* Neuroablation
Accessory nerve lesions, 438
Accessory nerve palsy, 438
Accident
   and disease, 648–649
   injury with, 647–649
Acculturation, 18
Acetabular dysplasia, 362
Acetaminophen, 64
   for chronic pain, 547
   for herpes simplex, 314
   for joint pain, 478
   for malignant pain, 83, 393
   for tension headache, 259
   used in children, 106
Acetylcholine, 26, 448
Acetylsalicylic acid. *See* Aspirin
Achilles reflex, 166
   absence of, 168
Achilles tendinitis, 488
Actinotherapy, 157–158
Activity
   changes in, 43–44
   diaries, 44
   level of, 213, 215–216
   Pattern Indicators, 572
Acupuncture, 182–183
   conflicting results of, 183–184
   history of, 182
   in modification of pain perception, 537
   in pain treatment, 183–184
   for postherpetic neuralgia, 471
   in surgical procedures, 184–185
   TENS, 157
Acute illness model, 225
Acyclovir, 313, 463
Adaptive copers, 229
Adductores brevis muscle pain, 503–505
Adductores longus muscle pain, 503–505
A-delta fibers, 10, 298, 550
   in TENS, 566

A-delta nociceptors, 446–447
Adenine arabinosidem 463–646
Adenomyosis, 375
Adenosine monophosphate, 464
Adenosine triphosphate (ATP), 510
Adjunctive treatment techniques, 174–189. *See also specific techniques*
Adjuvant drugs, 395
Affective responses, measurement of, 573–576
Afferent nerve, orofacial, 299
Afferent pain fibers, 10–11
Afferent pain pathways, 551
Afferent pain signals, 39
Agonist-antagonist analgesics, 65–67
Agorphobia, 92
AIDS, neuropathy with, 426
Akathisia, 94
Alcohol
   abuse of, 4647
   as neurolytic agent, 398
   celiac block with, 420
Alcoholic neuropathy, 426
Alcoholism, with dysthymic pain, 198–199
Alexithymia, 199, 542
Alfentanil, 553
Algometers, 491
Alkaloids, 252–253
Allergic hepatotoxicity, 94
Allergies, 240–241
Allopurinol, 485
Alpha motor neurons, 29
Alprazolam (Xanax), 97
Amantadine, 94, 464
American Academy of Pain Medicine, survey of, 228
American Pain Society, 665
Amitriptyline (Elavil), 65, 74–75, 83, 88, 90
   for acute pain, 74
   with analgesics, 77
   with migraine, 75, 256
   for myofascial pain syndrome, 527
   for neuralgia, 279
   for postherpetic neuralgia, 293, 467, 468
Amoxapine (Asendin), 88–89
Amphetamines, 86, 98
Amputations, 127–128
   phantom pain with, 455–459

685

686 Index

Amputations—continued
  preoperative preparation for, 457–458
Amyloidosis, 426
Amyotrophic lateral sclerosis, 323, 327
  affecting cervical spine, 330
Analgesia
  acupuncture, 184–185
  patient-controlled, 396
  placebo, 185–189
  stimulation, 137, 140, 566
Analgesic loading, 560
Analgesics. See also specific drugs
  centrally acting, 59–67
  for chronic pain, 544–547
  classification of, 544t
  doctor as, 543–544
  for dysthymic pain, 204
  guidelines for use of, 54–55
  for herpes zoster, 462
  interactions of with lithium, 93
  interactions of with neuroleptics, 95
  intramuscular administration of, 557
  intravenous administration of, 556–557
  for joint pain, 478
  for migraine, 254
  in modification of pain perception, 537
  narcotic, 546t, 547. See also Narcotics
    guidelines for use of, 544t
    for malignant pain, 394–395
    used in children, 107t
  for neuropathies, 428
  oral administration of, 558
  in Pain Therapy Centers, 659
  patient-controlled administration of, 558–560
  peripherally acting, 55–58
  for postherpetic neuralgia, 467
  potentiation of, 107
  subcutaneous administration of, 557–558
  with TENS, 137
  for tension headache, 259
  transdermal administration of, 558
  used in children, 107–108t
Anatomic variations, 514–516
Androgens, 377
Anemia, 513
Anergia, 198
Anesthesia dolorosa, 140
Anesthetics, 116
Anger, suppression of, 199
Anhedonia, 198
Ankle
  fracture of, 35
  trauma to, 441
  weakness of, 35
Ankylosing spondylitis, 76, 332, 360, 485
  in cervical spine, 324
  early stages of, 341
  treatment for, 478
Annulus fibrosus innervation, 357
Anserine bursitis, 487–488
Anteriolisthesis subluxation, 164
  with spondylolysis, 165
Anterior interosseous nerve, 32
Anterior interosseous nerve syndrome, 432–433
Anterolateral cordotomy, 419–420
Anthranilic acids, 58

Anthropological variations, 19–20
Antianxiety drugs, 84–86. See also specific drugs
  treatment approaches with, 96–98
Antibiotics, 463
Anticholinergics, 384
Anticipated consequences, 224
Anticonvulsants, 91
  for herpes zoster, 464
  mechanism of, 77
  for migraine, 256
  for neuralgias, 280, 467–468
  for neuropathies, 428
Antidepressants, 46, 69–70
  commonly used, 89t
  for dysthymic pain, 205–206
  effects of, 91
  in elderly, 112
  for herpes zoster, 464
  for migraine, 256
  for myofascial pain syndrome, 599
  for neuropathies, 428
  nonresponse to, 91
  in pain centers, 659, 673
  for postherpetic neuralgia, 467–468
  for tension headache, 259–260
  tricyclic, 65, 69, 88–91. See also Tricyclics
    for acute pain, 70–74
    as analgesic adjuncts, 77
    for chronic pain, 74–77
    mechanisms of action of, 77
    used in children, 107
Antiemetics, 254
Antihypertensive medication, 182
Anti-inflammatory agents, 55–58. See also Nonsteroidal anti-inflammatory drugs
  for postherpetic neuralgia, 467
Antimalarials
  for rheumatoid arthritis, 483
  for spondyloarthropathies, 485–486
Antinociceptive fibers, 566
Antinuclear antibodies, 477
Antiparkinsonism agents, 94
Antipsychotic drugs, 80–82t
Antipyretics, 56, 393
Antispasmodics, 384
Antiviral agents, 463, 467
Anxiety, 4, 46, 69
  with benzodiazepines, 97
  chronic, 97–98
  ethnic factors in, 18
  maintenance treatment for, 98
  psychological evaluation and, 39
Anxiolytics, 97–98
Aphasia, 15
Appendicitis, 378
Aquatics, 151
Arachidonic acid
  cascade, 366
  metabolism of, 555
Arachnoiditis, 369
Arachnoidopathy, 369
Arm abduction, 516
Arm pain, 495–499
  trigger points of, 496, 498
Arnold-Chiari malformations, 326

Arthritis
　assistive devices for, 160
　crystal-induced, 483–484, 485
　of elbow, 433
　gouty, 330
　of TMJ, 307
　tricyclics for, 76–77
Arthritis Impact Measurement Scales (AIMS), 577
Arthropathies, 357–364. See also specific conditions
Articular dysfunction, 520
Articular pain, 476
Ascorbic acid, 512
Aspirin, 55–56, 64
　adverse effects of, 57–58
　for cancer pain, 83, 393
　for chronic pain, 547
　dosages of, 57
　drug interactions of, 57
　effects and uses of, 56–57
　hypersensitivity to, 57
　for joint pain, 478
　for tension headache, 259
　used in children, 105–106
Assistive devices, 159–160
Association bundles, 15
Asthenopia, 249
Ataxia, 97, 277
Atlantoaxial joint, 321
Atlanto-occipital joint, 321
Auditory relay nucleus, 14
Augmentative neurosurgery, 417, 421–422
Auranofin, 483
Auriculotemoral nerve damage, 314–315
Aurothiomalate, 482
Autogenic relaxation, 179, 411
Autoimmune disease, 488
Automobile accidents, enigmatic pain from, 521–522
Autonomic activity, parameters of, 664
Autonomic nervous system
　visceral afferent blockade of, 123
　visceral efferent blockade of, 121–123
Autonomic responses, 15
Avoidance learning, 44
Avulsion, of spinal root, 126–128
Avulsion injuries, 126–128
Axillary nerve entrapment, 437
Axonal disorders, 29
Azathioprine, 483

B fibers, 10
Babinski's reflex, 326
Back. See also Back pain
　brace for, 360
　physical examination of, 345–346
　tenderness of, 346
Back pain. See also Spinal pain
　arthropathies and, 357–364
　chronic, 76
　　characteristics of, 675t
　cognitive aspects of, 42
　coping strategies for, 577
　low, 76
　　assessment method for, 335–351
　　categories of, 166–168
　　chronic uncomplicated, 167
　　differential diagnosis of, 335–356

　　documentation of structural lesion of, 351–356
　　manipulation for, 164
　　mechanical, 343–349
　　neurologic signs and symptoms of, 349–350
　　nonmechanical, 341–342
　　spinal manipulation for, 166–168
　　tricyclics for, 76
　muscular, 499–503
　　trigger points of, 500–501
　neuropathies and nerve root lesions with, 365–371
　nonorganic, 341t
　referred, 341
　screening tests for, 342
　spinal surgery for, 317–319
　uncomplicated, 166
Back Pain Classification Scale, 575–576, 579
Back schools, 593–594
Baclofen (Lioresal)
　for migraine, 256
　for postherpetic neuralgia, 468
　for trigeminal neuralgia, 277, 289
Bacterial infections, 513
　of cervical spine, 359
Barbiturates, 253
　interactions of with MAOIs, 92
Bariba society, 19
Basal body temperature, 513
Basilar artery migraine, 244–245
Beck Depression Scale, 74
　in pain centers, 672
Behavior. See also Pain behavior
　direct observations of, 570–571, 584
　extinction of, 211
　measurement and observation of, 570–573
　self-monitoring of, 584
Behavior modification, 210. See also Contingency management
　for cancer pain management, 412–413
　for dysthymic pain, 205
　in Pain Therapy Centers, 661
　techniques of, 211–212
Behavioral analysis, 43
　activity changes and, 43–44
　avoidance learning and, 44
　deactivation and, 44
　interpersonal relationships and family response in, 44–45
　learning history in, 44
　vocational, financial, and litigation issues in, 45–46
Behavioral conceptualizations, 212–213
Behavioral contracts, 216
Behavioral rating scales, 638
Belladonna alkaloids, 253
Bellergal, 256, 261
Bell's palsy, evaluation of, 26
Benign orgasmic cephalgia, 245
Benzodiazepines, 84–86
　with analgesics, 555
　for dysthymic pain, 204
　interactions with, 96
　mechanisms of action of, 86
　pretreatment evaluation with, 96–97
　properties and side effects of, 96
　sudden discontinuation of, 96
　for tension headache, 260
　treatment techniques of, 97–98
Benzoin tincture, 314
6,7-Benzomorphans, 61

Beta blockers, 448
　for migraine, 254–255, 261
　for post-traumatic headache, 260
Biceps brachii muscle pain, 497
Biceps femoris muscle pain, 505
Biceps reflex, 166, 322
Bicipital tendinitis, 487
Bicycle, stationary, 151
Bicycle ergometers, 611–612
Biofeedback, 159, 210
　for back pain, 319
　for cancer pain, 411
　for chronic pain, 543
　efficacy of, 273
　electromyographic, 153, 159, 269, 270–271, 411
　for headache in children, 260
　long-term effects of, 272–273
　with migraine, 75
　in modification of pain perception, 537
　for phantom pain, 458
　with relaxation training, 178–179
　thermal, 159
　for TMJ disease, 294
　training in, 269–270
　　for headache management, 269–271
Biphasic respiratory depression, 563
Bladder
　dysfunction of with spinal opiates, 564
　obstruction of, 384
　pain of in males, 384
Blistex, 314
Blockage, definition of, 163
Boarding study, 620–625
　objectives of, 622
　recommendations for, 625–626
Boarding machine, improved, 626
Bolus demand dose, 560
Bone infections, 284
Bone scanning, 333–334
Bonica, John, 664
Bony demineralization, 450
Bony spur formation, in cervical spine, 324
Borderline personality disorder, 541
Bowstring sign, 347
BPCS. See Back Pain Classification Scale
Braces, 159
　for back, 360
　for knee, 160
Brachial neuralgia, 168
Brachial plexus block, 565
Brachialis muscle pain, 497
Brachioradialis reflex, 166
Bradykinins, 677
Brain
　abscess, 247
　electrical stimulation of, 140–141, 421–422
　lesions of, neurosurgical treatment of, 420
　tumor of, 247
Brainstem
　in pain perception, 16
　pain systems of, 12–14
Breathing technique, 179, 180–181
Brief Symptom Inventory, 579
Brompton's cocktail, 63, 86
Brucellosis, 332
Bruxism, 313

Bulbourethral glans, 383
Bupivacaine (Marcaine), 116
　for herpes zoster, 465
　for post-traumatic neuralgias, 310–311
Buprenorphine, 66
　patient-control administration of, 559
Buproprion (Wellbutrin), 90
Burning mouth syndrome, 285, 313
Burning tongue syndrome, 313
Bursitis
　anserine, 487–488
　subacromial, 487
　treatment of, 480
Burst TENS, 567
Buspirone (BuSpar), 98
Butorphanol, 63, 67
Butt life, 514
Buttock pain, 345–346
Butyrophenone, 83
　patient-control administration of, 560

C fibers, 10, 299, 391, 447, 536–537, 550
　blockade of, 446
　stimulation of, 183
　in TENS, 566
C1-C2 instability, 358
Cabot, Richard, on placebos, 188
Caffeine, 86
　mechanism of action of, 86
Calamine lotion, 462
Calcium antagonists (channel blockers)
　for cluster headache, 258
　for migraine, 255
　for neuropathies, 428
Calcium pyrophosphate dihydrate deposition disease, 484
Calisthenics, 151
Cancer, 403
　of face, 294
　mentality, 379
　narcotics for, 63
　pain related to, 391t
　　assessment of, 407–409
　　Brompton's mixture for, 86
　　case study of, 414
　　causes of, 403
　　cognitive response to, 404, 406
　　complications of, 406–407
　　comprehensive treatment packages for, 413
　　consequences of, 406
　　diminishers of, 406
　　neurosurgical treatment of, 417–422
　　overt behavioral responses to, 404–405
　　phenothiazines for, 83
　　physical management of, 390
　　precipitators of, 405–406
　　psychological management of, 402–415
　　self-monitoring of, 405
　　sensory-physiologic responses to, 405
　　staff education in managing, 412–413
　　treatment of, 403–404, 413–414
　of penis, 387
　peripheral neuropathies with, 427
Canes, 160
Capitis musculature, 321
Carbamazepine (Tegretol), 91, 93
　for herpes zoster, 464

for migraine, 256
for phantom pain, 458
for post-traumatic headache, 260
for trigeminal neuralgia, 276, 288–289
Carbidopa-levodopa (Sinemet), 93
Cardiovascular conditions, 342
CARF accreditation, 675, 676
Caridopalevodopa (Sinemet), 468
Carotidynia, 292–293
Carpal tunnel syndrome, 31, 32–33, 430
　clinical features of, 431
　pathology and treatment of, 432
Carpi radialis muscle pain, 499
Carpometacarpal joint stabilization, 160
Catastrophizing, 577
Catecholamines, 447
Category scales, 578
Caudal midbrain, 14
Causal priority, 224
Causalgia, 11, 121–122, 368, 370, 451, 454
　clinical signs and symptoms of, 445, 452–453t
　diagnosis of, 448
　gross anatomy and, 446
　microanatomy of, 446–447
　reactive, 391
　synapses and, 447–448
　theory of, 445–446
　treatment of, 448–449
Causalgia minor, 122
Celiac ganglion block, 123
Celiac plexus, 123
　block of, 399, 420
Central biasing mechanism, 157, 183
Central cord syndromes, 331
Central nervous system
　agents of, 86–88
　orofacial pain pathways of, *300*
　stimulants of, 98–99
Centromedian nucleus, 15
Cephalic vasomotor response feedback, 269, 271
Ceramid trihexosidase deficiency, 427
Cerebral cortex
　descending pathways of, 536–537
　memory regions of, 537
　pain and, 12
　pain perception and, 15–16
Cerebrospinal fluid
　blocking of, 240
　elevated pressure of and headache, 247
　opiates in, 561–562
Cervical cordotomy, 133
Cervical lordosis
　exercise for, 153
　loss of, 495
Cervical muscles, posterior, 495
Cervical nerve roots, 166
　avulsion of, 126
　blockade of, 119
　disorders of, 325
Cervical orthoses, 159
Cervical outflow, 446
Cervical radiculitis, 329
Cervical radiculopathies, 30–31
Cervical spine
　anatomy and biomechanics of, 321–322
　arthropathies of

　management of, 359–360
　pain of, 358–360
　clinical examination of, 324–326
　diagnostic studies of, 326
　disorders of, 333–334
　extrinsic neoplasms of, 327–328
　infections of, 332–333
　inflammatory disease of, 359
　intrinsic motor and sensory disorders of, 327
　lesions of, 359
　medical history of, 324
　nerve root irritations of, 329–330
　osteoarthritis of, 328–329
　pain syndromes of, 326–333
　　acute, 168
　　differential diagnosis and management of, 320–334
　　spinal manipulation for, 168–169
　pathology of, 323–324
　rheumatoid arthritis of, 331–332
　spondylosis of, 247, 314
　stiffness of, 358–359
　traction of, 154, 360
　trauma to, 330–331
　vascular supply of, 323
Charcot-like joints, 481
Chassaignac's tubercle, 119, 122
Cheiralgia paresthetica, 34
Chemical hypophysectomy, 134
Chemical neurolysis, 398–399
Chemistry battery, 526
Chest pain syndrome, 23
Chickenpox, 132, 460
Childbirth
　acupuncture analgesia with, 185
　attitude toward pain of, 19
Children
　contingency management in, 219
　dose selection for, 105
　drugs used in pain management in, 104–109
　headaches in, 260
　underprescribing in, 104
Chiropractic subluxation, 163
Chlamydia infections, 377–378
Chlonazepam (Clonopin), 84–86
Chloral hydrate, 92
Chlordiazepoxide (Librium), 77, 84–86, 97
Chlorimipramine (Anafranil), 76–77
Chlorphenesin (Maolate), 289
Chlorpromazine (Thorazine), 80, 83, 88, 95, 154, 158
Chlorprothixene (Taractan), 468
Chondrocalcinosis, 360
Chondrosarcoma, 284, 328
Chordomas, 328
Chordotomy. *See* Cordotomy
Chronic Illness Problem Inventory, 573
Chronic pain. *See also* Chronic pain syndromes
　all-or-none hypothesis in, 4
　antianxiety agents for, 84–86
　anxiety with, 46
　behavior modification for, 205
　behavioral/psychosocial evaluation of, 229
　central nervous system, 86
　characteristics of, 298t
　classification system of, 229–230, 365, 637
　　critique of, 601–602
　　pros and cons of, 600–601

Chronic pain—*continued*
  cognitive aspects of, 4–5
    evaluation of, 42–43
  cognitive-behavioral perspective on, 222–235
  components of, 3–5
  depression with, 540–541
  diagnosis and ligitimization of, 21
  of enigmatic origin, 521–522
  interacting factors in, 509
  litigation and compensation for, 21–22, 45–46, 543
  medical/physical evaluation of, 227–229
  multidisciplinary approach to, 6
  nerve blocks for management of, 115–124
  neuroleptics for, 95–96
  operational definition of, 3–4
  pain therapy centers for, 656–678
  patient profile for, 197–200
  pharmacologic management of
    in children, 104–109
    in elderly, 109–113
  phenothiazines for, 83
  predisposing central factors to, 368
  psychological evaluation in, 38–50
  recovery from
    and financial compensation for, 21–22
    and litigation, 45–46
  in relatives of dysthymic and depressed patients, 201
  sick role with, 20–21
  social and cultural factors in, 17–24
  social consequences of, 17
  Social Security classification of, 637
  Social Security Disability and, 637–638
  specialists, 652–653
  treatment of
    goals and expectations of, 43
    successful, 21
  tricyclics for, 74–77, 90–91
Chronic pain syndromes, 23
  contributing components of, 40
  early identification of, 603
  early intervention in, 592, 594–596
  intractable benign, 369, 371t
  management of, 2
  prevention of, 594–596
  tricyclics for, 74–77
Ciguatera, 327
Cimetidine (Tagamet), 96
Cingulotomy, 133, 420
  for postherpetic neuralgia, 470
Circumcision, 19, 387
Claims adjusters, 231–232
CLBP. *See* Back pain, low
Clinic staff, 231
Clonazepam (Klonopin), 64, 91, 449
  for trigeminal neuralgia, 289
Clonidine, 256
Clorazepate (Tranxene), 97
Cluster headache, 75, 240, 245–246
  chlorpromazine for, 83
  chronic, 245–246, 256–257
  chronic paroxysmal, 257
  episodic, 256
  pain with, 292–293
    facial, 311
  treatment of, 256–257
    preventive, 257–259

symptomatic, 257
  trigger factors in, 245
  variant, 246
Cobalamin, 512
Cocaine, 86, 280
Codeine, 64
  for chronic pain, 547
  interactions of with MAOIs, 92
  for joint pain, 478
  for malignant pain, 393
  structure of-activity of, 61
Cognitive Behavior Therapy Package (CTP), 413
Cognitive distortions, 576–577
Cognitive restructuring, for cancer pain, 412
Cognitive theory, 39
Cognitive therapeutic techniques
  for cancer pain, 411–413
  for headache, 271
Cognitive-behavioral approach, 46, 222–223, 230–232
  in assessment of chronic pain, 227–230
  assumptions of, 224–225
  components of, 232–235
  conceptualization of chronic pain in, 223–226
  objective of, 225–226, 230
  treatment techniques of, 230–232
Cognitive-behavioral rehearsal, 233
Cognitive-verbal response, 584
  measurement of, 573–582
Colchicine, 484
Cold. *See also* Therapeutic cold
  lasers, 158
  sores, 313
Collagen
  disorders of, 314
  distensibility of, 148, 151
Commissural myelotomy, 419
Communication of symptoms
  cultural and anthropolic influences on, 18–20
  ethnic influences on, 18
Communication skills, 226
Compensation. *See also* Disability; Workers' compensation
  behavioral analysis and, 45–46
  formula for, 646
    for injury arising out of employment, 649–650
    for injury by accident, 647–649
    for personal injury, 646–647
  influence of, 21–22
  neurosis, 21–22, 337
  prevention and early intervention and, 602–604
Complex repetitive discharges, 28
Compression neuropathies, 430
Compressive root lesions, 31
Computed tomography
  for back pain diagnosis, 342
  of cervical spine, 326, 333
  for chronic myofascial pain, 526
  in gynecologic pain diagnosis, 374
  for headache, 242
  for low back pain diagnosis, 335–336, 352–353
  for malignant pain, 390
COMT, 448
Conditioning effects, 212–213
Condyloma acuminata, 387–388
Connective tissue diseases, 486–487
  pain with, 475
Consensual vascular response, 149

Contingency management, 210. *See also* Behavior modification
  conditions for effective use of, 212
  definition of, 210–211
  future trends in, 219
  issues and needs in, 218–219
  primary paradigms of, 211–212
  in reduction of overt pain behavior, 213–218
  self-applied, 218
Contingent reinforcement, 412
Contraceptives, oral, 376
Contrast materials, 352
Conversion hysteria, 23. *See also* Hysteria
Conversion V pattern, 540
Cooling devices, 151
Coping strategies, 234
  for cancer pain, 412
  inadequate skills for, 523
  measurement of, 577–578
Coping Strategies Questionnaire, 577, 581, 584
Cordotomy, 317, 365, 398
  anterolateral, 419–420
  open, 420
  percutaneous, 397
  for phantom pain, 458
  for postherpetic neuralgia, 470
Corgard, 255
Corona radiata, 15
Corpus luteum cysts, 375–376
Corsets, 159, 360
Cortical receptor area, 15
Corticosteroids
  for chronic pain, 547
  depot, 480
  for herpes zoster, 463
  for inflammatory vascular disease, 293
  intra-articular, 481
  for joint pain, 479–480
  for osteoarthritis, 481
  for polymylagia rheumatica, 488
  for rheumatoid arthritis, 483
  for spondyloarthropathies, 485–486
Corticothalamic fibers, 14
Cost containment, 676–677
Costovertebral-costotransverse subluxation, 165
Counseling, for phantom pain, 458–459
Counterirritation techniques, 470–471
Courage, traditions of, 19
Couvade, 19
Cracked tooth syndrome, 285
Cranial nerves, 321. *See also specific nerves*
  sympathetic, 11
Cranial neuritides, 247–248
Craniofacial pain, musculoskeletal, 281–284
C-reactive protein tests, 513
Crohn's disease, 485
Cross-talk, 304, 368
Crutches, 160
Crying, 535
Cryoanalgesia, 470, 567
Cryosurgery, 388
Cryotherapy, 150–151
Crystal-induced arthritis, 483–484
  treatment for, 484–485
Crystal-induced arthropathies, 480
Cubital tunnel syndrome, 433
  treatment of, 434

Cultural framework, 17
Culture
  components of, 18–19
  influence of, 18
Cumulative trauma disorders, 614
  case history of, 616–617
  causative factors in, 614–616
  control program for, 617
  expert system for, 617–620
  process of, 616
Cyanocobalamin, 512
Cycling, 151, 153
Cyclobenzaprine (Flexeril), 77
Cyclo-oxygenase enzyme system inhibition, 56, 555
Cyclophosphamide, 293, 483
Cyproheptadine (Periactin), 256, 258
  in children, 260
Cystotoscopy, 384
Cytomegalovirus, 460
Cytosine arabinoside, 463

Dallas Spinal Pain Program, 22
Danazol (Danocrine), 261
Dartmouth Pain Questionnaire, 573
De Quervain's extensor tenosynovitis, 436
De Quervain's tendinitis, 34, 487
Deactivation, 44
Deafferentation pain, 75–76, 125, 304
  blocking of, 392
  clinical diagnosis of, 129–130
  deep brain stimulation for, 140–141
  evaluation of, 391
  neurosurgical treatment of, 126–134
Deafferentation syndromes, 77, 83–84
  hypersensitivity states, 370
Death benefits, 651
Decompression
  of cervical nerve roots, 330
  of posterior interosseous nerve, 436
  for trigeminal neuralgias, 311
Deep brain stimulation, 140–141
  risks of, 141
Deep relaxation, 411. *See also* Relaxation training
Deep-heating devices, 149–150
Dejerine-Roussy syndrome. *See* Thalamic syndrome
Deltoid muscle pain, 495–497
Dementia, drug-induced, 112–113
Denervation
  for trigeminal neuralgia, 289
  of vagus nerve, 292
Denonvilliers' fascia, 380
Dentinal sensation, 302
Dependence, fear of, 535
Depolarization, spontaneous, 27
Depression, 4, 23, 69, 540
  behavioral indicators of, 42
  with cancer pain, 403
  with chronic pain, 24, 540–541
  defective neurotransmission and, 246
  definition of, 70
  dysthymic pain disorder and, 197–208
  evaluation of, 46
  major, 70, 200
    dysthymic pain disorder and, 201–202
  MAOIs for, 92
  MMPI scale for, 576

Depression—*continued*
  neuroleptics for, 96
  pain perception and, 537
  patterns of, 241t
  psychological evaluation and, 39
  psychotic, 541
  screening for, 48
  treatment for, 74
Dermatomes, distribution of, 358
Dermatomyositis, 35
Descending pathways, 15
Desipramine (Norpramin, Pertofrane), 74, 90, 206
  with analgesics, 77
Dexamethasone
  concentrations of, 91
  nonsuppression of, 202, 204
  suppression test (DST), 91, 201, 598
Dexedrine, 98
Dextroamphetamine, 86
  half-life of, 99
Dextromethorphan, 92
Dextropropoxyphene, 478
Dextrose, 117
Diabetes
  neuropathy in, 368, 425–426
    radiating leg pain with, 343
    treatment of chronic pain with, 74
  postherpetic neuralgia with, 466
  with relaxation training, 182
  tricyclics with, 75
Diagnostic and Statistical Manual of Mental Disorder, Third Edition, 46
  critique of, 602
  depressive disorder diagnosis in, 70
  diagnostic criteria of for major depression, 200
  scheme of, 601
Diagnostic nerve blocks, 391–392
Diaphragm, innervation of, 322
Diathermy, 149–150
Diazepam (Valium), 64, 75, 84–86, 97–98
Dichloralphenazone, 253
Diclofenac, 527
Dietary restrictions, for headache in children, 260
Diffuse idiopathic skeletal hyperostosis (DISH) syndrome, 332
Diflunisal, 58, 555
Dihydroergotamine, 254, 260
Diltiazem (Cardizem), 255
Dimenhydrinate (Dramamine), 527
Diphenhydramine, 94
Diphenylhydantoin, 277
Diphenylmethane derivatives, 84
Diphenylpropylamines, 61
Disability
  adjudication process for, 637
  benefits, 650–651
  compensation, 22, 535. *See also* Compensation
  behavioral analysis and, 45–46
  definition of, 3, 635
  insurance, 21
  prevention and early intervention and, 602–604
  secondary gain of, 535–536
  specialists, 652–653
Disabled patient, 229
Discomfort, in workplace, 614
Discriminative stimuli, 211–212
Disk herniation, 168–169, 325, 329, 344
  in cervical spine, 324
Diskectomy, 361
Diskography, 318
Displacement suggestions, 410
Dissociation, 410
Dissociative visualization, 181
Distraction techniques, 169–170
Disulfiram (Antabuse), 96
DNA synthesis, 512
Doctor shopping, 542
Doctor-patient relationship, 543–544
Dopa, 447
Dopamine, 447
  blockade of, 83
  deactivation of, 98
  system malfunction of, 537
Dorsal column stimulation, 470
Dorsal gray horn, 12–13
Dorsal rhizotomy, 418
  for postherpetic neuralgia, 470
Dorsal root entry zone (DREZ), 126
Dorsal root ganglia, 11
Dorsolateral funiculus, 12
Douglas bag method, 611
Doxepin, 65, 70, 90
  with analgesics, 77
  for facial pain, 76
  for headache, 75, 256
Doxepin hydrochloride, 527
DREZ. *See* Dorsal root entry zone
DREZ caudalis electrode, 131
DREZ lesions, 129–132
  dorsal horn area involved in, *129*
  for postherpetic neuralgia, 470
  results of, *134*
  thoracic, 132–133
DREZ operation, 128–130, 132–133, 448
DRGs, 667
Droperidol, 559
Drug(s)
  abuse of, 46–47
  interactions of in elderly, 111–113
  profile, 46–47
Drug-clearing organs, 554
DSM-III. *See* Diagnostic and Statistical Manual of Mental Disorders, Third Edition
DST. *See* Dexamethasone suppression test
Dynamic myelography, 352
Dysesthesias
  postsympathectomy, 451
  treatment of, 428
Dysesthetic chronic pain, 370
Dysfunctional patient, 229
Dysmenorrhea, 374–377
Dyspareunia, 378
  with endometriosis, 376
Dysthymic pain disorders
  biologic markers in, 199
  clinical features of, 198
  controlled studies of, 200–204
  definition of, 197
  demographics of, 198
  depressive features of, 198–199
  family history in, 199
  in geriatric patients, 203–204
  nosologic considerations of, 200

patient profile for, 197–200
premorbid traits in, 198
prognosis for, 208
psychodynamic features of, 199–200
treatment of, 204–208
treatment response of, 206–207
Dystonia, 94

Eagle's syndrome, 293–294, 315
Early intervention
  compensation and disability program impact on, 602–604
  legal disincentive to, 604
  in myofascial syndromes, 598–600
  with pain-prone patient, 594–596
Early recognition, 592–606
Ectopic pregnancy, 374
Education, 593–594. See also Patient education
  about lifting and fitness, 596
  in cognitive-behavioral approach, 232–233
  on cumulative trauma disorders, 617
  for phantom pain, 458–459
Educational development time, 641, 642–643t
Efferent sympathetic fibers, 11
Efflurage, 155
Effort syndrome, 23
Ehlers-Danlos syndrome, 314
Einstein, Albert, 158
Elbow
  entrapments, 32–34
  neuropathy at, 33
Elderly
  contingency management in, 219
  dosage and drug interactions in, 111–113
  dysthymic pain disorder in, 203–204
  homeostasis in, 110
  older, 109
  orthostatic hypotension in, 112
  overprescribing in, 104
  pharmacokinetics of pain medication in, 110–111
  pharmacologic management of pain in, 109–113
  polypharmacy in, 112–113
  prescribing guidelines for, 111–112
Electrical stimulation
  vs. acupuncture, 184
  of brain, 421–422
  effects of, 144
  implanted devices for, 142–143
  indications for, 141–142
  in modification of pain perception, 537–538
  patient management in, 141–142
  percutaneous testing of, 141–142
  for phantom pain, 458
  of spinal cord, 421
  stimulation waveforms in, 143–144
  techniques of, 136–144
  transcutaneous, 157. See also Transcutaneous electrical nerve stimulation
Electroconvulsive therapy (ECT), 540–541
Electrode migrations, spontaneous, 138, 139
Electrode placement sites, 157
Electrodiagnosis, 26–37
  case studies of, 36–37
  clinical applications of, 30–35
  examination with, 36–37
  of low back pain, 354–355

Electrolytes
  disorders of, 27
  low levels of, 513
Electromagnetic radiation, 150
Electromyographic abnormalities, 30
  with cervical radiculopathies, 31
  in median nerve, 32
Electromyographic biofeedback, 153, 159, 269
  for cancer pain, 411
  vs. cephalic vasomotor biofeedback, 271
  for headache, 270
Electromyography, 26–27
  of cervical spine, 326
  in ergononmics analysis, 611
  insertional activity and, 27
  in low back pain diagnosis, 355
  for measuring physiologic variables of pain, 582–583
  for physiologic response of pain, 584
  of resting muscle, 27–28
  of voluntary muscle contraction, 28
Electrostimulation. See Electrical stimulation
Elongated styloid proces. See Eagle's syndrome
EMG. See Electromyography
EMG biofeedback. See Electromyographic biofeedback
Emotional decompression, 182
Emotional disorders, 246
Emotional distress, reduction of, 5
Emotional factors, 23
Emotional state, 3–4
Emotionally expressive groups, 535
Encephalitis, 240
Endocrine dysfunction, 512–513
Endometriosis, 376–377
Endoperoxide intermediates, 555
Endorphin receptors, 421
Endorphin system
  endogenous, 421
  in modification of pain perception, 537
β-Endorphins, 177–178
Endorphins, 183, 367, 677
  with depression and chronic pain, 199
  increased levels of, 188, 422
  research on, 676
Endurance exercises, 153
Enkephalins, 367
  increased levels of, 422
Enteropathic arthritis, 485
Enthesopathy, 485
Entrapment neuropathies, 424, 430–441
Entrapment syndromes, 371
  evaluation of, 31–35
Environment
  in cumulative trauma disorders, 615
  influence of on behavior, 225
Enzyme dysfunction, 510–512
Epicondylitis, 499
  lateral, 487
Epicritic pain, 10
Epididymal orchitis, 385–386
Epididymal pain, 385–386
Epididymis, 382–383
Epidural neurolysis, 398–399
Epidural spinal blocks, 118
  for postherpetic neuralgia, 469
Epidural steroids, 118
Epidural venography, 355

Epileptogenic foci, development of, 304
Epinephrine, 447
　with anesthetic, 116
Epstein-Barr virus, 460
Ergonomic deficiencies, 613–614
　examples of, 618–620
Ergonomic survey, 628–634
Ergonomics, 608–610
　analysis, 610–614
　of boarding, 620–626
　definition of, 608
Ergot derivatives, 468
Ergotamine alkaloids
　contraindications for, 253
　for migraine, 253, 292
Ergotamine tartrate
　inhalant forms of, 261
　for migraine, 252–253, 261
Escape/avoidance response, 215
Estrogen-progestin therapy, 377
Ethical codes, 18–19
Ethnic factors, 17–18, 534
Euphoria, 62
Evoked potentials, 355
Exaggeration reaction, 337, 339–341
Excessive force, 613–614
Exercise, 151
　in contingency management, 215
　for general activity, 151
　goal-specific, 152–153
　in pain centers, 672, 673
　therapeutic, 147
Exertional factors, 636
Extension subluxation, 164
Extensores digitorum muscle pain, 499, 507
Extinction, 211
Extra-articular pain syndromes, 482, 487–488
Extracranial surgery, 311
Extrapyramidal symptoms, 94
Eyestrain, 249

F wave, 29
　ulnar nerve latency, 33
Fabry's disease, 427
Facet joint
　block, 123–124
　　for low back pain diagnosis, 354–355
　denervation of, 123–124
　pain of, 123
Facet syndrome, 123, 167
Facial bone tumors, 284
Facial carcinoma, 294
Facial nerve, 298
Facial neuralgias, 275–280, 281
　antidepressants for, 76
Facial pain
　atypical, 285
　　treatment for, 75–76, 292
　with postherpetic infection, 130–131
　treatment of, 79
Facial sensation, anatomical organization of, 130–131
Facial trauma, 277–278
Failed back syndrome, 137–139, 317, 369
　procedures leading to, 318
Fallopian tube, implantation in, 374
Familial pain model, 24

Family
　disruption of with mother's incapacitation, 22–23
　education, 678
　as factor in pain etiology, 24
　history of, 47
　interactions in, 580–581
　problems of, 24
　in rehabilitation, 606
　relationships with loss of work, 22–23
　response of to pain behaviors, 44–45
Fasciculation potentials, 28
Fasciculus proprius, 12
Fatigue, 4
　in workplace, 614
Feedback conferences, 41
Feedback endorphin system, pain- blocking, 367
Feedback loop, 367
　negative, 183
Femoral motor conduction studies, 34
Femoral nerve
　entrapment of, 34–35
　stretch of, 347, 348
　syndromes of, 440
Femur, prosthetic replacement of, 363
Fenoprofen (Nalfon), 58, 479
Fentanyl, 553–554
　patient-control administration of, 559
Fever, reduction of, 56
Fever blisters, 313
Fibrillation potentials, 27
Fibrillations, 27
Fibro-osseous tunnel, 430
Fibrositis (fibromyalgia), 283, 338, 519–520
　massage for, 155
　treatment of, 527
Field blocks, 565–566
Financial compensation. See Compensation
Finkelstein's test, 34, 436
Finsen, Niels, 157
Fitz-Hugh and Curtis syndrome, 378
Fixation, 163
　spinal, 165
Fixed sacroiliac syndrome, 167
Flexion subluxation, 164
Flexor pollicis longus nerve, 32–33
Flexores digitorum muscle pain, 499
Floggings, 533
Fluoroscopy, 117, 119
Fluphenazine (Prolixin), 83, 91
　for neuralgia, 279, 293, 468, 478
Focal tenderness, 491
Folate, 512
Follicular cysts, 375
Foot orthoses, 160
Foramina stenosis, 325
Foraminal encroachment subluxation, 165
Fordyce theory, 222–223
Forearm suppination, 516–517
Forrestier's disease, 332
Fractionation, 177
Fractures
　in cervical spine, 324
　of TMJ, 307–308
Freud, Sigmund, 24
Frey's syndrome, 314–315
Friction, in massaging, 155

Index

Frontal lobotomy, 470
Function versus pain orientation, 522–523
Functional bowel syndrome, 534
Functional capacity, 3
Functional disability
    questionnaires, 583–584
    self-reports of, 572–573
Functional limitation, definition of, 3
Functional status, 3
    enhancement of, 5
    at home and at work, 4

GABA (γ-aminobutyric acid), 86, 96
Ganglionitis, viral, 461
Gastrocnemium muscle pain, 505
Gate control theory, 39, 136–137, 157, 223, 225, 664
    acupuncture and, 183
    and deafferentation pain, 304
    pain perception and, 537
    phantom pain and, 456–457
Geniculate neuralgia, 279
    treatment for, 292
Genitourinary pain
    gynecologic, 373–379
    in male genitalia, 380–388
Giant cell arteritis, 488
Glaucoma, 249
Glossodynia, 285, 313
Glossopharyngeal nerve, 298
Glossopharyngeal neuralgia, 279–280
    headache and, 248
    treatment of, 292
Gluteus maximum pain, 503
Gluteus medius muscle pain, 503
Gluteus minimus muscle pain, 503
Glycerol, 290–291
Gold compounds, 485–486
Gonococcal infections, 377–378
Gout, 330, 441, 484, 512–513
    carpal tunnel syndrome in, 432
    treatment for, 478
Grasp, sustained strong, 517
Gray rami, 446
Grid laser technique, 158
Grief
    with chronic pain, 541
    pain as symbol of, 19
Guillain-Barré syndrome, 427
    evaluation of, 29
    neuropathy with, 426
Guilt, control of, 199
Guyon's canal, nerve compression at, 33
Gynecologic pain, 373. See also specific causes of
    causes of, 374–379
    diagnostic tools in, 373–374
    psychological response to, 379
Gyri, 15

H reflex, 29
    abnormalities of, 31
Halazepam (Paxipam), 97
Hallucinations, 15, 23
    with migraine, 244
Hallucis longus muscle pain, 507
Haloperidol (Haldol), 83, 91
Hamilton Rating Scale for Depression, 201

Hamstring tightness, 346
Hansen's disease, 368
Headache Scale, 579
Head, Henry, 10–11
Head compression test, 325
Head pain
    acute, 492–495
    nerve block for, 120
Head trauma, 240
Headache. See also Migraine
    Ad Hoc Committee on the Classification of (1962), 251–252
        classification scheme of, 265
        formation of, 264
    age at onset of, 238–239
    allergies and, 240–241
    antianxiety agents for, 84
    assessment of, 266–268
    associated symptoms of, 239–240
    of cervical origin, 168
    characteristics of patients with, 203
    in children, 260
    classification of, 243, 251–252, 265
    cognitive techniques for treatment of, 271
    course and frequency of, 239
    of delusional, conversion, or hypochondriacal states, 266
    differential diagnosis of, 238–249
    emotional factors in, 23, 240
    facial pain with, 311
    family history of, 240
    general treatment considerations of, 252
    history of, 238–241
    laboratory and radiographic studies of, 241–243
    lithium carbonate for, 79
    location of pain in, 239
    lower-half, 293
    manipulation for, 164
    medical examination for, 266
    medical management of, 251–262
    medication history and, 241
    with medication overuse and dependency
        treatment of, 261
    nerve block for, 120
    neuroleptics for, 95
    occupational and work-related factors in, 240
    operant pain-control techniques for, 271–272
    pain pathways for, 238
    patient interview for, 266–267
    phenothiazines for, 83
    physical and neurologic examination for, 241
    precipitating factors of, 240
    prevalence of, 238
    prodromal symptoms of, 239
    psychological management of, 264–273
        issues in, 272–273
    psychophysiology of, 268
    relaxation techniques for, 178
    self-monitoring in, 267–268, 272
    severity and pain characteristics of, 239
    special drug techniques for, 260–261
    tension vs. noncephalic pain, 203
    with TMJ derangements, 306
    treatment of
        efficacy of, 270
        in inpatient units, 261–262
    tricyclics for, 75
    types of, 243–249. See also under specific types

Headache, types of—*continued*
   defining characteristics of, 264–266
   with vascular dysfunction, 292–293
Head-forward posture, 516
Health care practitioner
   cognitive-behavioral, 231
   cultural influences of, 20
   stereotyping by, 17, 20
Health Locus of Control Scale, 672
Hearing deficits, 15
Heart, pain from, 11
Heart rate, at work, 623–624
Heat. *See also* Therapeutic heat
   distant effects of, 149
   local effects of, 148
   with massage, 155
Heating devices, 149, 406
   for deep-heating, 149–150
   superficial, 149
Heating lamps, 149
Heating pads, 149, 406
Heel life, 514
Hemicrania continua, 246
Hemilaminectomy, 418–419
Hemimandibulectomy, 312
Hemipelvis, small, 514–515
Hemiplegic migraine, 245
Hendler Back Pain Scale, 657
Hepatotoxicity, 485
Herniated nucleus pulposus, *346*
Heroin, 63
   CNS effects of, 61–62
   legalization of, 63–64
   structure of-activity of, 61
Herpecin-L, 314
Herpes simplex
   orofacial pain with, 313–314
   in pelvic infection, 377
Herpes zoster
   acute, 278, 460–461. *See also* Postherpetic neuralgia
      clinical manifestations of, 461–462
      complications of, 462
      diagnosis of, 462
      treatment for, 462–465
   end stage, 367
   neoplasms and, 461
   thoracic radiculopathy with, 360
Herpesvirus type 1, 513
Herpesvirus varicellae, 460
Hip
   arthropathies of, 361–364
      treatment for, 362–364
   pathology of, radiating leg pain with, 342–343
   replacement, total, 363
   revision, total, 364
   sciatic nerve injuries with surgery of, 439–440
Histamine desensitization, 258
Histamine cephalgia, 245
HI-TENS, 157
HLA histocompatibility antigen, 485
Hoffmann's sign, 326
Ho-Ku point, 183
Homunculus, 15
Honeymooner's palsy, 435
Honor, traditions of, 19
Hook swinging ceremony, 19

Hormonal abnormalities, 245
Horner's syndrome, 122, 240, 245, 249, 280
Horton's cephalgia, 245
Hospice nurses, 65
Hot lasers, 158
Hot pack, 148
Hot water bottle, 149
Household responsibilities, 22–23
Hubbard tanks, 159
Human *Papillomavirus* (HPV), 388
Human-environment relationships, 608–610. *See also* Ergonomics
Hydrocele, 386
Hydrocollator packs, 149
Hydrocortisone, 436
Hydromorphone, 64
Hydrotherapy, 158–159
Hydroxocobalamin, 512
Hydroxyapatite deposition disease, 484
Hydroxychloroquine, 487
Hydroxyzine (Vistaril), 84–86
   with analgesics, 555
   mechanisms of action of, 86
   with methadone, 65
   for migraine, 254
Hyperalgesia, 137, 448
   treatments for, 449
Hyperesthesia zones, 164
Hyperextensive trauma, 314
Hyperirritability syndrome, posttraumatic, 514
Hyperkalemia, 27
Hyperpathia, 133
   with postherpetic neuralgia, 466–467
Hyperprolactinemia, 94
Hyperreflexia, 326, 327
Hypersensitivity, 370
   with postherpetic neuralgia, 466–467
   treatments for, 449
Hyperthyroidism, 432
Hypertrophic arthropathy, 123
Hypnoanalgesia, 174
   applications for, 175
   mechanism of, 177–178
   strategies of, 175–177
Hypnoanesthesia, 174
   mechanisms of, 177
Hypnoplasty, 176–177
Hypnosis, 174–178, 408–409
   for cancer pain, 410–411
      effectiveness of, 410–411
   efficacy of, 174–175
   in modification of pain perception, 537
   for phantom pain, 458
Hypnotic amnesia, 177
Hypnotic displacement, 176
Hypnotic dissociation, 176
Hypnotic reinterpretation, 176
Hypnotic suggestion, 175–176
Hypnotic time disorientation, 176
Hypobaric agent injection, 117–118
Hypochondriasis, 23, 533–534, 540, 542
   with dysthymic pain, 198
Hypoglycermia, 513
Hypokalemia, 27
Hypometabolism, 513
Hypomobility, 165

Hypophysectomy, 134, 398, 420
　chemical, 134
Hypotension, orthostatic, 112
Hypothalamic-pituitary-adrenal (HPA) axis suppression, 479–480
Hypothalamotomy, posteriomedial, 133
Hypothalamus, dysfunction of, 257
Hypothyroidism
　carpal tunnel syndrome in, 432
　with relaxation training, 182
Hypoventilation, 551
　with morphine, 547
Hysterectomy, 375
　abdominal, 377, 378
Hysteria, 23, 540
　in diagnosis, 48
　scale, 575–576

IASP. See International Association for the Study of Pain
IBQ scale. See Illness Behavior Questionnaire
Ibuprofen (Motrin), 58, 555
ICDA-IX classification system, 601
Ice massage, 673
Ice therapy, 470–471
Idoxuridine, 464
Illness behavior, 575
Illness Behavior Questionnaire, 575–576, 582, 584
Imagery training
　for chronic pain, 543
　in modification of pain perception, 537
　in Pain Therapy Centers, 660
Imipramine (Tofranil), 74–75, 83, 88, 90
　for arthritic disorders, 76
　in chronic pain syndrome, 77
　for headache, 75
　for low back pain, 76
Immunosuppression, 293
Impairment, 635
　definition of, 3
　ratings, 674
Imprimine, 77
Inadequacy syndrome, 23
Incisura, 14
Indolamines, 447
Indomethacin (Indocin), 58
　for crystal-induced arthritis, 484
　headache and, 241, 254, 256
　for joint pain, 479
Indoprofen, 555
Industrial accident prevention programs, 593–594
Infections, chronic, 513–514
Inflammatory demyelinating polyneuropathy, 426–427
Inflammatory headache, 247–249
Inflammatory vascular disease, 293
Information processing, 224
Infraspinatus muscle
　pain of, 497
　weakness of, 120
Initiation rituals, 19–20
Injection and stretch techniques, 518–519
Injury
　by accident, 674–649
　arising out of employment, 649–650
　compensation for, 21–22
　of head and neck, 126–127
　personal, 646–647
　return to work following, 21–22
　work-related, 21–22
Insertional activity, 27
Insomnia, 198, 201
Insular cortex, 15
Insulin pump, 427
Insulinoma, 427
Insurance companies, 232
Intercostal nerve
　block of, 115, 119, 564–565
　destruction of, 121
　manipulation for pain in, 171–172
Intercostal neuralgia, 115
Interdisciplinary team, 231–232
Interferon, 464
Intermittent reinforcement schedules, 605
Internal capsule, 14–15
International Association for the Study of Pain, 2, 665
　definition of pain by, 2–3
　pain classification by, 3, 6–9, 227, 229
Interossei muscle pain
　of foot, 507
　of hand, 499
Interosseous space subluxation, 165
Interosseus nerve, anterior, 32
Interpersonal relationships, 44–45
Interpersonally distressed patient, 229
Interpolaris, 13
Interspinous ligaments, 358
Intervertebral disk. See also Disk herniation
　calcification of, 360
　degeneration of, 360
　herniation of, in cervical spine, 324
　rupture of, 361
Intracellular muscle potentials, 26
Intracranial aneurysm, 249
Intracranial vertebral artery, 323
Intrathecal neurolysis, 398
Iohexol, 352
Iopamidol, 352
Iron deficiency, 313
Irritability, 4
Ischemic compression, 518
Isokinetic exercises, 152
Isometheptene mucate, 253–254
Isometric exercises, 152
Isotonic exercise, 152

Job
　demands, reduction of, 625
　difficulty of and pain, 623
　fitness for, 625
　performance rates in cumulative trauma disorders, 615–616
Job training time, 641
Job-related injury, 649–650
Joint pain, 475–476. See also specific joints
　with crystal-induced arthritis, 483–485
　diagnosis of, 476–478
　drug therapy for, 478–480
　with osteoarthritis, 480–481
　with rheumatoid arthritis, 481–483
　with spondyloarthropathies, 485–486
Joints. See also Joint pain
　dysfunctions of, 166
　　somatic, 163

Joints—continued
    manipulation of, 156, 166
Jump sign, 282

Kallicrein system mediation, 56
Kappa receptors, 62
Ketamine, 63
Ketobemidone, 553
Ketoprofen (Orudase), 58
Ketorolac, 555
Kidneys, 380
    pain from in males, 383–384
Klippel-Feil syndrome, 330
Knee orthoses, 148, 160

La belle indifference, 542
Laboratory tests, for myofascial chronic pain syndrome, 525–526
Laciniate ligament sectioning, 441
Lactobacillus, 513
Laminectomy, 138–139
    repeat, 369
Laparoscopy, 378
    in gynecologic pain diagnosis, 374
Lasers, 147, 158
    for penile pain, 388
    techniques for, 158
Latency, 29
    side-to-side comparisons, 29
Lateral cutaneous nerve entrapment, 440–441
Lateral femoral cutaneous nerve
    block of, 121
    entrapment of, 34, 121
Lateral flexion subluxation, 164
Laterolisthesis subluxation, 165
Latissimus dorsi muscle pain, 497
Lawyers, 231–232
Learning
    behavior and, 212, 213
    history, 44
    theory, 223
        placebo effect and, 187–188
Leg pain
    distribution of, 349
    muscle pain of, 503–507
    radiating, etiology of, 342–343
Leiomyoma, 375
Leriche's syndrome, 255
Les hommes douloureux, 542
Leukotrienes, 366
Levator scapulae muscle pain, 495
Levorphanol, 64
Lidocaine (Xylocaine), 86
    with epinephrine, 116
    for myofascial trigger points, 518–519
    for neuropathies, 428
Life adjustment problems, 403
Ligament of Struthers entrapment, 433
Ligamentous cervical spine injuries, 331
Lissauer, tract of, 12
Listening, 231
Lithium, 93–94
    toxicity, 93
Lithium battery technology, 143
Lithium carbonate, 69, 79
    for cluster headache, 257–258
    mechanisms of action of, 79–80
    treatment outcomes of, 78–79t
Litigation
    behavioral analysis and, 45–46
    influence of, 21–22
    prevention and early intervention and, 602–604
    process of, 737
    reaction, 336–339
    vs. Workers' Compensation, 644–645
Litigation neurosis, 337
Liver damage, 106
Loading (drug), 560
Lock out interval, 560
Long association bundles, 15
Long second metatarsal, 515–516
Long thoracic nerve lesions, 439
Long-handled reachers, 160
Longshore and Harbor Workers Compensation Act, 644
Lorazepam (Ativan), 97
LO-TENS, 157
Lower back losers, 542
Lower extremity muscle pain, 503–507
    trigger points of, *504, 506*
Lumbago, 342, 344
Lumbar arachnoiditis, 138
Lumbar facet denervation, 123–124
Lumbar paraspinal muscle pain, 502–503
Lumbar selective nerve root block, 119–120
Lumbar spine
    arthropathy of, 360–361
    examination of, 345
    manipulation of, 170, *171*
        for lordosis, 170–171
        in seated position, 171
    sympathetic block of, 122–123
Lumbar traction, 154–155
Lumbosacral orthoses, 159–160
Lumbosacral radiculopathy, 31, 136
    deep brain stimulation for, 140
Lumbosacral spine arthropathy, 360–361
Lungissimus muscle, stretch of, 502
Lupus-like syndromes, 476
Luschka's joints, 321

Machines, redesign of, 625
Magnetic resonance imaging
    for back pain diagnosis, 342
    of cervical spine, 326, 333
    for chronic myofascial pain, 526
    for headache, 242–243
    for low back pain diagnosis, 336, 353
    for malignant pain, 390
Male genitalial
    anatomy of, 380–383
    sources of pain in, 383–388
Malignant pain. *See also* Cancer; Tumors
    assessment of, 391, 404–408
    diagnostic nerve blocks for, 391–392
    individualized pharmacologic tailoring for, 392–396
    neurologic evaluation for, 391
    neurosurgical treatment of, 417–422
    physical evaluation of, 390–392
    physical management of, 390–400
        orchestration of, 399–400
    psychological management of, 402–415
        approaches in, 408–414

Malingering, 21, 337
Malnutrition, neuropathy in, 426
Malocclusion, 294
Maloxone, 183
Management of Pain, 664
Mandible, neoplasm in, 284
Mandibular nerve, 298
Manipulation, 156, 157
    definition of, 163
    goal of, 169
    preparation for, 170
    spinal, 163–172
Man-machine systems, 608–610
MAP approach, 229
Maprotiline (Ludiomil), 77, 88–89, 206
Marcaine, 353–354
Marital relationships, 580
Masochism, 199
Massage, 147, 155, 518
Masseter muscle pain, 493
Masticatory muscles, 492–493
Materials handling, 610
    excessive force in, 613–614
    redesign of, 617
Maxillary nerve, 298
Maxillofacial pain, sources of, 303–304
MBHI scale. See Millon Behavioral Health Inventory
McArdle's disease, 492
McGill Pain Questionnaire, 391, 578, 579–582, 584, 594
    in pain centers, 672
Meatal stenosis, 387
Mechanical hypersensitivity, 449
Meckel's cavity, 13
Meclofenamate, 479
Meclofenamate sodium (Meclomen), 254
Medial lemniscus, 14
Medial nerve entrapment, 31
Median nerve entrapment, 32–33, 430–433
    in proximal forearm, 32–33
Medicaid, 671
Medical benefits, 651–652
Medical consultants, 231
Medical electrodiagnostics, 26–37
Medical witnesses, 645–646
Medication(s)
    consumption patterns of, 595
    experimental, 677
    in pain centers, 659, 672–673
Meditative techniques, 179
Medulla, pain perception and, 12
Medullary tractotomy, 130, 131, 420, 470
Mefanamic acid (Ponstel), 58
Melantonin, 245
Melzack theory, 222
Meningitis, 240
Menstrual cycle, pain with. See Dysmenorrhea
Menstrual migraine, 261
Mental injuries, categories of, 674
Mental stress, 615
Mental-mental injuries, 647
Mental-physical injuries, 674
Meperidine (Demerol), 74, 82
    in children, 106
    congeners of, 64
    for malignant pain, 394
    patient-control administration of, 559

pharmacology of, 553–554
Mepivacaine, 310
Meralgia paresthetica, 34, 121, 440–441
Mesonephros, 376
Metabolic dysfunction, 512–513
Metanephros, 376
Metatarsalgia, 160
Metenkephalin, 245
Methadone (Dolophin), 65, 77
    congeners of, 64–65
    pharmacology of, 553
Methotrexate, 483, 486
Methotrimeprazine (Levoprome), 75, 80, 83, 95
Methylphenidate (Ritalin), 86, 98–99
Methylprednisolone acetate (Depo-Medrol, Depo-Predate), 117
Methysergide, 255, 258
Metoclopramide (Reglan), 261
Metoprolol (Lopressor), 254
Metrizamide, 352
Metronidazole, 426
Microvascular decompression, 291–292
    of trigeminal nerve, 277
Microwave diathermy, 150
Midazolam, 555
Midbrain, periaqueductal gray of, 15
Midrin, 253–254
Migraine, 243–244. See also Headache
    basilar artery, 244–245
    biofeedback for, 159
    characteristics of, 265
    classic, 244
    common, 244
    complicated, 244–245
    cyclic, 78–79
    differentiation of from headache, 239
    facial pain with, 311
    hemiplegic, 245
    neuroleptics for, 95
    ophthalmoplegic, 245
    precipitating factors in, 240
    prophylaxis for, 83
    relation of to tension headache, 251
    relaxation techniques for, 178
    treatment of
        preventive, 254–256
        resistant to, 78
        symptomatic, 252–254
    tricyclics for, 75
    with vascular dysfunction, 292–293
Millon Behavioral Health Inventory, 575–576, 582, 584, 657
Mini-Mental State examination, 46
Minimum effective analgesic concentration (MEAC), 558–559
Minnesota Multiphasic Personality Inventory, 407, 570, 573–575, 579
    for chronic pain patients, 540
    in pain centers, 672
    for preadmission evaluation to pain centers, 657
    in prevention, 594
    profile subgroups of, 581, 584
    in psychological evaluation, 38, 41, 47–48
    scales of, 576
    Welch code of, 50
Misonidazole, 426
Mixed headache syndrome, 247
MMPI. See Minnesota Multiphasic Personality Inventory
Mobilization, 156

700 Index

Mobilization—*continued*
  definition of, 163
Monakow's area, 13
Monoamine oxidase, 77, 447
  catecholamine release and, 86
  exciters, 448
  inhibitors, 69, 448
    for acute and chronic pain, 77–79
    drug interactions of, 92
    drug selection of, 92
    for dysthymic pain, 206
    for headache, 260
    hypertensive crisis with, 92
    mechanisms of action of, 79–80
    pretreatment evaluation of, 92
    properties and side effects of, 91–92
    treatment outcomes of, 78–79t
    treatment techniques of, 92
  for migraine, 256
Mononeuropathies, 427
Monoradiculopathy, 118
Mood
  disturbances of, 46
  fluctuations of, 70
Moral codes, 18–19
Morphinans, 61
Morphine, 555
  administration techniques for, 396
  CNS effects of, 61–62
  depression, 62
  endogenous, in modification of pain perception, 537
  gastrointestinal effects of, 62
  patient-control administration of, 559
  pharmacodynamics of, 61
  pharmacology of, 552, 554
  respiratory depression with, 563
  spinal, 421
  structure of, 60–61
Morphine congeners, 63–64
Morphine sulfate, 82, 547
Morphine-type agonist-antagonist analgesics, 66
Motion palpation, 166
Motion recording and analysis, 611
Motor behaviors. *See also* Behavior
  assessment of, 583
  automated measurement devices for, 571–572
  measurement of, 570–573
  self-monitored observations of, 572
  self-reports of, 572–573
Motor conduction studies, 29
Motor deficits, 15
Motor disorders, 327
Motor latency studies, 29
Motor loss, 350
Motor pain behavior, 213, 215
Mourning, pain as symbol of, 19
Movement, passive, 156–157
Mucosal diseases, 285
Multiaxial Assessment of Pain (MAP), 227
Multidimensional Pain Inventory (MPI), 229
Multiple sclerosis
  affecting cervical spine, 327, 330
  trigeminal neuralgia with, 276, 288
Munchausen syndrome, 541
Mural thrombosis, 437

Muscle
  contraction of, 28
  contract-relax cycle, 518
  loading, 624–625
  pain, myofascial, 490–507. *See also* Myofascial pain syndrome(s)
  resting potentials of, 27–28
  wasting of, 350
Muscle contraction headache, 239, 246–247
  characteristics of, 265
  relaxation technique for, 270
  and vascular headache, 265–266
Muscle relaxants, 259, 294
Muscle relaxation. *See also* Progressive muscle relaxation; Relaxation training
  for cancer pain, 411
  progressive, 179–180, 664
Muscle spasm, 327
  in lower back, 346
  paravertebral, 168
  stretching exercises for, 152–153
Muscle syndrome, 167
Muscle tension headache. *See* Muscle contraction headache; Tension headache
Muscle-relaxing exercises, for TMJ disease, 294
Muscular rheumatism, 283
Musculocutaneous nerve entrapment, 34, 438
Musculocutaneous sensory conduction, 34
Musculoskeletal dysfunction, 163. *See also specific disorders*
  orofacial, 314
Myalgia, 283
  torticollis, 168
Myelitis, 366
Myelography
  for back pain diagnosis, 342
  for cervical spine pain, 333–334
  for low back pain diagnosis, 335–336, 351–352
Myeloradicular arteries, 323
Myelotomy, commissural, 419
Myofacial pain dysfunction, 305
Myofascial pain syndromes(s), 282–283
  chronic, 509–527
    vs. acute and recurrent, 521
    causes of, 521–522
    conditions similar to, 519–520
    financial distress with, 522
    function vs. pain orientation in, 522–523
    inactivation of trigger points in, 517–519
    industrial cases of, 527
    intensification of, 522
    laboratory tests and imaging for, 525–526
    management approach to, 520–523, 526–527
    mechanical factors in, 514–517
    patient education in, 527
    patient history of, 523–525
    perpetuating factors of, 510–517
    physical examination for, 525
    systemic factors in, 510–514
  distribution of pain of, 491
  history of onset of, 491
  prevention and early intervention in, 598–600
  psychological factors in, 599
  single-muscle
    acute, 492–507
    pathogenesis of trigger points of, 492

recognition of, 490–492
  stretching exercises for, 152. See also Stretch and spray treatment
Myofascial therapy, 526
Myofascial trigger points (TrPs), 490–492, 509, 519
  of clavicular division, 493
  development of, 521
  exercise and, 523
  location of, 494
  pathogenesis of, 492
  perpetuating factors in, 510–517
  sensitivity of, 583
  in shoulder and upper extremity, 495–499
  of sternal division muscles, 493
  treatment of, 527
Myomectomy, 375
Myopathies, 27, 35
Myospastic cycle, 309
Myotonic discharges, 28

Nadolol (Corgard), 254
Nail brittleness, 450
Nalbuphine, 63, 67
  patient-control administration of, 559
  side effects of, 564
Nalorphine, 61
  derivatives of, 65
Nalorphine-type agonist-antagonist analgesics, 66–67
Naloxone, 61
  increased levels of, 188
  interactions of with MAOIs, 92
  side effects of, 563–564
Naprosyn sodium (Anaprox), 256
Naproxen (Naproxyn), 58, 555
Naproxen sodium, 254
Narcissistic personality disorder, 541
Narcotics. See also Morphine; Opiates
  abuse of, 77
  addiction to, 552
  agonists of, 63–65, 552
    hepatic metabolism of, 554
    pharmacokinetic and pharmacodynamic values for, 553
  as analgesics
    interactions of with MAOIs, 92
    interactions of with neuroleptics, 95
    potentiation of, 82–83
    used in children, 107t
  antagonists of, 65–67
  for chronic pain, 545–547
  continuous spinal or epidural infusion of, 396
  in elderly, 112
  epidural administration of, 562–563
  escalation of dosage of, 77
  intraventricular, 421
  for malignant pain, 393–395
  new administration techniques for, 395–396
  for phantom pain, 458
  pharmacokinetics of, 396
  pharmacology of, 552–554
  potentiation of, 86
  subcutaneous infusion of, 395
  sublingual delivery of, 395
  synthetic, structure of-activity of, 61
  transdermal delivery of, 395–396
Nausea and vomiting, 564

NCS. See Nerve conduction, tests
Neck, 320
  acute trauma to, 359
  anatomy and biomechanics of, 321–323
  clinical examination of, 324–325
  collars, 159
  hypermobility of, 495
  neurologic status of, 325–326
  pain in, 320. See also Cervical spine pain
    acute, 492–495
    manipulation for, 164
    with osteophytes, 358–359
    referred from muscle of, 492
    rheumatoid arthritis of, 331–332
  vascular supply of, 323
Needles, for nerve block, 116–117
Negative reinforcement, 211, 215
Neodymium YAG laser therapy, 388
Neoplasms, on ventrolateral spinal cord, 12. See also Cancer; Tumors
Neospinothalamic tracts, 12, 550
Neotrigeminothalamic pathway, 300
Nerve blocks, 536. See also specific types of
  basic equipment for, 116–117
  in chronic pain management, 115–116
  diagnostic, 391–392
  for herpes zoster, 464–465
  local infiltration, 469
  localized, 218
  peripheral, 564–566
  for postherpetic neuralgia, 469–470
  specific types of, 117–124
Nerve conduction
  tests, 28–29, 433
    in low back pain diagnosis, 355
    proximal, 29–30
  velocity, 29, 326
Nerve entrapment syndromes, 31–35
  nerve block for, 120, 121
Nerve excitability studies, 26
Nerve roots
  blocks of, 354
  compression of in spine, 168, 329
  infiltration of in low back pain diagnosis, 353–354
  inflammation of, 366
  irritation of
    of cervical spine, 329–330
    with intervertebral disk rupture, 361
  reflexes and, 166
  section of. See Rhizotomy
  stimulation of, 29
Neural blockade, 5
Neural crosstalk phenomenon, 304, 368
Neural stimulation techniques, 136–144. See also Electrical stimulation; Transcutaneous electrical nerve stimulation; specific nerves and techniques
Neuralgias, 365, 371. See also specific types of
  brachial, 168
  causes of, 369–370
  definition of, 369
  facial, 79, 275–281
    atypical, 76
  of head, 275–281
  headache and, 247–248
  intercostal, nerve block for, 115

Neuralgias—continued
  migrainous, 245
  occipital, 120, 168
  orofacial pain with, 310–311
  postherpetic, 74, 278–279, 460–471
  post-traumatic, 310–311
  treatment for, 74, 79, 293
  trigeminal, 13
    benzodiazepines for, 97
Neurectomy
  peripheral, 277, 417–418
  for trigeminal neuralgia, 289
Neuritis, 366–367
Neuroablation, 536
  by chemical neurolysis, 398–399
  neurosurgical procedures of, 397–398
  for postherpetic neuralgia, 470
Neuroanatomic deficits, 13
Neuroanatomic pain pathway, 536–537
Neurobiotaxis, 12
Neuroforamen, 118–119
  S1, 120
Neurogenic claudication, 168
Neurogenic thoracic outlet syndrome, 437
Neuroleptics, 80–84. See also specific drugs
  for cancer pain, 83
  commonly used, 94t
  drug interactions of, 95
    with tricyclics, 89
  nonresponse to, 96
  pretreatment evaluation of, 95
  properties and side effects of, 94–95
  selection of, 95
  treatment techniques with, 95–96
Neurologic disorders
  phenothiazines for, 83
  tricyclics for, 74–75
Neurolytic agents, 398–399
Neurolytic blocks, 470
  drugs for, 117
  sites of, 398t
Neuromas
  phantom tooth syndrome with, 311
  projected pain of, 304
Neuromuscular junction, 26
Neuropathies
  definition of, 365
  drug-induced, 426
  entrapment and compression, 424, 430–441
  evaluation of, 29
  painful, 74–75, 365–369
  peripheral, 35, 424–428
  radial sensory, 436
  radiating leg pain with, 343
  treatment of, 74, 370–371
Neuropharmacologic theory, 157
Neuropsychological testing, 46
Neurosurgery, 365. See also specific procedures
  ablation techniques, 397–398, 417–420
  augmentative, 421–422
  for deafferentation pain, 126–134
  for orofacial pain, 288–294
Neurosynaptic transmitters, 447–448
Neurotic bodily pain, 369
Neurotic triad, 540
Neurotoxins, 327

Neurotransmission
  of brain and spinal cord, 86
  in modification of pain perception, 537
  serotonergic and noradrenergic, 79
Neurotransmitters
  defect in and depression, 246
  noxiousness of, 11
  synthesis of, 511–512
Nifedipine (Procardia), 255
Nigrostrial system blockade, 94
Nitrofurantoin, 426
Nociception
  definition of, 297
  modulation of, 551
  orofacial, 299–301, 314
  peripheral, 365
  turning off of, 367
  types of neurons in, 300
Nociceptive fibers, 298
Nociceptive impulses, 550
  stratifiction of response to, 552t
  transmission, modulation, and perception of, 566
Nociceptive pain, 55, 126
Nociceptive receptors, 10
Nomifensine (Merital), 90
  with analgesics, 77
Nonarticular rheumatism, 283
Noncompliance, minimization of, 42
Nonsteroidal anti-inflammatory drugs, 55–56, 366
  for acute pain, 555
  adverse effects of, 57–58
  for arthritic disorders, 76
  caffeine with, 86
  for children, 105–106
  for chronic pain, 547
  for cluster headache, 258
  for crystal-induced arthritis, 484–485
  effects and uses of, 56–57
  for extraparticular pain syndromes, 487–488
  for joint and connective tissue pain, 475–476, 478–479, 487
  for malignant pain, 393–395
  with massage, 156
  for migraine, 254, 256
  for myofascial pain syndrome, 527
  for osteoarthritis, 481
  for post-traumatic headache, 260
  for rheumatoid arthritis, 482
  for spondyloarthropathies, 485–486
  for tension headache, 259
  types of, 58. See also specific agents
Norepinephrine, 447
  availability of, 91–92
  deactivation of, 98
  reuptake of, 89
Normeperidine, 64
Norms, cultural, 19
Nortriptyline (Aventyl), 90–91, 256
  with analgesics, 77
Nuclectomy, percutaneous, 318
Nucleus oralis, 13
Nuprin Pain Report, 264
Nutrition therapies, 677
Nutritional inadequacies, 510–512

Observational assessment, 42
Obturator hernias, 35

Obturator nerve entrapment, 35
Occipital nerve blockade, 120
Occipital neuralgia, 120, 168, 280
Occipital muscle, referred pain in, 493
Occular headaches, 249
Occupational Access System (OASYS), 638
Occupational function, 636
Occupational injury, 649–650
Occupational role, 22–23
  behavioral analysis and, 45–46
Occupational skills, transferability of, 636–638
Occupational stresses, 608–609
Occupational therapists, 45, 231
Odontalgia, 285
Odontogenic pain, 284–285
Oligoarticular arteritis, 488
On-Demand Analgesia Computer (ODAC), 559
Operant conditioning model, 223, 225
Operant pain-control techniques, 271–272
Operant theory, foundations of, 223–224
Ophthalmic herpes zoster, 465
Ophthalmicus, herpes zoster, 461, 462
  treatment of, 463
Ophthalomoplegia syndromes, 249
Ophthalmoplegic migraine, 245
Opiates, 59
  agonists of, 59
    partial, 555
  antagonists of, 59
    structure of, 61
  for chronic pain, 547
  for crystal-induced arthritis, 484
  endogenous, 183
  interaction of with tricyclics, 89
  intrathecal and epidural, 560–562
    administration of, 562–563
    side effects of, 563–564
  for joint and connective tissue pain, 476
  for postherpetic neuralgia, 469
  receptors of, 59, 62–63
  spinal, side effects of, 563–564
  tolerance of, 563
  used in children, 106–107
Opioids
  chronic use of, 46
  clinical uses of, 60
  continuous spinal or epidural infusion of, 396
  endogenous, stimulation of, 188
  history and use of, 59–60
  phamacology of, 552
  pharmacodynamics of, 61
  pharmacokinetics of, 396
  physiologic effects of
    analgesic, 62
    on central nervous system, 61–62
    gastrointestinal, 62
  street users of, 61–62
  structure-activity relationships of, 60–61
  used in children, 106–107
Optic neuritis, 249
Orabase, 313
Oral irritants, 313
Oral surgery, 311
Orofacial analgesic systems, 302–303
Orofacial central pathways
  first-order neurons in, 299–300
  second-order neurons in, 300–301
  thrid-order neurons in, 301
Orofacial nociception, 299–301, 314
Orofacial nociceptor fibers, 298
Orofacial pain. See also specific types of
  dental management of, 297–315
  differential diagnosis of, 275–286
  medical/neurosurgical management of, 288–294
  of mucosal origin, 285
  of psychological origin, 285–286
  rare causes of, 314–315
  treatment of, 298–301
Orofacial peripheral nerves, 298
Orthopedic ulcer, 338
Orthotics, 159–160
Osteoarthritis, 76, 368, 480–481
  of cervical spine, 328–329
  coping strategies for pain of, 577
  orthoses for, 160
  of temporomandibular joint, 283–284, 307
  treatment of, 480–481
Osteoid osteoma, 359
Osteopenia, 360
Osteophytes, of cervical spine, 325, 329, 358–359
Osteoporosis, 321, 324
Osteoradionecrosis, 284
Osteosarcomas, 328
Otitis, 311
Otolaryngological disorders, 311
Ovarian pregnancies, 374
Ovaries
  neoplasia of, 376
  pain of, 375–376
Overexertion, 613–614
Overgeneralization, 577
Oxazepam (Serax), 97
  with analgesics, 555
Oxicams, 58
Oxycodone, 64, 393
Oxygen consumption, measurement of, 611
Oxygen, for cluster headache, 257
OXYLOG, 611
Oxyphenbutazone, 58

Pacemakers, implanted, 137
Pacinian corpuscle, encapsulated, 10
PAG stimulation. See Periaqueductal gray matter, stimulation of
Paget's disease, 324
Pain, 3–4. See also Chronic pain; Pain behaviors
  acute, anatomy and neurophysiology of, 550–552
  adaptive aspects of, 533
  axes of, 3, 7–9
  behavioral conceptualization of, 212–213
  behaviors stimulating, 406
  brainstem systems of, 12–14, 16
  cerebral cortex, 15
  characteristics of, 298t
  classification system of, 3, 6–9, 227, 366t
    critique of, 601–602
    pros and cons of, 600–601
  cognitive component of, 4–5, 405–406
  compensation and litigation factors in, 21–22
  cultural and anthropoligic influences on, 17–20
  definitions of, 2, 6, 297
    of functional capacity, 3
    of International Association for the Study of Pain, 2–3

Pain, definitions of—*continued*
    operational, 3–5
    psychological, 2
  descending pathways and, 15
  descriptors of, 476, 579–582, 584
  diminishers of, 406
  early recognition of, 592–606
  efforts to diagnose and ligitimize, 23–24
  emotional component of, 4, 23, 406
  emotional descriptions of, 18
  environmental factors in, 406
  ethnic influences in, 18
  etiology of, 7, 8t, 23
  experience of, 212
  factors affecting report of, 408
  family considerations in, 23–24
  gate control theory of, 39. *See also* Gate control theory
  IASP taxonomy of, 7–9, 227
  induction technique for, 177
  intensity of, 7, 8t
    rating of, 662
  interethnic differences in response and attitudes to, 18
  internal capsule and, 14–15
  legal aspects of, 21–22, 635–638
  life adjustment problems and, 403
  list classification of, 7
  malignant, 544–545
  neurophysiological-behavioral continuum of, 2
  nomenclature, 602
  occupational role in, 22–23
  pathways of, 536–538
    modulation of, 396–397
  patient response to, 116
  pattern of occurrence of, 7, 8t
  peripheral structures of, 10–12
  phantom, 455–459
  physiologic precipitants of, 406
  postsurgical, pharmacologic therapy for, 82–83. *See also* Postoperative pain
  practitioner's culture, influence on, 20
  precipitators of, 405–406
  psychogenic, 539
    effects of, 40
  psychological aspects of, 2–3, 23, 69
  psychological evaluation in, 38–50
  quality of, 405
  quantification of medical-physical findings on, 227–229
  quantification of psychosocial/behavioral data on, 229
  receptors of, 10, 298, 357. *See also* Nociceptive receptors
  referred, 11–12, 344
    in male genitalia, 383
    orofacial, 303–304
    trigger points for, 155
  region of, 7
  reinforcement of nonpharmacologic control methods of, 216
  secondary gain with, 535–536, 542
  as sensory and emotional experience, 2–3
  sensory model of, 222–223
  sensory pathways of, 10–12, 16
  sick role and, 20–21
  social/cultural factors in, 17–24
  somatic, 16
  spinal cord and, 12, 16
  subjectivity of, 2
  suppression mechanism of, 183
  system in, 7, 8t
  temporal classification of, 366t
  thalamus and, 14, 133
  threshold, 537
  tolerance of, 164
  treatment of organization involved in advancement of, 684
    variables in, 476
  types of, 536
  visceral, 11, 16
    pathways of, 12, 15
Pain assessment interviews, 596
Pain Behavior Scale, 572–573
Pain behaviors, 3–4
  contingency management in reduction of, 210–219
  elimination of, 5
  evaluation of, 39–40
  family interaction effects on, 580–581
  measurement of, 583
    scales for, 584
  psychometric and behavioral evaluation tools for, 638
  reinforcement of, 43, 44–45
  relationships and family response to, 44–45
  sociocultural variables of, 533–535
Pain centers. *See* Pain clinics; Pain Therapy Centers
Pain clinics, 543
  academic parameters of, 668, 669–670, 675–676
  administrative parameters of, 667–669, 675
  analysis of
    in future, 675–678
    in past, 664–668
    in present, 668–675
  assessment and treatment at, 656–663
  clinical parameters of, 668, 671–675, 677–678
  economic parameters of, 668, 670–671, 676–677
  factors in development of, 665–667
  follow-up in, 674
  goals in, 674
  impairment ratings in, 674
  marketing of, 671
  parameters of, 667–668
  pretreatment evaluations in, 671–672
  program duration and cost of, 670
  services of, 670
  staff specialities of, 670
  survey of, 679–682
  treatment modalities in, 672–673
Pain cocktails, 527. *See also* Brompton's cocktail
Pain diaries, 595
Pain fibers, 12
Pain games, 23
Pain history, 41–42, 48
Pain management professionals, 652–653, 675–676
Pain orientation versus function, 522–523
Pain patient
  adaptive aspects of pain in, 533
  approach to, 532–533
  personality and secondary gain factors in, 535–536
  sociocultural variables of pain behavior in, 533–535
Pain perception
  cognitive factors in, 39
  measurement scales for, 578–580, 584
  modification of, 536–538
Pain proneness, 24, 542
  disorders of, 197
  identification of, 603
  prevention and early intervention with, 594–596
Pain Rating Index (PRI), 578–579

Pain Syndromes, Questionnaire for, 201
Pain Therapy Centers, 656–657
  assessment in, 657–658
  behavior modification in, 661
  medical regulation at, 659
  patient education in, 660–661
  physical reactivation in, 658–659
  preadmission evaluation for, 657–658
  psychological rehabilitation in, 660
  relaxation training in, 659–660
  treatment in, 658–661
    results of, 661–663
  vocational rehabilitation in, 661
Pain Visual Analog Scale, 391
Pain-related medication, 213, 216. See also specific agents
Pain-tension cycle, breaking of, 660
Paleospinothalamic tract, 12, 550
Palpation, of motion, 166
Panic attacks, 92
Papaver somniferum, 59
Papillomavirus strains, 388
Paraffin wax, 149
Paranoid schizophrenia, 95–96
Paraovarian cysts, 376
Paraphimosis, 387
Paraplegia, 129–130
Parasitic infestation, 514
Parasympathetics nerves, 11
Pariental operculum, 15
Parietal lobe, 15
Paroxysmal hemicrania, chronic, 257
Parsons, Talcott, 20
Patellar reflex, 166
Patellofemoral syndrome, 160
Patient education, 593–594, 678
  for myofascial pain syndrome, 527
  in pain centers, 672
  in Pain Therapy Centers, 660–661
Patient history, 596–598
Patients
  follow up of, 674, 677
  involvement of, 234
  semi-structured interview of, 596
  uptime of, 571
Patient-controlled analgesia (PCA) technique, 558–560
Pectoralis major and minor muscle pain, 499
Pelvic tilt exercises, 153
Pelvis
  autonomic innervation of, 383
  inflammatory disease of, 377–378
  pain of, in females, 373–379
Pemoline (Cylert), 98
Penicillamine, 482–483, 485–486
Penis, 381–382
  cancer of, 387
  inflammation of, 387–388
  pain from, 387–388
Pentazocine (Talwin), 63, 66–67, 393–394
Penthidine, 61
Periapical peridontitis, 285
Periaqueductal gray matter, 15
  stimulation of, 140–141, 183
    devices for, 143
  in trigeminal nociceptive neuron suppression, 302–303
Periarticular pain syndromes, 476

Pericarditis, 486
Pericarotid syndrome, 293
Perineum, 383
Periodontal abscess, 285
Peripheral denervation, 289
Peripheral nerves
  blocks of, 118
    brachial plexus, 565
    field, 565–566
    of greater occipital nerve, 120
    intercostal nerve, 121, 564–565
    mechanisms of, 157
    for postherpetic neuralgia, 469
    of selective root, 118–120
    of suprascapular nerve, 120–121
    in surgical wound perfusion, 565
  entrapment syndromes of, 31–35
  neuropathy of, 28, 424
    causes of, 425
    differential diagnosis of, 425–427
    symptoms and signs of, 424–425
    treatment of, 427–428
  polyneuropathy of, 35
  stimulation of, 136–137
Periventricular gray electrodes, 140–141
Peroneal nerve
  entrapment of, 35
  lesions of, 439
Peroneus brevis muscle pain, 505–507
Peroneus longus muscle pain, 505–507
Perphenazine (Trilafon), 80
Personal injury, 646–647
Personal injury lawyers, 232
Personality disorders, 541
Peyronie's disease, 387
Phantom limb pain, 77, 128, 369, 457
  deep brain stimulation for, 140
Phantom pain
  clinical cases of, 455–456
  etiology of, 456–457
  time course of, 457
  treatment of, 457–459
Phantom tooth syndrome, 311–312
Pharmacologic tailoring, 392–396
Phencyclidine, 63
Phenelzine (Nardil), 77–79, 92, 256
Phenobarbital, 64
Phenol, 398
Phenothiazine, 75, 254, 464, 467–468
  for acute pain, 80–83
  for chronic pain, 83
  derivatives of, 82
  mechanisms of action of, 83–84
Phenoxybenzamine, 448
Phentolamine, 448
Phenylbutazone (Butazolidin), 58
  for crystal-induced arthritis, 484
  interactions of with lithium, 93
  for joint pain, 479
4-Phenypiperidines, 61
Phenytoin (Dilantin), 64, 256, 260, 289, 464, 468
  use of in children, 107
Physical activity, as cancer pain treatment, 403–404. See also Exercise
Physical demands, 639–640
Physical examination, 596–598

Physical medicine, 147, 148. *See also specific types of*
   forms of, 148–160
   goals of, 147–148
Physical reactivation, 658–659
Physical stress, 615
Physical therapists, 593
Physical therapy, 218
   for osteoarthritis, 481
   in pain clinics, 673
   for phantom pain, 459
   for rheumatoid arthritis, 483
Physical-mental injuries, 674
Physiologic capacity, 610
Physiologic responses
   contributing factors in, 612–613
   ergonomic analysis of, 611–613
Physiologic variables, measurement of, 582–583
Piperazine agents, 94
Piriformis muscle pain, 503
Piroxicam (Feldene), 58
Placebo(s)
   analgesia, 185–189
   definition and origin of term, 186
   effect of, 185
      maximization of, 188–189
   ethical considerations with, 188
   mechanism of action of, 187–188
   in modification of pain perception, 537
   response to, 186–187, 365
   stimulation, 137
   studies of pain relief with, 186
Plantar fasciitis, 160
Platelet aggregation inhibition, 57
Plexopathies, 35
Pneumatic counterpressure pumps, 155
Pneumothorax
   prevention of, 121
   with stellate ganglion block, 122
Podophyllin, 388
Point stimulation laser technique, 158
Polio, 323
Polymylagia rheumatica, 488
Polymyositis, 27, 35, 314
Polyneuropathies, 430
   peripheral, 35
Polypharmacy, in elderly, 112–113
Porphyria, 427
Positive flip test, 347, *348*
Positive reinforcement, 211, 215
Positive sharp waves, 27
Postcordotomy dysesthesia, 140
Posterior facet syndrome, 167
Posterior interosseous nerve syndrome, 34, 435–436
Postherpetic neuralgia, 278–279, 460, 465–466
   pathophysiology of, 466
   symptoms and pain characteristics of, 466–467
   treatment for, 293, 467–471
      neurosurgical, 130–133
Postisometric relaxation, 517–518
Postlaminectomy syndrome, 137
Post-lumbar puncture headache, 247
Postoperative pain
   anatomy and neurophysiology of, 550–552
   cryoanalgesia for, 567
   intrathecal and epidural opiates for, 560–564
   pathophysiology of, 551–552

peripheral nerve blocks for, 564–566
pharmacologic therapy for, 82–83
systemic analgesics for
   methods of administration of, 555–560
   pharmacology of, 552–555
transcutaneous electrical nerve stimulation for, 566–567
Post-traumatic cephalgia, 260
Post-traumatic headaches, 248
Post-traumatic neuralgias, 310–311
Post-traumatic stress disorder, 541
Post-traumatic sympathetic dystrophy, 122
Postural stress, 516
Postural training, 360
Posture
   analysis of, 625
   alignment of, 167
   exercises for, 153
   extreme, 613
   targeting and analysis of, 611
Prazepam (Centrax), 97
Preauricular pain, 306
Prednisolone, 463
Prednisone, 257, 483
Pregnancy
   carpal tunnel syndrome in, 432
   ectopic, 374
   TENS and, 137
Presacral neurectomy, 377
Pressure perception, 10
   in brainstem, 13–14
Prevention
   compensation and disability program impact on, 602–604
   legal disincentive to, 604
   of myofascial syndromes, 598–600
   with pain-prone patient, 594–596
   patient history and examination in, 596–598
   primary, 592–594
   secondary, 592
   tertiary, 604–606
Priapism, 387
Primary care
   pain disorders seen in, 538–540
   pain patient in, 533–538
      approach to, 532–533
      management of, 543–547
      psychiatric disorders in, 540–543
Probenecid, 485
Problem-solving, 231
   skills for, 226
Prochlorperazine (Compazine), 80, 254
Profile of Mood States (POMS), 407
Progressive muscle relaxation, 179, 180, 664
   for cancer pain, 411
Projected pain. *See* Referred pain
Promazine (Sparine), 80, 82–83
Promethazine (Phenergan), 80, 82, 254, 555
Pronator syndrome, 32–33, 433
Prontor muscle weakness, 433
Propiomazine (Largon), 80, 82
Propoxyphene, 64, 467, 478
Propoxyphene hydrochloride, 393
Propranolol (Inderal), 75, 254
   interaction of with tricyclics, 89
Proprioception, loss of, 14
Proprionic acid derivatives, 58
Prosopalgia, 285

Prostaglandin synthetase inhibitors, 374, 375
Prostaglandins, 55, 366
    aspirin and, 56
    blockage of, 374–375
    excessive, 378
Prostate, 380–381
    obstruction of, 384–385
    pain from, 384–385
Prostatitis, 384–385
Prostatodynia, 385
Prostatosis, 385
Proteins, serum abnormalities of, 427
Protopathic pain, 10–11
Proximal conduction studies, 29–30
Proximal median nerve entrapment, 432–433
Pruritis, 564
Pseudogout, 478, 484
Pseudounipolar neurons, 13
Psoriatic arthritis, 485
Psychasthenia scale, 576
Psychiatric disorders, 2
Psychogenic pain, 23, 266
    effects of, 40
    in spine, 336
Psychological dysfunction, 46
Psychological evaluation, 38–39
    components of, 41–47
    concepts underlying, 39
    guidelines for reporting on, 48–50
    indications for, 39
    Minnesota Multiphasic Personality Inventory in, 47–48
    overview of, 41
    in pain centers, 671–672
    patient preparation for, 40
    purposes of, 39–40
Psychological factors, 23
    drug treatments for. See Psychopharmacologic agents
    in malignant pain management, 402–415
Psychological rehabilitation, 660
Psychological stress, 514
Psychological testing, 570–584. See also specific techniques and tests
    of chronic pain patients, 536
Psychometric evaluation tools, 638
Psychomotor agitation, 200
Psychomotor retardation, 200
Psychopharmacologic agents, 69. See also specific agents
    outcomes of, 69–88
    treatment approaches with, 88–99
Psychophysical scaling procedures, 578–580
Psychophysiology research, 664
Psychosis, neuroleptics for, 95–96
Psychosocial Adjustment to Illness Scale, 672
Psychosocial history, 49
Psychosomatic spinal pain, 336, 337–338
Psychostimulants, 86–88
    treatment approach to, 98–99
Psychotherapeutics techniques
    for cancer pain, 409–410
    in pain centers, 673
    for painful neuropathies, 370–371
    for phantom pain, 458–459
    for postherpetic neuralgia, 471
Psychotomimetic reactions, 65
Psychotropic drugs, 69
    for depression, 540

diagnostic indications for, 88t
in joint pain treatment, 476
Pterygoid muscle, 495
    pain of, 493
Public service announcements, 593
Puboprostatic ligaments, 380
Pulpal nerve fibers, 302
Pulpitis, 285
Pulsed ultrasound, 150
Pulse-train TENS, 567
Pulvinar lesions, 133
Punishment
    in behavior control, 211
    pain as, 19
PVG electrodes. See Periventricular gray electrodes
Pyrazoles, 58
Pyridoxine, 511–512
Pyroles, 58

Quadratus lumborum muscle pain, 502
Quadriceps femoris muscle pain, 505
Quality assurance programs, 674, 676
Quervain's disease. See De Quervain's tendinitis

Radial motor conduction studies, 34
Radial nerve
    compression of, 34, 435
    entrapment of, 33–34
        high, 435
        below or at elbow, 435–436
    palsy, 435
Radial sensory conduction studies, 34
Radial sensory neuropathy, 436
Radicular pain, of cervical origin, 168–169
Radicular syndrome
    acute
        bilateral, 348
        criteria for diagnosis of, 349t
        unilateral, 344–347
    chronic
        bilateral, 349
        unilateral, 348–349
    neurologic changes in, 350t
Radiculitis, 366
Radiculoneuritis, 366, 368
Radiculopathies, 368, 520
    cause of, 358
    electrodiagnostic studies of, 30–31
    evaluation of, 29
    thoracic, 360
Radiofrequency denervation, 120
Radiofrequency electrocoagulation, 291
    for neuralgia, 289–290, 292
Radiofrequency electrodes, 117, 123, 142–143
Radiofrequency lesions, 119, 121
Radiofrequency receiver, 142
Radiography, 526
Raeder's paratrigeminal neuralgia, 280–281, 315
    headaches with, 249
Range of movement exercises, 152
Rational restructuring, 226
Raynaud's phenomenon
    with carpal tunnel syndrome, 431
    migraine and, 244, 255
    with ulnar nerve entrapment, 434
Recreational therapy, 673

Rectus abdominis muscles, trigger points of, 503
Rectus femoris muscle trigger points, 505
Referred pain, 11–12, 344
  in male genitalia, 383
  in myofascial pain syndrome, 491–492
  orofacial, 303–304
  trigger points for, 155
Referring physicians, 231–232
Reflex activity, changes in, 349–350
Reflex sympathetic dystrophy, 293, 370, 454
  acute stage of, 444
  atrophic stage of, 445
  clinical signs and symptoms of, 444–445, 452–453t
  diagnosis of, 449
  dystrophic stage of, 444–445
  gross anatomy of, 446
  microanatomy of, 446–447
  sympathetic blocks for, 465
  synapses and, 447–448
  theory of, 445–446
  treatment of, 449–451
Reflex vasodilation, 149
Reglan (metoclopramide hydrochloride), 254
Rehabilitation, 617
  benefits, 652
  of chronic pain syndrome patient, 604–606
  in cognitive-behavioral approach, 230
  with dysthymic pain disorder, 207–208
  family participation in, 606
  goal of, 605
  programs for in pain centers, 676
  psychological, 660
  skills for, 577
  vocational, 661
  and vocational prognosis, 638
Reil, island of, 15
Reimbursement, 667, 670–671
Reinforcers, in behavior modification, 216–217
Reiter's syndrome, 477, 485
  treatment for, 478, 486
Relapse prevention, 234
Relaxation
  with biofeedback, 159
  exercises for, 153
  response, 178
  skills, 226
Relaxation training, 172–183, 210
  adverse patient reactions to, 181–182
  for cancer pain, 411
  for cervical spine arthropathy, 360
  contraindications for, 182
  for headache management, 268–269
  integrative approach to, 179–181
  in modification of pain perception, 537
  in Pain Therapy Centers, 659–660
  for phantom pain, 458
Religion, 19
Religious ceremonies, 20
REM sleep abnormality, 199, 202
Renal pain, in males, 383–384
Renal pelvis, 380
Repolarization abnormalities, 94
Research, 676
Reserpine, 241
Residual functional capacity, 636

Respiratory depression
  delayed, 563–564
  with spinal opiates, 563–564
Rest reinforcers, 215
Resting behavior, 44
Resting muscle activity, 27–28
Resting potentials, 26, 27–28
Reticular formation, 12–14
  zones of, 301
Reticular nuclei, 14
Retrolisthesis subluxation, 165
Rexed layers, 126–128
  DREZ lesions in, 131
Rexed's laminae, 12
Reye's syndrome, 106
Rheumatic disease
  extra-articular manifestations of, 477
  failures at managing pain of, 475
  laboratory analyses for, 477–478
  pain associated with, 475
  treatment of, 475–476
Rheumatoid arthritis, 35, 76, 481–482
  of cervical spine, 324, 331–332
  drug treatment for, 482–483
  dysthymic pain disorder and, 202–203
  physical therapy for, 483
  step-care approach to, 483
  tarsal tunnel syndrome with, 441
  of TMJ, 307
  treatment for, 478
Rheumatoid factors, 477, 488
Rheumatoid synovitis, 436
Rhizotomy, 365, 397
  for cancer pain management, 418–419
  for phantom pain, 458
  for postherpetic neuralgia, 469–470
Rib cage
  manipulation for distortion of, 171–172
  nerve block for fracture of, 121
  pain of, 169
Roosevelt, Franklin D., 21
Root tension, 346
Rotational subluxation, 164
Rotator cuff tendinitis, 487

S1 motor roots, 29
Sacral nerve roots, traumatic avulsion of, 127
Sacral rhizotomy, 418–419
Sacral selective nerve root block, 120
Sacroiliac joint
  arthropathy of, 361
  manipulations of, 170
  mechanical derangement of, 167
  subluxation of, 165
Sadomasochist, 542
Salicylates
  for crystal-induced arthritis, 484
  glomerular filtration rate and, 57
  for joint pain, 478
  for osteoarthritis, 481
  for rheumatoid arthritis, 482
Salicylic acid, 56
Salicylism, 57
  in children, 105
Salivary duct obstruction, 313

Salivary glands
   inflammation of, 312–313
   stones of, 313
Salivation, depression of, 313
Salpingo-oophorectomy, 377–378
Saturday night palsy, 33
Scaleni muscle pain, 495
Scalp trauma, 120
Scanning laser technique, 158
Scapular winging, 438–439
Schizophrenia scale, 48, 574
Sciatic nerve, 439
   lesions of, 439–440
   stimulation of, 136
Sciatic scoliosis, 345–346
Sciatica, 342
SCL–90. *See* Symptom Checklist–90 scale
Scleroderma, 35
Scotoma, 244
Scrotum, 382
   pain of, 384, 386–387
Seated postural stress, 516
Sedative-hypnotics, 46
   abuse of, 46
   interaction of, 89, 92–93
Sedatives, 84–85. *See also specific agents*
   as adjuncts to analgesics, 555
   antidepressants, 205–206
Seizures, 64
Selective abstraction, 577
Selective nerve root blockade, 118–119
   technique for, 119–120
Self-actualization, 22
Self-esteem
   with dysthymic pain, 200
   occupational role and, 22–23
   psychogenic pain and, 23
Self-hypnosis, 175
   for cancer pain, 409, 410
   techniques of, 177
Self-management, 230–231
Self-monitoring, 226
Self-reports, 572–573
Self-sacrifice, 198
Seminal vesicles, 383
Sensations, hypnotic replacement of, 176
Sensory conduction studies, 29
Sensory impulse pathways, 12–16
Sensory loss, 350
Sensory model, 222–223
Sensory nerve roots, cervical, 321, 322
Sequestra, 284
Serositis, 486, 487
Serotonin, 447
   availability of, 91–92
   blockade of, 89
   in migraine, 78
   tooth pulp and, 302
Serotoninergic systems, 537
Serratus anterior muscle pain, 499–502
Serratus posterior superior muscle pain, 502
Sex hormones, 241
Sexual activity, frequency of, 45
Sexual dysfunction, 45
Shingles, 132, 460–461
   clinical manifestations of, 461–462
   complications of, 462
   diagnosis of, 462
   treatment for, 462–465
Short leg, 514–515
Short upper arm, 515
Shortwave diathermy, 149–150
Shoulder elevation, 516
Shoulder pain, 495–499
   trigger points of, 496, 498
Sialadenitis, 312–313
Sialogogues, 313
Sick role, 20–21
   adoption of, 542
   family response to, 22
Sickness Impact Profile (SIP), 572–573, 584
   functional impairment scores, 577, 580
Side posture manipulation and rotation with extension, 170–171
Sigma receptors, 62–63
   stimulation of, 65
Sinus disease, 294
Sinusitis, 284, 294
   facial pain with, 311
Sjörgren's syndrome, 427, 486–487
Skeletal muscles
   energy of, 510
   spasm of with malignant infiltration, 395
Skeletal traction, 331
Skills acquisition, in cognitive-behavioral approach, 233
Skills training, for cancer pain management, 412–413
Skull x-rays, 241–242
Sleep abnormalities, 199, 202
SLR testing, 346–347
Sluder's syndrome, 280
SMAC profile, 477
Social history, 47
Social influences, 18
Social modeling, 210
Social Security Act of 1935, 21
Social Security Administration, 602
   chronic pain classification of, 637
   Commission on Pain Evaluation of, 602, 603
   recommendations of, 638
   sequential evaluation process of, 635–636
Social Security Disability Insurance program, 21
   pain and, 635–638
Sociocultural factors, 533–535
Socioeconomic class, 18
Sodium serum concentrations, 26
Soldiers, effort syndrome in, 23
Soleus muscle pain, 505
Somatic dysfunction, 163
Somatic pain, 16
   classification of, 10–11
Somatic preoccupation, 3–5
Somatic stimulation, 183
Somatoform disorders, 542–543
Somatosensory cortex, 301
Somatosensory-evoked potentials, 29–30
South American cultures, 19
Spa treatments, 147
Spastic torticollis, 314
Spermatic cord structures, 382
Sphenopalatine ganglion surgery, 258

Sphenopalatine neuralgia, 280
Sphenous nerve entrapment, 440
Spinal arteries, 323
Spinal blocks, 117–118
Spinal cord
   anatomy of, 126
   central canal of, 12
   cervical, 322–323
   compression of, 321, 323, 327, 331
   cysts of, 323
   electrical stimulation of, 137–140, 421
   inflammation of, 366
   injury to, 331
      deep brain stimulation for, 140
      fibrillations with, 27
   ischemia of, 323, 327
   in pain pathway, 536
   trauma to, 126–130
Spinal fixation, 164–165
Spinal ganglia, 11
Spinal gating mechanism, 566
Spinal joint pain, pathophysiology of, 357–358
Spinal manipulation, 156, 163–164
   contraindications for, 166, 172
   criteria for, 165
   indications for, 166–169
   pain tolerance and, 164
   short lever, high-velocity, 170
   spinal biomechanics and, 164–166
   types of, 169–172
Spinal nerve root blockade, 118
Spinal opiates, 563–564
Spinal radicular lesions, 156
Spinal root avulsion, 126–128
Spinal stenosis, 168
Spinal surgery, 317–319, 536
   unnecessary, 318–319
Spine. See also Cervical spine; Lumbar spine; Spinal cord; Spinal manipulation; Vertebral disk
   biomechanics of, 164
   kinetic vertebral motion unit subluxations and, 165–166
   pain of
      arthropathies and, 357–364
      differential diagnosis and management of, 320–334
      neuropathies and nerve root lesions with, 365–371
      nonorganic, classification of, 336–337
      psychogenic, 336, 338
      psychosomatic, 336, 337–338
      situational, 336–337, 338–341
      tolerance of, 164
   static vertebral motor distortions and, 164–165
Spinothalamic pathways, 12, 12–13
Spinothalamic tracts, 536, 550
Splenii muscle, 495
Spondyloarthropathies, 485–486
   characteristics of, 477
   treatment of, 480
Spondylolisthesis, 167–168, 344
Spondylolysis, 165
Spondylosis, 247
Spurling's test, 325
SSDI program. See Social Security Disability Insurance program
Standing postural stress, 516
Staphylococcal infection, 332
Static loading, 614
Stellate ganglion block, 122

nerve blocks for, 465
Stenosis, 168
Stereotaxic mesencephalotomy, 133
Sternocleidomastoid muscle
   innervation of, 321
   pain of, 493
   weakness of, 438
Steroids
   epidural depository, 118
   for herpes zoster, 463, 465
   for migraine, 254
   for reflex sympathetic dystrophy, 450–451
   for tarsal tunnel syndrome, 441
Stereotyping, 17, 20
Stevens-Johnson syndrome, 485
Stiff neck syndrome, 495
Stimulants, 87–88
   of CNS, 98–99
   mechanism of action of, 86
Stimulation. See also Electrical stimulation; Transcutaneous electrical nerve stimulation
   analgesia, 140
      mechanisms of, 137
   devices for, implanted, 142–143
   gate theory and, 136
   waveforms, 137, 143–144
Stimuli, discriminative, 211–212
Stoicism, 20, 534, 535
Strengthening exercises, 152
Streptococcal infection, 332
Stress, 49
   concentration of, 614
   mechanical, 516–517
   mental, 615
   modification of, 47
   pain as time out from, 43
   physical, 615
   psychological, 514
   in psychological evaluation, 47
   reduced concentration of, 625
   thermal, 626
Stress Audit, 672
Stretch and spray treatment, 152, 493, 495, 497, 502, 503, 517
Stretching exercises, 152–153
Stroke, 27
Subarachnoid hemorrhage, 249
Subarachnoid spinal blocks, 117–118
Subdural hematomas, 247
Subluxation, 163
   anterolisthesis, 164–165
   extension, 164
   flexion, 164
   foraminal encroachment, 165
   interosseous space, 165
   lateral flexion, 164
   laterolisthesis, 165
   retrolisthesis, 165
   rotational, 164
   sacroiliac, 165
   of vertebral motion unit, 165–166
Submandibular lymphadenitis, 313
Suboccipital craniectomy, 291
Suboccipital muscles, 495
Subscapularis muscle pain, 497
Substance P, 536
Suggestion, power of, 187

Suicide
  causes of, 460
  ideation, 200–201
Sulfinpyrazone, 485
Sulindac (Clinoril), 58
Supinator muscle pain, 499
Supracapular neuropathy, 437–438
Suprascapular nerve entrapment, 34, 120
Suprasegmental reflex responses, 550
Supraspinatus muscle
  pain of, 497
  weakness of, 120
Suprofen (Suprol), 58
Surgical wound perfusion, 565
Swimming, 151
Sympathectomy, 11, 122
  for causalgia, 445
  chemical, 451
  for phantom pain, 458
  for postherpetic neuralgia, 470
  surgical, 449
Sympathetic blockade, 121–123
  effectiveness of, 116
  ganglionic, 392
  by neuromas, 304
  for neuropathies, 428
  for postherpetic neuralgia, 469–470
Sympathetic denervation, 446
Sympathetic dystrophy, post-traumatic, 122
Sympathetic nerves, 11
  hyperactivity of, 121–122
  pathway of, 446
Sympathetically maintained pain (SMP), 445–447
Sympathomimetic agents, 92
Sympathomimetic amines, 89
Symptoms Checklist–90 scale, 575–577, 582, 584, 672
Synapses, 447–448
Synovial fluid
  analysis of, 477
  viscosity of, 148
Syringomyelia, 12, 330
Systemic lupus erythematosus, 486
  treatment of, 480
Szondi Experimental Diagnostic of Drives, 201

Tardive dyskinesia, 91, 94–95
Tardy ulnar nerve palsy, 368, 433
  treatment of, 434
Tarsal tunnel syndrome, 31, 35, 441
  anterior, 35
  causes of, 441
Taut band of muscle, 491, 519
T-cells, 537
Telescoping, 457
Temporal arteritis, 247
Temporalis muscle pain, 493
Temporomandibular dysfunction
  with arthritides, 307
  differential diagnosis and treatment of, 305–306
  with fractures, 307–308
  internal derangements in, 306–307
  neuromuscular pathologies in, 308–310
  with tumors, 307
Temporomandibular joint
  clicks, 306
  degeneration of, 288

disease of, 294, 305
  etiologic theories of, 308–309
  myospastic cycle in, 309
  workup for, 309–310
inflammation of, 314
internal derangements of, 306–307
osteoarthritis of, 283–284
pain and dysfunction syndrome of, 281–282
pain of, 281–282
referred pain from, 304
structure of, 305–306
Temporomandibular joint syndrome
  antidepressants for, 75–76
  treatment of, 79
Tendinitis, 487–488
Tennis elbow, 34, 499
Tenomyositis, 283
Tenosynovitis, 436, 441, 485
  treatment of, 480
TENS. See Transcutaneous electrical nerve stimulation
Tension headache, 168
  antianxiety agents for, 84
  vs. noncephalic pain, 203
  relation of to migraine, 251
  treatment of, 259
    for chronic, 259–260
    symptomatic, 259
  tricyclics for, 75
Tension points, 156
Tentorium cerebelli, 14
Terminally ill, management of, 65
Testicles, 382–383
  pain of, 385–386
  trauma to, 386
Testicular torsion, 385
Tetracaine (Pontocaine), 116–117
Tetrahydrocannabinol, 547
Thalamic nuclei, 14
  relay, 15
Thalamic syndrome, 14
  deep brain stimulation for, 140
  neurosurgical treatment of, 133–134
Thalamocortical loop, 14
Thalamotomy, 294, 420, 458
Thalamus
  infarction of, 293
  lesions of, 133
  pain and, 12, 74, 293
  pain perception and, 14, 16
  stimulation of for postherpetic neuralgia, 470
  trigeminal pathways to, 13–14
Theca-lutein cysts, 375, 376
Therapeutic cold, 147, 150–150
Therapeutic heat, 147–148
  contraindications for, 149
  heating devices for, 149–150
  indications for, 149
  physiologic effects of, 148–149
Therapeutic light treatment, 157–158
Therapeutic modalities. See also specific treatments and techniques
  adjunctive techniques, 174–189
  analgesic/anti-inflammatory medications, 54–67
  cognitive-behavioral perspective on, 222–235
  in dysthymic pain disorder, 197–208
  nerve blocks in, 115–124

Therapeutic modalities—*continued*
   neural stimulation techniques, 136–144
   neurosurgical treatments, 125–134
   pharmacologic pain management, special factors in, 104–113
   physical medicine in, 147–160
   psychopharmacologic agents, 69–99
   to reduce overt pain behavior, 210–219
   spinal manipulation in, 163–172
Therapeutic orphan, 104
Thermal biofeedback, 159, 269
   for headache, 270
Thermal hypersensitivity, 449–450
Thermal stress, reduced, 626
Thermocoagulation, 133
Thermography, 355, 526
Thermoneurolysis, peripheral, 311
Thiamine, 511
Thoracic fibers cascade, 11
Thoracic iliocostalis muscle pain, 502
Thoracic microtrauma, 169
Thoracic nerve root blocks, 119
Thoracic outlet syndrome, 33, 314, 436
   neurogenic, 437
   vascular, 436–437
Thoracic paraspinal muscle pain, 502–503
Thoracic radiculopathies, 31, 360
Thoracic spine
   arthropathy of, 360
   manipulation of, 171, *172*
   pain of, 169
Thoracic sympathetic nerves, 11
Thoracoabdominal pain, 131–133
Thrombophlebitis, 441
Thromboxane, 56–57
Thromboxane A2, 56
Thymidine analogs, 464
Thyroid function tests, 93
Thyroid supplementation, 513
Tibial H reflex latency, 31
Tibial nerve entrapment, 35, 441
Tibialis anterior muscle pain, 505
Tic douloureux. *See* Trigeminal neuralgia
Timolol (Tenormin), 254
Tinel's sign, 34
Tissue typing, 477
TMPDS. *See* Temporomandibular joint, pain and dysfunction syndrome of
Tolmetin (Tolectin), 58, 106
Tolosa-Hunt syndrome, 249
Tongue thrusting, 313
Tonsilitis, 311
Tooth. *See also* Phantom tooth syndrome
   anatomy of, *301*
   dentine, 302
   innervation of, 301–303
   pulp, 301–302
   referred pain and, 303–304
   sensitivity of, 301–302
Toothache, 284–285
Tort system, 644–645
Torticollis, 168, 327
Touch perception, 13–14
Toxins
   affecting nervous system, 327
   neuropathy with, 426, 428
Traction, 153–155
   contraindications for, 154
   injuries with, 439
Traction headache, 247–249
Tractotomy, 365
   medullary, 420
Traditions, cultural, 19
Training time, 642–643t
Tranquilizers. *See also specific drugs*
   for chronic pain, 464, 467–468, 547
   major, 80–84
Transcutaneous electrical nerve stimulation, 137, 157, 218, 396–397
   vs. acupuncture, 184
   adverse effects of, 157
   applied physiology of, 566
   contraindications and precautions for, 137
   in modification of pain perception, 538
   for neuropathies, 428
   in pain centers, 673
   for phantom pain, 458
   for postherpetic neuralgia, 470
   practical considerations for, 566–567
   trial of, 136
Transmembrane potentials, 26
Tranylcypromine (Parnate), 77, 92
Trapezius muscles, 493
Trauma
   to cervical spine, 330–331
   to neck, 359
Traumatic arthritis, 307
Traumatic neuromas, 304
Treatments
   goals and expectations of, 43
   noncompliance with, 42
   role of, 5
Triceps brachii muscle pain, 497
Triceps musculature, examination of, 325
Triceps reflex, 166
Tricyclics, 65, 69
   for acute pain, 70–74
   as analgesic adjuncts, 77
   for chronic pain, 74–77
   for depression, 540–541
   drug interactions of, 89
   drug selection of, 90
   for dysthymic pain, 206
   in elderly, 112
   glycemic control with, 75
   for herpes zoster, 464
   mechanisms of action of, 77
   in modification of pain perception, 538
   for myofascial pain syndrome, 527
   for neuropathies, 428
   in Pain Therapy Centers, 659
   for phantom pain, 459
   for postherpetic neuralgia, 467–468
   pretreatment evaluation with, 89–90
   properties of, 88–89
   side effects of, 88–89, 206t
   for tension headache, 259–260
   treatment techniques of, 90–91
      outcomes for, 70–74t
   used in children, 107
Trifluoperazine (Stelazine), 80
Trigeminal gangliolysis, 277
Trigeminal gasserian ganglion, 13

Trigeminal herpes zoster, 278
  nerve block for, 465
Trigeminal innervation, 299
Trigeminal nerve, 298, 299
  dental branch damage of, 310
  divisions of, 298
Trigeminal neuralgia, 13, 275, 288
  atypical, 276, 291–292
  benzodiazepines for, 97
  control of, 304
  extracranial surgery for, 311
  headache and, 247
  idiopathic, 275–276
  prevalence of, 276
  secondary, 275–278
  symptomatic, 276
  treatment of, 74, 276–277
    medical, 288–289, 291, 310–311
    neurosurgical, 289–291
Trigeminal neuropathy, 292
Trigeminal nociceptive neurons, suppression of, 302–303
Trigeminal nucleus claudalis, 130–131
Trigeminal sensory complex, 13–14, 300
  projected pain of, 304
Trigeminal thalamic pathways, 14
Trigeminal tractotomy, 279, 294
Trigger points, 155. See also Myofascial trigger points (TrPs)
Trimipramine (Surmotil), 75
Trunk muscle pain, 499–503
  trigger points of, 500–501
Tryptophan, 92
L-Tryptophan, 447
Tuberculosis, of cervical spine, 332
Tuberoinfundibular system blockade, 94
Tumors
  of cervical spine, 324, 328
  of facial bones, 284
  metastatic to vertebral body, 359
  ovarian, 376
  of TMJ, 307
Tunica vaginalis, 382
Tyramine, 92
Tyramine-restricted diet, 240t

Ulnar nerve entrapment/compression, 33, 433–434
    below elbow, 434–435
    treatment of, 434
Ultrasonography, 150
  in gynecologic pain diagnosis, 373–374
  in low back pain diagnosis, 355–356
  for postherpetic neuralgia, 471
  of scrotum, 386
Ultraviolet light treatments, 157–158
Upper extremity pain, 495–499
Uremic neuropathy, 427
Ureters, 380
  obstruction of, 384
  pain of, in males, 383–384
  spasms in, 384
Urethra, male, 381
  pain in, 385
Urethral strictures, 385
Urethroscopy, 385
Urinary bladder
  male, 380–381
    pain in, 384

spasms, 384
Urinary retention, 564
Uterus
  pain in, 374–375
  tumors of, 375
Uveitis, 249

Vagus nerve, 298
Vail's syndrome, 280
Vapocoolant spray, 151
  for back muscle pain, 502
  for myofascial trigger points, 515
  with stretching exercises, 152
  for trapezius muscle pain, 493
Varicoceles, scrotal, 386–387
Vas deferens, 382
Vascular disease
  inflammatory, 293
  orofacial pain with, 311
  treatment for, 292–293
Vascular headache, 243–246
  and muscle contraction, 265–266
Vascular insufficiency, 327
Vascular shunts, 432
Vascular thoracic outlet syndrome, 436–437
Vasoconstriction
  with cold therapy, 150–151
  local, for nerve blocks, 116
Vasodilation, with heating, 148–149
Vasomotor instability, 450
Vasospastic angina, 244
Vastus intermedius trigger points, 505
Vastus lateralis muscle trigger points, 505
Vastus medialis trigger points, 505
Venography, epidural, 355
Ventral posterolateral nucleus, 536
Ventral tract, 12
Verapamil (Isoptin, Calan), 244
Verbal pain behavior, 213, 214–215
Verbal pain descriptors, 476, 584
  measurement scales for, 581–582
  ratio scales of, 579–580
Vertebral disks. See also Spine
  degeneration of, 321, 328–330
  herniation of. See Disk herniation
  rupture of, 321
Vertebral ligaments, innervation of, 357–358
Vertebral motion unit subluxations, 165–166
Vertebral motor distortions, static, 164–165
Vibrating belts, 155
Vidian neuralgia, 280
Viral disease, 513–514
Visceral afferent blockade, 123
Visceral efferent blockade, 121–123
Visceral pain, 11, 16
  pathways of, 12, 15
Visual analogue scales, 578
Visual field deficits, 15
Visual-evoked potentials, 30
Vitamin A, 512
Vitamin B, 511–512
  deficiencies of, 285, 313
  for postherpetic neuralgia, 468
Vitamin C, 512
Vitamin D, 512
Vitamin E, 468, 512

Vitamins. *See also specific vitamins*
   deficiencies of, 510–511
   fat-soluble, 512
   inadequacy of, 510–511
   sutdies of, 526
   water-souble, 511–512
Vocational counselors, 45, 231
Vocational evaluation, 677
Vocational history, 49
Vocational preparation time, 641
Vocational prognosis, 636–638
Vocational rehabilitation, 527, 661, 673
Vocational relevance concept, 636
Vocational skills, transferability of, 636–637, 638
Vocational stress, 516–517
Voluntary motor system pathways, 15
Voluntary muscle contraction, 28

Wakefield Depression Scale, 579
Walking, 151
   endurance, 153
War, stress of, 23
Water, immersion in, 158–159
Watson-Schwartz test, 427
WDR neurons, 444, 446, 447, 466
Weber's syndrome, 13
Wegener's granulomatosis, 285
Weight reduction, for osteoarthritis, 481
Weight-bearing relief, 159–160
Well behaviors, 45
   nonverbal, 215
   reinforcement of, 661
   verbal, 215
Wellness programs, 594
West Haven-Yale Multidimensional Pain Inventory, 573
Whiplash, 337
Whipple's disease, 485
White rami communicantes, 446
Wide dynamic range neurons. *See* WDR neurons
Wisconsin Brief Pain Inventory (BPI), 407
Women, self-esteem of with incapacitation, 22–23
Work. *See also* Job; Workplace
   history, 45
   rehabilitation at, 207–208
   return to, 22, 43

   role in, 22–23
Workalholism, 198
Workers' Compensation, 45, 334, 602, 604, 644
   compensation formula for, 646–650
   death benefits of, 651
   disability benefits of, 650–651
   medical benefits of, 651–652
   medical witnesses in, 645–646
   pain centers and, 671
   rehabilitation benefits of, 652
   specialists and, 652–653
   vs. tort-based systems, 644–645
   unusualness requirement of, 647–648
Workers' Compensation Board, 338
Workers' compensation laws, 21
Workplace
   conditions of, 640
   cumulative trauma disorders in, 615–620
   ergonomic deficiencies in, 613–614
   ergonomics in, 608–614
      analysis of, 610–614
      of boarding, 620–626
   modification of, 617
   physical demands of, 639–640
   physical stresses of, 608–610
   training time in, 641
Worried well patients, 533–534
Wrist
   median nerve entrapment at, 31, 32–33
   orthoses, 160
   radial nerve compression at, 34
   splinting of
      for carpal tunnel syndrome, 432
      for wrist-drop, 435
   ulnar nerve entrapment at, 434
Wrist-drop, 435

Xerostomia, 285, 313
X-rays, 351

Zoster immune globulin, 464
Zoster non herpete, 461
Zung depression scores, 75
Zygoapophyseal joints, 321, 322, 358
Zylocaine, 313

GERALD E. SWANSON, M.D.
9601 UPTON ROAD
MINNEAPOLIS, MN 55431
TELE: 881-6869